The American Psychiatric Publishing
Textbook of Mood Disorders

Editorial Board

The American Psychiatric Publishing
Textbook of Mood Disorders

EDITED BY

DAN J. STEIN, M.D., PH.D.

DAVID J. KUPFER, M.D.

ALAN F. SCHATZBERG, M.D.

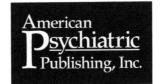

Washington, DC
London, England

Manufactured in the United States of America on acid-free paper
09 08 07 06 05   5 4 3 2 1
First Edition

Typeset in Adobe's Frutiger and Janson Text.

American Psychiatric Publishing, Inc.
1000 Wilson Boulevard
Arlington, VA 22209-3901
www.appi.org

Library of Congress Cataloging-in-Publication Data

The American Psychiatric Publishing textbook of mood disorders / edited by Dan J. Stein, David J. Kupfer, Alan F. Schatzberg.-- 1st ed.
    p. ; cm.
 Includes bibliographical references and index.
 ISBN 1-58562-151-X (hardcover : alk. paper)
 1. Affective disorders.
 [DNLM: 1. Mood Disorders. WM 171 A5115 2005] I. Title: Textbook of mood disorders. II. Stein, Dan J. III. Kupfer, David J., 1941- IV. Schatzberg, Alan F. V. American Psychiatric Publishing.

 RC537.A545 2005
 616.85'27--dc22

                                                                 2005008198

British Library Cataloguing in Publication Data

A CIP record is available from the British Library.

Contents

P A R T   1

Symptomatology and Epidemiology

Dan J. Stein, M.D., Ph.D., Section Editor

P A R T   2

Pathogenesis of Mood Disorders

Pedro L. Delgado, M.D., Section Editor

P A R T   3

Investigating Mood Disorders

Husseini K. Manji, M.D., Section Editor

P A R T   4

Somatic Interventions for Mood Disorders

Mark S. George, M.D., Section Editor

P A R T   8

Additional Perspective on Mood Disorders

David J. Kupfer, M.D., Section Editor

Contributors

Berry Anderson, R.N.
Clinical Research Nurse, Medical University of South Carolina, Charleston, South Carolina

Tanya J. Bennett, M.D.
Staff Psychiatrist, Eating Disorders Program, Menninger Clinic; Instructor in Psychiatry, Baylor College of Medicine, Houston, Texas

Susan Bentley, D.O.
National Research Service Award Primary Care-Psychiatry Fellow, Department of Psychiatry and Behavioral Sciences, University of Washington School of Medicine, Seattle, Washington

Wade Berrettini, M.D., Ph.D.
Karl E. Rickels Professor of Psychiatry and Director, Center for Neurobiology and Behavior, University of Pennsylvania School of Medicine, Philadelphia, Pennsylvania

Antje Bittner, Dipl.Psych.
Research Associate, Institute of Clinical Psychology and Psychotherapy, Technische Universität Dresden, Dresden, Germany

Pierre Blier, M.D., Ph.D.
Endowed Chair, Mood Disorders Research, Institute of Mental Health Research, Royal Ottawa Hospital; Professor, Departments of Psychiatry and Cellular and Molecular Medicine, University of Ottawa, Ottawa, Ontario, Canada

Daryl E. Bohning, Ph.D.
Professor of Radiology, Medical University of South Carolina, Charleston, South Carolina

Robert Boland, M.D.
Associate Professor of Psychiatry and Human Behavior, Brown Medical School, Providence, Rhode Island

Jeffrey Borckardt, Ph.D.
Instructor, Department of Psychiatry, Medical University of South Carolina, Charleston, South Carolina

David A. Brent, M.D.
Academic Chief, Child and Adolescent Psychiatry, and Professor of Psychiatry, Pediatrics, and Epidemiology, Western Psychiatric Institute and Clinic, University of Pittsburgh School of Medicine, Pittsburgh, Pennsylvania

Daniel J. Buysse, M.D.
Professor of Psychiatry, Clinical Neuroscience Research Center, Department of Psychiatry, University of Pittsburgh School of Medicine, Pittsburgh, Pennsylvania

Joseph R. Calabrese, M.D.
Professor of Psychiatry and Co-Director, Bipolar Disorders Across the Life Cycle Interventions and Services Research Center, Case University School of Medicine, University Hospitals of Cleveland, Cleveland, Ohio

Colleen E. Carney, Ph.D., C.Psych.
Research Associate, Duke University Medical Center, Durham, North Carolina

Kenneth Carpenter, Ph.D.
Assistant Professor of Clinical Psychology in Psychiatry, Columbia University, Department of Psychiatry, New York State Psychiatric Institute, New York, New York

Bruce K. Christensen, Ph.D., C.Psych.
Head, Neuropsychology Lab, and Assistant Professor of Psychiatry, Centre for Addiction and Mental Health, Clarke Site, University of Toronto, Toronto, Ontario, Canada

Dianne Currier, Ph.D.
Staff Associate, Department of Psychiatry, Columbia University, New York, New York

Carrie Davies, B.S.
Research Assistant, New York State Psychiatric Institute, New York, New York

Pedro L. Delgado, M.D.
Professor and Chairman, Department of Psychiatry, and Associate Dean for Faculty Development, School of Medicine, the University of Texas Health Sciences Center at San Antonio, San Antonio, Texas

D.P. Devanand, M.D.
Professor of Clinical Psychiatry and Neurology, College of Physicians and Surgeons, Columbia University; and Co-Director, Memory Disorders Center, New York State Psychiatric Institute, New York, New York

Mary Amanda Dew, Ph.D.
Professor of Psychiatry, Psychology, and Epidemiology; Director, Clinical Epidemiology Program; and Associate Director, Advanced Center for Interventions and Services Research for Late Life Mood Disorders, University of Pittsburgh School of Medicine and Medical Center, Pittsburgh, Pennsylvania

Andrea F. DiMartini, M.D.
Associate Professor, Department of Psychiatry, University of Pittsburgh School of Medicine and Medical Center, Pittsburgh, Pennsylvania

Graham J. Emslie, M.D.
Professor of Psychiatry and Division Chief, Child and Adolescent Psychiatry, University of Texas Southwestern Medical Center at Dallas, Dallas, Texas

Benjamin H. Flores, M.D.
Clinical Instructor and Research Scientist, Department of Psychiatry and Behavioral Sciences, Stanford University School of Medicine, Stanford, California

Ellen Frank, Ph.D.
Professor of Psychiatry and Psychology, Department of Psychiatry, University of Pittsburgh School of Medicine, Western Psychiatric Institute and Clinic, Pittsburgh, Pennsylvania

Edward S. Friedman, M.D.
Professor of Psychiatry, University of Pittsburgh, Pittsburgh, Pennsylvania

Glen O. Gabbard, M.D.
Brown Foundation Chair of Psychoanalysis; Professor, Director of Psychotherapy Education; Director, Baylor Psychiatry Clinic, Baylor College of Medicine, Houston, Texas

Mark S. George, M.D.
Distinguished Professor of Psychiatry, Radiology, and Neurology; and Director of the Brain Stimulation Laboratory and the Center for Advanced Imaging Research, Medical University of South Carolina, Charleston, South Carolina

Anne Germain, Ph.D.
Assistant Professor of Psychiatry, Sleep and Chronobiology Program, Department of Psychiatry, University of Pittsburgh School of Medicine, Pittsburgh, Pennsylvania

Renee D. Goodwin, Ph.D., M.P.H.
Assistant Professor of Epidemiology, Department of Epidemiology, Mailman School of Public Health, Columbia University, New York, New York

Todd D. Gould, M.D.
Laboratory of Molecular Pathophysiology, National Institute of Mental Health, Bethesda, Maryland

Deborah Hasin, Ph.D.
Professor of Clinical Public Health (Epidemiology) (in Psychiatry), New York State Psychiatric Institute, Columbia University, York, New York

Jennifer L. Hughes, B.A.
Research Study Coordinator, University of Texas Southwestern Medical Center at Dallas, Dallas, Texas

Frank Jacobi, Ph.D.
Epidemiology and Health Services Research (Head), Institute of Clinical Psychology and Psychotherapy, Technische Universität Dresden, Dresden, Germany

G. Eric Jarvis, M.D., M.Sc.
Assistant Professor, Department of Psychiatry, Division of Social and Transcultural Psychiatry, McGill University, Culture and Mental Health Research Unit, Sir Mortimer B. Davis—Jewish General Hospital, Montreal, Quebec, Canada

Wayne J. Katon, M.D.
Professor and Vice-Chair, Department of Psychiatry and Behavioral Sciences, University of Washington School of Medicine, Seattle, Washington

Paul E. Keck Jr., M.D.
Professor of Psychiatry, Pharmacology and Neuroscience; Vice Chairman for Research, Department of Psychiatry, University of Cincinnati College of Medicine, Mental Health Care Line and General Clinical Research Center, Cincinnati Veterans Affairs Medical Center, Cincinnati, Ohio

Beth D. Kennard, Psy.D.
Associate Professor of Psychiatry, University of Texas Southwestern Medical Center at Dallas, Dallas, Texas

Ronald C. Kessler, Ph.D.
Professor, Department of Health Care Policy, Harvard Medical School, Boston, Massachusetts

Laurence J. Kirmayer, M.D.
James McGill Professor and Director, Division of Social and Transcultural Psychiatry, McGill University, Culture and Mental Health Research Unit, Sir Mortimer B. Davis—Jewish General Hospital, Montreal, Quebec, Canada

Daniel N. Klein, Ph.D.
Professor, Departments of Psychology and Psychiatry and Behavioral Science, Stony Brook University, Stony Brook, New York

Susan G. Kornstein, M.D.
Professor of Psychiatry and Obstetrics and Gyneceology; Executive Director, Mood Disorders Institute; Executive Director, Institute for Women's Health, Department of Psychiatry, Medical College of Virginia Campus, Virginia Commonwealth University, Richmond, Virginia

F. Andrew Kozel, M.D., M.S.
Assistant Professor of Psychiatry and VA Psychiatry Research and Neuroscience Fellow, Medical University of South Carolina, Charleston, South Carolina

K. Ranga Rama Krishnan, M.B., Ch.B.
Chairman and Professor of Psychiatry and Behavioral Sciences, Duke University Medical Center, Durham, North Carolina

David J. Kupfer, M.D.
Thomas Detre Professor and Chair, Department of Psychiatry, University of Pittsburgh School of Medicine, Western Psychiatric Institute and Clinic, Pittsburgh, Pennsylvania

Natalie Lester, B.S.
Vanderbilt University School of Medicine, Nashville, Tennessee

Xiangbao Li, M.D.
Visiting Research Scientist and Research Fellow, Department of Psychiatry, Medical University of South Carolina, Charleston, South Carolina

Husseini K. Manji, M.D.
Laboratory of Molecular Pathophysiology, National Institute of Mental Health, Bethesda, Maryland

J. John Mann, M.D.
The Paul Janssen Professor of Translational Neuroscience (in Psychiatry and Radiology), Columbia University; Chief of Neuroscience, New York State Psychiatric Institute, New York, New York

John C. Markowitz, M.D.
Research Psychiatrist, New York State Psychiatric Institute; Clinical Professor of Psychiatry, Weill Medical College of Cornell University; Adjunct Associate Professor of Clinical Psychiatry, Columbia University College of Physicians and Surgeons, New York, New York

Helen S. Mayberg, M.D.
Professor, Psychiatry and Neurology, Emory University School of Medicine, Atlanta, Georgia

Taryn L. Mayes, M.S.
Clinical Research Coordinator, University of Texas Southwestern Medical Center at Dallas, Dallas, Texas

Meghan E. McDevitt-Murphy, Ph.D.
Postdoctoral Fellow, Department of Psychiatry and Human Behavior, Brown University Medical School, Providence, Rhode Island

Susan L. McElroy, M.D.
Professor of Psychiatry and Neuroscience; Director, Psychopharmacology Research Program, Department of Psychiatry, University of Cincinnati College of Medicine, Cincinnati, Ohio

Brian R. McFarland, M.A.
Doctoral Student, Department of Psychology, Stony Brook University, Stony Brook, New York

Francisco A. Moreno, M.D.
Associate Professor, Department of Psychiatry, University of Arizona College of Medicine, Tucson, Arizona

Chiwen Mu, M.D., Ph.D.
Visiting Research Scientist and Research Fellow, Department of Psychiatry, Medical University of South Carolina, Charleston, South Carolina

David J. Muzina, M.D.
Director, Bipolar Disorders Clinic and Adult Inpatient Psychiatry, Department of Psychiatry and Psychology, Cleveland Clinic Foundation, Cleveland, Ohio

Larissa Myaskovsky, Ph.D.
Postdoctoral Fellow in Clinical Epidemiology, Department of Psychiatry, University of Pittsburgh School of Medicine and Medical Center, Pittsburgh, Pennsylvania

Ziad Nahas, M.D.
Assistant Professor of Psychiatry, Medical University of South Carolina, Charleston, South Carolina

Harold W. Neighbors, Ph.D.
Professor of Health Behavior and Health Education, School of Public Health, and Faculty Associate, Research Center for Group Dynamics, Institute for Social Research, University of Michigan, Ann Arbor, Michigan

Randolph M. Nesse, M.D.
Professor of Psychiatry and Psychology; Research Professor, Research Center for Group Dynamics, Institute for Social Research; and Director, ISR Evolution and Human Adaptation Program, University of Michigan, Ann Arbor, Michigan

Mitchell S. Nobler, M.D.
Medical Director, Electroconvulsive Therapy Service, Department of Biological Psychiatry, New York State Psychiatric Institute; and Associate Professor of Clinical Psychiatry, Department of Psychiatry, College of Physicians and Surgeons of Columbia University, New York, New York

Eric A. Nofzinger, M.D.
Associate Professor of Psychiatry, Sleep Neuroimaging Research Program, Department of Psychiatry, University of Pittsburgh School of Medicine, Pittsburgh, Pennsylvania

Edward Nunes, M.D.
Professor of Clinical Psychiatry, Columbia University, Department of Psychiatry, New York State Psychiatric Institute, New York, New York

Robert A. Padich, Ph.D.
Senior Scientific Communications Associate, Eli Lilly and Company, Indianapolis, Indiana

Cynthia R. Pfeffer, M.D.
Professor of Psychiatry, Weill Medical College of Cornell University, New York Presbyterian Hospital, White Plains, New York

William Zeigler Potter, M.D., Ph.D.
Vice President, Clinical Neuroscience, Merck Research Laboratories, Blue Bell, Pennsylvania (previously: Distinguished Medical Fellow, Eli Lilly and Company, Indianapolis, Indiana)

Jorge A. Quiroz, M.D.
Laboratory of Molecular Pathophysiology, National Institute of Mental Health, Bethesda, Maryland

Frederic M. Quitkin, M.D., D.M.Sc.
Professor of Clinical Psychiatry, Columbia University College of Physicians and Surgeons, and Research Psychiatrist, New York State Psychiatric Institute, New York, New York

Grazyna Rajkowska, Ph.D.
Professor, Department of Psychiatry and Human Behavior, University of Mississippi Medical Center, Jackson, Mississippi

Steven P. Roose, M.D.
Professor of Clinical Psychiatry, College of Physicians and Surgeons, Columbia University; and Director, Neuro-psychiatric Research Clinic, New York State Psychiatric Institute, New York, New York

Joshua Z. Rosenthal, M.D.
Fellow, Department of Psychiatry, University of Maryland Medical System, Baltimore, Maryland

Norman E. Rosenthal, M.D.
Clinical Professor of Psychiatry, Georgetown Medical School, Washington, D.C.

Eric Rubin, M.D., Ph.D.
Assistant Professor of Psychiatry, Columbia University, Department of Psychiatry, New York State Psychiatric Institute, New York, New York

Matthew V. Rudorfer, M.D.
Acting Chief, Adult Treatment and Preventive Interventions Research Branch, Division of Services and Intervention Research, National Institute of Mental Health, Bethesda, Maryland

A. John Rush, M.D.
Professor and Vice-Chairman for Research, Betty Jo Hay Distinguished Chair in Mental Health, Rosewood Corporation Chair in Biomedical Science, Department of Psychiatry, The University of Texas Southwestern Medical Center, Dallas, Texas

Harold A. Sackeim, Ph.D.
Chief, Department of Biological Psychiatry, New York State Psychiatric Institute; and Professor of Clinical Psychology in Psychiatry and Radiology, Departments of Psychiatry and Radiology, College of Physicians and Surgeons of Columbia University, New York, New York

Alan F. Schatzberg, M.D.
Kenneth T. Norris, Jr., Professor and Chairman, Department of Psychiatry and Behavioral Sciences, Stanford University School of Medicine, Stanford, California

Zindel V. Segal, Ph.D., C.Psych.
Professor of Psychiatry and Psychology, Centre for Addiction and Mental Health (CAMH), Clarke Site, University of Toronto, Toronto, Ontario, Canada

Stuart N. Seidman, M.D.
Assistant Professor of Clinical Psychiatry, Department of Psychiatry, College of Physicians and Surgeons of Columbia University; and the New York State Psychiatric Institute, New York, New York

Stewart A. Shankman, Ph.D.
Assistant Professor, Department of Psychology, University of Illinois at Chicago, Chicago, Illinois

M. Tracie Shea, Ph.D.
Associate Professor, Department of Psychiatry and Human Behavior, Brown University Medical School; Providence VA Medical Center, Providence, Rhode Island

Richard C. Shelton, M.D.
James G. Blakemore Professor, Department of Psychiatry, and Professor, Department of Pharmacology, Vanderbilt University School of Medicine, Nashville, Tennessee

Jaskaran B. Singh, M.D.
Laboratory of Molecular Pathophysiology, National Institute of Mental Health, Bethesda, Maryland

Diane M.E. Sloan, Pharm.D.
Director of Clinical Services, Medesta Associates; Senior Medical Director, CardinalHealth, Inc., Wayne, New Jersey

Dan J. Stein M.D., Ph.D.
Professor and Chair, Department of Psychiatry, University of Cape Town, Cape Town, South Africa

Jonathan W. Stewart, M.D.
Professor of Clinical Psychiatry, Columbia University College of Physicians and Surgeons, and Research Psychiatrist, New York State Psychiatric Institute, New York, New York

Michael H. Stone, M.D.
Professor of Clinical Psychiatry, Columbia College of Physicians and Surgeons, New York, New York

Stephen M. Strakowski, M.D.
Professor of Psychiatry, Psychology, and Neuroscience; Professor of Biomedical Engineering; Director, Divison of Bipolar Disorders Research; and Director, Center for Imaging Research, University of Cincinnati College of Medicine, Cincinnati, Ohio

Holly A. Swartz, M.D.
Assistant Professor of Psychiatry, Department of Psychiatry, University of Pittsburgh School of Medicine, Western Psychiatric Institute and Clinic, Pittsburgh, Pennsylvania

Galen E. Switzer, Ph.D.
Associate Professor of Medicine and Psychiatry, Department of Medicine, University of Pittsburgh School of Medicine and Medical Center, Pittsburgh, Pennsylvania; Co-Chief, Measurement Core, the Veterans Administration Center for Health Equity Research and Promotion, Pittsburgh, Pennsylvania

Michael E. Thase, M.D.
Associate Professor of Psychiatry, University of Pittsburgh, Pittsburgh, Pennsylvania

Marianna I. Tovt-Korshynska, M.D., Ph.D.
Associate Professor, Department of Internal and Family Medicine, Uzhgorod National State University School of Postgraduate Study, Uzhgorod, Ukraine

Philip S. Wang, M.D., Dr.P.H.
Assistant Professor, Department of Health Care Policy, Harvard Medical School; Division of Pharmacoepidemiology and Pharmacoeconomics, Brigham and Women's Hospital, Harvard Medical School, Boston, Massachusetts

V. Robin Weersing, Ph.D.
Assistant Professor, Child Study Center, Yale University School of Medicine, New Haven, Connecticut

David R. Williams, Ph.D., M.P.H.
Harold W. Cruse Collegiate Professor of Sociology and Professor of Epidemiology, School of Public Health; and Research Professor, Institute for Social Research, University of Michigan, Ann Arbor, Michigan

Hans-Ulrich Wittchen, Ph.D.
Professor, Chairman, and Director, Institute of Clinical Psychology and Psychotherapy, Technische Universität Dresden, Dresden, Germany; Max Planck Institute, Munich, Germany

Shirley Yen, Ph.D.
Assistant Professor (Research), Department of Psychiatry and Human Behavior, Brown University Medical School, Providence, Rhode Island

Carlos A. Zarate, M.D.
Laboratory of Molecular Pathophysiology, National Institute of Mental Health, Bethesda, Maryland

Preface

MOOD DISORDERS are the bread and butter of clinical psychiatry. Depression is the second most disabling of all medical disorders worldwide, and it is predicted to top the burden-of-disease tables by 2020. Suicide as a result of untreated or treatment-resistant mood disorder remains—appropriately—a major public health concern. Bipolar disorder accounts for a significant proportion of psychiatric hospitalizations. Mood disorders may result from general medical disorders, and they may also be an important risk factor for onset or adverse outcome of these medical conditions.

Fortunately, work on mood disorders continues to advance. Current classification systems provide reliable diagnosis, and they have also provided a useful base from which to conduct the epidemiological studies that have demonstrated the prevalence and morbidity of mood disorders. The explosion of modern neuroscience has provided new insights into the underlying neuronal circuits, and their associated molecular systems, that underpin mood symptoms. A range of new pharmacotherapies and psychotherapies have been introduced that are effective in both primary and specialist settings.

In view of the importance of mood disorders and the continuous progress in the field, we thought that a comprehensive text focusing on these conditions would be a timely contribution. We are delighted that so many leading experts in mood disorders agreed to contribute to this volume; this has allowed us to bring together a series of comprehensive and up-to-date reviews of the phenomenology, pathogenesis, pharmacotherapy, and psychotherapy of each of the major mood disorders in one volume. We are hopeful that this comprehensive text will be useful for clinicians in their day-to-day practice.

We would like to thank several people who made this volume possible. First, we would like to thank the Section Editors; each of the sections could stand as a volume on its own. Second, we are grateful to the contributors who sacrificed valuable research time in the hope that this volume would make their work more easily accessible. Third, the editorial team at American Psychiatric Publishing, Inc., made working on this volume an absolute pleasure, and we owe a particular debt of gratitude to Robert E. Hales, M.D., for his insightful advice and to Tina Coltri-Marshall for her tireless manuscript tracking assistance. Finally, we wish to acknowledge our families, who have been strongly supportive despite our frequent absences.

Dan J. Stein, M.D., Ph.D.

David J. Kupfer, M.D.

Alan J. Schatzberg, M.D.

PART 1

Symptomatology and Epidemiology

SECTION EDITOR: DAN J. STEIN, M.D., PH.D.

1

Historical Aspects of Mood Disorders

MICHAEL H. STONE, M.D.

What doth ensue but moody and dull melancholy, kinsman to grim and comfortless despair, and at her heels a huge infectious troop of pale distemperatures and foes to life?

Shakespeare, *Comedy of Errors* V, i, 79–82

THERE IS NO REASON to suppose that human nature has changed from the time we emerged, long before recorded history, as the intellectually gifted, language-capable, warlike primate *Homo sapiens*. A corollary to this premise is that mania and depression are two of the many manifestations of the human potential, even though their outward display and the names assigned to the varieties of mood have changed from one time frame to the next. The systematic *study* of mood disorders occupies only a small fraction of our 100,000-year history as *H. sapiens*, going back only some 2,500 years to the time of the ancient Greeks. Before that, we find only sporadic references in Hindu and biblical literature to persons who experienced bursts of fury, elation, or dejection or brief periods of what appear to us as psychotic depression.

In the Old Testament, for example, a few stories allude to disturbances of mood. When King Saul and his army were defeated by the Philistines, he begged his armorbearer to kill him. The man refused, so Saul took his own life (1 Sam. 18:11). Earlier, Saul had tried to kill David, apparently out of envy at David's having managed to kill Goliath. Nearer to our idea of "mood swings" is the story of King Samuel's mother, Hannah, who at first had been bitter and depressed because she had been unable to conceive. Her husband, Elkanah, asked her: "Why weepest thou? Why eatest thou not? And why is thy heart grieved? Am I not better to thee than ten sons?" (1 Sam. 2:1). But her "vegetative signs of depression" (if that is what they were) rapidly cleared up when she became pregnant. When she gave birth, she exclaimed: "Mine horn is exalted in the Lord; my mouth is enlarged over mine enemies." The 3,000-year gap between her time and ours makes it difficult to know if we can legitimately claim that this was a shift from dysthymia to hypomania.

TABLE 1–1.   The four elements and their corresponding temperaments

Element	Bodily fluid	Season	Planet/Other	Temperament
Earth	Black bile	Autumn	Saturn	Melancholic
Air	Blood	Spring	Jupiter	Sanguine
Fire	Yellow bile	Summer	Sun, Mars	Choleric
Water	Phlegm	Winter	Moon, Venus	Phlegmatic

During the time of the Buddha in the sixth century B.C., the legend arose concerning a certain princess who could not accept her infant's death. She would carry the dead baby from place to place, beseeching others to help her restore it to health. No one knew what to do with the crazed woman. Someone finally suggested that she seek out the Buddha. After she told him her story, he instructed her to gather poppy seeds—only they had to come from the houses of families who had never been touched by death. Of course, there were no such homes. When she returned to the abode of the Buddha, she began to realize the inner meaning of his words. As though awakening from a dream, so the story goes, she regained her sanity and buried the cold body of her dead child; afterward, she became a disciple of the Buddha (Stone 1997, p. xiii). The princess's story has some of the earmarks of what we might call psychotic depression. Whether her condition meets our criteria for that diagnosis must remain undecided, although it does seem clear that she had a severe mood disorder of a depressive type (Stone 1997).

Origins of Mania and Melancholy

Homer's *Iliad* begins with the account of Achilles' wrath—his Μηνις (mānis)—at being cheated out of his prize, the maiden Briseis; it is this word by which we designate our *mania*, even though the current concept answers more to the notion of abnormal elation than to wrath or fury. The same semantic disconnect occurs with the word *melancholy*, which we still use as a term denoting severe forms of sadness or depression, even though the term derives from Greek words meaning *black* and *bile*.

Ironically, despite the advances in psychiatry during the last century, including those in the area of mood disorders, the diagnostic labels for moods and temperaments have scarcely changed since Hippocrates' time. Writing in the sixth century B.C., the Greek-Sicilian philosopher

Empedocles and the physician Hippocrates both adhered to the four-element theory of the composition of all things in nature: *earth, air, fire,* and *water*. The Greeks were not the first to elaborate this theory, which existed earlier in Egypt, India, and China.[1] In the Old Testament, similar allusions to these elements (water, wind, fire, and earth) are mentioned (e.g., in Psalms 104:3, 5). The theory was not "medicalized," however, until Hippocrates' time, when excesses in the constitution of our bodies of one of these elements were cited as the cause of various diseases. This theory is illustrated in Table 1–1.

Even now, when it is clear that these "elements" play no causative role in mood disorders, the temperament words are still in use, although it is currently more common to refer to the "sanguine" type as hypomanic and to the "choleric" type as irritable. *Sanguine* and *choleric*, medical terms still used in the late nineteenth century, are now seldom encountered except in novels.

Arguably, the first to elaborate a coherent theory for the relations between the extremes of mood—mania and melancholy—was Aretaeus of Cappadocia (1856), a contemporary of Galen of Pergamum, in the first century A.D. On the topic of *melancholy*, Aretaeus commented:

> If black bile be determined upwards toward the stomach and diaphragm, it forms melancholy.... It is a lowness of spirit without fever; and it appears to me that melancholy is the commencement of mania. For in those who are mad, the understanding is turned sometimes to anger and sometimes to joy, but in the melancholics—to sorrow and despondency only.... Unreasonable fear also seizes them, if the disease tend to increase, when the dreams are true, terrifying and clear.... But if the illness become more urgent, hatred, avoidance of the haunts of men, vain lamentations; they complain of life, and desire to die. (pp. 298–300)

The allusion to the area below the diaphragm is important; the Greek word was *hypochondrium*, and because this subdiaphragmatic region was believed to be the seat of melancholic disposition, the term *hypochondriac* came into use (and remains in use) to describe melancholic per-

[1]The Chinese spoke of five elements: *Jin, Mù, Shui, Ho, Tu:* gold, wood, water, fire, and earth—with fire being equated with anger and irritability (see also Appendix).

sons who, among their other worries, fret excessively over bodily complaints.

Aretaeus's chapter on mania is titled "Περι Μανιης (Peri Manias)," but he uses the word *mania* not so much in our sense of manic illness as for *madness* in general. In his description, use of the term *mania* differs from current use. "The modes of mania/madness are infinite in species," he writes, "but one in genus." He adds,

> Those prone to the disease are such as are naturally passionate, irritable, of active habits, of an easy disposition, joyous, puerile; likewise those whose disposition inclines to the opposite condition, namely, such as are sluggish, sorrowful, slow to learn, but patient in labour…those likewise are more prone to melancholy who have formerly been in a mad condition [lit.: εκμαινονται: who were "mad" or "manic"]. (p. 301)

Aretaeus's description of "the manic" here resembles that of the (less severe) hyperthermic or the (more severe) hypomanic temperaments, followed by his description of a melancholic temperament. He pictures both as part of the same illness, showing that he was a "lumper," diagnostically, rather than a "splitter." This two-sides-of-the-same-coin theory of the mood disorders remained the dominant view for much of the next two millennia.

The views of Galen (131–200 A.D.) parallel those of Aretaeus. Galen described three forms of melancholy, one of which involved the accumulation of black bile below the rib cage (i.e., in the hypochondriac region), with symptoms of abdominal pain, flatulence, and belching, along with psychological symptoms. Black bile was a kind of psychic force, besides being a bodily substance, in Greco-Roman medicine (Berrios and Mumford 1995, p. 468). This viewpoint was not to change until the anatomical dissections of the Renaissance, the discoveries of which could no longer support the ancient humoral theories.

The following examples are clinical vignettes of melancholy described by Galen:

> I knew a man from Cappadocia who had gotten a crazy idea in his head, and once that happened, he fell into a state of melancholy. The idea was truly absurd: His family saw him crying, and they asked him why he was so sad. He told them, sighing profusely the while, that he was afraid that the whole world was about to collapse. His sadness, he went on, came from the king (of whom the poets speak) who carries the world—and is called Atlas: Atlas was growing tired of carrying the world for so long a time. Whence the risk that the heavens would fall and destroy the world.
>
> [A]nd you have heard me speak about the man who, while in the presence of other people, had passed wind—and who then, out of shame, wasted away and died. (*Commentaries* VIII, Epistle VI, cited in Postel and Quetel 1994, p. 19; my translation)

If Freud could be transported back in time, he would have understood the man as a depressed person projecting onto the god Atlas his own sense of mounting fatigue and powerlessness. But we see no hint of possible psychodynamics or of the symbolic expression of unacceptable feelings throughout the ancient period or, indeed, throughout most psychological writings for the next 1,500 years.

It becomes clear, through the works of Hippocrates, Aretaeus, and Galen, that *mania* was for Homer the name of a mere symptom and a temporary state; for the medical writers, it was the name of a distinct malady or illness of some lasting duration. *Melancholy* was used more often for a malady, although in the case of melancholy brought about by lovesickness, this could be either brief (if the impediments to the romance quickly eliminated) or (in the case of unrequited love or an unavailable object) protracted.

In the fifth century A.D., Caelius Aurelianus divided mania into two broad types: 1) a temporary form with lucid intervals and 2) a continuous form (Postel and Quetel 1994, p. 12). In either case, the condition affected the young and apparently men more often than women. Precipitants might be falling in love, anger, sadness, shock, or fear. Some patients were described who thought themselves to be a god, a famous actor, or the "center of the world" (similar to our full-blown manic psychosis).

Caelius Aurelianus seems to have agreed with Aretaeus and Galen that mania and melancholy were related maladies. As for treatment, he recommended that the "manic patient be placed in a room that is neither too bright nor too dark, that is disturbed neither by noises nor by pictures, and that is on the ground floor, given that manic patients sometimes hurl themselves out of windows" (*Chronicles* 1, 155ff, cited in Postel and Quetel 1994, p. 14).

A case of a woman whose melancholy, similar to Galen's case earlier in this chapter, stemmed from the conviction that her hand was crushed from holding in it the whole world, which would crumble if she bent her finger, was cited by the sixth-century A.D. writer Alexander of Tralles. He also maintained that phrenitis, a condition characterized by agitation with fever, was caused by yellow bile that expanded in the brain, leading to inflammation (Postel and Quetel 1994, p. 9). Alexander subscribed to the belief that melancholy was a form of mania (*hanc passionem furoris speciem*); however, writing in Latin, his word for *mania* also was the general word for *madness: furor* (the origin of our *fury*). It is easy to understand how the concepts of mania and madness got conflated: the person who believes he or she is a god, and whose movements are agitated and wild, seems decidedly more "crazy" or "mad" than an immobile and lugubrious person obsessed with the worry that Atlas has grown tired of holding up the world.

Mood Disorder in the Medieval Period

Following the Arab conquests and the spread of Islam after the death of Muhammad in the seventh century, knowledge of Greco-Roman medicine passed into the hands of Muslim physicians in the Near East and in Persia. In this medieval period, the two opposite mood states, still understood as manifestations of one underlying disorder, were now conflated under the term *melancholy*. There was a chain of influences, from Rufus of Ephesus to Ishaq ibn Amran (in the eleventh century) to Constantin the African, who thought that black bile, originating in the brain, could diffuse down into the body, ending up below the diaphragm (i.e., in the hypochondriac region), where it might even mix with other humors, such as yellow bile. This could provoke several subtly different symptoms. Melancholy, therefore, could exist in many different forms. Sadness and anxiety need not be the predominant manifestations. This led Jacques Despar in the fifteenth century to write, in his commentary on Avicenna, that physicians used the term *melancholy* as a common term both for melancholy, properly speaking, and for mania, given that both represent an alienation of the spirit caused by the black bile emanating from the "median brain ventricle."

Born in Bukhara in 981, Avicenna (Abu 'Alī al-Husayn ibn 'Abd Allāh *ibn Sīnā*)) showed his brilliance from an early age (he memorized the 6,300 verses of the Qur'an by age 10); on becoming a physician, Avicenna (1999) wrote a compendium—*The Canons of Medicine*—that was to become the standard text for the next 500 years. He carried forward the humoral theory of mood disorders, stating that "when melancholy is composed of laughter and leaping about, or is admixed with argumentativeness or combativeness, we call it *mania*. But we wouldn't call it mania unless it stem from yellow bile, nor do we refer to melancholy, narrowly speaking, unless it come from black bile" (Liber 3, tract. 4 of the Latin translation: Basel, 1556; my translation).

Toward the end of the thirteenth century and in the fourteenth century, the topic of *love* entered the nosography of Arab medicine. This can be schematized as a sequence of events, as follows: perception of the love object leads to the anticipation of pleasure, which affects one's powers of judgment, such that one estimates that the pleasure would be maximal. This estimate is retained in the imaginative powers of memory, and one's cognitive faculty busies itself continually with finding the means of attaining the love object. This painstaking reflection can at times lead to so profound a preoccupation as to end in madness. The madness in question was that of lovesick-ness or, as the Arabs called it, *ishk*. The responsibility for the illness is attributed to the (faulty) powers of judgment, which led to the conviction that the object of one's desire was the *only* person in the world who could satisfy that desire. The object is "therefore" irreplaceable; its loss, a fatal threat. The (profoundly melancholic) mood disorder that accompanies lovesickness could be either temporary or lasting and ultimately fatal—temporary, if the love object somehow became available (in which case the spirits immediately lifted), and lasting and dangerous, if the love object were unattainable. This theme repeats itself interminably in later dramatic works (the hero in Goethe's *The Sorrows of Young Werther* of the late eighteenth century; the heroine in Alexandre Dumas fils's *La Dame aux Camélias*—the inspiration for Violetta in Verdi's *La Traviata*).

Of course, this focus on lovesickness was not original: it had been described in ancient times, and Aretaeus himself had mentioned the condition in his chapter on melancholy. He told of a young man "dejected and spiritless from being unsuccessful with a certain girl, and appeared melancholic." When she ultimately accepted him, he "ceased from his dejection, and dispelled his passion and sorrow; and with joy he awoke from his lowness of spirits (χαρμη δε εξενηψε της δυσθυμιης)" (p. 300). Aretaeus's word *dysthymia* for "lowness of spirits" presages our current use of the term to designate a mild form of characterological depression.

This brings to mind the famous example from Avicenna, retold by Hajal (1994). The story illustrates the clinical acumen of Avicenna, who was called on to cure the nephew of the king in a province of Persia through which the physician was then traveling. Suspecting *ishk* as the diagnosis, and feeling the man's pulse, Avicenna asked this man, who was familiar with the area, to name aloud all the districts of the city. At mention of a certain district, the man's pulse fluttered. Avicenna then asked that he name all the streets and then the houses of the streets and their inhabitants. Putting together the names of just those places and families that caused the pulse to quicken, Avicenna concluded that the man was in love with a certain woman. Although greatly embarrassed, the man acknowledged this. When Avicenna informed the king, it turned out that the two were cousins. But their marrying each other was not forbidden, and the king quickly arranged the marriage, after which the lovesickness subsided at once.

As these examples make clear, the melancholy of lovesickness, although it may be characterized by alterations of mood and thought akin to our conception of depression, is different from the depressive forms of manic-depressive illness in that this syndrome can occur in many persons, not just in those with a biological and heritable predisposition to severe depression. I am prepared to believe, however, that persons with unipolar or bipolar illness may be more vulnerable to romantic disappointment, developing much more severe reactions (e.g., depression with vegetative signs, stalking behaviors) than would occur in persons without these disorders in a similar context.

As for the "vegetative signs of depression" in our current nosology, a contemporary of Avicenna, Ishaq ibn Amram, enumerated the following symptoms of melancholy: a general slowing down, immobility, mutism, sleep troubles, poor appetite, agitation, taciturnity, demoralization, worry, anxiety, sadness, and the risk of suicide. Amram's definition is closely in line with our conception of (serious) depression. However, *melancholy* was for the most part a very broad term in this era, covering both transitory conditions such as (the curable forms of) lovesickness and the more chronic and severe conditions resembling our endogenous depression (whether unipolar or bipolar). The more general descriptions of melancholy collected in the seventeenth century by Richard Burton (see "Reformation and Renaissance: Prelude to the Enlightenment" section later in this chapter) derived in good measure from the ninth-century Egyptian-Jewish physician Isaac Judaeus, whose works were translated into Latin in 1080.

The church fathers expressed their views on melancholy, including lovesickness—writing, of necessity, less from personal experience than from the cold logic of reason. The scholastic theologian and logician Saint Thomas Aquinas (1225–1274), for example, considered *sadness* the most dangerous of the passions: it "leads the body to melancholy and weighs down the soul." "Because sadness results from the presence of an evil," he stated, "it interferes with the movement of the Will, and gets in the way of enjoyments of its action," reminiscent of the abulia (loss of will) often noted in depressed persons. As for a remedy of sadness, Thomas Aquinas theorized (hopefully, it would seem) that "feelings belonging to the present are stronger than the memory of the past, and love of the Self is stronger than the love of others—so that in the end, joy pushes back Sadness" (*Summa Theologica* I, IIae, 2.38a, 1–3n).

Reformation and Renaissance: Prelude to the Enlightenment

We find little difference, let alone originality, in works devoted to mood disorders until the days of the Reformation. The scientific advances (notably, the Copernican discovery that the Earth was not the center of the universe) and the challenge to the authority of the Church (whose granting of indulgences was rightfully criticized) promoted freedom of thought. The aforementioned anatomical dissections of the Renaissance overturned the old theory of humors. These changes facilitated a new look at mood disorders.

Theory gradually changed, but adherence to humoral theory persisted for a time; of course, the names—mania and melancholy—live on.

Timothy Bright (1551–1615) was a physician in Elizabethan times whose treatise on melancholy (Bright 1586) still reflects Galenic theory, mentioning that "black bile riseth by excessive heate in such parts where it is engendered" (p. 31). Bright's monograph influenced Shakespeare, in whose works we find *melancholy* mentioned 69 times; mania, never.

Richard Burton (1577–1639), the dean of divinity at Oxford and author of *The Anatomy of Melancholy* (Burton 1621), a massive encyclopedia on the subject going back to ancient times, was himself melancholic. In personality, Burton was described as solitary, gloomy, self-deprecatory, guilt-ridden (despite a blameless life), bitter, and morbidly shy. Cox-Maksimov (1996) considers *The Anatomy of Melancholy* a philosophical, not a medical, work. For Burton, melancholy was a concept both broad and vague, occupying a middle ground between *folly* and *madness*. Yet a melancholic person might shift, under various circumstances, from one pole to the other. Burton pictured the body as composed of spirits and humors. The *spirits* were natural, vital, and animal, originating in the liver, heart, and brain, respectively. (In everyday speech, we still speak of the heart as the seat of emotion.) The solid parts of the body were the *humors*, as reflected in his comment: "For anger stirres choler, heats the blood and vitall spirits. Sorrow, on the other side, refrigerates the Body…overthrows appetite, hinders concoction [i.e., digestion], and perverts the understanding" (Burton 1621, p. 239). As Brink (1979) pointed out, Burton saw a connection between loss of attachment and subsequent mood disorder, anticipating the seminal work of John Bowlby (1980).

George Cheyne (1671–1743) was an English physician who wrote what is considered the earliest example of a book about one's own mental illness, which was apparently a mixture of melancholy (or, perhaps, dysthymia; he used the phrase *lowness of spirits*), "vapours," and hypochondriacal and hysterical distempers (Cheyne 1733). The combination of melancholy and intestinal distress that Cheyne described, along with his tendency to overindulge in alcohol and his morbid obesity (he came to weigh 32 stone, or 448 lbs!) and shortness of breath, all point not to any severe mental illness, as we understand the term, but to biliary disease and Pickwickian syndrome. Thus, his ascriptions, in regard to his illness, to the humors of black and yellow bile ironically ring true.

Cheyne is the one figure from the past writing on mood disorders whose "melancholy" really did relate to the biliary system.

Medical writers in the seventeenth century generally accepted the idea that melancholy and mania were aspects of the same disorder. This was so with Thomas Willis (1672; of the eponymous circle of arteries supplying the brain), who saw mania as a common sequel to melancholy: "post melancholiam, sequitur agendum de Mania, quae isti in tantum affinis est, ut hi affectus saepe vices commutent, et alteruter in alterum transeat" (p. 485). Here, he acknowledges that the one state could turn into the other and back again.

The French writer Antoine-Charles Lorry (1765) continued to endorse a humoral origin to melancholy, viewing it as a disease emanating from the liver, the repository of black and yellow bile. But he agreed with Willis about the unitary theory of melancholy and mania and their interchangeability, even referring at time to *"mania-melancholia"* as one word (Marneros 2001, p. 230).

The English physician Richard Mead (1673–1754), besides accepting the interchangeability of the two mood states, also posited that the phases of the moon affected various bodily functions and mental disorders, including the "furor of maniacs" (Mead 1746, p. 42). His impressions, ignored for some centuries, gained credence in modern times, in connection with certain bipolar patients who experienced exacerbations of their irritability and depression around the time of the full moon (Stone 1976).

Taking a cue from Mead, the French encyclopedist Denis Diderot (1713–1784) wrote the following in his article on mania:

> It is absolutely necessary to reduce mania and melancholy to one species of illness, and to view them at one glance, because experiments and one's daily observations teach us that the one and the other are of the same origin and of the same cause—which is to say, an excessive congestion of the blood in the brain (the weakest and softest part of the body), such that melancholy can be understood as the beginning stage of mania, and mania as the last stage of melancholy. (cited by Beauchêne 1993, Vol. 4, p. 1110; my translation)

A possible dissenting voice from this era was that of Vincenzo Chiarugi (1759–1820), who opposed the physical restraint of mental patients even before Philippe Pinel (1745–1826) did, although it is Pinel who has gotten credit for removing the chains from the "insane." Director of the Hospital of Bonifacio in Florence, Italy, Chiarugi (1795) was a systematizer, creating a kind of DSM of the eighteenth century. Mania, for Chiarugi, "signifies raving madness. The mania is like a tiger or a lion, and in this re-

spect may be considered a state opposite to true melancholy" (p. 301; my translation) It is not clear whether Chiarugi thought the two conditions were of different origin altogether (which would be a departure from the usual view) or merely wished to underscore the opposite nature of their clinical manifestations.

As for the treatment of melancholy and mania, advice and methods scarcely changed from the time of the ancient Egyptians, the predecessors of the ancient Greeks. For melancholy (in the narrower sense of a depressive illness), the cure consisted of pleasant music and games, recreations of all sorts, voluptuous paintings in the patients' rooms, beautiful gardens, excursions to lovely places, and so forth—that is, everything likely to cheer a patient up. For mania, opposite measures were taken of a sort that would induce calmness and reduce agitation. Various and exotic potions, including tartar emetic and digitalis, also were prescribed, many of which are cataloged at the end of Cheyne's treatise (1733) and later rejected as worthless by the physician John Ferriar (1761–1815), of Manchester, England, one of the first to recommend isolation of violent manic patients rather than restraint (Ferriar 1816, pp. 96ff).

The first breath of originality in this field comes from Leopold Elder von Auenbrugger (1722–1809), famous for his invention of auscultation by the stethoscope. He also described a cure for mania via administration of camphor (Auenbrugger 1776) to 11 patients. The camphor was given orally, rather than by injection (as was done a century and a half later by Ladislas Meduna), and may have produced seizures: the patients did foam at the mouth ("spuma circa oris labia colligebatur," p. 132) and undergo violent movements. Ferriar used camphor in some of his manic patients, but he obtained no beneficial results and abandoned it. Auenbrugger's method seems to anticipate the use of shock treatment developed in the 1920s and 1930s. There is some debate as to whether his camphor doses, given every 2 hours, *did* produce genuine seizures (as cited by Rudorfer et al. 2003) or not (Fink 2001). The words in the original are suggestive—*corporis motus:* "motions of the body." What is clear, however, is that the method was essentially forgotten for a century and a half.

Enlightenment Period

Toward the latter part of the eighteenth century, there was a marked change in the way mental illness was understood. Hitherto, the tendency was to view the mentally ill as anatomically incorrect specimens in whom the four elements and their corresponding humors were improperly distributed: those with too much black bile had melancholia, those with too much yellow bile had cholera, and so on. The erratic behavior of the uterus caused hysteria, purely a woman's disease, and so on. Occasionally, a more modern voice was heard, such as that of Charles LePois (1618), who claimed that men also could have hysteria and that financial worries and disappointments in love could lead to mental illness, irrespective of one's humoral balance. Comparatively little attention was paid to the subtle differences of individual people or to their early family backgrounds.

One of the first signs of attitudinal change was found in the writings of an obscure author, Christian Spiess (1796), which embody both the spirit of the Enlightenment, with its emphasis on direct observation, empiricism, and classification, and the spirit of romanticism, with its emphasis on sympathetic interest in the individual. Spiess wrote 10 biographies of mental patients, each reading like a brief novel of 30–70 pages. One of the biographies concerns a young woman who developed what we would call a psychotic depression after her infant was killed by the nuns of the convent she entered after her husband had gambled his money away and was then killed in a duel. The woman would fashion a "baby" out of rags, which she then fondled and cradled. I have given a fuller synopsis elsewhere (Stone 1997, pp. 56–57).

Black bile is not mentioned here; only the overwhelming life circumstances that the author assumes were the precipitants of her breakdown are described.

Pinel, considered by many to be the father of modern psychiatry, was "perhaps the last great man to use melancholia and mania in the classical sense" (Berrios 1995, p. 389). For Pinel, *melancholia* was a type of madness characterized by delusions limited to certain spheres of thinking. As Berrios points out, Pinel's use of the term is so broad as to encompass all form of chronic psychosis, including what we would now call schizophrenia (Berrios 1995). The following excerpts give the flavor of Pinel's approach to the subject and also show his acceptance of the one-illness model concerning the interchangeability of moods:

> The circumstances typical for succumbing to Melancholy are: sadness, fear, overwork…violent passionate love, abuse of intoxicants.… One has a marked tendency toward inactivity, but the affections of the soul are susceptible to great violence: love is carried to the level of madness; anger, to the level of frenzy…a gloomy taciturnity is often interrupted by bursts of gaiety of almost a convulsive nature. (Pinel 1798, p. 22; my translation)

Further on, he comments on mania:

> Mania has an affinity with melancholy and hypochondriasis, which makes one suppose that the site of these conditions is the epigastric region—since that is the center from which the episodes of mania spread. Some [patients] show an excess of joviality and break out into immoderate laughter; others show a gush of tears for no reason, or else an intense sadness.… In other cases you will see a sparkling look and an exuberant loquacity, which foretell the next explosion of a manic episode. (p. 25; my translation)

Pinel also described an intermittent or a periodic form of mania, adding that the various species of mania were not related to unhappy love, domestic woes, and the like but stemmed from the constitution of the individual. He also thought that gifted men with ardent imagination, capable of the strongest feeling and most energetic passion, were the closest to a "manic disposition" (Pinel et al. 1992). This description resembles the *hyperthermic temperament* (as an attenuated form of bipolar constitution) mentioned by Akiskal (1995).

Pinel's pupil Jean-Etienne Esquirol (1772–1840) brought about significant changes in the nosology of the day. He criticized the term *melancholia* as too broad and vague and advocated instead a term he coined to designate a *délire partielle*, or partial madness that was compartmentalized in just one area of life. Later, he called these encapsulated syndromes *monomanias* and suggested the term *lypémanie* (Esquirol 1838) for the monomania involving sadness of mood, which Esquirol considered a disorder of the emotions, not primarily of the intellect. Many of his contemporaries were in agreement with him, including James Cowles Prichard (1786–1848) in England and Benjamin Rush (1745–1813) in America. Pinel and his younger contemporary at the Salpêtrière, Georget (1820), while acknowledging the disturbance of emotion in melancholy and mania, saw disturbed thoughts as the culprit in setting in motion the subsequent mood disorder. As Georget explained it: "Fury or mania…is an intensification of nervous and muscular forces, excited by a false perception, a reminiscence or a false idea.…Outbreaks of mania are veritable paroxysms of madness [*délire*], which vary in their duration and in the frequency of their recurrence" (p. 107; my translation).

Lypémanie (from the Greek: "sad-madness") never caught on as a label (for what we would now call unipolar or bipolar depression) but neither did Rush's neologism, *tristemania* (Rush 1812). Prichard also emphasized the emotional aspect of melancholy and "raving madness" (mania), referring to these monomanias under the heading of "moral insanity." By *moral*, he meant the emotions, in a similar way to our use of the word *morale*—one's general spirits. For Prichard (1835), morbid irascibility and destructiveness of property also were among the examples of moral insanity; thus, many have now mistaken his *moral insanity* to be the equivalent of the modern term *psychopathy*. But our psychopathic patient, whose feelings are deranged in quite a different way from the person with severe mood disorder, is only one species of moral insanity: the two labels are not coextensive.

A little before the invention of the camera, etchings were occasionally made of mental patients. The famous etching of the woman with lypemania appears opposite page 408 in Volume 1 of Esquirol's 1838 text. Another well-known representation is Etching 3 of the depressed man in Ideler's 1841 book of biographical sketches of mental patients. Ideler's sketches, like those of Spiess, are lengthy and filled with the kind of detail about the patient's early life that modern-day psychiatrists consider routine and indispensable.

Mood Disorders in the Early Modern Period

Psychiatry, in particular its nosology, began to take on a modern appearance in the middle of the nineteenth century. Esquirol's dissatisfaction with the term *melancholy* that led him to substitute *lypémania* was shared by an ever-greater number of physicians. Esquirol (1838, pp. 22–24) also described, under the heading of "monomania," cases of what we now call *seasonal affective disorder*, including that of a woman who was active and eager for society during the winter but who became slothful, indecisive, and sedentary every spring and summer. Delasiauve (1856), on the staff of the Bicêtre Hospital in Paris, had already begun to use the word *depression* in place of *melancholy*, one of the first instances in psychiatry, although Samuel Johnson (1709–1784) had spoken of depression in the 1750s as a synonym for "low spirits" (Rousseau 2000).

Apropos of "low spirits," even by the 1820s, the English alienist Francis Willis had redefined mood disorders as either the "high state" or the "low state." "Both are apparently free," he mentioned, "from any bodily disease, and liable to pass one into the other; and in both, the greater number of sufferers, although they may be incurable, are easily, by good management, rendered tractable and comfortable in themselves. I conceive these two states are the MANIA and MELANCHOLIA of the ancients" (F. Willis 1823, p. 214).

A further detachment from the older terminology was effected by Wilhelm Griesinger, professor of psychiatry at Berlin's Charité Hospital (whose previous head had been Ideler). Griesinger, the teacher of Emil Kraepelin

(1856–1926), was an internist as well and is considered the father of biological psychiatry because of the conviction that there must be brain changes that corresponded to mental disorders and by virtue of the efforts he made to discover these organic changes. He also believed that the conditions of contemporary society contributed to the physical, mental, and moral degeneration of people, especially in the industrialized nations. There are echoes here of Jean-Jacques Rousseau's admiration for the "noble savage"—untainted (supposedly) by the complexities of modern life. Griesinger also belonged to the early generation of psychiatrists who went beyond being mere keepers of asylums to become professionals whose clinical work was amplified by research and teaching.

The taxonomy of Griesinger (1871), for whom only one fundamental form of insanity existed, the symptoms of which might change over time, consisted of the following: hypochondriasis; melancholy in the strict sense; depression with either apathy, destructiveness, or continual excitement of the will; psychic exaltation; rage (*tobsucht*); madness (*wahnsinn*); psychic weakness; partial madness (*partielle Verrücktheit*); and dementia (*allgemeine Verrücktheit*). The new term for depression was *Schwermut* (literally: heavy mood). The differentiation we now make between, say, schizophrenia and manic depression—as genetically separate entities—was not to come until later. In this way, Griesinger was in agreement with Zeller (1844) about madness, or psychosis as Zeller called it, being a global species unto itself.

Griesinger also described seasonal affective disorder, as had Esquirol, although Griesinger said that the melancholic phase began in the late autumn or winter (Angst and Marneros 2001).

Two French psychiatrists made signal contributions to the study of mood disorders that served as forerunners of the modern concept of manic-depressive illness. These contributions were, for all intents and purposes, simultaneous. Both represented a shift from the anatomical view of mind/brain as championed by Griesinger (who may have been the source of their inspiration [Angst and Marneros 2001]) toward the symptom-based or syndromal view. The latter was made possible, as Berrios (1988) mentioned, by the new psychological theories that acknowledged three separate faculties of the mind: the *intellectual*, the *emotional*, and the *volitional*. The philosopher Immanuel Kant had earlier elaborated a similar tripartite model of the mind, consisting of *thought*, *affect*, and *behavior*, a compartmentalization that allowed for the idea of a *partial* insanity (Hare 1981) and that contributed to Pinel's division of mania into a variant without delusion (his *folie raison-nante*) and a variant with delusion (mania proper). This paved the way for a division in the taxonomy of psychopathology along these three lines: it was now legitimate to posit that the emotions could, in certain cases, play the major and defining role in a mental illness (Berrios 1985). The importance of the emotions was augmented by the romantic movement of the late eighteenth century, as we saw with Christian Spiess and Karl Ideler. Other representatives included Pierre Maine de Biran (1803) and Jacques Moreau de Tours (1852). As for the two French psychiatrists, it is customary to speak first of Jules Falret, then of Jules Baillarger, because Falret's paper may have preceded Baillarger's by about a week. Both had been trained by Esquirol. Falret had mentioned in an 1851 lecture a special form of insanity he called "circular": *folie circulaire*, in which (manic) excitement alternated with *affaisement* or depression; lucid intervals typically occurred between the episodes (Falret 1854; Haustgen 1995). Baillarger (1854) spoke of *la folie à double forme*, in which there were two regular periods, one of depression and one of excitation. Each episode could last a few days or up to 2 years. The transition was often abrupt, as Haustgen (1995) mentions, such that one might go to bed melancholic and awaken manic. Baillarger thought that the lucid intervals of which his rival spoke were not important; the double-form attacks—if their periods were short—are the forerunners of our rapid-cycling bipolar disorder.

Falret thought that his *folie circulaire* was hereditary, more common in women, and detectable sometimes in attenuated forms, similar to our cyclothymic personality, in which the patient oscillated between lethargy and sadness and vivacity or "hypomania," without experiencing the extremes of either mood state. It was a generation later that Kahlbaum (1882) actually used the term *cyclothymia* or that Mendel (1881) coined the term *hypomania* (Brieger and Marneros 1997). As Angst and Marneros (2001) stated, Carl Jung (1904) described a hypomanic (or even milder "hyperthermic") state, under the heading *manische Verstimmung*, that ran a fairly stable course and might be associated with social restlessness, alcohol abuse, and delinquency. Jung's observation here mirrors his interest in subtle forms of abnormality that belong to the domain of personality, as in his descriptions of the introvert and extravert (Jung 1921), which can be seen as attenuated forms of the corresponding major psychoses (schizoid and hypomanic personalities). That some patients showed personality characteristics that partook of both depressive and manic traits but that fell short of full-blown "bipolar" illness was described by Kahlbaum's pupil (and cousin of his first wife) Ewald Hecker (1877). Hecker's cyclothymia consisted of brief depressions interspersed with mild excitements of short duration (a few days), similar to our bipolar II manic depression (Koukopoulos 2003). Subtle distinctions were made between *Mischbilder* (rapid alter-

nation between the two states) and *Mischzustände* (see discussion of Weygandt in last paragraph of this section), in which hypomanic and depressive features were present simultaneously (Maggini et al. 2000). Weygandt's insight served as a stimulus to Kraepelin's unified manic-depressive disorder concept, now more commonly called *bipolar disorder* (Salvatore et al. 2002).

Toward the end of the nineteenth century, Kraepelin (1883), the great systematizer in psychiatry, completed his textbook, which went through many editions from 1883 to 1909. He described the mood disorders under the rubric of manic-depressive insanity. For Kraepelin, this was a unitary concept; he did not make a distinction between unipolar and bipolar forms. In successive editions, he depicted various "mixed states" of manic depression. Marneros (2001) mentions several of these: manic stupor (*Stumpfheit*) in 1893; mania with inhibition (*Hemmung*) in 1899; depression with exaltation in 1904; and depressive anxious mania or inhibited mania in 1913. In this domain, Kraepelin was indebted to the earlier work of Germany's first professor of psychiatry, Johann Christian Heinroth (1818), who devoted several chapters to *gemischte Gemuthstörungen* (mixed mood disturbances) in his textbook. Included are descriptions of mixed states of exaltation and mental "weakness," as well as mixed mental disorders resembling our schizoaffective psychosis (Marneros 2001).

As for the signature clinical signs of mania, Kraepelin enumerated flight of ideas, euphoria, and hyperactivity, whereas for depression, the main signs were inhibition of thought, depressed mood, and weakness of volition (Marneros 2001). To the extent that Falret had emphasized the longitudinal course as part of the diagnosis of his *folie circulaire*, he is more in harmony with Kraepelin, for whom the time factor was an important dimension of diagnosis. Baillarger's syndromal view put him in greater harmony with DSM-IV (American Psychiatric Association 1994) (Haustgen 1995). For a time, Kraepelin made a distinction between manic-depressive insanity and involutional melancholia. The latter, occurring after age 45, he at first ascribed to the aging process rather than to the factors (including genetic ones) that underlay the various forms of manic depression. But, as Berrios (1995) pointed out (p. 393), Kraepelin abandoned the notion of involutional melancholia once it became clear to him that those who had this condition had manifested earlier in their lives the more usual forms of manic depression.

In the sixth edition of the textbook (1899), Kraepelin proposed a two-psychosis classification, differentiating manic depression from dementia praecox (Hare 1981). This was a departure from the *Einheitspsychose* of Zeller and the unitary psychosis of Griesinger. Now there was a cognitive psychosis alongside the mood psychosis—in line with Kant's tripartite model of the mind (our current concept of psychopathy represents the third, and volitional, psychosis). The typical (although not invariable) downhill course of dementia praecox was an important distinguishing feature. Ironically, the reformulation of Kraepelin's dementia praecox into the *schizophrenia* of Eugen Bleuler (1911) was as broad a concept as the unitary psychosis of the mid-1850s. Bleuler described the composer Robert Schumann, for example, as a schizophrenic person, although now his illness is seen to fall clearly within the manic-depressive spectrum: bipolar, with more depressive than manic episodes (Ostwald 1985, p. 303).

What helped place Kraepelin's division between manic depression and schizophrenia on stronger ground was the study of genetic factors in mental illness. Kraepelin himself suspected the importance of such factors but did not live to see his impressions confirmed. In 1921, he expressed the view that environmental stress factors might trigger attacks of manic or depressive episodes (more so at the beginning of the illness) but that "permanent internal changes" (i.e., innate) were the real cause of the malady (Kraepelin 1921, pp. 180–181). The twin and adoption studies in the 1930s and beyond were to bolster the genetic hypothesis. The monozygotic twin concordance in a 1935 study of 90 pairs, in which at least one twin had an affective disorder, for example, was 69% (Rosanoff et al. 1935).

At the close of the nineteenth century, Wilhelm Weygandt (1899), a pupil of Kraepelin, wrote a monograph on mixed manic-depressive states, including mania with thought poverty, agitated depression, and depression with flight of ideas. In a sense, the notion of mixed states represents a reawakening or reemphasis of the Greco-Roman authors (namely, Hippocrates and Aretaeus), who, as we have seen, wrote of melancholia going into mania and of states in which the symptoms of each co-occurred.

Developments in the Twentieth Century

Among the many accomplishments in the field of mood disorders in the last century, two that stand out are 1) the establishment of a more precise differentiation between manic-depressive and schizophrenic conditions and 2) the development of pharmacological agents that have a good measure of specificity for the treatment of mood disorders. Although clinicians in Europe were better about making the appropriate diagnostic distinctions, those in the United States overdiagnosed schizophrenia and underdiagnosed mania well through the 1960s and 1970s. The

availability of lithium and the publication of DSM-III (American Psychiatric Association 1980) helped set matters straight.

Credit for the discovery of lithium's usefulness in reducing the irritability and hyperexcitability of manic patients goes to the Australian physician Cade (1949). Lithium salts had been used in the 1890s in the treatment of periodic depression (Haenel 1986) but had almost no effect on the field; Cade's work lifted lithium out of obscurity and gave it a prominent place in our pharmacopoeia. Lithium is regarded as the first specific pharmacotherapeutic agent for a psychiatric illness (Vestergaard and Licht 2001). Mogens Schou (1957) in Denmark did much to widen the awareness and the use of lithium in the treatment of mania; the drug finally became available in the United States in 1969, whereafter it made good sense for psychiatrists to pay attention to diagnostic signs that might discriminate between mania and schizophrenia. This played a large role in reducing the tendency to lump all psychoses together as "schizophrenia."

A decade before the advent of lithium, convulsive therapy had been introduced to the treatment first of schizophrenia and then of affective disorders.

The pioneer in this form of somatic therapy was the Hungarian neuropsychiatrist Ladislas Meduna (1937), who used injections of camphor intramuscularly; later, he used intravenous injections of pentylenetetrazol. These methods induced seizures, which were followed by improvement in the patient's clinical picture. The use of camphor, an unwitting rediscovery of what Auenbrugger had used in the eighteenth century, was inspired by the supposition (albeit erroneous) that schizophrenia and epilepsy were "antagonistic" conditions (Fink 2001), such that induction of the one would be curative of the other.

Shock therapy has been refined and remains an important tool in the therapy for the "endogenous" mood disorders, especially those not responsive to pharmacotherapy (Goodwin and Jamison 1990, p. 660). As mentioned by Fink, the psychotropic drugs of the 1950s and 1960s have largely replaced the use of convulsive therapy (including the electroconvulsive therapy [ECT] developed in the 1920s by Cerletti and Bini in Italy [Rudorfer et al. 2003]).

The tricyclic antidepressants had been developed by the mid-1950s (Kuhn 1958). Their use and the use of antidepressants of other chemical classes (including the serotonin reuptake blockers, which, since the 1980s, have largely eclipsed their predecessors) have contributed to the waning of enthusiasm for ECT, despite the efficacy of the latter in remediating severe forms of mood disorders. The history of antidepressant therapy, including the use of monoamine oxidase inhibitors, is discussed in detail by Ban (2001).

A major controversy emerged in the middle of the twentieth century concerning manic-depressive illness: Did manic-depressive illness represent one broad entity, as Kraepelin had argued? Or was it more properly divisible into two entities—unipolar and bipolar—as Leonhard (1957) had proposed? (Angst and Perris 1968; Perris 1966). Leonhard emphasized the variable of clinical course: if manic and depressive episodes occurred in the same patient, then the condition was considered *bipolar*. This was "true manic-depressive illness" (Perris 1992). Recurrent episodes of either mania or (psychotic) depression, without episodes of an opposite type, were considered *unipolar*. Evidence from family pedigree studies was adduced to support Leonhard's hypothesis. The risk of bipolar illness in the first-degree relatives of probands with unipolar depression, in most studies between 1966 and 1982, significantly lower than for unipolar depression (Perris 1992). Because one cannot predict, from a first episode of psychotic depression, how the patient will track over time, Perris recommended that the term *unipolar* be reserved for persons experiencing at least three such episodes (granting that any episode after the third could still turn out to be manic).

The controversy about unipolar versus bipolar conditions has not yet been put to rest, but current research, such as that carried out by Hagop Akiskal (2003) and his colleagues, lends support once again to a broad bipolar spectrum, given that within the spectrum of bipolarity, "the most common manifestations are depressive in nature" (p. 2). Akiskal's work also points to a spectrum of bipolar disorders, ranging from bipolar I (manic episodes as intense as the depressive episodes) to bipolar II (serious depressions but only hypomanic episodes) to cyclothymia (Bourgeois et al. 1991) and, blending into the quasi-normal population, "hyperthermic" temperament. The latter is characterized by joviality, sociability, optimism, self-confidence, and adventurousness (Akiskal 1995, p. 6)—similar to the concept of extraversion and representing, presumably, mild genetic loading for bipolarity. Increasing evidence indicates that at least an important subgroup of patients with borderline personality disorder also should be included within the spectrum of "soft" bipolar disorders (Akiskal et al. 1983; Deltito et al. 2001).

Beyond this point, history blends into current events. To become familiar with where the field of mood disorders is now, the reader is well advised to consult the comprehensive text of Goodwin and Jamison (1990), in which all aspects of mood disorders—descriptive, genetic, diagnostic, prognostic, and therapeutic—are covered extensively and brilliantly.

References

Akiskal HS: Le spectre bipolaire: acquisitions et perspectives cliniques [The bipolar spectrum: research and clinical perspectives]. Encephale 21 (spec no 6):3–11, 1995

Akiskal HS: Validating "hard" and "soft" phenotypes within the bipolar spectrum: continuity or discontinuity? J Affect Disord 73:1–5, 2003

Akiskal HS, Hirschfeld RMA, Yerevanian BI: The relationship of personality to affective disorders. Arch Gen Psychiatry 40:801–810, 1983

American Psychiatric Association: Diagnostic and Statistical Manual of Mental Disorders, 3rd Edition. Washington, DC, American Psychiatric Association, 1980

American Psychiatric Association: Diagnostic and Statistical Manual of Mental Disorders, 4th Edition. Washington, DC, American Psychiatric Association, 1994

Angst J, Marneros A: Bipolarity from ancient to modern times: conception, birth and rebirth. J Affect Disord 67:2–19, 2001

Angst J, Perris C: Nosologie endogener depressionen: vergleich der ergebnissen zweier untersuchungen [On the nosology of endogenous depression: comparison of the results of two studies]. Arch Psychiatr Nervenkr 210:373–386, 1968

Aretaeus of Cappadocia: Τα Σωζομενα [The Extant Works]. Translated and edited by Adams F. London, Sydenham Society, 1856

Auenbrugger L: Experimentum Nascens de Remedio Specifico sub Signo Specifico in Mania Virorum [An Experiment Arising out of a Specific Cure Under the Specific Signs of Mania in Men]. Vienna, Austria, Joseph Kurzbök, 1776

Avicenna (Abu 'Alī al-Husayn ibn 'Abd Allāh ibn Sīnā): The Canon of Medicine (al-Qānūn fi'l-tibb). Translated by Gruner OC, Shah MH; Adapted by Bakhtiar L. Chicago, IL, KAZI Publications, 1999

Baillarger J: De la folie à double forme [Concerning the madness of double form]. Ann Med Psychol (Paris) 6:367–391, 1854

Ban TA: Pharmacotherapy of depression: a historical analysis. J Neurol Transm 108:707–716, 2001

Beauchêne H: Histoire de la Psychopathologie [History of Psychopathology], 2nd Edition. Paris, Presse Universitaires de France, 1993

Berrios GE: The psychopathology of affectivity: conceptual and historical aspects. Psychol Med 15:745–758, 1985

Berrios GE: Melancholia and depression during the 19th century: a conceptual history. Br J Psychiatry 153:298–304, 1988

Berrios GE: Mood disorders, in A History of Psychiatry: The Origin and History of Psychiatric Disorders. Edited by Berrios GE, Porter R. New York, NYU Press, 1995, pp 384–408

Berrios GE, Mumford D: Somatoform disorders, in A History of Psychiatry: The Origin and History of Psychiatric Disorders. Edited by Berrios GE, Porter R. New York, NYU Press, 1995, pp 451–475

Bleuler E: Dementia Praecox, oder die Gruppe der Schizophrenien [Dementia Praecox, or the Group of Schizophrenias]. Leipzig, Germany, Franz Deuticke, 1911

Bourgeois M, Verdoux H, Peyre F: Unipolaires et bipolaires: les deux maladies de l'humeur [Unipolar and bipolar disorders: 2 mood disorders]. Ann Med Psychol (Paris) 149:502–511, 1991

Bowlby J: Attachment and Loss: Loss, Sadness and Depression, Vol 3. New York, Basic Books, 1980

Brieger P, Marneros A: Dysthymia and cyclothymia: historical origins and contemporary development. J Affect Disord 45:117–126, 1997

Bright T: A Treatise of Melancholy. London, William Stansby, 1586

Brink A: Depression and loss: a theme in Robert Burton's "Anatomy of Melancholy" (1621). Can J Psychiatry 24:767–772, 1979

Burton R (written under the pseudonym Democritus Junior): The Anatomy of Melancholy. London, John Lichfield & James Short, 1621

Cade JFJ: Lithium salts in the treatment of psychotic excitement. Aust N Z J Psychiatry 33:527–531, 1949

Cheyne G: The English Malady, or a Treatise of Nervous Diseases of All Kinds…With the Author's Own Case at Large. London, G Strahan, 1733

Chiarugi V: Abhandlung über den Wahnsinn, überhaupt und insbesondere nebst einer Centurie von Beobachtungen [A Treatise on Madness, in General and Especially, Together With a Hundred Observations]. Leipzig, Germany, GD Meyer, 1795 [translation of Della Pazzia in Genere, e in Specie, 1793/1794]

Cox-Maksimov DCT: Burton's Anatomy of Melancholy: philosophically, medically and historically, part I. Hist Psychiatry 7:201–224, 1996

Delasiauve LJF: Du diagnostic différentiel de la lypémanie [Concerning the differential diagnosis of lypemania]. Ann Med Psychol (Paris) 146:271–280, 1856

Deltito J, Martin L, Riefkohl J, et al: Do patients with borderline personality disorder belong to the bipolar spectrum? J Affect Disord 67:221–228, 2001

Esquirol J-E: Des Maladies Mentales [On Mental Disorders]. Paris, J-B Baillière, 1838

Falret J-P: Mémoire sur la folie circulaire [A report on the circular madness]. Bulletin de l'Académie de Médicine 19:382–415, 1854

Ferriar J: Medical Histories and Reflections. Philadelphia, PA, Dobson, 1816

Fink M: Convulsive therapy: a review of the first 55 years. J Affect Disord 63:1–15, 2001

Georget E: De la Folie: Considérations sur cette Malade, son Siége et ses Symptomes [On Madness: Considerations Concerning This Condition, Its Basis and Its Symptoms]. Paris, Crevot, 1820

Goodwin FK, Jamison KR: Manic-Depressive Illness. New York, Oxford University Press, 1990

Griesinger W: Die Patholigie und Therapie der psychischen Krankheiten [Pathology and Treatment of Psychical Illnesses], 3rd Edition. Braunschweig, Germany, Friedrich Wreden, 1871

Haenel T: Historical notes on the therapy of depression. Schweiz Med Wochenschr 116:1652–1659, 1986

Hajal F: Diagnosis and treatment of lovesickness: an Islamic medieval case study. Hosp Community Psychiatry 45:647–650, 1994

Hare E: The two manias: a study of the evolution of the modern concept of mania. Br J Psychiatry 138:89–99, 1981

Haustgen T: Aspects historiques des troubles bipolaires dans la psychiatrie française [Historical aspects of bipolar disorders in French psychiatry]. Encephale Suppl 6:13–20, 1995

Hecker E: Die cyclothymie: eine cirkulare Gemüthserkrankung [Cyclothymia: an emotional disorder of a circular type]. Zeitschrift für praktische Ärzte 7:6–15, 1877

Heinroth JCA: Lehrbuch der Störungen des Seelenlebens, oder der Seelenstörung und ihrer Behandlung vom rationaler Standpunkt aus entworfen [A Textbook of the Disorders of Mental Life or of Mental Disturbance and Its Treatment Outlined From a Rational Standpoint]. Leipzig, Germany, Vogel, 1818

Ideler KW: Biographieen Geisteskranker in ihrer psychologischen Enwicklung [The Biographies of the Mentally Ill in Their Psychological Development]. Berlin, EH Schröder, 1841

Jung CG: Über manische Verstimmung [Manic mood disturbance]. Allgemeine Zeitschrift für Psychiatrie 61:15–39, 1904

Jung CG: Psychologische Typen [Psychological Types]. Zürich, Rascher, 1921

Kahlbaum KL: Über cyclishces Irresein [Concerning cyclical madness]. Der Irrenfreund 10:145–157, 1882

Koukopoulos A: Ewald Hecker's description of cyclothymia as a cyclical mood disorder: its relevance to the modern concept of bipolar-II. J Affect Disord 73:199–205, 2003

Kraepelin E: Compendium der Psychiatrie [A Compendium of Psychiatry]. Leipzig, Germany, Abel, 1883

Kraepelin E: Psychiatrie: Ein Lehrbuch für Studierende und Ärzte. Achte, vollständig umgearbeitete Auflage [A Textbook for Students and Physicians: 8th and Completely Revised Edition], 4 Vols. Leipzig, Germany, J A Barth, 1909

Kraepelin E: Manic-Depressive Insanity. Edinburgh, E&S Livingstone, 1921

Kuhn R: The treatment of depressive states with G22355 (imipramine hydrochloride). Am J Psychiatry 115:459–464, 1958

Leonhard K: Aufteilung der endogenen Psychosen [The Distribution of the Endogenous Psychoses]. Berlin, Germany, Akademie, 1957

LePois C: Selectiorum Observatiorum [On Some Particular Observations]. Pont-a-Mousson, France, Carolus Mercator, 1618

Lorry A-C: De Melancholia et Morbis Melancholiis [On Melancholia and on Melancholic Disorders], 2 Vols. Paris, Guillaume Caveller, 1765

Maggini C, Salvatore P, Gerhard A, et al: Psychopathology of stable and unstable mixed states: a historical review. Compr Psychiatry 41:77–82, 2000

Maine de Biran P: Influence de l'Habitude sur la Faculté de Penser [The Influence of Habit on the Faculty of Thought]. Paris, Henrichs, 1803

Marneros A: Origin and development of concepts of bipolar mixed states. J Affect Disord 67:229–240, 2001

Mead R: De Imperio Solis ac Lunae in Corpora Humana et Morbis inde Oriundis [On the Power of the Sun and the Moon on the Human Body and on the Illnesses Arising Therefrom]. London, John Brindley, 1746

Meduna L: Die Konvulsionstherapie der Schizophrenie [Convulsion-Therapy for Schizophrenia]. Halle, Germany, K Marhold, 1937

Mendel E: Die Manie [Mania]. Vienna, Urban & Schwarzenberg, 1881

Moreau de Tours JP: L'Identité de l'État de Rêve et de la Folie [The Identity of the Dream State and of Madness]. Paris, Baillière, 1852

Ostwald P: Schumann: The Inner Voices of a Musical Genius. Boston, MA, Northeastern University Press, 1985

Perris C: A study of bipolar (manic-depressive) and unipolar recurrent depressive psychoses. Acta Psychiatr Scand Suppl 194, 1966

Perris C: The distinction between unipolar and bipolar mood disorders: a 25-years perspective. Encephale 18 (spec no 1): 9–13, 1992

Pinel P: (An VI). Nosographie Philosophique, ou la Méthode d'Analyse Appliquée à la Médecine [A Philosophic Discourse on Illness, or the Method of Analysis Applied to Medicine]. Paris, Maradan, 1798

Pinel P, Allen DF, Postel J: On periodic or intermittent mania. Hist Psychiatry 3:351–370, 1992

Postel J, Quetel C (eds): Nouvelle Histoire de la Psychiatrie [A New History of Psychiatry]. Paris, Dunod, 1994

Prichard JC: A Treatise on Insanity and Other Disorders Affecting the Mind. London, Sherwood, Gilbert & Piper, 1835

Rosanoff AJ, Handy LM, Plesset IR: The etiology of manic-depressive syndromes with special reference to their occurrence in twins. Am J Psychiatry 91:247–286, 1935

Rousseau G: Depression's forgotten genealogy: notes toward a history of depression. Hist Psychiatry 11 (41 pt 1):71–106, 2000

Rudorfer MV, Henry ME, Sackheim HA: Electroconvulsive therapy, in Psychiatry. Edited by Tasman A, Kay J, Lieberman JA. New York, Wiley, 2003, pp 1865–1901

Rush B: Medical Inquiries and Observations Upon Diseases of the Mind. Philadelphia, PA, Kimber & Richardson, 1812

Salvatore P, Baldessarini RJ, Centorrino F, et al: Weygandt's "On the Mixed States of Manic-Depressive Insanity": a translation and commentary on its significance in the evolution of the concept of bipolar disorder. Harv Rev Psychiatry 10: 255–275, 2002

Schou M: Biology and pharmacology of the lithium ion. Pharmacol Rev 9:17–58, 1957

Spiess CH: Biographien der Wahnsinnigen [Biographies of the Mentally Ill]. Leipzig, Germany, [no publisher given], 1796

Stone MH: Madness and the moon revisited: possible influence of the full moon in a case of atypical mania. Psychiatr Ann 6:47–50, 1976

Stone MH: Healing the Mind. New York, WW Norton, 1997

Vestergaard P, Licht RW: 50 Years with lithium treatment in affective disorders: present problems and priorities. World J Biol Psychiatry 2:18–26, 2001

Weygandt W: Über die Mischzustände des manisch-depressiven Irreseins [Concerning the Mixed States of the Manic-Depressive Illness]. München, Germany, JF Lehmann, 1899

Willis F: A Treatise on Mental Derangement, Containing the Substance of the Gulstonian Lectures of May, 1822. London, Longman, Hurst, Rees, Orme & Brown, 1823

Willis T: De Anima Brutorum [On the Animal Soul]. Oxford, UK, R Davis, 1672

Zeller E: Die Einheitspsychose [The unitary psychosis]. Allgemeine Zeitschrift für Psychiatrie 1:1–79, 1844

Appendix: Mood Disorders as Understood in Chinese Medicine

Abundant references are found in Chinese medical literature to mania (*K'uang*, the character that indicates "mad, wild, violent") and depression (*Dian* or *Tien*, the character that embraces "craziness" or "epilepsy"). The more technical dictionary words are *Tsao K'uang* for mania and *Yū Ch'ou* for depression. The characters for the latter signify "grief-sad," or melancholy.

Mania and depression are considered two separate entities; a disorder involving mood swings from one pole to the other is seldom mentioned (Jiang 2003). Mania is seen as belonging to the element of fire (*ho*), akin to the Greek equating of fire with yellow bile and the choleric temperament. Mania could result from an excess of *yang qi* (the male spirit), whereas depression is often seen as the result of depletion of *yang qi*, leading to the relatively *yin* (female principle) state, in which the *yang qi* has, in effect, become exhausted. Insufficient exercise and eating too many sugary or fatty foods are thought to slow down the function of the liver and spleen, leading to depression (Trebichavska 2003). Those interested in a more detailed exposition of the Chinese approach to mood disorders, to the bodily organs that are implicated, and to the respective cures should consult the Internet article "Mental Disorders" (2002).

References

Jiang Y-P: The TCM diagnosis and treatment of bipolar disorder, part one. Acupuncture Today 4 (9), 2003. Available at: http://www.acupuncturetoday.com/archives2003/sep/09jiang.html.

Mental Disorders: Mood (affective) patterns/disorders. 2002. Available at: http://tcm.health-info.org/Common%20Diseases/Bipolar.htm.

Trebichavska D: Treating depression with traditional Chinese medicine and nutrition. 2003. Available at: http://www.healthtransformations.net/depression.htm.

CHAPTER

Classification of Mood Disorders

DANIEL N. KLEIN, PH.D.
STEWART A. SHANKMAN, PH.D.
BRIAN R. McFARLAND, M.A.

IN THIS CHAPTER, we provide an overview of current systems and issues in the classification of mood disorders. We begin with a brief discussion of the two official systems for classifying mood disorders: DSM-IV-TR (American Psychiatric Association 2000) and ICD-10 (World Health Organization 1992). Next, we discuss the boundaries between mood disorders, normal variations in mood, and selected groups of nonmood psychiatric disorders. Then, we review several subtyping distinctions that have been proposed within the mood disorders, with an emphasis on categories and specifiers included in DSM-IV-TR (some of which are discussed in greater detail in Chapter 32, by Rosenthal and Rosenthal; Chapter 33, by Stewart et al.; and Chapter 34, by Flores and Schatzberg, in this volume).

Finally, we review the issue of categorical versus dimensional classification systems and the related question of whether the various forms of mood disorders are discrete entities or regions on a continuum.

Current Classification Systems: DSM-IV-TR and ICD-10

The terms *mania* and *melancholia* and clinical descriptions of what we currently recognize as major mood disorders can be traced back to the ancient Greeks. However, modern views of mood disorders did not crystallize until the nineteenth century, with the work of French and German psychiatrists such as Falret, Baillarger, Kahlbaum, and Kraepelin (see Stone, Chapter 1, in this volume).

The two major classification systems in use today are DSM-IV-TR and ICD-10. Each system has its own particular history. However, both were significantly influenced by the development of explicit diagnostic criteria with clearly specified inclusion, exclusion, and duration criteria in the 1970s by the Washington University group (Feighner et al. 1972) and the Research Diagnostic Criteria (RDC; Spitzer et al. 1978). This approach was first introduced into an official classification system in DSM-III (American Psychiatric Association 1980). Its influence rapidly spread beyond the United States, and it was eventually adopted in ICD-10.

Although DSM-IV-TR and ICD-10 use somewhat different frameworks for organizing their sections on mood disorders, considerable overlap exists in their categories and subtypes and the specific diagnostic criteria used. As a result, a high level of concordance exists between the diagnoses assigned by the two systems (Andrews et al. 1999). However, the two systems do differ in some respects. For example, the DSM-IV-TR criteria for a major depressive episode require a minimum of 5 from a list of 9 symptoms, at least one of which must be depressed mood or loss of interest or pleasure. In contrast, the ICD-10 criteria for a depressive episode require at least 4 from a list of 10 symptoms (the 9 symptoms in DSM-IV-TR plus loss of confidence and self-esteem), and at least 2 of these symptoms must include depressed mood, decreased interest or pleasure, or decreased energy and fatigue. The ICD-10 subtypes depressive episodes according to the presence or absence of somatic symptoms, which is similar, but not identical, to the DSM-IV-TR melancholia specifier. In addition, ICD-10 does not include mood disorders due to general medical conditions or substance-induced mood disorders in the mood disorder category but instead classifies them as organic mental disorders and substance use disorders, respectively. Finally, DSM-IV-TR includes some specifiers that are not included in ICD-10 (e.g., atypical, seasonal).

The introduction of explicit diagnostic criteria has been associated with a significant increase in interrater reliability. Although it remains uncertain how reliable diagnosis is in routine clinical practice, it is clear that the higher-order mood disorder categories can be applied with a relatively high degree of interrater reliability and that even most of the lower-order subtypes and specifiers can be used with fair reliability (Holzer et al. 1996). The greater question concerns validity. The validity of a diagnostic system ultimately hinges on its ability to distinguish conditions with differing etiologies. However, the etiologies of almost all forms of mood disorders are currently unknown; hence, these disorders are defined on the basis of clinical data. As a result, the mood disorders are more aptly described as clinical syndromes than as disorders.

In the absence of knowledge of etiology, psychopathological syndromes generally have been evaluated with the construct validation framework developed by Robins and Guze (1970) and extended by others, which includes identifying a cluster of correlated symptoms, distinguishing it from other disorders, establishing predictive utility with respect to longitudinal course and treatment response,

showing familial aggregation, and identifying distinctive neurobiological and/or psychosocial correlates. Although considerable construct validation has accrued for bipolar disorder and major depressive disorder (MDD) since the introduction of the Feighner criteria 30 years ago, progress toward elucidating the etiology and pathogenesis of these conditions has been limited. As a result, dissatisfaction with existing classification systems is increasing, and recognition of the need for major revisions is growing (Van Praag 1998). However, there are currently few clear suggestions and no consensus regarding alternative classification systems.

Boundaries

In this section, we briefly review the relations and boundaries between the mood disorders and schizophrenia, anxiety disorders, and normality. Because of space limitations, several other important, and often problematic, boundaries are not considered, such as those involving personality disorders (especially borderline and depressive personality), substance use disorders, eating disorders, somatoform disorders, and general medical conditions.

Schizophrenia and Schizoaffective Disorder

The boundary between schizophrenia and the major mood disorders was established by Kraepelin, who argued that although the two conditions had overlapping symptoms, the former was characterized by a chronic, unremitting course, whereas the latter was characterized by a periodic course with a return to premorbid functioning between episodes. Although this distinction has been challenged, it has been supported by studies indicating that schizophrenia and the major mood disorders are relatively stable over time and differ with respect to familial aggregation and long-term outcome. Nonetheless, determining precisely where to place the boundary between the mood disorders and schizophrenia is difficult, and it has been necessary to develop intermediate categories such as schizoaffective disorder for patients with features of both conditions.

During the middle of the twentieth century, the definition of schizophrenia used in the United States was much broader than the one used in Europe, whereas the definition of mood disorders was correspondingly narrower. However, follow-up studies of broadly diagnosed schizophrenic patients in the United States found that many had relatively good outcomes and that these "good prognosis" patients often were characterized by affective symptoms and a family history of mood disorders. By the late 1970s, a literature accumulated indicating that patients with "schizoaffective" or "good prognosis" schizophrenia appeared to be more like patients with major mood disorders than like patients with more classical forms of schizophrenia on family history and course (Pope and Lipinski 1978). In light of these data, DSM-III significantly shifted the boundary between schizophrenia and the mood disorders, substantially narrowing the former category and expanding the latter.

This approach has continued through DSM-IV-TR; most patients who have psychotic features (whether mood-congruent or mood-incongruent) during a manic or major depressive episode are given a mood disorder diagnosis (see Flores and Schatzberg, Chapter 34, in this volume). The category schizoaffective disorder, which is placed in the "Schizophrenia and Other Psychotic Disorders" section of DSM-IV-TR, is reserved for patients who experience concurrent mood disorder episodes and psychotic symptoms but also have psychotic symptoms in the absence of prominent mood symptoms (e.g., after the mood disorder has remitted). This definition departs from most other definitions of schizoaffective disorder, which emphasize the presence of contemporaneous mood and psychotic symptoms (e.g., RDC, ICD-10). However, the definition is supported by evidence that schizoaffective patients who continue to experience psychotic symptoms in the absence of prominent mood symptoms tend to have relatively poor outcomes and an elevated rate of schizophrenia in their first-degree relatives (Kendler et al. 1995a). Schizoaffective disorder is divided into bipolar and depressive subtypes because some evidence (albeit inconsistent) suggests that the former bears a greater resemblance to bipolar disorder, whereas the latter is intermediate between schizophrenia and MDD on family history and course (Lapensée 1992).

Anxiety Disorders

There has been a long-standing debate in the literature as to whether depressive and anxiety disorders are distinct conditions or variants of a single disorder or whether a third category of anxious depression exists that is distinct from both pure depression and pure anxiety. Many studies in both clinical and community samples have documented high rates of comorbidity between mood disorders and anxiety disorders. More than 50% of the individuals with MDD or dysthymic disorder meet criteria for an anxiety disorder, and more than 50% of the individuals with anxiety disorders meet criteria for MDD or dysthymia (Mineka et al. 1998). All of the specific anxiety disorders have high comorbidity with depression (T.A. Brown et al. 2001). Although most studies have focused on nonbipolar

disorders, there is also evidence of high comorbidity between bipolar disorder and anxiety disorders (Freeman et al. 2002).

The high comorbidity between depression and anxiety may be due to shared genetic factors, particularly in the case of MDD and generalized anxiety disorder (GAD) (Kendler et al. 1995b), and shared psychosocial causes, such as childhood and adult adversity (G.W. Brown et al. 1996). However, there is also evidence indicating that the mood and anxiety disorders are at least partially distinct. For example, family studies indicate that MDD and anxiety disorders are independently transmitted (Klein et al. 2003), and twin studies suggest substantial genetic independence between MDD and most anxiety disorders (Kendler et al. 1995b).

The age at onset of anxiety disorders is typically earlier than the onset of MDD, which has led some investigators to hypothesize that anxiety disorders predispose to the development of mood disorders (Mineka et al. 1998). However, this sequence does not hold for all disorders. For example, dysthymic disorder typically precedes the onset of comorbid panic disorder, obsessive-compulsive disorder, and posttraumatic stress disorder (T.A. Brown et al. 2001).

Clark and Watson (1991) proposed a framework for describing the complex association between depression and anxiety. Their tripartite model parses the domain of anxiety and depression into three dimensions: general distress, anhedonia, and physiological hyperarousal. According to the model, depression and anxiety are both characterized by a high level of distress. However, depression is uniquely characterized by a high level of anhedonia, whereas anxiety is uniquely characterized by a high level of physiological hyperarousal. One implication of the model is that the distinction between depression and anxiety can be sharpened by emphasizing the two specific dimensions—anhedonia and physiological hyperarousal—and deemphasizing symptoms reflecting general distress (e.g., negative affect, insomnia, difficulty concentrating). The tripartite model has been supported by numerous studies (Mineka et al. 1998). However, to take into account the heterogeneity of anxiety disorders, it will be necessary to specify factors other than physiological hyperarousal that can distinguish particular anxiety disorders from depression and from one another (Mineka et al. 1998).

Normal Variations in Mood

The distinction between mood disorders and normal variations in mood, responses to stress, and unhappiness is complex because it is influenced by a variety of cultural, social, and economic factors and has changed over time.

Some investigators believe that mood disorder symptoms are continuously distributed throughout the population, with no clear boundary between normality and disorder. Among those who accept a boundary between mood disorders and normality, investigators disagree about where it should be placed. Some investigators believe that the current boundaries are too broad and include some individuals with transient responses to stress and demoralization. This argument is based on evidence that antidepressant medication is generally no more effective than placebo for mild cases of depression (Kocsis 1993) and the belief that the prevalence of mood disorders identified in community surveys is unreasonably high (Narrow et al. 2002). Other investigators believe that the current boundaries are too strict, pointing to evidence that many individuals with subthreshold depressive symptoms experience significant functional impairment but do not meet full criteria for a mood disorder (see Stewart et al., Chapter 33, in this volume).

The problem of the boundary between mood disorders and normality encompasses at least three different issues. First, when is dysphoria an expectable response to stress, and when does it indicate disorder? DSM-IV-TR defines mood disorders syndromally, with minimal assumptions about etiology: if a period of depression meets criteria for a mood disorder, it is diagnosed regardless of whether it is associated with stress. The one major exception involves bereavement. On the basis of evidence that approximately one-third of individuals meet criteria for MDD 2 months after the death of a spouse (Zisook and Shuchter 1991), DSM-IV-TR requires that such symptoms be diagnosed as uncomplicated bereavement unless the episode lasts longer than 2 months or is characterized by marked impairment, worthlessness, suicidal ideation, psychomotor retardation, or psychotic symptoms. However, some investigators believe that it is arbitrary to view depression as a normative response to bereavement but not to other significant losses, such as divorce or abandonment. Indeed, a wide variety of types of losses are associated with elevated risk for MDD, and more than 80% of individuals in the community with a major depressive episode have experienced a severe life event or major difficulty in the 6–12 months before onset (G.W. Brown and Harris 1989).

Second, the distinction between transient periods of elated mood and hypomanic episodes is problematic, particularly because hypomania is often ego-syntonic and can be socially and vocationally adaptive. This issue has become increasingly important with the growing interest in the soft bipolar spectrum (see Stewart et al., Chapter 33, in this volume). Unfortunately, little systematic research is available on where to draw the line between normal good mood and hypomania.

Third, the boundary between mood disorders and variants of temperament and personality such as neuroticism is also uncertain. This issue is particularly relevant for mild chronic mood disorders such as dysthymic and cyclothymic disorder, in which mood symptoms appear to be part of the individual's personality. Establishing this boundary is especially challenging in light of evidence that some personality or temperament dimensions may be precursors of, or predisposing factors to, mood disorders (Klein et al. 2002).

Subtypes and Forms of Mood Disorders

When Kraepelin distinguished dementia praecox from manic-depressive illness, his view of the latter was relatively broad, including most recurrent mood disorders and encompassing a wide range of severity. Much of the subsequent debate in the classification of mood disorders has revolved around whether to accept or reject this unitary view. In particular, the debate has focused on three distinctions: unipolar-bipolar, psychotic-neurotic, and endogenous-reactive.

Unipolar-Bipolar Distinction

One of the most influential challenges to the unitary perspective was proposed in the 1950s by Leonhard, who argued for a distinction between patients who had both manic and depressive episodes (bipolar) and those who had only manic or depressive episodes (unipolar). In the 1960s, Leonhard's proposal received strong confirmation from independent studies by Angst in Switzerland, Perris in Sweden, and Winokur in St. Louis, Missouri. However, because almost all patients with manias in these studies also had experienced depressive episodes, the few unipolar manic patients were combined with the bipolar patients, and the basis for the distinction shifted to the presence or absence of a history of mania. The unipolar-bipolar distinction is the backbone of the DSM-IV-TR classification of mood disorders, although MDD is used instead of the term *unipolar depression*.

The unipolar-bipolar distinction is supported by several lines of evidence:

1. The rate of bipolar disorder is elevated in the first-degree relatives of probands with bipolar disorder, but the rate of bipolar disorder in the relatives of unipolar probands is similar to that in the general population (Winokur et al. 1995).

2. Genetic factors play a larger role in bipolar disorder than in MDD (McGuffin et al. 2003).
3. The prevalence of bipolar disorder is approximately equal in both sexes, whereas unipolar disorder is about twice as common in women as in men (Perris 1992; see also Goodwin et al., Chapter 3, in this volume).
4. Patients with bipolar disorder have an earlier onset, a greater number of total mood disorder episodes, and possibly lower rates of chronicity than do patients with unipolar disorder (Winokur et al. 1993).

In addition, although findings conflict, bipolar patients tend to have hypersomnia and psychomotor retardation and are more likely to have psychotic symptoms during depressive episodes, whereas unipolar patients are more prone to experience insomnia, psychomotor agitation, anxiety, and hypochondriasis (Perris 1992). Moreover, several studies have found that patients with bipolar disorder in remission show higher levels of extraversion and lower levels of neuroticism than do patients with unipolar disorder in remission (Klein et al. 2002). Finally, antidepressant medications may be more likely to precipitate manic or hypomanic episodes in patients with bipolar disorder than in patients with unipolar disorder (Altschuler et al. 1995).

Despite these differences, the unipolar-bipolar distinction is not universally accepted (Akiskal et al. 2000). For example, some investigators have advocated a version of the unitary model that views the two disorders as falling along a continuum, with bipolar disorder being a more severe form of illness (Gershon et al. 1982). The two conditions clearly overlap—both are associated with elevated rates of unipolar disorder in relatives (Perris 1992), and both mania and depression are influenced by some of the same genes (McGuffin et al. 2003). However, recent twin study data indicated that most of the genetic variance between manic and depressive episodes is distinct (McGuffin et al. 2003). This is consistent with Johnson and Kizer's (2002) suggestion that bipolar and unipolar depressions are determined by the same processes and that another set of processes is responsible for manic episodes.

Research on the unipolar-bipolar distinction is complicated by the fact that approximately 10% of the individuals with MDD eventually develop manic or hypomanic episodes (Coryell et al. 1995). Thus, a small subgroup of unipolar depressions in most studies is probably misdiagnosed, which could obscure differences between the two subtypes and account for inconsistent findings in this area.

The belief that unipolar mania is rare has been questioned recently (Johnson and Kizer 2002). Studies have suggested that 16%–20% of the patients with bipolar disorder in community and clinical samples have no history of depressive episodes. However, at this point, it does not appear that the differences between individuals with bipolar and unipolar mania are meaningful enough to warrant distinguishing these subgroups (Yazici et al. 2002).

Kraepelin noted that many patients have complex admixtures of manic and depressive symptoms, either simultaneously (mixed states) or in rapid alternation (rapid cycling). DSM-IV-TR includes both of these presentations. In approximately 31% of manic episodes, prominent depressive symptoms are also evident (McElroy et al. 1992). Mixed (or dysphoric) mania is important clinically because it is associated with a poorer outcome and treatment response, especially to lithium (McElroy et al. 1992). DSM-IV-TR classifies patients who have both a full manic and a full depressive syndrome nearly every day for at least 1 week as having a mixed episode. This is a fairly conservative definition, and some investigators prefer a broader definition requiring fewer depressive symptoms (McElroy et al. 1992). DSM-IV-TR also includes a specifier for rapid-cycling bipolar disorder. Dunner and Fieve (1974) define rapid cycling as four or more manic, hypomanic, or depressive episodes within a 12-month period. Approximately 15% of bipolar patients experience rapid cycling (Coryell et al. 1992), the vast majority of whom are women. Like dysphoric mania, rapid cycling is associated with a poorer outcome and response to treatment (Bauer et al. 1994). Because most patients with rapid cycling also have periods of nonrapid cycling (Coryell et al. 1992), it is probably best conceptualized as a phase in the course of some bipolar disorders rather than as a distinct subtype.

Bipolar II and the Bipolar Spectrum

Kraepelin believed that mania can exist along a continuum of severity, ranging from episodes characterized by gross impairment and psychosis to milder episodes that shade into normal joy and exuberance. Fieve and Dunner (1975) distinguished between bipolar I disorder, which is characterized by manic and major depressive episodes, and bipolar II disorder, which is characterized by hypomanic and major depressive episodes. This definition was adopted in DSM-IV-TR, which distinguishes hypomania from mania by requiring that the episode not be severe enough to cause marked impairment or to necessitate hospitalization and that no psychotic features be present. In turn, DSM-IV-TR distinguishes hypomania from a normal good mood by requiring a minimum duration of 4 days, an unequivocal change in functioning, and that the disturbance in mood and change in functioning be observable by others. Some investigators believe that the 4-day duration criterion is too strict and should be reduced to 1–2 days (Akiskal et al. 2000).

It is unclear whether bipolar II should be considered a variant of bipolar I disorder, a variant of MDD, a mid-region in a continuum between bipolar I disorder and MDD, or a third distinct disorder. The data are most consistent with the view that bipolar II is a distinct condition, albeit with some overlap with bipolar I disorder and MDD. There are two main sources of support for its distinctiveness. Family studies indicate that the rate of bipolar II disorder is higher in the relatives of probands with bipolar II disorder than in the relatives of probands with bipolar I disorder and MDD (Coryell 1996). In addition, follow-up studies indicate that the distinction between bipolar I, bipolar II, and MDD is relatively stable over time (Coryell et al. 1995). However, some evidence also shows overlap between bipolar I and II disorders. Although the rate of bipolar I disorder in the relatives of bipolar II probands is lower than in the relatives of bipolar I probands, it is higher than in the relatives of MDD probands (Coryell 1996). Moreover, although only a small proportion of patients with bipolar II disorder develop manic episodes, the rate is higher than for patients with MDD (Coryell et al. 1995). Finally, bipolar II disorder overlaps with MDD in that it is much more prevalent in women, and patients with bipolar II disorder experience more frequent and longer periods of depression than do bipolar I patients (Judd et al. 2003).

DSM-IV-TR also includes the category of cyclothymic disorder, a milder form of bipolar disorder characterized by a long-standing pattern of recurrent hypomanic and depressive periods that are too brief to meet criteria for hypomanic and major depressive episodes. Although the literature is limited, cyclothymic disorder appears to have familial links to bipolar I and II disorders (Klein et al. 1985). In addition, patients with cyclothymia frequently develop hypomanic and major depressive episodes, qualifying for a diagnosis of bipolar II disorder, although full-blown manic episodes are much rarer (Akiskal et al. 1977). Finally, there have been proposals to extend the bipolar spectrum to include patients who develop manic or hypomanic episodes during treatment with antidepressant medication (bipolar III), a group that DSM-IV-TR classifies as having a substance-induced mood disorder, and patients with MDD and a hyperthymic temperament (i.e., hypomanic personality) (bipolar IV) (Akiskal et al. 2000).

Psychotic-Neurotic and Endogenous-Reactive Distinctions

The psychotic-neurotic and endogenous-reactive distinctions have sometimes been used interchangeably. The major debate with respect to both distinctions is whether they represent two distinct forms of mood disorder or the poles of a single dimension of severity. It has generally been assumed that bipolar disorder belongs in the psychotic and endogenous subgroups (Parker 2000). Hence, the debate has focused on the much larger, and more heterogeneous, population of persons with nonbipolar depression. In this section, we consider the concepts of psychotic, endogenous (or melancholic), neurotic, and reactive depression separately.

Psychotic Depression

The term *psychotic depression* has been used in two different ways: 1) to refer to depressive episodes with psychotic symptoms and 2) to refer to severe depressive episodes that may or may not have psychotic symptoms. DSM-IV-TR uses *psychotic features* in the former, more circumscribed, sense. In DSM-IV-TR, psychotic features can be noted for manic, mixed, and major depressive episodes. However, the validity of the psychotic-nonpsychotic distinction has received less attention in bipolar disorder and appears to have fewer correlates than it does for MDD (Keck et al. 2003).

The distinction between MDD with and without psychotic features is supported by differences in a number of areas. Psychotic depression has a poorer response to placebo and antidepressant medication and generally requires electroconvulsive therapy or combined treatment with antidepressants and neuroleptics (see Flores and Schatzberg, Chapter 34, in this volume). In addition, psychotic depression is characterized by greater psychomotor disturbance, neuropsychological deficits, hypothalamic-pituitary-adrenal (HPA) axis dysregulation, and electroencephalogram sleep abnormalities. Moreover, several studies have reported that the relatives of probands with psychotic depression have higher rates of bipolar disorder and MDD than do the relatives of probands with nonpsychotic MDD, although negative findings also have been reported. Finally, MDD with psychotic features has a poorer long-term outcome than nonpsychotic MDD (Schatzberg and Rothschild 1992).

A key question is whether these differences are specifically associated with the presence of psychotic features or are more broadly attributable to greater severity. Some evidence indicates that the differences persist even after controlling for severity of depressive symptoms, but most studies have not addressed this confound. However, evidence that the psychotic subtype runs in families (Coryell 1997) and is relatively stable over repeated episodes (Coryell et al. 1995) supports the distinctiveness of the subtype.

DSM also distinguishes between psychotic features that are mood congruent or mood incongruent according to whether the content of the delusions and hallucinations is consistent with a manic or depressed mood (i.e., themes of grandiosity or themes of guilt, disease, and nihilism, respectively). Although it is unclear whether bipolar disorder and MDD with mood-incongruent and mood-congruent psychotic features are distinct subtypes, some studies have reported that mood-incongruent psychotic features predict a poorer course and outcome (Fennig et al. 1996).

Endogenous Depression (Melancholia)

The endogenous-reactive distinction developed from the view that some depressions were caused by internal biological factors and others by external environmental factors. Thus, endogenous depression was presumed to be characterized by greater biological abnormalities, better response to somatic treatments, greater familial aggregation, and a lower rate of stressful life events. In addition, because the psychotic-neurotic and endogenous-reactive distinctions often were used synonymously, endogenous depression also was assumed to be associated with less personality disturbance and to have a more episodic (less chronic) course. However, DSM-III and subsequent DSM editions eschewed the etiological implications of the term *endogenous* and renamed the construct *melancholia*. It is included as a specifier for major depressive episodes in the context of both bipolar disorder and MDD.

Clinical descriptions of endogenous, or melancholic, depression have emphasized a particular constellation of symptoms, including psychomotor disturbance (especially retardation), lack of reactivity to the environment, terminal insomnia, weight loss, distinct quality of depressed mood, diurnal variation of mood with worsening in the morning, anhedonia, guilt, and psychotic features. This profile has been supported by numerous studies that used factor analysis and cluster analysis and consistently found that these symptoms, or patients with these symptoms, tend to cluster together (Rush and Weissenburger 1994).

In contrast, studies comparing MDD patients with and without melancholia on external variables that would be expected to distinguish the two groups have been less consistent. Moreover, melancholia consistently has been shown to be associated with greater symptom severity, even when considering only nonmelancholic depressive symptoms (Zimmerman and Spitzer 1989). Hence, to the extent that the predicted differences are obtained, they may be due to severity differences rather than because melancholia is a distinct subtype.

Studies have found that patients with melancholia have greater biological abnormalities, such as failure to suppress cortisol on the dexamethasone suppression test (DST) and decreased rapid eye movement latencies, al-

though these findings vary somewhat depending on the criteria used to define melancholia (Rush and Weissenburger 1994). Early studies reported that melancholic features predicted response to electroconvulsive therapy and tricyclic antidepressants. However, these findings generally have not been replicated in studies conducted over the past several decades (Rush and Weissenburger 1994; Zimmerman and Spitzer 1989). Interestingly, several studies have reported that melancholia is associated with a lower placebo response rate (e.g., Peselow et al. 1992).

Family studies have yielded mixed findings (Rush and Weissenburger 1994; Zimmerman and Spitzer 1989). Several studies have found a higher rate of MDD in the relatives of melancholic than nonmelancholic probands, but other studies have failed to find a difference. In addition, no evidence indicates that the relatives of melancholic probands have a higher rate of melancholia. The lack of specificity of familial aggregation of melancholia is consistent with a quantitative, rather than a qualitative, distinction. Indeed, Kendler (1997) found support for a multiple threshold model in which melancholia was on the same continuum with, but was simply a more severe form than, nonmelancholic MDD. Interestingly, several studies have reported that nonmelancholic probands have a higher rate of alcoholism in their relatives, which is consistent with the view that they represent a more heterogeneous, and possibly characterological, form of depression (Zimmerman and Spitzer 1989). Studies examining differences between melancholic and nonmelancholic depressed patients on stressful life events have yielded mixed, although predominantly negative, findings (Rush and Weissenburger 1994; Zimmerman and Spitzer 1989). Similarly, research on childhood adversity in melancholic and nonmelancholic MDD has produced conflicting results (Harkness and Monroe 2002; Parker et al. 1997). Studies of personality disturbance and disorders also have been mixed, with some reporting that nonmelancholic patients have greater personality disturbance (Kendler 1997) and others obtaining no difference (Tedlow et al. 2002). Melancholia does not appear to be associated with a more episodic, or less chronic, course (Kendler 1997; Rush and Weissenburger 1994). Finally, the melancholic subtype is unstable across repeated episodes (Coryell et al. 1995), raising the question of whether it characterizes a particular type of episode rather than a type of patient.

Despite the mixed support for the validity and clinical utility of the melancholia subtype, recent taxometric studies have found preliminary evidence that melancholia (or at least a depressive subtype with prominent vegetative symptoms) is a discrete category (see the section "Discrete Entities or Regions on a Continuum" later in this chapter). This is consistent with the view that melancholia may be a valid subtype but that it is not optimally assessed with existing approaches. For example, Parker (2000) argued that current approaches to diagnosing melancholia place undue emphasis on patients' reports of symptoms rather than clinical observation of behavioral signs. He believes that psychomotor retardation is particularly crucial for identifying melancholia and that it must be assessed through clinical observation. Parker and Hadzi-Pavlovic (1996) developed an observational rating scale to assess aspects of psychomotor retardation (the CORE system) and reported strong support for the validity of melancholia with this approach. However, Joyce et al. (2002) found that the CORE system did not perform much better than DSM-IV-TR criteria in predicting putative correlates of melancholia.

Neurotic and Reactive Depression

The traditional counterparts to the psychotic and endogenous or melancholic subtypes have been the neurotic and reactive subtypes, respectively. Like psychotic and endogenous depression, the neurotic and reactive subtypes can be viewed as distinct but have often been used interchangeably. Neither category is included in DSM-IV-TR, although some aspects of neurotic depression have been preserved in the categories of atypical depression and dysthymic disorder (see Stewart et al., Chapter 33, in this volume), and adjustment disorder with depressed mood overlaps with the least severe segment of reactive depression.

Neurotic depression is a confusing construct because it has multiple meanings, including mild, chronic, and associated with "neurotic" (anxiety and personality disorder) features (Klerman et al. 1979). Each of these uses of the term refers to a somewhat different, albeit overlapping, group of patients, resulting in a very heterogeneous category. To bring some uniformity to the definition, Winokur (1985) proposed explicit criteria for neurotic-reactive depression that emphasized nonendogenous depressive symptoms, personality problems, and a stormy lifestyle. Several studies subsequently reported that patients meeting these criteria were less likely to have abnormal results on the DST and more likely to have a family history of alcoholism and a chronic course at 3-year follow-up. However, it is unclear whether these findings are better explained by the existence of a specific neurotic-reactive subtype or by the presence of comorbid personality disorder. Recently, Parker (2000) proposed an approach to classifying nonmelancholic depressions on the basis of temperament dimensions such as anxiety and irritability that overlaps with the criteria proposed by Winokur (1985) and with earlier cluster-analytic typologies of depression.

Reactive depression refers to depressive episodes precipitated by stressful life events. This subtype was included in the RDC under the rubric of situational MDD. This subtype is associated with several major difficulties. First, although severe stress almost certainly plays a causal role in many cases of depression (G.W. Brown and Harris 1989), it is very difficult to determine its role in individual cases. Second, the concept of reactive depression may not give sufficient consideration to the role of preexisting vulnerabilities (Parker 2000). Third, the role of stress may change over the course of depression, playing a greater role in the onset of a first episode than in recurrences (Post 1992).

A few studies have compared patients with RDC situational depression with those with other forms of MDD, but few differences have been identified (e.g., Coryell et al. 1994). Interestingly, however, there appears to be a higher rate of MDD in the relatives of probands with situational than nonsituational MDD (Coryell et al. 1994), raising the possibility that severe stress may be a marker for a subgroup with a heightened vulnerability to mood disorders. Although the use of the term reactive depression has faded, there continues to be some interest in use of more sophisticated conceptual frameworks and methods to delineate a subtype of stress-related depression (see Monroe and Hadjiyannakis 2002).

Atypical Depression

The atypical subtype, one segment of the large and heterogeneous group formerly referred to as neurotic depression, was introduced in DSM-IV (American Psychiatric Association 1994) as a specifier for major depressive episodes (in the context of both bipolar disorder and MDD) and dysthymic disorder. The concept of atypical depression was developed by West and Dally in London in the late 1950s to describe a group of depressed patients with prominent phobic anxiety, histrionic traits, a lack of melancholic features, and a favorable response to monoamine oxidase inhibitors (MAOIs). It was subsequently modified by investigators at Columbia University in New York City and defined by the presence of mood reactivity, reversed vegetative symptoms (hypersomnia and weight gain), leaden paralysis, and rejection sensitivity (see Stewart et al., Chapter 33, in this volume).

Despite the implications of its name, atypical depression is actually quite common in clinical and community samples (Angst et al. 2002; Posternak and Zimmerman 2002). Patients with atypical depression are more likely to be female, tend to have a younger age at onset and more comorbidity (particularly with anxiety and personality disorders), and have a more chronic course compared with patients with nonatypical depression (Angst et al. 2002; Posternak and Zimmerman 2002). The strongest support for the atypical subtype stems from its relatively specific pharmacological response profile, with atypical patients responding to MAOIs but not to tricyclic antidepressants (see Stewart et al., Chapter 33, in this volume).

The validity of the atypical subtype remains controversial. Several recent studies have reported that some of the key clinical features used to define atypical depression (particularly mood reactivity) are not correlated with the other features, raising questions about the current definition of the syndrome (Parker et al. 2002; Posternak and Zimmerman 2002). In addition, the treatment implications of the atypical subtype may have diminished with the widespread use of newer antidepressants such as the selective serotonin reuptake inhibitors (SSRIs) and the decline in use of the tricyclics. However, one recent study found that the SSRIs are no more effective than tricyclics for this subgroup (McGrath et al. 2000). Thus, MAOIs still may be the preferred pharmacological treatment, although cognitive therapy appears to be an equally efficacious psychosocial alternative (Jarrett et al. 1999).

Chronic and Recurrent Depression

In the past several decades, recognition has been growing that the mood disorders are recurrent, and often chronic, conditions. Because previous course has important implications for prognosis and long-term treatment, DSM-IV-TR includes several categories, subtypes, and specifiers that provide a detailed picture of previous course. These include the distinction between MDD, single episode, and MDD, recurrent; a specifier for chronic major depressive episode; a specifier for the presence or absence of full interepisode recovery in individuals with recurrent episodes of mood disorder; and the category of dysthymic disorder. The specifiers for chronic major depressive episode and presence or absence of full interepisode recovery can be applied to both bipolar disorder and MDD, although here we focus on their use in MDD.

The distinction between single-episode and recurrent MDD is well supported and has important etiological and clinical implications. More than any other clinical feature, the recurrent subtype predicts a greater familial aggregation of MDD (Sullivan et al. 2000), suggesting that it may provide a useful means of parsing MDD into more homogeneous subgroups for both neurobiological and psychosocial research on the etiology and development of depression. From a clinical perspective, recurrent major depressive episodes predict a greater likelihood of relapse and recurrence (Mueller et al. 1999), which suggests the need for maintenance treatment.

A chronic major depressive episode is defined as an episode that meets full criteria for a minimum of 2 years. Although research on the validity of the chronic major depressive episode specifier is limited, chronic major depressive episodes may require a longer duration of treatment to respond (Keller et al. 1998).

The course specifier "with or without full interepisode recovery" is used to describe the degree of remission between episodes in recurrent major mood disorders. Partial recovery from a major depressive episode is common and is associated with increased risk of relapse and poorer long-term course (Judd et al. 2000).

Along with MDD, dysthymic disorder is one of the two main categories of nonbipolar depression included in DSM-IV-TR. Dysthymic disorder is characterized by a relatively mild level of symptomatology; a chronic, persistent course; and an insidious onset (see Stewart et al., Chapter 33, in this volume). Like atypical depression, it covers a portion of the broad territory formerly referred to as *neurotic depression*. It has been argued that dysthymic disorder is better conceptualized as a personality disorder than as a mood disorder because of its chronic course and typically early onset. The high rate of comorbidity with Axis II personality disorders is consistent with this view. However, several lines of evidence also support a close link between dysthymic disorder and MDD. Individuals with dysthymic disorder have an elevated rate of MDD in their relatives (Klein et al. 1995) and respond to antidepressant treatment; the vast majority develop a superimposed major depressive episode at some point in their lives (Klein et al. 2000), a phenomenon referred to as *double depression*.

Given the close link between dysthymic disorder and MDD, one might conceptualize the two conditions as lying on a severity continuum, with MDD as the more severe condition. However, this view is inconsistent with family study data indicating that the relatives of patients with dysthymic disorder have a significantly higher rate of dysthymia, and a similar or higher rate of MDD, compared with the relatives of patients with episodic MDD (Klein et al. 1995, 2004). Instead, from the standpoint of familial liability, dysthymic disorder is either a distinct form of depression or a *more* severe variant of MDD.

DSM-IV-TR includes early- (before age 21 years) and late-onset (at age 21 years or older) subtypes of dysthymic disorder. This distinction is supported by evidence from several studies indicating that early-onset dysthymia is associated with greater comorbidity and a higher familial loading of mood disorders (Klein et al. 1999). However, it is noteworthy that early-onset MDD and bipolar disorder have similar correlates (Schürhoff et al. 2000; Weissman et al. 1984), suggesting that an age at onset specifier may have general utility across categories of mood disorders.

Although it appears useful to distinguish the various forms of chronic depression in DSM-IV-TR from non-chronic forms of MDD, it is less clear that elaborate distinctions between chronic forms of depression are necessary. For example, in two studies, McCullough and colleagues (2000, 2003) reported almost no meaningful differences in clinical features, comorbidity, early adversity, family history, and response to treatment among large samples of patients with chronic MDD, double depression, and recurrent MDD with incomplete recovery between episodes.

Other DSM-IV Specifiers

DSM-IV-TR also includes several other episode and course specifiers. The seasonal pattern specifier can be applied to major depressive episodes in the context of bipolar disorder or recurrent MDD. Seasonal affective disorder (SAD) refers to a characteristic pattern of onset and remission at certain times of the year, typically with depression beginning in the fall or winter and remitting in the spring (see Rosenthal and Rosenthal, Chapter 32, in this volume). SAD occurs primarily in women, and its prevalence varies with distance from the equator. The depressive episodes are characterized by anergia and reversed vegetative symptoms such as hypersomnia and increased appetite. When evident in bipolar disorder, seasonal pattern is more likely to be associated with hypomanic than manic episodes. The hallmark characteristic of SAD is its positive (and very fast) response to exposure to bright light.

The postpartum onset specifier can be applied to manic or major depressive episodes with an onset within 4 weeks after childbirth. It was long believed that this was a period of increased risk, but more recent studies indicate that childbirth does not generally convey greater risk than other major life changes (Whiffen and Gotlib 1993) and that the risk factors for postpartum and nonpostpartum mood disorders are similar (Jones and Craddock 2001). Thus, the evidence for the validity of this specifier is weak. However, postpartum mood episodes are clinically important because of their implications for the infants' welfare. This is of particular concern when psychotic features are present. Moreover, psychotic features during postpartum mood episodes are associated with a high risk of recurrence in subsequent deliveries.

The catatonic features specifier can be applied to manic or major depressive episodes to note the presence of prominent catatonic behaviors such as immobility, mutism, posturing, negativism, rigidity, and echophenomena. Research on this specifier is limited, although the available evidence suggests that catatonic features are frequently linked with mania (Taylor and Fink 2003). Catatonia is often misdiagnosed as schizophrenia; hence, the inclusion of this specifier encourages clinicians to consider a differential diagnosis of mood disorder.

Non-DSM Subtypes

In this section, we briefly discuss several subtyping systems that have been used to reduce the heterogeneity of nonbipolar depression in research but are not included in DSM. The first, and most widely used, is the primary-secondary distinction. Developed by the Washington University group (Feighner et al. 1972), this system classifies MDD on the basis of whether its onset was temporally prior to that of other major psychiatric disorders experienced by the individual. The distinction is based solely on temporal ordering; assumptions about etiology or the primary focus of treatment (i.e., principal diagnosis) are not considered. Although the primary-secondary distinction was widely used in the 1970s and 1980s, interest in it has diminished for several reasons. First, there has been variation in which nonmood disorders were considered as potentially primary (e.g., only those in the Feighner et al. criteria, all psychiatric disorders, major medical illnesses). Second, differences between primary and secondary MDD have not been consistently replicated. Finally, the temporal ordering of disorders may simply reflect differences in the typical age at onset of various conditions (Grove and Andreasen 1992).

Because primary depression is still quite heterogeneous, Winokur developed a subtyping system based on family history to create more homogeneous subgroups of primary MDD. Winokur's system consists of three subgroups: 1) pure depressive disease, defined by the presence of a family history of mood disorder but not alcoholism or antisocial personality disorder; 2) depressive spectrum disease, defined by a family history of alcoholism or antisocial personality regardless of family history of mood disorder; and 3) sporadic depression, defined by a negative family history for mood disorder, alcoholism, and antisocial personality. Winokur and his colleagues reported that patients with pure depressive disease had greater HPA axis dysregulation and better response to somatic antidepressant treatments, whereas patients with depressive spectrum disease had greater personality disturbance, more stressful life events and suicide attempts, and more frequent but shorter and less severe episodes. However, attempts to replicate these findings in other centers have yielded mixed results (Grove and Andreasen 1992; Winokur 1997).

Several subtyping systems based on personality and cognitive style have been proposed. Investigators from the psychoanalytic (Blatt 1974) and cognitive (Beck 1983) traditions independently distinguished between a subtype of depression characterized by interpersonal concerns involving care and approval and a second subtype characterized by concerns about self-definition and self-worth. Blatt referred to the two groups as *anaclitic* and *introjective*, respectively, whereas Beck labeled them as *sociotropic* and *autonomous*, respectively. Each subgroup was hypothesized to be vulnerable to developing MDD when exposed to life events that "matched" their focus of concern (interpersonal loss for the anaclitic or sociotropic group; threats to autonomy and achievement for the introjective or autonomous group). In addition, both theorists posited that the two groups had different patterns of symptomatology when depressed: anaclitic or sociotropic individuals are characterized by helplessness, tearfulness, and mood reactivity, whereas introjective or autonomous individuals are characterized by guilt, worthlessness, anhedonia, and social withdrawal. However, empirical studies testing these hypotheses have provided only mixed support (Klein et al. 2002).

Abramson et al. (1989) proposed the existence of a hopelessness subtype of nonbipolar depression. They argued that in the presence of negative life events, individuals with cognitive styles that lead them to 1) attribute negative events to stable and global causes, 2) anticipate that the events will lead to negative consequences, and 3) believe that they are unworthy will become hopeless. Hopelessness, in turn, is the proximal cause of the hopelessness subtype of depression that is characterized by sadness, psychomotor retardation, suicidality, apathy, low energy, sleep disturbance, poor concentration, and negative cognitions. A large-scale prospective test of this model is ongoing (Abramson et al. 2002).

Subthreshold Mood Disorders

Subthreshold forms of mood disorder are attracting increasing attention because of their high prevalence and association with significant functional impairment (see Stewart et al., Chapter 33, in this volume). These subthreshold conditions have been given a variety of labels (Pincus et al. 1999). For example, they have been defined as syndromes, such as minor depressive disorder (similar to MDD, but with fewer symptoms), recurrent brief depressive disorder (similar to MDD, but briefer and occurring at least once a month) (Angst et al. 1990), and mixed anxiety-depressive disorder (a combination of anxiety and depressive symptoms that do not meet criteria for an anxiety or a mood disorder diagnosis), all of which are included in DSM-IV-TR Appendix B as conditions requiring further study. Subthreshold mood disorders also have been defined simply on the basis of symptom counts that fall short of diagnostic thresholds and by scores on self-report inventories. An advantage of using syndromes is that this approach often considers the course, as well as the number, of subthreshold symptoms, which is important in light of evidence that frequency of subthreshold episodes is associated with degree of impairment (Maier et al. 1997). However, the symptom count approach is consistent with evidence of a linear relation between the number of subthreshold symptoms and impairment, family history of MDD, and risk for subsequent MDD (Kendler and Gardner 1998).

Some studies have reported that subthreshold and full-threshold mood disorders are closely related. Unfortunately, some of these studies have included individuals with partially remitted full-threshold mood disorders in the subthreshold group, confounding comparisons between the subthreshold and full-threshold conditions (Solomon et al. 2001). Nonetheless, family studies indicate that the relatives of probands with subthreshold depression and no history of full-threshold mood disorders have a higher rate of MDD than do the relatives of control subjects but a lower rate of MDD than do the relatives of probands with MDD (Kendler and Gardner 1998). Similarly, Lewinsohn et al. (2000) found an elevated rate of bipolar disorder in the relatives of probands with subthreshold bipolar disorder. Interestingly, the rate of subthreshold mood disorders does not appear to be elevated in the relatives of probands with subthreshold depression or subthreshold bipolar disorder, indicating that they are not distinct conditions (e.g., Lewinsohn et al. 2000). Finally, several studies have reported that individuals with subthreshold depression are at increased risk for developing a first-in-lifetime onset of MDD (e.g., Horwath et al. 1992). These data indicate that subthreshold mood disorders are not a distinct entity but instead lie on a continuum with full-threshold mood disorders. However, subthreshold mood disorders are probably heterogeneous, with some subgroups being more closely related to full-threshold mood disorders than others are.

Categories Versus Dimensions

The controversy over categorical versus dimensional models of mood disorders subsumes two distinct, but overlapping, questions: 1) Are the mood disorders discrete entities? and 2) Should the current categorical classification system be replaced with a dimensional system?

Discrete Entities or Regions on a Continuum

Whether mood disorders are discrete entities or regions on a continuum has been debated for much of the past century (Parker 2000). This topic is not merely of academic interest because the answer may provide clues regarding the nature of etiological factors, indicate which assessment approaches and statistical models provide optimal power, and help refine the definition of disorders and subtypes.

Several statistical techniques have been used to address the issue of discreteness. Unfortunately, most have significant limitations. For example, cluster analysis and latent class analysis are two of the more widely used approaches, but both generate clusters or classes even when the data are continuous (Klein and Riso 1993). Meehl (1995) developed an alternative approach referred to as *taxometrics* that is increasingly being used to test whether discrete latent entities (or taxons) can account for the covariation among a set of observed variables. Two of the advantages of this approach are that it can determine whether the data are consistent with the existence of a latent taxon and that it includes several different procedures that can be used to check for consistency across methods.

A growing number of studies have used taxometric procedures to test whether depression in general, and various subtypes of depression, is consistent with a taxonic latent structure (Haslam and Kim 2002). Several studies have failed to find evidence that the latent structure of depression in general is taxonic (e.g., Ruscio and Ruscio 2000). However, several other studies have reported evidence that there may be a form of depression characterized by melancholic or vegetative symptoms that has a taxonic latent structure (e.g., Ambrosini et al. 2002).

In considering the question of discreteness, several issues must be kept in mind. First, it is important to be clear about exactly what depression is discrete with respect to. Mood disorders may be discrete with respect to some boundaries but not others, some types of mood disorders may be discrete but others are not, and there may even be dimensionality (e.g., variations in severity) within discrete classes (Haslam and Kim 2002). This has important implications for sampling because a sufficient number of individuals with the relevant boundary condition or subtype must be included in the study. Second, most taxometric studies of mood disorders to date have focused on cross-sectional symptomatology. Taxometric studies may be more powerful and informative if they also include longitudinal data and potential endophenotypic indicators such as genetic and neurobiological variables that may be closer to the level of etiology (Beauchaine 2003). Third, as Beauchaine (2003) noted, the failure to detect a taxon

does not necessarily mean that a disorder is continuous because current taxometric procedures are only capable of detecting large effects and may be greatly limited if indicators with suboptimal precision and validity are used. Finally, identifying a taxon does not provide any information about the significance or nature of the underlying causal processes. This requires further research examining the association between taxon membership and etiologically relevant external variables (Haslam and Kim 2002).

Categorical or Dimensional Classification

Although psychiatric classification systems typically have used a categorical format, many investigators believe that dimensional systems are more appropriate. This debate is frequently confounded with the issue of discreteness because proponents of categorical models tend to assume that psychiatric disorders are discrete entities, whereas advocates of dimensional models generally believe that psychiatric disorders are regions on a continuum. However, whether a disorder is discrete or not ultimately depends on the nature of the underlying etiological processes. Because the etiologies of almost all psychiatric disorders are unknown, psychiatric classification is based on clinical features. Hence, the discrete versus continuous and categorical versus dimensional debates address different levels of analysis (Beauchaine 2003). As a result, one might reasonably advocate a categorical approach to classification on the pragmatic grounds that it is an efficient means of summarizing and communicating information about clinical syndromes and guiding decision making for treatment and policy without necessarily believing that the disorders will ultimately prove to be etiologically discrete. Indeed, this is the position taken by DSM-IV-TR, which has a categorical format but does not assume that each mental disorder is a discrete entity. At the same time, it is also reasonable to believe that although most disorders will ultimately prove to be discrete, dimensional models are more useful at present when so little is known about etiology because dimensional models do not require arbitrary assumptions about boundaries (Klein and Riso 1993).

Most studies that used dimensional approaches to depression have simply summed the number of depressive symptoms. However, some investigators have suggested separating depressive symptoms and behavior into key functional domains that may more closely reflect underlying biological abnormalities (e.g., Van Praag 1998). Clark and Watson's (1991) tripartite model is an important step in this direction. However, it is unlikely that dimensional classification systems that rely entirely on symptoms will be sufficient because depressive symptoms wax and wane over time and are not stable across episodes, and concordance between patients' reports of symptoms and behavioral ratings by trained observers is poor. Hence, as Angst and Merikangas (2001) and Shankman and Klein (2002) have argued, dimensional models also must consider key course variables such as the frequency and duration of episodes (recurrence and chronicity).

It is important for any dimensional alternative to the current classification system for mood disorders to show that it either has greater validity than the present system or is equally valid but more parsimonious. For example, a simple threefold classification consisting of polarity (presence or absence of mania or hypomania), by severity (subthreshold, mild, moderate, severe, psychotic features) and by course (single nonchronic episode, recurrent episodes with full interepisode recovery, chronic), might provide a more parsimonious typology that preserves most of the information in the existing classification system (e.g., Klein et al. 2004).

References

Abramson LY, Metalsky GI, Alloy LB: Hopelessness depression: a theory-based subtype of depression. Psychol Rev 96:358–372, 1989

Abramson LY, Alloy LB, Hankin BL, et al: Cognitive vulnerability-stress models of depression in a self-regulatory and psychobiological context, in Handbook of Depression and Its Treatment. Edited by Gotlib IH, Hammen CL. New York, Guilford, 2002, pp 268–294

Akiskal HS, Djenderedijian AH, Rosenthal RH, et al: Cyclothymic disorder: validity criteria for inclusion in the bipolar affective group. Am J Psychiatry 134:1227–1233, 1977

Akiskal HS, Bourgeois ML, Angst J, et al: Re-evaluating the prevalence of and diagnostic composition within the broad clinical spectrum of bipolar disorders. J Affect Disord 59:S5–S30, 2000

Altschuler LL, Post RM, Leverich GS, et al: Antidepressant-induced mania and cycle acceleration: a controversy revisited. Am J Psychiatry 152:1130–1138, 1995

Ambrosini PJ, Bennett DS, Cleland CM, et al: Taxonicity of adolescent melancholia: a categorical or dimensional construct. J Psychiatr Res 36:247–256, 2002

American Psychiatric Association: Diagnostic and Statistical Manual of Mental Disorders, 3rd Edition. Washington, DC, American Psychiatric Association, 1980

American Psychiatric Association: Diagnostic and Statistical Manual of Mental Disorders, 4th Edition. Washington, DC, American Psychiatric Association, 1994

American Psychiatric Association: Diagnostic and Statistical Manual of Mental Disorders, 4th Edition, Text Revision. Washington, DC, American Psychiatric Association, 2000

Andrews G, Slade T, Peters L: Classification in psychiatry: ICD-10 versus DSM-IV. Br J Psychiatry 174:3–5, 1999

Angst J, Merikangas KR: Multi-dimensional criteria for the diagnosis of depression. J Affect Disord 62:7–15, 2001

Angst J, Merikangas KR, Scheidegger P, et al: Recurrent brief depression: a new subtype of affective disorder. J Affect Disord 19:87–98, 1990

Angst J, Gamma A, Sellaro R, et al: Toward validation of atypical depression in the community: results of the Zurich cohort study. J Affect Disord 72:125–138, 2002

Bauer MS, Whybrow PC, Gyulai L, et al: Testing definitions of dysphoric mania and hypomania: prevalence, clinical characteristics and inter-episode stability. J Affect Disord 32:201–211, 1994

Beauchaine TP: Taxometrics and developmental psychopathology. Dev Psychopathol 15:501–527, 2003

Beck AT: Cognitive therapy of depression: new approaches, in Treatment of Depression: Old and New Approaches. Edited by Clayton P, Barrett J. New York, Raven, 1983, pp 265–290

Blatt SJ: Levels of object representation in anaclitic and introjective depression. Psychoanal Study Child 29:107–157, 1974

Brown GW, Harris TO: Depression, in Depression in Life Events and Illness. Edited by Brown GW, Harris TO. New York, Guilford, 1989, pp 49–93

Brown GW, Harris TO, Eales MJ: Social factors and comorbidity of depressive and anxiety disorders. Br J Psychiatry 168 (suppl 30):50–57, 1996

Brown TA, Campbell LA, Lehman CL, et al: Current and lifetime comorbidity of the DSM-IV anxiety and mood disorders in a large clinical sample. J Abnorm Psychol 110:585–599, 2001

Clark LA, Watson D: Tripartite model of anxiety and depression: evidence and taxonomic implications. J Abnorm Psychol 100:316–336, 1991

Coryell W: Bipolar II disorder: a progress report. J Affect Disord 41:159–162, 1996

Coryell W: Do psychotic, minor, and intermittent depressive disorders exist on a continuum? J Affect Disord 45:75–83, 1997

Coryell W, Endicott J, Keller M: Rapidly cycling affective disorder: demographics, diagnosis, family history, and course. Arch Gen Psychiatry 49:126–131, 1992

Coryell W, Winokur G, Maser JD, et al: Recurrently situational (reactive) depression: a study of course, phenomenology and familial psychopathology. J Affect Disord 31:203–210, 1994

Coryell W, Endicott J, Maser JD, et al: Long-term stability of polarity distinctions in the affective disorders. Am J Psychiatry 152:385–390, 1995

Dunner DL, Fieve RR: Clinical factors in lithium carbonate prophylaxis failure. Arch Gen Psychiatry 30:229–233, 1974

Feighner JP, Robins E, Guze SB, et al: Diagnostic criteria for use in psychiatric research. Arch Gen Psychiatry 26:57–63, 1972

Fennig S, Bromet EJ, Karant MT, et al: Mood-congruent versus mood-incongruent psychotic symptoms in first-admission patients with affective disorder. J Affect Disord 37:23–29, 1996

Fieve RR, Dunner DL: Unipolar and bipolar affective states, in The Nature and Treatment of Depression. Edited by Flach FF, Draghi SS. New York, Wiley, 1975, pp 145–160

Freeman MP, Freeman SA, McElroy SL: The comorbidity of bipolar and anxiety disorders: prevalence, psychobiology, and treatment issues. J Affect Disord 68:1–23, 2002

Gershon ES, Hamovit J, Guroff JJ, et al: A family study of schizoaffective, bipolar I, bipolar II, unipolar, and normal control probands. Arch Gen Psychiatry 39:1157–1167, 1982

Grove WM, Andreasen NC: Concepts, diagnosis and classification, in Handbook of Affective Disorders, 2nd Edition. Edited by Paykel ES. Edinburgh, Churchill Livingstone, 1992, pp 25–41

Harkness KL, Monroe SM: Childhood adversity and the endogenous versus nonendogenous distinction in women with major depression. Am J Psychiatry 159:387–393, 2002

Haslam N, Kim H: Categories and continua: a review of taxometric research. Genet Soc Gen Psychol Monogr 128:271–320, 2002

Holzer CE III, Nguyen HT, Hirschfeld RMA: Reliability of diagnosis in mood disorders. Psychiatr Clin North Am 19:73–84, 1996

Horwath E, Johnson J, Klerman GL, et al: Depressive symptoms as relative and attributable risk factors for first-onset major depression. Arch Gen Psychiatry 49:817–823, 1992

Jarrett RB, Schaffer M, McIntire D, et al: Treatment of atypical depression with cognitive therapy or phenelzine: a double-blind placebo-controlled trial. Arch Gen Psychiatry 56:431–437, 1999

Johnson SL, Kizer A: Bipolar and unipolar depression, in Handbook of Depression and Its Treatment. Edited by Gotlib IH, Hammen CL. New York, Guilford, 2002, pp 141–165

Jones I, Craddock N: Familiality of the puerperal trigger in bipolar disorder: results of a family study. Am J Psychiatry 158:913–917, 2001

Joyce PR, Mulder RT, Luty SE, et al: Melancholia: definitions, risk factors, personality, neuroendocrine markers, and differential antidepressant response. Aust N Z J Psychiatry 36:376–383, 2002

Judd LL, Paulus MJ, Schettler PJ, et al: Does incomplete recovery from first lifetime major depressive episode herald a chronic course of illness? Am J Psychiatry 157:1501–1504, 2000

Judd LL, Akiskal HS, Schettler PJ, et al: The comparative clinical phenotype and long term longitudinal episode course of bipolar I and II: a clinical spectrum or distinct disorders? J Affect Disord 73:19–32, 2003

Keck PE Jr, McElroy SL, Havens JR, et al: Psychosis in bipolar disorder: phenomenology and impact on morbidity and course of illness. Compr Psychiatry 44:263–269, 2003

Keller MB, Gelenberg AJ, Hirschfeld RMA, et al: The treatment of chronic depression, part 2: a double-blind, randomized trial of sertraline and imipramine. J Clin Psychiatry 59:598–607, 1998

Kendler KS: The diagnostic validity of melancholic major depression in a population-based sample of female twins. Arch Gen Psychiatry 54:299–304, 1997

Kendler KS, Gardner CO Jr: Boundaries of major depression: an evaluation of DSM-IV criteria. Am J Psychiatry 155:172–177, 1998

Kendler KS, McGuire M, Gruenberg AM, et al: Examining the validity of DSM-III-R schizoaffective disorder and its putative subtypes in the Roscommon Family Study. Am J Psychiatry 152:755–764, 1995a

Kendler KS, Walters EE, Neale MC, et al: The structure of genetic and environmental risk factors for six major psychiatric disorders in women: phobia, generalized anxiety disorder, panic disorder, bulimia, major depression, and alcoholism. Arch Gen Psychiatry 52:374–383, 1995b

Klein DN, Riso LP: Psychiatric disorders: problems of boundaries and comorbidity, in Basic Issues in Psychopathology. Edited by Costello CG. New York, Guilford, 1993, pp 19–66

Klein DN, Depue RA, Slater JF: Cyclothymic disorder in the adolescent offspring of parents with bipolar affective disorder. J Abnorm Psychol 94:115–117, 1985

Klein DN, Riso LP, Donaldson SK, et al: Family study of early onset dysthymia: mood and personality disorders in relatives of outpatients with dysthymia and episodic major depression and normal controls. Arch Gen Psychiatry 52:487–496, 1995

Klein DN, Schatzberg AF, McCullough JP, et al: Early versus late-onset dysthymic disorder: comparison in outpatients with superimposed major depressive episodes. J Affect Disord 52:187–196, 1999

Klein DN, Schwartz JE, Rose S, et al: Five-year course and outcome of early onset dysthymic disorder: a prospective, naturalistic follow-up study. Am J Psychiatry 157:931–939, 2000

Klein DN, Durbin CE, Shankman SA, et al: Depression and personality, in Handbook of Depression and Its Treatment. Edited by Gotlib IH, Hammen CL. New York, Guilford, 2002, pp 115–140

Klein DN, Lewinsohn PM, Rohde P, et al: Family study of comorbidity between major depressive disorder and anxiety disorders. Psychol Med 33:703–714, 2003

Klein DN, Shankman AS, Lewinsohn PM, et al: Family study of chronic depression in a community sample of young adults. Am J Psychiatry 161:646–653, 2004

Klerman GL, Endicott J, Spitzer R, et al: Neurotic depressions: a systematic analysis of multiple criteria and meanings. Am J Psychiatry 136:57–61, 1979

Kocsis JH: DSM-IV "major depression": are more stringent criteria needed? Depression 1:24–28, 1993

Lapensée MA: A review of schizoaffective disorder, I: current concepts. Can J Psychiatry 37:335–346, 1992

Lewinsohn PM, Klein DN, Seeley JR: Bipolar disorder during adolescence and young adulthood in a community sample. Bipolar Disord 2:281–293, 2000

Maier W, Gänsicke M, Weiffenbach O: The relationship between major and subthreshold variants of unipolar depression. J Affect Disord 45:41–51, 1997

McCullough JP, Klein DN, Keller MB, et al: Comparison of DSM-II-R chronic major depression and major depression superimposed on dysthymia (double depression): a study of the validity and value of differential diagnosis. J Abnorm Psychol 109:419–427, 2000

McCullough JP, Klein DN, Borian FE, et al: Chronic forms of DSM-IV major depression: validity of the distinctions: a replication. J Abnorm Psychol 112:614–622, 2003

McElroy SL, Keck PE Jr, Pope HG Jr, et al: Clinical and research implications of the diagnosis of dysphoric or mixed mania or hypomania. Am J Psychiatry 149:1633–1644, 1992

McGrath PJ, Stewart JW, Janal MN, et al: A placebo-controlled study of fluoxetine versus imipramine in the acute treatment of atypical depression. Am J Psychiatry 157:344–350, 2000

McGuffin P, Rijsdijk F, Andrew M, et al: The heritability of bipolar affective disorder and the genetic relationship to unipolar depression. Arch Gen Psychiatry 60:497–502, 2003

Meehl PE: Bootstraps taxometrics: solving the classification problem in psychopathology. Am Psychol 50:266–275, 1995

Mineka S, Watson D, Clark LA: Comorbidity of anxiety and unipolar mood disorders. Annu Rev Psychol 49:377–412, 1998

Monroe SM, Hadjiyannakis K: The social environment and depression: focusing on severe life stress, in Handbook of Depression and Its Treatment. Edited by Gotlib IH, Hammen CL. New York, Guilford, 2002, pp 314–340

Mueller TI, Leon AC, Keller MB, et al: Recurrence after recovery from major depressive disorder during 15 years of observational follow-up. Am J Psychiatry 156:1000–1006, 1999

Narrow WE, Rae DS, Robins LN, et al: Revised prevalence based estimates of mental disorders in the United States: using a clinical significance criterion to reconcile 2 surveys. Arch Gen Psychiatry 59:115–123, 2002

Parker G: Classifying depression: should paradigms lost be regained? Am J Psychiatry 157:1195–1203, 2000

Parker G, Hadzi-Pavlovic D: Melancholia: A Disorder of Movement and Mood. New York, Cambridge University Press, 1996

Parker G, Gladstone G, Wilhelm K, et al: Dysfunctional parenting: over-representation in non-melancholic depression and capacity of such specificity to refine sub-typing depression measures. Psychiatry Res 73:57–71, 1997

Parker G, Roy K, Mitchell P, et al: Atypical depression: a reappraisal. Am J Psychiatry 159:1470–1479, 2002

Perris C: Bipolar-unipolar distinction, in Handbook of Affective Disorders, 2nd Edition. Edited by Paykel ES. Edinburgh, Churchill Livingstone, 1992, pp 57–75

Peselow ED, Sanfilipo MP, Difiglia C, et al: Melancholic/endogenous depression and response to somatic treatment and placebo. Am J Psychiatry 149:1324–1334, 1992

Pincus HA, Wakefield W, McQueen LE: "Subthreshold" mental disorders: a review and synthesis of studies on minor depression and other "brand names." Br J Psychiatry 174:288–296, 1999

Pope HG, Lipinski JF: Diagnosis in schizophrenia and manic-depressive illness. Arch Gen Psychiatry 35:811–828, 1978

Post RM: Transduction of psychosocial stress into the neurobiology of recurrent affective disorder. Am J Psychiatry 149:999–1010, 1992

Posternak M, Zimmerman M: Partial validation of the atypical features subtype of major depressive disorder. Arch Gen Psychiatry 59:70–76, 2002

Robins E, Guze SB: Establishment of diagnostic validity in psychiatric illness: its application to schizophrenia. Am J Psychiatry 126:983–987, 1970

Ruscio J, Ruscio AM: Informing the continuity controversy: a taxometric analysis of depression. J Abnorm Psychol 109:473–487, 2000

Rush AJ, Weissenburger JE: Melancholic symptom features and DSM-IV. Am J Psychiatry 151:489–498, 1994

Schatzberg AF, Rothschild AJ: Psychotic (delusional) major depression: should it be included as a distinct syndrome in DSM-IV? Am J Psychiatry 149:733–745, 1992

Schürhoff F, Bellivier F, Jouvent R, et al: Early and late onset bipolar disorders: two different forms of manic-depressive illness? J Affect Disord 58:215–221, 2000

Shankman SA, Klein DN: Dimensional diagnosis of depression: adding the dimension of course to severity, and comparison to the DSM. Compr Psychiatry 43:420–426, 2002

Solomon A, Haaga DAF, Arnow BA: Is clinical depression distinct from subthreshold depressive symptoms? A review of the continuity issue in depression research. J Nerv Ment Dis 189:498–506, 2001

Spitzer RL, Endicott J, Robins E: Research Diagnostic Criteria: rationale and reliability. Arch Gen Psychiatry 35:773–782, 1978

Sullivan PF, Neale MC, Kendler KS: Genetic epidemiology of major depression: review and meta-analysis. Am J Psychiatry 157:1552–1562, 2000

Taylor MA, Fink M: Catatonia in psychiatric classification: a home of its own. Am J Psychiatry 160:1233–1241, 2003

Tedlow J, Smith M, Neault N, et al: Melancholia and Axis II comorbidity. Compr Psychiatry 43:331–335, 2002

Van Praag HM: The diagnosis of depression in disorder. Aust N Z J Psychiatry 32:767–772, 1998

Weissman MM, Wickramaratne P, Merikangas KR, et al: Onset of major depression in early adulthood: increased familial loading and specificity. Arch Gen Psychiatry 41:1136–1143, 1984

Whiffen VE, Gotlib IH: Comparison of postpartum and non-postpartum depression: clinical presentation, psychiatric history, and psychosocial functioning. J Consult Clin Psychol 61:485–494, 1993

Winokur G: The validity of neurotic-reactive depression: new data and reappraisal. Arch Gen Psychiatry 42:1116–1122, 1985

Winokur G: All roads lead to depression: clinically homogeneous, etiologically heterogeneous. J Affect Disord 45:97–108, 1997

Winokur G, Coryell W, Keller M, et al: A prospective follow-up of patients with bipolar and primary unipolar affective disorder. Arch Gen Psychiatry 50:457–465, 1993

Winokur G, Coryell W, Keller M, et al: A family study of manic-depressive (bipolar I) disease: is it a distinct illness separable from primary unipolar depression? Arch Gen Psychiatry 52:367–373, 1995

World Health Organization: International Statistical Classification of Diseases and Related Health Problems, 10th Revision. Geneva, World Health Organization, 1992

Yazici O, Kora K, Üçok A, et al: Unipolar mania: a distinct disorder? J Affect Disord 71:97–103, 2002

Zimmerman M, Spitzer RL: Melancholia: from DSM-III to DSM-III-R. Am J Psychiatry 146:20–28, 1989

Zisook S, Shuchter SR: Depression through the first year after the death of a spouse. Am J Psychiatry 148:1346–1352, 1991

CHAPTER

3

Epidemiology of Mood Disorders

RENEE D. GOODWIN, PH.D., M.P.H.

FRANK JACOBI, PH.D.

ANTJE BITTNER, DIPL.PSYCH.

HANS-ULRICH WITTCHEN, PH.D.

MOOD DISORDERS are among the most pressing public health problems worldwide. Mood disorders are common and are associated with significant functional impairment, lower quality of life, and decline in social functioning. Epidemiologic research is needed in order to understand and quantify the magnitude and dispersion of morbidity associated with mood disorders in the population. Data from epidemiologic studies are also critical to informing the planning of health services in the community. It is projected that major depression will be responsible for the largest burden of disease of any illness by the year 2020 (Murray and Lopez 1996).

Epidemiologic studies provide information on the distribution of mood disorders in the general population. This includes both the prevalence and the incident rates and is generally known as *descriptive epidemiology*. Epidemiologic research also provides unique information on the risk factors and correlates of mood disorders in the

general population. This information is unavailable from clinical studies with patient or selected samples. Specifically, because of selection bias, individuals who seek help differ from those who do not and cannot be considered representative of all who suffer from the disorder within the community (Bijl et al. 2003). This is especially pertinent to the study of mood disorders because it has been repeatedly demonstrated that the majority of individuals with mood disorders will not seek help or receive psychiatric treatment (Goldberg and Huxley 1980). Therefore, epidemiology provides critical information on the natural history, course, and outcomes of mood disorders that is essentially impossible to obtain from any other source.

This chapter will provide an introduction to methodological aspects of epidemiologic research in mood disorders, as well as an overview of international results on prevalence, course, comorbidity, risk factors, and correlates of mood disorders in the general adult population.

Criteria for and Assessment of Mood Disorders

Development of Diagnostic Criteria

Epidemiology of mood disorders is a relatively young field. The history of psychiatric epidemiology and the epidemiology of mood disorders is generally classified into three generations of studies (Dohrenwend and Dohrenwend 1982). Distinction between generations is made via progress and developments in methodology over the years.

In first-generation studies, cases were identified and the prevalence of mood disorders was assessed by using agency records as well as informants such as physicians, general practitioners, and clergy members. In these studies, which date back to the mid-1800s, community members were not directly interviewed. In the mid-1900s, second-generation studies began. The major methodological advance in the second generation was direct interview of representative samples of adults in the community. Psychopathology was assessed in these studies by using two techniques. First, global ratings of psychopathology were assessed in a written questionnaire completed by the participant. This method did not produce diagnoses. Second, information from participants was obtained via direct interview by a clinician, resulting in a diagnosis (Streiner 1998). Yet at this point the development of diagnostic criteria was incomplete, and lack of standardized assessment instruments led to poor reliability between clinicians. Therefore, the results were limited. During this period, diagnostic categories were relatively nonspecific compared with current diagnoses. For example, mild forms of depression were generally grouped under the same heading as anxiety disorders, generally termed *neuroses*. Bipolar disorders and more severe depression were categorized as *affective psychoses*.

In subsequent decades, objective, explicit diagnostic criteria were developed because of the inadequacy of psychometrics of measurement of psychiatric diagnoses in community studies. These included the Research Diagnostic Criteria (RDC) (Spitzer et al. 1978) and then DSM-III (American Psychiatric Association 1980) and later DSM-III-R, DSM-IV, DSM-IV-TR (American Psychiatric Association 1987, 1994, 2000) criteria and ICD-9 and ICD-10 (World Health Organization 1977, 1992). Along with the development and implementation of diagnostic criteria, standardized diagnostic interviews were produced with the goal of assessing and diagnosing specific mental disorders in general population samples with instruments that have high interrater reliability. Still, first- and second-generation studies resulted in the first available evi-

TABLE 3–1.   Selected assessment instruments

Examples of semistructured interviews (for use by interviewers with clinical experience)

- Present State Examination (PSE; Wing et al. 1974)
- Schedule for Affective Disorders and Schizophrenia (SADS; Endicott and Spitzer 1978)
- Schedules for Clinical Assessment in Neuropsychiatry (SCAN; Wing et al. 1990)
- Structured Clinical Interview for DSM-IV (SCID; First et al. 1997)

Examples of standardized interviews (for use by lay interviewers)

- Diagnostic Interview Schedule (DIS; Robins et al. 1981)
- Composite International Diagnostic Interview (CIDI; Robins et al. 1988 and several modified/updated versions)
- Revised Clinical Interview Schedule (CIS-R; Lewis et al. 1992)

Note.   In some recent studies, mandatory standardized assessment is accompanied by clinical severity ratings, preferably administered by clinically trained interviewers; thus, the dichotomy of these approaches is not absolute.

dence that mental disorders were common and that most people with mental disorders did not have access to treatment (Tohen et al. 2000). Therefore, despite lack of data on diagnoses, these studies made a sizable impact by demonstrating that mental disorders were an important public health problem.

Third-generation studies include those that have used standardized interviews based on diagnostic criteria and produced diagnoses of specific mental disorders in representative community samples (Table 3–1). Third-generation studies have facilitated a much broader and in-depth understanding of the size and burden of mood disorders, and of other mental disorders, among adults in the population. The methodological advances characterizing third-generation studies have led to an increase in community-based research in the United States and developed countries worldwide over the past 20 years. Briefly, the Epidemiologic Catchment Area (ECA) Study is considered the benchmark of third-generation studies (Eaton and Kessler 1981; Eaton et al. 1984; Regier et al. 1990) and was among the first major psychiatric epidemiologic studies to assess prevalence of mental disorders among adults in the community using standardized instruments (i.e., the Diagnostic Interview Schedule [DIS; Robins et al. 1981]) and direct interview of participants by trained lay interviewers. This study provided fairly reliable estimates of the prevalence and correlates of mental disorders as well as the use of mental health services in five community samples, though these results were not nationally representative. Subsequent to the ECA Study, there have been several methodological advances in diagnostic assessment procedures. One result of this progress was the merging of the DIS with international instruments including the Present State Examination (PSE; Wing et al. 1974), which led to the development of the World Health Organization (WHO)-Composite International Diagnostic Interview (CIDI; Wittchen 1994; World Health Organization 1990). The National Comorbidity Survey (NCS; Kessler et al. 1994), which used the CIDI, followed the ECA Study as the first study in which the prevalence of mental disorders, morbidity, and service use was assessed in a nationally representative sample of adults ages 15–54 in the United States.

Validity Issues in the Assessment of Mood Disorders

Substantial advances have been made in the measurement of mood disorders in epidemiologic studies using semi-structured and standardized assessments. Yet several critical methodological issues remain unresolved. Among the most important issues is the lack of resolution regarding the validity of diagnostic assessment in epidemiologic studies. Sizable differences in prevalence rates for mood disorders have been found across studies using different assessment tools (e.g., Narrow et al. 2002; Regier et al. 1998). As such, the degree to which the assessment technique is valid-and whether and to what extent the results of a specific study are more influenced by the type of specific tool used rather than the true prevalence of disorder-remains unclear.

Assessment of mood disorders is challenging for a number of reasons (Table 3-2). Standardized measurement techniques (e.g., M-CIDI; Wittchen and Pfister 1997) demonstrate good-excellent reliability and validity in the assessment of depressive disorders, although the validity of the currently used methods for measurement of bipolar disorder is less clear and may benefit from further investigation (Kessler et al. 1998, 2000, 2003; Wittchen 1994).

Among the most frequently debated issues in assessment in epidemiologic studies is whether standardized interviews or semistructured interviews offer superior results. This controversy may remain unresolved until evidence can demonstrate that clinical methods lead to results superior to those obtained using standardized interviews from a psychometric perspective. To date, standardized measures offer results that are more psychometrically sound in some respects (e.g., disclosure vs. bias due to social acceptability). Other unsettled methodological topics include the decision to include measures of severity

TABLE 3–2.   Obstacles to the measurement of mood disorders in community samples

In mood disorders, valid assessment is difficult for various reasons:

- Mood disorders are episodic and chronic. Therefore, prevalence estimates and accuracy of measurement are influenced by the time of assessment, both in terms of the recency of the episode and whether the episode is current. As time since last episode increases, there is some evidence that recall bias may result in inaccurately low estimates (Andrews 1999).

- Mood disorder symptoms wax and wane. If a mood disorder is assessed during a period when the number of symptoms is elevated but does not meet diagnostic criteria, this again may lead to artificially low estimates of the burden of depression in the community. It has been shown that even subclinical depression is associated with substantial impairment, increased service utilization, and suicidal ideation.

- To differentiate between bipolar disorder and depression, lifetime assessment of major depression is necessary to rule out pure mania and make an accurate differential diagnosis.

of psychiatric disorder, the need for more extensive information on disability and help-seeking, more in-depth probing and rating procedures within interviews, obtaining information to be used in health economics research, and the increasingly recognized need for and importance of longitudinal epidemiologic data to identify causal risk factors for disorder onset and severity and to increase understanding of the course of mood disorders across the life span.

Epidemiology of Mood Disorders: International Findings

Lifetime and Current Prevalence Rates in the General Population

Major Depression and Dysthymia

The prevalence rates of major depression and dysthymia in a selection of recent epidemiological surveys are displayed in Table 3–3. As the table shows, a substantial percentage (20%–40%) of unipolar depression cases also meet criteria for a comorbid diagnosis of dysthymia. Numerous studies have highlighted the finding that major depression and dysthymia are commonly comorbid (Bland 1997; Kessler 1995). Lifetime prevalence rates of comorbid depression and dysthymia range from 1.5% to 2.5% in the general adult population (Bland 1997).

TABLE 3–3. Epidemiologic studies of adults that included assessment of mood disorders

Study	Author	Place	Diagnostic system	Instrument	Age (years)	N
ECA	Robins and Regier 1991	United States, 5 cities	DSM-III	DIS	>18	18,572
	Robins and Regier 1991		DSM-III-R	Interview		
DMHDS	McGee et al. 1990	New Zealand	DSM-III	DISC-C	15	943
	Feehan et al. 1994		DSM-III-R	DIS-III-R	18	930
Basel	Wacker et al. 1992	Switzerland	DSM-III-R ICD-10	CIDI	18–65	470
CHDS	Fergusson et al. 1993	New Zealand	DSM-III-R	DISC-C, DISC-P	15	986
NCS	Kessler et al. 1994, 1996, 1997, 2003	United States	DSM-III-R	CIDI	15–54	8,098
OHS	Boyle et al. 1996; Offord et al. 1996	Canada	DSM-III-R	CIDI	15–64	9,953
Spanish population	Canals et al. 1997	Spain	DSM-III-R	SCAN	18	290
NPMS	Jenkins et al. 1997	United Kingdom	ICD-10	CIS-R	16–65	10,108
NEMESIS	Bijl et al. 1998	The Netherlands	DSM-III-R	CIDI	18–64	7,076
MAPSS	Vega et al. 1998	United States	DSM-III-R	CIDI	18–59	3,012
Toronto	De Marco 2000	Canada	DSM-III-R	CIDI	18–55	1,393
FINHCS	Lindeman et al. 2000	Finland	DSM-III-R	CIDI	15–75	5,993
DFS	Becker et al. 2000	Germany	DSM-IV	F-DIPS	18–25	2,068
TACOS	Meyer et al. 2000	Germany	DSM-IV	CIDI	18–64	4,075
Oslo	Kringlen et al. 2001	Norway	DSM-III-R	CIDI	18–65	2,066
GHS-MHS	Wittchen and Jacobi 2001; Jacobi et al. 2002, 2004	Germany	DSM-IV	CIDI	18–65	4,181
ODIN study	Ayuso-Mateos et al. 2001	Europe, 5 countries	DSM-IV ICD-10	SCAN	18–64	8,764
ANMHS	Andrews et al. 2001	Australia	DSM-IV ICD-10	CIDI	18+	10,641
SF-Study	Turner and Gil 2002	United States	DSM-IV	CIDI	19–21	1,803

TABLE 3–3. Epidemiologic studies of adults that included assessment of mood disorders *(continued)*

Study	Author	Place	Diagnostic system	Instrument	Age (years)	N
DEPRES Study	Angst et al. 2002	Europe, 6 countries	DSM-IV	MINI	16+	78,458
ECAS-SP	Andrade et al. 2000, 2002, 2003	Brazil	DSM-III-R	CIDI	18+	1,464
CPPS	Andrade et al. 2003	Chile	DSM-III-R	CIDI	15+	2,978
GISSH	Andrade et al. 2003	Japan	DSM-III-R	CIDI	20+	1,029
EPM	Andrade et al. 2000, 2003	Mexico	DSM-III-R	CIDI	18–54	1,734
MHP-T	Andrade et al. 2000, 2003	Turkey	DSM-III-R	CIDI	18–54	6,095
Czech CIDI Survey	Andrade et al. 2003	Czech Republic	DSM-IV	CIDI	18–79	1,534
NCS-R	Kessler et al. 2003	United States	DSM-IV	CIDI	18+	9,090

Note. CIDI=Composite International Diagnostic Interview; DIS=Diagnostic Interview Schedule; DIS-III-R=Diagnostic Interview Schedule; DISC-C=Diagnostic Interview Schedule for Children—Child Version; DISC-P=Diagnostic Interview Schedule for Children—Parent Version; K-SADS=Schedule for Affective Disorders and Schizophrenia for School-Age Children; CAPA=Child and Adolescent Psychiatric Assessment; SCAN=Schedules for Clinical Assessment in Neuropsychiatry; CIS-R=Revised Clinical Interview Schedule; CAPI=Computer-Assisted Personal Interview of the Munich Version of the Composite International Diagnostic Interview–M-CIDI; F-DIPS=Diagnostisches Interview psychischer Störungen (Forschungsversion); MINI=Mini International Neuropsychiatric Interview.

Sociodemographic Correlates

Data on the sociodemographic characteristics associated with major depression among adults in the community have been relatively consistent across studies.

Age.   Results consistently show a mean age at first onset of depression in early adulthood (i.e., in the late 20s). For instance, the mean age at onset of depression was 27.4 in the ECA Study. Consistent with Weissman and colleagues' (1996) earlier cross-national study in which the mean age at onset ranged from 24.8 to 34.8, in the International Consortium of Psychiatric Epidemiology studies, the median age at onset of major depression in all countries was between the early and mid-30s (Andrade et al. 2003). De Graaf et al. (2003) found a mean age at onset of major depression of 29.9 years in the Netherlands Mental Health Survey and Incidence Study (NEMESIS), with females having a younger age at onset compared with males.

Gender.   Major depression occurs twice as frequently among female adults as among males (Brown and Harris 1978; Kessler et al. 1998; Weissman et al. 1993). This is one of the most consistent findings in the epidemiology of mood disorders. The reason for this gender difference is unknown, although it remains among the most intensely studied and frequently debated issues. Hypothesized explanations include hormonal differences, personality factors, social or environmental factors, and exposure to stressful life events (see also Williams and Neighbors, Chapter 9, in this volume). This is especially intriguing because the gender difference in prevalence of depression is reversed among children—with boys having higher rates—and the shift emerges during adolescence and continues throughout adulthood. Evidence has indicated that no gender difference exists in the prevalence of depression among prepubescent boys and girls (Angold and Rutter 1992; Cyranowski et al. 2000; Kashani et al. 1983). One possible explanation for the gender difference later in adolescence and into adulthood is a preponderance of negative life events among females (data have shown higher reporting of negative events among females than among males) (Cyranowski et al. 2000). In contrast to the gender difference in onset, there does not appear to be a significant gender difference in recurrence rates (Emslie et al. 1997).

Marital status.   Overall, epidemiological studies have found that rates of depression are higher among those never married or previously married compared with those currently married. Interestingly, Weissman et al. (1996) found that the two countries with the lowest rates of divorce had the lowest rates of depression (Korea and Tai-

wan) and that the association between separation or divorce and depression was higher in men than in women. In the National Comorbidity Survey (NCS), adults who were married and never married had significantly lower rates of depression than those who were divorced, separated, or widowed (Kessler et al. 1997). In the replication study (NCS-R), never having been married was a risk factor for past-year major depression, whereas previously having been married was a risk factor for lifetime depression (Kessler et al. 2003).

Race/ethnicity.   Findings are mixed on the association between depression and race/ethnicity among adults in the community. In the NCS, Kessler et al. (1997) found a marginally higher rate of depression among those with minority racial status. A more recent study of a household probability sample among adults in the United States (Dunlop et al. 2003) found higher rates of major depression among black and Hispanic adults, compared with white adults, but after confounders were controlled, Hispanic and white adults had similar rates, whereas black adults had lower rates. Factors associated with major depression are more common among minority groups; therefore, it appears that the higher rate of major depression in minorities is largely due to factors such as greater health burdens and lack of health care resources. Yet the association between race/ethnicity and depression remains unclear and in need of further study.

Socioeconomic status.   Epidemiological studies have been relatively consistent in showing an association between low socioeconomic status (SES) and increased rates of depression (Kessler et al. 1997; Weissman and Myers 1978; Williams and Neighbors, Chapter 9, in this volume). Results from the NCS showed an association between depression and the lowest income (Kessler et al. 1997), and unemployment was a risk factor for depression in the ECA Study. Yet Weissman and Myers (1978) found current rates of depression higher among lower SES groups and lifetime rates of depression more elevated among higher SES groups in the ECA Study. Measurement differences may account for this discrepancy. Again, the nature of the observed relation between lower SES and increased depression is not known. It may be that one causes the other or that common factors are associated with increased risk for both. More recent studies show that even low SES during childhood (Gilman et al. 2003) is associated with increased risk for depression during adulthood.

Urban or rural residence.   Findings are mixed, but most data suggest that major depression is less common in rural than in urban settings (Patten et al. 2003). The reason for this difference is not well understood, but it has been suggested that factors such as crime, availability of illicit substances, unemployment, and stressful life events may contribute.

Cohort Effects: Are Depression Rates Increasing?

A remarkable and consistent increase in prevalence rates of major depression across studies has been reported over the past three decades. Consequently, there is an ongoing debate about whether there has been a "true" secular increase in the prevalence of depression worldwide over the past quarter century or whether the observed increase is mainly a result of methodological artifacts induced by the use of more sensitive diagnostic criteria and increased willingness of respondents to report psychiatric symptoms (Neugebauer et al. 1980; Paykel 2000). Klerman and Weissman (1989) reanalyzed epidemiological and family genetic data showing that there has indeed been a secular increase in depression; these investigators presented considerable evidence that this increase appears to be continuing (WHO World Mental Health Survey Consortium 2004). Subsequently, numerous authors have generally confirmed these trends. For example, Kessler et al. (2003) showed large and significant differences between rates of depression in successive birth cohorts (18–29 years, 30–44 years, 45–59 years, 60 years or older) in the NCS-R, suggesting that the prevalence of depressive disorders has increased substantially in recent years. However, the issue is far from being definitively resolved. In addition to methodological changes, variations in the diagnostic criteria used to assess depression over the past several decades make direct comparability of rates over decades, and comparison, difficult. Therefore, it is not entirely clear to what degree such cohort findings are influenced by other methodological biases (e.g., recall bias in younger participants, more comfort with admitting depressive symptoms among younger cohorts).

Course of Major Depression

The course of major depression varies widely depending on a range of factors. Differences in course may relate to factors such as age at onset, severity of symptoms, and symptomatology (e.g., subclinical vs. clinical). Gender, age, and severity of symptoms have been linked with the course of depression in terms of chronicity, with earlier onset and more severe symptoms related to a more chronic course (Emslie et al. 1997; Goodyer et al. 1997).

Challenges to the investigation of the course of major depression include the following:

- Cross-sectional studies have shown that retrospective recall is not reliable (e.g., Andrews et al. 1999), so longitudinal studies are needed.
- Longitudinal epidemiological studies that have used DSM criteria are lacking.
- Longitudinal study participants are not yet old enough to allow for studies of course of depression across the life span.
- Information is needed on the trajectory from youth to older adulthood, which will require the sustained funding of several ongoing studies for decades.

Evidence to date suggests that depression may begin relatively early in life (i.e., adolescence) (Oldehinkel et al. 1999) or during early adulthood (up to age 30), by which age most have developed their first episode. Also, some evidence indicates that preceding disorders, such as primary anxiety and depression, may be associated with a considerable risk of experiencing major depression overall, as well as at an earlier age, as compared with subjects without a primary disorder (Bittner et al. 2004).

Further evidence shows that in most cases, major depression runs a recurrent course across the life span. Most participants with major depression in the NCS (72.3%) reported having more than one episode, which also suggests that the disorder is recurrent (Kessler et al. 1997). Estimates from the Netherlands Mental Health Survey and Incidence Study (NEMESIS; Spijker et al. 2002) and the German National Health Interview and Examination Survey–Mental Health Survey (GHS-MHS; Jacobi 2004), however, seem to be somewhat lower (40%–50%). Evidence from prospective studies generally confirms the high risk of recurrence and also provides clues for factors influencing course. Murphy et al. (2000a, 2000b) found that major depression was associated with greater chronicity and recurrence than were anxiety disorders in a 40-year prospective study on the prevalence of major depression in a Canadian sample. In an investigation of a 15-year follow-up period of a prospective study of young adults in the community in Switzerland, Merikangas et al. (2003) found that the co-occurrence of anxiety and depression was more methodologically stable than depression alone (or anxiety alone) and that patterns of stability were similar for subthreshold- and threshold-level disorders.

In sum, research has demonstrated that the course and outcome of major depression in the community are heterogeneous. Severity of major depression ranges from mild to severe and life-threatening, and course varies from single lifetime episode to multiple, recurrent episodes across the life span. Evidence suggests that there may be key determinants of the course of depression (e.g., age at onset, family history, comorbid anxiety disorders) across the life span. Although longitudinal epidemiologic studies of depression from youth and throughout adulthood are now increasing, much further research is needed to understand the course of depression throughout adulthood and to uncover the potential role of treatment in modifying course.

Psychiatric Comorbidity

Psychiatric comorbidity has been found to be the rule, rather than the exception, among adults with major depression in the community. Note, however, that some controversy remains as to what degree these comorbidity findings are merely an artifact of increasing sophistication in the recent diagnostic classification systems (Wittchen 1996). Findings suggest that approximately three of four adults with lifetime major depression meet criteria for at least one other mental or substance use disorder (Angst 1996; Kessler et al. 1996; Merikangas et al. 1996; Regier et al. 1998). Here, we present a brief overview of patterns of psychiatric comorbidity among adults in the community.

Findings have consistently shown that comorbidity in depression is highest with anxiety disorders, followed by substance use disorders, as shown in several reports from the NCS. Rates and patterns of comorbidity are relatively consistent cross-nationally. For instance, Weissman et al. (1996) found that the most common disorders comorbid with depression included alcohol abuse or dependence, panic disorder, obsessive-compulsive disorder, and drug abuse or dependence. More recently, de Graaf et al. (2003) examined comorbidity between mood and other psychiatric disorders and found that in a representative sample of 7,076 adults ages 18–64 years in the Netherlands, 46% of the men and 57% of the women with mood disorders had lifetime anxiety disorders and 43% and 15%, respectively, had substance use disorders. Moreover, other analyses have shown that comorbid depression and anxiety disorders are associated with even greater morbidity in terms of social impairment, occupational disability, and suicidal ideation and behavior (e.g., Angst et al. 2002b; Hagnell and Gräsbeck 1990; Kessler 1995; Murphy 1990; Roy-Byrne et al. 2000).

Risk Factors for Major Depression

Epidemiological research is the key to the identification of risk factors for mental disorders. Cross-sectional epidemiological studies can be used to describe correlates of major depression, but identification of true risk factors is not possible in cross-sectional studies because of reliance on retrospective recall, with some exceptions for fixed

factors such as race and gender. In most cases, longitudinal data are needed to identify potential risk factors and examine them prospectively. In this section, we provide an overview of available data on identified risk factors and evaluate their implications, and later we identify needed areas of future research.

Demographic Characteristics

As described earlier, specific demographic characteristics are differentially associated with the prevalence of and risk for depression onset in adults in the community. Among the most striking is female gender, although the mechanisms of this association are not clear. Several theories, both biological and environmental, have been proposed to explain this finding (see Kornstein and Sloan, Chapter 41, in this volume). Closer examination of the relation between gender and risk of depression onset throughout development suggests that the mechanism of this association may be found in social or environmental factors. This suggestion has been made because the gender difference in prevalence changes between childhood (higher among boys than girls) and puberty (higher rate among females than males). Investigators have suggested that hormonal changes may account for this difference. However, no study has been able to link hormonal changes with depression, specifically in this age group, and furthermore, the same gender effect is not seen in conjunction with hormonal changes in other age groups (e.g., menopause). Therefore, researchers suspect that changes in social and environmental exposures may play the most prominent role in this discrepancy. Specifically, females have significantly higher rates of exposure to factors such as stressful life events and trauma throughout the life span (Klose and Jacobi 2004), although these factors do not seem to account fully for gender differences in depression (Fergusson et al. 2002).

Familial Transmission

Family studies have contributed enormously to our understanding of the familial nature of major depression. Specifically, family studies have shown that family history of major depression is associated with a significantly increased risk of major depression (Klein et al. 2001; Lieb et al. 2002a; Merikangas et al. 1988; Nomura et al. 2001; Warner et al. 1999; Weissman and Wickramaratne 2000; Weissman et al. 1987, 1997; Wickramaratne et al. 2000; Winokur et al. 1992). Family history has also been associated with increased severity of depression, compared to those without a family history. The majority of family studies to date, however, have been based on clinical samples, making the degree to which these results are generalizable to the community unclear. For instance, it may be that these studies include only individuals with severe depression, not mild depression, leading to results that may be relevant only to severe depression. Still, this is not necessarily the case, considering that the few community-based family studies to date generally support findings from clinically based results. Specifically, Lieb et al. (2002) demonstrated a link between parental history of depression and increased risk of depression in offspring in a community-based longitudinal study. Findings from this study also revealed that parental depression was associated with earlier onset and greater depression severity in offspring. Other community-based studies have found consistent results (Klein et al. 2003). Additionally, there is increased interest and evidence of the interaction between family history of depression and environmental influences leading to risk of depression. For instance, Kendler et al. (1998) showed that stressful life events are associated with a significantly greater risk of depression among those with a family history of depression compared to those without such a history. Future community-based family studies are needed if we are to understand whether and to what degree findings from clinically based family studies are informative about the familial nature of major depression in the general population.

Early Adverse Life Events

Early childhood trauma and adverse life events are associated with increased risk of onset and severity of depression among adults in the community. Specifically, several studies have demonstrated a link between childhood physical and sexual abuse and neglect and increased risk of depression in adulthood (Bifulco and Brown 1998; Brown and Harris 1993; Brown et al. 1993a, 1993b; Dinwiddie et al. 2000; Fergusson et al. 1996, 2002; Jaffee et al. 2002; Kessler et al. 1997; MacMillan et al. 2001). Longitudinal studies have also demonstrated consistent links between loss events, especially parental loss by separation or death, and elevated risk of depression during adulthood. Moreover, evidence suggests that loss events may be specifically associated with heightened vulnerability to depression, whereas other traumatic life events (e.g., neglect) may be more strongly linked with anxiety disorders or other mental disorders in adulthood (Brown 1993; Deadman et al. 1989; Miller and Ingham 1983).

Comorbidity as a Risk Factor for Depression

Studies have consistently shown that a lifetime history of any mental disorder strongly increases the risk for first onset of major depression and increases the likelihood of persistence, severity, and recurrence of the disorder. Specifically, anxiety disorders have been shown to precede and predict the onset of major depression in numerous cross-sectional (e.g., Kessler et al. 1998) and longitudinal studies (e.g., Pine et al. 2001; Stein et al. 2001; Wittchen et al. 2000; Woodward and Fergusson 2001). With the possible exception of panic disorder, most studies have found that the onset of all anxiety disorders precedes the onset of incident major depression. For instance, several studies have shown that anxiety disorder onset occurs in most cases of anxiety-depression comorbidity (e.g., Lewinsohn et al. 1997; Merikangas et al. 1996; Regier et al. 1998), and other studies have found that all Axis I disorders predict onset of major depression (Hettema et al. 2003). Previous epidemiological studies also showed that dysthymia and schizophrenia (Horwath et al. 1992) were both associated with increased risk for onset of depression in the ECA.

Research has shown that the link between prior symptoms and risk for major depression spans all developmental stages. Canals et al. (2002) examined predictors of depression onset at age 18 and found that 80% of those with depression onset at 18 had symptoms of major depression between ages 11 and 14. These findings support a continuity of depression from adolescence to young adulthood, with subclinical scores on the Children's Depression Inventory (CDI; Kovacs 1985) as an early indicator of long-term risk. This study also found early symptoms of anxiety to be a predictor of depression at age 18, but only among boys. Reinherz et al. (2000) found that internalizing variables such as anxiety and depression were specific predictors of depression onset and that a past episode of depression or anxiety disorder predicted onset of depression in early adulthood (Lewinsohn et al. 1995). Similarly, anxious and depressive behaviors at ages 6 and 9, as reported by parents and teachers, were found to be predictors of subsequent depression, yet the self-report of anxiety and depression at age 9 appeared to be a depression-specific risk factor for males only (Reinherz et al. 2000). Self-esteem also has been found to predict onset of major depression and dysthymia more accurately in girls than in boys. Specifically, low self-esteem at age 14 was a risk factor for depression among females (Canals et al. 2002).

Negative Life Events

Stressful life events are among the best-documented risk factors for major depression among adults in the community (see also Williams, Chapter 9, in this volume). Stressful or negative life events in interpersonal relationships, family, health, work and financial status have been consistently linked with onset of depression (Kessler 1997). These associations exist across age groups and males and females, although there is some evidence of gender differences noted in the strength of linkages between specific events and risk of depression.

While there is some evidence that the link is causal, the mechanism of the link between stressful life events and depression remains unclear, as do the role of specific types of events. Brown and colleagues (1995) have investigated the use of four dimensions of stressful life events (loss, entrapment, humiliation and danger). Relatively few studies have used this model to examine the specificity of these types of events in predicting depression, but preliminary evidence suggests that specific types of events (loss, humiliation) more strongly predict depression (Kendler et al. 2003), compared with anxiety disorders. Other lines of research have suggested an interaction between stressful life events and genetic/familial vulnerability to depression, coping styles (Mazure and Maciejewski 2003), and personality traits (Maier et al. 1995) in the degree of risk of depression conferred by exposure to stressful life events. For instance, genetic vulnerability to depression has also been found to moderate the influence of negative life events on risk of depression (Caspi et al. 2003; Kendler et al. 1995). In addition, previous studies have also shown that the degree to which exposure to stressful life events increases the risk of depression may be influenced by underlying personality traits. For instance, several studies have shown that individuals with high neuroticism, compared with low, are significantly more likely to develop major depression after exposure to stressful life events (Kendler et al. 1995; Ormel et al. 1991; van Os et al. 1999). More work is needed to understand these pathways.

Bipolar Disorder

In comparison with the measurement of major depression in major epidemiological studies, research in the epidemiology of bipolar disorder has been more limited by methodological challenges. Thus, comparatively fewer data on the epidemiology of bipolar disorder are available.

Prevalence rates of bipolar disorders in selected third-generation epidemiological surveys are presented in Table 3–4; rates in women and men are about the same (lifetime 1%–2% in most studies). The differences between lifetime and current (12-month) rates are smaller than in unipolar depressions, which could indirectly indicate a higher rate of chronicity. It should be noted that in this chapter bipolar I and bipolar II disorders are grouped together, but, by far, most of the epidemiological studies on bipolar illness have examined bipolar I disorder.

The key challenges lie in several areas. First, methodological problems are inherent in the diagnosis of bipolar disorder in general and especially by lay interviewers. Given the complexity of the disease, diagnosis of bipolar disorder is a challenge in almost any setting, and this issue is compounded by the use of lay interviewers in epidemiological studies. For example, hypomanic symptoms can be difficult to differentiate from ordinary good mood, especially when they have occurred years prior. Second, the diagnosis of bipolar disorder necessitates reliance on retrospective recall because both depressive and manic or hypomanic states must be present, and memory and judgment about these events may be skewed. Third, considerable changes have been made in the diagnostic criteria for the disorder over time, and debate is ongoing about the conceptualization of bipolar disorder. Therefore, with few exceptions, measurement of bipolar disorder in epidemiological studies has been questionable, and some ongoing longitudinal studies have omitted assessment of bipolar disorder. Furthermore, bipolar disorder is thought to be relatively rare; thus, unless a study's sample size were extremely large, inclusion would not be fruitful because cell sizes would be too small for analysis.

Prevalence of Bipolar Disorder

Lifetime prevalence of bipolar disorder has been reported as 0.5%–1.6% (Bland et al. 1988; Canino et al. 1987; Chen et al. 1993; Hwu et al. 1989; Kessler et al. 1997; Lee et al. 1990; Wells et al. 1989; Wittchen et al. 1992). A range from 0.7% (past 2 weeks) to 1.2% (lifetime) prevalence was found among five sites in the ECA (Weissman et al. 1988). Kessler et al. (1997) reported a 12-month prevalence of 0.37% and a lifetime prevalence of 0.45% after reinterview with the Structured Clinical Interview for DSM-IV (SCID), whereas the CIDI rate was 1.5% in the NCS. Subsequent validation studies used the SCID to reinterview positive cases and found an adjusted rate (excluding false-positive cases) of 0.9%. Note, however, that the CIDI included a limited number of symptoms of mania and hypomania (for description, see Kessler et al. 1997), and this may have biased results toward detection of a particular type of bipolar phenomenology. In an earlier cross-national comparison study, Weissman et al. (1996) found that the prevalence of bipolar disorder across countries—ranging from 0.3% in Taiwan to 1.5% in New Zealand—was more consistent than the prevalence of major depression across countries.

TABLE 3–4. Rates of mood disorders in epidemiologic studies

Study	Author	Time frame	Total	Major depression	Hypo-mania	Manic episode	Bipolar disorder	Bipolar I disorder	Bipolar II disorder
ECA	Weissman et al. 1991	Point	2.4	—	—	—	—	—	—
		1 year	3.7	2.7	—	—	—	0.7	0.3
		Lifetime	7.8	4.9	—	—	—	0.8	0.5
Basel	Wacker et al. 1992	Lifetime	19.4	6.6 (9.1)	—	—	0.4	—	—
NCS	Kessler et al. 1994	1 year	11.3	10.3	—	1.3	—	—	—
		Lifetime	19.3	17.1	—	1.6	—	—	—
NPMS	Jenkins et al. 1997	1 week	—	2.3	—	—	—	—	—
NEMESIS	Bijl et al. 1998	1 month	3.9	2.7	—	—	0.6	—	—
		1 year	7.6	5.8	—	—	1.1	—	—
		Lifetime	19.0	15.4	—	—	1.8	—	—
Toronto	De Marco 2000	1 year	—	10.4	—	—	—	—	—
		Lifetime	—	24.4	—	—	—	—	—
FINHCS	Lindeman et al. 2000	1 year	—	9.3	—	—	—	—	—
DFS	Becker et al. 2000	Point	1.9	1.2	—	—	—	0.3	0.0
		Lifetime	12.8	10.6	—	—	—	0.7	0.1
TACOS	Meyer et al. 2000	Lifetime	12.3	10.0	0.3	—	0.4	0.4	0.1
Oslo	Kringlen et al. 2001	1 year	—	7.3	—	—	0.9	—	—
		Lifetime	—	17.8	—	—	1.6	—	—
BGS	Wittchen and Jacobi 2001	1 month	6.3	—	—	—	0.6	—	—
		1 year	11.9	—	—	—	0.8	—	—
		Lifetime	18.6	—	—	—	1.0	—	—
ODIN study	Ayuso-Mateos et al. 2001	Point	—	6.6	—	—	—	—	—
ANMHS	Andrews et al. 2001	1 month	—	3.2	—	—	—	—	—
		1 year	—	6.3	—	—	—	—	—
SF-Study	Turner and Gil 2002	1 year	—	11.6	—	—	—	—	—
		Lifetime	—	17.4	—	—	—	—	—
ECAS-SP	Andrade et al. 2003	1 month	—	3.9	—	—	—	—	—

TABLE 3–4. Rates of mood disorders in epidemiologic studies (*continued*)

Study	Author	Time frame	Total	Major depression	Hypo-mania	Manic episode	Bipolar disorder	Bipolar I disorder	Bipolar II disorder
CPPS	Andrade et al. 2003	1 year	—	5.8	—	—	—	—	—
		Lifetime	—	12.6	—	—	—	—	—
	Andrade et al. 2003	1 month	—	3.3	—	—	—	—	—
		1 year	—	5.6	—	—	—	—	—
		Lifetime	—	9.0	—	—	—	—	—
GISSH	Andrade et al. 2003	1 month	—	0.9	—	—	—	—	—
		1 year	—	1.2	—	—	—	—	—
		Lifetime	—	3.0	—	—	—	—	—
EPM	Andrade et al. 2003	1 month	—	2.2	—	—	—	—	—
		1 year	—	4.5	—	—	—	—	—
		Lifetime	—	8.1	—	—	—	—	—
MHP-T	Andrade et al. 2003	1 month	—	3.1	—	—	—	—	—
		1 year	—	3.5	—	—	—	—	—
		Lifetime	—	6.3	—	—	—	—	—
Czech CIDI Survey	Andrade et al. 2003	1 month	—	1.0	—	—	—	—	—
		1 year	—	2.0	—	—	—	—	—
		Lifetime	—	7.8	—	—	—	—	—
NCS-R	Kessler et al. 2003	1 year	—	6.6	—	—	—	—	—
		Lifetime	—	16.2	—	—	—	—	—

Note. ECA=Epidemiologic Catchment Area Study; NYCLS=New York Child Longitudinal Study; DMHDS=Dunedin Multidisciplinary Health and Development Study; CHDS=Christchurch Health and Development Study; NCS=National Comorbidity Survey; MECA=Methods for the Epidemiology of Child and Adolescent Mental Disorders Study; GSMS=The Great Smoky Mountains Study; MAPSS=Mexican American Prevalence and Services Survey; OHS=Ontario Health Survey; ZESCAP=Zürich Epidemiological Study of Child and Adolescent Psychopathology; NEMESIS=Netherlands Mental Health Survey and Incidence Study; FINHCS=Finnish Health Care Survey; ECAS-SP=The Epidemiologic Catchment Area Study in the city of Sao Paulo; CPPS<=Chile Psychiatric Prevalence Study; GISSH=The Gifu Interview Survey on Stress, Lifestyle and Health; EPM=Epidemiology of Psychiatric Comorbidity Project; MHP-T=Mental Health Profile of Turkey; NPMS=National Psychiatric Morbidity Surveys; EDSP=Early Developmental Stages of Psychopathology; BJS=Bremer Jugendstudie; GHS-MHS=German Health Survey—Mental Health Supplement; DFS=Dresdner Frauenstudie; TACOS=Transitions in Alcohol Consumption and Smoking; ODIN study=European Outcome of Depression International Network study; ANMHS=Australian National Mental Health Survey; ANMHS (child+adolescent)=Australian National Mental Health Survey (child and adolescent component); SF-Study=South Florida Study; NCS-R=National Comorbidity Survey Replication.

Bipolar Spectrum Disorders

The lifetime prevalence rates of bipolar spectrum disorders are considerably higher: 3%–6% across countries and a variety of cultures (Angst 1998; Kessler et al. 1997; Weissman et al. 1996). Newer trends in the epidemiology of bipolar spectrum disorders suggest that at least 5% of the general population have disabling bipolar disorder that may be in the "soft" bipolar realm (Akiskal et al. 2003). The bipolar spectrum is thought to include mania, hypomania, recurrent brief hypomania, sporadic brief hypomania, and cyclothymia. Evidence of bipolar spectrum disorders is commonly found in clinical samples (Akiskal and Mallya 1987; Akiskal et al. 1983; Cassano et al. 1992) and in the community (Angst 1995). The Zurich Cohort Study provided extensive data on the epidemiology of bipolar spectrum disorders, in which Angst (1998) documented a 5.5% prevalence of DSM-IV hypomania/mania and a 2.8% rate of brief hypomania (lasting 1–3 days). For instance, findings from the Zurich Cohort Study suggested that "brief hypomania" should be added to the diagnostic classification, in part supported by associations with major depression and suicidality, which is thought to represent a subgroup of the bipolar spectrum.

Reliance on retrospective recall to diagnose bipolar disorder has led to attempts to calculate conversion rates for those symptoms detected as depressive—in estimating that a specific percentage will convert into bipolar disorder. Yet these calculations have not been universally agreed on in terms of rate of conversion (5%–10% of major depressive disorders convert to bipolar disorder). The heterogeneity of the disorder, in symptomatology, phenomenology, and course, has challenged the reliability and usefulness of this sort of formula, and therefore lifetime prevalence rates are more commonly relied on than all incidence rates.

Sociodemographic Characteristics Associated With Bipolar Disorder

Age

A bimodal age at onset has been noted in most studies, with the most frequent age at onset occurring between ages 18 and 44 and a generally accepted decline in risk after age 50. Kessler et al. (1997) found a higher prevalence in 15- to 34-year-olds compared with 35- to 54-year-olds in the NCS. Earlier onset has been frequently noted in more recent cohorts (Bland et al. 1988; Canino et al. 1987; Wells et al. 1989; Wittchen et al. 1992) and may be the result of a secular increase of illness (Sharma and Markar 1994), selection bias associated with household sampling, or another methodological issue.

Gender

In contrast to major depression, there appear to be relatively few gender differences in bipolar disorder, a finding that has been supported by large population studies, across various countries and cultures with little exception. Specifically, the majority of studies have not found gender differences in the prevalence of bipolar disorder (Burke et al. 1990; Chen et al. 1993; Egeland and Hostetter 1983; Hwu et al. 1989; Kessler et al. 1997; Lee et al. 1990; Weissman et al. 1991; Wells et al. 1989). It is of interest that absence of depressive episodes in bipolar disorder was much more common among males (38.9%) compared with females (4.1%) in the NCS.

Socioeconomic Status

Results of epidemiological studies have been mixed, with several results showing a link between low SES and bipolar disorder (Kessler et al. 1997; Smith and Weissman 1992). Kessler et al. (1997) also found a marginally significant association between poor education and bipolar disorder. In slight contrast, clinical studies have consistently reported an association between higher SES and bipolar disorder (Krauthammer and Klerman 1979; Weissman and Myers 1978; Winokur and Tanna 1969; Woodruff et al. 1971). Therefore, these findings may have been affected by selection bias of various types (for review, see Goodwin and Jamison 1990).

Race/Ethnicity

Findings on the link between race/ethnicity and bipolar disorder have been relatively weak and inconsistent. No association was found between race and bipolar disorder in the ECA Study, and a marginally statistically significant preponderance of bipolar disorder was found among nonwhite participants in the NCS (Kessler et al. 1997). Several studies have been unable to investigate the relation between bipolar disorder and race/ethnicity because of limited racial/ethnic variation of the sample.

Marital Status

As with depression, being unmarried is associated with higher rates of bipolar disorder. Kessler et al. (1997) found a marginal association between being unmarried and bipolar disorder, whereas Weissman et al. (1991) found higher rates of bipolar disorder among those never married, separated or divorced, and widowed compared with married adults.

Urban or Rural Residence

Findings on an association between urban or rural residence and bipolar disorder have been mixed (Weissman et al. 1991). In two ECA sites—St. Louis, Missouri, and Durham, North Carolina—where both urban and rural participants were included and compared, significantly higher rates of bipolar disorder were found in urban settings. Similarly, Kessler et al. (1997) found a marginally statistically significant association between urban residence and bipolar disorder in the NCS. More research is needed to draw a more definitive conclusion on this issue.

Course of Bipolar Disorder

Although bipolar disorder is thought to be a chronic condition (Coryell and Winokur 1992), most available information comes from clinical samples not representative of the course of bipolar disorder and bipolar spectrum disorder in the community. Little epidemiological evidence is available on the course of bipolar disorder, largely because of the methodological challenges mentioned earlier, as well as some additional obstacles to the accurate and reliable measurement needed to describe course. Additional challenges to measuring the course of bipolar disorder in the community include prospective measurement of onset, episodes, remission, and periods when subclinical symptoms may be present. Because there have been few prospective studies of bipolar disorder in the community, reliance on retrospective recall of first onset and past episodes has been much more common than in research on depression or other mental disorders.

Because diagnosis of bipolar disorder is largely defined by history or course of symptomatology and related phenomenology rather than current state, retrospective recall is essential to diagnosis in the absence of prospectively collected data. Critical information that is usually available only retrospectively includes 1) onset of various symptoms, 2) periods of spontaneous remission or remission in response to treatment, and 3) chronicity of course. These problems are compounded by the difficulty in relying on reports that either are provided during active phases of the disorder or involve retrospective recall about those phases.

Relatively consistent data suggest that bipolar disorders first manifest in early adulthood (early 20s) (Angst 1998; Marneros et al. 1989a, 1989b, 1989c; Wittchen et al. 1998a). The mean age at onset of bipolar disorder has been reported at age 21 in both the NCS and the ECA Study (Kessler et al. 1997; Weissman et al. 1991). Consistent with data from clinical samples (Abrams et al. 1979; Andreasen et al. 1988; Fogarty et al. 1994), 20% of the

adults with bipolar disorder in the NCS denied lifetime depressive episodes (Kessler et al. 1997). In one prospective epidemiological study of young persons in the community (Lieb et al. 2000; Wittchen et al. 1998b), 2.3% of the participants reported one episode of hypomania, and 1.5% reported a full DSM-IV manic episode (Early Developmental Stages of Psychopathology). The mean age at onset was 14.9 for hypomania and 14.5 for mania. In contrast, retrospectively reported ages at onset in the GHS-NHS, which included adults ages 18–65 in the community, were 20.5 for hypomania and 23.8 for mania, suggesting the possibility of either skewed recall or cohort effects (Jacobi et al. 2002). Yet it is unclear whether more recent reports reflecting earlier age at onset are due to cohort changes or methodological differences.

Another unresolved dilemma that warrants further epidemiological research is whether the advent and increasingly widespread use of mood-stabilizing agents, such as lithium and valproate, has resulted in a lowering of the rates of bipolar disorder in epidemiological studies. Overall, compared with clinical studies, community-based studies seem to report a considerably earlier age at onset, with frequent onset even in adolescence and young adulthood (Lewinsohn et al. 2000).

Comorbidity of Bipolar Disorder

Bipolar disorder and bipolar spectrum disorders have been found to be associated with extremely high rates of psychiatric comorbidity in the community (Regier et al. 1990; Robbins 1991). Most cases of bipolar disorder are characterized by either comorbidity or multimorbidity, with "pure" bipolar disorder appearing quite rarely. For instance, in the NCS, Kessler et al. (1997) found that 92.1% of the participants with bipolar disorder also met lifetime criteria for any anxiety disorder, 90.1% had any affective disorder, 71.0% had any substance use disorder, 59.4% had conduct disorder, and 29.0% had adult antisocial behavior. Interestingly, 59.3% with bipolar disorder said that another disorder began prior to onset of bipolar disorder. Anxiety disorders were the most common comorbidity with bipolar disorder in the NCS, whereas substance use disorders showed the highest rates of comorbidity in treated samples. The reason for this discrepancy is not known. It may be a result of higher levels of impairment and use of mental health services among those with substance use disorders, or it may be that anxiety disorders are more commonly associated with the symptom profile used to diagnose bipolar disorder in the NCS. In the NCS, prior onset of anxiety disorders, cocaine use, stimulant abuse or dependence, conduct disorder, and adult antisocial behavior were associated with increased risk for subsequent onset of bipolar disorder. Angst and Dobler-Mikola (1985) showed similarly high rates of comorbidity and multimorbidity in bipolar spectrum disorders in the Zurich Cohort Study. These data are suggestive of potential pathways between bipolar disorder and other mental disorders, but much additional research into these patterns with prospectively collected longitudinal data is needed to accurately document and untangle the nature of these links.

Risk Factors for Bipolar Disorder

Compared with major depression, significantly fewer studies have examined the risk and protective factors for bipolar disorder. Given the relative scarcity of longitudinal studies with bipolar disorder outcomes in adulthood, the available data on true causal risk factors for bipolar disorder remain in their relative infancy. Although correlates of bipolar disorder, such as age, female gender, and even comorbid psychiatric disorders and stressful life events, have been documented in numerous studies, relatively few studies have used prospective measurement of longitudinal data to document the temporal sequence of onset, compared with available clinical data on this subject. Most available data on risk factors for bipolar disorder come from family and genetic studies, although these have not been conducted with epidemiological samples. Therefore, it is not known whether these results are generalizable. For instance, previous data suggest that family history of bipolar disorder is associated with a strong increased risk for the disorder. Yet these data are based on clinically derived samples. As a result, whether this increased risk applies to only severe cases of bipolar disorder or to all cases regardless of severity or treatment status is unknown. These findings need replication in community-based samples before they can be considered reflective of bipolar disorder in the community. More recent epidemiological studies, mainly from Lewinsohn et al. (2000), suggest that childhood or adolescent major depression is associated with increased risk for bipolar disorder in young adulthood. Future research will be needed to add to and expand these findings.

Family Genetic Transmission

Increased risk for bipolar disorder among individuals whose family members have bipolar disorders has been noted. However, replication is needed in epidemiological samples to determine whether this is true in the general population or only in select cases. Understanding the interaction between environmental and genetic factors in the risk for mood disorders is a pressing issue that needs to be addressed in future research. In addition, although numerous studies have shown strong evidence that mood disorders are familial, no data are available to date showing specific genes that increase the risk for bipolar disorder or major depression. One exception to date is a study by Caspi et al. (2003), which found that a functional polymorphism in the promoter region of the serotonin transporter gene moderated the influence of stressful life events on depression.

Conclusion

Mood disorders are among the most common mental disorders among adults in the population, with some evidence that the prevalence is increasing with successive cohorts. Major depression is expected to account for the leading burden of disease by the year 2020 (Murphy and Lopez 1996; Wang and Kessler, Chapter 4, in this volume). Growing evidence suggests that bipolar disorder is more common, especially in terms of bipolar spectrum disorders, than previously thought, and debate regarding the diagnostic criteria for these disorders continues. In this chapter, we have reviewed prevalence rates, correlates, comorbidity, course, and risk factor research in mood disorders to provide a basic epidemiological overview of this area.

Research on bipolar disorder in the general population has been fraught with methodological challenges, although an increasing number of recent studies have provided consistent evidence on prevalence, demographic correlates, and comorbidity; previously, the source of this information was limited to clinical samples. Contributions have been made to this area among youths in recent years, but an area that remains sparse is risk factors for bipolar disorders. Similarly, relatively little is known about the natural course of bipolar disorders across the life span. Comparatively, more data are available on the course of and risk factors for major depression, although more evidence is needed here as well. Specific areas of interest include gender differences and related differences in risk factors, course, and phenomenology of early- and late-onset major depression, as well as physiological and genetic factors. It is important to note that prospective, longitudinal, community-based studies, which involve following up large samples from birth or early childhood far into adulthood, to examine mood disorders specifically are needed to identify true risk factors. Thus, commitments to funding such investigations for decades will be needed. Otherwise, our knowledge of risk factors may be limited, and possibly skewed, if based solely on retrospective or cross-sectional community-based studies, or even prospectively followed up clinical samples. The identification of risk factors and the distinction between modifiable risk factors, risk markers, and variable markers for disease are therefore essential. If the development of preventive interventions is to be realized, intervention will be effective only if it is made on modifiable risk factors. Increased focus on identification of specific and modifiable risk factors, as compared with general factors such as social class, will be increasingly important in order to develop interventions targeted at high-risk groups. Furthermore, as increasing information becomes available on risk factors for bipolar disorder and major depression, it will be exciting to determine whether any specificity in risk factors exists for these disorders.

In addition to environmental risk factors, family and genetic studies drawn from epidemiological samples are needed to understand whether previous findings on the familiality of mood disorder are generalizable to depression and bipolar disorder as they occur in the general population or whether these findings apply differently to severe and nonsevere disorders (or clinical vs. community samples). Additional research on gene–environment interaction risk factors should play a critical role in using a multidisciplinary perspective on the relative contributions of each of these factors to the onset, recurrence, and level of morbidity of the range of these disorders.

Unresolved issues in the investigation of major depression include 1) the reason for the gender difference; 2) the role of the increase in use of antidepressants or psychotherapeutic treatment in the prevalence and course (e.g., remission, recurrence) in the community; 3) the role of genetic factors in the risk of depression, as well as the interaction between genetic and environmental risk factors; 4) physiological correlates of depression; and 5) routes to possible community-based prevention of major depression. In terms of bipolar disorder, increased information from epidemiological studies is needed, particularly in the areas of 1) risk factors; 2) the role of treatment in the overall prevalence and prevention of chronicity of the disorder on a population level; and 3) course of bipolar and bipolar spectrum disorders in the community, including spontaneous remission.

Important questions related to the prevalence of mood disorders include the following: 1) What will the changing demographics of the population (e.g., an increase in percentage of population composed of older age groups) do to the prevalence of major depression worldwide? and 2) What should be the significance of widespread availability and use of antidepressant medications for prevalence rates in the next decade? Lifetime rates may not change, but theoretically, rates of current depression should decline at some point if medication is being

used properly (prescribed and taken). Still, current data suggest that only a minority of adults with major depression in the community seek and receive antidepressant treatment or any attention from a health care professional for depression.

Future epidemiological research in mood disorders that includes a blending of epidemiological sampling and survey methods with more recently developed and sophisticated measurement done in clinical settings is needed next to push the field forward. For instance, little is currently known about factors that appear to increase the risk for bipolar disorder, as well as the heritability and familial risk of bipolar disorder. These data are derived almost exclusively from patient samples. Although the data are extremely informative and have led to great advances in our knowledge of this disorder as a clinical entity, including biological, physiological, and behavioral correlates, it is not known to what degree these findings are generalizable to the community. Adaptation and integration of neuroimaging techniques in the investigation of population-based longitudinal studies would be novel. Clearly, logistic and financial obstacles to this type of study exist, but such studies may be needed to obtain the desired information. In addition, investigation of physiological correlates of mood disorders according to physical or physician diagnoses (e.g., lung function, cardiac tests), as well as challenge studies, are needed. In terms of risk factor research, the identification and delineation of statistical predictors of mood disorders into risk factors, risk markers, and variable markers may be the most important and useful information, in terms of future directions of research in etiology and prevention.

Epidemiology in other fields is actively focused on developing community-based recommendations and interventions. For instance, nutritional recommendations derived from risk of cancer, resulting from cancer epidemiology research, are given to the population as a whole. Yet psychiatric epidemiology has not been as active in this respect. Despite the burden of disease associated with mood disorders, significantly less attention has been paid in preventive intervention and treatment delivery and reimbursement, compared with other conditions (e.g., heart disease). This may be partially because of a focus on broad risk factors (e.g., low SES), which makes intervention less feasible. In thinking ahead about identifying modifiable risk factors for prevention efforts, it will be important to think about primary and secondary prevention for mood disorders. Primary prevention deals with attempts to prevent or delay incident cases or first onset of a disease, and secondary prevention deals with efforts aimed at preventing secondary morbidity in the presence of disease (e.g., prevention of onset of alcohol abuse in a person with major depression). Despite great advances in efficacy and range of available treatments, only a relatively small percentage of those with mood disorders are seen in clinical settings, and even fewer receive treatment. As can be seen from this review, the burden of disease in mood disorders is not limited to the disorder alone but extends to high rates of comorbidity, recurrence, and (as covered in Chapter 4 of this volume) the social burden of disease associated with mood disorders on both individual and society.

References

Abrams R, Taylor MA, Hayman MA, et al: Unipolar mania revisited. J Affect Disord 1:59–68, 1979

Akiskal HS, Mallya G: Criteria for the "soft" bipolar spectrum: treatment implications. Psychopharmacol Bull 23:68–73, 1987

Akiskal HS, Walker P, Puzantian VR, et al: Bipolar outcome in the course of depressive illness: phenomenologic, familial, and pharmacologic predictors. J Affect Disord 5:115–128, 1983

Akiskal HS, Hantouche EG, Allilaire JF, et al: Validating antidepressant-associated hypomania (bipolar III): a systematic comparison with spontaneous hypomania (bipolar II). J Affect Disord 73:65–74, 2003

American Psychiatric Association: Diagnostic and Statistical Manual of Mental Disorders, 3rd Edition. Washington, DC, American Psychiatric Association, 1980

American Psychiatric Association: Diagnostic and Statistical Manual of Mental Disorders, 3rd Edition, Revised. Washington, DC, American Psychiatric Association, 1987

American Psychiatric Association: Diagnostic and Statistical Manual of Mental Disorders, 4th Edition. Washington, DC, American Psychiatric Association, 1994

American Psychiatric Association: Diagnostic and Statistical Manual of Mental Disorders, 4th Edition, Text Revision. Washington, DC, American Psychiatric Association, 2000

Andrade L, Caraveo-Anduaga JJ, Berglund P, et al: Cross-national comparisons of the prevalences and correlates of mental disorders. Bulletin of the World Health Organization 78:413–426, 2000

Andrade L, Walters EE, Gentil V, et al: Prevalence of ICD-10 mental disorders in a catchment area in the city of São Paulo, Brazil. Soc Psychiatry Psychiatr Epidemiol 37:316–325, 2002

Andrade L, Caraveo-Anduaga JJ, Berglund P, et al: The epidemiology of major depressive episodes: results from the International Consortium of Psychiatric Epidemiology (ICPE) Surveys. Int J Methods Psychiatr Res 12:3–21, 2003

Andreasen NC, Grove WM, Coryell WH, et al: Bipolar versus unipolar and primary versus secondary affective disorder: which diagnosis takes precedence? J Affect Disord 15:69–80, 1988

Andrews G, Anstey K, Brodaty H, et al: Recall of depressive episode 25 years previously. Psychol Med 29:787–791, 1999

Andrews G, Henderson S, Hall W: Prevalence, comorbidity, disability and service utilisation. Br J Psychiatry 178:145–153, 2001

Angold A, Rutter M: The effects of age and pubertal status on depression in a large clinical sample. Development and Psychopathology 4:5–28, 1992

Angst J: The epidemiology of depressive disorders. Eur Neuropsychopharmacol 5 (suppl):95–98, 1995

Angst J: Comorbidity of mood disorders: a longitudinal prospective study. Br J Psychiatry 168 (suppl 30):31–37, 1996

Angst J: The emerging epidemiology of hypomania and bipolar II disorder. J Affect Disord 50:143–151, 1998

Angst J, Dobler-Mikola A: The Zurich study: a prospective epidemiological study of depressive, neurotic, and psychosomatic syndromes, IV: recurrent and nonrecurrent brief depression. Eur Arch Psychiatry Neurol Sci 234:408–416, 1985

Angst J, Gamma A, Gastpar M, et al: Gender differences in depression, epidemiological findings from the European DEPRES I and II studies. Eur Arch Psychiatry Clin Neurosci 252:201–209, 2002a

Angst J, Sellaro R, Merikangas KR: Multimorbidity of psychiatric disorders as an indicator of clinical severity. Eur Arch Psychiatry Clin Neurosci 252:147–154, 2002b

Ayuso-Mateos JL, Vázquez-Barquero JL, Dowrick C, et al: Depressive disorders in Europe: prevalence figures from the ODIN study. Br J Psychiatry 179:308–316, 2001

Becker E, Türke V, Neumer S, et al: Incidence and prevalence rates of mental disorders in a community sample of young women: results of the "Dresden Study," in Public Health Research and Practice: Report of the Public Health Research Association Saxony 1998-1999. Edited by Heess-Erler G, Manz R, Kirch W. Regensburg, Germany, S Roderer Verlag, 2000, pp 259–291

Bifulco A, Brown GW: Cognitive coping response to crises and onset of depression. Soc Psychiatry Psychiatr Epidemiol 31:163–172, 1998

Bijl RV, van Zessen G, Ravelli A, et al: The Netherlands Mental Health Survey and Incidence Study (NEMESIS): objectives and design. Soc Psychiatry Psychiatr Epidemiol 33:581–586, 1998a

Bijl RV, Ravelli A, van Zessen G: Prevalence of psychiatric disorder in the general population: results of the Netherlands Mental Health Survey and Incidence Study (NEMESIS). Soc Psychiatry Psychiatr Epidemiol 33:587–595, 1998b

Bijl RV, de Graaf R, Hiripi E, et al: The prevalence of treated and untreated mental disorders in five countries. Health Aff (Millwood) 22:122–133, 2003

Bittner A, Goodwin RD, Wittchen H-U, et al: What characteristics of primary anxiety disorders predict subsequent major depression? J Clin Psychiatry 65:618–626, 2004

Bland RC: Epidemiology of affective disorders: a review. Can J Psychiatry 42:367–377, 1997

Bland RC, Orn H, Newman SC: Lifetime prevalence of psychiatric disorders in Edmonton. Acta Psychiatr Scand 338 (suppl):24–32, 1988

Boyle MH, Offord DR, Campbell D, et al: Mental health supplement to the Ontario Health Survey: Methodology. Can J Psychiatry 41:549–558, 1996

Brown GW: Life events and affective disorder: replications and limitations. J Psychosom Med 55:248–259, 1993

Brown GW, Harris TO: Social Origins of Depression: A Study of Psychiatric Disorder in Women. London, Tavistock, 1978

Brown GW, Harris TO: Aetiology of anxiety and depressive disorders in an inner-city population, 1: early adversity. Psychol Med 23:143–154, 1993a

Brown GW, Harris TO, Eales MJ: Aetiology of anxiety and depressive disorders in an inner-city population, 2: comorbidity and adversity. Psychol Med 23:155–165, 1993b

Brown GW, Harris TO, Hepworth C: Loss, humiliation and entrapment among woman developing depression: a patient and non-patient comparison. Psychol Med 25:7–21, 1995

Burke KC, Burke JD, Regier DA, et al: Age at onset of selected mental disorders in five community populations. Arch Gen Psychiatry 47:511–518, 1990

Canals J, Domènech E, Carbajo G, et al: Prevalence of DSM-III-R and ICD-10 psychiatric disorders in a Spanish population of 18-year-olds. Acta Psychiatr Scand 96:287–294, 1997

Canals J, Domenech-Llaberia E, Fernandez-Ballart J, et al: Predictors of depression at eighteen: a 7-year follow-up study in a Spanish nonclinical population. Eur Child Adolesc Psychiatry 11:226–233, 2002

Canino GJ, Bird HR, Shrout PE, et al: The prevalence of specific psychiatric disorders in Puerto Rico. Arch Gen Psychiatry 44:727–735, 1987

Caspi A, Sugden K, Moffitt TE, et al: Influence of life stress on depression: moderation by a polymorphism in the 5-HTT gene. Science 301:386–389, 2003

Cassano GB, Savino M, Perugi G, et al: Major depressive episode: unipolar and bipolar II. Encephale 18 (Spec No 1): 15–18, 1992

Chen CN, Wong J, Lee N, et al: The Shatin Community Mental Health Survey in Hong Kong, II: major findings. Arch Gen Psychiatry 50:125–133, 1993

Coryell W, Winokur G: Course and outcome, in Handbook of Affective Disorders, 2nd Edition. Edited by Paykel ES. New York, Guilford, 1992, pp 89–108

Cyranowski JM, Frank E, Young E, et al: Adolescent onset of the gender difference in lifetime rates of major depression: a theoretical model. Arch Gen Psychiatry 57:21–27, 2000

Deadman JM, Dewey MJ, Owens RG, et al; Threat and loss in breast cancer. Psychol Med 19:677–681, 1989

de Graaf R, Bijl RV, Beekman AT, et al: Temporal sequencing of lifetime mood disorders in relation to comorbid anxiety and substance use disorders: findings from the Netherlands Mental Health Survey and Incidence Study. Soc Psychiatry Psychiatr Epidemiol 38:1–11, 2003

De Marco RR: The epidemiology of major depression: Implications of occurence, recurrence, and stress in a Canadian community sample. Can J Psychiatry 45:67–74, 2000

Dinwiddie S, Heath AC, Dunne MP, et al: Early sexual abuse and lifetime psychopathology: a co-twin-control study. Psychol Med 30:41–52, 2000

Dohrenwend BP, Dohrenwend BS: Perspectives on the past and future of psychiatric epidemiology: The 1981 Rema Lapouse Lecture. Am J Public Health 72:1271–1279, 1982

Dunlop DD, Song J, Lyons JS, et al: Racial/ethnic differences in rates of depression among preretirement adults. Am J Public Health 93:1945–1952, 2003

Eaton WW, Kessler LG: Rates of symptoms of depression in a national sample. Am J Epidemiol 114:528–538, 1981

Eaton WW, Holzer CE 3rd, Von Korff M, et al: The design of the Epidemiologic Catchment Area surveys: the control and measurement of error. Arch Gen Psychiatry 41:942–948, 1984

Egeland JA, Hostetter AM: Amish Study, I: affective disorders among the Amish, 1976–1980. Am J Psychiatry 140:56–61, 1983

Emslie GJ, Rush AJ, Weinberg WA, et al: A double-blind, randomized, placebo-controlled trial of fluoxetine in children and adolescents with depression. Arch Gen Psychiatry 54:1031–1037, 1997

Endicott J, Spitzer RL: A diagnostic interview: the Schedule for Affective Disorders and Schizophrenia. Arch Gen Psychiatry 35:837–844, 1978

Feehan M, McGee R, Raha S, et al: DSM-III-R disorders in New Zealand 18-year-olds. Aust N Z J Psychiatry 28:87–99, 1994

Fergusson DM, Horwood J, Lynskey MT: Prevalence and comorbidity of DSM-III-R diagnoses in birth cohort of 15-year-olds. J Am Acad Child Adolesce Psychiatry 32:1127–1134, 1993

Fergusson DM, Horwood LJ, Lynskey MT: Childhood sexual abuse and psychiatric disorder in young adulthood, II: psychiatric outcomes of childhood sexual abuse. J Am Acad Child Adolesc Psychiatry 35:1365–1374, 1996

Fergusson DM, Swain-Campbell NR, Horwood LJ: Does sexual violence contribute to elevated rates of anxiety and depression in females? Psychol Med 32:991–996, 2002

First MB, Spitzer RL, Gibbon M, et al: Structured Clinical Interview for DSM-IV Axis I Disorders, Research Version, Non-Patient Edition (SCID-I/NP). New York, Biometrics Research, 1997

Fogarty F, Russell JM, Newman SC, et al: Epidemiology of psychiatric disorders in Edmonton: mania. Acta Psychiatr Scand Suppl 376:16–23, 1994

Gilman SE, Kawachi I, Fitzmaurice GM, et al: Socio-economic status, family disruption and residential stability in childhood: relation to onset, recurrence and remission of major depression. Psychol Med 33:1341–1355, 2003

Goldberg D, Huxley P: Mental Illness in the Community: The Pathway to Psychiatric Care. London, Tavistock, 1980

Goodwin FK, Jamison KJ: Manic-Depressive Illness. New York, Oxford University Press, 1990

Goodyer IM, Herbert J, Secher SM, et al: Short-term outcome of major depression, I: comorbidity and severity at presentation as predictors of persistent disorder. J Am Acad Child Adolesc Psychiatry 36:179–187, 1997

Hagnell O, Gräsbeck A: Comorbidity of anxiety and depression in the Lundby 25-year prospective study: the pattern of subsequent episodes, in Comorbidity of Mood and Anxiety Disorders. Edited by Maser JD, Cloninger CR. Washington, DC, American Psychiatric Press, 1990, pp 139–152

Hettema JM, Prescott CA, Kendler KS: The effects of anxiety, substance use and conduct disorders on risk of major depressive disorders. Psychol Med 33:1423–1432, 2003

Horwath E, Johnson J, Weissman MM, et al: The validity of major depression with atypical features based on a community study. J Affect Disord 26:117–126, 1992

Hwu H-G, Yeh E-K, Chang L-Y: Prevalence of psychiatric disorders in Taiwan defined by the Chinese Diagnostic Interview Schedule. Acta Psychiatr Scand 79:136–147, 1989

Jacobi F: Prevalence patterns, help-seeking and burden of various types of affective disorders. J Affect Disord 78 (suppl 1):39–40, 2004

Jacobi F, Wittchen H-U, Hölting C, et al: Estimating the prevalence of mental and somatic disorders in the community: aims and methods of the German National Health Interview and Examination Survey. Int J Methods Psychiatr Res 11:1–18, 2002

Jacobi F, Wittchen H-U, Hölting C, et al: Prevalence, comorbidity and correlates of mental disorders in the general population: results from the German Health Interview and Examination Survey (GHS). Psychol Med 34:597–611, 2004

Jaffee SR, Moffitt TE, Caspi A, et al: Differences in early childhood risk factors for juvenile-onset and adult-onset depression. Arch Gen Psychiatry 59:215–222, 2002

Jenkins R, Bebbington PE, Brugha TS, et al: The National Psychiatric Morbidity Surveys of Great Britain: strategy and methods. Psychol Med 27:765–774, 1997

Jenkins R, Lewis G, Bebbington PE, et al: The National Psychiatric Morbidity Surveys of Great Britain: initial findings from the Household Survey. Psychol Med 27:775-789, 1997

Kashani JH, McGee RO, Clarkson SE, et al: Depression in a sample of 9-year-old children, prevalence and associated characteristics. Arch Gen Psychiatry 40:1217–1223, 1983

Kendler KS, Kessler RC, Walters EE, et al: Stressful life events, genetic liability, and onset of an episode of major depression in women. Am J Psychiatry 152:833–842, 1995

Kendler KS, Karkowski L, Prescott CA: Stressful life events and major depression: risk period, long-term contextual threat and diagnostic specificity. J Nerv Ment Dis 186:661–669, 1998

Kendler KS, Hettema JM, Butera F, et al: Life event dimensions of loss, humiliation, entrapment, and danger in the prediction of onsets of major depression and generalized anxiety. Arch Gen Psychiatry 60:789–796, 2003

Kessler RC: Epidemiology of psychiatric comorbidity, in Textbook in Psychiatric Epidemiology. Edited by Tsuang M, Tohen M, Zahner GEP. New York, Wiley, 1995, pp 179–197

Kessler RC: The effects of stressful life events on depression. Annu Rev Psychol 48:191–214, 1997

Kessler RC, Walters EE: Epidemiology of DSM-III-R major depression and minor depression among adolescents and young adults in the National Comorbidity Survey. Depress Anxiety 7:3–14, 1998

Kessler RC, McGongale KA, Zhao S, et al: Lifetime and 12-month prevalence of DSM-III-R psychiatric disorders in the United States: results from the National Comorbidity Survey. Arch Gen Psychiatry 51:8–19, 1994

Kessler RC, Nelson CB, McGonagle KA, et al: Comorbidity of DSM-III-R major depressive disorder in the general population: results from the US National Comorbidity Survey. Br J Psychiatry 168 (suppl 30):17–30, 1996

Kessler RC, Zhao S, Blazer DG, et al: Prevalence, correlates, and course of minor depression and major depression in the National Comorbidity Survey. J Affect Disord 45:19–30, 1997

Kessler RC, Stang P, Wittchen H-U, et al: Lifetime panic-depression comorbidity in the National Comorbidity Survey. Arch Gen Psychiatry 55:801–808, 1998

Kessler RC, Stang P, Wittchen H-U, et al: Lifetime comorbidities between social phobia and mood disorders in the U.S. National Comorbidity Survey. Psychol Med 29:555–567, 1999

Kessler RC, Wittchen H-U, Abelson J, et al: Methodological issues in assessing psychiatric disorders with self-reports, in The Science of Self-Report: Implications for Research and Practice. Edited by Stone AA, Turkkan JS, Bachrach CA, et al. Mahwah, NJ, Lawrence Erlbaum, 2000, pp 229–255

Kessler RC, Berglund P, Demler O, et al: The epidemiology of major depressive disorder: results from the National Comorbidity Survey Replication (NCS-R). JAMA 289:3095–3105, 2003

Klein DN, Lewinsohn PM, Seeley JR, et al: Family study of major depressive disorder in a community sample of adolescents. Arch Gen Psychiatry 58:13–20, 2001

Klein DN, Lewinsohn PM, Rohde P, et al: A family study of comorbidity between major depressive disorder and anxiety disorders. Psychol Med 33:703–714, 2003

Klerman GL, Weissman MM: Increasing rates of depression. JAMA 261:2229–2235, 1989

Klose M, Jacobi F: Can gender differences in the prevalence of mental disorders be explained by sociodemographic factors? Arch Women Ment Health 7:133–148, 2004

Kovacs M: The Children's Depression Inventory. Psychopharmacol Bull 21:995–998, 1985

Krauthammer C, Klerman GL: Mania secondary to thyroid disease. Lancet 1(8120):827–828, 1979

Kringlen E, Torgersen S, Cramer V: A Norwegian psychiatric epidemiological study. Am J Psychiatry 158:1091–1098, 2001

Lee CK, Kwak YS, Yamamoto J, et al: Psychiatric epidemiology in Korea; part I: gender and age differences in Seoul. J Nerv Ment Dis 178:242–246, 1990

Lewinsohn PM, Klein DN, Seeley JR: Bipolar disorders in a community sample of older adolescents: prevalence, phenomenology, comorbidity, and course. J Am Acad Child Adolesc Psychiatry 34:454–463, 1995

Lewinsohn PM, Zinbarg RE, Seeley JR, et al: Lifetime comorbidity among anxiety disorders and between anxiety disorders and other mental disorders in adolescents. J Anxiety Disord 11:377–394, 1997

Lewinsohn PM, Klein DN, Seeley JR: Bipolar disorder during adolescence and young adulthood in a community sample. Bipolar Disord 2 (3 pt 2):281–293, 2000

Lewis G, Pelosi AJ, Araya R, et al: Measuring psychiatric disorder in the community: a standardized assessment for use by lay interviewers. Psychol Med 22:465–486, 1992

Lieb R, Isensee B, von Sydow K, et al: The Early Developmental Stages of Psychopathology Study (EDSP): a methodological update. Eur Addict Res 6:170–182, 2000

Lieb R, Isensee B, Höfler M, et al: Parental major depression and the risk of depression and other mental disorders in offspring: a prospective-longitudinal community study. Arch Gen Psychiatry 59:365–374, 2002

Lindeman S, Hämäläinen J, Isometsä E, et al: The 12-month prevalence and risk factors for major depressive episode in Finland: representative sample of 5993 adults. Acta Psychiatr Scand 102:178–184, 2000

Maciejewski PK, Prigerson HG, Mazure CM: Sex differences in event-related risk for major depression. Psychol Med 31:593–604, 2001

MacMillan HL, Fleming JE, Streiner DL, et al: Childhood abuse and lifetime psychopathology in a community sample. Am J Psychiatry 158:1878–1883, 2001

Maier W, Minges J, Lichtermann D, et al: Personality patterns in subjects at risk for affective disorders. Psychopathology 28 (suppl 1):59–72, 1995

Marneros A, Deister A, Rohde A: Unipolar and bipolar schizoaffective disorders: a comparative study, I: premorbid and sociodemographic features. Eur Arch Psychiatry Neurol Sci 239:158–163, 1989a

Marneros A, Rohde A, Deister A: Unipolar and bipolar schizoaffective disorders: a comparative study, II: long-term course. Eur Arch Psychiatry Neurol Sci 2239:164–170, 1989b

Marneros A, Deister A, Rohde A, et al: Unipolar and bipolar schizoaffective disorders: a comparative study, III: long-term outcome. Eur Arch Psychiatry Neurol Sci 239:171–176, 1989c

Mazure CM, Maciejewski PK: A model of risk for major depression: effects of life stress and cognitive style vary by age. Depress Anxiety 17:26–33, 2003

McGee R, Feehan M, Williams S, et al: DSM-III disorders in a large sample of adolescents. J Am Acad Child Adolesc Psychiatry 29: 611–619, 1990

Merikangas KR, Prusoff BA, Weissman MM: Parental concordance for affective disorders: psychopathology in offspring. J Affect Disord 15:279–290, 1988

Merikangas KR, Angst J, Eaton W, et al: Comorbidity and boundaries of affective disorders with anxiety disorders and substance misuse: results of an international task force. Br J Psychiatry 168 (suppl 30):58–67, 1996

Merikangas KR, Ahang H, Avenevoli S, et al: Longitudinal trajectories of depression and anxiety in a prospective community study: the Zurich Cohort Study. Arch Gen Psychiatry 60:993–1000, 2003

Meyer C, Rumpf H-J, Hapke U, et al: Lebenszeitprävalenz psychischer Störungen in der erwachsenen Allgemeinbevölkerung [Lifetime prevalence of mental disorders in general adult population. Results of TACOS study]. Nervenarzt 71:535–542, 2000

Miller PM, Ingham JG: Dimensions of experience. Psychol Med 13:417–429, 1983

Murphy JM: Diagnostic comorbidity and symptom co-occurrence: the Stirling County Study, in Comorbidity of Mood and Anxiety Disorders. Edited by Maser JD, Cloninger CR. Washington, DC, American Psychiatric Press, 1990, pp 153–176

Murphy JM, Laird NM, Monson RR, et al: A 40-year perspective on the prevalence of depression: the Stirling County Study. Arch Gen Psychiatry 57:209–215, 2000a

Murphy JM, Laird NM, Monson RR, et al: Incidence of depression in the Stirling County Study: historical and comparative perspectives. Psychol Med 30:505–514, 2000b

Murray CJL, Lopez AD (eds): The Global Burden of Disease: A Comprehensive Assessment of Mortality and Disability for Diseases, Injuries, and Risk Factors in 1990 and Projected to 2020. Geneva, World Health Organization, 1996

Narrow WE, Rae DS, Robins LN, et al: Revised prevalence estimates of mental disorders in the United States: using a clinical significance criterion to reconcile 2 surveys' estimates. Arch Gen Psychiatry 59:115–123, 2002

Neugebauer R, Dohrenwend BP, Dohrenwend BS: Formulation of hypotheses about the true prevalence of functional psychiatric disorders among adults in the United States, in Mental Illness in the United States. Edited by Dohrenwend BP. New York, Praeger, 1980, pp 45–94

Nomura Y, Warner V, Wickramaratne P: Parents concordant for major depressive disorder and the effect of psychopathology in offspring. Psychol Med 31:1211–1222, 2001

Offord DR, Boyle MH, Campbell D, et al: One-year prevalence of psychiatric disorder in Ontarians 15 to 64 years of age. Can J Psychiatry 41:559–563, 1996

Oldehinkel AJ, Wittchen H-U, Schuster P: Prevalence, 20-month incidence and outcome of unipolar depressive disorders in a community sample of adolescents. Psychol Med 29:655–668, 1999

Ormel J, Wohlfarth T: How neuroticism, long-term difficulties, and life situation change influence psychological distress: a longitudinal model. J Pers Soc Psychiatry 60:744–755, 1991

Patten SB, Stuart HL, Russell ML, et al: Epidemiology of major depression in a predominantly rural health region. Soc Psychiatry Psychiatr Epidemiol 38:360–365, 2003

Paykel ES: Not an age of depression after all? Incidence rates may be stable over time. Psychol Med 30:489–490, 2000

Pine DS, Cohen P, Brook J: Adolescent fears as predictors of depression. Biol Psychiatry 50:721–724, 2001

Regier DA, Farmer ME, Rae DS, et al: Comorbidity of mental disorders with alcohol and other drug abuse: results from the Epidemiologic Catchment Area (ECA) Study. JAMA 264:2511–2518, 1990

Regier DA, Kaelber CT, Rae DS, et al: Limitations of diagnostic criteria and assessment instruments for mental disorders: implications for research and policy. Arch Gen Psychiatry 55:109–115, 1998

Reinherz HZ, Giaconia RM, Hauf AM, et al: General and specific childhood risk factors for depression and drug disorders by early adulthood. J Am Acad Child Adolesc Psychiatry 39:223–231, 2000

Robins LN, Regier DA: Psychiatric Disorders in America: The Epidemiologic Catchment Area Study. New York, Free Press, 1991

Robins LN, Helzer JE, Croughan J, et al: National Institute of Mental Health Diagnostic Interview Schedule. Arch Gen Psychiatry 38:381–389, 1981

Robins LN, Wing J, Wittchen H-U, et al: The Composite International Diagnostic Interview: an epidemiological instrument suitable for use in conjunction with different diagnostic systems and in different cultures. Arch Gen Psychiatry 45:1069–1077, 1988

Robins LN, Locke BZ, Regier DA: An overview of psychiatric disorders in America, in Psychiatric Disorders in America: The Epidemiologic Catchment Area Study. Edited by Robins LN, Regier DA. New York, Free Press, 1991, pp 328–366

Roy-Byrne PP, Stang P, Wittchen HU, et al: Lifetime panic-depression comorbidity in the National Comorbidity Survey: association with symptoms, impairment, course and help-seeking. Br J Psychiatry 176:229–235, 2000

Sharma R, Markar HR: Mortality in affective disorder. J Affect Disord 31:91–96, 1994

Smith AL, Weissman MM: Epidemiology, in Handbook of Affective Disorders, 2nd Edition. Edited by Paykel ES. New York, Guilford, 1992, pp 111–129

Spijker J, de Graaf R, Bijl RV, et al: Duration of major depressive episodes in the general population: results from The Netherlands Mental Health Survey and Incidence Study (NEMESIS). Br J Psychiatry 181:208–213, 2002

Spitzer RL, Endicott J, Robins E: Research Diagnostic Criteria: rationale and reliability. Arch Gen Psychiatry 35:773–782, 1978

Stein MB, Fuetsch M, Muller N, et al: Social anxiety disorder and the risk of depression: a prospective community study of adolescents and young adults. Arch Gen Psychiatry 58:251–256, 2001

Streiner DL: Let me count the ways: measuring incidence, prevalence, and impact in epidemiological studies. Can J Psychiatry 43:173–179, 1998

Tohen M, Bromet E, Murphy JM, et al: Psychiatric epidemiology. Harv Rev Psychiatry 8:111–125, 2000

Turner RJ, Gil AG: Psychiatric and substance use disorders in South Florida. Arch Gen Psychiatry 59:43–50, 2002

Van Os J, Jones PB: Early risk factors and person-environment relationships in affective disorder. Psychol Med 29:1099–1067, 1999

Vega WA, Kolody B, Aguilar-Gaxiola S, et al: Lifetime prevalence of DSM-III-R psychiatric disorders among urban and rural mexican americans in California. Arch Gen Psychiatry 55:771–778, 1998

Wacker HR, Müllejans R, Klein KH, et al: Identification of cases of anxiety disorders and affective disorders in the community according to ICD-10 and DSM-III-R by using the composite international diagnostic interview (CIDI). Int J Methods Psychiatr Res 2:91–100, 1992

Warner V, Weissman MM, Mufson L, et al: Grandparents, parents, and grandchildren at high risk for depression: a three-generation study. J Am Acad Child Adolesc Psychiatry 38:289–296, 1999

Weissman MM, Myers J: Affective disorders in a V.S. urban community: the use of research diagnostic criteria in an epidemiological survey. Arch Gen Psychiatry 35:1304–1311, 1978

Weissman MM, Wickramaratne P: Age at onset and familial risk in major depression. Arch Gen Psychiatry 57:513–514, 2000

Weissman MM, Gammon GD, John K, et al: Children of depressed parents: increased psychopathology and early onset of major depression. Arch Gen Psychiatry 44:847–853, 1987

Weissman MM, Leaf PJ, Tischler GL, et al: Affective disorders in five United States communities. Psychol Med 18:140–153, 1988

Weissman MM, Bruce LM, Leaf PJ, et al: Affective disorders, in Psychiatric Disorders in America: The Epidemiologic Catchment Area Study. Edited by Robins LN, Regier DA. New York, Free Press, 1991, pp 53–80

Weissman MM, Bland RC, Joyce PR, et al: Sex differences in rates of depression: cross-national perspectives. J Affect Disord 29:77–84, 1993

Weissman MM, Bland RC, Canino GJ, et al: Cross-national epidemiology of major depression and bipolar disorder. JAMA 276:293–299, 1996

Weissman MM, Warner V, Wickramaratne P, et al: Offspring of depressed parents: 10 years later. Arch Gen Psychiatry 54:932–940, 1997

Wells KB, Stewart A, Hays RD: The functioning and well-being of depressed patients: results from the Medical Outcomes Study. JAMA 262:916–919, 1989

WHO World Mental Health Survey Consortium: Prevalence, severity, and unmet need for treatment of mental disorders in the World Health Organization World Mental Health Surveys. JAMA 291:2581–2590, 2004

Wickramaratne PJ, Greenwald S, Weissman MM: Psychiatric disorders in the relatives of probands with prepubertal-onset or adolescent-onset major depression. J Am Acad Child Adolesc Psychiatry 39:1396–1405, 2000

Wing JK, Cooper JE, Sartorius N: The Measurement and Classification of Psychiatric Symptoms: An Instruction Manual for the Present State Examination and CATEGO Programme. London, Cambridge University Press, 1974

Wing JK, Babor T, Brugha T, et al: SCAN: Schedules for Clinical Assessment in Neuropsychiatry. Arch Gen Psychiatry 47:589–593, 1990

Winokur G, Coryell W: Familial subtypes of unipolar depression: a prospective study of familial pure depressive disease compared to depression spectrum disease. Biol Psychiatry 32:1012–1018, 1992

Winokur G, Tanna VL: Possible role of X-linked dominant factor in manic depressive disease. Dis Nerv Syst 30:89–94, 1969

Wittchen H-U: Reliability and validity studies of the WHO-Composite International Diagnostic Interview (CIDI): a critical review. J Psychiatr Res 28:57–84, 1994

Wittchen H-U: Critical issues in the evaluation of comorbidity of psychiatric disorders. Br J Psychiatry 168 (suppl 30):9–16, 1996

Wittchen H-U, Jacobi F: Die Versorgungssituation psychischer Störungen in Deutschland. Eine klinisch-epidemiologische Abschätzung anhand des Bundes-Gesundheitssurveys 1998. Bundesgesundheitsblatt-Gesundheitsforschung-Gesundheitsschutz 44: 993–1000, 2001

Wittchen HU, Pfister H (eds): Manual und Durchführungsbeschreibung des DIA-X/M-CIDI [Manual of DIA-X/M-CIDI]. Frankfurt, Germany, Swets & Zeitlinger, 1997

Wittchen HU, Essau CA, von Zerssen D, et al: Lifetime and six-month prevalence of mental disorders in the Munich Follow-Up Study. Eur Arch Psychiatry Clin Neurosci 241:247–258, 1992

Wittchen H-U, Nelson CB, Lachner G: Prevalence of mental disorders and psychosocial impairments in adolescents and young adults. Psychol Med 28:109–126, 1998a

Wittchen H-U, Perkonigg A, Lachner G, et al: Early Developmental Stages of Psychopathology Study (EDSP): objectives and design. Eur Addict Res 4:18–27, 1998b

Wittchen H-U, Carter RM, Pfister H, et al: Disabilities and quality of life in pure and comorbid generalised anxiety disorder and major depression in a national survey. Int Clin Psychopharmacol 15:319–328, 2000

Woodruff RA Jr, Guze WB, Clayton PJ: Unipolar and bipolar primary affective disorder. Br J Psychiatry 119:33–38, 1971

Woodward LJ, Fergusson DM: Life course outcomes of young people with anxiety disorders in adolescence. J Am Acad Child Adolesc Psychiatry 40:1086–1093, 2001

World Health Organization: International Classification of Diseases, 9th Revision. Geneva, World Health Organization, 1977

World Health Organization: International Statistical Classification of Diseases and Related Health Problems, 10th Revision. Geneva, World Health Organization, 1992

World Health Organization: Compositie International Diagnostic Interview (CIDI). Geneva, World Health Organization, 1993

Global Burden of Mood Disorders

PHILIP S. WANG, M.D., DR.P.H.
RONALD C. KESSLER, PH.D.

IN THIS CHAPTER, we review the literature on the global burden of mood disorders. Interest in the costs of illness—not only direct treatment costs but also human costs—has increased dramatically over the past decade as part of the larger movement to rationalize the allocation of treatment resources to maximize benefit in relation to cost. Much of the current interest in mood disorders, and especially depression, among health policy-makers is based on the fact that depression consistently has been found in these studies to be among the most costly health problems in the world. Bipolar disorder also has been ranked as a very costly illness in recent cost-of-illness studies. As reviewed here, several factors account for these results, which have important implications for the design of treatment programs for mood disorders.

Mood Disorders Are Among the Most Burdensome Conditions Worldwide

Over the past several decades, evidence has been accumulating that mood disorders, including major depression (Broadhead et al. 1990; Coryell et al. 1993; Rohde et al. 1990; Tweed 1993; Wells et al. 1989; Zeiss and Lewinsohn 1988), bipolar disorder (Calabrese et al. 2003; Coryell et al. 1993; Dion et al. 1988; Lish et al. 1994; MacQueen et al. 2001), and dysthymia (Cassano et al. 1990; Hays et al. 1995; Klein et al. 1988; Stewart et al. 1988), impose substantial societal burdens. Even highly prevalent subsyndromal levels of affective symptomatology have been associated with significantly reduced function-

Preparation of this chapter was supported, in part, by National Institute of Mental Health grants K01 MH01651, R01 MH61941, R01 MH69772 (P.S.W.), and K05 MH00507 (R.C.K.) and by Robert Wood Johnson Foundation grant 048123 (P.S.W.).

ing (Judd et al. 1994, 1996; Rapaport and Judd 1998). However, some of these investigations were conducted in small or specialized populations, and few placed the burdens from mood disorders into perspective by comparing them with the burdens from other conditions. For these reasons, two studies represent watersheds in our understanding of just how large and serious the burdens from mood disorders truly are.

The first is the Global Burden of Disease study from the World Health Organization (WHO). First published in 1996, the Global Burden of Disease study quantified the burdens from a wide variety of conditions in terms of disability-adjusted life-years (DALYs) (Murray and Lopez 1996). It found that worldwide depression is responsible for more disability than any other condition during the middle years of life, with no other disease or condition accounting for even half of the total burden imposed by depression in this part of the age range. Furthermore, the Global Burden of Disease study identified bipolar disorder as the sixth leading cause of disability in this age group. Importantly, depression and bipolar disorder remained in the top 10 causes of lost DALYs across important subgroups, including men, women, developed countries, and developing regions of the world (Murray and Lopez 1996).

The second study, the Medical Outcomes Study, used the 36-item Short-Form Health Survey (SF-36; Wells et al. 1989) to assess the functioning of more than 11,000 patients with a variety of chronic medical illnesses. Like the Global Burden of Disease study, the Medical Outcomes Study identified depression as being at least as disabling as other general medical conditions. In addition, the Medical Outcomes Study (Wells et al. 1992), along with other investigations (Friedman et al. 1995; Leader and Klein 1996), observed that dysthymia may impose functional burdens at least as great as, if not greater than, those from depression. A related finding was that disease burdens are additively heightened during periods in which dysthymia is complicated by major depressive episodes.

Components of Burdens From Mood Disorders: The Increasing Relevance of Economic Costs

Burden of illness researchers have found that the negative effects of mood disorders run not only deep but also quite broad, in terms of both the domains typically disrupted and the members and stakeholders in society affected (McGuire et al. 2002). For afflicted individuals, burdens include significant clinical morbidity; increased mortality,

particularly from suicide; loss of quality of life; and diminished functioning in the realms of activities of daily living, education, work, marital relationships, family and other social relationships; mood disorders also have been observed to impose burdens on not only afflicted individuals but also their families, caregivers, and communities (Goodwin and Jamison 1990; Harwood et al. 1984; Hirschfeld et al. 2003; Jacob et al. 1987; Klerman and Weissman 1992; Mueser et al. 1992; Perlick et al. 1999; Rice et al. 1990; Stoudemire et al. 1986; Wells and Sherbourne 1999). Several excellent recent reviews of the literature on these effects of mood disorders are available (Bauer et al. 2002; Hirschfeld et al. 2000; Simon 2003).

Although economic costs are but one component of the total burdens from illness, they are increasingly becoming a focus of attention in the United States because of the prominent role of employers in purchasing health insurance and the interests of employers in the workplace costs of illness. These data are needed to inform the social policy debate concerning the extent to which there should be health insurance coverage for mental disorders. Policy-makers, benefits managers, health plan administrators, employers, and other stakeholders increasingly need to make difficult decisions regarding how to allocate limited health care resources, even in the most economically advantaged societies. Economic data, including data on the costs of illness and the cost-effectiveness of treatments, have become high priorities to help make adequately informed decisions.

Three categories of costs typically have been included in cost-of-illness research to estimate the overall economic burdens from diseases (Greenberg et al. 1993; Jarvinen et al. 1988). First are the direct treatment costs, consisting of resources spent on inpatient, outpatient, partial hospitalization, residential, pharmacological, and other treatments. Second are the indirect economic costs arising from any increase in mortality attributable to the illness. Third are indirect economic burdens arising from morbidity, particularly those that cause reductions in afflicted individuals' productive capacities.

Recent estimates of the economic burdens attributable to mood disorders have been staggering. Greenberg and colleagues (1996) estimated that the economic costs from depression are $53 billion each year in the United States. These investigators also identified which types of costs are most responsible for these heavy economic burdens. Economic losses due to work impairment from depression are responsible for the lion's share, or $33 billion annually. Direct treatment costs, however, are responsible for much less, or $12 billion annually. Economic costs from increased mortality due to suicides contribute $8 billion annually (Greenberg et al. 1996). Further breakdown of the economic losses due to work impairment indicated that depression-related absenteeism accounts for $24.5 billion annually and that depression-related impairment while at work ("presenteeism") accounts for $8.5 billion annually (Greenberg et al. 1996). Similar findings have been reported for bipolar illness, in terms of both the large magnitude and the relative distribution among subtypes of economic costs. For example, Wyatt and Henter (1995) estimated that the total economic costs from bipolar disorder are $45 billion each year in the United States. Again, economic losses due to work impairment from bipolar disorder account for the largest proportion (nearly $18 billion annually), whereas direct treatment costs and mortality due to suicides accounted for less (about $8 billion each).

Note that the true economic costs of mood disorders to society are almost certainly larger than those suggested in the previous paragraph (Greenberg et al. 1993). We have reviewed estimates for only depression and bipolar disorder but not other common mood syndromes such as dysthymia or subthreshold affective conditions. In addition, the cost estimates in the studies of economic effects do not capture the potentially devastating long-term consequences that mood disorders can have on education and professional attainment (Kessler et al. 1995). Current cost-of-illness studies are also predicated on assigning a value to life based on the productive contribution a person makes to society (i.e., a human capital model). In addition to not accounting for nonmonetary costs such as pain, suffering, and decrements in quality of life due to depression, such models place no value on the contributions of individuals not employed in the labor market, such as children, those engaged primarily in nonwage household work, and elderly retirees.

Reasons for the High Costs of Mood Disorders

With estimated costs as high as those cited in the previous section, it is critical to examine the components that account for them. One set of reasons is that mood disorders are among the most commonly occurring chronic diseases and tend to strike far earlier in the life course than other conditions with comparable prevalence. Furthermore, the prevalence of mood disorders appears to be increasing in recent cohorts. A second set of reasons, which we alluded to earlier, is that mood disorders are associated with very large decrements in multiple aspects of work performance. This leads to large aggregate losses, again because mood disorders tend to strike before or

during prime working years. The chronicity of mood disorders further adds to these substantial losses in productivity (Kessler et al. 1995). A final set of reasons is that few people with mood disorders receive adequate care, despite the availability of effective treatments that could otherwise lead to improved clinical and work outcomes. In the next subsections, we review the evidence regarding each of these three sets of reasons.

High Prevalence of Depression and Associated Impairments

Mood disorders are very common in the general population, as described in more detail elsewhere in this book (see Goodwin et al., Chapter 3). Importantly, mood disorders are also very common in working populations (Eaton et al. 1990; Kessler et al. 1994, 2003b) and have powerful negative effects on work performance. For example, in the Epidemiologic Catchment Area (ECA) study, major depression was associated with a 27 times greater likelihood of work loss from emotional problems compared with having none of the DSM disorders assessed, and 44% of the depressed workers had missed 1 or more days from work for emotional problems in the prior 3 months (Kouzis and Eaton 1994). In the National Comorbidity Survey (NCS; Kessler and Frank 1997), depression was associated with a significant risk for not only sickness absence days but also days in which the respondent was at work but performing poorly (work cutback days). In fact, more recent research (Stewart et al. 2003) suggests that depression's impairment of on-the-job performance (presenteeism) may be larger than previously thought and may outweigh its effects on absenteeism. The nationally generalizable Midlife Development in the United States (MIDUS) survey in 1997 (Kessler et al. 2001b) found that depression was one of the five most impairing medical conditions in the United States in terms of work loss and work cutback and that of these five conditions, depression was by far the most prevalent. In the WHO Collaborative Study on Psychological Problems in General Health Care (Sartorius and Ustun 1995) survey of 25,000 primary care patients in 14 countries, 48% of the depressed respondents reported moderate to severe occupational role impairment and an average of 7.7 days of work impairment in the past month (Ormel et al. 1994).

Fewer investigations have examined the work impairments associated with other mood disorders, but those that have did observe comparably large decrements in work performance. In the nationally generalizable U.S. National Health Interview Survey (NHIS), those with bipolar disorder were found to be 40% less likely to be gainfully employed (Zwerling et al. 2002). Among primary care samples, patients with bipolar disorder have been observed to be seven times more likely to miss work (Olfson et al. 1997).

Mixed Efficacy of Treatment in Reducing Burdens From Mood Disorders

Substantial evidence shows that various treatment modalities have efficacy in reducing the clinical symptoms of mood disorders. This evidence is not reviewed here because it is covered and critiqued in several other chapters of this text. In addition, growing evidence indicates that existing treatments can reduce other important burdens from mood disorders. Given the size of the economic burdens due to mood disorders, we largely limit our review to the evidence that existing treatments can mitigate these costs. In doing so, we focus on what is known about the effects of treatments for mood disorders on the two largest cost drivers—namely, health care utilization costs and lost work productivity.

Effects of Treatment on Reducing the High Health Care Utilization Costs Associated With Mood Disorders

Mood disorders have been observed to be associated with very large health care costs. For example, investigators have consistently reported high rates of use of general medical services among patients with depression in numerous observational studies (Simon and Katzelnick 1997). Patients with bipolar disorder also have been observed to use more general medical and specialty mental health services and have total health care costs that are 2.5-fold greater than those for sex- and age-matched general medical patients (Simon and Unutzer 1999).

Such findings from nonexperimental studies originally raised hopes that treatments for mood disorders might have the additional benefit of significant "cost offsets," in which the direct costs of treating mood disorders might be completely offset or even outweighed by cost savings from lower use of other general medical services. Such cost offsets, to the extent that they exist, could then serve as powerful policy levers to increase support for expanded treatment of mood disorders.

Unfortunately, economic analyses of recent depression treatment effectiveness trials (reviewed later in this chapter) have consistently shown that although interventions do lead to improvements in clinical and functional outcomes relative to usual care, they also lead to generally higher overall costs (i.e., the interventions fail to be the "dominant" strategy) (Katon et al. 1995, 1996; Katzelnick

et al. 2000; Lave et al. 1998; Schulberg et al. 1996; Von Korff et al. 1998). At most, interventions for depression have led to partial offsets, in which reductions in non-depression general medical use only somewhat offset the greater costs from use of depression treatments among intervention patients. These findings suggest that the large cost offsets anticipated on the basis of earlier observational data may not serve as the economic impetus for increased treatment of mood disorders as was once hoped for.

Effects of Treatment on Reducing Work Impairments Associated With Mood Disorders

Several lines of evidence have been useful for identifying whether treating mood disorders can have an effect on their associated work impairments. First, evidence shows that improvements in clinical symptoms of mood disorders are also associated with improvements in work impairments. Respondents in the cross-sectional NCS (Kessler and Frank 1997) whose depression remitted no longer had significant increases in either sickness absence or work cutback relative to respondents who were never depressed. Longitudinal naturalistic studies (Hays et al. 1995; Ormel et al. 1990, 1991, 1993; Von Korff et al. 1992) also have been conducted to identify whether changes in the severity of work impairment occur synchronously with changes in severity of depression. One of these studies (Von Korff et al. 1992) of high utilizers of general medical health care found that depressed patients who failed to improve retained high levels of work impairment that were unchanged from baseline; in contrast, those with severe depression that improved reduced their impairment days per year from 79 to 51, and those with moderate depressions that improved reduced their impairment days from 62 to 18. Other investigators (Ormel et al. 1990, 1991, 1993) have reported similar patterns of synchronous change between depression symptom severity and work impairment severity in primary care samples.

All of the studies described so far assessed work impairment through patient self-reports, leaving open the possibility of information biases from mood disorders, such as a "pessimism" bias among depressed respondents (Morgado et al. 1991). For this reason, calibration studies documenting good consistency between self-reports and objective ratings of work performance (Kessler et al. 2003a; Revicki et al. 1994) have been important. The few longitudinal naturalistic studies of synchrony of change that have used objective measures of work functioning also have been reassuring. One study merged biweekly objective productivity records on a large sample of insurance claims adjusters over a several-year period with health insurance claims data from the same period. It found that productivity dropped substantially in the half year prior to the onset of treated episodes of depression but that this decline improved over the course of treatment. This study also identified that the indirect costs from lost productivity were substantially greater than the direct costs of treatment, raising the possibility that treating depression might actually be cost-saving.

Results from these time series suggested that treatment of mood disorders improved work outcomes, but the possibility remains that such naturalistic studies were confounded (e.g., difficulty getting along with supervisors could have led to both exacerbations of mood disorders and work impairments). For this reason, researchers also have examined data from treatment trials to investigate the synchrony of change in severity of mood disorders and work impairments. One secondary analysis of six uncontrolled trials (Mintz et al. 1992) found that patients with remitted depression had significantly less serious work impairment than did those not remitting, and improvements were more common with longer durations of treatment. Remission of work impairment lagged behind depression symptom improvement; furthermore, the association between depression symptom severity and serious work impairment was greatest at higher levels of depression severity. Relapse of depression also was associated with a return of serious work impairment. Most (Bergner et al. 1981; Berndt et al. 1998; Finkelstein et al. 1996; Kocsis et al. 1988; Mauskopf et al. 1996; McHorney et al. 1994; Weissman et al. 1978) but not all (Barge-Schaapveld et al. 1995; Friedman et al. 1995) of the other uncontrolled treatment trials have reported similar synchrony between changes in depression severity and work functioning. (Note: the stronger effects for longer treatments and among more severely depressed patients observed earlier [Friedman et al. 1995] could explain the lack of synchrony in trials of shorter duration [Barge-Schaapveld et al. 1995] and in milder depressions [Friedman et al. 1995].)

A final line of evidence is important for ruling out that the improvements in productivity observed in uncontrolled trials are simply a result of placebo effects rather than the treatments themselves. In one reanalysis of placebo-controlled clinical trials conducted among patients with depression (Mintz et al. 1992), all four trials showed a significant benefit of treatment on reducing serious work impairment compared with placebo. Other placebo-controlled clinical trials in patients with major depression (Mynors-Wallis et al. 1995) have reported similar results, as have placebo-controlled trials of early-onset primary dysthymia (Kocsis et al. 1997) and other chronic depressive syndromes (Agosti et al. 1991).

Although Effective Treatments Are Available, Few With Mood Disorders Receive Adequate Care

The data reviewed above suggest that available treatments, if applied correctly, would be efficacious in terms of reducing the burdens from mood disorders, particularly those from lost work productivity. In spite of this, epidemiological data on the use and quality of treatments in real-world settings have consistently shown that very few of those with mood disorders achieve critical milestones on the pathway to receiving adequate care.

One important component of the problem is the failure to seek help in a timely manner. In a recent reanalysis of the NCS, respondents with mood disorders, including depression and dysthymia, typically waited a decade after the onset of their disorders before making any contact with providers (Wang et al. 2003). Patients with bipolar disorder responding to a National Depressive and Manic-Depressive Association survey reported typically waiting 5 years or more after onset before seeking any help (Lish et al. 1994). This survey also identified another important source of delays—namely, the failure of professionals to correctly diagnose mood disorders even after patients present to them (i.e., on average, patients did not receive a diagnosis of bipolar disorder until they had consulted their third professional, and an additional 5 years typically elapsed between initial treatment contacts and receiving bipolar diagnoses) (Lish et al. 1994).

Epidemiological data have consistently shown that the initiation and quality of treatments for mood disorders are lacking as well. The National Institute of Mental Health (NIMH) Clinical Research Branch Collaborative Program on the Psychobiology of Depression Study in the 1980s reported that only a minority of depressed patients received adequately intensive treatment, both while in the community before the study (Keller et al. 1982) and, surprisingly, even after entering the Collaborative Depression Study (Keller et al. 1986). Newer classes of medications with greater tolerability have become widely available in the subsequent decades and may be responsible for a substantial increase in the proportion of individuals with mood disorders who begin pharmacotherapy. One recent investigation found that between 1987 and 1997, this proportion rose from one-third to nearly three-fourths for patients with depression (Olfson et al. 2002).

Despite this increase in the proportion of individuals with mood disorders who initiate treatment, recent studies have found that treatments for mood disorders continue to fail to meet minimal standards for adequacy. In the NCS Replication (NCS-R) conducted between 2001 and 2002, only 21.7% of the respondents with major depression were receiving adequate treatment (Kessler et al. 2003b). This result confirmed other studies conducted in the second half of the 1990s that found that only 17% (Wang et al. 2000) to 30% (Young et al. 2001) of people with depression received depression treatments that met minimal standards of adequacy. Rates of adherence to evidence-based recommendations also have been low in recent studies of treatments for bipolar disorder. One investigation in the United States found that more than one-third of visits to psychiatrists by patients with bipolar disorder did not result in prescriptions for mood stabilizers and that nearly one-fourth resulted in prescriptions for antidepressants without mood stabilizers (Blanco et al. 2002). These findings of widespread poor-quality treatment for mood disorders in the real world are troubling because a growing body of literature (Katon et al. 1995, 1996; Wells et al. 2000) suggests that to be effective, treatments for mood disorders must conform to evidence-based recommendations (American Psychiatric Association 1994, 2000; Depression Guideline Panel 1993) concerning modality, intensity, duration, and follow-up.

Such low figures might be of less concern if inadequate treatments were largely restricted to those with mild or unimpairing mood disorders that do not necessarily require care (Narrow et al. 2002). However, results from several studies argue against this possibility. Even among the subgroup of individuals in the NCS with the most serious occupational and social impairments from their mood disorders, about half received no treatment in the prior year (Kessler et al. 2001a), and only 21.8% received treatment that met minimal standards of adequacy (Wang et al. 2002b). A decade later, in the NCS-R, estimates among those with severe and very severe depressions were similar: only 24.6% and 39.1%, respectively, received minimally adequate care (Kessler et al. 2003b).

Interventions to Enhance the Adequacy of Care Can Reduce Burdens of Mood Disorders

In the last two sections, we show that although randomized, controlled clinical trials do provide evidence that treatments for mood disorders improve burdens from work impairments, they potentially lack external validity in real-world populations and settings. This problem arises because patient samples in randomized, controlled trials are often atypical of the patients seen in the community because of strict exclusion criteria. The highly controlled conditions in randomized, controlled trials are also unrepresentative of the usual regimens and the routine conditions in many practice settings. The result of these two issues is that routine care for mood disorders is likely to be far less effective than the treatments used in randomized, controlled trials. Clearly, improving the burdens imposed by mood disorders will require enhancing the adequacy of care in typical populations and settings.

Major strides toward this goal have been made during the past decade. Mental health services researchers have developed a new generation of treatment "effectiveness" trials that still involve randomizing patients to different trial arms but also retain the naturalistic practice conditions in usual-care settings. The first effectiveness trials conducted focused on depression in primary care settings because most depression treatment takes place in primary care settings (Regier et al. 1993) and because the quality of depression treatment in primary care is often especially poor (Wells et al. 1994, 1996). Coupled with the goal of identifying effective interventions with lasting effects, effectiveness trials have sought to work with existing primary care resources and structures and to create feasible quality improvements that can then be widely disseminated. Investigators at Group Health Cooperative (Katon et al. 1995, 1996) first pioneered the development of a collaborative care model of depression treatment in primary care. Their multifaceted intervention included patient education, collaboration between an on-site psychiatrist and the primary care physician, and surveillance of patient outcomes and medication adherence.

In subsequent effectiveness trials, investigators have tried to enhance the feasibility of interventions by identifying optimal levels of intensity that balance the effectiveness of interventions with the likelihood that successful interventions will find widespread acceptance and uptake. For example, the investigators at Group Health Cooperative (Katon et al. 1999) subsequently developed a stepped collaborative care model, which focused greater resources on patients with persistent depressions. Other investigators (Katzelnick et al. 2000; Simon et al. 2000) have developed less intensive interventions that involve telephone-based treatment coordination from a trained nonphysician. Some investigators (Rost et al. 2000; Wells et al. 2000) have tested primary care quality improvement strategies that can be used in the large majority of managed care settings that fall outside the staff-model health maintenance organizations used in earlier effectiveness trials. More recently, this effectiveness research has been expanded to new populations (e.g., the elderly [Unutzer et al. 2002], racial and ethnic minorities [Miranda et al. 2003], and those with comorbid general medical illnesses [Koike et al. 2002]), to new mental disorders (Katon et al. 2002), and to intervention effects on new outcomes such as employment and work productivity (Schoenbaum et al. 2002; Smith et al. 2002).

These effectiveness trials have fairly consistently shown that interventions to enhance the care of mood disorders led to significantly improved clinical outcomes compared with usual care (Katon et al. 1995, 1996, 1999; Katzelnick et al. 2000; Koike et al. 2002; Miranda et al. 2003; Simon et al. 2000; Unutzer et al. 2002; Wells et al. 2000). However, with regard to the economic burdens from mood disorders, effectiveness trial results have been more mixed. As mentioned earlier, interventions to enhance the care of mood disorders have led to greater health care costs from use of depression treatments, costs that were only partially offset by savings in nondepression health care use (Katon et al. 1995, 1996; Katzelnick et al. 2000; Lave et al. 1998; Schulberg et al. 1996; Von Korff et al. 1998). Results concerning the effects of enhanced depression treatment specifically on work outcomes also have been mixed. One reanalysis (Simon et al. 1998) of data from two effectiveness trials found that interventions tended to improve functional impairments and lost work productivity but that these differences did not reach statistical significance. However, as the investigators pointed out, this outcome may have been partly a result of the relatively short duration of the interventions and follow-up (4–7 months). As mentioned earlier, improvement in occupational functioning may lag behind improvements in mood symptoms, and sustained remissions may be necessary to achieve good occupational outcomes (Mintz et al. 1992). Results from one effectiveness trial (Wells et al. 2000) partially confirmed this possibility. Patients were given enhanced depression care that lasted 6 months and were then followed up for 12 months. The investigators found that among depressed patients initially employed, a significantly greater proportion of the patients receiving enhanced depression care were still working at 12 months compared with those receiving usual care.

Balancing the Reductions in Burdens With the Increased Costs of Enhanced Care for Mood Disorders

As indicated in the previous sections, adequately treating mood disorders could ease the heavy burdens imposed by mood disorders, including the enormous losses in terms of labor outcomes. However, such care also would clearly add to direct treatment costs. Formal decision and economic analytic techniques have been developed to help balance these and determine the net costs compared with

the benefits (Woods and Baker 2002). Data from randomized, controlled clinical trials are most often used to estimate the efficacy and costs of treatments in such analyses, but randomized, controlled clinical trials are often conducted under highly controlled conditions and among atypical patients. Therefore, investigators have sought other sources of data on the costs and effectiveness of regimens used by typical populations in routine practice and under real-world conditions. Some cost-effectiveness analyses have drawn estimates from administrative claims databases, although such analyses are subject to selection bias because of the observational nature of the data sources.

Recent effectiveness trials of interventions to enhance treatment for mood disorders may be the optimal source of estimates for studies that seek to identify the net costs and benefits of treating mood disorders. One analysis (Simon et al. 2001a) that was based on a depression effectiveness trial estimated that each depression-free day added by the intervention had an incremental cost of only $21. Although the interventions used in other depression effectiveness trials have varied in terms of their levels of intensity and costs (Coulehan et al. 1997; Katon et al. 1995, 1996; Katzelnick et al. 2000; Lave et al. 1998; Schoenbaum et al. 2001; Schulberg et al. 1996; Simon et al. 2001b; Von Korff et al. 1998), economic analyses of these interventions generally have found comparable results, with the incremental costs per depression-free day ranging from approximately $10 to $35.

Such results are already encouraging, but it is important to point out that these economic analyses of effectiveness trials did not take into account the important potential benefits of enhanced treatment on lost work productivity. For this reason, one study (Kessler et al. 1999) used data from two nationally representative general population samples of workers to attempt to make a crude lower-bound estimate of the possible workplace cost savings associated with enhanced treatment. Dollar values were assigned to reports of work loss and cutback according to respondents' earnings, and instrumental variable methods were used to estimate the effect of change in depression symptom severity on change in the salary-equivalent dollar value of work impairments. Treatment effect sizes in the range found in effectiveness trials led to average decreases in work loss and work cutback over a year of treatment per treated worker of between $1,100 and $1,800. These potential benefits are substantial in the face of estimated incremental treatment costs per depression-free day, again raising the intriguing possibility that enhanced treatment of mood disorders may actually be cost-saving.

Ongoing Initiatives and Future Research Needs

The ability of society to provide medical treatments for all its citizens and for all their illnesses has unfortunately become increasingly strained as a result of the proliferation of costly therapies for chronic conditions (Burner et al. 1992). Triage rules based on the principles of cost-effectiveness analysis and cost-benefit analysis (Weinstein and Fineberg 1980) have been developed and applied with growing frequency to deal with this problem. Mood disorders are not exempt from such analyses, making it crucial to provide policy-makers, benefits managers, health care purchasers, and other stakeholders with up-to-date and accurate information on the enormous burdens and the cost-effectiveness of treatments for mood disorders.

Two very-large-scale research programs are currently under way that can help document the true burdens from mood disorders and provide decision makers with this critically needed information. In the United States, the NCS (Kessler and Walters 2002) is nearing completion and will include the NCS-R of 10,000 new adult respondents, the NCS-2 re-interviews of respondents to the original NCS a decade earlier, and the NCS-Adolescents (NCS-A), which included 10,000 adolescents. The NCS contains a broad range of measures of role impairment and disability, including assessments designed to capture specific aspects of role impairments (e.g., the WHO Disability Assessment Schedule) as well as global measures (e.g., use of a "willingness to pay" approach). This will allow the NCS program to provide nationally generalizable information on the social costs of mood disorders that is both comprehensive and detailed.

The WHO World Mental Health (WMH) initiative is another ongoing research program that is a direct outgrowth of the WHO Global Burden of Disease study (Kessler and Walters 2002). When complete, it will involve a quarter of a million respondents from more than 24 countries worldwide. Critics of the original Global Burden of Disease study have pointed out that the levels of disability from illnesses were assigned by panels of clinical experts, potentially undermining the persuasive power of Global Burden of Disease findings regarding the preeminent burdens from mood disorders. In response, the WMH initiative surveys directly measure respondents' role impairments and disabilities with the same wide range of specific and global measures as used in the NCS. Importantly, measurement of functioning and disability in the NCS and WMH programs is done across mental and physical disorders, allowing for rigorous comparisons of the burdens of mood disorders with those from other conditions.

Although economic burdens are but one component of the total burdens from mood disorders, their enormous sizes may allow them to serve as particularly effective policy levers for expanding and enhancing the care of mood disorders. For this reason, developing and applying accurate measures of the economic burdens from mood disorders, particularly impairments in work performance, remain high priorities. Toward this end, self-reported measures such as the WHO Health and Work Performance Questionnaire have been developed to directly quantify the magnitude of different types of work impairments. Initial studies have confirmed the validity of the Health and Work Performance Questionnaire compared with objective measures of work performance (Kessler et al. 2003a), the feasibility of implementing Health and Work Performance Questionnaire assessments across occupations and sites (Wang et al. 2002a), and the particularly burdensome nature of mood disorders on work performance relative to other chronic conditions (Wang et al. 2003). The WHO Health and Work Performance Questionnaire also has been included as part of both the NCS and the WMH survey.

The paradox of widespread underuse and poor-quality use of treatments for mood disorders in the face of such enormous burdens needs to be addressed. In part, this will require additional effectiveness and cost-effectiveness research. Several models for enhancing the care of depression in primary care already have been shown to be effective and cost-effective. However, expanding effectiveness research to identify optimal strategies for new mood disorders, settings, populations, and with potentially more cost-efficient interventions is also needed (Miranda and Gonzalez 2002).

Ultimately, however, considerable effort still will be needed to increase the uptake and dissemination of effective interventions for mood disorders once they have been identified. Despite the consistently positive findings in effectiveness trials, there has been widespread reluctance to implement enhanced depression treatment programs in primary care. Several reasons have begun to emerge as potential explanations for this reluctance.

At the physician level, one critically important barrier is that of competing demands, in which the limited time and resources of primary care physicians must be spent attending to not only mental disorders but also multiple general medical illnesses (Klinkman 1997; Williams 1998). At the health care system level, a related barrier is that programs to improve the treatment of mood disorders must compete with other disease specialty quality improvement initiatives, such as the now numerous programs to improve the detection and treatment of arthritis, asthma, diabetes, low back pain, migraine headaches, seasonal allergies, and urge incontinence. Even innovative practices will adopt only a few such programs, and the current chaotic cross-marketing of quality improvement initiatives is likely to dampen interest in all initiatives, including programs for mood disorders. At the level of purchasers, a third barrier to implementation of programs of enhanced treatment for mood disorders has been the failure of the "value-based purchasing" movement to motivate employers to purchase health care from plans that deliver the highest-quality care. In part, this failure derives from the unfortunate reality that common metrics to rate the quality of care (e.g., the Health Plan Employer Data and Information Set [National Committee for Quality Assurance 1997] and the Consumer Assessment of Health Plans Study [Crofton et al. 1999]) fail to inform employers what their return on investment would be if enhanced care programs for mood disorders were purchased.

Overcoming these barriers will likely require multiple strategies operating at different levels of the problem, including interventions that target providers, purchasers, patients, communities, and public policy (Ford et al. 2002; Wells et al. 2002). Several large-scale efforts in these areas are already under way. The new Robert Wood Johnson Foundation initiative on primary care treatment of depression is addressing the lack of widespread adoption of enhanced depression treatment programs in the United States, in part by designing and evaluating innovative incentive programs for primary care physicians to detect and treat depression (Pincus et al. 2003). The Harvard Health Performance Initiative is seeking to address barriers at the purchaser level by creating competitive pressure for high-quality care of mood disorders. Creating this purchaser demand requires making a strong business case that enhanced treatment has a positive effect on the outcomes most relevant to employers, such as sickness absence, job performance, job-related accidents, turnover, and the return on investment. Toward this end, the NIMH-funded Harvard Work Outcomes Research and Cost-Effectiveness Study (WORCS) recently has been launched and will identify the effectiveness of an enhanced depression care intervention in work outcomes among multiple large national employers. Economic analyses of the WORCS trial will subsequently identify the cost-effectiveness and return on investment of enhanced depression care, explicitly from the perspective of employers. The NIMH Working Group on Overcoming Barriers to Reducing the Burden of Affective Disorders was recently charged with outlining critically needed interventions at these and other levels. At the community level, the NIMH Strategic Plan on Mood Disorders includes essential interventions to change public attitudes, reduce social stigma, improve treatment access, and ensure adherence to treatments for mood disorders (Bruce et al. 2002). Furthermore, at the level of public policy, the NIMH Strategic Plan on Mood Disorders also includes important policy that needs to be implemented, including parity legislation and policies affecting managed care, the uninsured, Medicaid, and federal Medicare programs (Scheffler et al. 2002). The success of these and other ongoing efforts is clearly crucial for ultimately reducing the staggering burdens caused by mood disorders.

References

Agosti V, Stewart JW, Quitkin FM: Life satisfaction and psychosocial functioning in chronic depression: effect of acute treatment with antidepressants. J Affect Disord 23:35–41, 1991

American Psychiatric Association: Practice Guideline for the Treatment of Patients With Bipolar Disorder. Washington, DC, American Psychiatric Association, 1994

American Psychiatric Association: Practice Guideline for the Treatment of Patients With Major Depressive Disorder, 2nd Edition. Washington, DC, American Psychiatric Association, 2000

Barge-Schaapveld DQ, Nicolson NA, van der Hoop RG, et al: Changes in daily life experience associated with clinical improvement in depression. J Affect Disord 34:139–154, 1995

Bauer M, Unutzer J, Pincus HA, et al: Bipolar disorder. Ment Health Serv Res 4:225–229, 2002

Bergner M, Bobbitt RA, Carter WB, et al: The Sickness Impact Profile: development and final revisions of a health status measure. Med Care 19:787–805, 1981

Berndt ER, Finkelstein SN, Greenberg PE, et al: Workplace performance effects from chronic depression and its treatment. J Health Econ 17:511–535, 1998

Blanco C, Laje G, Olfson M, et al: Trends in the treatment of bipolar disorder by outpatient psychiatrists. Am J Psychiatry 159:1005–1010, 2002

Broadhead WE, Blazer DG, George LK, et al: Depression, disability days, and days lost from work in a prospective epidemiologic survey. JAMA 264:2524–2528, 1990

Bruce ML, Smith W, Miranda J, et al: Community-based interventions. Ment Health Serv Res 4:205–214, 2002

Burner ST, Waldo DR, McKusick DR: National health expenditures projections through 2030. Health Care Financ Rev 14:1–29, 1992

Calabrese JR, Hirschfeld RM, Reed M, et al: Impact of bipolar disorder on a U.S. community sample. J Clin Psychiatry 64:425–432, 2003

Cassano GB, Perugi G, Maremmani I, et al: Social adjustment in dysthmia, in Dysthymic Disorder. Edited by Burton SW, Akiskal HS. London, Gaskell, 1990, pp 78–85

Coryell W, Scheftner W, Keller M, et al: The enduring psychosocial consequences of mania and depression. Am J Psychiatry 150:720–727, 1993

Coulehan JL, Schulberg HC, Block MR, et al: Treating depressed primary care patients improves their physical, mental, and social functioning. Arch Intern Med 157:1113–1120, 1997

Crofton C, Lubalin JS, Darby C: Consumer Assessment of Health Plans Study (CAHPS): foreword. Med Care 37:MS1–MS9, 1999

Depression Guideline Panel: Clinical Practice Guideline, Number 5. Depression in Primary Care, Vol 2: Treatment of Major Depression (AHCPR Publ No 93-0551). Rockville, MD, Agency for Health Care Policy and Research, 1993

Dion GL, Tohen M, Anthony WA, et al: Symptoms and functioning of patients with bipolar disorder six months after hospitalization. Hosp Community Psychiatry 39:652–657, 1988

Eaton WW, Anthony JC, Mandel W, et al: Occupations and the prevalence of major depressive disorder. J Occup Med 32:1079–1087, 1990

Finkelstein SN, Berndt ER, Greenberg PE, et al: Improvement in subjective work performance after treatment of chronic depression: some preliminary results. Chronic Depression Study Group. Psychopharmacol Bull 32:33–40, 1996

Ford DE, Pincus HA, Unutzer J, et al: Practice-based interventions. Ment Health Serv Res 4:199–204, 2002

Friedman RA, Markowitz JC, Parides M, et al: Acute response of social functioning in dysthymic patients with desipramine. J Affect Disord 34:85–88, 1995

Goodwin FK, Jamison KJ: Manic-Depressive Illness. New York, Oxford University Press, 1990

Greenberg PE, Stiglin LE, Finkelstein SN, et al: The economic burden of depression in 1990. J Clin Psychiatry 54:405–418, 1993

Greenberg PE, Kessler RC, Nells TL, et al: Depression in the workplace: an economic perspective, in Selective Serotonin Reuptake Inhibitors: Advances in Basic Research and Clinical Practice. Edited by Feighner JP, Boyer WF. New York, Wiley, 1996, pp 327–363

Harwood H, Napolitano DM, Christensen PL, et al: Economic Costs to Society of Alcohol and Drug Abuse and Mental Illness, 1980. Report to the Alcohol, Drug Abuse, and Mental Health Administration. Research Triangle Park, NC, Research Triangle Institute, 1984

Hays RD, Wells KB, Sherbourne CD, et al: Functioning and well-being outcomes of patients with depression compared with chronic general medical illnesses. Arch Gen Psychiatry 52:11–19, 1995

Hirschfeld RM, Montgomery SA, Keller MB, et al: Social functioning in depression: a review. J Clin Psychiatry 61:268–275, 2000

Hirschfeld RM, Lewis L, Vornik LA: Perceptions and impact of bipolar disorder: how far have we really come? Results of the National Depressive and Manic-Depressive Association 2000 survey of individuals with bipolar disorder. J Clin Psychiatry 64:161–174, 2003

Jacob M, Frank E, Kupfer DJ, et al: Recurrent depression: an assessment of family burden and family attitudes. J Clin Psychiatry 48:395–400, 1987

Jarvinen D, Rice DP, Kelman S: Cost of Illness Studies: An Annotated Bibliography 1988. Rockville, MD, U.S. Department of Health and Human Services, Public Health Service, Alcohol, Drug Abuse, and Mental Health Administration, 1988

Judd LL, Rapaport MH, Paulus MP, et al: Subsyndromal symptomatic depression: a new mood disorder? J Clin Psychiatry 55 (suppl):18–28, 1994

Judd LL, Paulus MP, Wells KB, et al: Socioeconomic burden of subsyndromal depressive symptoms and major depression in a sample of the general population. Am J Psychiatry 153:1411–1417, 1996

Katon W, Von Korff M, Lin E, et al: Collaborative management to achieve treatment guidelines: impact on depression in primary care. JAMA 273:1026–1031, 1995

Katon W, Robinson P, Von Korff M, et al: A multifaceted intervention to improve treatment of depression in primary care. Arch Gen Psychiatry 53:924–932, 1996

Katon W, Von Korff M, Lin E, et al: Stepped collaborative care for primary care patients with persistent symptoms of depression. Arch Gen Psychiatry 56:1109–1115, 1999

Katon WJ, Roy-Byrne P, Russo J, et al: Cost-effectiveness and cost offset of a collaborative care intervention for primary care patients with panic disorder. Arch Gen Psychiatry 59:1098–1104, 2002

Katzelnick DJ, Simon GE, Pearson SD, et al: Randomized trial of a depression management program in high utilizers of medical care. Arch Fam Med 9:345–351, 2000

Keller MB, Klerman GL, Lavori PW, et al: Treatment received by depressed patients. JAMA 248:1848–1855, 1982

Keller MB, Lavori PW, Klerman GL, et al: Low levels and lack of predictors of somatotherapy and psychotherapy received by depressed patients. Arch Gen Psychiatry 43:458–466, 1986

Kessler RC, Frank RG: The impact of psychiatric disorders on work loss days. Psychol Med 27:861–873, 1997

Kessler RC, Walters EE: The National Comorbidity Survey, in Textbook in Psychiatric Epidemiology. Edited by Tsuang MT, Tohen M. New York, Wiley, 2002, pp 343–362

Kessler RC, McGonagle KA, Zhao S, et al: Lifetime and 12-month prevalence of DSM-III-R psychiatric disorders in the United States: results from the National Comorbidity Survey. Arch Gen Psychiatry 51:8–19, 1994

Kessler RC, Foster CL, Saunders WB, et al: Social consequences of psychiatric disorders, I: educational attainment. Am J Psychiatry 152:1026–1032, 1995

Kessler RC, Barber CB, Birnbaum HG, et al: Depression in the workplace: effects on short-term disability. Health Aff (Millwood) 18:163–171, 1999

Kessler RC, Berglund PA, Bruce ML, et al: The prevalence and correlates of untreated serious mental illness. Health Serv Res 36:987–1007, 2001a

Kessler RC, Greenberg PE, Mickelson KD, et al: The effects of chronic medical conditions on work loss and work cutback. J Occup Environ Med 43:218–225, 2001b

Kessler RC, Barber C, Beck A, et al: The World Health Organization Health and Work Performance Questionnaire. J Occup Environ Med 45:156–174, 2003a

Kessler RC, Berglund P, Demler O, et al: The epidemiology of major depressive disorder: results from the National Comorbidity Survey Replication. JAMA 289:3095–3105, 2003b

Klein DN, Taylor EB, Dickstein S, et al: Primary early onset dysthymia: comparison with primary nonbipolar nonchronic major depression on demographic, clinical, familial, personality, and socioenvironmental characteristics and short-term outcome. J Abnorm Psychol 97:387–398, 1988

Klerman GL, Weissman MM: The course, morbidity and costs of depression. Arch Gen Psychiatry 49:831–834, 1992

Klinkman MS: Competing demands in psychosocial care: a model for the identification and treatment of depressive disorders in primary care. Gen Hosp Psychiatry 19:98–111, 1997

Kocsis JH, Frances AJ, Voss C, et al: Imipramine and social-vocational adjustment in chronic depression. Am J Psychiatry 145:997–999, 1988

Kocsis JH, Zisook S, Davidson J, et al: Double-blind comparison of sertraline, imipramine, and placebo in the treatment of dysthymia: psychosocial outcomes. Am J Psychiatry 154:390–395, 1997

Koike AK, Unutzer J, Wells KB: Improving the care for depression in patients with comorbid medical illness. Am J Psychiatry 159:1738–1745, 2002

Kouzis AC, Eaton WW: Emotional disability days: prevalence and predictors. Am J Public Health 84:1304–1307, 1994

Lave JR, Frank RG, Schulberg HC, et al: Cost-effectiveness of treatments for major depression in primary care practice. Arch Gen Psychiatry 55:645–651, 1998

Leader JB, Klein DK: Social adjustment in dysthymia, double depression and episodic major depression. J Affect Disord 37:91–101, 1996

Lish JD, Dime-Meenan S, Whybrow PC, et al: The National Depressive and Manic-Depressive Association (DMDA) survey of bipolar members. J Affect Disord 31:281–294, 1994

MacQueen GM, Young LT, Joffe RT: A review of psychosocial outcome in patients with bipolar disorder. Acta Psychiatr Scand 103:163–170, 2001

Mauskopf JA, Simeon GP, Miles MA, et al: Functional status in depressed patients: the relationship to disease severity and disease resolution. J Clin Psychiatry 57:588–592, 1996

McGuire T, Wells KB, Bruce ML, et al: Burden of illness. Ment Health Serv Res 4:179–185, 2002

McHorney CA, Ware JE Jr, Lu JF, et al: The MOS 36-item Short-Form Heath Survey (SF-36), III: tests of data quality, scaling assumptions, and reliability across diverse patient groups. Med Care 32:40–66, 1994

Mintz J, Mintz LI, Arruda MJ, et al: Treatments of depression and the functional capacity to work. Arch Gen Psychiatry 49:761–768, 1992 [published erratum appears in 50:241, 1993]

Miranda J, Gonzalez JJ: Research on reducing burden of affective disorders for special populations: introduction and general recommendation. Ment Health Serv Res 4:223–224, 2002

Miranda J, Duan N, Sherbourne C, et al: Improving care for minorities: can quality improvement interventions improve care and outcomes for depressed minorities? Results of a randomized, controlled trial. Health Serv Res 38:613–630, 2003

Morgado A, Smith M, Lecrubier Y, et al: Depressed subjects unwittingly over-report poor social adjustment which they reappraise when recovered. J Nerv Ment Dis 179:614–619, 1991

Mueser KT, Bellack AS, Blanchard JJ: Comorbidity of schizophrenia and substance abuse: implications for treatment. J Consult Clin Psychol 60:845–856, 1992

Murray CJL, Lopez AD: The Global Burden of Disease: A Comprehensive Assessment of Mortality and Disability From Diseases, Injuries and Risk Factors in 1990 and Projected to 2020. Cambridge, MA, Harvard University Press, 1996

Mynors-Wallis LM, Gath DH, Lloyd-Thomas AR, et al: Randomised controlled trial comparing problem solving treatment with amitriptyline and placebo for major depression in primary care. BMJ 310:441–445, 1995

Narrow WE, Rae DS, Robins LN, et al: Revised prevalence estimates of mental disorders in the United States: using a clinical significance criterion to reconcile 2 surveys' estimates. Arch Gen Psychiatry 59:115–123, 2002

National Committee for Quality Assurance: HEDIS 3.0: Narrative—What's in It and Why It Matters. Annapolis Junction, MD, National Committee for Quality Assurance, 1997

Olfson M, Fireman B, Weissman MM, et al: Mental disorders and disability among patients in a primary care group practice. Am J Psychiatry 154:1734–1740, 1997

Olfson M, Marcus SC, Druss B, et al: National trends in the outpatient treatment of depression. JAMA 287:203–209, 2002

Ormel J, Van Den Brink W, Koeter MW, et al: Recognition, management, and outcome of psychological disorders in primary care: a naturalistic follow-up study. Psychol Med 20:909–923, 1990

Ormel J, Koeter MW, Van Den Brink W, et al: Recognition, management, and course of anxiety and depression in general practice. Arch Gen Psychiatry 48:700–706, 1991

Ormel J, Von Korff M, Van Den Brink W, et al: Depression, anxiety, and social disability show synchrony of change in primary care patients. Am J Public Health 83:385–390, 1993

Ormel J, Von Korff N, Ustun TB, et al: Common mental disorders and disability across cultures: results from the WHO Collaborative Study on Psychological Problems in General Health Care. JAMA 272:1741–1748, 1994

Perlick D, Clarkin JF, Sirey J, et al: Burden experienced by caregivers of persons with bipolar affective disorder. Br J Psychiatry 175:56–62, 1999

Pincus HA, Hough L, Houtsinger JK, et al: Emerging models of depression care: multi-level ('6 P') strategies. Int J Methods Psychiatr Res 12:54–63, 2003

Rapaport MH, Judd LL: Minor depressive disorder and subsyndromal depressive symptoms: functional impairment and response to treatment. J Affect Disord 48:227–232, 1998

Regier DA, Narrow WE, Rae DS, et al: The de facto U.S. Mental and Addictive Disorders Service System: Epidemiologic Catchment Area prospective 1-year prevalence rates of disorders and services. Arch Gen Psychiatry 50:85–94, 1993

Revicki DA, Irwin D, Reblando J, et al: The accuracy of self-reported disability days. Med Care 32:401–404, 1994

Rice DP, Kelman S, Miller LS, et al: The Economic Costs of Alcohol and Drug Abuse and Mental Illness: 1985. Rockville, MD, Alcohol, Drug Abuse, and Mental Health Administration, 1990

Rohde P, Lewinsohn P, Seeley J: Are people changed by the experience of having an episode of depression? A further test of the scar hypotheses. J Abnorm Psychol 99:264–271, 1990

Rost K, Nutting PA, Smith J, et al: Designing and implementing a primary care intervention trial to improve the quality and outcome of care for major depression. Gen Hosp Psychiatry 22:66–77, 2000

Sartorius N, Ustun TB: Mental Illness in Primary Care: An International Study. New York, Wiley, 1995

Scheffler R, Durham M, McGuire T, et al: Policy intervention. Ment Health Serv Res 4:215–222, 2002

Schoenbaum M, Unutzer J, Sherbourne C, et al: Cost-effectiveness of practice-initiated quality improvement for depression: results of a randomized controlled trial. JAMA 286:1325–1330, 2001

Schoenbaum M, Unutzer J, McCaffrey D, et al: The effects of primary care depression treatment on patients' clinical status and employment. Health Serv Res 37:1145–1158, 2002

Schulberg HC, Block MR, Madonia MJ, et al: Treating major depression in primary care practice: eight-month clinical outcomes. Arch Gen Psychiatry 53:913–919, 1996

Simon GE: Social and economic burden of mood disorders. Biol Psychiatry 54:208–215, 2003

Simon GE, Katzelnick DJ: Depression, use of medical services and cost-offset effects. J Psychosom Res 42:333–344, 1997

Simon GE, Unutzer J: Health care utilization and costs among patients treated for bipolar disorder in an insured population. Psychiatr Serv 50:1303–1308, 1999

Simon GE, Katon W, Rutter C, et al: Impact of improved depression treatment in primary care on daily functioning and disability. Psychol Med 28:693–701, 1998

Simon GE, Von Korff M, Rutter C, et al: Randomised trial of monitoring, feedback, and management of care by telephone to improve treatment of depression in primary care. BMJ 320:550–554, 2000

Simon GE, Katon WJ, VonKorff M, et al: Cost-effectiveness of a collaborative care program for primary care patients with persistent depression. Am J Psychiatry 158:1638–1644, 2001a

Simon GE, Manning WG, Katzelnick DJ, et al: Cost-effectiveness of systematic depression treatment for high utilizers of general medical care. Arch Gen Psychiatry 58:181–187, 2001b

Smith JL, Rost KM, Nutting PA, et al: Impact of primary care depression intervention on employment and workplace conflict outcomes: is value added? J Ment Health Policy Econ 5:43–49, 2002

Stewart JW, Quitkin FM, McGrath PJ, et al: Social functioning in chronic depression: effect of 6 weeks of antidepressant treatment. Psychiatry Res 25:213–222, 1988

Stewart WF, Ricci JA, Chee E, et al: Cost of lost productive work time among US workers with depression. JAMA 289:3135–3144, 2003

Stoudemire A, Frank R, Hedemark N, et al: The economic burden of depression. Gen Hosp Psychiatry 8:387–394, 1986

Tweed DL: Depression-related impairment: estimating concurrent and lingering effects. Psychol Med 23:373–386, 1993

Unutzer J, Katon W, Callahan CM, et al: Collaborative care management of late-life depression in the primary care setting: a randomized controlled trial. JAMA 288:2836–2845, 2002

Von Korff M, Ormel J, Katon W, et al: Disability and depression among high utilizers of health care: a longitudinal analysis. Arch Gen Psychiatry 49:91–100, 1992

Von Korff M, Katon W, Bush T, et al: Treatment costs, cost offset, and cost-effectiveness of collaborative management of depression. Psychosom Med 60:143–149, 1998

Wang PS, Berglund P, Kessler RC: Recent care of common mental disorders in the United States: prevalence and conformance with evidence-based recommendations. J Gen Intern Med 15:284–292, 2000

Wang PS, Beck AL, McKenas DK, et al: The effects of efforts to increase response rates on a workplace chronic condition screening survey. Med Care 40:752–760, 2002a

Wang PS, Demler O, Kessler RC: Adequacy of treatment for serious mental illness in the United States. Am J Public Health 92:92–98, 2002b

Wang PS, Beck A, Berglund P, et al: Chronic medical conditions and work performance in the HPQ calibration surveys. J Occup Environ Med 45:1303–1311, 2003

Weinstein MC, Fineberg HV: Clinical Decision Analysis. Philadelphia, PA, WB Saunders, 1980

Weissman MM, Prusoff BA, Thompson WD, et al: Social adjustment by self-report in a community sample and in psychiatric outpatients. J Nerv Ment Dis 166:317–326, 1978

Wells KB, Sherbourne CD: Functioning and utility for current health of patients with depression or chronic medical conditions in managed, primary care practices. Arch Gen Psychiatry 56:897–904, 1999

Wells KB, Stewart A, Hays RD, et al: The functioning and well-being of depressed patients: results from the Medical Outcomes Study. JAMA 262:914–919, 1989

Wells KB, Burnam MA, Rogers W, et al: Course of depression for adult outpatients: results from the Medical Outcomes Study. Arch Gen Psychiatry 49:788–794, 1992

Wells KB, Katon W, Rogers B, et al: Use of minor tranquilizers and antidepressant medications by depressed outpatients: results from the Medical Outcomes Study. Am J Psychiatry 151:694–700, 1994

Wells KB, Sturm R, Sherbourne CD, et al: Caring for Depression. Cambridge, MA, Harvard University Press, 1996

Wells KB, Sherbourne C, Schoenbaum M, et al: Impact of disseminating quality improvement programs for depression in managed primary care: a randomized controlled trial. JAMA 283:212–220, 2000

Wells KB, Miranda J, Bauer MS, et al: Overcoming barriers to reducing the burden of affective disorders. Biol Psychiatry 52:655–675, 2002

Williams JBW: Competing demands: does care for depression fit in primary care? J Gen Intern Med 13:137–139, 1998

Woods SW, Baker CB: Cost-effectiveness of the newer generation of antidepressants, in Neuropsychopharmacology: The Fifth Generation of Progress. Edited by Davis K, Charney D, Coyle J, et al. Philadelphia, PA, American College of Neuropsychopharmacology, 2002, pp 1119–1137

Wyatt RJ, Henter I: An economic evaluation of manic-depressive illness—1991. Soc Psychiatry Psychiatr Epidemiol 30:213–219, 1995

Young AS, Klap R, Sherbourne CD, et al: The quality of care for depressive and anxiety disorders in the United States. Arch Gen Psychiatry 58:55–61, 2001

Zeiss AM, Lewinsohn PM: Enduring deficits after remission of depression: a test of the "scar" hypotheses. Behav Res Ther 26:151–158, 1988

Zwerling C, Whitten PS, Sprince NL, et al: Workforce participation by persons with disabilities: the National Health Interview Survey Disability Supplement, 1994 to 1995. J Occup Environ Med 44:358–364, 2002

CHAPTER

Rating Scales for Mood Disorders

MARY AMANDA DEW, PH.D.

GALEN E. SWITZER, PH.D.

LARISSA MYASKOVSKY, PH.D.

ANDREA F. DiMARTINI, M.D.

MARIANNA I. TOVT-KORSHYNSKA, M.D., PH.D.

RATING SCALES FOR mood disorders in adults encompass a broad array of measurement and assessment strategies, including diagnostic interview schedules, clinician or observer evaluations and checklists, and self-report questionnaires. They include scales to assess unipolar depressive conditions, as well as scales for mania and bipolar illness, and they have been used to examine these conditions across the adult life span. Rating scales are tools to aid clinical judgment and decision making and to assist in the systematic examination of research hypotheses about the occurrence, treatment, and prevention of psychopathology. Although the accuracy of clinical decisions and research conclusions depends on more than the assessment tools that are used, it is equally true that clinical and research accuracy can be seriously undermined by failure to use reliable, valid indices of respondents' clinical status.

What may have optimal reliability and validity in one context may be of questionable utility or lack feasibility in another setting. For example, the evaluation of depression in psychiatric inpatients is carried out in very different circumstances and under a different set of time and personnel constraints than the evaluation of depression in, say, a primary care setting or in a community-based sample. The goals of evaluation both within and across these settings and populations are also likely to differ markedly. These goals may include the following:

Preparation of this chapter was supported, in part, by grants MH59229 and MH52247 from the National Institute of Mental Health and a National Institutes of Health Scholarship to Dr. Tovt-Korshynska.

- Screening individuals to identify those requiring a more detailed evaluation
- Determining the differential diagnosis of mood disorders
- Evaluating potential research participants to ensure that only individuals with certain conditions or symptom levels are enrolled in research protocols
- Evaluating the severity of mood-related symptoms
- Monitoring individuals' responses to treatment or intervention efforts

At present, no single rating scale for mood disorders is equally appropriate in all settings and populations *and* capable of providing data equally useful for achieving all evaluation goals. Given the large number of scales that are currently available, then, a central issue is how best to select from among them to achieve one's immediate clinical and research aims.

With this goal in mind, we first provide an overview of the basic properties and defining characteristics of different classes of rating scales for mood disorders. We then summarize the range of rating scales in current use for the assessment of depression, dysthymia, mania, and bipolar illness. Finally, we provide guidelines for the selection of scales to administer in various settings and populations to achieve the user's clinical and/or research goals.

Defining Characteristics of Rating Scales for Mood Disorders

The term *rating scale* refers broadly to measurement instruments in which an observer or evaluator assigns a numerical value, either explicitly or implicitly, to certain judgments or assessments (Rosenthal and Rosnow 1991). In the case of psychiatric phenomena, the observer may be a clinician or health care provider, or the respondent may be reporting on his or her own status. The numerical value assigned to each judgment may be explicitly required to fall along a continuum denoting, for example, the degree of severity with which a symptom or condition is experienced. Alternatively, a nominal judgment may be required; for example, the categorization of a symptom or condition as present or absent. (Such nominal judgments or categorizations can ultimately be assigned quantitative values, e.g., 1=present, 0=absent.)

Figure 5–1 shows a typology of rating scales for mood disorders in adults that reflects this basic distinction in measurement: these scales can be classified as either categorical or dimensional measures. Categorical (or diagnostic) measures yield diagnostic judgments regarding the

presence of one or more mood disorders, including major depression, dysthymia, bipolar I and II disorder, and cyclothymia. Such diagnostic instruments—also called *schedules* or *interviewer-administered examinations*—adhere to current classification systems, or nosologies, such as DSM-IV-TR (American Psychiatric Association 2000) and ICD-10 (World Health Organization 1992). They typically diagnose a range of other disorders in addition to mood disorders.

Dimensional instruments—also called *symptom inventories*, *clinical rating scales*, or *screening scales*, depending on their design—yield information about an individual's relative level of symptomatology or distress. These instruments allow such distress to be placed along a continuum of symptom frequency or severity (e.g., more or less depressed). As shown in Figure 5–1, dimensional scales can be further distinguished by whether they rely on a clinician to rate the individual's symptoms or whether the individual rates his or her own symptoms. Most clinician-rated instruments focus on only one mood condition, such as depression or mania. In comparison, self-report measures include those specific to one component of mood, as well as more global measures that assess multiple areas of distress. The global measures typically include one or more subcomponents that consider distinct elements of mood.

The central distinction between categorical and dimensional measures (regardless of whether the latter are clinician- or self-rated) reflects fundamental differences not only in the major outcome of the assessment (diagnosis vs. severity ratings) but also in the conceptualization of mental illnesses, including mood disorders. Proponents of the diagnostic approach argue that discrete categorization of mental illness is necessary from practical and theoretical standpoints. For example, such decisions are required to determine rates of caseness, or prevalence, of different mental disorders in the population. Prevalence rates, in turn, are essential for objectives such as formulating policy and justifying the funding of mental health services. On an individual patient level, diagnostic information is typically required to determine eligibility for mental health services, insurance, and/or social service assistance. In addition, it has been asserted that a diagnostic typology, founded on consistent decision rules, will produce more precise assessments of mental illness than will dimensional systems (First 2002; Regier et al. 1984). A central argument is that mental illness is more than a matter of degree of severity along a continuous dimension: conditions such as major depression and mania are qualitatively distinct from normal human functioning (Clementz and Iacono 1993; for further discussion, see Klein et al., Chapter 2, in this volume).

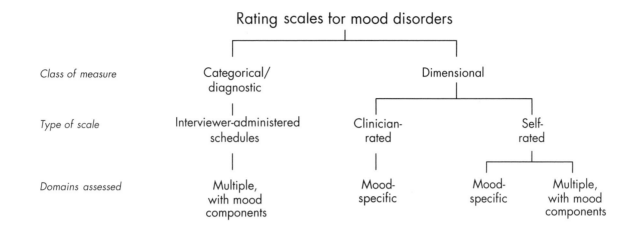

Rating scales for mood disorders

FIGURE 5–1.   Typology of rating scales for mood disorders in adults.

In contrast, proponents of a dimensional approach suggest that the diagnostic perspective relies inappropriately heavily on biomedical models that view individuals as either diseased or not and that view mental illness as reflecting biological and genetic rather than social etiologies (Mirowsky and Ross 1989, 2002; Wheaton 2001; see also Klein et al., Chapter 2, in this volume). Mirowsky and Ross argued that discrete measurement of nondiscrete psychological phenomena is weak from several perspectives. First, it disregards useful information about the degree and characteristics of psychological distress. From a conceptual perspective, depression, for example, is more accurately considered to be on a continuum on which cut points would serve as only artificial boundaries. Second, discrete measurement can confound understanding of symptoms, causes, and consequences of distress. Dimensional approaches, in contrast, are more amenable to testing models of the nature (e.g., prototypical features) of psychopathology and its correlates (Rogers 2001). Finally, diagnostic schedules and a categorical measurement approach yield assessments that are relatively insensitive to changes in psychological status, such as those expected during treatment (Murphy 2002). Many dimensional measures show high sensitivity to change.

Clearly, to select an appropriate rating scale, potential users must become familiar with arguments on both sides of the categorical and dimensional distinction, as well as carefully consider the goals to be achieved with the selected scale. Thus, as noted earlier, in some circumstances, a determination of "caseness" is critical. In other circumstances, monitoring a patient's or research participant's degree of distress is of utmost importance. For example,

during the treatment of depression or bipolar illness, the central issue most likely will be adequate detection of symptom change rather than the repeated reassessment of whether formal diagnostic criteria are met. Hence, not only one's conceptual perspective but also the specific goals of the assessment will ultimately influence the selection of scales for various contexts. We discuss additional issues to consider in the selection of categorical or dimensional rating scales later in this chapter (see section "Selection of Rating Scales for Mood Disorders").

In addition to the broad differences in perspective underlying categorical and dimensional measures, these classes of rating scales also differ in who collects the data, the time needed to collect them, and the data collection format. Dimensional scales encompass measures that require different types of raters, whereas diagnostic schedules all require extensively trained interviewers. (Some computerized versions of diagnostic schedules have been developed to eliminate the need for an interviewer, but none is in widespread use or has well-established psychometric properties.) Because diagnostic schedules were originally designed to replicate traditional clinical examinations (but with greater precision and reliability), trained mental health professionals were required in the earliest of these assessments, and they continue to be required for many schedules in use today. However, other currently available schedules can be conducted by trained lay interviewers without clinical expertise. In contrast, dimensional scales vary greatly in whether the rater must have clinical experience or prior training in administering the measure. In addition, as noted earlier, the rater may be the patient or research participant.

Diagnostic schedules examine the respondent's current status but also may review past months or years (or even the entire lifetime). Dimensional measures focus on the respondent's experiences currently or in the recent past (the last 2–4 weeks, at most). This difference is one of many factors that contribute to the fact that diagnostic schedules take considerably more time to administer than dimensional scales. Interviews with diagnostic schedules may be as short as 45–60 minutes, or as long as several hours, depending on the nature of the respondent's mental health problems. However, if only the components of a diagnostic schedule that pertain to mood disorders are used, and if the interview considers only the present rather than the respondent's past, the interview duration usually can be considerably reduced. In contrast, most clinician-rated dimensional rating scales take 30 minutes or less, and they vary in whether they require an actual interview. Some rely on the clinician's past observations or on collateral information from medical records or family members. Finally, self-report rating scales tend to be the most brief. Some are as brief as 1–2 minutes; the longest mood-specific measures require about 20 minutes. (A few of the multicomponent measures that assess domains in addition to mood are more lengthy.) Of course, the depth of information collected with a 2-minute scale will differ dramatically from that obtained with lengthier measures. This relates, once more, to the need to consider the fundamental goals or purpose of using a particular measure.

The format and sequencing of questions differ in categorical (diagnostic) and dimensional rating scales. Diagnostic schedules follow algorithms that, in general, allow for the determination of symptom presence, duration, and functional impairment required by a given diagnosis. Questions follow a specific order, but not all questions may be asked. For example, if a respondent answers negatively to certain questions, some avenues of additional questioning will be skipped. Diagnostic schedules typically group together all questions pertaining to a specific disorder. Each disorder section, or module, generally begins with a few "stem" questions to ascertain whether the respondent meets basic conditions required by the diagnosis. If the respondent does not meet these conditions, the interviewer skips the remaining items and proceeds to the next module. The wording of all questions is consistently in the direction such that a positive response indicates that a given symptom or condition is present (or has occurred).

In contrast, the format and administration of dimensional measures is usually invariant: all items are asked of all respondents, regardless of their response to any given item. Clinician- or observer-rated dimensional instruments generally order items so that logical groups of similar types of symptoms or experiences (e.g., all somatic symptoms of depression) are inquired about before proceeding to the next symptom type. Self-rated dimensional scales, in contrast, often deliberately mix different types of symptoms, and the wording of items is not always in the direction such that a positive answer would indicate that a symptom was present. Both an at-random ordering of items and the strategy of negative or reverse wording of some items are used to avoid problems of response biases and response styles (as, for example, in the case of the responder who answers affirmatively to every item or to every item within a certain class).

Finally, the scope of diagnostic and dimensional mood disorder scales differs. Most diagnostic instruments assess most or all DSM-IV-TR Axis I and/or equivalent ICD-10 mental disorders. The full range of mood disorders is typically included. In contrast, dimensional instruments are quite varied. As noted earlier, clinician-rated scales usually focus on only a single illness or condition (e.g., unipolar depression). Self-report dimensional instruments include highly focused measures as well as global, multicomponent scales.

Despite the many differences between diagnostic and dimensional rating scales (as well as between clinician- and self-rated dimensional scales), all of these scales collect systematic information that ultimately can be evaluated quantitatively. Although diagnostic schedules are more complex to administer than most dimensional rating scales, our discussion in the following two sections of this chapter will clarify the settings and circumstances in which greater complexity may be warranted compared with situations in which a dimensional approach is optimal.

Overview of Rating Scales for Mood Disorders in Current Use

In this section, we describe the range of rating scales available within each of the categories delineated in Figure 5–1. We first consider categorical, diagnostic measures. Then, within the dimensional class, we discuss clinician-rated measures of depression and mania, followed by self-rated measures. Rather than providing a lengthy narrative on the nature and typical applications of each instrument, we present this information in tabular format. This will allow our commentary to focus on similarities and differences among the many measures.

We included rating scales in our review if they met several criteria. First, they must be in active, current use. For older instruments designed 10–30 years ago, we required that they continue to be used in new research protocols and to be cited frequently in the published literature of the last decade. Relatively new instruments would not yet have had the opportunity to be used in many studies. For these, we required that they appear to be receiving accelerating use since their initial publication. Second, we included only those instruments for which published reliability and validity data exist (although there is wide variability in how much data are available). Third, we included measures that assess one or more mood disorders broadly defined; we did not consider scales designed only to differentiate subtypes of depression (e.g., the Newcastle Scales; Carney et al. 1965) or to assess subcomponents of the experience of depression or mania (e.g., the presence of psychosis in inpatients, as assessed by the Brief Psychiatric Rating Scale; Overall 1988).

Diagnostic Schedules

Table 5–1 describes key characteristics of 10 diagnostic schedules. Most assess a range of disorders; the table lists the specific mood disorder diagnoses that are determined and the diagnostic systems that may be applied. The table notes whether each schedule covers current and/or lifetime disorders. Administration characteristics are summarized, including whether the schedule is semi- or fully structured, its typical duration, and the type of evaluator required. The last column of Table 5–1 provides an approximate rating of how widely used each instrument has been in the last 10 years according to the number of published citations it has received (ISI Web of Science citation indices).

Many of the diagnostic schedules are second- and third-generation versions of measures used in earlier decades. For example, the Composite International Diagnostic Interview (Robins et al. 1988) evolved from earlier versions of the Diagnostic Interview Schedule (Robins et al. 1981) and the Present State Examination (PSE; Wing et al. 1974). The Schedules for Clinical Assessment in Neuropsychiatry (Wing et al. 1990) also evolved (and expanded on) the PSE. The Primary Care Evaluation of Mental Disorders (PRIME-MD; Spitzer et al. 1994) arose from the Structured Clinical Interview for DSM-III-R (Spitzer et al. 1990) and DSM-IV (SCID; First et al. 1997), which itself grew out of the Schedule for Affective Disorders and Schizophrenia (Endicott and Spitzer 1978). Murphy (2002) and Robins (2002) provide detailed accounts of the evolution of current measures.

Except for the Geriatric Mental State Examination (GMSE; Copeland et al. 1988), the diagnostic schedules in Table 5–1 are designed for use across the adult life span. Most assess the full range of mood disorders diagnosed within the DSM-IV-TR or ICD-10 systems, in-

cluding major depressive disorder (MDD), dysthymia, manic episodes, bipolar disorder, and cyclothymia. Several of the briefer measures evaluate only a subset of mood disorders—most commonly, MDD and dysthymia. All yield current diagnoses, and many yield at least some lifetime diagnostic information.

The schedules vary in whether they are semi- or fully structured and hence in the type of evaluator that is required. Semistructured measures allow evaluators more latitude in conducting the assessment, primarily because they can ask their own questions to clarify a respondent's answer to an item. Thus, these measures require clinician-interviewers with the experience to judge when and what type of additional probing is needed. Fully structured measures also permit additional probes, but these probes consist of specific questions that do not allow for any deviation. Under a fully structured approach, then, lay interviewers without clinical expertise can be trained to administer the interview. The time needed to complete the interviews varies markedly. The Diagnostic Interview for Genetic Studies (Nurnberger et al. 1994) may take as much as 3–4 hours of interview time and, for this reason, has been largely limited to use in research settings. The PRIME-MD, the Mini-International Neuropsychiatric Interview (MINI; Sheehan et al. 1998), and the Symptom-Driven Diagnostic System for Primary Care (SDDS-PC; Broadhead et al. 1995) are quite brief, and even though they provide diagnoses, they might be more appropriately considered as screening instruments.

The most frequently used diagnostic schedules are of moderate duration, assess a full range of disorders, and include current and lifetime diagnoses. Less frequently used schedules include those that focus on specific populations (the GMSE for geriatric samples, the PRIME-MD and the SDDS-PC for primary care samples) or that include only a subset of mood disorder diagnoses (e.g., the Clinical Interview Schedule—Revised and the MINI).

We have not included detailed information about the psychometric properties of each diagnostic schedule. Partly because of the cost of administering the diagnostic schedules (in terms of time and personnel), fewer reliability and validity data have been published compared with those available for many dimensional measures. In addition, except for the newest measures, most psychometric studies examined earlier versions of the schedules designed for DSM-III (American Psychiatric Association 1980), DSM-III-R (American Psychiatric Association 1987), or ICD-9 (World Health Organization 1977) rather than the versions in current use. Psychometric work has focused primarily on reliability.

The reliability of an instrument refers to its consistency or stability (Rosenthal and Rosnow 1991). Consis-

TABLE 5–1. Diagnostic schedules assessing mood disorders within currently used diagnostic systems

Instrument	Mood domains assessed	Diagnostic criteria	Time frame	Format	Duration of assessment (min)	Evaluator	Studies using measure[a]
Geriatric Mental State Examination (GMSE; versions A3, B3; Copeland et al. 1988)	MDD, dysthymia, mania	ICD-10, DSM-III-R, DSM-IV, descriptive syndromes	Current, some historical information	Semistructured	20–50	Trained clinician	Some
Diagnostic Interview Schedule (DIS, DIS-IV; Robins et al. 1981, 1996)	All[b]	DSM-III, DSM-III-R, DSM-IV	Current, lifetime	Fully structured	45–90	Trained lay interviewer	Many
Composite International Diagnostic Interview (CIDI, CIDI—University of Michigan version; Kessler et al. 1994; Robins et al. 1988)	All	ICD-10, DSM-IV	Current, lifetime	Fully structured	75–180	Trained lay interviewer	Many
Schedules for Clinical Assessment in Neuropsychiatry (SCAN; Wing et al. 1990)	All	ICD-10, DSM-III-R, DSM-IV, descriptive syndromes	Current, lifetime	Semistructured	90–180	Trained clinician	Many
Clinical Interview Schedule—Revised (CIS-R; Lewis et al. 1992)	Depressive episode	ICD-10, descriptive syndromes	Current	Fully structured	30	Trained lay interviewer	Some
Diagnostic Interview for Genetic Studies (DIGS; Nurnberger et al. 1994)	All	DSM-III, DSM-III-R, DSM-IV	Current, lifetime	Semistructured	60–240	Trained clinician	Some
Primary Care Evaluation of Mental Disorders (PRIME-MD; Spitzer et al. 1994)	MDD, dysthymia	DSM-III-R, DSM-IV	Current	Fully structured	5–10 (patient form) +8–10 (clinician evaluation)	Health professional, minimal training	Many
Symptom-Driven Diagnostic System for Primary Care (SDDS-PC; Broadhead et al. 1995)	MDD	DSM-IV	Current	Fully structured	5 (patient form) +5–10 for each of 7 modules[c]	Health professional, minimal training	Few
Structured Clinical Interview for DSM-IV Axis I Disorders (SCID-I; First et al. 1997)	All	DSM-III-R, DSM-IV	Current, lifetime	Semistructured	45–90	Trained clinician	Many
Mini-International Neuropsychiatric Interview (MINI; Sheehan et al. 1998)	MDD, dysthymia, mania	DSM-III-R, DSM-IV, ICD-10	Current, lifetime (mania only)	Fully structured	15	Health professional, minimal training	Some

Note. MDD=major depressive disorder.

[a]Based on numbers of ISI Web of Science citations 1994–2003; many=450+, some=200–449, few=<200.

[b]All mood diagnoses available within the diagnostic systems used.

[c]Modules are completed on the basis of screen results.

tency can be evaluated across time, across observers or raters, and among items (all of which are purported to measure the same underlying concept). Given the polythetic nature of the diagnostic systems in use today, the latter area of reliability is of limited relevance to the instruments in Table 5–1. Diagnostic schedules have shown generally adequate test-retest reliability, although it is usually considerably higher in clinical than in community samples (Üstün and Tien 1995). Reliability studies for the SCID are representative in this regard: the SCID multisite test-retest studies found that overall reliability for current episodes of disorder was fair to good in patient samples (mean $\kappa=0.61$) but poor in nonpatients (mean $\kappa=0.37$) (J.B. Williams et al. 1992). In patients, test-retest reliability was better for bipolar disorder ($\kappa=0.84$), adequate for MDD ($\kappa=0.64$), and poor for dysthymia ($\kappa=0.40$). Test-retest reliabilities for lifetime diagnoses tend to be somewhat better than for current diagnoses (Nunes et al. 1996; J.B. Williams et al. 1992). A major contributor to reduced test-retest reliability for the SCID and all other diagnostic schedules in Table 5–1 is attenuation, or the tendency of respondents to report fewer symptoms during the second interview compared with the initial evaluation (Robins 1985).

Interrater reliability for the instruments in Table 5–1 has been found to be strong. For example, κ coefficients for the SCID ranged from moderate ($\kappa>0.75$) to very high ($\kappa>0.85$) across nine investigations (Rogers 2001). The high interrater reliability is most likely because diagnostic instruments have a structured format. However, it also may be inflated by the method of data collection. Most often, either two evaluators observe and rate the same videotaped interview or one evaluator conducts the interview while the second one observes it. Under both approaches, the evaluators' ratings are not truly independent.

In contrast to reliability, evidence for diagnostic instruments' validity is weaker. An instrument's validity concerns the extent to which the instrument measures what it is intended to measure (Rosenthal and Rosnow 1991). Of the various types of validity, criterion, convergent, and discriminant validity are particularly pertinent for diagnostic schedules. Criterion validity implies an independent "gold standard" with which to compare the results of a diagnostic schedule. One criterion used for this purpose is the diagnosis reached after a traditional clinical interview. Use of this standard suggests poor criterion validity for today's diagnostic schedules (Rogers 2001). Yet because structured diagnostic schedules were designed to improve on the weaknesses of unstructured, traditional interviews, validating instruments against these approaches is increasingly seen as inappropriate (Murphy

2002). Alternatives have been proposed (e.g., Spitzer's 1983 "LEAD" standard [Longitudinal data collection with Expert consensus based on All Data available]), but they have not often been implemented and—when used—have not yielded evidence of strong validity for today's diagnostic schedules.

The schedules fare better with respect to convergent and discriminant validity. These types of validity pertain, respectively, to whether a measure correlates strongly with measures designed to assess similar concepts and does not correlate strongly with measures of conceptually unrelated concepts. Evaluation of these validities has included direct comparisons between diagnostic schedules and comparisons to dimensional scales. Good convergent validity, for example, would be suggested by 1) similarity in resulting diagnoses across schedules and/or 2) strong correlations with dimensional measures of similar areas of symptomatology. The instruments in Table 5–1 appear reasonably strong with respect to convergent and discriminant validities, particularly for mood disorders (Rogers 2001; Üstün and Tien 1995).

Dimensional Instruments

There are many more dimensional scales than diagnostic schedules for mood disorders. Consistent with the typology in Figure 5–1, we consider clinician-rated (or observer-rated) scales for depression and mania separately from self-report scales. For each, we provide two summary tables (Tables 5–2 through 5–5) of all mood-specific measures that met our inclusion criteria. The first summary tables (Table 5–2 and 5–4) show key descriptive characteristics of each scale (e.g., its scope, rating format, and administration time), and we report how widely each has been used during the past 10 years. Finally, we include global ratings of each scale's reliability and validity. We assigned these ratings on the basis of the approach used by McDowell and Newell (1996) in their review of health-related rating scales. Two ratings—thoroughness of the psychometric testing and strength of results—for reliability and for validity are provided. Thoroughness of testing can be independent of the strength of the findings for an instrument's reliability and/or validity.

The second summary tables provided for both clinician- and self-rated scales (Tables 5–3 and 5–5) specific to mood disorders show specific reliability and validity coefficients obtained for each scale across studies evaluating it. This table lists the upper and lower bounds of three types of reliability and three types of validity coefficients, as well as whether the scale has been found to be responsive to change. Although these data contributed to our own global ratings of reliability and validity for each scale,

TABLE 5–2. Dimensional rating scales: clinician- or observer-rated measures of mood disorder symptomatology

Instrument	Scope	No. of items[a]	Item response format and time frame	Administration time and context	Evaluator	Major uses of scale	Studies using measure[b]	Reliability: thoroughness/results[c]	Validity: thoroughness/results[c]
Depression and dysthymia									
Hamilton Rating Scale for Depression (Ham-D; Hamilton 1960, 1967)[d]	Depressive symptoms	17, 21, 24	2 items: 0=absent, 2=clearly present Remainder: 0=absent, 4=most severe Past several days or week	20–30 min, based on interview plus any data from collateral sources	Clinician	Evaluate severity; monitor treatment response	Many	+++/+++	+++/++
Raskin Depression Rating Scale (Three-Area Severity of Depression Scale; Raskin et al. 1969)	Depressive symptoms (in persons screened for depression)	3	1=absent, 5=severe Present time	10–15 min, based on interview, nurse report, any collateral data	Clinician	Evaluate severity; monitor treatment response	Few	+/+	+/?
Zung Depression Status Inventory (Zung DSI; Zung 1972)	Depressive symptoms	20	1=none, 4=severe Present time	10 min, based on interview and clinical observation	Clinician	Evaluate severity	Few	+/+	+/+
Montgomery-Åsberg Depression Rating Scale (MADRS; Montgomery and Åsberg 1979)	Depressive symptoms	10	0=absent, 6=severe Any time frame; rater notes time frame considered	10–15 min, based on interview and observation of patient	Clinician or trained health professional	Evaluate severity; monitor treatment response	Many	++/++	++/+++
Bech-Rafaelsen Melancholia Scale (Bech and Rafaelsen 1980)	Depressive symptoms	11	0=absent, 4=most severe Last 3 days	10–15 min, based on interview	Clinician	Evaluate severity; monitor treatment response	Few	++/++	+/+
Clinical Interview for Depression (Paykel 1985)	Depressive symptoms	36	35 items: 1=absent, 7=extremely severe 1 item: 1=absent, 4=severe Past week	30–45 min, based on interview	Clinician or trained health professional	Evaluate severity; monitor treatment response	Few	+/+	+/+
Inventory of Depressive Symptomatology—Clinician Administered (IDS-C; Rush et al. 1986, 1996)[e]	Depressive signs and symptoms	28, 30	0=absent, 3=severe Past week	30–45 min, based on interview	Clinician	Evaluate severity; monitor treatment response	Some	+/++	+/++

TABLE 5–2. Dimensional rating scales: clinician- or observer-rated measures of mood disorder symptomatology (*continued*)

Instrument	Scope	No. of items[a]	Item response format and time frame	Administration time and context	Evaluator	Major uses of scale	Studies using measure[b]	Reliability: thoroughness/results[c]	Validity: thoroughness/results[c]
Cornell Dysthymia Rating Scale (Mason et al. 1993)	Chronic, mild depressive symptoms	20, 27	0=not at all, 4=severe Last 2 weeks (or since last rating)	20 min, based on interview plus any data from collateral sources	Clinician	Evaluate severity; monitor treatment response	Few	+/+	+/+
Mania									
Manic-State Rating Scale (MSRS; Beigel et al. 1971)	Manic symptoms	26	Each item rated twice: Frequency: 0=none, 5=all the time Intensity: 1=very minimal, 5=very marked During last nursing shift	15 min, based on interview and observation	Clinician or trained nursing staff	Evaluate severity; monitor treatment response	Some	++/++	++/+
Rating of Mania (Petterson et al. 1973)	Manic behaviors	9	0=absent, 5=extreme During interview	30 min, based on interview	Clinician	Evaluate severity; monitor treatment response	Few	++/+	++/+
Modified Manic State Rating Scale (MMSRS; Blackburn et al. 1977)	Manic symptoms	28	0=absent, 5=continuous and gross During interview	Duration not noted; based on interview	Clinician	Evaluate severity; monitor treatment response	Few	+/+	+/+
Young Mania Rating Scale (YMRS; Young et al. 1978)	Manic symptoms	11	7 items: 0=absent, 4=extreme 4 items: 0=absent, 8=extreme Last 48 hours	15–30 min, based on interview	Clinician	Evaluate severity; monitor treatment response	Many	++/+	++/++
Bech-Rafaelsen Mania Scale (Bech et al. 1978)	Manic symptoms	11	0=normal, 4=severe/extreme Past several days or week	15–30 min, based on interview	Clinician	Evaluate severity; monitor treatment response	Some	++/++	+/+

TABLE 5–2. Dimensional rating scales: clinician- or observer-rated measures of mood disorder symptomatology *(continued)*

Instrument	Scope	No. of items[a]	Item response format and time frame	Administration time and context	Evaluator	Major uses of scale	Studies using measure[b]	Reliability: thoroughness/ results[c]	Validity: thoroughness/ results[c]
Mania Diagnostic and Severity Scale (MADS; Secunda et al. 1985)	Manic symptoms	23[f]	Mixed format During episode	Total duration not noted; based on interviews and observations	Clinician (11 items); nursing staff (12 items)	Evaluate severity; monitor treatment response	Some	+/+	+/+
Clinician-Administered Rating Scale for Mania (CARS-M; Altman et al. 1994)	Manic symptoms	15	14 items: 0=absent, 5=extreme; 1 item: 0=absent, 4=extreme Past week	Duration not noted; based on interview and any collateral data	Clinician	Evaluate severity; monitor treatment response	Some	+/+	+/+
Bipolar spectrum									
Clinical Global Impression Scale for Use in Bipolar Illness (CGI-BP; Spearing et al. 1997)	Bipolar spectrum symptoms	3	Severity (1 item); 1=normal, 7=very ill; Change (2 items); 1=very much improved, 7=very much worse During current episode	Duration not noted; based on constructing recent life chart for patient	Clinician	Evaluate severity; monitor treatment response	Some	+/+	0/0
Structured Clinical Interview for Mood Spectrum (SCI-MOODS; Fagiolini et al. 1999)	Bipolar spectrum symptoms	140	Symptom occurred vs. did not occur Lifetime	Duration not noted; based on interview	Clinician	Evaluate lifetime occurrence	Few	+/++	+/+

[a]For scales with multiple versions, the number of items in each is noted.

[b]Based on numbers of ISI Web of Science citations 1994–2003: for depression scales, many=450+, some=100–449, few=<100, for mania and bipolar spectrum scales, many=100+, some=30–99, few=<30.

[c]For thoroughness of psychometric testing, 0=no reported evidence of reliability or validity; +=very basic information only; ++=several types of test or several studies have reported reliability and validity; +++=all major forms of reliability/validity testing have been reported. For strength of results, 0=no numerical results reported; ?=results uninterpretable; +=weak reliability/validity; ++=adequate reliability/validity; +++=excellent reliability/validity.

[d]Numerous scales have been developed that are modifications of the Ham-D (see Williams 2001). We have not included additional versions unless they represent substantial revisions of the original scale (e.g., the Bech-Rafaelsen Melancholia Scale). A self-rated version, the Carroll Rating Scale for Depression, is described in Table 5–4.

[e]There is also a self-report version; it is included in Table 5–4.

[f]This measure is composed of three separately administered scales.

our ratings took into account not merely the range of co-efficients obtained but also the central tendency or average coefficients usually achieved. Finally, we provide an additional table summarizing information for several prominent self-report psychiatric symptom scales that, although not specific to mood disorders, include subscales for depression and/or mania. (Because much of these scales' psychometric data do not pertain specifically to mood disorders, we do not separately list data for specific types of psychometric evaluations.)

Clinician-Rated Scales

Seventeen measures are in active, current use to assess mood disorder symptoms, including 8 depression scales, 7 mania scales, and 2 scales of bipolar spectrum symptoms (see Tables 5–2 and 5–3). All were originally designed for patient samples (usually in inpatient settings). Most are now used routinely in outpatient settings. Except for the two bipolar scales, the measures focus on symptoms specific to a single pole of the mood disorder spectrum. They vary considerably in total number of items; most have 10–20 items. Items are generally rated in terms of severity on 4- to 6-point scales and cover a time frame of the past few days or week. The exception to this is the Structured Clinical Interview for Mood Spectrum (SCI-MOODS; Fagiolini et al. 1999), which evaluates the lifetime presence of bipolar spectrum symptoms.

The scales themselves generally take 30 minutes or less for the rater to complete, although additional time is implicit in the need either to conduct interviews, to observe the patient, or to collect collateral data. This additional time may be significant. For example, although the Clinical Global Impression Scale for Use in Bipolar Illness (Spearing et al. 1997) has only three items, the rater must first construct a recent life chart of the patient's symptom course. Although most of the scales require a trained mental health professional, two depression scales (the Montgomery-Åsberg Depression Rating Scale [MADRS; Montgomery and Åsberg 1979] and the Clinical Interview for Depression; Paykel 1985) and two mania scales (the Manic-State Rating Scale [MSRS; Beigel et al. 1971] and the Mania Diagnostic and Severity Scale [MADS; Secunda et al. 1985]) allow other health professionals to serve as raters on all or part of the scale. Unlike the diagnostic schedules, no observer-rated scales for mood disorders use lay assessors because the range of information needed to complete the ratings requires clinical expertise for integration.

With the exception of the SCI-MOODS, which evaluates symptom occurrence, all of the clinician-rated scales yield a total score indicating the overall severity of the mood condition. Most also have been used to monitor response to treatment in clinical trials. By far, the most frequently used depression scale for both purposes is the Hamilton Rating Scale for Depression (Ham-D; Hamilton 1960), although the MADRS also has been extensively used. It is noteworthy that all of the depression scales were developed 20–45 years ago. With the exception of the Inventory of Depressive Symptomatology (Rush et al. 1986, 1996), none have been substantially revised since their initial development, despite changes in both DSM and ICD descriptions of mood disorders and their diagnostic criteria. We discuss this issue from the perspective of scale selection later in the chapter (see section "Selection of Rating Scales for Mood Disorders"). Mania and bipolar spectrum scales show a more recent history of development. Among them, by far the most frequently used is the Young Mania Rating Scale (YMRS; Young et al. 1978), probably in part because it was designed to be easily administered in conjunction with the Ham-D.

Table 5–2 shows marked differences among the scales in our ratings of the thoroughness and strength of their reliability and validity evaluations. Among the depression scales, only the Ham-D and the MADRS have been thoroughly evaluated *and* show relatively strong psychometric properties. The MADRS, in particular, has been found to be very responsive to change, although the Ham-D is strong in this regard as well. The remainder of the clinician-rated scales are considerably weaker in both the extent and the results of psychometric evaluation. For mania and bipolar scales, these weaknesses may reflect the fact that these scales are newer. Yet it is striking that some of the oldest depression and mania scales (that, by virtue of their inclusion in this review, remain in active use) have weak and/or poorly documented psychometric properties (e.g., the Raskin Depression Rating Scale [Raskin et al. 1969], the Zung Depression Status Inventory [Zung 1972], the Modified MSRS [Blackburn et al. 1977], the MADS [Secunda et al. 1985]).

Table 5–3 allows for easy identification of the areas in which reliability and validity of specific scales are stronger or weaker. Interrater reliability is essential for clinician-rated scales, and all of the scales have been examined and found to be generally satisfactory in this regard. However, only about half have received internal consistency reliability testing, and fewer than one-third have undergone test-retest reliability studies.

With respect to validity, the depression scales have been more thoroughly evaluated in criterion and convergent validity than in discriminant validity. The scales have shown good evidence of validity in these areas. When discriminant validity has been examined, the depression

TABLE 5–3. Reliability and validity data on clinician-rated scales of mood disorder symptomatology

Instrument	Reliability			Criterion	Validity		Responsive to change
	Interrater	Internal consistency	Test-retest[a]		Convergent	Discriminant	
Hamilton Rating Scale for Depression	0.46–0.95 (items) 0.78–0.96 (total score)	0.48–0.95	0.70–0.72	With clinical ratings, r=0.84–0.90 Distinguished severity[b]	0.50–0.90	0.45	Yes
Raskin Depression Rating Scale	0.34–0.74 (items) 0.88 (total score)	—	—	—	—	—	Yes
Zung Depression Status Inventory	0.91 (items)	0.81	—	Distinguished diagnosis[c]	—	—	—
Montgomery-Åsberg Depression Rating Scale	0.57–0.76 (items) 0.65–0.97 (total score)	0.86	—	With clinical ratings, r=0.70–0.89 Distinguished severity	0.22–0.94	0.37–0.42	Yes
Bech-Rafaelsen Melancholia Scale	0.75–0.93 (total score)	—	0.98	With clinical ratings, r=0.35–0.77	0.69–0.97	0.42	Yes
Inventory of Depressive Symptomatology	0.96 (items)	0.67–0.94	—	Distinguished severity	0.83–0.95	—	Yes
Cornell Dysthymia Rating Scale	0.92 (items)	0.72–0.90	—	With clinical ratings, r=0.42–0.65	0.26–0.90	0.22–0.44	Yes
Clinical Interview for Depression	0.81–0.82 (items)	—	—	—	0.53–0.73	—	Yes
Manic-State Rating Scale	0.60–0.97 (items)	—	—	0.58 (days hospitalized) Distinguished severity	0.25–0.99	—	Yes
Rating of Mania	0.48–1.00 (items) 0.68–0.88 (total score)	—	—	0.50 (days hospitalized)	0.65–0.89	—	Yes
Modified Manic-State Rating Scale	0.37–0.47 (items) 0.79–0.81 (total score)	—	—	With clinical ratings, r=0.65–0.80	0.65–0.80	—	—
Young Mania Rating Scale	0.36–0.95 (items) 0.84–0.93 (total score)	0.80	—	With clinical ratings, r=0.82 Distinguished severity	0.71–0.88	—	Yes
Bech-Rafaelsen Mania Scale	0.80–0.95 (items) 0.97–0.99 (total score)	0.93	—	—	—	—	Yes

TABLE 5–3. Reliability and validity data on clinician-rated scales of mood disorder symptomatology (*continued*)

Instrument	Reliability			Validity			
	Interrater	Internal consistency	Test-retest[a]	Criterion	Convergent	Discriminant	Responsive to change
Mania Diagnostic and Severity Scale	0.85–0.91 (items)	—	—	Distinguished diagnosis	—	—	Yes
Clinician-Administered Rating Scale for Mania	0.66–0.94 (items) 0.93 (total score)	0.88, 0.63 (mania and psychotic scales)	0.78, 0.95 (mania and psychotic scales)	Distinguished diagnosis	0.94	—	Yes
Clinical Global Impression Scale for Use in Bipolar Illness	0.64–0.91 (items)	—	—	—	—	—	—
Structured Clinical Interview for Mood Spectrum	0.86–0.96 (domains)	0.79–0.92	0.93–0.94	Mania items distinguished diagnosis	—	—	—

[a]Generally days or weeks apart.
[b]Distinguished severity=discriminated between patient groups with different severities of depression.
[c]Distinguished diagnosis=discriminated between patient groups with different psychiatric diagnoses.

TABLE 5–4. Self-rated scales of mood disorder symptomatology

Instrument	Scope and population[a]	No. of items[b]	Item response and time frame	Administration time	Clinical cut point and score range	Major uses of scale	Studies using measure[c]	Reliability: thoroughness/results[d]	Validity: thoroughness/results[d]
Depression									
Beck Depression Inventory (BDI; Beck et al. 1961); First revision (BDI-IA; Beck et al. 1986); Second revision (BDI-II; Beck and Steer 1993); BDI-Primary Care (PC; Beck et al. 1997)	Depressive symptom severity	7 (PC), 13, 21	0=least severe/absent, 3=most severe BDI-I: past week BDI-II: past 2 weeks	2 min (PC) 10–15 min (longer versions)	7-item: 4+ range=0–21 13-item: 5+ range=0–39 21 item: 10+ range=0–63	Screen; evaluate severity; monitor treatment response	Many	+++/+++	+++/+++
Zung Self-Rating Depression Scale (Zung SDS; Zung 1965, 1974)	Depressive symptom severity	20	1=a little of the time, 4=most of the time (alternative wordings for lower anchor of scale: 1=none of the time, 1=none or a little of the time, 0=none of the time) Present	5–10 min	50+ range=25–100 (sum/80×100)	Screen; evaluate severity	Many	++/++	+++/++
Center for Epidemiologic Studies Depression Scale (CES-D) and short forms (Kohout et al. 1993; Radloff 1977)	Depressive symptom severity	10, 11, 20	0=rarely/none of the time, 3=most or all of the time Past week	5–10 min	20-item: 16+ range=0–60 10-item: 4+ range=0–30	Screen; evaluate severity	Many	++/++	+++/++
Carroll Rating Scale for Depression (CDS; Carroll 1998; Carroll et al. 1981)	Depressive symptom severity	5, 12, 52, 61	0=absent, 1=present Past few days	2 min (screen) 20 min (longer versions)	12-item: 6+ range=0–12	Screen; evaluate severity; monitor treatment response	Some	++/++	++/++
Depression Adjective Check Lists (DACL; Lubin 1965); State-Trait DACL (Lubin 1994)	Dysphoria, psychological distress	32, 34	0=absent, 1=present State: today Trait: today and generally	5 min	None	Evaluate severity	Few	+++/++	++/++

TABLE 5–4. Self-rated scales of mood disorder symptomatology (continued)

Instrument	Scope and population[a]	No. of items[b]	Item response and time frame	Administration time	Clinical cut point and score range	Major uses of scale	Studies using measure[c]	Reliability: thoroughness/results[d]	Validity: thoroughness/results[d]
Geriatric Depression Scale (GDS; Yesavage and Brink 1983) and short form (GDS-15; Sheikh and Yesavage 1986)	Depressive symptom presence (adults age 65 or older)	15, 30	0=absent, 1=present Past week	15-item: 5–7 min 30-item: 10–15 min	15-item: 3+, 4+ range=0–15 30-item: 11+ range=0–30	Screen; evaluate severity	Many	+++/+++	++/++
Inventory of Depressive Symptomatology—Self-Report (IDS-SR; Rush et al. 1986, 1996)	Depressive symptom severity (in- and outpatients)	28, 30	0=absent, 3=severe Past week	20–25 min	18+ range=0–90 (30-item version)	Screen; evaluate severity; monitor treatment response	Some	+/++	++/++
Inventory to Diagnose Depression (IDD; Zimmerman et al. 1986)	Depressive symptom severity and duration	22	0=no disturbance, 4=severe Past week, plus duration of endorsed symptoms	10–15 min	Uses algorithm based on DSM-III-R	Screen; evaluate severity	Some	+/+	+/+
Edinburgh Postnatal Depression Scale (Cox et al. 1987)	Depressive symptom severity (postpartum women)	10	0=absent, 3=severe, most of time Past week	5 min	13+ range=0–30	Screen; evaluate severity; monitor treatment response	Many	+/+	++/++
MOS Depression Screener (Burnam et al. 1988)	Depressive and dysthymic symptom severity	8	6 items: 0=rarely, 3=most or all days 2 items: 0=no, 1=yes Past week	2–5 min	0.06 (logistic regression) range=0–1 (regression)	Screen	Some	0/0	+/+
Depression Scale (DEPS; Salokangas et al. 1995)	Depressive symptom severity	10	0=not at all, 3=extremely Last month	5 min	9+ range=0–30	Screen; evaluate severity	Few	+/+	+/+

TABLE 5–4. Self-rated scales of mood disorder symptomatology (continued)

Instrument	Scope and population[a]	No. of items[b]	Item response and time frame	Administration time	Clinical cut point and score range	Major uses of scale	Studies using measure[c]	Reliability: thoroughness/results[d]	Validity: thoroughness/results[d]
Patient Health Questionnaire—Depression Scale (PHQ-9; Kroenke et al. 2001)	Depressive symptom severity	9	0=not at all, 3=nearly every day; Past 2 weeks	2–5 min	10+ range=0–27	Screen; evaluate severity; monitor treatment response	Few	++/++	++/+
Depression—Arkansas Scale (D-ARK; Smith et al. 2002)	Depressive symptom severity	11	1=not at all, 4=nearly every day; Last month	5–10 min	None	Evaluate severity	Few	+/+	++/++
PHQ Two-Item Screener (PHQ-2; Kroenke et al. 2003)	Presence of depressive symptoms	2	0=not at all, 3=every day; Past 2 weeks	<1 min	3+ range=0–6	Screen	Few	0/0	+/+
Mania									
Self-Rating Manic Inventory (SRMI; Shugar et al. 1992)	Manic symptom severity	48	0=false, 1=true; Any time frame (user may specify)	Not noted	18+ range=0–48	Screen; evaluate severity; monitor treatment response	Few	++/++	+/+
Altman Self-Rating Mania Scale (Altman et al. 1997)	Manic symptom severity	13	0=absent, 4=extreme; Last week	5 min	4-item mania subscale: 6+ range=0–24	Screen; evaluate severity	Few	+/+	+/+
Bipolar spectrum									
Internal State Scale (ISS; Bauer et al. 1991)	Bipolar spectrum symptom severity	17	Visual Analog Scale, 0=low severity/frequency, 100=high severity/frequency; Last 24 hours	10–15 min	None	Screen; evaluate severity; monitor treatment response	Some	+/++	+/+

TABLE 5–4. Self-rated scales of mood disorder symptomatology (continued)

Instrument	Scope and population[a]	No. of items[b]	Item response and time frame	Adminis-tration time	Clinical cut point and score range	Major uses of scale	Studies using measure[c]	Reliability: thorough-ness/results[d]	Validity: thorough-ness/ results[d]
Mood Disorder Questionnaire (MDQ; Hirschfeld et al. 2000)	Bipolar spectrum symptom presence	15	13 items: 0=absent, 1=present 1 item: yes/no for lifetime symptom co-occurrence 1 item: 4-point scale from no problem to serious functional impairment Lifetime	5 min	13 items: 7+ (range=0–13) *and* "yes" for co-occurrence and moderate or serious functional impairment	Screen	Few	+/+	+/+
MOODS-SR (Dell'Osso et al. 2002)	Bipolar spectrum symptom severity	140	Symptom occurred vs. did not occur Lifetime	Not noted	None	Evaluate lifetime occurrence	Few	+/+	+/+

[a]Unless otherwise noted, the population appropriate for each scale consists of all adults.

[b]For scales with multiple versions, the number of items in each is noted.

[c]Based on numbers of ISI Web of Science citations 1994–2003: for depression scales, many=450+, some=100–449, few=<100; for mania and bipolar spectrum scales, many=100+, some=30–99, few=<30.

[d]For thoroughness of psychometric testing, 0=no reported evidence of reliability or validity; +=very basic information only; ++=several types of test or several studies have reported reliability/validity; +++=all major forms of reliability/validity testing have been reported. For strength of results, 0=no numerical results reported; ?=results uninterpretable; +=weak reliability/validity; ++=adequate reliability/validity; +++=excellent reliability/validity.

TABLE 5–5. Reliability and validity data for self-rated scales of mood disorder symptomatology

Instrument	Reliability		Validity				Responsive to change
	Internal consistency	Test-retest[a]	Criterion		Convergent	Discriminant	
			Sensitivity, Specificity[b]	Other			
Beck Depression Inventory (BDI)	0.73–0.95 (full version) 0.78–0.86 (short form) 0.85–0.88 (BDI-PC)	0.48–0.86	Full version: cut point of 10+ sensitivity: 85%–93% specificity: 40%–97% Short form: cut point of 5+ sensitivity: 92%–98% specificity: 61%–65% BDI-PC: cut point of 4+ sensitivity: 91%–97% specificity: 91%–99%	With clinical ratings, $r=0.20$–0.96 For short form with clinical ratings, $r=0.55$–0.67 Distinguished severity[c] Distinguished diagnosis[d]	0.40–0.89	0.14	Yes
Zung Self-Rating Depression Scale	0.59–0.95	0.61	Cut point of 50+ sensitivity: 31%–97% specificity: 55%–95%	With clinical ratings, $r=0.20$–0.95 Distinguished severity Did not distinguish diagnosis	0.54–0.86	0.74	No
Center for Epidemiologic Studies Depression Scale	0.76–0.91 (full version) 0.80–.92 (short form)	0.32–0.70 0.83 (short form)	Full version: cut point of 16+ sensitivity: 60%–99% specificity: 53%–100% Short form: cut point of 4+ sensitivity: 97%–100% specificity: 84%–92%	With clinical ratings, $r=0.28$–0.85 Distinguished diagnosis	0.51–0.82	0.61–0.72	Yes
Carroll Rating Scale for Depression	0.95 (61-item) 0.90 (12-item)	0.97 (revision)	Brief version: cut point of 6+ sensitivity: 73%–100% specificity: 79%–93%	With clinical ratings, $r=0.57$–0.84 Distinguished severity	0.66–0.86	0.26	Yes
Depression Adjective Check Lists	0.82–0.94 (state) 0.79–0.91 (trait)	0.19–0.59 (state) 0.44–0.84 (trait)	—	With clinical ratings, $r=0.71$–0.72 Distinguished severity	0.27–0.77	—	Yes
Geriatric Depression Scale	0.80–0.99	0.85–0.98	Cut point of 11+ sensitivity: 75%–100% specificity: 64%–95% Short form, cut point of 3+ sensitivity: 67%–100% specificity: 72%–73%	With clinical ratings, $r=0.62$–0.83 Distinguished severity	0.85–0.88	—	—

TABLE 5–5. Reliability and validity data for self-rated scales of mood disorder symptomatology *(continued)*

| Instrument | Reliability | | Validity | | | | Responsive to change |
| | Internal consistency | Test-retest[a] | Criterion | | Convergent | Discriminant | |
			Sensitivity, Specificity[b]	Other			
Inventory of Depressive Symptomatology—Self-Report	0.77–0.94	—	Cut point of 18+ sensitivity: 100% specificity: 94%	With clinical ratings, r=0.85 Distinguished severity	0.83–0.93	—	Yes
Inventory to Diagnose Depression	0.92	0.56–0.98	See Table 5–4 for cut point sensitivity: 90% specificity: 75%–100%	With clinical ratings, r=0.80–0.81 Distinguished severity Distinguished diagnosis	0.87	—	—
Edinburgh Postnatal Depression Scale	0.81–0.87	—	Cut point of 13+ sensitivity: 75%–95% specificity: 78%–96%	With clinical ratings, r=0.79–0.80	0.67–0.79	—	Yes
MOS Depression Screener	—	—	Major depressive disorder or dysthymia, cut point of 0.06+ sensitivity: 66%–93% specificity: 63%–95%	—	—	—	—
Depression Scale	0.88	—	Cut point of 9+ sensitivity: 74%–75% specificity: 85%–88%	Distinguished severity	—	—	—
Patient Health Questionnaire—Depression Scale	0.86–0.89	0.84	Cut point of 10+ sensitivity: 88% specificity: 88%	Distinguished severity	0.73	0.33–0.37	—
Depression-Arkansas Scale	0.86	—	—		0.70–0.83	0.25–0.45	—
PHQ Two-Item Screener	—	—	Cut point of 3+ sensitivity: 83% specificity: 90%	Distinguished severity	—	—	—
Internal State Scale	0.81–0.92 (subscales)	—	—	Distinguished diagnosis	0.44–0.84	—	Yes
Self-Rating Manic Inventory	0.94	0.73–0.93	Cut point of 18+ sensitivity: 71% specificity: 89%	Distinguished diagnosis	0.63–0.89	—	Yes

TABLE 5–5. Reliability and validity data for self-rated scales of mood disorder symptomatology *(continued)*

| Instrument | Reliability | | Validity | | | | |
| | | | Criterion | | | | |
	Internal consistency	Test-retest[a]	Sensitivity, Specificity[b]	Other	Convergent	Discriminant	Responsive to change
Altman Self-Rating for Mania Scale	—	0.86	Cut point of 6+ sensitivity: 86% specificity: 88%	With clinical ratings, $r=-0.22$–0.41 Distinguished diagnosis	0.72–0.77	—	—
Mood Disorder Questionnaire	0.84–0.90 (symptom items)	—	See Table 5–4 for cut point sensitivity: 28%–73% specificity: 90%–97%	—	—	—	—
Mood Spectrum Self-Report (MOODS-SR)	—	0.97[e]	—	Distinguished diagnosis	—	—	—

Note. Reliability and validity data refer to the full version of each scale unless another version is specified.
[a]Generally days or weeks apart.
[b]Sensitivity and specificity for detecting major depressive disorder or mania unless otherwise noted.
[c]Distinguished severity=discriminated between patient groups with different severities of depression.
[d]Distinguished diagnosis=discriminated between patient groups with different psychiatric diagnoses.
[e]The authors evaluated the correlation between one administration of the MOODS-SR and one administration of the SCI-MOODS (the clinician-administered version of the MOODS-SR).

scales are also strong in this area. Most mania scales have had their criterion validity evaluated, although not as extensively as for the depression scales. Convergent validity, when examined, has been adequate. However, mania scales have not been considered with regard to discriminant validity. Most of the clinician-rated scales for mood disorders have been tested and found to show responsiveness to symptom change during treatment.

Self-Rated Scales

In this section, we focus on mood-specific scales and comment more briefly on multicomponent scales with subscales that assess elements of mood. Tables 5–4 and 5–5 provide descriptive and psychometric information, respectively, for the 19 mood-specific scales that met our inclusion criteria. Fourteen assess depression, 2 assess mania, and 3 assess bipolar spectrum symptoms. All were designed to be administered in a paper-and-pencil format. Most were originally designed for patient samples, but virtually all have now been used in a variety of patient and community-based samples. Like the clinician-rated dimensional measures, most were designed to evaluate symptom severity and to detect changes in severity over time or across treatment groups. However, unlike clinician-rated scales, some self-rated scales were designed exclusively to screen individuals (i.e., to make an initial "rough cut" among respondents who may have clinically significant symptoms vs. those unlikely to be in distress). Thus, measures such as the Medical Outcomes Study (MOS) Depression Screener (Burnam et al. 1988), the Patient Health Questionnaire Two-Item Screener (Kroenke et al. 2003), and the Mood Disorder Questionnaire (Hirschfeld et al. 2000) are useful primarily in situations in which a more detailed clinical or research evaluation is planned for respondents who have positive results on these screening measures. Most of the self-rated measures—even those not originally created for screening purposes—now have been evaluated to determine optimal cut point scores that identify individuals likely to meet mood disorder diagnostic criteria. Table 5–5 provides data on the sensitivity and specificity of scales' cut points for identifying cases, under the general category of criterion validity.

Like the clinician-rated measures, most self-rated scales focus on symptoms specific to a single pole of the mood disorder spectrum. However, fewer self-rated than clinician-rated scales are available for mania. This is likely because of the long-standing view that individuals experiencing manic symptoms will be unable to report on their symptoms accurately because of either agitation, unwillingness to cooperate, or lack of insight required to make valid judgments.

This view has been challenged in recent years (Altman 1998), and growing evidence indicates that self-report mania scales have adequate reliability and validity.

The self-rated scales of mood disorder symptoms tend to be the most brief of all measures discussed in this chapter, requiring at most about 15 minutes and sometimes as little as 1 minute to complete. Some of the scales have multiple versions that vary in number of items, which may facilitate their use even when little time is available for administration. Generally, the shortest of the versions are appropriate only for screening purposes. Most scales require respondents to rate items on 3- or 4-point scales of severity during the past few days or weeks.

Although many of the self-rated scales in active use were developed as long ago as the earliest clinician-rated scales, an important difference is that some self-rated scales have undergone major revisions since their initial publication to reflect changes in the conceptualization of mood disorders and changes in diagnostic criteria. Often, however, reevaluation of their psychometric properties has lagged behind these revisions. Thus, most of the data on reliability and validity for scales with multiple revisions pertain to earlier rather than the most recent versions. When revisions were minor, one would not expect psychometric properties to change significantly. However, a few scales have undergone more substantial changes. For example, the Beck Depression Inventory, Second Revision (BDI-II; Beck et al. 1993), altered the original 1-week time frame to 2 weeks. The Zung Self-Rating Depression Scale revision (Zung SDS; Zung 1974) modified a few items, and the labels for the item rating scale anchors have varied somewhat across the literature in which the scale was used. Little psychometric data are available for the BDI-II (most pertain to the BDI-I Beck et al. 1961). For the Zung SDS, it is often unclear as to whether reliability and validity evaluations were based on the original or the revised measure and which anchors for ratings were used.

By far the most frequently used self-rated depression measures are the BDI, the Zung SDS, and the Center for Epidemiologic Studies Depression Scale (CES-D; Radloff 1977). Two measures designed for subgroups of the adult population, the Edinburgh Postnatal Depression Scale (Cox et al. 1987) and the Geriatric Depression Scale (GDS; Yesavage and Brink 1982–1983), are also widely used. The mania and bipolar spectrum scales have been used less extensively to date, but they are relatively new measures. A dominant self-report scale for mania or bipolar spectrum symptoms has not yet emerged.

In general, the level and degree of psychometric evaluation have been more extensive for the self-rated measures than for the clinician-rated measures. However, as for the clinician-rated measures, marked differences are seen among the self-rated scales in the thoroughness and strength of their psychometric evaluations. As shown in Table 5–4, the BDI is the only measure to receive high marks across the board, although a variety of other widely used measures show generally strong properties as well. Several of the newer measures, especially those designed only as screens, have received quite poor psychometric evaluations to date.

Table 5–5 provides a more detailed summary of the psychometric information available. Internal consistency reliability is particularly important for self-rated measures, and it is generally high for most measures. Test-retest reliability has been considered somewhat less often and is more variable across the scales. In the area of validity, all but 1 of the 19 measures have had some aspect of criterion validity evaluated. Most have had convergent validity established through examining correlations with other symptom-based self-report measures. Fewer depression scales, and none of the mania or bipolar spectrum scales, have been evaluated for discriminant validity. Fewer self-rated measures than clinician-rated measures have been examined with respect to responsiveness to change, and one measure (the Zung SDS) is unable to detect change consistently. The areas of convergent and discriminant validity have been particularly problematic for self-rated measures. They are often weak or show mixed evidence in these areas: they are able to detect distress in general, but they do not necessarily detect distress and symptomatology specific to depression or mania as opposed to other types of distress (e.g., anxiety) (McDowell and Newell 1996). This is perhaps their chief weakness.

Finally, Table 5–6 summarizes the characteristics of 10 self-rated multicomponent scales that include subscales to assess depressive and manic symptoms. All include depression items, and 2 include mania items as well. Except for the Hospital Anxiety and Depression Scale (HADS; Zigmond and Snaith 1983), all were designed for use in general community samples. Many are available in a variety of longer and shorter versions. Administration time ranges from a few minutes to more than 1 hour. Their major use in terms of mood disorder symptomatology is to evaluate severity, although some have been evaluated for their ability to screen individuals (usually for the presence of MDD) (J.W. Williams et al. 2002). A few have been used to monitor response to mood disorder treatments. Most of these measures have strong to reasonably good psychometric evaluations and results. The strongest in this regard are the General Health Questionnaire (Goldberg 1972), the Hopkins Symptom Checklist (Derogatis et al. 1974) and its related scales, and the HADS.

Selection of Rating Scales for Mood Disorders

We have alluded to a variety of factors that are relevant for scale selection. Here, we summarize key considerations in the following areas: scales' ability to assign diagnoses or make fine distinctions in severity of symptoms, scope or range of coverage of the mood disorder spectrum, psychometric strengths and liabilities, demonstrated use for clinical or research purposes and in populations of interest, and feasibility of administration.

Diagnoses Versus Severity of Symptomatology

General issues relevant to the choice of categorical or dimensional scales were discussed earlier in this chapter. From a practical perspective, selection of a scale from one broad category or the other should depend on the assessment goal. For example, if the goal is to describe differences between cases and noncases or to isolate risk factors for a particular disorder, a diagnostic instrument would be appropriate. If the goal is to assess the degree of impairment or to describe the comorbidity and intensity of symptoms, a dimensional instrument would be more suitable. What is known or suspected about the distribution of psychiatric disorders in the population to be studied should have a role in the selection. The prevalence and incidence of some mood disorders such as bipolar illness are low in the general population (Dew et al. 2003). Alternatively, even for more common conditions such as MDD, the planned sample size may be too small to yield many cases. In either situation, studies that use a diagnostic approach may have difficulty generating enough cases to examine in relation to other variables.

In some circumstances, the optimal approach to scale selection might be a combined, or multimethod, strategy that draws on the relative strengths of both diagnostic and dimensional instruments and thus maximizes the quality of information gathered (Üstün and Tien 1995). One multimethod approach uses both types of instruments in a sequential process first to screen and then to diagnose disorders in individuals whose symptoms meet initial criteria. With this approach, the ability of dimensional scales to provide reliable estimates of clinically significant or lesser degrees of distress in the population could be combined with the ability of diagnostic measures to provide finer-grained estimates of disorder near the diagnostic cut point.

TABLE 5–6. Global self-rated instruments with mood components

Instrument	Mood domains assessed and population[a]	No. of items[b]	Item response and time frame	Administration time	Clinical cut point and score range[c]	Major uses of scale (relevant to mood symptoms)	Studies using measure[d]	Reliability: thoroughness/results[e]	Validity: thoroughness/results[e]
General Health Questionnaire (GHQ; Goldberg 1972)	Depression	12, 20, 28, 30, 60	0=not at all, 4=much more than usual (usual) scoring: 0=absent, 1=present Past few weeks	2–10 min	12-item: 3+ 20-item: 4+ 28-, 30-item: 5+ 60-item: 12+ range=count, with 0–1 scoring	Screen; evaluate severity; monitor treatment response	Many	+++/+++	+++/+++
Hopkins Symptom Checklist (HSCL; Derogatis et al. 1974); Symptom Checklist-90-R (SCL-90-R; Derogatis 1983); Brief Symptom Inventory (BSI; Derogatis and Melisaratos 1983)	Depression	HSCL: 38, 53 SCL-90-R: 90 BSI: 58	HSCL: 1=not at all, 4=extremely distressed SCL-90-R, BSI: 0=not at all, 4=extremely distressed Past week or past 2 weeks	10–20 min	HSCL: 43+ range=25–100	Screen; evaluate severity; monitor treatment response	Many	+++/+++	+++/++
Millon Clinical Multiaxial Inventory (MCMI; Millon 1977; Millon et al. 1994)	Dysthymia, depression, hypomania, mania, cycloid	175	0=false, 1=true Present	Not noted	None	Evaluate severity	Some	++/++	++/++
Mental Health Inventory (MHI; Veit and Ware 1983)	Depression	5, 18, 38	6=none of the time, 1=all of the time Past month	2–20 min	None	Evaluate severity	Some	++/++	++/++
Hospital Anxiety and Depression Scale (HADS; Zigmond and Snaith 1983)	Depression (nonpsychiatric medical patients)	14	1=absent, 3=severe Past week	5–10 min	8+, 11+ range=0–21	Screen; evaluate severity	Many	+++/+++	+++/++
Multiple Affect Adjective Checklist—Revised (MAACL-R; Zuckerman and Lubin 1985)	Depression	132	0=absent, 1=present State: today Trait: today and generally	5–10 min	None	Evaluate severity	Few	+/+	+/+

TABLE 5–6.　Global self-rated instruments with mood components (continued)

Instrument	Mood domains assessed and population[a]	No. of items[b]	Item response and time frame	Administration time	Clinical cut point and score range[c]	Major uses of scale (relevant to mood symptoms)	Studies using measure[d]	Reliability: thoroughness/results[e]	Validity: thoroughness/results[e]
Minnesota Multiphasic Personality Inventory—2 (MMPI-2; Butcher et al. 1989)	Depression, mania	567	0=false, 1=true Present	60–90 min	None	Evaluate severity	Many	+++/++	+++/++
Profile of Mood States (POMS, POMS short form; McNair et al. 1992)	Depression	30, 65	0=not at all, 3=extremely Past week	5–10 min	None	Evaluate severity; monitor treatment response	Many	++/++	++/++
Depression Anxiety Stress Scales (DASS; Lovibond and Lovibond 1993)	Depression	21, 42	0=did not apply to me at all; 3=applied to me very much or most of the time Past week	10–15 min	None	Evaluate severity	Some	++/++	++/++
Patient Health Questionnaire (PHQ; Spitzer et al. 1994)	Depression	27	0=not at all, 3=nearly every day Past 2 weeks; past month	5–10 min	See PHQ-9 in Table 5–4	Screen; evaluate severity	Few	++/++	++/+

[a]Unless otherwise noted, the population appropriate for each scale consists of all adults.

[b]For scales with multiple versions, the number of items in each is noted.

[c]Cut point for detecting major depressive disorder.

[d]Based on numbers of ISI Web of Science citations 1994–2003: many=450+, some=100–449, few=<100.

[e]For thoroughness of psychometric testing, 0=no reported psychometric testing; +=very basic information only; ++=several types of test or several studies have reported reliability/validity; +++=all major forms of reliability/validity testing have been reported. For strength of results, 0=no numerical results reported; ?=results uninterpretable; +=weak reliability/validity; ++=adequate reliability/validity; +++=excellent reliability/validity.

Scope

The diagnostic schedules vary in whether they include all or a subset of currently diagnosed mood disorders. The dimensional scales also vary in their coverage of the mood spectrum. A more subtle difference among the dimensional scales pertains to the range of symptoms (even at one pole of the mood spectrum) that may be included. Some scales were developed specifically because of a perceived lack in coverage by existing measures of the full range of symptoms. For example, the Ham-D was designed to assess core depressive symptoms, and it spawned the development of measures such as the Bech-Rafaelsen Melancholia Scale (Bech and Rafaelsen 1980) and the Clinical Interview for Depression (Paykel 1985). Both of these measures significantly expanded the range of symptoms that were assessed by incorporating items from other measures.

Recently developed dimensional scales may include different items than older scales because of changes in diagnostic criteria. Measures of mania are good examples of this (Livianos-Aldana and Rojo-Moreno 2001; Poolsup et al. 1999). Several measures developed prior to the DSM-IV (American Psychiatric Association 1994) conceptualization of mania do not include attributes now seen as integral to psychopathology in this area. For example, the Bech-Rafaelsen Mania Scale (Bech et al. 1978) does not assess risk-taking behaviors, whereas the MSRS does not assess sleep disturbance or lability of mood. The most widely used mania scale, the YMRS, was designed to have a broader scope than an earlier measure (the Rating of Mania; Petterson et al. 1973) but to be more brief and explicit in its severity ratings than the MSRS. Recently, however, the YMRS also has been seen as deficient in covering some symptom areas, and it has been argued that the MSRS remains the most thorough evaluation of the phenomenology of mania (Akiskal et al. 2003).

Psychometric Strengths and Liabilities

In general, rating scales for mood disorders have stronger evidence for their reliability than for their validity. This is particularly the case for categorical, diagnostic instruments, for which questions persist about levels of validity and even how best to assess validity (Murphy 2002). Dimensional scales tend to be more evenly balanced in terms of relative strengths in the domains of reliability and validity: most have had some evaluation of multiple aspects of both domains. However, some clinician-rated scales and some self-report scales are clearly in the "top tier" in terms of psychometric strengths, including the clinician-rated Ham-D and MADRS and the self-rated

BDI-I, GDS, General Health Questionnaire, Hopkins Symptom Checklist and related scales, and HADS. It is noteworthy that all of these are either measures of depression or multicomponent scales with depression subscales. No measures of mania or bipolar spectrum symptoms show thoroughly established or uniformly strong reliability and validity. Some more recently developed measures look promising, including the Clinician-Administered Rating Scale for Mania (Altman et al. 1994) and the Self-Rating Manic Inventory (Shugar et al. 1992). However, they have yet to be used in many studies.

Demonstrated Use for Intended Purpose and in Populations of Interest

In the beginning of this chapter, we listed a series of goals for which scales may be selected. The typology in Figure 5–1 and the data provided in Tables 5–1 through 5–6 allow for quick determination of whether a given measure can be used to achieve one or more of these goals. Within a given class of measures (e.g., self-rated dimensional measures), some have been found to achieve multiple goals, including screening, evaluating overall symptom severity, and monitoring response to treatment. Others have a narrower range of applications. Unless a key aim is to provide evidence regarding a new area of use, it usually would be a mistake to select a scale that has not been shown to be capable of achieving the assessment goal at hand.

An often more difficult issue is whether a scale will be useful in a particular population of interest. The difficulty arises because 1) scales are usually initially developed and tested in a single population, rather than through a multicultural or multipopulation approach, and 2) even within a single population, scales are rarely evaluated equally thoroughly among the many possible subgroups that might be of interest (e.g., gender, age, racial/ethnic groups). Most instruments are based on middle-class western European or North American assumptions about mental illness and "norms" about how psychiatric symptoms are expressed. To the extent that other cultural groups express distress differently, then even the most technically accurate translation of many of our scales into other languages will not be adequate for truly capturing the nature of mood disorder symptoms in these other groups. Examples of differences particularly important to mood include evidence that the expression and meaning of somatic complaints vary in populations of Hispanic and European heritage (Escobar et al. 1983) and evidence that Asian language speakers may differ from English language speakers in willingness to endorse items pertaining to positive or negative mood (Iwata et al. 1998).

Even within more homogeneous cultural groups, psychosocial and medical status characteristics (e.g., age, education, motivation for completing the scale) are likely to necessitate careful consideration of which scales may be more or less useful for sensitively evaluating mood without being confounded by other variables. For example, some instruments (e.g., the BDI) may be less appropriate for less educated populations because the scales have relatively complex response options. Other instruments (e.g., those that include a relatively high proportion of somatic symptom items) may be inappropriate for physically ill or disabled groups in whom such symptoms may reflect medical status rather than emotional distress (Dew 1998).

Feasibility of Administration

Feasibility issues include the burden to potential respondents and the financial cost per respondent of gathering the information. Community respondents may be reluctant to complete a lengthy assessment (e.g., a diagnostic schedule) because of both the time involved and their concerns about confidentiality. Selecting scales that minimize the time burden is therefore critical, yet choosing the class of measures that are generally the most brief (self-report scales) may not be optimal for overcoming reticence resulting from confidentiality concerns. Clinician-administered dimensional scales that allow for rapport to be established may ultimately provide a higher quality of information, to the extent that they can overcome respondents' reluctance through gentle progress in the assessment. Treated populations may have had more experience with the types of questions asked in mood disorder scales and thus may be less reluctant to answer questions. Yet depending on the nature or severity of their illnesses, they may have more difficulty in completing certain types of assessments such as self-report scales or in completing scales that are very lengthy and have complex questioning sequences.

Another important feasibility consideration is the cost of the assessment modality and of the services of the person who will administer the assessment. Clinician interviewers are most costly, followed by trained nonclinician interviewers and self-rated scales. Even the use of nonclinician lay interviewers can become expensive in the context of administering diagnostic schedules because they must receive extensive training and careful monitoring.

In terms of the format of data gathering, in-person assessments are generally the most costly, followed by telephone interviews and paper-and-pencil self-rated scales. Self-rated scales are dependent on the respondent's ability to read and understand questions and thus may not always

be appropriate. Both diagnostic schedules and clinician-rated dimensional instruments were originally designed solely for in-person assessments, but they have been modified and found to be ably administered by telephone in many circumstances (e.g., Fenig et al. 1993). The use of computers and related technologies to aid in recording responses to both interviews and self-administered questionnaires also has become more prevalent, and these approaches can efficiently collect rating scale information in various settings (Kobak et al. 1996; Robins 2002).

Conclusion

A large array of rating scales for mood disorders have been developed, particularly for the assessment of depression. Future work is needed to develop and refine a more complete set of measures for mania and bipolar spectrum symptoms. Across the full range of mood disorder rating scales—including diagnostic schedules, clinician-rated dimensional scales, and self-rated scales—the strength of psychometric information has been steadily increasing. Nevertheless, numerous gaps remain, particularly with respect to validity. Moreover, at present, no single rating scale for mood disorders is equally appropriate in all settings and populations. The future of psychometrics, including item bank development and increasing use of computerized adaptive testing, eventually may provide a unified assessment approach that shows greater flexibility across diverse circumstances (McHorney 1999; Weiss, in press). In the meantime, however, clinicians may choose from a wealth of rating scales for mood disorders to maximize their ability to meet today's clinical and research goals.

References

Akiskal HS, Azorin JM, Hantouche EG: Proposed multidimensional structure of mania: beyond the euphoric-dysphoric dichotomy. J Affect Disord 73:7–18, 2003

Altman E: Rating scales for mania: is self-rating reliable? J Affect Disord 50:283–286, 1998

Altman EG, Hedeker DR, Janicak PG, et al: The Clinician-Administered Rating Scale for Mania (CARS-M): development, reliability, and validity. Biol Psychiatry 36:124–134, 1994

Altman EG, Hedeker D, Peterson JL, et al: The Altman Self-Rating Mania Scale. Biol Psychiatry 42:948–955, 1997

American Psychiatric Association: Diagnostic and Statistical Manual of Mental Disorders, 3rd Edition. Washington, DC, American Psychiatric Association, 1980

American Psychiatric Association: Diagnostic and Statistical Manual of Mental Disorders, 3rd Edition, Revised. Washington, DC, American Psychiatric Association, 1987

American Psychiatric Association: Diagnostic and Statistical Manual of Mental Disorders, 4th Edition. Washington, DC, American Psychiatric Association, 1994

American Psychiatric Association: Diagnostic and Statistical Manual of Mental Disorders, 4th Edition, Text Revision. Washington, DC, American Psychiatric Association, 2000

Bauer MS, Crits-Christoph P, Ball WA, et al: Independent assessment of manic and depressive symptoms by self-rating: scale characteristics and implications for the study of mania. Arch Gen Psychiatry 48:807–812, 1991

Bech P, Rafaelsen OJ: The use of rating scales exemplified by a comparison of the Hamilton and the Bech-Rafaelsen Melancholia Scale. Acta Psychiatr Scand 62 (suppl 285):128–131, 1980

Bech P, Rafaelsen OJ, Kramp P, et al: The Mania Rating Scale: scale construction and inter-observer agreement. Neuropharmacology 17:430–431, 1978

Beck AT, Steer RA: Beck Depression Inventory Manual. San Antonio, TX, Psychological Corporation, Harcourt, Brace, 1993

Beck AT, Ward CH, Mendelson M, et al: An inventory for measuring depression. Arch Gen Psychiatry 4:561–571, 1961

Beck AT, Steer RA, Brown CK: Beck Depression Inventory—Second Edition Manual. San Antonio, TX, Psychological Corporation, Harcourt Brace Jovanovich, 1986

Beck AT, Guth D, Steer RA, et al: Screening for major depression disorders in medical inpatients with the Beck Depression Inventory for Primary Care. Behav Res Ther 35:785–791, 1997

Beigel A, Murphy DL, Bunney WE: The Manic-State Rating Scale: scale construction, reliability, and validity. Arch Gen Psychiatry 25:256–262, 1971

Blackburn IM, Loudon JB, Ashworth CM: A new scale for measuring mania. Psychol Med 7:453–458, 1977

Broadhead WE, Leon AC, Weissman MM: Development and validation of the SDDS-PC screen for multiple mental disorders in primary care. Arch Fam Med 4:211–219, 1995

Burnam MA, Wells KB, Leake B, et al: Development of a brief screening instrument for detecting depressive disorders. Med Care 26:775–789, 1988

Butcher JN, Dahlstrom WG, Graham JR, et al: Minnesota Multiphasic Personality Inventory-2 (MMPI-2): Manual for Administration and Scoring. Minneapolis, University of Minnesota Press, 1989

Carney MWP, Roth M, Garside RF: The diagnosis of depressive syndromes and the prediction of ECT response. Br J Psychiatry 111:659–674, 1965

Carroll BJ: Carroll Depression Scales—Revised: Technical Manual. Toronto, Ontario, Multi-Health Systems, 1998

Carroll BJ, Feinberg M, Smouse PE, et al: The Carroll Rating Scale for Depression, I: development, reliability and validation. Br J Psychiatry 138:194–200, 1981

Clementz BA, Iacono WB: Nosology and diagnosis, in Psychopathology in Adulthood. Edited by Bellack AS, Hersen M. Needham Heights, MA, Allyn & Bacon, 1993, pp 3–20

Copeland JRM, Dewey ME, Henderson AS, et al: The Geriatric Mental State (GMS) used in the community: replication studies of the computerised diagnosis AGECAT. Psychol Med 8:219–223, 1988

Cox JL, Holden JM, Sagovsky R: Detection of postnatal depression: development of the 10-item Edinburgh Postnatal Depression Scale. Br J Psychiatry 150:782–786, 1987

Dell'Osso L, Armani A, Rucci P, et al: Measuring mood spectrum: comparison of interview (SCI-MOODS) and self-report (MOODS-SR) instruments. Compr Psychiatry 43:69–73, 2002

Derogatis LR: The SCL-90 Manual II. Towson, MD, Clinical Psychometric Research, 1983

Derogatis LR, Melisaratos N: The Brief Symptom Inventory: an introductory report. Psychol Med 13:595–605, 1983

Derogatis LR, Lipman RS, Rickels K, et al: The Hopkins Symptom Checklist (HSCL): a self-report symptom inventory. Behav Sci 19:1–15, 1974

Dew MA: Psychiatric disorder in the context of physical illness, in Adversity, Stress and Psychopathology. Edited by Dohrenwend BP. New York, Oxford University Press, 1998, pp 177–218

Dew MA, Martire LM, Hall M: Depression: epidemiology and risk factors, in Advances in the Management and Treatment of Depression. Edited by Potokar J, Thase ME. London, Martin Dunitz, 2003, pp 1–39

Endicott J, Spitzer RL: A diagnostic interview: the Schedule for Affective Disorders and Schizophrenia. Arch Gen Psychiatry 35:837–844, 1978

Escobar JI, Gomez J, Tuason VB: Depressive phenomenology in North and South American patients. Am J Psychiatry 140:47–51, 1983

Fagiolini A, Dell'Osso L, Pini S, et al: Validity and reliability of a new instrument for assessing mood symptomatology: the Structured Clinical Interview for Mood Spectrum (SCI-MOODS). Int J Methods Psychiatr Res 8:71–82, 1999

Fenig S, Levav I, Kohn R, et al: Telephone vs. face-to-face interviewing in a community psychiatric survey. Am J Public Health 83:896–898, 1993

First MB: DSM-IV and psychiatric epidemiology, in Textbook in Psychiatric Epidemiology, 2nd Edition. Edited by Tsuang MT, Tohen M. New York, Wiley-Liss, 2002, pp 333–342

First MB, Gibbon M, Spitzer RL, et al: Structured Clinical Interview for DSM-IV Axis I Disorders. Washington, DC, American Psychiatric Press, 1997

Goldberg DP: The Detection of Psychiatric Illness by Questionnaire. Oxford, England, Oxford University Press, 1972

Hamilton M: A rating scale for depression. J Neurol Neurosurg Psychiatry 23:56–62, 1960

Hamilton M: Development of a rating scale for primary depressive illness. Br J Soc Clin Psychol 6:278–296, 1967

Hirschfeld RMA, Williams JBW, Spitzer RL, et al: Development and validation of a screening instrument for bipolar spectrum disorder: the Mood Disorder Questionnaire. Am J Psychiatry 157:1873–1875, 2000

Iwata N, Umesue M, Egashira K, et al: Can positive affect items be used to assess depressive disorders in the Japanese population? Psychol Med 28:153–158, 1998

Kessler RC, McGonagle KA, Zhao S, et al: Lifetime and 12-month prevalence of DSM-III-R psychiatric disorders in the United States: results of the National Comorbidity Survey. Arch Gen Psychiatry 51:8–19, 1994

Kobak KA, Greist JH, Jefferson JW, et al: Computer-administered clinical rating scales. A review. Psychopharmacology 127:291–301, 1996

Kohout FJ, Berkman LF, Evans DA, et al: Two shorter forms of the CES-D (Center for Epidemiological Studies Depression) depression symptoms index. J Aging Health 5:179–193, 1993

Kroenke K, Spitzer RL, Williams JBW: The PHQ-9: validity of a brief depression severity measure. J Gen Intern Med 16:606–613, 2001

Kroenke K, Spitzer RL, Williams JBW: The Patient Health Questionnaire-2: validity of a two-item depression screener. Med Care 41:1284–1292, 2003

Lewis G, Pelosi AJ, Araya R, et al: Measuring psychiatric disorder in the community: a standardized assessment for use by lay-interviewers. Psychol Med 22:465–486, 1992

Livianos-Aldana L, Rojo-Moreno L: Rating and quantification of manic syndromes. Acta Psychiatr Scand 104 (suppl 409):2–33, 2001

Lovibond SH, Lovibond PF: Manual for the Depression Anxiety Stress Scales (DASS). Australia, Psychology Foundation Monograph, University of New South Wales, 1993

Lubin B: Adjective checklists for measurement of depression. Arch Gen Psychiatry 12:57–62, 1965

Lubin B: State Trait-Depression Adjective Check Lists: Professional Manual. Odessa, FL, Psychological Assessment Resources, 1994

Mason BJ, Kocsis JH, Leon AC, et al: Measurement of severity and treatment response in dysthymia. Psychiatr Ann 23:625–631, 1993

McDowell I, Newell C: Measuring Health: A Guide to Rating Scales and Questionnaires. New York, Oxford University Press, 1996

McHorney CA: Health status assessment methods for adults: past accomplishments and future challenges. Annu Rev Public Health 20:309–335, 1999

McNair DM, Lorr M, Droppleman LF: Manual for the Profile of Mood States. San Diego, CA, EdITS, 1992

Millon T: Manual for the Millon Clinical Multiaxial Inventory. Minneapolis, MN, National Computer Systems, 1977

Millon T, Millon C, Davis R: Millon Clinical Multiaxial Inventory-III Manual. Minneapolis, MN, National Computer Systems, 1994

Mirowsky J, Ross CE: Psychiatric diagnosis as reified measurement. J Health Soc Behav 30:11–25, 1989

Mirowsky J, Ross CE: Measurement for a human science. J Health Soc Behav 43:152–170, 2002

Montgomery SA, Åsberg M: A new depression scale designed to be sensitive to change. Br J Psychiatry 134:382–389, 1979

Murphy JM: Symptom scales and diagnostic schedules in adult psychiatry, in Textbook in Psychiatric Epidemiology, 2nd Edition. Edited by Tsuang MT, Tohen M. New York, Wiley-Liss, 2002, pp 273–332

Nunes EV, Goehl L, Seracini A, et al: A modification of the Structured Clinical Interview for DSM-III-R to evaluate methadone patients. Am J Addict 5:241–248, 1996

Nurnberger JI Jr, Blehar MC, Kaufmann CA, et al: Diagnostic interviews for genetic studies: rationale, unique features, and training. Arch Gen Psychiatry 51:849–859, 1994

Overall JE: The Brief Psychiatric Rating Scale (BPRS): recent developments in ascertainment and scaling. Psychopharmacol Bull 24:97–99, 1988

Paykel ES: The Clinical Interview for Depression: development, reliability and validity. J Affect Disord 9:85–96, 1985

Petterson U, Fyro B, Sedvall G: A new scale for the longitudinal rating of manic states. Acta Psychiatr Scand 49:248–256, 1973

Poolsup N, Li Wan Po A, Oyebode F: Measuring mania and critical appraisal of rating scales. J Clin Pharm Ther 24:433–443, 1999

Radloff LS: The CES-D Scale: a self-report depression scale for research in the general population. Appl Psychological Measurement 1:385–401, 1977

Raskin A, Schulterbrandt J, Reatig N, et al: Replication of factors of psychopathology in interview, ward behavior and self-report ratings of hospitalized depressives. J Nerv Ment Dis 148:87–98, 1969

Regier DA, Myers JK, Kramer M, et al: The NIMH Epidemiologic Catchment Area program: historical context, major objectives, and study population characteristics. Arch Gen Psychiatry 41:934–941, 1984

Robins LN: Epidemiology: reflections on testing the validity of psychiatric interviews. Arch Gen Psychiatry 42:918–924, 1985

Robins LN: Birth and development of psychiatric interviews, in Textbook in Psychiatric Epidemiology, 2nd Edition. Edited by Tsuang MT, Tohen M. New York, Wiley, 2002, pp 257–271

Robins LN, Helzer JE, Croughan J, et al: The National Institute of Mental Health Diagnostic Interview Schedule. Its history, characteristics and validity. Arch Gen Psychiatry 45:381–389, 1981

Robins LN, Wing JK, Wittchen H-U, et al: The Composite International Diagnostic Interview. An epidemiologic instrument suitable for use in conjunction with different diagnostic systems and in different cultures. Arch Gen Psychiatry 45:1069–1077, 1988

Robins LN, Marcus L, Reich W, et al: Diagnostic Interview Schedule, Version IV. St. Louis, MO, Department of Psychiatry, Washington University School of Medicine, 1996

Rogers R: Handbook of Diagnostic and Structured Interviewing. New York, Guilford, 2001

Rosenthal R, Rosnow RL: Essentials of Behavioral Research: Methods and Data Analysis, 2nd Edition. New York, McGraw-Hill, 1991

Rush AJ, Giles DE, Schlesser MA, et al: The Inventory for Depressive Symptomatology (IDS): preliminary findings. Psychiatry Res 18:65–87, 1986

Rush AJ, Gullion CM, Basco MR, et al: The Inventory of Depressive Symptomatology (IDS): psychometric properties. Psychol Med 26:477–486, 1996

Salokangas RKP, Poutanen O, Stengård E: Screening for depression in primary care: development and validation of the Depression Scale, a screening instrument for depression. Acta Psychiatr Scand 92:10–16, 1995

Secunda SK, Katz MM, Swann A, et al: Mania: diagnosis, state measurement and prediction of treatment response. J Affect Disord 8:113–121, 1985

Sheehan DV, Lecrubier Y, Sheehan KH, et al: The Mini-International Neuropsychiatric Interview (M.I.N.I.): the development and validation of a structured diagnostic psychiatric interview for DSM-IV and ICD-10. J Clin Psychiatry 59 (suppl 20):22–33, 1998

Sheikh JI, Yesavage JA: Geriatric Depression Scale (GDS): recent evidence and development of a shorter version. Clin Gerontol 5:165–173, 1986

Shugar G, Schertzer S, Toner BB, et al: Development, use, and factor analysis of a self-report inventory for mania. Compr Psychiatry 33:325–331, 1992

Smith GR, Kramer TL, Hollenberg JA, et al: Validity of the Depression-Arkansas (D-ARK) Scale: a tool for measuring major depressive disorder. Ment Health Serv Res 4:167–173, 2002

Spearing MK, Post RM, Leverich GS, et al: Modification of the Clinical Global Impressions (CGI) Scale for Use in Bipolar Illness (BP): the CGI-BP. Psychiatry Res 73:159–171, 1997

Spitzer RL: Psychiatric diagnosis: are clinicians still necessary? Compr Psychiatry 25:399–411, 1983

Spitzer RL, Williams JBW, Gibbon M, et al: Structured Clinical Interview for DSM-III-R. Washington, DC, American Psychiatric Press, 1990

Spitzer RL, Williams JBW, Kroenke K, et al: Utility of a new procedure for diagnosing mental disorders in primary care: the PRIME-MD 1000 Study. JAMA 272:1749–1756, 1994

Üstün TB, Tien AY: Recent developments for diagnostic measures in psychiatry. Epidemiol Rev 17:210–220, 1995

Veit CT, Ware JE Jr: The structure of psychological distress and well-being in general populations. J Consult Clin Psychol 51:730–742, 1983

Weiss DJ: Computerized adaptive testing for effective and efficient measurement in counseling and education. Measurement and Evaluation in Counseling and Development 37:70–84, 2004

Wheaton B: The role of sociology in the study of mental health...and the role of mental health in the study of sociology. J Health Soc Behav 42:221–234, 2001

Williams JBW: Standardizng the Hamilton Depression Rating Scale: past, present, and future. Eur Arch Psychiatry Clin Neurosci 251 (suppl 2):11/6–11/12, 2001

Williams JBW, Gibbon M, First MB, et al: The Structured Clinical Interview for DSM-III-R (SCID), II: multisite test-retest reliability. Arch Gen Psychiatry 49:630–636, 1992

Williams JW Jr, Noël PH, Cordes JA, et al: Is this patient clinically depressed? JAMA 287:1160–1170, 2002

Wing JK, Cooper JE, Sartorius N: Measurement and Classification of Psychiatric Symptoms: An Instruction Manual for the PSE and CATEGO Program. London, Cambridge University Press, 1974

Wing JK, Babor T, Brugha T, et al: SCAN: Schedules for Clinical Assessment in Neuropsychiatry. Arch Gen Psychiatry 47:589–593, 1990

World Health Organization: International Classification of Diseases, 9th Revision. Geneva, World Health Organization, 1977

World Health Organization: The ICD-10 Classification of Mental and Behavioral Disorders: Clinical Descriptions and Diagnostic Guidelines. Geneva, World Health Organization, 1992

Yesavage JA, Brink TL: Development and validation of a geriatric depression screening scale: a preliminary report. J Psychiatr Res 17:37–49, 1982–1983

Young RC, Biggs JT, Ziegler VE, et al: A rating scale for mania: reliability, validity and sensitivity. Br J Psychiatry 133:429–435, 1978

Zigmond AS, Snaith RP: The Hospital Anxiety and Depression Scale. Acta Psychiatr Scand 67:361–370, 1983

Zimmerman M, Coryell W, Corenthal C, et al: A self-report scale to diagnose major depressive disorder. Arch Gen Psychiatry 43:1076–1081, 1986

Zuckerman M, Lubin B: Manual for the MAACL-R: The Multiple Affect Adjective Checklist—Revised. San Diego, CA, EdITS, 1985

Zung WWK: A self-rating depression scale. Arch Gen Psychiatry 12:63–70, 1965

Zung WWK: The Depression Status Inventory: an adjunct to the Self-Rating Depression Scale. J Clin Psychol 28:539–543, 1972

Zung WWK: The measurement of affects: depression and anxiety, in Psychological Measurements in Psychopharmacology. Edited by Pichot P. Basel, Switzerland, S Karger, 1974, pp 170–188

PART 2

Pathogenesis
of Mood Disorders

SECTION EDITOR: PEDRO L. DELGADO, M.D.

Neurochemistry of Mood Disorders

PEDRO L. DELGADO, M.D.

FRANCISCO A. MORENO, M.D.

THE ROLE OF neurotransmitters and neuromodulators in the pathophysiology of mood disorders has been the subject of intensive study for many decades. As is often the case, early theories were overly simplistic, and as the scientific base of knowledge increased, so did the complexity of subsequent theories. In the 1960s and 1970s, it seemed as though mood disorders would turn out to be simple "chemical imbalances" of monoamine neurotransmitters such as serotonin (5-HT), norepinephrine (NE), and dopamine (DA) (Coppen 1967; Schildkraut 1965). As the twentieth century drew to a close, increasing knowledge of the effects of stress on neuroplasticity (Sapolsky 2000) and the molecular events that follow neurotransmitter–receptor interactions (Hyman and Nestler 1996; Manji et al. 2001) led to more complicated models for mood disorders based on the emerging awareness of the importance of neuroplasticity to the pathophysiology of mood disorders and to the mechanisms underlying treatment efficacy (Duman 2004; Gould and Tanapat 1999; Nestler and Duman 1996; Santarelli et al. 2003). It has become clear that a full understanding of the biology of mood disorders must incorporate knowledge of a much broader range of neurochemicals than the monoamines, take into account the possible toxicity of stressful life events and general health status, consider the role of multiple genetic influ-

ences that confer vulnerability, and, finally, be able to explain how these effects converge to alter the structure and function of the brain's emotion and cognition circuits, culminating in the symptoms that define mood disorders.

In this chapter, we focus on the neurochemistry of mood disorders, reviewing data supporting a role for selected neurochemical systems in their pathophysiology. Most of the data presented focus on human studies because significant questions persist regarding the adequacy of animal models.

Anatomical Considerations

The pathophysiology of mood disorders cannot be fully understood without considering the interaction between neurochemistry and the neuroanatomical structure of the brain's emotion systems. For example, before one can link a molecular event to a change in behavior, one has to understand how that event alters the physiology of individual neurons and interactions between groups of neurons that form circuits. Although molecular and cellular events are important to understand, it is the multicellular interactions in the brain that are the immediate underpinnings of behavior, cognition, and emotion. Neurochemical systems modulate emotion and cognition by either direct innervation (e.g., monoamines) via generalized dissemination through the bloodstream or local release and direct diffusion. Monoamine systems have attracted the interest of researchers in part because they are almost exclusively organized as large *systems* of single-source divergent neurons (Bloom 1995) able to coordinate neural activity across many parts of the brain simultaneously.

The brain's emotion and cognition circuits play a central role in mediating the symptoms that define mood disorders. By and large, the relevant areas and circuits entail the structures historically referred to as the *limbic system* (Maclean 1949), although it is now thought that the original concept of the limbic system as emotion circuits separate and distinct from cognition circuits was not accurate; these circuits overlap and interact (LeDoux 2000). The emotion and cognition circuits most relevant to mood disorders are composed of predominantly local circuits within and long hierarchical circuits between specific regions of the brain, including the prefrontal cortex (PFC), cingulate gyrus, amygdala, hippocampus, insula, ventral striatum, and thalamus (Phillips et al. 2003) (see also Rajkowska, Chapter 11, and Mayberg, Chapter 13, in this volume). Mood disorders most likely result from either dysfunction of the neurons that make up these emotion and cognition circuits or dysfunction of the neurochemical systems that modulate their function. Regardless of where the primary dysfunction lies, it is important to keep in mind that these brain structures and circuits are the proximal mediators of the alterations in emotions, cognitions, and behaviors that define mood disorders (LeDoux 2000; Maclean 1949; Phillips et al. 2003).

Serotonin System in Mood Disorders

Anatomy and Physiology of the Serotonin System

Serotonin is synthesized from the essential amino acid tryptophan in two enzymatic steps. The rate-limiting step in the synthesis of serotonin is the conversion of tryptophan to 5-hydroxytryptophan by the enzyme tryptophan hydroxylase. Plasma tryptophan cannot passively cross the blood-brain barrier and is transported by the large neutral amino acid transporter protein. The tryptophan hydroxylase enzyme is poorly saturated; therefore, increases and decreases in tryptophan availability as well as changes in the ratio of tryptophan to large neutral amino acid can influence the rate of serotonin synthesis and lead to corresponding changes in brain serotonin and 5-hydroxyindoleacetic acid (5-HIAA). Brain serotonin is metabolized by monoamine oxidase–A (MAO-A) into 5-HIAA. Once released into the synaptic cleft, serotonin is taken back up into the neuron by the serotonin transporter (SERT).

The serotonin system is the largest cohesive neurotransmitter system in the brain, and serotonin neurons innervate all areas of the brain. The system has two major subdivisions: the ascending and the descending arms. The descending arm projects to the spinal cord and is involved in pain perception. Limbic brain regions (hippocampus, amygdala, and temporal lobes) and those nuclei involved in sensory transmission (thalamus) are some of the most heavily innervated areas. Some serotonin release may be independent of cell firing, accounting for some of the discrepancies between measures of serotonin levels and changes in firing rate of serotonin neurons after stress (Adell et al. 1997; Jacobs and Azmitia 1992).

Signaling for the serotonin system is complex; humans have as many as 14 distinct subtypes of serotonin receptors, designated 5-HT_{1A}, 5-HT_{1B}, 5-HT_{1D}, 5-HT_{1E}, 5-HT_{1F}, 5-HT_{2A}, 5-HT_{2B}, 5-HT_{2C}, 5-HT_{3}, 5-HT_{4}, 5-HT_{5A}, 5-HT_{5B}, 5-HT_{6}, and 5-HT_{7} (Kroeze et al. 2002). 5-HT_{1A}, 5-HT_{1B}, and 5-HT_{1D} receptors are found presynaptically and serve to provide inhibitory feedback inhibition on firing rate (5-HT_{1A}) and release (5-HT_{1B} [mouse] and 5-HT_{1D} [human]) of serotonin. Most of the subtypes also have been reported postsynaptically, and the physiological effects include both inhibitory and excitatory actions. From the perspective of mood disorders, the most important serotonin receptors include the 5-HT_{1A}, 5-HT_{2}, 5-HT_{4}, 5-HT_{6}, and 5-HT_{7} subtypes. 5-HT_{2C} receptor agonists decrease, whereas 5-HT_{2C} receptor antagonists increase mesocorticolimbic DA function. The serotonin system exerts both phasic and tonic control of mesocorticolimbic DA function through 5-HT_{2C} receptors, but it does not appear to play a major role in regulating nigrostriatal DA function (Di Matteo et al. 2001).

Preclinical studies in laboratory animals showed that altering the function of the serotonin system alters many of the behaviors and somatic functions that form the core symptoms of clinical depression, including appetite, sleep, sexual function, pain sensitivity, body temperature, and circadian rhythms (Maes and Meltzer 1995). Serotonin neurons have an intrinsic pacemaker-like activity and fire at nearly constant rates during the daytime and then go completely silent during rapid eye movement (REM) sleep. Serotonin neuronal firing is relatively constant, but serotonin release is quite stress responsive. Physical stresses, such as foot shock, immobilization, and forced swimming, as well as nonphysical stress paradigms increase serotonin release in many brain areas (Adell et al. 1997).

Along with its role as a classical neurotransmitter, serotonin also has neurotrophic factor–like actions, maintaining the structural integrity of those neurons innervated by it (Azmitia 1999; Duman 2004). Serotonin receptors and the SERT are found on glial cells. Astrocytes and glial cells release a neurotrophic factor, $S100\beta$, in response to stimulation of $5\text{-}HT_{1A}$ receptors. When serotonin input to the adult rat hippocampus is disrupted, a loss of neuronal synapses occurs within 10–14 days. Stimulation of $5\text{-}HT_{1A}$ receptors leads to a restoration of lost synapses and to an increase in dendritic growth. This finding suggests that serotonin may have important effects on maintaining synaptic connections in several brain regions, such as the hippocampus (Duman 2004).

Static and Postmortem Studies of the Serotonin System

Various static markers for serotonin have frequently but not consistently been found abnormal in depressed patients. Decreased plasma free and/or total tryptophan levels or a decreased ratio of tryptophan to competing large neutral amino acids has been reported in drug-free depressed patients (Maes and Meltzer 1995). Decreased lumbar and ventricular cerebrospinal fluid (CSF) tryptophan has been reported. However, not all studies have confirmed these findings, and plasma tryptophan can be reduced by glucocorticoids, tricyclic antidepressants, and salicylates as well as some dietary manipulations. Additionally, several drugs and some cytokines increase tryptophan pyrrolase activity, shunting tryptophan away from the serotonin pathway and toward the production of quinolinic acid, reducing both plasma tryptophan levels and serotonin synthesis (Badawy 1977).

One of the most consistent findings in biological psychiatry has been the association of decreased CSF 5-HIAA with impulsivity, aggression, and violent suicide (Asberg et al. 1976). Most authors conclude that a subgroup of depressed patients (35%) fall into a low CSF 5-HIAA group and that patients with low CSF 5-HIAA are more prone to impulsive, violent suicide, although the finding is not specific to mood disorders (Asberg and Forslund 2000).

Measurement of platelet SERT number and function has been used as a proxy for SERT function in the brain. Many studies of serotonin uptake by the SERT on platelets have found decreased uptake in drug-free depressed patients compared with healthy control subjects, even though the SERT number appears to be normal (Healy et al. 1990).

Various studies have assessed markers for neurochemical function in the postmortem brains of people with a history of depression or of suicide victims (see also Raj-

kowska, Chapter 11, in this volume). These studies are inherently limited because of the difficulty in obtaining reliable clinical information about diagnoses and course of illness, especially, alcohol or illicit drug use. Postsuicide studies are especially problematic because they often include people without psychiatric diagnoses or those with schizophrenia or bulimia.

Postmortem studies have reported a decreased number of SERT in the frontal cortex of suicide victims (Stanley et al. 1982) and in the hippocampus and occipital cortex of depressed patients (Perry et al. 1983). SERT binding also was decreased in the PFC of suicide victims (Arango et al. 2003) and patients with antemortem depression (Mann et al. 2000). [^{3}H]Paroxetine binding to the SERT was not altered in the midbrain of depressed suicide victims (Bligh-Glover et al. 2000).

Increased platelet $5\text{-}HT_2$ receptors in blood from depressed or suicidal patients have been reported, although many studies have not replicated these findings, and a recent review has raised important questions about the inconsistent methodology used in prior studies (Muller-Oerlinghausen et al. 2004). Most investigators have found increased $5\text{-}HT_2$ binding in the postmortem brains of some depressed patients and suicide victims (Rosel et al. 2004) compared with postmortem brains from nondepressed age-, sex-, and time to autopsy–matched individuals. In contrast, a recent positron emission tomography (PET) study (Mintun et al. 2004) found decreased $5\text{-}HT_{2A}$ receptors in antidepressant-free depressed patients.

Several postmortem studies in suicide victims reported a reduction in $5\text{-}HT_{1A}$ receptors in the dorsal raphe and median raphe (Arango et al. 2001). PET studies have reported a reduction in the binding of the selective $5\text{-}HT_{1A}$ receptor ligand [^{11}C]WAY-100635 in the raphe nuclei and in several cortical regions in depressed subjects compared with healthy control subjects (Drevets et al. 1999; Sargent et al. 2000). Parsey et al. (2002) found higher $5\text{-}HT_{1A}$ binding in the dorsal raphe, amygdala, anterior cingulate, medial PFC, and orbital PFC in healthy control women compared with men, suggesting that sex differences exist for $5\text{-}HT_{1A}$ binding.

The SERT gene (*SLC6A4*) is located on chromosome 17 (17q11.1–12). A functional polymorphism of the promoter region of the SERT gene (5-HTTLPR) has a 44–base pair insertion and deletion. In the presence of the insertion, the allele is labeled *l* for long, and in the absence of the insertion, the allele is labeled *s* for short (Lesch et al. 1996). The gene frequency is 57% for *l* and 43% for *s* in Caucasians. In humans, the 5-HTTLPR genotypes are distributed according to Hardy-Weinberg equilibrium: 32% *ll*, 49% *ls*, and 19% *ss* (Lesch et al. 1996). In vitro studies show that the *l* allele is associated with a two to three times greater basal transcriptional activity and higher activity in response to cyclic adenosine monophosphate (cAMP) and protein kinase C than the *s* allele.

Studies that used brain imaging to measure SERT number relative to genotype have reported inconsistent results (Heinz et al. 2000; van Dyck et al. 2004). Postmortem studies also have been inconsistent (Little et al. 1998; Mann et al. 2000), as have studies investigating the association of 5-HTTLPR genotypes with depression or suicide (Du et al. 1999; Mann et al. 2000; Ohara et al. 1998) (see also Berrettini, Chapter 14, in this volume). Recent data suggest that people with the *ss* genotype are more likely to experience depression or suicidal ideation with repeated stress than are those with *ll* or *ls* genotypes (Caspi et al. 2003).

Neuroendocrine Challenges of the Serotonin System

Release of serotonin increases release of various pituitary hormones, including prolactin, corticotropin, and growth hormone. Various compounds have been used to stimulate serotonin release or serotonin receptors' these compounds include tryptophan; 5-hydroxytryptophan; fenfluramine; clomipramine; and azaspirodecanedione drugs such as buspirone, ipsapirone, gepirone, and tandospirone. The most consistent finding from this research is that the prolactin response to intravenous tryptophan, fenfluramine, and clomipramine is blunted in most depressed patients compared with control subjects (Delgado et al. 1992). Less consistent effects have been seen with the 5-HT_1 receptor agonist *m*-chlorophenylpiperazine (m-CPP) or azaspirodecanediones.

Serotonin Depletion Challenges

The idea to use neurotransmitter depletion as a research tool dates to the 1950s. The discovery of the synthetic pathways for monoamines made it possible to deplete them by pharmacologically blocking a step in synthesis or limiting the availability of an essential amino acid precursor. It was known that a subset of people taking the nonselective monoamine-depleting agent reserpine for hypertension developed clinical symptoms of depression (Freis 1954). In order to be more selective, several reversible synthesis inhibitors were developed and studied in humans; these included *p*-chlorophenylalanine (PCPA), a reversible inhibitor of tryptophan hydroxylase, the rate-limiting step in the synthesis of serotonin (Koe and Weissman 1966), and α-methyl-*p*-tyrosine (AMPT), a reversible inhibitor of tyrosine hydroxylase, the rate-limiting enzyme in NE and DA synthesis (Engelman et al. 1968).

In a study of nonpsychiatric patients with serotonin-producing carcinoid tumors, PCPA reduced serotonin metabolism and led to lethargy, irritability, anxiety, depression, and psychosis, although most subjects showed little behavior change (W. T. Carpenter 1970). Two landmark studies showed that PCPA administration rapidly reversed the antidepressant effects of tranylcypromine (Shopsin et al. 1976) or imipramine (Shopsin et al. 1975). Depressed patients experienced a depressive relapse within 24 hours of the initiation of PCPA treatment and a return to remission within 24 hours of discontinuation. PCPA use was discontinued in the late 1970s because of concerns over tolerability and safety.

In part because of the absence of acceptable pharmacological agents, precursor depletion challenges became the most extensively studied method of serotonin depletion. Brain serotonin synthesis is acutely sensitive to tryptophan availability because the enzyme tryptophan hydroxylase is poorly saturated. In humans, oral administration of a 15–amino acid, tryptophan-free drink reduces plasma tryptophan by 80% within 5 hours of the drink (Delgado et al. 1990) and decreases CSF 5-HIAA by 25% when measured by continuous CSF sampling (L.L. Carpenter et al. 1998) or single lumbar puncture (Moreno et al. 2000). PET imaging with [^{11}C]α-methyltryptophan showed that tryptophan depletion reduced the rate of brain serotonin synthesis by 80%–90% within 5 hours of amino acid drink consumption (Nishizawa et al. 1997). Tryptophan depletion decreased 5-HT_2 receptor binding in various cortical regions, as measured with PET (Yatham et al. 2001), and it specifically altered brain metabolic activity (Neumeister et al. 2004) and electroencephalographic activity (P. Moore et al. 1998).

The most consistent behavioral effects of tryptophan depletion have been reported in depressed patients who responded to and continued to take potent serotonin reuptake inhibitor antidepressants during the depletion challenge. Many studies have shown that in this patient group, tryptophan depletion can transiently reverse antidepressant response, causing a short-lived return of core depressive symptoms during the time corresponding with the maximal depletion (Aberg-Wistedt et al. 1998; Bremner et al. 1997; Delgado et al. 1990, 1999; Neumeister et al. 2004; Spillmann et al. 2001). Similar depressive responses have been reported in light therapy–treated patients with seasonal affective disorder (Lam et al. 1996; Neumeister et al. 1997). In contrast to the robust effects seen in patients taking potent serotonin reuptake inhibitor antidepressants, patients who responded to and continued taking noradrenergic antidepressants such as desipramine (Delgado et al. 1999) and patients with bipolar disorder taking lithium (Benkelfat et al. 1995; Hughes et al. 2000; Johnson et al. 2001) were less likely to experience depressive symptoms during tryptophan depletion. Tryptophan depletion in healthy subjects receiving fluoxetine resulted in no mood effects (Barr et al. 1997).

Tryptophan depletion in medication-free depressed patients has yielded more variable results. The majority of studies have reported that most nondepressed, medication-free people with a history of major depression experienced moderate depressive symptoms during tryptophan depletion (Moreno et al. 1999; Smith et al. 1997), although not all investigators have found this outcome (Leyton et al. 1997; Neumeister et al. 2004). In contrast, symptomatic, medication-free patients with major depression did not have worse symptoms during tryptophan depletion (Berman et al. 2002; Delgado et al. 1994). Medication-free patients with panic disorder (Goddard et al. 1994), obsessive-compulsive disorder (Barr et al. 1992), or Tourette's disorder (Rasmusson et al. 1997) also showed no depressive symptoms during tryptophan depletion. Tryptophan depletion also did not induce depression in nondepressed, abstinent cocaine abusers (Satel et al. 1995) or alcoholic patients (Petrakis et al. 2001). Cue exposure during tryptophan depletion caused an increased craving for cocaine in cocaine abusers (Satel et al. 1995) but not for alcohol in alcoholic patients (Petrakis et al. 2001); however, nondepressed subjects with coexisting alcohol dependence and major depression showed an increase in cue-induced craving for alcohol during tryptophan depletion (Pierucci-Lagha et al. 2004).

Tryptophan depletion causes either no change or transient, mild, nonclinical increases in negative mood in healthy young men (Young et al. 1985). Healthy people with a multigenerational family history of a major mood disorder appear to be more likely to experience negative mood states or impaired cognition during tryptophan depletion compared with those without such a family history (Sobczak et al. 2002). Healthy women may have greater mood responses than do men (Ellenbogen et al. 1996), consistent with the finding that women show a greater reduction in serotonin synthesis during tryptophan depletion (Nishizawa et al. 1997).

Genetic differences in the serotonin system may contribute to mood response to tryptophan depletion. In healthy women, mood response to tryptophan depletion was greatest in those homozygous for the *s* genotype (Neumeister et al. 2002), whereas in depressed patients, mood response was greatest in those homozygous for the *l* genotype (Moreno et al. 2002). Patients with co-occurring alcohol dependence and major depression showed a mood response to tryptophan depletion similar to that of the depressed patients, with the effect being seen predominantly in those homozygous for the *l* polymorphism (Pierucci-Lagha et al. 2004).

The results of tryptophan depletion challenge studies are summarized in Table 6–1. These data suggest that both trait and state variables affect the likelihood of a depressive response to depletion. These data show that decreased serotonin neurotransmission may contribute to vulnerability to depression (trait) but may not directly mediate the actual symptoms of depression, suggesting that reduced serotonin function *may* be necessary but is clearly not sufficient to induce the symptoms of major depression (Delgado 2004).

Norepinephrine System in Mood Disorders

Anatomy and Physiology of the Norepinephrine System

The synthesis of NE is dependent on availability of the precursor amino acid tyrosine and phenylalanine. Tyrosine, one of eight large neutral amino acids, is competitively transported across the blood-brain barrier from the serum to the CSF by a large, neutral amino acid carrier. Tyrosine is converted to L-dihydroxyphenylalanine (L-dopa) by the rate-limiting enzyme for NE synthesis, tyrosine hydroxylase. L-Dopa is then rapidly decarboxylated to DA. DA is taken up into vesicles and metabolized to NE by DA β-hydroxylase. Vesicular NE is then transported to nerve terminals, where release of NE into the synaptic cleft occurs during neuronal firing in a calcium-dependent process. Synaptic NE is rapidly taken back up into presynaptic terminals by the NE transporter (NET) or into DA terminals by the DA transporter (DAT) (Torres et al. 2003). NE is then either transported back into vesicles or metabolized intraneuronally by MAO-A, producing 3,4-dihydroxyphenylglycol (DHPG) or 3,4-dihydroxymandelic acid (DHMA). These compounds are then metabolized further into the primary NE metabolites 3-methoxy-4-hydroxyphenylglycol (MHPG) or 3-methoxy-4-hydroxymandelic acid (VMA).

NE neurons in the central nervous system (CNS) originate from several distinct nuclei in the brain stem and project rostrally to almost all areas of the mid- and forebrain, dorsoventrally to the cerebellum, and caudally to the lumbar segments of the spinal cord (Ungerstedt 1971). About half of all CNS NE cell bodies originate from the locus coeruleus (LC) in the dorsal pons (Grant and Redmond 1981). A natural loss of LC neurons occurs with aging. NE mediates its effects on target neurons via receptors classified into three groups according to G-protein coupling: the β-adrenergic subtype (G_s coupled; β_1, β_2); the α_2-adrenergic subtype (G_i coupled; α_{2a}, α_{2b},

TABLE 6-1.   Depressive symptoms during neurotransmitter depletion

Population	Subpopulation	Tryptophan[a]	NE or DA[b]	Placebo[c]
Subjects with major depressive disorder	SSRI responders[d]	+++	No	No
	NE reuptake inhibitor responders[d]	No	+++	No
	Mirtazapine responders	+++	+++	−
Subjects with seasonal affective disorder	Light therapy responders	+++	+++	No
	Untreated depressed	No	No	No
	Untreated remitted	+++	+++	No
Subjects with bipolar disorder	Lithium responders	No	No	No
Healthy subjects	Men	±	±	No
	Women	±	±	No
	Healthy subjects taking fluvoxamine	No	No	
	Healthy subjects with positive family history	+	+	No

Note. NE=norepinephrine; DA=dopamine; SSRI=selective serotonin reuptake inhibitor; +++=statistically significant increase in clinically significant depressive symptoms compared with placebo; No=no statistically significant mood effects compared with placebo condition; for placebo condition, no describes absence of effect; SAD=seasonal affective disorder; ±=inconsistent results: some studies report mild symptoms, and some report no symptoms; +=statistically significant increase in mild depressive symptoms compared with placebo.
[a]Tryptophan depletion: via ingestion of a 100-g tryptophan-free 15–amino acid drink.
[b]NE or DA depletion: via ingestion of α-methyl-*p*-tyrosine (AMPT) 1 g three times a day or tyrosine- and phenylalanine-free amino acid drink.
[c]Placebo: for amino acid drink depletions, a balanced amino acid drink; for AMPT depletion, diphenhydramine.
[d]SSRI or NE reuptake inhibitor responder: results in patients having achieved and for 2 consecutive weeks maintained a 50% reduction in Hamilton Rating Scale for Depression score from baseline.

α_{2C}); and the α_1-adrenergic subtype (G_x coupled; α_{1a}, α_{1b}) (Bylund 1988).

The NE system modulates the function of the PFC. The PFC is densely innervated by both NE and DA systems. The PFC is involved in the process of using working memory to regulate behavior and attention, allowing for inhibition of inappropriate responses. Lesions of the NE system impair several other functions of the PFC, including maintenance of sustained and shifting attention. Deficits induced by NE depletion or lesions of the PFC can be reversed by administration of drugs that stimulate α_2-adrenergic receptors on PFC neurons (Friedman et al. 1999). The LC is also activated by a variety of stressful and aversive conditions, and this is thought to contribute to some of the behavioral symptoms of stress as well as being an adaptive response (Valentino et al. 1993).

The NE system also plays an important role in the acquisition of emotionally arousing memories. For example, when people are asked to describe their memory of prewritten vignettes with or without emotionally charged content, recall for details of the memory that included emotionally arousing material is significantly greater than recall for an emotionally neutral one (Cahill et al. 1994).

This effect can be blocked by propranolol (Cahill et al. 2000), a β-adrenergic antagonist that crosses the blood-brain barrier, but not by nadolol (van Stegeren et al. 1998), a β-adrenergic antagonist that does not enter the CNS. These and other data have led to the hypothesis that NE modulates the amygdala in such a way as to strengthen memory consolidation and fear conditioning, playing an essential role in conveying emotional significance to memories of prior experience (Cahill et al. 2001).

Static and Postmortem Studies of the Norepinephrine System

Many studies have investigated plasma, urine, and CSF levels of NE and/or its main metabolite, MHPG, in patients with mood disorders and healthy control subjects. The results of these studies have been inconsistent and frequently negative (Ressler and Nemeroff 1999). Many investigators had hoped that direct measurement in the CSF would uncover the much-sought-after abnormality in NE function, but the data also have been inconsistent and mostly negative, possibly because of the many methodological issues involved (Linnoila et al. 1983).

Many studies also have investigated NE receptors on platelets and lymphocytes. Increased platelet α_2-adrenergic receptor numbers have been reported with only some ligands in patients with mood disorders compared with healthy subjects. Studies of peripheral α_2-adrenergic receptor responsiveness also have been contradictory, as have studies measuring lymphocyte β-adrenergic receptors. Conversely, studies measuring the cAMP response to stimulation of β-adrenergic receptors by β-adrenergic agonists have more consistently reported a blunted response in depressed patients when compared with healthy subjects (Ressler and Nemeroff 1999).

Postmortem analysis of brain tissue from suicide victims has found increased density and affinity of α_2 adrenoceptors in the frontal cortex (Callado et al. 1998) and LC (Ordway et al. 2003). When compared with healthy control subjects, depressed patients showed an increased blood flow response to intravenous clonidine in the right superior PFC when measured with $[^{15}O]H_2O$ PET (Fu et al. 2001), consistent with a greater density and affinity of α_2 receptors in this region.

Postmortem studies also showed that some individuals with depression or suicide had decreased neuronal density in the LC compared with control subjects (Rajkowska, Chapter 11, in this volume). Studies measuring tyrosine hydroxylase activity have reported inconsistent results. Reduced binding of radiolabeled nisoxetine, a ligand for the NE reuptake transporter, has been reported in the postmortem LC tissue from suicide victims and patients with depression (Klimek et al. 1997).

Neuroendocrine Challenges of the Norepinephrine System

Several different types of neuroendocrine challenge–type studies have been aimed at assessing NE function in mood disorders. The most consistent data were obtained by investigating growth hormone response to α_2-adrenergic receptor agonists such as clonidine. Many studies have noted that the growth hormone response to clonidine is blunted in drug-free depressed patients (Schittecatte et al. 1994). Unfortunately, a blunted growth hormone response to clonidine is not specific to patients with major depression because it is also reported in patients with panic disorder, generalized anxiety disorder, social phobia, obsessive-compulsive disorder, alcohol dependence, Gilles de la Tourette syndrome, and schizoaffective disorder.

Norepinephrine Depletion Challenges

Many studies have been performed that attempted to understand the role of NE in depression through depletion of NE. However, selective NE depletion is not currently feasible. Therefore, all published studies aimed at depleting NE in humans also have depleted DA and therefore would most appropriately be described as catecholamine depletion studies. Two methods of catecholamine depletion have been widely used: 1) pharmacological inhibition of tyrosine hydroxylase and 2) depletion of the precursor amino acids tyrosine and phenylalanine. Table 6–1 summarizes the results of catecholamine depletion studies.

Tyrosine hydroxylase is competitively inhibited by AMPT. In humans, 3 g/day of AMPT reduces urinary MHPG by 70% and CSF levels of homovanillic acid (HVA) by 61% with no change in 5-HIAA (Bunney et al. 1971). Maximum reduction of catecholamine metabolites occurs within 48–72 hours and returns to normal within 3–4 days after discontinuation of AMPT (Engelman et al. 1968).

AMPT administered daily for several months to patients with various general medical problems was not noted to cause significant changes in mood in most subjects (Engelman et al. 1968), although sedation is a common initial side effect, and insomnia can occur for a few days after discontinuation (Bunney et al. 1971; McCann et al. 1995). In an open treatment trial of AMPT in patients with essential hypertension, 6 of 20 hypertensive patients had a history of a depressive episode. Three of these 6 became agitated while taking AMPT, requiring drug discontinuation (Engelman et al. 1968). AMPT reduced manic symptoms in 5 of 7 bipolar patients in the manic phase, but unexpectedly, 2 of these manic patients had an increase in manic symptoms (Brodie et al. 1971; Bunney et al. 1971). In the same study, 3 of 4 psychotic depressed patients became more depressed during AMPT treatment (Brodie et al. 1971; Bunney et al. 1971). AMPT had no effect on the antidepressant response to imipramine in 3 patients with major depression who had responded to imipramine and continued to take it during the AMPT exposure (Shopsin et al. 1975).

The most prominent mood effects of AMPT have been in depressed patients who received and continued to take an antidepressant with potent effects on NE reuptake inhibition (Delgado et al. 1993; Miller et al. 1996). Patients who achieved and maintained a treatment response to desipramine were more likely to have a temporary return of depressive symptoms during exposure to 3 g/day of AMPT than were those successfully treated with fluoxetine or sertraline (Delgado et al. 1993; Miller et al. 1996). These findings are the mirror image of the results with the use of rapid plasma tryptophan depletion (Delgado et al. 1999).

Similar to the results with tryptophan depletion, the symptoms of unmedicated, currently depressed patients did not worsen during exposure to 3 g/day of AMPT. Severity of depression did not alter the behavioral response to depletion, which suggests that the lack of response was not easily explained by postulating a "floor" or "ceiling" effect (Berman et al. 2002; Miller et al. 1996).

Studies in healthy volunteers with no personal or family history of depression showed that depletion alone could not bring about depressive symptoms (Krahn et al. 1999). However, in patients who had recovered from recurrent episodes of major depression and who were medication-free, most of the patients experienced a transient return of depressive symptoms in response to catecholamine depletion (Berman et al. 1999).

Tyrosine or phenylalanine depletion produces mild depressive feelings in healthy individuals; subjects report feeling less "content" and have a greater bias for emotionally negative words (McLean et al. 2004) or report diminished ratings of "feel good" (Harmer et al. 2001).

Dopamine System in Mood Disorders

Anatomy and Physiology of the Dopamine System

Inside DA neurons, tyrosine is converted to L-dopa by tyrosine hydroxylase. L-Dopa is then decarboxylated to DA by L-aromatic amino acid decarboxylase. Because of the high activity of this enzyme and the low L-dopa levels in the brain, L-dopa loading can induce dramatic increases in the production of DA. Synaptic DA is rapidly taken back up into DA presynaptic terminals by the DAT or into NE terminals by the NET (Torres et al. 2003).

DA cell bodies located in the ventral mesencephalon account for most DA cell bodies and project widely throughout the CNS. These cell bodies give rise to the nigrostriatal, mesocortical, and mesolimbic DA projections. DA cell bodies projecting to the hypothalamus and pituitary arise from a different brain region and are referred to as the *tuberoinfundibular* and *tuberohypophyseal neurons*. These cell bodies arise primarily from the arcuate nucleus. The tuberohypophyseal neurons project ventrally to the neurointermediate lobe of the pituitary, and the tuberoinfundibular neurons project to the hypothalamus and the hypothalamic-hypophyseal portal system. Dopaminergic tuberoinfundibular projections are involved in the tonic inhibition of prolactin secretion and the stimulation of growth hormone release.

DA binds to two broad classes of receptors sometimes referred to as the D_1-like (D_1 and D_5) and the D_2-like (D_2, D_3, D_4). All DA receptors linked to adenylate cyclase signaling pathways and the D_1-like receptors stimulate, and the D_2-like receptors inhibit, adenylate activity. The D_1-like receptor group mainly activates G proteins (G_s or G_{olf}), which stimulate adenylyl cyclases and elevate cytosolic cAMP levels. The D_2-like receptor group mainly activates the inhibitory G proteins (G_i), which decrease cytosolic cAMP levels (Chen and Zhuang 2003).

The D_3, D_4, and D_5 receptors are more localized within certain areas of the CNS, tending to be found in limbic areas, whereas the D_1 and D_2 receptors tend to be present in a much broader range of brain areas and are the predominant subtype found in the striatum (Sokoloff and Schwartz 1995). The D_2 and D_3 receptors are found both pre- and postsynaptically. The presynaptic D_3 receptor functions as an autoreceptor, providing negative feedback inhibition of DA release at some terminals (Langer 1997). Postsynaptic DA receptors are expressed by a wide array of neurons.

As for other monoamine neurons, the DA system is organized in a fashion that suggests that its primary function is modulation of neuronal activity in target projection areas. The nigrostriatal pathway is involved mainly in modulation of motor function, the mesolimbic pathway in reward and motivation, and the mesocortical pathway in working memory and attention (Chen and Zhuang 2003). DA released from mesolimbic neurons projecting to the nucleus accumbens is thought to play a central role in mediating aspects of the reinforcing properties of a variety of drugs of abuse and pleasurable behaviors (Koob 1996; Naranjo et al. 2001). DA release in the PFC and core of the nucleus accumbens also occurs with aversive stimuli or stress (Claustre et al. 1986). However, in the nucleus accumbens shell, DA release is unchanged or decreased by the aversive stimulus followed by an increase soon after the stimulus ends (Di Chiara et al. 1999). These data suggest that DA's role in hedonic responses, stress, and motivation is complicated and may relate to differences in DA function in discrete brain areas (Naranjo et al. 2001).

Some investigators have hypothesized that dysfunction of DA neurotransmission may be involved in depression and especially in mania (Bridges et al. 1976; Willner 1983). This hypothesis is based on the observations that some DA agonists such as L-dopa, amphetamine, methylphenidate, and bromocriptine have been associated with the development of mania and that DA antagonists are efficacious in the treatment of mania. Furthermore, medications such as bupropion and nomifensine, both of which enhance DA activity, are effective antidepressants. Finally, the role of the DA system in motivation and hedonic responses has led to an interest in whether the DA system plays a role in mood disorders (Naranjo et al. 2001; Willner 1983).

Static and Postmortem Studies of the Dopamine System

The DA metabolite HVA has been measured in the CSF, and inconsistent results have been reported (Roy et al. 1989). Postmortem studies also have been equivocal (Willner 1995). Decrease in CSF levels of HVA appears to be most pronounced in patients with psychomotor retardation, and CSF HVA levels are elevated in manic patients, although the relation of these differences to locomotor activity cannot be ruled out (Willner 1995).

Postmortem and brain imaging studies have reported inconsistent results in the DA receptor number and DAT binding in depressed patients and in the brains of people who committed suicide.

Neuroendocrine Challenges of the Dopamine System

Neuroendocrine challenge strategies also have been used to assess DA function in depressed patients. However, tuberoinfundibular and tuberohypophyseal DA neurons are regulated differently and may not provide an accurate index of the functional state of the mesolimbic or meso-cortical DA projections (K.E. Moore et al. 1987; Willner 1995). Neuroendocrine responses to apomorphine have been inconsistent, and responses to L-dopa and bromocriptine are normal in depressed patients (Willner 1995).

A rapid but transient improvement in mood has been reported in some depressed patients after acute administration of amphetamine. It has been suggested that the pretreatment improvement in mood following administration of amphetamine in depressed patients may predict subsequent antidepressant response. Additionally, compared with healthy control subjects, depressed patients may have a blunted euphoric response to amphetamine (Naranjo et al. 2001). However, cocaine, which has some of the most potent effects on the release of DA, does not improve mood in most depressed patients (Post et al. 1974).

Neuropeptides in Mood Disorders

Many of the neuropeptides are co-localized and co-released with neurotransmitters such as NE, serotonin, DA, or γ-aminobutyric acid (GABA). For example, neuropeptide Y is mainly located in inhibitory interneurons and commonly co-released with GABA (Baraban and Tallent 2004). In some cases, more than one neuropeptide

is co-localized with a classical neurotransmitter. When expressed in neurons, neuropeptides are stored and released from large dense-core vesicles in a slower manner than classical neurotransmitters (Baraban and Tallent 2004). Neuropeptides are also expressed in all three major classes of glial cell, including oligodendrocytes, microglia, and astrocytes (Ubink et al. 2003). The exact function of co-released neuropeptides is not clear, although they seem to regulate neuronal excitability. In the sections that follow, we review endogenous opioids, somatostatin, and neuropeptide Y. Corticotropin-releasing hormone is discussed in Seidman, Chapter 7, in this volume.

Opioids

The discovery of endogenously occurring opioids and the characterization of opiate receptors stimulated research into their behavioral effects, including the role of these substances in "stress" responses in laboratory animals (Gold et al. 1988). The effects of opioids on mood in depressed and manic patients have been widely studied. Initial results were promising, but subsequent placebo-controlled trials have found no significant antidepressant effects of many synthetic and natural opioids (Berger and Nemeroff 1987). There continues to be an interest in the possible use of some opiate agonists in patients with refractory depression (Stoll and Rueter 1999).

Neuroendocrine effects of opiates, opioids, and opiate antagonists also have been investigated in humans. Some investigations have assessed the effects of methadone and β-endorphin on plasma cortisol levels and the effects of morphine and methadone on plasma prolactin levels. Neuroendocrine response to morphine, methadone, and fentanyl has frequently been blunted in depression; however, the neuroendocrine effects of opiates and opioids may be mediated through catecholamine, serotonin, or histaminergic neurotransmitter systems (Berger and Nemeroff 1987).

Somatostatin

Somatostatin is a tetradecapeptide that was first isolated and characterized in the early 1970s. Initially, somatostatin was identified for its noted effect on inhibiting the release of growth hormone (somatotropin). Somatostatin is found in significant concentrations in the hypothalamus, amygdala, and nucleus accumbens in the human brain. Somatostatin receptors are localized in the deep layers of the cortex, cingulate cortex, claustrum, LC, and limbic system (Bissette and Myers 1992).

Somatostatin is involved in the regulation of a variety of behaviors and vegetative functions in animals, which has led to the hypothesis that it is involved in mood disorders. It is involved in the regulation of slow-wave sleep and REM sleep, food consumption, locomotor activity, analgesia, and learning. Somatostatin also is involved in the regulation of other hormones and neurotransmitters, including thyrotropin-releasing hormone, insulin, glucagon, cholecystokinin, secretin, motilin, calcitonin, parathyroid hormone, DA, NE, serotonin, and acetylcholine (ACH) (Rubinow et al. 1988).

Compared with healthy subjects, depressed patients have been noted to have decreased CSF levels of somatostatin. This finding has been replicated in six other studies, but it is not specific to depressed patients (Bissette and Myers 1992).

Neuropeptide Y

Neuropeptide Y is a 36–amino acid peptide localized primarily in the LC, paraventricular nucleus of the hypothalamus, septohippocampal neurons, nucleus of the solitary tract, and ventral lateral medulla. Neuropeptide Y is also found in the amygdala, hippocampus, cerebral cortex, basal ganglia, and thalamus (Broberger and Hoekfelt 2001). Most neuropeptide Y neurons are short interneurons. It is often co-localized with NE, somatostatin, GABA, and galanin. Neuropeptide Y has effects on pituitary hormone release, autonomic function, and various behaviors in laboratory animals that suggest its possible role in mood disorders (Wahlestedt et al. 1989). Neuropeptide Y mediates its effects through three receptor subtypes: NPY1, NPY2, and NPY3 (Gehlert 1994).

Reduced neuropeptide Y levels have been found in the CSF of patients with major depression (Heilig et al. 2004), and a negative correlation exists between neuropeptide Y levels and ratings of anxiety in depressed patients (Heilig and Widerlov 1995). Neuropeptide Y levels in the cortex are increased by the antidepressant drugs imipramine and zimelidine (Heilig et al. 1988) as well as by electroconvulsive therapy (Wahlestedt et al. 1990). Neuropeptide Y administration has been reported to exert anxiolytic or sedative effects in rats (Heilig et al. 1988).

Central Role of Neuroplasticity in the Pathophysiology of Mood Disorders and Their Treatment

Several converging lines of data suggest that the brain's mechanisms for adaptation to stress may play a fundamental role in the pathophysiology of mood disorders and that antidepressant and mood-stabilizing drugs may medi-

ate their therapeutic effects by targeting these processes (see also Singh et al., Chapter 12, in this volume). Central to this hypothesis are the data showing that certain brain structures—especially the hippocampus—are adversely affected by various forms of environmental stress (Sapolsky 1996; Watanabe et al. 1992). In the mammalian hippocampus, neuronal dendrite branching (arborization) and the formation of new neurons continue into adulthood, and the rates of neurogenesis and arborization are reduced by stress and enhanced by serotonin and NE (Duman 2004; Gould 1999; Santarelli et al. 2003).

Clinical data are consistent with the hypothesis that neuroplastic mechanisms may be involved in mood disorders. Most forms of mood disorders are chronic, with high rates of relapse and recurrence. Additionally, with each subsequent episode of illness, patients with depression are more likely to have future episodes, and later episodes are less likely to be associated with antecedent stressful events; thus, these episodes may be more spontaneous (Kendler et al. 2000). Some genetic factors may predispose to poor stress tolerance; people with the *ss* polymorphism of the 5-HTTLPR are more likely to develop depression or suicidal ideation with recurrent stress (Caspi et al. 2003). Furthermore, structural imaging studies suggested an association between depression and reduced hippocampal volume (Campbell et al. 2004; Sheline et al. 1999) and reduced gray matter volume in the anterior cingulate, gyrus rectus, and orbitofrontal cortex (Ballmaier et al. 2004) (see also Mayberg, Chapter 13, in this volume). Postmortem studies confirm the presence of cellular dysfunction in various limbic structures, including the orbitofrontal cortex and anterior cingulate (Rajkowska, Chapter 11, in this volume).

Monoamine neurotransmitters have both short- and long-term effects on postsynaptic neurons. The long-term effects have increasingly become the focus of attention because they correspond more closely to the temporal pattern of therapeutic response. Increases in synaptic NE and serotonin change the long-term expression of a variety of gene products (Hyman and Nestler 1996), including the production of brain-derived neurotrophic factor (BDNF) (Duman 2004). Mood stabilizers may share certain common effects on neuroplastic mechanisms in bipolar disorder (Manji 2003). Increased BDNF has been hypothesized to be a possible final common pathway for how NE- and serotonin-enhancing drugs mediate their therapeutic effects in depression (Duman 2004). The increase in BDNF and signal transduction mediated by serotonin and NE could be explained by effects of serotonin on 5-HT_{1A} and 5-HT_2 receptors and of NE on either b_1- or α_1-adrenergic receptors (Duman 2004). 5-HT_{2A} receptors may play a complex role in the response to stress. In most cortical areas, 5-HT_{2A} receptors increase BDNF, whereas in the hippocampus, they decrease BDNF (Duman 2004).

Conclusion

Several research findings over the past 15 years have led to a broader focus for research into the biology of mood disorders and have suggested the need for more complex theoretical models. First, it has become increasingly clear that both for the general category of mood disorders and for the more specific subcategories of major depression (Kendler et al. 2003) and bipolar disorder (Belmaker 2004; Manji and Lenox 2000), a single etiology is unlikely. Second, research has implicated dysfunction in emotion-mediating circuits (Campbell et al. 2004; Drevets 2001; Rajkowska 2000; Sheline et al. 1999), but evidence for a primary neurochemical dysfunction has been lacking.

Investigation of various neurotransmitter systems and neuromodulators in patients with mood disorders has identified several differences between patients and healthy control subjects; however, many of these findings are nonspecific or could be a result of stress. For example, animal studies suggested that decreased function of 5-HT_{1A} or 5-HT_2 receptors could be the result of increased cortisol (Cavus and Duman 2003; Lopez et al. 1999). To ensure that neurochemical findings are specific to mood disorders, future studies need to compare patients who have mood disorders with stressed but otherwise healthy people or with other psychiatrically ill patients who do not have mood disorders.

In addition, some of the neurochemical abnormalities summarized in this chapter could serve to increase vulnerability to mood disorders or to act as a trigger for an individual episode. In other words, the data suggest that the neurochemical "abnormalities" summarized in this chapter may not be either necessary or sufficient to explain the illness.

This seems increasingly to be the case for some of the serotonin abnormalities. For example, most people with the *ss* genotype of the 5-HTTLPR do not have major depression; however, when this genotype is present, there is a greater likelihood of major depression after stressful life events (Caspi et al. 2003). Most people with low CSF levels of 5-HIAA do not have major depression, although it is more commonly found in this group than in healthy control subjects. Data on tryptophan depletion and catecholamine depletion suggest the same finding. Most people can show normal mood states when serotonin or NE and DA are depleted; however, some patients with mood disorders rapidly develop depressive symptoms during depletion.

These data converge to suggest that the central pathology in mood disorders may reside in the neurons of the brain circuits underlying emotion. These "sick" neurons may be unable to tolerate diminished serotonin or NE and DA modulation, whereas people with healthier neurons are able to sustain relatively more normal function in the face of diminutions in these key modulating neurotransmitters.

If this hypothesis proves to be correct, then research attention needs to focus increasingly on the integrity of the brain's emotion circuits in patients with mood disorders. In particular, given the likelihood that stressful life events contribute to the pathophysiology of mood disorders, understanding why and how some people are more vulnerable than others to the adverse effects of stress should become a greater focus of attention. As this work unfolds, future chapters on the neurochemistry of mood disorders may very well be reviewing an entirely new set of molecules relevant to cellular integrity and adaptation.

References

Aberg-Wistedt A, Hasselmark L, Stain-Malmgren R, et al: Serotonergic "vulnerability" in affective disorder: a study of the tryptophan depletion test and relationships between peripheral and central serotonin indexes in citalopram-responders. Acta Psychiatr Scand 97:374–380, 1998

Adell A, Casanovas JM, Artigas F: Comparative study in the rat of the actions of different types of stress on the release of 5-HT in raphe nuclei and forebrain areas. Neuropharmacology 36:735–741, 1997

Arango V, Underwood MD, Boldrini M, et al: Serotonin 1A receptors, serotonin transporter binding and serotonin transporter mRNA expression in the brainstem of depressed suicide victims. Neuropsychopharmacology 25:892–903, 2001

Arango V, Huang Y-y, Underwood MD, et al: Genetics of the serotonergic system in suicidal behavior. J Psychiatr Res 37:375–386, 2003

Asberg M, Forslund K: Neurobiological aspects of suicidal behaviour. Int Rev Psychiatry 12:62–74, 2000

Asberg M, Traskman L, Thoren P: 5-HIAA in the cerebrospinal fluid: a biochemical suicide predictor? Arch Gen Psychiatry 33:1193–1197, 1976

Azmitia EC: Serotonin neurons, neuroplasticity, and homeostasis of neural tissue. Neuropsychopharmacology 21 (2 suppl): 33S–45S, 1999

Badawy AA: The functions and regulation of tryptophan pyrrolase. Life Sci 21:755–768, 1977

Ballmaier M, Toga AW, Blanton RE, et al: Anterior cingulate, gyrus rectus, and orbitofrontal abnormalities in elderly depressed patients: an MRI-based parcellation of the prefrontal cortex. Am J Psychiatry 161:99–108, 2004

Baraban SC, Tallent MK: Interneuron Diversity Series: Interneuronal neuropeptides—endogenous regulators of neuronal excitability. Trends Neurosci 27:135–142, 2004

Barr LC, Goodman WK, Price LH, et al: The serotonin hypothesis of obsessive compulsive disorder: implications of pharmacologic challenge studies. J Clin Psychiatry 53:17–28, 1992

Barr LC, Heninger GR, Goodman W, et al: Effects of fluoxetine administration on mood response to tryptophan depletion in healthy subjects. Biol Psychiatry 41:949–954, 1997

Belmaker RH: Bipolar disorder. N Engl J Med 351:476–486, 2004

Benkelfat C, Seletti B, Palmour RM, et al: Tryptophan depletion in stable lithium-treated patients with bipolar disorder in remission. Arch Gen Psychiatry 52:154–155, 1995

Berger P, Nemeroff C: Opioid peptides in affective disorders, in Psychopharmacology: The Third Generation of Progress. Edited by Meltzer HY. New York, Raven, 1987, pp 637–646

Berman RM, Narasimhan M, Miller HL, et al: Transient depressive relapse induced by catecholamine depletion. Arch Gen Psychiatry 56:395–403, 1999

Berman RM, Sanacora G, Anand A, et al: Monoamine depletion in unmedicated depressed subjects. Biol Psychiatry 51:469–473, 2002

Bissette G, Myers B: Minireview: somatostatin in Alzheimer's disease and depression. Life Sci 51:1389–1410, 1992

Bligh-Glover W, Kolli TN, Shapiro-Kulnane L, et al: The serotonin transporter in the midbrain of suicide victims with major depression. Biol Psychiatry 47:1015–1024, 2000

Bloom FE: Introduction to preclinical neuropsychopharmacology, in Psychopharmacology: The Fourth Generation of Progress. Edited by Bloom FE, Kupfer DJ. New York, Raven, 1995, pp 1–7

Bremner J, Innis RB, Salomon RM, et al: Positron emission tomography measurement of cerebral metabolic correlates of tryptophan depletion-induced depressive relapse. Arch Gen Psychiatry 54:364–374, 1997

Bridges PK, Bartlett JR, Sepping P, et al: Precursors and metabolites of 5-hydroxytryptamine and dopamine in the ventricular cerebrospinal fluid of psychiatric patients. Psychol Med 6:399–405, 1976

Broberger C, Hoekfelt T: Hypothalamic and vagal neuropeptide circuitries regulating food intake. Physiol Behav 74:669–682, 2001

Brodie HK, Murphy DL, Goodwin FK, et al: Catecholamines and mania: the effect of alpha-methyl-para-tyrosine on manic behavior and catecholamine metabolism. Clin Pharmacol Ther 12:218–224, 1971

Bunney WE, Brodie H, Murphy DL, et al: Studies of alpha-methyl-para-tyrosine, L-dopa, and L-tryptophan in depression and mania. Am J Psychiatry 127:872–881, 1971

Bylund DB: Subtypes of alpha 2-adrenoceptors: pharmacological and molecular biological evidence converge [see comment]. Trends Pharmacol Sci 9:356–361, 1988

Cahill L, Prins B, Weber M, et al: Beta-adrenergic activation and memory for emotional events. Nature 371:702–704, 1994

Cahill L, Pham CA, Setlow B: Impaired memory consolidation in rats produced with beta-adrenergic blockade. Neurobiol Learn Mem 74:259–266, 2000

Cahill L, McGaugh JL, Weinberger NM: The neurobiology of learning and memory: some reminders to remember. Trends Neurosci 24:578–581, 2001

Callado LF, Meana JJ, Grijalba B, et al: Selective increase of alpha2A-adrenoceptor agonist binding sites in brains of depressed suicide victims. J Neurochem 70:1114–1123, 1998

Campbell S, Marriott M, Nahmias C, et al: Lower hippocampal volume in patients suffering from depression: a meta-analysis. Am J Psychiatry 161:598–607, 2004

Carpenter LL, Anderson GM, Pelton GH, et al: Tryptophan depletion during continuous CSF sampling in healthy human subjects. Neuropsychopharmacology 19:26–35, 1998

Carpenter WT: Serotonin now: clinical implications of inhibiting its synthesis with para-chlorophenylalanine. Ann Intern Med 73:607–630, 1970

Caspi A, Sugden K, Moffitt TE, et al: Influence of life stress on depression: moderation by a polymorphism in the 5-HTT gene. Science 301:386–389, 2003

Cavus I, Duman RS: Influence of estradiol, stress, and 5-HT2A agonist treatment on brain-derived neurotrophic factor expression in female rats. Biol Psychiatry 54:59–69, 2003

Chen L, Zhuang X: Transgenic mouse models of dopamine deficiency [see comment]. Ann Neurol 54 (suppl 6):S91–S102, 2003

Claustre Y, Rivy JP, Dennis T, et al: Pharmacological studies on stress-induced increase in frontal cortical dopamine metabolism in the rat. J Pharmacol Exp Ther 238:693–700, 1986

Coppen A: The biochemistry of affective disorders. Br J Psychiatry 113:1237–1264, 1967

Delgado PL: How antidepressants help depression: mechanisms of action and clinical response. J Clin Psychiatry 65:25–30, 2004

Delgado PL, Charney DS, Price LH, et al: Serotonin function and the mechanism of antidepressant action: reversal of antidepressant-induced remission by rapid depletion of plasma tryptophan. Arch Gen Psychiatry 47:411–418, 1990

Delgado PL, Price LH, Heninger GR, et al: Neurochemistry of affective disorders, in Handbook of Affective Disorders, 2nd Edition. Edited by Paykel ES. Edinburgh, Churchill Livingstone, 1992, pp 219–253

Delgado PL, Miller HL, Salomon RM, et al: Monoamines and the mechanism of antidepressant action: effects of catecholamine depletion on mood of patients treated with antidepressants. Psychopharmacol Bull 29:389–396, 1993

Delgado PL, Price LH, Miller HL, et al: Serotonin and the neurobiology of depression: effects of tryptophan depletion in drug-free depressed patients. Arch Gen Psychiatry 51:865–874, 1994

Delgado PL, Miller HL, Salomon RM, et al: Tryptophan-depletion challenge in depressed patients treated with desipramine or fluoxetine: implications for the role of serotonin in the mechanism of antidepressant action. Biol Psychiatry 46:212–220, 1999

Di Chiara G, Loddo P, Tanda G: Reciprocal changes in prefrontal and limbic dopamine responsiveness to aversive and rewarding stimuli after chronic mild stress: implications for the psychobiology of depression. Biol Psychiatry 46:1624–1633, 1999

Di Matteo V, De Blasi A, Di Giulio C, et al: Role of 5-HT(2C) receptors in the control of central dopamine function. Trends Pharmacol Sci 22:229–232, 2001

Drevets WC: Neuroimaging and neuropathological studies of depression: implications for the cognitive-emotional features of mood disorders. Curr Opin Neurobiol 11:240–249, 2001

Drevets WC, Frank E, Price JC, et al: PET imaging of serotonin 1A receptor binding in depression. Biol Psychiatry 46:1375–1387, 1999

Du L, Faludi G, Palkovits M, et al: Frequency of long allele in serotonin transporter gene is increased in depressed suicide victims. Biol Psychiatry 46:196–201, 1999

Duman RS: Depression: A Case of Neuronal Life and Death? Biol Psychiatry 56:141–145, 2004

Ellenbogen MA, Young SN, Dean P, et al: Mood response to acute tryptophan depletion in healthy volunteers: sex differences and temporal stability. Neuropsychopharmacology 15:465–474, 1996

Engelman K, Horwitz D, Jequier E, et al: Biochemical and pharmacologic effects of alpha-methyltyrosine in man. J Clin Invest 47:577–594, 1968

Freis ED: Mental depression in hypertensive patients treated for long periods with large doses of reserpine. N Engl J Med 251:1006–1008, 1954

Friedman JI, Adler DN, Davis KL: The role of norepinephrine in the pathophysiology of cognitive disorders: potential applications to the treatment of cognitive dysfunction in schizophrenia and Alzheimer's disease. Biol Psychiatry 46:1243–1252, 1999

Fu CH, Reed LJ, Meyer JH, et al: Noradrenergic dysfunction in the prefrontal cortex in depression: an [15O] H2O PET study of the neuromodulatory effects of clonidine. Biol Psychiatry 49:317–325, 2001

Gehlert DR: Subtypes of receptors for neuropeptide Y: implications for the targeting of therapeutics. Life Sci 55:551–562, 1994

Goddard AW, Sholomskas DE, Walton KE, et al: Effects of tryptophan depletion in panic disorder. Biol Psychiatry 36:775–777, 1994

Gold PW, Goodwin FK, Chrousos GP: Clinical and biochemical manifestations of depression: relation to the neurobiology of stress (1) [see comment]. N Engl J Med 319:348–353, 1988

Gould E: Serotonin and hippocampal neurogenesis. Neuropsychopharmacology 21:46S–51S, 1999

Gould E, Tanapat P: Stress and hippocampal neurogenesis. Biol Psychiatry 46:1472–1479, 1999

Grant SJ, Redmond DE Jr: The neuroanatomy and pharmacology of the nucleus locus coeruleus. Prog Clin Biol Res 71:5–27, 1981

Harmer CJ, McTavish SFB, Clark L, et al: Tyrosine depletion attenuates dopamine function in healthy volunteers. Psychopharmacology 154:105–111, 2001

Healy D, Theodorou AE, Whitehouse AM, et al: 3H-imipramine binding to previously frozen platelet membranes from depressed patients, before and after treatment. Br J Psychiatry 157:208–215, 1990

Heilig M, Widerlov E: Neurobiology and clinical aspects of neuropeptide Y. Crit Rev Neurobiol 9:115–136, 1995

Heilig M, Wahlestedt C, Ekman R, et al: Antidepressant drugs increase the concentration of neuropeptide Y (NPY)-like immunoreactivity in the rat brain. Eur J Pharmacol 147:465–467, 1988

Heilig M, Zachrisson O, Thorsell A, et al: Decreased cerebrospinal fluid neuropeptide Y (NPY) in patients with treatment refractory unipolar major depression: preliminary evidence for association with preproNPY gene polymorphism. J Psychiatr Res 38:113–121, 2004

Heinz A, Jones DW, Mazzanti C, et al: A relationship between serotonin transporter genotype and in vivo protein expression and alcohol neurotoxicity. Biol Psychiatry 47:643–649, 2000

Hughes JH, Dunne F, Young AH: Effects of acute tryptophan depletion on mood and suicidal ideation in bipolar patients symptomatically stable on lithium. Br J Psychiatry 177:447–451, 2000

Hyman SE, Nestler EJ: Initiation and adaptation: a paradigm for understanding psychotropic drug action. Am J Psychiatry 153:151–162, 1996

Jacobs BL, Azmitia EC: Structure and function of the brain serotonin system. Physiol Rev 72:165–229, 1992

Johnson L, El-Khoury A, Aberg-Wistedt A, et al: Tryptophan depletion in lithium-stabilized patients with affective disorder. Int J Neuropsychopharmacol 4:329–336, 2001

Kendler KS, Thornton LM, Gardner CO: Stressful life events and previous episodes in the etiology of major depression in women: an evaluation of the "kindling" hypothesis. Am J Psychiatry 157:1243–1251, 2000

Kendler KS, Prescott CA, Myers J, et al: The structure of genetic and environmental risk factors for common psychiatric and substance use disorders in men and women. Arch Gen Psychiatry 60:929–937, 2003

Klimek V, Stockmeier C, Overholser J, et al: Reduced levels of norepinephrine transporters in the locus coeruleus in major depression. J Neurosci 17:8451–8458, 1997

Koe BK, Weissman A: p-Chlorophenylalanine: a specific depletor of brain serotonin. J Pharmacol Exp Ther 154:499–516, 1966

Koob GF: Hedonic valence, dopamine and motivation. Mol Psychiatry 1:186–189, 1996

Krahn LE, Lin SC, Klee GG, et al: The effect of presynaptic catecholamine depletion on 6-hydroxymelatonin sulfate: a double blind study of alpha-methyl-para-tyrosine. Eur Neuropsychopharmacol 9:61–66, 1999

Kroeze WK, Kristiansen K, Roth BL: Molecular biology of serotonin receptors structure and function at the molecular level. Curr Top Med Chem 2:507–528, 2002

Lam RW, Zis AP, Grewal A, et al: Effects of rapid tryptophan depletion in patients with seasonal affective disorder in remission after light therapy. Arch Gen Psychiatry 53:41–44, 1996

Langer SZ: 25 years since the discovery of presynaptic receptors: present knowledge and future perspectives [see comment]. Trends Pharmacol Sci 18:95–99, 1997

LeDoux JE: Emotion circuits in the brain. Annu Rev Neurosci 23:155–184, 2000

Lesch K-P, Bengel D, Heils A, et al: Association of anxiety-related traits with a polymorphism in the serotonin transporter gene regulatory region. Science 274:1527–1531, 1996

Leyton M, Young SN, Blier P, et al: The effect of tryptophan depletion on mood in medication-free former patients with major affective disorder. Neuropsychopharmacology 16:294–297, 1997

Linnoila M, Karoum F, Miller T, et al: Reliability of urinary monoamine and metabolite output measurements in depressed patients. Am J Psychiatry 140:1055–1057, 1983

Little KY, McLaughlin DP, Zhang L, et al: Cocaine, ethanol, and genotype effects on human midbrain serotonin transporter binding sites and mRNA levels. Am J Psychiatry 155:207–213, 1998

Lopez JF, Liberzon I, Vazquez DM, et al: Serotonin 1A receptor messenger RNA regulation in the hippocampus after acute stress. Biol Psychiatry 45:934–937, 1999

Maclean PD: Psychosomatic disease and the "visceral brain"; recent developments bearing on the Papez theory of emotion. Psychosom Med 11:338–353, 1949

Maes M, Meltzer HY: The serotonin hypothesis of major depression, in Psychopharmacology: The Fourth Generation of Progress. Edited by Bloom FE, Kupfer DJ. New York, Raven, 1995, pp 933–944

Manji H: Depression, III: treatments. Am J Psychiatry 160:24, 2003

Manji HK, Lenox RH: The nature of bipolar disorder. J Clin Psychiatry 61:42–57, 2000

Manji HK, Moore GJ, Chen G: Bipolar disorder: leads from the molecular and cellular mechanisms of action of mood stabilisers. Br J Psychiatry 178:S107–S119, 2001

Mann J, Huang Y-y, Underwood MD, et al: A serotonin transporter gene promoter polymorphism (5-HTTLPR) and prefrontal cortical binding in major depression and suicide. Arch Gen Psychiatry 57:729–738, 2000

McCann UD, Thorne D, Hall M, et al: The effects of L-dihydroxyphenylalanine on alertness and mood in alpha-methyl-para-tyrosine-treated healthy humans: further evidence for the role of catecholamines in arousal and anxiety. Neuropsychopharmacology 13:41–52, 1995

McLean A, Rubinsztein JS, Robbins TW, et al: The effects of tyrosine depletion in normal healthy volunteers: implications for unipolar depression. Psychopharmacology 171:286–297, 2004

Miller HL, Delgado PL, Salomon RM, et al: Effects of alpha-methyl-para-tyrosine (AMPT) in drug-free depressed patients. Neuropsychopharmacology 14:151–157, 1996

Mintun MA, Sheline YI, Moerlein SM, et al: Decreased hippocampal 5-HT$_{2A}$ receptor binding in major depressive disorder: in vivo measurement with [18F]altanserin positron emission tomography. Biol Psychiatry 55:217–224, 2004

Moore KE, Demarest KT, Lookingland KJ: Stress, prolactin and hypothalamic dopaminergic neurons. Neuropharmacology 26:801–808, 1987

Moore P, Gillin J, Bhatti T, et al: Rapid tryptophan depletion, sleep electroencephalogram, and mood in men with remitted depression on serotonin reuptake inhibitors. Arch Gen Psychiatry 55:534–539, 1998

Moreno FA, Gelenberg AJ, Heninger GR, et al: Tryptophan depletion and depressive vulnerability. Biol Psychiatry 46:498–505, 1999

Moreno FA, McGavin C, Malan T Jr, et al: Tryptophan depletion selectively reduces CSF 5-HT metabolites in healthy young men: results from single lumbar puncture sampling technique. Int J Neuropsychopharmacol 3:277–283, 2000

Moreno FA, Rowe DC, Kaiser B, et al: Association between a serotonin transporter promoter region polymorphism and mood response during tryptophan depletion. Mol Psychiatry 7:213–216, 2002

Muller-Oerlinghausen B, Roggenbach J, Franke L: Serotonergic platelet markers of suicidal behavior—do they really exist? J Affect Disord 79:13–24, 2004

Naranjo CA, Tremblay LK, Busto UE: The role of the brain reward system in depression. Prog Neuropsychopharmacol Biol Psychiatry 25:781–823, 2001

Nestler EJ, Duman RS: Relevance of intracellular signal transduction pathways to psychiatry, in American Psychiatric Press Review of Psychiatry, Vol 15. Edited by Dickstein L, Riba MB, Oldham JM. Washington, DC, American Psychiatric Press, 1996, pp 279–309

Neumeister A, Praschak-Rieder N, Hesselmann B, et al: Effects of tryptophan depletion on drug-free patients with seasonal affective disorder during a stable response to bright light therapy. Arch Gen Psychiatry 54:133–138, 1997

Neumeister A, Konstantinidis A, Stastny J, et al: Association between serotonin transporter gene promoter polymorphism (5HTTLPR) and behavioral responses to tryptophan depletion in healthy women with and without family history of depression. Arch Gen Psychiatry 59:613–620, 2002

Neumeister A, Nugent AC, Waldeck T, et al: Neural and behavioral responses to tryptophan depletion in unmedicated patients with remitted major depressive disorder and controls. Arch Gen Psychiatry 61:765–773, 2004

Nishizawa S, Benkelfat C, Young SN, et al: Differences between males and females in rates of serotonin synthesis in human brain. Proc Natl Acad Sci USA 94:5308–5313, 1997

Ohara K, Nagai M, Tsukamoto T, et al: Functional polymorphism in the serotonin transporter promoter at the SLC6A4 locus and mood disorders. Biol Psychiatry 44:550–554, 1998

Ordway GA, Schenk J, Stockmeier CA, et al: Elevated agonist binding to alpha$_2$-adrenoceptors in the locus coeruleus in major depression. Biol Psychiatry 53:315–323, 2003

Parsey RV, Oquendo MA, Simpson NR, et al: Effects of sex, age, and aggressive traits in man on brain serotonin 5-HT$_{1A}$ receptor binding potential measured by PET using [C-11]WAY-100635. Brain Res 954:173–182, 2002

Perry EK, Marshall EF, Blessed G, et al: Decreased imipramine binding in the brains of patients with depressive illness. Br J Psychiatry 142:188–192, 1983

Petrakis IL, Trevisan L, Boutros NN, et al: Effect of tryptophan depletion on alcohol cue-induced craving in abstinent alcoholic patients. Alcohol Clin Exp Res 25:1151–1155, 2001

Phillips ML, Drevets WC, Rauch SL, et al: Neurobiology of emotion perception, I: the neural basis of normal emotion perception. Biol Psychiatry 54:504–514, 2003

Pierucci-Lagha A, Feinn R, Modesto-Lowe V, et al: Effects of rapid tryptophan depletion on mood and urge to drink in patients with co-morbid major depression and alcohol dependence. Psychopharmacology 171:340–348, 2004

Post RM, Kotin J, Goodwin FK: The effects of cocaine on depressed patients. Am J Psychiatry 131:511–517, 1974

Rajkowska G: Postmortem studies in mood disorders indicate altered numbers of neurons and glial cells. Biol Psychiatry 48:766–777, 2000

Rasmusson AM, Anderson GM, Lynch KA, et al: A preliminary study of tryptophan depletion on tics, obsessive-compulsive symptoms, and mood in Tourette's syndrome. Biol Psychiatry 41:117–121, 1997

Ressler KJ, Nemeroff CB: Role of norepinephrine in the pathophysiology and treatment of mood disorders. Biol Psychiatry 46:1219–1233, 1999

Rosel P, Arranz B, Urretavizcaya M, et al: Altered 5-HT2A and 5-HT4 postsynaptic receptors and their intracellular signalling systems IP$_3$ and cAMP in brains from depressed violent suicide victims. Neuropsychobiology 49:189–195, 2004

Roy A, de Jong J, Linnoila M: Cerebrospinal fluid monoamine metabolites and suicidal behavior in depressed patients: a 5-year follow-up study. Arch Gen Psychiatry 46:609–612, 1989

Rubinow DR, Davis CL, Post RM: Somatostatin in neuropsychiatric disorders. Prog Neuropsychopharmacol Biol Psychiatry 12:137–155, 1988

Santarelli L, Saxe M, Gross C, et al: Requirement of hippocampal neurogenesis for the behavioral effects of antidepressants. Science 301:805–809, 2003

Sapolsky RM: Why stress is bad for your brain. Science 273:749–750, 1996

Sapolsky RM: Glucocorticoids and hippocampal atrophy in neuropsychiatric disorders. Arch Gen Psychiatry 57:925–935, 2000

Sargent PA, Kjaer KH, Bench CJ, et al: Brain serotonin-$_{1A}$ receptor binding measured by positron emission tomography with [11C]WAY-100635: effects of depression and antidepressant treatment. Arch Gen Psychiatry 57:174–180, 2000

Satel SL, Krystal JH, Delgado PL, et al: Tryptophan depletion and attenuation of cue-induced craving for cocaine. Am J Psychiatry 152:778–783, 1995

Schildkraut JJ: The catecholamine hypothesis of affective disorders: a review of supporting evidence. Am J Psychiatry 122:509–522, 1965

Schittecatte M, Charles G, Machowski R, et al: Effects of gender and diagnosis on growth hormone response to clonidine for major depression: a large-scale multicenter study. Am J Psychiatry 151:216–220, 1994

Sheline YI, Sanghavi M, Mintun MA, et al: Depression duration but not age predicts hippocampal volume loss in medically healthy women with recurrent major depression. J Neurosci 19:5034–5043, 1999

Shopsin B, Gershon S, Goldstein M, et al: Use of synthesis inhibitors in defining a role for biogenic amines during imipramine treatment in depressed patients. Psychopharmacol Commun 1:239–249, 1975

Shopsin B, Friedman E, Gershon S: Parachlorophenylalanine reversal of tranylcypromine effects in depressed patients. Arch Gen Psychiatry 33:811–819, 1976

Smith KA, Clifford EM, Hockney RA, et al: Effect of tryptophan depletion on mood in male and female volunteers: a pilot study. Hum Psychopharmacol 12:111–117, 1997

Sobczak S, Riedel WJ, Booij I, et al: Cognition following acute tryptophan depletion: difference between first-degree relatives of bipolar disorder patients and matched healthy control volunteers. Psychol Med 32:503–515, 2002

Sokoloff P, Schwartz JC: Novel dopamine receptors half a decade later. Trends Pharmacol Sci 16:270–275, 1995

Spillmann MK, Van der Does A, Rankin MA, et al: Tryptophan depletion in SSRI-recovered depressed outpatients. Psychopharmacology 155:123–127, 2001

Stanley M, Virgilio J, Gershon S: Tritiated imipramine binding sites are decreased in the frontal cortex of suicides. Science 216:1337–1339, 1982

Stoll AL, Rueter S: Treatment augmentation with opiates in severe and refractory major depression. Am J Psychiatry 156:2017, 1999

Torres GE, Gainetdinov RR, Caron MG: Plasma membrane monoamine transporters: structure, regulation and function. Nat Rev Neurosci 4:13–25, 2003

Ubink R, Calza L, Hokfelt T: "Neuro"-peptides in glia: focus on NPY and galanin. Trends Neurosci 26:604–609, 2003

Ungerstedt U: Stereotaxic mapping of the monoamine pathways in the rat brain. Acta Physiol Scand Suppl 367:1–48, 1971

Valentino RJ, Foote SL, Page ME: The locus coeruleus as a site for integrating corticotropin-releasing factor and noradrenergic mediation of stress responses. Ann N Y Acad Sci 697:173–188, 1993

van Dyck CH, Malison RT, Staley JK, et al: Central serotonin transporter availability measured with [123I]beta-CIT SPECT in relation to serotonin transporter genotype. Am J Psychiatry 161:525–531, 2004

van Stegeren AH, Everaerd W, Cahill L, et al: Memory for emotional events: differential effects of centrally versus peripherally acting beta-blocking agents. Psychopharmacology 138:305–310, 1998

Wahlestedt C, Blendy JA, Kellar KJ, et al: Electroconvulsive shocks increase the concentration of neocortical and hippocampal neuropeptide Y (NPY)-like immunoreactivity in the rat. Brain Res 507:65–68, 1990

Wahlestedt C, Ekman R, Widerlov E: Neuropeptide Y (NPY) and the central nervous system: distribution effects and possible relationship to neurological and psychiatric disorders. Prog Neuropsychopharmacol Biol Psychiatry 13:31–54, 1989

Watanabe Y, Gould E, McEwen BS: Stress induces atrophy of apical dendrites of hippocampal CA3 pyramidal neurons. Brain Res 588:341–345, 1992

Willner P: Dopamine and depression: a review of recent evidence, I: empirical studies. Brain Res Rev 6:211–224, 1983

Willner P: Dopaminergic mechanisms in depression and mania, in Psychopharmacology: The Fourth Generation of Progress. Edited by Bloom FE, Kupfer DJ. New York, Raven, 1995, pp 921–931

Yatham LN, Liddle PF, Shiah IS, et al: Effects of rapid tryptophan depletion on brain 5-HT(2) receptors: a PET study. Br J Psychiatry 178:448–453, 2001

Young SN, Smith SE, Pihl RO, et al: Tryptophan depletion causes a rapid lowering of mood in normal males. Psychopharmacology 87:173–177, 1985

7

Psychoneuroendocrinology of Mood Disorders

STUART N. SEIDMAN, M.D.

INCREASED INTEREST IN the relation between hormone axes (and the neural circuits that regulate them) and mood disorders is primarily a result of the following observations: 1) in addition to being the regulator of hormonal systems, the brain is a primary target organ of hormones—and activation leads to emotional and behavioral outcomes; 2) neural circuits that regulate hormone axes are intimately involved in the pathophysiology of mood disorders; and 3) endocrinopathies commonly affect mood and behavior (Halbreich 1997).

A primary role of hormones is to coordinate behavior with other physiological events in the body (e.g., sexual behavior with fertility, food seeking with the appropriate metabolic state). Modern endocrinological investigations have explored the mechanism of hormonal influence on central nervous system (CNS) processes, such as cerebral blood flow, receptors, enzymes, cell membranes, and signal transduction (McEwen 1998; Mong and Pfaff 2003). As it has become clear that hormones target the CNS and affect behavior, the use of exogenous hormones to treat

psychiatric disorders has gained momentum (see Seidman, Chapter 19, in this volume). Indeed, accumulating evidence suggests the following: Thyroid hormone may be an effective adjunct to antidepressant medication and, further, may accelerate the rate of antidepressant response; gonadal steroids (i.e., testosterone in men and estrogen in women) may be effective antidepressants in selected groups of elderly depressed individuals; and antiglucocorticoids and dehydroepiandrosterone (DHEA) may have some antidepressant properties.

The relation between hormone axis physiology and psychiatric symptoms and syndromes is complex and bidirectional. That is, endocrinopathies are associated with reversible psychiatric syndromes, and primary psychiatric conditions are associated with hormonal dysregulations (Prange 1998). Indeed, the primary goal of some of the pioneers in biological psychiatry, such as Manfred Bleuler and Edward Sachar, was to relate psychopathology to endocrine dysregulation. Although this approach was overshadowed by the dramatic advances in the psychopharma-

The author thanks Donald F. Klein, M.D., for his comments on an earlier version of this manuscript, Steven P. Roose, M.D., for his support of the research, and the Partnership for Gender-Specific Medicine and the National Institute of Mental Health (grant K23 MH1740) for salary support.

cological approach, important contributions continue to be made that suggest that hormone axis dysregulation may be etiologically related to affective illness (Holsboer 2001).

Endocrinopathies that are associated with state-dependent psychiatric symptoms include the following: 1) male hypogonadism with loss of libido, low mood, and low energy; 2) hypothyroidism with depression and cognitive dysfunction; 3) hyperthyroidism with anxiety, irritability, and psychomotor agitation; 4) acromegaly with hypersomnia and loss of libido; 5) Cushing's syndrome and Addison's disease with dysphoric mood; 6) hypercortisolemia with euphoria and psychosis; and 7) hyperprolactinemia with low libido (Halbreich 1997; Prange 1998; Seidman and Walsh 1999). Bleuler's demonstration that hormone replacement led to improvement in psychiatric symptoms led to major efforts to assess endocrinological functioning in psychiatric patients.

Psychoendocrine investigators subsequently found hormonal dysregulations associated with psychiatric conditions, particularly with respect to the hypothalamic-pituitary-adrenal (HPA) and hypothalamic-pituitary-thyroid (HPT) axes in affective disorders (Rubin et al. 1987, 1989; Steiger et al. 1993). That changes in neuroendocrine function have been shown so consistently in major depressive disorder (MDD) suggests that neuroendocrine axes are intimately involved in the pathophysiology of this disorder and may even be the substrate for the fundamental defect (Nemeroff 2002). Two hypotheses relating to hormones and neuropsychiatry have emerged: 1) psychotropic drugs may be able to target the neuronal circuits that regulate neuroendocrine function; and 2) psychotropic effects of gonadal steroids, corticosteroids, thyroid hormones, brain-secreted hormones (neurosteroids), and neuroregulatory peptides may play a role in the treatment of mood disorders. In this chapter, I explore the role of the HPA, HPT, and hypothalamic-pituitary-gonadal (HPG) axes in mood disorders, primarily MDD.

Endocrine Psychophysiology

The hypothalamus is situated in a critical location at the base of the brain; from this "primitive" region, it readily influences all signals that flow out into the periphery. The hypothalamus integrates disparate information about the internal and external milieu and is the primary coordinator of mass-sustained organismic functions (e.g., osmolality, body temperature, circadian rhythms, appetite, libido, and motivational state, which may be experienced as mood) (Kasckow et al. 2003). The hormone axes are a critical component of hypothalamic-regulated homeo-

static adaptations to the challenges of survival (e.g., response to life-threatening stimuli, reproduction). As such, hormones have potent and wide-ranging behavioral effects that are complemented by metabolic effects in the promotion of an adaptive response.

Highly differentiated glandular cells secrete hormones into the bloodstream, and these messengers then travel to adjacent or distant targets. Secretion is stimulated by the action of a neurohormone, which is a secretory product of a hypothalamic neuroendocrine transducer cell. The concentration of hormones is typically very small, and discrete mechanisms have developed to facilitate their actions. Hormones act via activation of specific membrane-bound, intracellular, or nuclear receptors, which trigger tissue-specific changes in functional activity of the target cell.

The same hormone can have different effects by acting at different sites (i.e., they are pleiotropic). This makes them especially well suited for modulating complex behaviors and for integrating such behaviors with a metabolic state. To do this, they must interact with the CNS in ways separate from those that serve merely a self-regulatory function (e.g., negative feedback). In addition, it should be remembered that hormonal effects are generally tonic and diffuse, setting the "gain" on a system, and have a much longer duration of action than neurotransmitters. This allows for more subtle influence on integrated behavioral responses.

Hypothalamic-Pituitary-Adrenal Axis

Hypothalamic-Pituitary-Adrenal Axis Physiology

Perceived threats activate the HPA axis, which regulates the adaptive response. A cascade begins in the CNS that involves pituitary release of corticotropin and culminates with adrenal release of glucocorticoids, which modulate metabolism, reproduction, inflammation, and immunity, as well as hippocampal neurogenesis and apoptosis (Plotsky et al. 1998; Thrivikraman et al. 2000). Activation also modulates cognitive processes (e.g., sensory processing, stimulus habituation, and memory), pain, and sleep (Wolkowitz et al. 2001).

The CNS is the main controller of the HPA axis. Corticotropin-releasing hormone (CRH) is released in synergy with arginine vasopressin (AVP) (Arborelius et al. 1999). During acute stress, multiple brain regions with afferent projections to the hypothalamus are activated:

- Cholinergic and serotonergic inputs provide the primary stimulatory control.

- Noradrenergic innervation from the brain stem, pontine locus coeruleus, amygdala, cerebral cortex, and hippocampus may be either stimulatory (at low levels, α_1-adrenoceptors) or inhibitory (at high levels, β-adrenoceptors).
- γ-Aminobutyric acid (GABA) agonists have inhibitory effects.
- Opioids have mixed effects.
- The neuropeptides, such as substance P, cholecystokinin, and neurophysin, have neuromodulatory effects that are not well characterized (Plotsky et al. 1998).

When stimulated, both CRH and AVP are released into the portal plexus blood system and transported to the pituitary gland. CRH stimulates the pituitary release of proopiomelanocortin (POMC)-derived peptides (corticotropin and endorphin) into the peripheral circulation, and corticotropin stimulates the adrenal release of cortisol. There is a negative feedback by corticosteroids acting through specific glucocorticoid receptors in the CNS. Two types of corticosteroid receptors have been identified: 1) MR-I, the high-affinity mineralocorticoid receptor, which is predominantly hippocampal, and 2) GR-II, the lower-affinity glucocorticoid receptor, which is distributed throughout the brain. Such a dual-receptor system for a single class of hormones is a flexible way to regulate the diverse physiological functions of corticosteroids (Holsboer 2003; Plotsky et al. 1998). CRH activates the locus coeruleus noradrenergic circuit (thereby increasing general arousal and selective attention) and, at the same time, inhibits vegetative functions (e.g., appetite, libido) (Wolkowitz et al. 2001).

Finally, DHEA and its metabolite, DHEA sulfate [together abbreviated "DHEA(S)"], and androstenedione are androgenic steroids secreted by the adrenal cortex. Although not potent androgens themselves, they are converted in target organs to testosterone and dihydrotestosterone. This is likely of significant androgenic consequence in women (Wolkowitz et al. 2000). DHEA(S) is also produced in situ in brain tissue and is therefore a "neurosteroid" (Rupprecht 2003).

Plasma and cerebrospinal fluid (CSF) DHEA(S) levels decline with age: at age 70, DHEA(S) levels are about 20% of those at age 20 (Feldman et al. 2002; Wolkowitz et al. 2000). In an 8-year population-based longitudinal study, DHEA(S) levels declined 5.2% per year in middle-aged men (Feldman et al. 2002). Many, but not all, studies have reported lowered levels of DHEA(S) or lowered ratios of DHEA(S) to cortisol in patients with depression, chronic fatigue syndrome, postpartum depression (PPD), and anxiety (Wolkowitz et al. 2000). Similarly, in many population-based studies of the elderly, DHEA(S) level has been positively correlated with cognitive and general functional abilities and negatively associated with mortality. Some investigators have, therefore, proposed DHEA(S) as a marker of "successful aging" (Ravaglia et al. 1997; Wolkowitz et al. 2000). There is speculation that DHEA(S) "buffers" the deleterious effects of excessive glucocorticoid exposure. For example, DHEA(S) has been shown to prevent or reduce hippocampal neurotoxicity induced by the glutamate agonist N-methyl-D-aspartate (NMDA), corticosterone, and oxidative stressors (Wolkowitz et al. 2000). Overall, the accumulating descriptive and epidemiological data suggest a relationship between DHEA(S) levels and functional abilities, memory, mood, and sense of well-being, but the literature contains many inconsistencies.

Hypothalamic-Pituitary-Adrenal Axis and Depression

HPA Axis Dysfunction and Mood

More than half of the patients with high levels of cortisol caused by Cushing's disease or exogenous glucocorticoids develop a reversible mood syndrome, and approximately 10% develop suicidal ideation or psychosis (Holsboer 2003; Plotsky et al. 1998; Starkman et al. 1981; Wolkowitz et al. 2001). Psychiatric symptoms of hypercortisolism (e.g., anergia, anhedonia, and depressed mood) are positively associated with urinary free cortisol levels and generally resolve, albeit slowly, after successful treatment with either surgery or antiglucocorticoid agents (Starkman et al. 1986). In a review of 28 case reports of antiglucocorticoid treatment of Cushing's syndrome, improvements in mood were apparent in many patients, although full response was erratic and often delayed. In the largest two series, the "antidepressant response rate" (which was not clearly defined) was 70%–73% (Wolkowitz and Reus 1999).

Investigators also have assessed the relation between DHEA(S) level and overall "well-being" and cognitive functioning. In some population-based studies, cognitive and general functional abilities were positively correlated with DHEA(S) levels in the elderly, but in other studies, the correlations were gender specific and/or negative (Ravaglia et al. 1997; Wolkowitz et al. 2000). In one study, neuropsychological evaluations and sex hormone assays were completed for 188 elderly female nursing home residents (mean age=87.8 years; standard deviation=7.0 years); DHEA(S) levels were inversely correlated with scores on multiple cognitive tests (Breuer et al. 2002).

MDD and HPA Axis Function

Further evidence that HPA axis functioning is related to depression comes from studies of patients with MDD and includes the following: 1) patients with MDD (compared with control subjects) have elevated cortisol in plasma, CSF, and urine (Carroll et al. 1981); 2) patients with MDD show a resistance to the normal suppression of cortisol and corticotropin secretion by dexamethasone (Sachar et al. 1970); 3) depressed patients have increased CSF CRH (Holsboer 2003; Plotsky et al. 1998); and 4) adrenal gland hypertrophy and increased sensitivity to corticotropin may be reversible state markers of depression (Rubin et al. 1995; Wolkowitz et al. 2001). This pattern of HPA axis dysregulation does not suggest any definitive mechanism, although Holsboer (2001) suggested that HPA axis dysregulation in MDD results from impaired signaling through corticosteroid receptors and that antidepressants work by normalizing this signaling. Alternatively, it is possible that HPA axis dysregulation is an MDD epiphenomenon or that other glucocorticoid–monoamine interactions are more central to MDD pathophysiology—particularly those that influence serotonergic and dopaminergic neurotransmission (Sachar et al. 1970; Wolkowitz et al. 2001).

Sachar and colleagues (1970) showed that in MDD-associated hypercortisolism, in contrast to Cushing's disease, the secretory *pattern* was dysregulated—that is, there were more secretory bursts, but between these bursts, cortisol levels returned to a normal baseline. This led to the introduction of the dexamethasone suppression test (DST), which detects resistance to glucocorticoid-mediated feedback, as a putative diagnostic marker of MDD. In the traditional test, 1 mg of dexamethasone was administered at 11:00 P.M., and blood was drawn for cortisol level the next day at 4:00 P.M. and 11:00 P.M. High plasma cortisol level (generally >5 g/dL) was associated with MDD. In the original studies (Carroll et al. 1981), DST nonsuppression was 90% sensitive and 50% specific for MDD, and the degree of nonsuppression generally correlated with severity of the depression and normalized following remission. This finding generated a great deal of research interest. Further studies have tempered the early enthusiasm for the DST: its specificity is generally less than 30% for MDD because DST nonsuppression occurs commonly in the setting of medical illnesses, medication use, malnutrition, and infection (Copolov et al. 1989).

A significant improvement has been achieved by combining the DST with CRH stimulation (Deuschle et al. 1998; Heuser et al. 1994; Schule et al. 2001). In this combined test, after administration of 1.5 mg of dexamethasone the previous night (11:00 P.M.) and 100 μg of intra-venous CRH the next day (3:00 P.M.), five specimens are drawn for cortisol at 3:00, 3:15, 3:30, 3:45, and 4:00 P.M. Cortisol is consistently high in patients with MDD and normalizes after remission. Importantly, those who remit and do not have a normalization of this combined DST/CRH test result are at high risk for relapse within the next 6 months (Deuschle et al. 1998; Heuser et al. 1994; Schule et al. 2001). In addition, HPA normalization precedes clinical recovery, and a return to an abnormal HPA system precedes clinical relapse—suggesting that HPA axis dysregulation is not a result of depressive illness (e.g., via stress or malnutrition) (Heuser et al. 1994).

Recent interest in the HPA axis and depression concerns the central regulator of the HPA axis—CRH—and its role *outside* the neuroendocrine system, primarily based on the work of three research groups (led by Gold et al. [1995], Holsboer [2003], and Nemeroff [2002]). In a rat model, CRH caused behavior changes that mimicked depression—and were reversed by CRH type 1 receptor antagonists. In humans, the following evidence from patients with MDD suggests that CRH is hypersecreted: 1) blunted corticotropin response to CRH (due, presumably, to CRH receptor downregulation), 2) elevated CRH in the CSF, 3) increased numbers of cells expressing CRH in postmortem hypothalamic brain tissue, and 4) reduced CRH receptor sites in the frontal cortex of depressed suicide victims (Arborelius et al. 1999). Finally, preliminary evidence supports antidepressant efficacy of a CRH receptor antagonist—irrespective of the patient's baseline HPA functioning and without interfering with the patient's HPA axis feedback regulation (Arborelius et al. 1999; Kunzel et al. 2003). Overall, although multiple lines of evidence support CRH dysregulation in MDD, it is unclear whether this defect is primary or a reflection of higher-level dysregulation (e.g., of monoamine systems).

HPA Axis Antidepressants

Antiglucocorticoids, CRH antagonists, and DHEA have been studied as antidepressants, although systematic research is limited (see Seidman, Chapter 19, in this volume).

Hypothalamic-Pituitary-Thyroid Axis

Hypothalamic-Pituitary-Thyroid Axis Physiology

Thyroid hormones regulate every organ system and are particularly important for food metabolism, temperature regulation, and development—including neuronal growth and synaptogenesis. The thyroid gland secretes two hormones: triiodothyronine (T_3) and thyroxine (T_4). Thyrotropin-releasing hormone (TRH) is a tripeptide produced primarily in the hypothalamus; TRH travels in the axon of its synthesizing neuron to the median eminence, where it is released into the hypophyseoportal blood supply, and stimulates the anterior pituitary release of thyrotropin. Serotonin is inhibitory and dopamine stimulatory to TRH release (Rubin 1989; Rubin et al. 1987). Thyrotropin is a 112–amino acid peptide that acts at membrane receptors in the thyroid gland to promote the synthesis and secretion of thyroid hormones. Thyrotropin release is controlled by TRH, along with thyroid hormone negative feedback, inhibitory influences of dopamine and somatostatin, and stimulatory influences of norepinephrine (Loosen et al. 1986; Marchesi et al. 1988; Mokrani et al. 2000).

In the blood, thyroid hormones are bound firmly but reversibly to proteins—primarily thyroid-binding globulin and to a lesser degree other proteins, such as transthyretin, albumin, and lipoproteins. The free hormone concentration determines the cellular effects. Thyroid hormones bind to the intranuclear thyroid receptor, which binds to DNA and regulates gene expression. Thyroid hormones also have effects on the cell's mitochondria. Hypo- and hyperthyroid states induce profound changes in noradrenergic, serotonergic, and GABA receptor density in particular brain regions. In addition, TRH directly influences neuronal excitability and cholinergic, noradrenergic, and dopaminergic neurotransmission (Ogasawara et al. 1996).

Hypothyroidism is classified into several grades:

1. Grade I, or clinical, hypothyroidism: thyroid hormone levels are decreased, and basal thyrotropin is increased.
2. Grade II hypothyroidism: thyroid hormone levels are in the normal range, but basal thyrotropin is increased.
3. Grade III hypothyroidism: thyroid hormone levels and basal thyrotropin are normal, but the thyrotropin response to TRH stimulation is increased.

It has been estimated that 5%–15% of the patients with subclinical (i.e., grades II or III) hypothyroidism progress to overt hypothyroidism each year, and 80% of the patients with antithyroid antibodies progress to overt hypothyroidism within 4 years (Prange 1998; Targum et al. 1982a).

Hypothalamic-Pituitary-Thyroid Axis and Depression

Thyroid Dysfunction and Mood

Given the direct CNS effects of TRH, thyrotropin, and thyroid hormones, it is not surprising that thyroid dysreg-

ulation can lead to psychiatric symptoms. Indeed, thyroid disorders can induce virtually every psychiatric condition, although there is no consistent association with a specific psychiatric disorder (Brownlie et al. 2000; Gunnarsson et al. 2001; Talbot-Stern et al. 2000). The symptoms most commonly associated with hypothyroidism include fatigue, memory impairment, irritability, and decreased libido, but psychosis, delirium, and suicidality are also reported (Chueire et al. 2003; Rack and Makela 2000). Hyperthyroidism is associated with emotional lability, irritability, insomnia, anxiety, weight loss, and psychomotor agitation (Demet et al. 2002), although it can also present with apathy, fatigue, and withdrawal.

Despite the clinical consensus that many patients with thyroid abnormalities have psychiatric—particularly depressive—symptoms, population-based studies do not uniformly support an increased prevalence of clinical mood disorders in such patients (Engum et al. 2002; Manciet et al. 1995; Mazur 1994). For example, in an epidemiological study in which 30,589 individuals ages 40–89 years were assessed with thyroid assays (thyrotropin and T_4) and self-rating scales for depression and anxiety (Hospital Anxiety and Depression Scale), those with evidence of clinical hypothyroidism (i.e., high thyrotropin and low T_4) had a significantly *lower* risk for self-reported depression compared with the euthyroid reference group (odds ratio [OR]=0.53; 95% confidence interval [CI]=0.31–0.91); neither subclinical hypothyroidism nor hyperthyroidism was associated with depression or anxiety (Engum et al. 2002; Marangell 2002).

MDD and HPT Axis Function

Approximately one-fourth of patients with mood disorders have thyroid dysfunction (Rubin 1989). The most commonly reported abnormalities in patients with MDD include 1) a state-dependent increase in circulating T_4, 2) a blunting of the response of thyrotropin to TRH infusion, and 3) a reduced nocturnal (midnight to 2:00 A.M.) thyrotropin surge (Rubin et al. 1987). Subclinical thyroid axis abnormalities also have been identified in patients with depression, particularly severe MDD (Berlin et al. 1999). Various measures of a hypofunctioning HPT axis have been reported to predict poor response to antidepressant treatment (Brady and Anton 1989; Joffe 1999; Joffe and Marriott 2000; Rao et al. 1996) and earlier depression recurrence (Joffe and Marriott 2000).

The TRH stimulation test involves obtaining a baseline thyrotropin level, administering intravenous TRH, and then measuring thyrotropin at regular intervals. A normal response is a thyrotropin rise of greater than 5 µU/mL above baseline. Serum thyrotropin level following TRH stimulation is blunted in about one-fourth of depressed patients and in hypothyroid patients and exaggerated in hyperthyroid patients and in about 10% of depressed patients (Loosen 1992; Staner et al. 2001; Targum et al. 1984). However, such blunting is also evident in many healthy elderly individuals and in other psychiatric disorders (e.g., eating disorders, alcohol dependence, posttraumatic stress disorder, panic disorder, obsessive-compulsive disorder, premenstrual syndrome, and schizophrenia), which makes this test of little use in the elderly or for differential diagnosis (Rubin 1989; Staner et al. 2001; Targum et al. 1989; Wahby et al. 1988). The preeminent theory regarding thyrotropin blunting in depression had been that TRH hypersecretion in depressed patients leads to a downregulation of TRH receptors (Unden et al. 1986), but contradictory evidence has led to a reconsideration of this hypothesis (Frye et al. 1999). Larger studies suggest that most depressed patients are euthyroid and, moreover, that overall this test is of little value with regard to depressive subtyping or prognosis (Rubin 1989).

A blunted nocturnal thyrotropin surge appears to be a more sensitive HPT axis probe in depressed patients. Bartalena and colleagues (1990) assessed thyrotropin secretion in 15 women (mean age=50 years) with untreated MDD and 15 healthy age-matched women. Morning thyrotropin values did not differ between the groups, but nocturnal (midnight to 2:00 A.M.) thyrotropin concentration was lower in the depressed group ($P<0.0005$), and the nocturnal thyrotropin surge was abolished in 14 of 15 depressed patients. Similar nocturnal HPT blunting was reported by Rubin et al. (1987) in 40 patients with MDD compared with 40 control subjects and by Peteranderl et al. (2002) in 10 patients with MDD and 10 matched control subjects. These data suggest that the loss of the nocturnal serum thyrotropin surge is a more sensitive indicator of HPT axis alterations in MDD than the TRH stimulation test.

Nocturnal HPT axis blunting appears to be correlated with nocturnal HPA axis blunting (Peteranderl et al. 2002; Rubin et al. 1987). Indeed, the following evidence suggests that HPT abnormalities in patients with depressive disorder may be a consequence of HPA abnormalities: 1) glucocorticoids inhibit thyrotropin secretion in both depressed and healthy individuals (Samuels and McDaniel 1997); and 2) a strong positive correlation exists between functional tests of HPT (i.e., TRH stimulation of thyrotropin release) and HPA (i.e., CRH stimulation of corticotropin release) axes in patients with depressive disorders—suggesting a common regulator (Holsboer et al. 1986).

Other data, however, support the independent dys-regulations of HPT and HPA axes in depressed patients. For example, Targum et al. (1982b) reported results of both TRH stimulation tests and DSTs in 54 patients with MDD and 19 nondepressed control subjects. One-third (18 of 54) of the depressed patients and no nondepressed subjects had a blunted thyrotropin response; 23 of 54 depressed subjects (43%) and 2 of 19 nondepressed subjects (11%) were DST nonsuppressors. Yet only 6 of 54 depressed patients (11%) had abnormal responses to *both* the DST and the TRH test. Similarly, Steiner et al. (1985) performed both tests on 61 psychiatric inpatients (42 with MDD, 19 with other psychiatric disorders). Twenty-two of 42 depressed patients (52%) and 4 of 19 patients with non-MDD psychiatric disorders (21%) had a blunted thyrotropin response; 18 of 42 depressed patients (43%) and 1 of 19 patients with non-MDD psychiatric disorders (5%) were DST nonsuppressors. Notably, in this group of more severely depressed patients, 13 of 42 (31%) had abnormal responses to both tests, and compared with the other depressed patients, these patients were older, were more severely depressed, and had longer episodes of illness and a later age at onset of their first episode.

It has been commonly reported that depressed patients have a relative increase in total or free T_4 and a relative decrease in T_3, yet several studies do not support these findings (Hendrick et al. 1998; Rubin 1989; Rubin et al. 1987). Total and free T_4 levels decline after patients achieve remission with antidepressant medication (Brady and Anton 1989; Konig et al. 2000), electroconvulsive therapy (Esel et al. 2002), or cognitive therapy (Joffe et al. 1996); however, not all studies have reported such changes (Amsterdam et al. 1996; Korner et al. 1987). Investigators have suggested that an HPT axis downregulation occurs at the hypothalamic level in MDD, and some treatments may be effective because they normalize this subtle dysregulation (Brady and Anton 1989). Alternatively, HPT axis normalization following remission may simply be secondary to HPA axis normalization.

Thyroid axis abnormalities often have been reported in patients with bipolar disorder, especially in patients with rapid cycling (Baumgartner et al. 1995; Whybrow et al. 1992). However, mood-stabilizing agents, including lithium, carbamazepine, and valproic acid, lower thyroid hormone levels (Baumgartner et al. 1995); thus, it is unknown whether these HPT axis abnormalities are medication induced.

HPT Axis Antidepressants and Mood Stabilizers

Thyroid supplementation has been studied as an adjunct to antidepressant medication and appears to accelerate the rate of TCA (Altshuler et al. 2001)—not SSRI (Appelhof et al.

2004)—antidepressant response, convert some treatment-resistant patients to responders (Joffe 1997), and stabilize some patients with refractory bipolar disorder (Whybrow et al. 1992) (see Seidman, Chapter 19, in this volume).

Hypothalamic-Pituitary-Gonadal Axis

Whereas women experience considerable monthly cyclic hormonal changes as well as a rapid decline in gonadal steroid hormone production at menopause, men rarely experience such rapid hormonal shifts. To assess HPG axis psychophysiology, we must therefore consider men and women separately because of the different hormonal physiologies.

Male Hypothalamic-Pituitary-Gonadal Axis Physiology

Male hypogonadism is generally diagnosed when the total testosterone level falls below a certain threshold, assumed by clinical consensus to be between 200 and 300 ng/dL. Sequelae of testosterone deficiency include reduced musculoskeletal mass, increased adipose deposition, and sexual dysfunction (Vermeulen 2003; Villareal and Morley 1994). Exogenous testosterone replacement consistently reverses these sequelae: body weight, fat-free muscle mass, and muscle size and strength increase; continued bone loss is prevented; and sexual function and secondary sex characteristics (e.g., facial hair) are restored and maintained (Burris et al. 1992; Luisi and Franchi 1980; Snyder et al. 2000; Villareal and Morley 1994).

Male HPG function declines progressively with age, and a substantial proportion of men older than 50 have testosterone levels lower than the threshold values used to define testosterone deficiency in younger men. Mild testosterone deficiency in elderly men, therefore, can be considered physiological (i.e., a para-aging phenomenon) or pathological (i.e., a deficit state). Because age-adjusted norms are not used, it is treated as pathological. Yet even if it is considered physiological, this "normative" decline may be clinically significant, as it is with the age-associated decline in female gonadal hormones.

Whether the age-dependent decline in androgen levels leads to health problems in men is being debated vigorously (McKinlay et al. 1989; Morales et al. 2000; Seidman 2003). Some investigators argue that age-associated testosterone deficiency, or "andropause," is responsible for many of the typical signs of male aging, such as erectile dysfunction, decreased lean body mass, skin alterations, osteoporosis, and increased visceral fat, as well as for neu-

ropsychiatric problems, such as fatigue, loss of libido, depression, irritability, insomnia, and memory impairment (Morales et al. 2000). Furthermore, some investigators believe that the application of a testosterone replacement strategy for older men with low or low-normal testosterone levels is especially promising for reversing such presumed "andropausal" sequelae (Morley 2000). Yet it has been difficult to correlate hormone levels with these age-related phenomena (McKinlay et al. 1989; Morales et al. 2000), and testosterone replacement in elderly men is not especially effective in reversing these symptoms (Snyder et al. 1999a, 1999b). Although testosterone replacement in elderly men has been reported to enhance upper limb strength (Bakhshi et al. 2000; Sih et al. 1997) and mass (Snyder et al. 1999a), improve bone mineral density (Snyder et al. 1999b), increase hematocrit (Hajjar et al. 1997), and reduce leptin levels (an effect that may improve visceral adiposity) (Sih et al. 1997), such effects appear to be weak and of questionable clinical significance. Moreover, few testosterone replacement studies have considered psychiatric symptoms of mild hypogonadism in elderly men (Gray 2005).

Male Hypothalamic-Pituitary-Gonadal Axis and Depression

Male Hypogonadism and Mood

There appears to be a clinical consensus among andrologists that testosterone replacement enhances mood in hypogonadal men (Morley 2001; Vermeulen 2003). Yet until recently, few testosterone replacement studies considered mood as an outcome to be systematically measured. Two influential clinical trials did include self-reported mood assessments during testosterone replacement: Wang et al. (2000) (N=243) and McNicholas et al. (2003) (N=208). In both of these studies, the investigators found that compared with hypogonadal baseline, testosterone replacement was associated with improved mood and "well-being" and reduced fatigue and irritability. Notably, Wang and colleagues (2004) recently reported that in the 123 men receiving testosterone replacement who were followed for 3 years, the improvements in mood persisted. Yet, importantly, no placebo controls (or placebo substitutions) were included in these studies; thus, whether the reported mood improvements might have been equally detectable in a group of hypogonadal men receiving placebo who thought they might be receiving testosterone is unknown.

Indeed, this negative picture emerges from the only two placebo-controlled testosterone replacement studies in which mood was systematically assessed (Sih et al. 1997;

Steidle et al. 2003). In both studies, despite describing mood as a primary outcome, the results were reported in a limited manner (i.e., one general sentence; no table, graph, or data, as was provided for all other outcomes). In neither study was a testosterone–placebo difference distinguishable with respect to mood. For example, Steidle and colleagues (2003) randomized 99 hypogonadal men to placebo and 307 hypogonadal men to different doses of testosterone replacement. Patients rated positive moods (alert, full of energy, friendly, well or good) and negative moods (angry, irritable, sad or blue, tired, nervous) on a 0–7 Likert scale. The one sentence describing the mood results is as follows: "Although all treatments resulted in mean improvements from baseline in both positive and negative mood scores, no significant differences among the treatment groups were observed" (Steidle et al. 2003, p. 2677).

Finally, two well-designed experiments have recently been reported in which men received chemical castration followed by controlled testosterone replacement, with careful characterization of ensuing mood changes. In the first study, Schmidt et al. (2004) examined the effects of a 1-month suppression of testosterone secretion with leuprolide, followed by double-blind, placebo-controlled testosterone replacement in 31 young men. The testosterone-deficient state was associated with reduced libido and with reduced feelings of being "emotionally charged" but had no demonstrable effect on mood. Notably, three men (10%) experienced clinically relevant depressive symptoms during the hypogonadal state, and these symptoms were reversed by testosterone replacement.

In the second study, Gray et al. (2005) administered leuprolide to 60 older men (ages 60–75) and randomly assigned them to receive one of five doses of weekly intramuscular testosterone (25, 50, 125, 300, or 600 mg) for 20 weeks. The testosterone–behavior relationship (i.e., dose-response) was most striking for overall sexual function ($P=0.003$) and waking erections ($P=0.024$); there was no testosterone–dose effect observed for the measures of mood used (Ham-D, $P=0.359$; Young Mania Rating Scale, $P=0.851$). These studies, taken together, provide compelling evidence that testosterone replacement consistently improves libido but does not have an effect on mood that is consistent throughout the male populaation.

Investigators also have used population-based studies to examine the relation between testosterone level and depressive symptoms. The Massachusetts Male Aging Study (MMAS) included a community-based sample of men ages 40–70 years ($N=1,709$) (Araujo et al. 1998). Participants completed a self-report depression inventory, the Center for Epidemiologic Studies Depression Scale (CES-D), and provided a morning blood sample for hormone measurement. In a multiple logistic regression

analysis, serum testosterone levels were not associated with CES-D–diagnosed depression (i.e., CES-D score ≥ 16; OR=0.90; 95% CI=0.75–1.09). However, in a follow-up analysis of these data, Seidman and colleagues (2001) included data regarding an androgen receptor (AR) genetic polymorphism. The AR gene has a polymorphic CAG repeat sequence whose length is inversely correlated with transactivation; inverse relations have been described between the number of CAG triplets in the AR gene and the risk of prostate cancer. In the MMAS cohort, a significant interaction was seen between AR CAG repeats, testosterone level, and CES-D score, suggesting that these HPG axis state and trait features may interact to produce depressive symptoms. That is, although neither testosterone level nor AR isotype alone was associated with CES-D–defined depression, in a model that used all three variables, AR isotype and testosterone together predicted depression (significant effect for the interaction term) (Seidman et al. 2001). Thus, this AR trait marker may define a vulnerable group in whom depression is expressed when testosterone levels decline below a particular threshold. This relationship between total testosterone, AR isotype, and depression was not detected in a community sample of 236 older men (median age 75 years) (T'sjoen et al. 2005). However, a similar vulnerability based on the interaction of these HPG markers has recently been described with regard to risk for Alzheimer's disease (Lehmann et al. 2004).

In the Rancho Bernardo Study (Barrett-Connor et al. 1999), adult residents of a southern California community were enrolled in a study of heart disease risk factors. In a 10-year follow-up study that included 82% of the surviving community residents, 856 men ages 50–89 years (mean age = 70 years) completed the Beck Depression Inventory (BDI) and had a morning blood sample drawn for hormone assays. Multiple linear regression analysis found a significant inverse correlation between BDI score and bioavailable, but not total, testosterone levels ($\beta = -0.302 \pm 0.11$; $P=0.007$). That is, men with lower free testosterone levels had higher BDI scores, which is indicative of increased depressive symptoms.

MDD and Male HPG Axis Function

Neuroendocrine studies of HPG axis functioning among men with MDD have been cross-sectional (i.e., mean testosterone levels in a group of depressed men are compared with levels in a group of nondepressed control subjects) and longitudinal (i.e., testosterone levels during acute depressive illness are compared with hormone levels after remission). Findings from such studies have been inconsistent, except that early-morning luteinizing hormone and testosterone release is blunted in men with melancholic depression (Rupprecht et al. 1988; Schweiger et al. 1999). Overall, comparable numbers of studies have reported lower testosterone levels in depressed men than in control subjects as have those showing no difference in testosterone levels between depressed and control subjects; none has found higher testosterone levels in the depressed state (Seidman 2003). Inconsistencies in this literature may be a result of small sample sizes, different diagnostic assessments of depression, and heterogeneity in depressive symptoms or diagnoses in different study samples. Considerable diurnal, seasonal, situational, and age-related variability in HPG axis functioning is also likely from study to study. However, data are most consistent with the interpretation that MDD has virtually no functional effect on the male HPG axis.

Clinical data suggest that the normative age-related decline in testosterone level, persisting over years, may lead to a chronic, low-grade, depressive illness such as dysthymia but not to MDD. In a sample of elderly depressed men who presented to a geriatric depression clinic, Seidman and colleagues (2002) reported that the median total testosterone level in 32 men with dysthymia (295 ng/dL; range=180–520 ng/dL) was significantly lower than that of 13 age-matched men with MDD (425 ng/dL; range=248–657 ng/dL) or 175 age-matched nondepressed men from the MMAS sample (423 ng/dL; range=9–1,021 ng/dL). Notably, 56% of these elderly dysthymic men had testosterone levels in the hypogonadal range (i.e., ≤300 ng/dL).

Two epidemiological studies provide indirect support for the hypothesis that the testosterone–mood relationship is curvilinear. In a study completed in Belgium, Delhez and colleagues (2003) evaluated morning hormone levels and self-reported psychiatric symptoms in 153 men ages 50–70 years. Using the Carroll Rating Scale (CRS) for depression, they found that free testosterone was negatively correlated with CRS score ($r=-0.17$). Yet when 25 frankly depressed subjects (CRS score >14) were *removed* from the analysis, the association was stronger ($r=-0.33$; $P<0.01$). In the Veterans' Experience Study, a representative sample of Vietnam-era veterans (mean age=38 years) were administered the Diagnostic Interview Schedule and provided morning blood samples for testosterone assay. Booth and colleagues (1999) found that the relation between testosterone level and depression was nonlinear: both those with very low and those with very high testosterone levels were more likely to be depressed.

Exogenous Testosterone Administration

Testosterone has variable and likely idiosyncratic effects on mood. It has not been shown by systematic research to be an antidepressant (see Seidman, Chapter 19, in this volume).

Female Hypothalamic-Pituitary-Gonadal Axis

Female HPG Axis and Depression

The lifetime prevalence of mood disorders in women is approximately twice that in men, a pattern that appears to begin with puberty (Weissman et al. 1988). It has been suggested that the sudden appearance of higher levels of estrogen at puberty alters the sensitivity of neurotransmitter systems in ways that may increase vulnerability to depression (Steiner et al. 2003). Furthermore, the cyclic flux of gonadal steroids gives rise to ongoing and chronic modifications of neurotransmitter systems that may precipitate mood problems in vulnerable women (Rubinow et al. 2002).

Premenopausal women.   The mood disorders occurring in women of reproductive age that have been of primary interest to psychoendocrine investigators include MDD, premenstrual dysphoric disorder (PMDD), and PPD. Studies of MDD in cycling women generally have not shown any consistent HPG axis dysregulation. This negative finding has been consistent across multiple studies of basal hormone levels and dynamic studies (i.e., stimulation tests) (Amsterdam et al. 1981, 1995; O'Toole and Rubin 1995; Unden et al. 1988; Young and Korszun 2002).

PMDD is a mood disorder in which a symptom complex resembling a major depressive episode occurs in most menstrual cycles. By definition, the mood episode is confined to the luteal phase and ends at or within a few days of the onset of menses. In a review that summarized both the extensive literature and the results of their own comprehensive work in this area, Rubinow and colleagues (2002) concluded that no luteal-phase-specific physiological abnormality is clearly seen in women with PMDD. Indeed, when they experimentally eliminated the typical late luteal hormonal milieu, women with PMDD experienced typical symptoms. There is suggestive evidence, however, that estrogen, progesterone, or neurosteroids may be correlated with symptom severity (Rubinow et al. 2002).

PPD also resembles MDD, but the onset is associated with parturition. It affects about 10% of women in the postpartum period and is particularly associated with a history of mood disorder, especially a previous episode of PPD (Rubinow et al. 2002). Compared with women matched for reproductive status, no consistent differences in gonadal steroid levels or HPG axis functioning have been found in women with histories of PPD. A hyperactive HPA axis characterizes women in the immediate postpartum period, and its persistence during PPD is not necessarily distinct from the well-established HPA axis dysregulation of nonpuerperal MDD (Rubinow et al. 2002; Steiner et al. 2003). Even so, Bloch et al. (2005) demonstrated such HPA dysregulation by comparing five women with PPD histories with seven control subjects under conditions of exposure to a gonadal steroid challenge consistent with pregnancy/postpartum.

Peri- and postmenopausal women.   Menopause is a state of relative gonadal steroid deficiency. The average age at onset of menopause is 50 years, and this is unrelated to menarche, body composition, diet, or socioeconomic status (Prior 1998; Steiner et al. 2003). In the years preceding menopause, the loss of ova and their associated follicles leads to ovarian resistance to follicle-stimulating hormone stimulation and to a reduction in the major ovarian estrogen, 12-β-estradiol. Although normative, menopause can be considered pathological, and, independent of age, this female hypogonadal state is associated with acceleration of age-related bone loss, vasomotor symptoms (e.g., hot flashes and night sweats), and urogenital dryness or atrophy (which can lead to dyspareunia).

The most commonly reported mood symptoms in perimenopausal women include irritability, tearfulness and crying spells, anxiety, labile mood, fatigue, reduced libido (or intensity of orgasm), and lack of motivation (Steiner et al. 2003). Such symptoms are linked to the precipitous withdrawal from high and erratic estradiol levels (Prior 1998). Despite clinic-based reports suggesting that menopause is associated with depressive symptoms, most population-based studies do not support an increased incidence of MDD (Avis et al. 1997; Birkhauser 2002; Maartens et al. 2002).

Peri- and postmenopausal women with depression have dysregulated HPG axes (O'Toole and Rubin 1995). In the first 4 years of menopause, as the estrogen feedback inhibition to the pituitary is severely reduced, depressed women have higher HPG axis activity (i.e., higher levels of FSH, LH, and LH-releasing-hormone–stimulated FSH) (O'Toole and Rubin 1995). In later menopause, HPG axis activity in depressed women becomes subnormal (O'Toole and Rubin 1995). Taken together, these data suggest that the depressive state may impair the ability to normally regulate the HPG axis.

Female HPG Axis Antidepressants

Gonadal hormones for female mood disorders, including hormone replacement therapy in peri- and postmenopausal women, are discussed elsewhere in this volume (Seidman, Chapter 19; Kornstein and Sloan, Chapter 41).

Conclusion

Neuroendocrine research strategies for mood disorders have evolved through distinct phases. Initially, the focus was on the psychiatric manifestations of endocrinopathies, and the therapeutic paradigm was hormone axis normalization. Second, functional tests, such as the DST, were studied as a way to biologically verify the diagnosis of MDD or the subtype (e.g., melancholia). Neither of these approaches has proven to be of lasting importance. Yet they provided the foundation for the current approach, which holds enormous promise with regard to the understanding of the etiology and phenomenology of mood disorders and, moreover, provides novel therapeutic options.

Specifically, the modern era of investigation of neuroendocrine dysregulation in patients with mood disorders provides a window into the pathophysiology of the underlying disease. Three observations are instructive: 1) study of HPA axis dysregulation in MDD led to the recognition of the role of CRH and eventually to the entirely novel therapeutic strategy of CRH antagonist treatment; 2) the fact that some hormone axis abnormalities precede a depressive episode, and in affected patients must normalize before full remission occurs, suggests an etiological relation between neuroendocrine regulation and MDD pathology and provides a novel approach to monitoring the course of illness; and 3) a minority of patients develop depressive symptoms in response to HPG axis changes, and this "trait" makes them vulnerable to depressive syndromes (e.g., women with PMDD, men with depression related to testosterone deficiency). The existence of such subgroups suggests that genotypic studies would have great potential for better understanding of disease pathophysiology and for targeted treatment. Further investigation in these areas of overlapping neuroendocrine and mood disorders research, as well as systematic clinical trials with exogenous hormonal treatments, holds great promise.

References

Altshuler LL, Bauer M, Frye MA, et al: Does thyroid supplementation accelerate tricyclic antidepressant response? A review and meta-analysis of the literature. Am J Psychiatry 158:1617–1622, 2001

Amsterdam JD, Winokur A, Caroff S, et al: Gonadotropin release after administration of GnRH in depressed patients and healthy volunteers. J Affect Disord 3:367–380, 1981

Amsterdam JD, Maislin G, Rosenzweig M, et al: Gonadotropin (LH and FSH) response after submaximal GnRH stimulation in depressed premenopausal women and healthy controls. Psychoneuroendocrinology 20:311–321, 1995

Amsterdam JD, Fava M, Maislin G, et al: TRH stimulation test as a predictor of acute and long-term antidepressant response in major depression. J Affect Disord 38:165–172, 1996

Appelhof BC, Brouwer JP, van Dyck R, et al: Triiodothyronine addition to paroxetine in the treatment of major depressive disorder. J Clin Endocrinol Metab 89:6271–6276, 2004

Araujo AB, Durante R, Feldman HA, et al: The relationship between depressive symptoms and male erectile dysfunction: cross sectional results from the Massachusetts Male Aging Study. Psychosom Med 60:458–465, 1998

Arborelius L, Owens MJ, Plotsky PM, et al: The role of corticotropin-releasing factor in depression and anxiety disorders. J Endocrinol 160:1–12, 1999

Avis NE, Crawford SL, McKinlay SM: Psychosocial, behavioral, and health factors related to menopause symptomatology. Womens Health 3:103–120, 1997

Bakhshi V, Elliott M, Gentili A, et al: Testosterone improves rehabilitation outcomes in ill older men. J Am Geriatr Soc 48:550–553, 2000

Barrett-Connor E, Von Muhlen DG, Kritz-Silverstein D: Bioavailable testosterone and depressed mood in older men: the Rancho Bernardo Study. J Clin Endocrinol Metab 84:573–577, 1999

Bartalena L, Placidi GF, Martino E, et al: Nocturnal serum thyrotropin (TSH) surge and the TSH response to TSH-releasing hormone: dissociated behavior in untreated depressives. J Clin Endocrinol Metab 71:650–655, 1990

Baumgartner A, von Stuckrad M, Muller-Oerlinghausen B, et al: The hypothalamic-pituitary-thyroid axis in patients maintained on lithium prophylaxis for years: high triiodothyronine serum concentrations are correlated to the prophylactic efficacy. J Affect Disord 34:211–218, 1995

Berlin I, Payan C, Corruble E, et al: Serum thyroid-stimulating-hormone concentration as an index of severity of major depression. Int J Neuropsychopharmcol 2:105–110, 1999

Birkhauser M: Depression, menopause and estrogens: is there a correlation? Maturitas 41 (suppl 1):S3–S8, 2002

Bloch M, Rubinow DR, Schmidt PJ, et al: Cortisol response to ovine corticotropin-releasing hormone in a model of pregnancy and parturition in euthymic women with and without a history of postpartum depression. J Clin Endocrinol Metab 90:695–699, 2005

Booth A, Johnson DR, Granger DA: Testosterone and men's depression: the role of social behavior. J Health Soc Behav 40:130–140, 1999

Brady KT, Anton RF: The thyroid axis and desipramine treatment in depression. Biol Psychiatry 25:703–709, 1989

Breuer B, Martucci C, Wallenstein S, et al: Relationship of endogenous levels of sex hormones to cognition and depression in frail, elderly women. Am J Geriatr Psychiatry 10:311–320, 2002

Brownlie BE, Rae AM, Walshe JW, et al: Psychoses associated with thyrotoxicosis—"thyrotoxic psychosis": a report of 18 cases, with statistical analysis of incidence. Eur J Endocrinol 142:438–444, 2000

Burris AS, Banks SM, Carter CS, et al: A long-term, prospective study of the physiologic and behavioral effects of hormone replacement in untreated hypogonadal men. J Androl 13:297–304, 1992

Carroll BJ, Feinberg M, Greden JF, et al: A specific laboratory test for the diagnosis of melancholia: standardization, validation, and clinical utility. Arch Gen Psychiatry 38:15–22, 1981

Chueire VB, Silva ET, Perotta E, et al: High serum TSH levels are associated with depression in the elderly. Arch Gerontol Geriatr 36:281–288, 2003

Copolov DL, Rubin RT, Stuart GW, et al: Specificity of the salivary cortisol dexamethasone suppression test across psychiatric diagnoses. Biol Psychiatry 25:879–893, 1989

Delhez M, Hansenne M, Legros JJ: Andropause and psychopathology: minor symptoms rather than pathological ones. Psychoneuroendocrinology 28:863–874, 2003

Demet MM, Ozmen B, Deveci A, et al: Depression and anxiety in hyperthyroidism. Arch Med Res 33:552–556, 2002

Deuschle M, Schweiger U, Gotthardt U, et al: The combined dexamethasone/corticotropin-releasing hormone stimulation test is more closely associated with features of diurnal activity of the hypothalamo-pituitary-adrenocortical system than the dexamethasone suppression test. Biol Psychiatry 43:762–766, 1998

Engum A, Bjoro T, Mykletun A, et al: An association between depression, anxiety and thyroid function—a clinical fact or an artefact? Acta Psychiatr Scand 106:27–34, 2002

Esel E, Turan T, Kula M, et al: Effects of electroconvulsive therapy on hypothalamic-pituitary-thyroid axis activity in depressed patients. Prog Neuropsychopharmacol Biol Psychiatry 26:1171–1175, 2002

Feldman HA, Longcope C, Derby CA, et al: Age trends in the level of serum testosterone and other hormones in middle-aged men: longitudinal results from the Massachusetts male aging study. J Clin Endocrinol Metab 87:589–598, 2002

Frye MA, Dunn RT, Gary KA, et al: Lack of correlation between cerebrospinal fluid thyrotropin-releasing hormone (TRH) and TRH-stimulated thyroid-stimulating hormone in patients with depression. Biol Psychiatry 45:1049–1052, 1999

Gold PW, Licinio J, Wong ML, et al: Corticotropin releasing hormone in the pathophysiology of melancholic and atypical depression and in the mechanism of action of antidepressant drugs. Ann N Y Acad Sci 771:716–729, 1995

Gray PB, Singh AB, Woodhouse LJ, et al: Dose-dependent effects of testosterone on sexual function, mood and visuospatial cognition in older men. J Clin Endocrinol Metab [Epub ahead of print, first published as doi:10.1210/jc.2005-0247], April 12, 2005

Halbreich U: Hormonal interventions with psychopharmacological potential: an overview. Psychopharmacol Bull 33:281–286, 1997

Hendrick V, Altshuler L, Whybrow P: Psychoneuroendocrinology of mood disorders: the hypothalamic-pituitary-thyroid axis. Psychiatr Clin North Am 21:277–292, 1998

Heuser I, Yassouridis A, Holsboer F: The combined dexamethasone/CRH test: a refined laboratory test for psychiatric disorders. J Psychiatr Res 28:341–356, 1994

Holsboer F: Stress, hypercortisolism and corticosteroid receptors in depression: implications for therapy. J Affect Disord 62:77–91, 2001

Holsboer F: Corticotropin-releasing hormone modulators and depression. Curr Opin Investig Drugs 4:46–50, 2003

Holsboer F, Gerken A, von Bardeleben U, et al: Human corticotropin-releasing hormone in depression—correlation with thyrotropin secretion following thyrotropin-releasing hormone. Biol Psychiatry 21:601–611, 1986

Joffe RT: Refractory depression: treatment strategies, with particular reference to the thyroid axis. J Psychiatry Neurosci 22:327–331, 1997

Joffe RT: Peripheral thyroid hormone levels in treatment resistant depression. Biol Psychiatry 45:1053–1055, 1999

Joffe RT, Marriott M: Thyroid hormone levels and recurrence of major depression. Am J Psychiatry 157:1689–1691, 2000

Joffe R[T], Segal Z, Singer W: Change in thyroid hormone levels following response to cognitive therapy for major depression. Am J Psychiatry 153:411–413, 1996

Kasckow JW, Aguilera G, Mulchahey JJ, et al: In vitro regulation of corticotropin-releasing hormone. Life Sci 73:769–781, 2003

Konig F, Hauger B, von Hippel C, et al: Effect of paroxetine on thyroid hormone levels in severely depressed patients. Neuropsychobiology 42:135–138, 2000

Korner A, Kirkegaard C, Larsen JK: The thyrotropin response to thyrotropin-releasing hormone as a biological marker of suicidal risk in depressive patients. Acta Psychiatr Scand 76:355–358, 1987

Kunzel HE, Zobel AW, Nickel T, et al: Treatment of depression with the CRH-1-receptor antagonist R121919: endocrine changes and side effects. J Psychiatr Res 37:525–533, 2003

Lehmann DJ, Hogervorst E, Warden DR, et al: The androgen receptor CAG repeat and serum testosterone in the risk of Alzheimer's disease in men. J Neurol Neurosurg Psychiatry 75:163–164, 2004

Loosen PT: The thyroid state of depressed patients. Clin Neuropharmacol 15 (suppl 1 pt A):382A–383A, 1992

Loosen PT, Garbutt JC, Tipermas A: The TRH test during dopamine receptor blockade in depressed patients. Psychoneuroendocrinology 11:327–336, 1986

Luisi M, Franchi F: Double-blind group comparative study of testosterone undecanoate and mesterolone in hypogonadal male patients. J Endocrinol Invest 3:305–308, 1980

Maartens LW, Knottnerus JA, Pop VJ: Menopausal transition and increased depressive symptomatology: a community based prospective study. Maturitas 42:195–200, 2002

Manciet G, Dartigues JF, Decamps A, et al: The PAQUID survey and correlates of subclinical hypothyroidism in elderly community residents in the southwest of France. Age Ageing 24:235–241, 1995

Marangell LB: Thyroid hormones and mood: are population data applicable to clinical cohorts? Acta Psychiatr Scand 106:1–2, 2002

Marchesi C, Chiodera P, De Risio C, et al: Dopaminergic control of TSH secretion in endogenous depression. Psychiatry Res 25:277–282, 1988

Mazur A: Do cortisol and thyroxin correlate with nervousness and depression among male army veterans? Biol Psychol 37:259–263, 1994

McEwen BS: Gonadal and adrenal steroids and the brain: implications for depression, in Hormones and Depression. Edited by Halbreich U. New York, Raven, 1998, pp 239–253

McKinlay JB, Longcope C, Gray A: The questionable physiologic and epidemiologic basis for a male climacteric syndrome: preliminary results from the Massachusetts Male Aging Study. Maturitas 11:103–115, 1989

McNicholas TA, Dean JD, Mulder H, et al: A novel testosterone gel formulation normalizes androgen levels in hypogonadal men, with improvements in body composition and sexual function. BJU Int 91:69–74, 2003

Mokrani M, Duval F, Diep TS, et al: Multihormonal responses to clonidine in patients with affective and psychotic symptoms. Psychoneuroendocrinology 25:741–752, 2000

Mong JA, Pfaff DW: Hormonal and genetic influences underlying arousal as it drives sex and aggression in animal and human brains. Neurobiol Aging 24 (suppl 1):S83–S88, discussion S91–S92, 2003

Morales A, Heaton JP, Carson CC: Andropause: a misnomer for a true clinical entity. J Urol 163:705–712, 2000

Morley JE: Testosterone treatment in older men: effects on the prostate. Endocr Pract 6:218–221, 2000

Morley JE: Testosterone replacement in older men and women. J Gend Specif Med 4:49–53, 2001

Nemeroff CB: New directions in the development of antidepressants: the interface of neurobiology and psychiatry. Hum Psychopharmacol 17 (suppl 1):S13–S16, 2002

O'Toole SM, Rubin RT: Neuroendocrine aspects of primary endogenous depression, XIV: gonadotropin secretion in female patients and their matched controls. Psychoneuroendocrinology 20:603–612, 1995

Ogasawara T, Itoh Y, Tamura M, et al: NS-3, a TRH-analog, reverses memory disruption by stimulating cholinergic and noradrenergic systems. Pharmacol Biochem Behav 53:391–399, 1996

Peteranderl C, Antonijevic IA, Steiger A, et al: Nocturnal secretion of TSH and ACTH in male patients with depression and healthy controls. J Psychiatr Res 36:189–196, 2002

Plotsky PM, Owens MJ, Nemeroff CB: Psychoneuroendocrinology of depression. hypothalamic-pituitary-adrenal axis. Psychiatr Clin North Am 21:293–307, 1998

Prange AJ Jr: Psychoendocrinology: a commentary. Psychiatr Clin North Am 21:491–505, 1998

Prior JC: Perimenopause: the complex endocrinology of the menopausal transition. Endocr Rev 19:397–428, 1998

Rack SK, Makela EH: Hypothyroidism and depression: a therapeutic challenge. Ann Pharmacother 34:1142–1145, 2000

Rao ML, Ruhrmann S, Retey B, et al: Low plasma thyroid indices of depressed patients are attenuated by antidepressant drugs and influence treatment outcome. Pharmacopsychiatry 29:180–186, 1996

Ravaglia G, Forti P, Maioli F, et al: Determinants of functional status in healthy Italian nonagenarians and centenarians: a comprehensive functional assessment by the instruments of geriatric practice. J Am Geriatr Soc 45:1196–1202, 1997

Rolf C, Nieschlag E: Potential adverse effects of long-term testosterone therapy. Baillieres Clin Endocrinol Metab 12:521–534, 1998

Rubin RT: Pharmacoendocrinology of major depression. Eur Arch Psychiatry Neurol Sci 238:259–267, 1989

Rubin RT, Poland RE, Lesser IM, et al: Neuroendocrine aspects of primary endogenous depression, IV: pituitary-thyroid axis activity in patients and matched control subjects. Psychoneuroendocrinology 12:333–347, 1987

Rubin RT, Poland RE, Lesser IM, et al: Neuroendocrine aspects of primary endogenous depression, V: serum prolactin measures in patients and matched control subjects. Biol Psychiatry 25:4–21, 1989

Rubin RT, Phillips JJ, Sadow TF, et al: Adrenal gland volume in major depression: increase during the depressive episode and decrease with successful treatment. Arch Gen Psychiatry 52:213–218, 1995

Rubinow DR, Schmidt PJ, Roca CA, et al: Gonadal hormones and behavior in women: concentrations versus context, in Hormones, Brain and Behavior. Edited by Pfaff D, Arnold AP, Etgen AM, et al. New York, Academic Press, 2002, Chapter 84, pp 37–73

Rupprecht R: Neuroactive steroids: mechanisms of action and neuropsychopharmacological properties. Psychoneuroendocrinology 28:139–168, 2003

Rupprecht R, Rupprecht C, Rupprecht M, et al: Different reactivity of the hypothalamo-pituitary-gonadal-axis in depression and normal controls. Pharmacopsychiatry 21:438–439, 1988

Sachar EJ, Hellman L, Fukushima DK, et al: Cortisol production in depressive illness: a clinical and biochemical clarification. Arch Gen Psychiatry 23:289–298, 1970

Samuels MH, McDaniel PA: Thyrotropin levels during hydrocortisone infusions that mimic fasting-induced cortisol elevations: a clinical research center study. J Clin Endocrinol Metab 82:3700–3704, 1997

Schule C, Baghai T, Zwanzger P, et al: Sleep deprivation and hypothalamic-pituitary-adrenal (HPA) axis activity in depressed patients. J Psychiatr Res 35:239–247, 2001

Schmidt PJ, Berlin KL, Danaceau MA, et: The effects of pharmacologically induced hypogonadism on mood in healthy men. Arch Gen Psychiatry 61:997–1004, 2004

Schweiger U, Deuschle M, Weber B, et al: Testosterone, gonadotropin, and cortisol secretion in male patients with major depression. Psychosom Med 61:292–296, 1999

Seidman SN: Testosterone deficiency and mood in aging men: pathogenic and therapeutic interactions. World J Biol Psychiatry 4:14–20, 2003

Seidman SN, Roose SP: The male hypothalamic-pituitary-gonadal axis: pathogenic and therapeutic implications in psychiatry. Psychiatr Ann 30:102–112, 2000

Seidman SN, Walsh BT: Testosterone and depression in aging men. Am J Geriatr Psychiatry 7:18–33, 1999

Seidman SN, Araujo AB, Roose SP, et al: Testosterone level, androgen receptor polymorphism, and depressive symptoms in middle-aged men. Biol Psychiatry 50:371–376, 2001

Seidman SN, Araujo AB, Roose SP, et al: Low testosterone levels in elderly men with dysthymic disorder. Am J Psychiatry 159:456–459, 2002

Sih R, Morley JE, Kaiser FE, et al: Testosterone replacement in older hypogonadal men: a 12-month randomized controlled trial. J Clin Endocrinol Metab 82:1661–1667, 1997

Snyder PJ, Peachey H, Hannoush P, et al: Effect of testosterone treatment on body composition and muscle strength in men over 65 years of age. J Clin Endocrinol Metab 84:2647–2653, 1999a

Snyder PJ, Peachey H, Hannoush P, et al: Effect of testosterone treatment on bone mineral density in men over 65 years of age. J Clin Endocrinol Metab 84:1966–1972, 1999b

Snyder PJ, Peachey H, Berlin JA, et al: Effects of testosterone replacement in hypogonadal men. J Clin Endocrinol Metab 85:2670–2677, 2000

Staner L, Duval F, Calvi-Gries F, et al: Morning and evening TSH response to TRH and sleep EEG disturbances in major depressive disorder. Prog Neuropsychopharmacol Biol Psychiatry 25:535–547, 2001

Starkman MN, Schteingart DE, Schork MA: Depressed mood and other psychiatric manifestations of Cushing's syndrome: relationship to hormone levels. Psychosom Med 43:3–18, 1981

Starkman MN, Schteingart DE, Schork MA: Cushing's syndrome after treatment: changes in cortisol and ACTH levels, and amelioration of the depressive syndrome. Psychiatry Res 19:177–188, 1986

Steidle C, Schwartz S, Jacoby K, et al: AA2500 testosterone gel normalizes androgen levels in aging males with improvements in body composition and sexual function. J Clin Endocrinol Metab 88:2673–2681, 2003

Steiger A, von Bardeleben U, Guldner J, et al: The sleep EEG and nocturnal hormonal secretion studies on changes during the course of depression and on effects of CNS-active drugs. Biol Psychiatry 17:125–137, 1993

Steiner M, Goldman SE, Gupta RN, et al: Specificity of the combined dexamethasone suppression and TRH/TSH tests in melancholia. Prog Neuropsychopharmacol Biol Psychiatry 9:655–659, 1985

Steiner M, Dunn E, Born L: Hormones and mood: from menarche to menopause and beyond. J Affect Disord 74:67–83, 2003

Talbot-Stern JK, Green T, Royle TJ: Psychiatric manifestations of systemic illness. Emerg Med Clin North Am 18:199–209, vii–viii, 2000

Targum SD, Sullivan AC, Byrnes SM: Compensatory pituitary-thyroid mechanisms in major depressive disorder. Psychiatry Res 6:85–96, 1982a

Targum SD, Sullivan AC, Byrnes SM: Neuroendocrine interrelationships in major depressive disorder. Am J Psychiatry 139:282–286, 1982b

Targum SD, Greenberg RD, Harmon RL, et al: The TRH test and thyroid hormone in refractory depression. Am J Psychiatry 141:463–469, 1984

Targum SD, Marshall LE, Magac-Harris K, et al: TRH tests in a healthy elderly population: demonstration of gender differences. J Am Geriatr Soc 37:533–536, 1989

Thrivikraman KV, Nemeroff CB, Plotsky PM: Sensitivity to glucocorticoid-mediated fast-feedback regulation of the hypothalamic-pituitary-adrenal axis is dependent upon stressor specific neurocircuitry. Brain Res 870:87–101, 2000

T'sjoen GG, De Vos S, Goemaere S, et al: Sex steroid level, androgen receptor polymorphism, and depressive symptoms in healthy elderly men. J Am Geriatr Soc 53:636–642, 2005

Unden F, Ljunggren JG, Kjellman BF, et al: Twenty-four-hour serum levels of T4 and T3 in relation to decreased TSH serum levels and decreased TSH response to TRH in affective disorders. Acta Psychiatr Scand 73:358–365, 1986

Unden F, Ljunggren JG, Beck-Friis J, et al: Hypothalamic-pituitary-gonadal axis in major depressive disorders. Acta Psychiatr Scand 78:138–146, 1988

Vermeulen A: Diagnosis of partial androgen deficiency in the aging male. Ann Endocrinol (Paris) 64:109–114, 2003

Villareal DT, Morley JE: Trophic factors in aging. Drugs Aging 4:492–509, 1994

Wahby VS, Ibrahim GA, Giller EL, et al: Relationship of age to TSH response to TRH in depressed men. Acta Psychiatr Scand 78:283–288, 1988

Wang C, Swerdloff RS, Iranmanesh A, et al: Transdermal testosterone gel improves sexual function, mood, muscle strength, and body composition parameters in hypogonadal men. Testosterone Gel Study Group. J Clin Endocrinol Metab 85:2839–2853, 2000

Wang C, Cunningham G, Dobs A, et al: Long-term testosterone gel (AndroGel) treatment maintains beneficial effects on sexual function and mood, lean and fat mass, and bone mineral density in hypogonadal men. J Clin Endocrinol Metab 89:2085–2098, 2004

Weissman MM, Leaf PJ, Tischler GL, et al: Affective disorders in five United States communities. Psychol Med 18:141–153, 1988 [published erratum appears in 18:792, 1988]

Whybrow PC, Bauer MS, Gyulai L: Thyroid axis considerations in patients with rapid cycling affective disorder. Clin Neuropharmacol 15 (suppl 1 pt A):391A–392A, 1992

Wolkowitz OM, Reus VI: Treatment of depression with antiglucocorticoid drugs. Psychosom Med 61:698–711, 1999

Wolkowitz OM, Brizendine L, Reus VI: The role of dehydroepiandrosterone (DHEA) in psychiatry. Psychiatr Ann 30:123–128, 2000

Wolkowitz OM, Epel ES, Reus VI: Stress hormone-related psychopathology: pathophysiological and treatment implications. World J Biol Psychiatry 2:115–143, 2001

Young EA, Korszun A: The hypothalamic-pituitary-gonadal axis in mood disorders. Endocrinol Metab Clin North Am 31:63–78, 2002

CHAPTER

Cognitive Processing Models of Depression

BRUCE K. CHRISTENSEN, PH.D., C.PSYCH.

COLLEEN E. CARNEY, PH.D., C.PSYCH.

ZINDEL V. SEGAL, PH.D., C.PSYCH.

IN THE 1960s, the field of psychology witnessed a paradigm shift away from strictly behavioral models to models that included cognitive mechanisms. A central tenet of cognitive mediator models is that information processing influences behavioral and emotional experiences and that human beings rely on an information-processing system to select, encode, manipulate, store, and retrieve information in a meaningful way. Moreover, these models emphasize the centrality of cognitive processing as a determinant of behavior and psychological functioning more generally. Consistent with this emphasis, distinct areas of experimental psychology have used a range of methodologies (e.g., neuropsychological testing, experimental cognition, and computer modeling) to understand how humans process cognitive material. As a result, the past 40 years have witnessed an unparalleled growth in the field's understanding and conceptualization of cognition and its related facets (e.g., cognitive neuroscience, artificial intelligence).

In the 1980s, Ingram and Kendall (1986) challenged clinical researchers to use what was known from cognitive science to understand the clinical processes involved in clinical depression. In this chapter, we examine clinical neuropsychological and experimental cognitive research and, in the spirit of Ingram and Kendall, how known cognitive impairments can inform our clinical understanding of depression.

In the first section of the chapter, we summarize findings from experimental studies of the impairments in information-processing speed, attention, memory, inhibition, and effortful processing among those with depression. We then briefly review several prominent cognitive models of depression. Finally, we discuss how understanding these cognitive deficits aids our understanding of both the thoretical and the clinical aspects of depression. The reader is referred elsewhere for reviews of cognitive processing models of bipolar mood disorder (Ball et al. 2003; Bearden et al. 2001).

131

Experimental Findings of Cognitive Deficits

Information-Processing Speed and Psychomotor Speed

Depressed individuals show a general decrease in speed of information processing (also referred to as *cognitive slowing* or *psychomotor slowing*), regardless of the emotional valence of information (Williams 1997). For example, they perform poorly on letter cancellation tasks, which require participants to cross out as many targets as possible within a time limit, whereas their performance on tests that are not time limited is similar to that of nondepressed persons (Mialet et al. 1996). Moreover, depressed individuals are more impaired by additional time restrictions on the same task. For example, although all participants perform worse in the paced rather than the unpaced versions of the Digit-Symbol Substitution Task (DSST), depressed persons' accuracy decreases more than control subjects' accuracy with additional time pressure (Raskin et al. 1982).

It is also recognized that a combination of motor and cognitive slowing contributes to reaction time deficits in depression (Knott et al. 1991). In choice reaction time tasks, depressed individuals have consistently longer latencies than do nondepressed individuals. Moreover, systematic variation of the motor (i.e., increasing motor complexity) and cognitive (i.e., increasing stimulus similarity in a discriminative response paradigm) task demands has indicated that both components contribute to depression-related reaction time increases (Cornell et al. 1984).

The clinical relevance of impaired speed of information processing is highlighted via its association with the severity of depression (Seppala et al. 1978). Furthermore, reaction times improve with amelioration of depression, and individuals whose mood significantly improved after antidepressant therapy had shorter choice reaction times (Seppala et al. 1978).

General Attention

Impaired attention is a cardinal feature of depression (Mialet et al. 1996), and subtle deterioration of attention may indicate the onset of an acute depressive episode (Hagerty et al. 1997). In addition, depressed individuals' self-reported ability to carry out common tasks that require attention, such as goal formulation and planning, is significantly worse when they are depressed than when they are in recovery (Williams et al. 2000). Neuropsychological and experimental evidence confirms that depressed individuals have diminished attentional capabilities (Mialet et al. 1996).

Depressed patients have deficits on neuropsychological tests that require high levels of attention (Cassens et al. 1990). For example, Zakzanis and colleagues (1998) conducted a meta-analysis of neuropsychological test results and found substantial deficits on attentionally demanding tasks such as letter cancellation tasks, the DSST, and the Trail-Making Test. In addition, depressed persons have significant deficits on the Continuous Performance Test (CPT), which is a task of sustained attention that requires participants to respond to targets among consecutively presented distractors. Individuals with depression fail to respond to the target stimuli more frequently than do nondepressed control subjects. Depressed individuals' deficits on the DSST, Trail Making Test, and CPT suggest significant impairments in selective and sustained attention. However, not all aspects of attention are equally impaired in depression. Preserved ability on tests of immediate auditory attention, or working memory (e.g., Digit Span Test), has been noted (Zakzanis et al. 1998).

Deficits on neuropsychological tests of attention may improve with clinical recovery. For example, patients with diurnal mood swings had significantly better performance on the DSST in the evenings, when they were less depressed (Moffoot et al. 1994). Furthermore, antidepressant medication can improve CPT performance within 48 hours (Buchsbaum et al. 1988); patients who received amoxapine for 2 days detected more targets and made fewer errors than did individuals who received a placebo (Buchsbaum et al. 1988). Although these studies suggest that attention improves with the resolution of depressive symptoms, results have been inconsistent. Moreover, none of these studies investigated changes in depressed persons' attentional abilities in a longitudinal fashion (i.e., from clinical depression through recovery).

Depressed individuals are also impaired on experimental tests of attention. Posner's test of covert orientation of visual attention (Posner 1980) can measure dissociable components of attention (orienting, maintaining, and shifting of visual attention). Although depressed individuals respond to correctly cued targets faster than to miscued targets, they are significantly slower than nondepressed individuals across conditions (Smith et al. 1995). Within this paradigm, varying the stimulus onset asynchrony between cue and target presentation enables one to separate the motor from the cognitive components of the response. The motor component can be inferred from the overall response times at different stimulus onset asynchronies, whereas the cognitive component can be measured by the response time difference between the invalid and valid cue conditions. Smith et al. (1995) found that the maximal detrimental effect of the invalid cue condition occurred at longer stimulus onset asynchronies for depressed individuals than for nondepressed individuals. Therefore, the cognitive components of attention (i.e., orienting, maintaining, and shifting) were delayed in depressed persons, independent of motor dysfunction (Smith et al. 1995).

Biased Attention

Clinically, individuals with depression consistently focus on negative aspects of themselves and situations (Gotlib and McCabe 1992). Depressed persons' attention is drawn toward negative information, and they often perceive an entire event as negative by focusing on minor negative components (Gotlib and McCabe 1992). Attentional bias toward negatively valenced stimuli, and/or away from positively valenced stimuli, has been demonstrated experimentally. For example, the emotional valence of information has been shown to affect depressed individuals' performance on the dichotic listening, visual dot probe, and emotional Stroop tasks (Gotlib et al. 1988; McCabe and Gotlib 1993; Williams and Nulty 1986).

Depressed individuals are distracted by the emotional valence of auditory information in the context of dichotic listening (Ingram et al. 1994; McCabe and Gotlib 1993). In a typical dichotic listening task, participants repeat or "shadow" stimuli presented to one ear while attempting to ignore different stimuli simultaneously presented to the other ear. By varying the valence of words presented in the unattended ear, one can measure the degree of attention participants allocate to irrelevant emotional stimuli. For example, depressed participants' reaction times to an intermittent light were significantly longer when negative-content stimuli were presented to the unattended ear (McCabe and Gotlib 1993). In contrast, no latency differences occurred across conditions in the nondepressed group. In addition, depressed participants no longer showed an attentional bias toward negative-content auditory stimuli with remission of symptoms (McCabe and Gotlib 1993).

Depressed individuals also have abnormal attentional allocation to visual emotional stimuli. The dot probe task provides a measure of shifts in selective attention toward the visuospatial location of emotional stimuli (MacLeod et al. 1986). In this task, word pairs are briefly presented, followed by a dot probe in the location of one of the preceding words. Clinically depressed individuals detect probes that appear in the same location as negative words faster than probes that appear in the same location as neutral words (Mogg et al. 1995). In a similar paradigm, the deployment-of-attention task (Gotlib et al. 1988), word pairs are briefly presented and replaced by green and red bars. Participants are told that one bar appears before the

other and are asked to indicate which bar was presented first. In fact, both bars are presented simultaneously; however, a bar appearing in an attended location will appear to occur sooner than that in an unattended location (Titchener 1908, as cited in Gotlib et al. 1988). Gotlib et al. (1988) found that depressed participants attended to negative words more often, and to positive words less often, than did the nondepressed participants. However, the primary difference was a positive attentional bias in nondepressed participants—that is, individuals with depression showed no evidence of selective attention to any one type of word (Gotlib et al. 1988; McCabe and Gotlib 1993).

The emotional version of the Stroop Test has been the most common method of assessing attentional bias in psychopathology (Williams et al. 1997). Abnormal results on this test have been seen in a variety of clinical populations, including general anxiety disorder, obsessive-compulsive disorder, posttraumatic stress disorder, specific phobia, and depression (Williams et al. 1997). In the emotional Stroop Test, the latency to name the color of positive and negative words is compared with the latency to name the color of neutral words (e.g., Gotlib and McCann 1984). Automatic processing of the word's semantic meaning interferes with the competing response of naming the ink color (Carter et al. 1992). In general, individuals with emotional disorders are slower to color-name emotional words that are relevant to their disorder, in comparison with color-naming of neutral words (Williams et al. 1996). Depressed persons are significantly slower to name the color of depressed-content words than neutral- or manic-content words, whereas nondepressed individuals do not differ in response latency across word types (Gotlib and McCann 1984). These findings have been replicated in participants with either subclinical or clinical depression. In addition, participants in an experimentally induced negative mood have longer reaction times to name the color of negative words than positive or neutral words (Gilboa and Gotlib 1997). Moreover, the magnitude of interference is affected by the nature of the stimuli and presentation method. Depressed individuals show greater interference for negative adjectives that are rated by participants as self-descriptive than for those rated as non-self-descriptive (Segal et al. 1995). Furthermore, exposure to a self-relevant priming phrase, such as "I often feel judged," disproportionately delays color-naming of a self-descriptive trait word if it is negative (Segal et al. 1995).

The Stroop interference effect frequently disappears after successful treatment (Williams et al. 1997). In a longitudinal study of individuals with clinical depression, Gotlib and Cane (1987) found normal response latencies to name the color of self-descriptive negative words following a reduction in depressive symptoms. Similarly,

Gilboa and Gotlib (1997) found no differences between previously dysphoric and never-dysphoric individuals in their performance on the emotional Stroop Test. Furthermore, color-naming interference on the emotional Stroop Test can differentiate patients who respond to treatment from those who do not. Patients who were significantly less depressed (i.e., treatment responders) following cognitive-behavioral therapy (CBT) showed less interference (posttreatment) for negative self-relevant material on the primed emotional Stroop Test (Segal and Gemar 1997). In contrast, individuals who remained depressed (i.e., treatment nonresponders) after CBT continued to show high levels of interference (Segal and Gemar 1997).

Memory

It is useful to conceptualize memory not as a unitary construct but as a system composed of several dissociable, but related, components. In this section, we review the separate aspects of memory that are differentially affected in depression. More specifically, we review evidence of deficits on tasks that involve long-term memory and explicit memory, as well as mood-congruent memory effects and autobiographical memory findings in those with depression. We suggest that the memory deficits found in major depressive disorder (MDD) reflect a pattern of reduced cognitive resources to initiate conscious and active search and retrieval functions.

General Memory Impairment

One of the ways that long-term and working memory are distinguishable from each other is on the basis of capacity; *long-term memory* has a large capacity for information gathered over the life span, whereas *working memory* involves short-term storage and has limited capacity. Those with MDD have deficits on long-term memory tasks but not on working memory tests (Burt et al. 1995). Deficits in working memory are typically seen only on delayed recall tasks. For example, on the Digit Span Test, the performance of depressed patients is no different from that of control subjects on immediate recall; however, on delayed recall (e.g., 20- to 30-second delay between the presentation of the numbers and the onset of repeating the numbers), those with depression are impaired relative to control subjects (Ilsley et al. 1995).

It also appears that the type of retrieval task affects the degree of memory impairment for those with MDD. Although individuals with depression are impaired on both *free recall* and *recognition* memory tasks, they show significantly more impairment on recall than on recognition tests (Calev and Erwin 1985). This disparity persists on tasks that are matched for level of difficulty and discriminatory power in nondepressed control subjects. Thus, those with depression may possess intact initial encoding processes, but the retrieval processes important for active recall are impaired (Ilsley et al. 1995).

Explicit and Implicit Memory

Two other dissociable forms of memory are explicit and implicit memory. *Explicit memory* refers to conscious remembering, whereas *implicit memory* is the recall of unconscious information. Implicit memory is typically assessed by priming (e.g., word-stem completion tasks) or procedural learning (e.g., mirror tracing) paradigms. Data from tasks such as these indicate that depressed persons have intact implicit memory (i.e., a word-stem completion task) but impaired explicit memory (i.e., a cued recall task) (Bazin et al. 1994). One interpretation to explain this finding is that the perceptual processing necessary for implicit memory is intact, but the cognitive resources required for effortful conscious recollection are compromised in depression (Roediger and McDermott 1992).

Mood-Congruent Memory

The emotional valence of to-be-remembered material significantly affects memory performance among those with depression. For both depressed and healthy participants, a match between the emotional valence of to-be-remembered material and the participants' mood produces superior recall relative to a situation in which there is a mismatch between emotional valence and mood (Dalgleish and Watts 1990). This phenomenon is called *mood-congruent memory*. Matt and colleagues (1992) found that those with MDD recalled 10% more negative stimuli than positive stimuli, whereas nondepressed participants recalled 8% more positive stimuli than negative stimuli, an effect that has been confirmed in a meta-analysis of 15 studies (Matt et al. 1992). Interestingly, for those with subclinical levels of depression, recall is equivalent for positively and negatively valenced material; furthermore, nondepressed participants who undergo a negative mood induction procedure preferentially recall negative material (Matt et al. 1992).

The mood-congruent memory bias is most evident for mood- or personally relevant descriptive words. Those with depression tend to recall more depression-related adjectives such as "hopeless," "guilty," or "worthless," relative to positive adjectives, although they do not show superior recall for all negative adjectives. For example, they do not show superior recall for physical threat–related negative words such as "assault" (Watkins et al.

1992), and studies with generally positive or negative words that are not trait related do not show the same consistent findings (Bellew and Hill 1990). Thus, the mood-congruent memory bias in depression is most related to adjectives descriptive of negative traits (Neshat-Doost et al. 1998). In fact, this effect becomes more pronounced when participants are required to indicate whether the adjective is personally descriptive or self-referent (Derry and Kuiper 1981).

Autobiographical Memory

Autobiographical memory refers to an individual's memory of his or her participation in a past situation. In an autobiographical recall paradigm, participants are presented with a set of neutral or valenced cue words and then are instructed to report the first memory that comes to mind. Individuals with MDD show increased mood-congruent recall for negative autobiographical memories and reduced recall for positive autobiographical memories when compared with nondepressed individuals. Clark and Teasdale (1982) found that those with a diurnal mood variation had the greatest probability of recalling unhappy memories at the time of day when they were most depressed, and happy memories were recalled at the time of day when they were less depressed. Thus, it appears that this phenomenon is a mood state effect rather than a result of being clinically depressed. Additionally, the mood-congruent effect is not attributable to those with MDD having more objectively sad or negative life experiences because nondepressed people had the same negative autobiographical memory bias after negative mood induction procedures (Teasdale and Taylor 1981).

In addition, autobiographical memory in depressed individuals tends to contain overly broad or generic aspects of personal experiences, whereas nondepressed individuals' recollections tend to be specific, personalized, and concrete (Williams 1997). Individuals who are more general in recalling negative events in their lives are also overly general in their recall of positive or neutral events (Williams 1996). This effect has been linked with poor problem solving (Evans et al. 1992), hopelessness, and difficulty viewing the future in any specific way (Williams 1997). It is also associated with a higher risk of suicide attempts and a greater number of depressive episodes (Kuyken and Brewin 1995).

Inhibition

Inhibition is the process of ignoring goal-irrelevant stimuli in favor of goal-relevant stimuli (Hasher and Zacks 1988). Those with depression have deficits in their ability to inhibit negative, self-referent material. On the Prose Distraction Task, participants are required to read a passage quickly while ignoring italicized distractor words. Those with depression take significantly longer to read stories with negative distractors relative to positive or neutral distractors (Lau et al. 1999). Interestingly, the nondepressed control participants read the passages with negative words more quickly than the passages with positive or neutral distractors, suggesting a possible protective positive bias. Those with anxiety disorders do not differ from control participants on inhibitory tasks; thus, general psychopathology cannot account for the inhibitory deficits for negative information found in MDD (Lau et al. 2000).

As reviewed earlier, those with MDD took longer to respond to light probes when negative but not positive or neutral words were presented in the unattended ear during a dichotic listening task (McCabe and Gotlib 1993). Thus, patients had difficulty inhibiting negative words from the unattended auditory channel. Similar results were found on an emotional Stroop Test when participants were required to name the color of ink for positive and negative adjectives when these adjectives were primed by emotional phrases (Segal et al. 1995). Those with depression had the slowest response for negative adjectives primed by negative phrases. Segal and colleagues interpreted these results as reflecting the presence of highly interconnected and easily activated semantic networks for negative information among depressed persons. Thus, for those with depression, inadequate inhibition of activated negative semantic networks results in increased interference scores on the emotional Stroop Test (Segal et al. 1995).

Conversely, on a motor response inhibition task, the Stop Signal Task (Logan et al. 1997), those with depression did not differ from nondepressed control subjects, even when the imperative stimuli were of a negative emotional valence (Lau et al. 1999). In this task, participants are required to either make a word and nonword discrimination ("go" condition) or, when signaled by a tone, inhibit their response to the imperative discrimination task ("stop" condition). Collectively, these results suggest that those with depression do not differ from nondepressed persons in their ability to inhibit motor responses but are deficient in suppressing attention to irrelevant negative stimuli (Lau et al. 1999).

Automatic Versus Effortful Processing

Depression is associated with impairments on tasks that require effortful, but not automatic, processing (Hartlage et al. 1993). *Effortful processing* requires volitional and conscious processing and also requires attentional resources (Beck and Clark 1997). *Automatic processing* is characterized by independence from attentional resources and is insensitive to voluntary control. Hartlage and colleagues (1993) concluded that those with depression have difficulty with tasks that require effortful processing of neutral material (e.g., tests of general intelligence, problem solving, general learning, semantically encoded word recall, and reading comprehension) but perform normally on tasks that require automatic processing. For example, depressed patients show impairments on effort-laden word learning (Cole and Zarit 1984) or free recall tasks (Golinkoff and Sweeney 1989) relative to nondepressed control subjects but not on more automatic tasks such as recognition memory.

The reason for this difficulty may be that attention is being focused on depression-related thoughts. Some evidence indicates that automatic processing of negative material occurs in those with depression. In event-related potential (ERP) studies, the ERP amplitudes in response to negative trait adjectives were significantly smaller in those with depression as compared with those not currently depressed (Blackburn et al. 1990). It is thought that lower amplitude of P300 in ERP studies is indicative of less effortful, or more automatic, processing because we experience greater amplitude in response to unexpected stimuli. The previously reviewed evidence for a mood-congruent recall bias also can be viewed as evidence for automatic processing of negative, self-referent material in active depressed states (Neshat-Doost et al. 1998).

Summary

Generally, those with depression have deficits in the areas of information-processing speed; attention; cognitive inhibition; effortful processing; and long-term, explicit, and autobiographical memory. More specifically, depressed individuals have superior memory for, pay more attention to, and show less inhibition of negative, self-referent information. These deficits are more pronounced with increasing severity of depressive symptoms, and they ameliorate with successful treatment of the depression. Many of these characteristics also return under conditions of dysphoric mood. Lastly, some evidence indicates that these deficits are particular to depression and not the result of psychopathology in general.

What, then, are the implications of these cognitive deficits for the understanding of MDD? From the preceding review of the cognitive deficits that characterize MDD, several themes emerge. First, persons with MDD have a processing bias for emotionally negative stimuli. Second, information-processing deficits are most pronounced for tasks requiring volitional effort and, conversely, are less pronounced for tasks involving automatic cognitive processes.

Third, cognitive deficits are present only during dysphoria and generally ameliorate with successful treatment.

In the following section, we summarize the main tenets of selected clinical theories of depression. We discuss the theoretical and clinical implications of these themes as a means of highlighting the ways in which data pertaining to the cognitive deficits associated with depression can aid in our understanding of its clinical features.

Theoretical Models of Depression

Schema Theory

The influential model of Beck (see Beck 1967) posits that dysfunctional cognitions, and underlying cognitive structures, cause depression. In this model, the three levels of cognitions are 1) a surface or manifest level (e.g., automatic, negative thoughts); 2) a deeper intermediate level characterized by irrational beliefs; and 3) the deepest level, which houses the foundation of dysfunctional cognition, schemas. *Schemas* are hypothetical structures that organize information in a meaningful and relatively enduring way. Schemas act as filters that guide attention, information processing, and memory. Schemas are believed to remain latent until activated in the face of emotional distress or dysphoria. When activated, schemas provide access to a complex system of negative, self-referent information processing, which then precipitates a depressive episode (Segal and Shaw 1986).

Associative Network Theory

Bower (1981) proposed an associative network theory to explain the cognitive-emotional activation underlying depression. He proposed that emotions have specific nodes in an associative (neural-like) network that, when activated, produce the experience of an emotion. Other aspects of the emotion, such as autonomic reactions, affective behaviors, and events or concepts related to the emotion, are connected to the original emotion node. Bower's theory is similar to Beck's schema theory in that it suggests that activation of emotional and related nodes enhances their accessibility; in this context, a person who was previously sad will be more likely to recall sad-related thoughts and experiences in the future.

Resource Allocation Model

Ellis and Ashbrook's (1988) resource allocation model postulates that cognitive resources are "taken up" by rumination about depressive symptoms, thus depriving the depressed individual of the resources necessary for cognitive processing. Some support exists for this model because depression is associated with "effort-related" deficits but does not appear to interfere with automatic processing (Hartlage et al. 1993). Further support is drawn from mood induction procedures, in which those induced into a sad mood have poorer performance on effort-laden tasks of attention and recall (Ellis et al. 1984). Providing active strategies for recall or attention allocation to those with depression removes the differences between depressed and nondepressed participants (Hertel and Rude 1991), suggesting that those with depression have difficulty in the *allocation* of resources for attention, encoding, or retrieval strategies.

Response Style Theory

The response style theory of depression posits that depressed patients respond to depressed mood by focusing on their depression symptoms and the resultant consequences of depressed mood (Nolen-Hoeksema 1991). Rumination has been shown to prolong negative mood and thinking, whereas responding to symptoms with a distractive response is associated with shortened episodes of depressed mood (Nolen-Hoeksema 1991). Those asked to perform ruminative tasks have greater activation of negative cognitions than do those involved in distracting tasks (Needles and Abramson 1990). Dysphoric participants who were instructed to ruminate on their feelings and personal aspects of themselves endorsed more negative interpretations of hypothetical situations than did dysphoric individuals who were instructed to focus their attention on things outside themselves and nondysphoric participants (Lyubomirsky and Nolen-Hoeksema 1995). In the same study, dysphoric participants who were instructed to ruminate were more pessimistic about positive events occurring in their future and offered more pessimistic explanations for interpersonal problems and hypothetical negative events. The rumination instruction also affected the dysphoric individuals' problem solving because they generated less effective solutions to interpersonal problems, whereas dysphoric individuals instructed to distract themselves generated as effective solutions and were as optimistic as nondysphoric participants.

Interacting Cognitive Subsystems

Whereas both Beck's and Bower's theories focus on a level of specific cognition as being important in depression, Teasdale suggests that focusing on the level of "meaning" causes problems. For example, if given the statement, "If I could always be right, then others would _____ me,"

people with depression would be apt to select "dislike" because they are biased toward negative appraisals of themselves. However, they are also inclined to select "like" because of the mapping onto personal worth schemas. Teasdale resolves this issue via his interacting cognitive subsystems hypothesis (Barnard and Teasdale 1991). That is, he suggests that there are two levels of meaning: a specific level and a more generic or holistic level. Emotion is thought to be associated with the generic level only. The specific level uses a propositional code to represent the specific meaning (e.g., Roger has brown hair). The holistic level uses a higher-order, generic code that does not map well onto language.

Therefore, while Bower suggests that negative mood increases the activation of stored negative constructs (thus precipitating increases in negative interpretations of experiences), Teasdale (Teasdale et al. 1995b) suggests that the depressogenic thinking is actually related to a shift in information processing from a specific to a more generic level. At this holistic level, interrelations between constructs or generic features of experience are encoded. Thus, this level encodes information in terms of its relation to generic, globally negative views of the self. Representations at this level encode the "interrelationships" and "prototypical patterns extracted from life experience" (Teasdale et al. 1995b).

Kindling and Episode Sensitization

Depression is most aptly viewed as a recurrent rather than a single-episode illness. Its course over time is characterized by increasing frequency of episodes and periods of recovery that become shortened with each subsequent episode (Sturt et al. 1984). On the basis of Post (1992), Segal and colleagues (1996) suggested that a "kindling" and "episode sensitization" approach might be an appropriate analogy for understanding the recurrence of MDD. *Kindling* refers to an event exceeding the threshold for activation, whereas *sensitization* refers to the lowering of thresholds with repeated experience, such that less activation is necessary to reach the threshold. Segal et al. (1996) posited that when individuals are depressed, an elaborate network of depression-related material becomes activated, thereby exerting a negatively biased influence on processing stimuli. This sets in motion a vicious cycle as it becomes harder to activate areas that could disconfirm negative thoughts, thereby maintaining a negative mood. Recurrence, then, can be conceptualized as a lowered activational threshold for depressogenic structures or schemas in the presence of dysphoric mood.

Segal et al. (1995) proposed that those with early negative life experiences and an accompanying experience of sadness also might experience concomitant activation of negative thoughts. Thus, the increased activation increases accessibility of sad-related thoughts (e.g., thoughts of worthlessness and hopelessness), such that patients begin to associate sadness with adversity. Over time, the so-called depression schema includes depression nodes that have become strongly associated and more generalized, so that many more contexts can activate the depressed mood and depressive thinking. A study of more than 2,000 female-female twin pairs found that the association between stressful life events and depression declines over time, but after about nine episodes, this relation weakens (Kendler et al. 2000). This evidence supports the kindling hypothesis but also suggests that this process is "saturable" because most changes to the threshold of activation occur in the first few episodes of depression. Post (1992) suggested that increased vulnerability to recurrence occurs at a neuronal level, and episodes leave a "neurobiological memory trace," which strengthens with each episode.

Differential Activation Hypothesis

Another way of viewing vulnerability to chronic and recurrent episodes of depression is through examination of the type of information processing that becomes activated in depression after a previous episode. The differential activation hypothesis (Teasdale 1988) posits that those who have experienced depression and processed information in negativistic terms are vulnerable for that mode of negativistic information processing to be activated during periods of lowered mood. Thus, those in mildly dysphoric moods are at risk for processing and distorting their current experience along depressogenic themes, which could lead to depression. This theory accounts for the finding that those remitted from depression do not report more negative beliefs than those not depressed, but when a dysphoric mood is induced experimentally, depressogenic processing is seen (for review, see Segal and Ingram 1994).

Cognitive Characteristics of Depression: Theoretical and Clinical Implications

Negative Processing Bias

A shared component of the reviewed theories is the presence of a negative processing bias. Overall, empirical findings suggest that depressed persons do indeed preferentially remember and attend to negative, self-referent

stimuli. These findings offer some support to Beck's schema activation hypothesis. One assumption of the schema activation model is that depressed mood should provide greater activation for mood-congruent, negative, self-referent schemas. Thus, we expect that the recall of personal memories during times of dysphoric mood reflects activation of the negative content of the schema (Teasdale and Barnard 1993). The finding of enhanced mood-congruent recall of negative personal memories has been found across many studies and occurs even in nondepressed participants after a negative mood induction procedure; thus, it cannot be attributable to more negative life events in those with depression.

Research also has supported depression-related attentional difficulties; more specifically, a negative attentional bias in those with depression, as evidenced by the greater cognitive effect of depression-related material (e.g., longer naming latency for negative words on the Stroop Test). Attention is one of the first steps in information processing in that it orients cognitive resources to stimuli that have been selected for more extensive processing. The information that those with depression attend to or select for further processing tends to be negative. The fact that depressed patients selectively attend to negative, self-referent information suggests that schemas may be self-perpetuating; that is, the information available becomes more congruent with the knowledge structures directing the search and selection processes. As a result, input that could disconfirm a negative self-schema is not readily attended to or accessible.

Beck's content specificity hypothesis (Beck 1967) posits that the automatic thoughts among those with depression are predominantly negative. The findings of a negative processing bias in depression also support this tenet. Negative processing might initiate a "downward spiral" in depression in the following manner: The thought "I'm going to fail" in response to an important test could generate feelings of depression or anxiety, which could stimulate avoidance behaviors that interfere with studying, which could then lead to poor performance on a test and confirmation of the original belief. The thoughts are automatic and compelling to the patient and negatively biased in content.

In addition to a bias toward negative information, depressed individuals are predisposed to favor self-referent information. Studies finding slower reaction times to name the color of depression-related (Williams et al. 1996) or self-descriptive (Segal et al. 1995) words on the Stroop Test support theories emphasizing a self- and depression-symptom focus. Such findings are also consistent with response style theory. In this theory, Nolen-Hoeksema (1991) describes rumination as a focus on depression symptoms and the personal consequences of such symptoms. A depression-related or self-referent bias in the cognitive structure of depressed patients could act as a mechanism underlying the ruminative features of depression. In this model, the self-focus of ruminative thinking does not permit outside information to interrupt or disconfirm beliefs; thus, the consequence of initiating this mode of ruminative thinking is prolonged negative mood. Similarly, Teasdale describes the ruminative process as a relatively closed loop of cognitive and somatic feedback that serves to confirm the presence of depression symptoms (Teasdale and Barnard 1993). Those instructed to distract themselves in rumination studies generate more effective solutions to problems, are more optimistic in their outlook, and do not show the negative processing bias of those instructed to ruminate (Nolen-Hoeksema 1991). The fact that depressed persons need distractive techniques to shift their focus away from self- and depression-related thoughts also may reflect a fundamental impairment of their inhibitory skills; that is, in the context of normal inhibition, these individuals may otherwise suppress ruminative thoughts voluntarily.

Experimental findings of a negative processing bias in depression support the kindling and episode sensitization hypothesis. In this model, depressed mood is thought to activate a network of depression-related material, thereby exerting a negative information-processing bias. While one is in this mode, information is processed negatively, and thereby the network is strengthened and the threshold of activation is lowered for future depressive episodes.

Teasdale et al. (2001) argued that CBT prevents relapse via a shift in process (e.g., away from an automatic and ruminative mode of processing) rather than a shift in content (e.g., modifying negative thoughts). Teasdale and colleagues suggested that it is not a change in accessibility of negative constructs but a change in higher-level mental models used to interpret experience. Teasdale et al. suggested that we do not have one "mind." Instead, we have several "minds" that become "switched on," the most dominant of which can be considered the "mind in place." They conceptualized depression as having a persistence of a particular mind in place. The finding that those with depression finish sentence completion tasks with negative words more often than do nondepressed participants, but only if the sentences are at a surface level of language form rather than a propositional level (e.g., the sentence implied relations between self-worth and success), supports this theory. To illustrate, when depressed participants complete the sentence, "If I could always be right, then others would _____ me," a negative activational explanation would expect the depressed person to complete it with a negative word such as "hate," but an inter-

acting cognitive subsystems explanation would expect those with depression to select "like" because of its loading on self-worth (Teasdale et al. 1995b). Indeed, those who have depression select "like" while in dysphoric states, in agreement with the interacting cognitive subsystems theory.

The clinical implication of the negative bias is that people with depression are bombarded by negative information, and their attention is diverted away from neutral or positive information. In CBT, the analogy that patients with depression see the world through gray-colored, as opposed to rose-colored, glasses is typically provided to illustrate biased attention to patients. This analogy may be particularly fitting because studies indicate that those with depression preferentially focus on negative material, whereas nondepressed people preferentially focus on positive material. The filtering of negative information reinforces underlying negative beliefs because no positive or potentially disconfirming information is attended to and, thus, cannot challenge the belief. CBT attempts to alter the biased filter. CBT provides a tool for attending to and processing more than just negative information. By monitoring automatic thoughts, patients who were previously unaware become cognizant of the negative processing bias and are later taught to challenge and consider more positive or realistic alternatives. Negative automatic thoughts are challenged via Socratic questioning or behavioral experiments, and patients are focused on information that potentially disconfirms negative beliefs to test the accuracy of their beliefs. Thus, patients are trained to consider more neutral or positive explanations as alternatives to the first thought that occurred in response to the situation, which, for depressed patients, is predominantly negatively biased. Furthermore, in CBT, depressed patients are instructed to engage in pleasurable and scheduled activities that could act as a distraction or otherwise promote the suppression of ruminative thoughts. CBT also can be conceptualized as "attentional training" because it trains patients to focus outside their symptoms and take in more information (e.g., more positive and/or neutral information) than before.

Other therapies, such as mindfulness-based cognitive therapy, are even more deliberate in their focus on attentional training. Mindfulness-based cognitive therapy is a relapse prevention treatment for patients whose MDD has remitted that teaches mindfulness as a method to increase awareness of the present. This is achieved through a daily practice of bringing attentional focus to the breathing and away from the stream of troublesome thoughts or general unawareness. In addition to the mindfulness component, a cognitive therapy component teaches patients about relapse prevention strategies. Mindfulness-based cognitive therapy trains people remitted from depression to observe and pay attention to their thoughts, thus creating an alternative filter that incorporates positive, negative, and neutral information.

Deficits in Effortful Processing

People with depression appear to have a generalized processing deficit in which processing is slow and effortful processing is impaired. Beck has suggested that the negative thoughts of those with depression are automatic and reflexive rather than effortful and deliberate. In Hartlage and colleagues' (1993) review of automatic and effortful processing in depression, they suggested that Beck's description of the content of automatic thoughts meets automatic processing criteria and is supported by findings of automatic activation of self-referent words in those currently depressed. Moreover, the prominence of automatic negative thoughts may be the direct consequence of impaired effortful systems to dampen or suppress their robust activation. Deficits in effortful processing are also consistent with response style theory because rumination is defined by both a negative processing bias and the automaticity of this process. Whereas effortful processing is difficult, rumination is reportedly automatic for those with depression. Possibly because those with depression have a preferential bias for depression-related and self-referent material, ruminating appears to be something that occurs quite naturally. When dysphoric participants were instructed to ruminate on their feelings and personal aspects of themselves, they generated less effective solutions to interpersonal problems, whereas dysphoric individuals instructed to distract themselves generated equally effective solutions as did nondysphoric participants (Lyubomirsky and Nolen-Hoeksema 1995).

The automaticity dimension is also consistent with resource allocation theory because controlled, effortful processing is presumed to require greater allocation of cognitive resources, and these tasks are impaired in depressed patients. In addition, providing active strategies for the allocation of recall or attentional resources to those with depression removes the differences between depressed and nondepressed participants (Hertel and Rude 1991). Teasdale and colleagues (2001) have argued that CBT prevents relapse via a shift in information processing (e.g., from an automatic and ruminative mode of processing to a more aware and controlled mode of processing) rather than via a shift in negative content (e.g., modifying negative thoughts).

An effortful-processing deficit has several clinical implications. First, it has implications for chronicity. If people with depression possess a bias for processing negative information and diminished capacity for effortful processing, their attempts to "solve the problem of depression" would result in unproductive rumination. In other words, the ruminative loop operates as a closed system, seemingly impermeable to attempts to disrupt it. CBT attempts to interrupt this process with the provision of tools, such as cognitive restructuring, to inhibit negative distractions, and to focus on more adaptive information. It teaches patients, "You are not your thoughts," as a method of decentering. As mentioned earlier, Beck's original clinical observations of automatic thoughts have implications for the theme of automatic processing. CBT attempts to train those with depression to monitor their thoughts and recognize the *automatic* nature of these thoughts. By training patients to stop, write down their thoughts, and challenge the veracity of their thoughts, cognitive restructuring breaks the momentum of automatic negative thinking and engages depressed patients in a more deliberate, effortful approach.

In CBT, interventions are designed with effortful-processing deficits in mind. For example, patients can be aided with effortful-processing deficits by daily homework assignments and preemptive problem solving to address potential problems with the completion of homework. Pleasurable and mastery-related activities are scheduled to increase motivation and offset tendencies toward low effort. Cognitive restructuring also may help to improve efficiency of information processing and problem solving and to redirect attention away from mood-congruent rumination. The cognitive-behavioral therapist designs homework experiments to ensure a high probability of success. Cognitive-behavioral therapists attempt to deal with reduced resources with repetitions at the end of the session, homework based on the topic discussed in session, and a recap at the beginning of the next session. Mindfulness-based cognitive therapy specifically trains people to respond differently to rumination: namely, to become aware and simply observe their thoughts rather than being led by them.

Mood-Dependent Characteristics

A final theme that emerges from our review of the cognitive characteristics of those with depression is that deficits are present only during periods of sad mood. Beck suggested that negativistic schemas are activated by a matching stimulus in the environment. The environment includes both external stimuli and internal stimuli that may activate schemas such as those relating to a negative self-concept and consequent negative emotions (Mischel and Shoda 1995). Thus, the activation of negativistic thinking in times of negative mood is consistent with Beck's ideas on activation. Beck further suggested that those with a history of depression may remain in a heightened "primed" state, such that depressogenic schemas are close to threshold at all times and less stressful internal or external events are necessary for activation. In Nolen-Hoeksema's model, the type of processing activated by sad mood (e.g., rumination) then perpetuates or maintains the depressed mood. Both Beck and Bower would predict that people susceptible to depression should show depression-related memory biases when depressed mood is activated. Findings of a negative processing bias during a sad mood supports Bower's proposal that the activation of the emotion and related nodes enhances their accessibility; thus, someone who is sad is more likely to recall sad-related thoughts and experiences. In particular, the evidence previously reviewed on studies that found increased recall of sad-related thoughts while in a sad mood (for review, see Matt et al. 1992) and increased sad-related thoughts during the most sad parts of the day for those with diurnal patterns of depression (Clark and Teasdale 1982) provides support for this idea.

According to the kindling and episode sensitization theory, even if the original depression episode is related to a negative life event, later triggers need only activate the original neurobiological substrate or depressogenic information processing rather than be related to an adverse life event. The finding that those remitted from depression do not report more negative beliefs than those without depression, but that when a dysphoric mood is induced experimentally, depressogenic processing is seen, is also consistent with the differential activation hypothesis. This theory asserts that previous episodes of depression create vulnerability for a negativistic mode of information processing when dysphoric mood states are experienced, and this could lead to depression. The finding that depressive thinking occurs only during dysphoric states is also consistent with the interacting cognitive subsystems theory because it posits that changes in mood create a shift in the schematic model used to interpret experience, such that while a person is in a dysphoric mood, information is processed in terms of its relation to self-worth.

Several studies have found that induced negative mood leads to impairments in information processing. For example, studies have found poorer recall (Ellis et al. 1984) and problems inhibiting irrelevant thoughts during tasks (Seibert and Ellis 1991) after negative-mood induction. Thus, findings from experimental research have suggested that negative mood leads to biases in attention, less efficient information processing, and memory difficulties, all of which are common clinical complaints of those with MDD.

In addition, the finding that recurrence may have a different etiological pathway than a first episode of depression has treatment implications. It may be more useful to tailor one treatment to target the factors maintaining a current depressive episode and use a different treatment to target the onset of relapse. Because relapse appears to be associated with the activation of a depressive mode of information processing, strategies that train people to disengage from this mode may be particularly helpful (Teasdale et al. 1995a). An example is a relapse prevention treatment that combines an attentional retraining or "mindfulness" skill with a CBT relapse prevention component (mindfulness-based cognitive therapy) (Segal et al. 2002). Mindfulness-based cognitive therapy teaches those remitted from depression to take a distanced or decentered approach to negative thoughts and feelings and has been shown to reduce relapse rates (Ma and Teasdale 2004). Mindfulness-based cognitive therapy also incorporates relapse prevention strategies from CBT that train patients to become aware of the signs or antecedents of depressogenic processing and respond proactively to preempt the activation of negativistic information processing or schemas.

Conclusion

In this review of the experimental literature on the cognitive deficits associated with depression, particular themes emerged. Namely, depression is characterized by a processing bias for emotionally negative stimuli, which is experienced as an automatic cognitive process and is primarily present during dysphoric mood states. In this chapter, points of convergence between experimental and clinical information-processing research were explored in the context of selected clinical theories of depression. This is meant as an illustration of how we can use the research on cognitive deficits associated with depression in both neuroscience and clinical psychological approaches to aid in our understanding of depression.

References

Ball J, Mitchell P, Malhi G, et al: Schema-focused cognitive therapy for bipolar disorder: reducing vulnerability to relapse through attitudinal change. Aust N Z J Psychiatry 37:41–48, 2003

Barnard P, Teasdale JD: Interacting cognitive subsystems: a systemic approach to cognitive-affective interaction and change. Cognition and Emotion 5:1–39, 1991

Bazin N, Perruchet P, De Bonis M, et al: The dissociation of explicit and implicit memory in depressed patients. Psychol Med 24:239–245, 1994

Bearden CE, Hoffman KF, Cannon TD: The neuropsychology and neuroanatomy of bipolar affective disorder: a critical review. Bipolar Disord 3:106–150, 2001

Beck AT: Depression: Causes and Treatment. Philadelphia, University of Pennsylvania Press, 1967

Beck AT, Clark DA: An information processing model of anxiety: reconsidering the role of automatic and strategic processes. Anxiety Research 1:23–36, 1997

Bellew M, Hill AB: Negative recall bias as a predictor of susceptibility to induced depressed mood. Pers Individ Dif 11:471–480, 1990

Blackburn IM, Roxborough HM, Muir WJ, et al: Perceptual and physiological dysfunction in depression. Psychol Med 20:95–103, 1990

Bower GH: Mood and memory. Am Psychol 36:129–148, 1981

Buchsbaum MS, Lee S, Haier R, et al: Effects of amoxapine and imipramine on evoked potentials in the Continuous Performance Test in patients with affective disorder. Neuropsychobiology 20:15–22, 1988

Burt DB, Zembar MJ, Niederehe G: Depression and memory impairment: a meta-analysis of the association, its pattern, and specificity. Psychol Bull 117:285–305, 1995

Calev A, Erwin PG: Recall and recognition in depressives: use of matched tasks. Br J Clin Psychol 24:127–128, 1985

Carter CS, Maddock RJ, Magliozzi J: Patterns of abnormal processing of emotional information in panic disorder and major depression. Psychopathology 25:65–70, 1992

Cassens GC, Wolfe L, Zola M: The neuropsychology of depression. J Neuropsychiatry Clin Neurosci 2:202–213, 1990

Clark DA, Teasdale JD: Diurnal variation in clinical depression and accessibility of memories of positive and negative experiences. J Abnorm Psychol 91:87–95, 1982

Cole KD, Zarit SH: Psychological deficits in depressed medical patients. J Nerv Ment Dis 172:150–155, 1984

Cornell DG, Suarez R, Berent S: Psychomotor retardation in melancholic and nonmelancholic depression: cognitive and motor components. J Abnorm Psychol 93:150–157, 1984

Dalgleish T, Watts FN: Biases of attention and memory in disorders of anxiety and depression. Clin Psychol Rev 10:589–604, 1990

Derry PA, Kuiper NA: Schematic processing and self-reference in clinical depression. J Abnorm Psychol 90:286–297, 1981

Ellis HC, Ashbrook PW: Resource allocation model of the effect of depressed mood states on memory, in Affect, Cognition, and Social Behavior. Edited by Fiedler K, Forgas J. Toronto, ON, Canada, Hogrefe, 1988, pp 25–43

Ellis HC, Thomas RL, Rodriguez IA: Emotional mood states and memory: elaborative encoding, semantic processing, and cognitive effort. J Exp Psychol Learn Mem Cogn 10:470–482, 1984

Evans J, Williams JMG, O'Loughlin S, et al: Autobiographical memory and problem-solving strategies of parasuicide patients. Psychol Med 22:399–405, 1992

Gilboa E, Gotlib IH: Cognitive biases and affect persistence in previously dysphoric and never-dysphoric individuals. Cognition and Emotion 11:517–538, 1997

Golinkoff M, Sweeney JA: Cognitive impairments in depression. J Affect Disord 17:105–112, 1989

Gotlib IH, Cane DB: Construct accessibility and clinical depression: a longitudinal investigation. J Abnorm Psychol 96:199–204, 1987

Gotlib IH, McCabe SB: An information-processing approach to the study of cognitive functioning in depression. Prog Exp Pers Psychopathol Res 15:131–161, 1992

Gotlib IH, McCann CD: Construct accessibility and depression: an examination of cognitive and affective factors. J Pers Soc Psychol 47:427–439, 1984

Gotlib IH, McLachlan AL, Katz AN: Biases in visual attention in depressed and nondepressed individuals. Cognition and Emotion 2:185–200, 1988

Hagerty BM, Williams RA, Liken S: Exploration of prodromal symptoms of major depression. Am J Orthopsychiatry 67:308–314, 1997

Hartlage S, Alloy LB, Vasquez C, et al: Automatic and effortful processing in depression. Psychol Bull 113:247–278, 1993

Hasher L, Zacks RT: Age and inhibition. J Exp Psychol Learn Mem Cogn 17:163–169, 1988

Hertel PT, Rude S: Depressive deficits in memory: focusing attention improves subsequent recall. J Exp Psychol Gen 120:301–309, 1991

Ilsley JE, Moffoot APR, O'Carroll RE: An analysis of memory dysfunction in major depression. J Affect Disord 35:1–9, 1995

Ingram RE, Kendall PC: Cognitive clinical psychology: implications of an information processing perspective, in Information Processing Approaches to Clinical Psychology. Edited by Ingram RE. Orlando, FL, Academic Press, 1986, pp 3–21

Ingram RE, Bernet CZ, McLaughlin SC: Attentional allocation processes in individuals at risk for depression. Cognit Ther Res 18:317–332, 1994

Kendler KS, Thornton LM, Gardner CO: Stressful life events and previous episodes in the etiology of major depression in women: an evaluation of the "kindling" hypothesis. Am J Psychiatry 157:1243–1251, 2000

Knott V, Lapierre Y, Griffiths L, et al: Event-related potentials and selective attention in major depressive illness. J Affect Disord 23:43–48, 1991

Kuyken W, Brewin CR: Autobiographical memory functioning in depression and reports of early abuse. J Abnorm Psychol 104:585–591, 1995

Lau MA, Christensen BK, Gemar M, et al: Inhibitory deficits for negative information in major depression. Paper presented at the 33rd Annual Convention of the Association for Advancement of Behavior Therapy, Toronto, Ontario, November 18–21, 1999

Lau MA, Christensen BK, Hawley LL, et al: Recovery of inhibitory deficits for negative information following cognitive behaviour therapy. Poster presented at the annual meeting of the Society for Research in Psychopathology, Boulder, CO, November 1–4, 2000

Logan GD, Schachar RJ, Tannock R: Impulsivity and inhibitory control. Psychol Sci 8:60–64, 1997

Lyubomirsky S, Nolen-Hoeksema S: Effects of self-focused rumination on negative thinking and interpersonal problem solving. J Pers Soc Psychol 69:176–190, 1995

Ma SH, Teasdale JD: Mindfulness-based cognitive therapy for depression: replication and exploration of differential relapse prevention effects. J Consult Clin Psychol 72:31–40, 2004

MacLeod C, Mathews A, Tata P: Attentional biases in emotional disorders. J Abnorm Psychol 95:15–20, 1986

Matt GE, Vazquez C, Cambell WK: Mood-congruent recall of affectively toned stimuli: a meta-analytic review. Clin Psychol Rev 12:227–255, 1992

McCabe SB, Gotlib IH: Attentional processes in clinically depressed subjects: a longitudinal investigation. Cognit Ther Res 17:359–377, 1993

Mialet JP, Pope HG, Yurgelun-Todd D: Impaired attention in depressive states: a non-specific deficit? Psychol Med 26:1009–1020, 1996

Mischel W, Shoda Y: A cognitive-affective system theory of personality: reconceptualizing situations, dispositions, dynamics, and invariance in personality structure. Psychol Rev 102:246–268, 1995

Moffoot APR, O'Carroll RE, Bennie J, et al: Diurnal variation of mood and neuropsychological function in major depression with melancholia. J Affect Disord 32:257–269, 1994

Mogg K, Bradley BP, Williams R: Attentional bias in anxiety and depression: the role of awareness. Br J Clin Psychol 34:17–36, 1995

Needles DJ, Abramson LY: Positive life events, attributional style, and hopelessness: testing a model of recovery from depression. J Abnorm Psychol 99:156–165, 1990

Neshat-Doost HT, Taghavi MR, Moradi AR, et al: Memory for emotional trait adjectives in clinically depressed youth. J Abnorm Psychol 107:642–650, 1998

Nolen-Hoeksema S: Responses to depression and their effects on the duration of depressive episodes. J Abnorm Psychol 100:569–582, 1991

Posner MI: Orienting of attention. Q J Exp Psychol 32:3–25, 1980

Post RM: Transduction of psychosocial stress into the neurobiology of recurrent affective disorder. Am J Psychiatry 149:999–1010, 1992

Raskin A, Friedman AF, DiMascio A: Cognitive and performance deficits in depression. Psychopharmacol Bull 18:196–202, 1982

Roediger HL, McDermott KB: Depression and implicit memory: a commentary. J Abnorm Psychol 101:587–591, 1992

Segal ZV, Gemar M: Changes in cognitive organization for negative self-referent material following cognitive behaviour therapy for depression: a primed Stroop study. Cognition and Emotion 11:501–516, 1997

Segal ZV, Ingram RE: Priming and construct activation in tests of cognitive vulnerability to unipolar depression. Clin Psychol Rev 14:663–695, 1994

Segal ZV, Shaw BF: Cognition in depression: a reappraisal of Coyne and Gotlib's critique. Cognit Ther Res 10:671–693, 1986

Segal ZV, Gemar M, Truchon C, et al: A priming methodology for studying self-presentation in major depressive disorder. J Abnorm Psychol 104:205–213, 1995

Segal ZV, Williams JM, Teasdale JD, et al: A cognitive science perspective on kindling and episode sensitisation in recurrent affective disorder. Psychol Med 26:371–380, 1996

Segal ZV, Williams JM, Teasdale JD: Mindfulness-Based Cognitive Therapy for Depression: A New Approach to Preventing Relapse. New York, Guilford, 2002

Seibert PS, Ellis HC: Irrelevant thoughts, emotional mood states, and cognitive task performance. Mem Cognit 19:507–513, 1991

Seppala T, Linnoila M, Mattila MJ: Psychomotor skills in depressed out-patients treated with L-tryptophan, doxepin, or chlorimipramine. Ann Clin Res 10:214–221, 1978

Smith MJ, Brebion G, Banquet JP, et al: Retardation of mentation in depressives: Posner's covert orientation of visual attention test. J Affect Disord 35:107–115, 1995

Sturt E, Kumarkura N, Der G: How depressing life is: lifelong morbidity risk for depression in the general population. J Affect Disord 6:104–122, 1984

Teasdale JD: Cognitive vulnerability to persistent depression. Cognition and Emotion 2:247–274, 1988

Teasdale JD, Barnard PJ: Affect, Cognition, and Change: Re-Modelling Depressive Thought. New York, Taylor & Francis, 1993

Teasdale JD, Taylor R: Induced mood and accessibility of memories: an effect of mood state or of induction variation? Br J Clin Psychol 20:39–48, 1981

Teasdale JD, Segal ZV, Williams JMG: How does cognitive therapy prevent depressive relapse and why should attentional control (mindfulness) training help? Behav Res Ther 33:25–39, 1995a

Teasdale JD, Taylor MJ, Cooper Z, et al: Depressive thinking: shifts in construct accessibility or in schematic mental models? J Abnorm Psychol 104:500–507, 1995b

Teasdale JD, Scott J, Moore RG, et al: How does cognitive therapy prevent relapse in residual depression? Evidence from a controlled trial. J Consult Clin Psychol 69:347–357, 2001

Watkins PC, Mathews A, Williamson DA, et al: Mood-congruent memory in depression: emotional priming or elaboration? J Abnorm Psychol 101:581–586, 1992

Williams JMG: Memory processes in psychotherapy, in Frontiers of Cognitive Therapy. Edited by Salkovskis PM. New York, Guilford, 1996, pp 114–134

Williams JMG: Depression, in Science and Practice of Cognitive Behaviour Therapy. Edited by Clark DM, Fairburn CG. New York, Oxford University Press, 1997, pp 259–283

Williams JMG, Nulty DD: Construct accessibility, depression and the emotional Stroop task: transient mood or stable structure? Pers Individ Dif 7:485–491, 1986

Williams JMG, Mathews A, MacLeod C: The emotional Stroop task and psychopathology. Psychol Bull 120:3–24, 1996

Williams JMG, Watts FN, MacLeod C, et al: Cognitive Psychology and Emotional Disorders, 2nd Edition. West Sussex, UK, Wiley, 1997

Williams JMG, Teasdale JD, Segal ZV, et al: Mindfulness-based cognitive therapy reduces overgeneral autobiographical memory in formerly depressed patients. J Abnorm Psychol 109:150–155, 2000

Zakzanis KK, Leach L, Kaplan E: On the nature and pattern of neurocognitive function in major depressive disorder. Neuropsychiatry Neuropsychol Behav Neurol 11:111–119, 1998

Social Perspectives on Mood Disorders

DAVID R. WILLIAMS, PH.D., M.P.H.

HAROLD W. NEIGHBORS, PH.D.

GROWING SCIENTIFIC EVIDENCE indicates that the prevalence of depressive disorders increased markedly in the last half of the twentieth century (Kasen et al. 2003; Kessler and Zhao 1999). Although debate persists regarding the underlying reasons for increasing rates of depression, it is implausible that they reflect marked changes in the genetic constitution of the population. Instead, changing environmental factors, including changes in social arrangements and role expectations, are likely to play a role. Given the substantial societal costs that are associated with mood disorders, including role impairment and disability, it is imperative that we develop an enhanced understanding of the social underpinnings of these disorders. In this chapter, we seek to provide an overview of factors in the social environment that can play a role as risk factors for the onset, course, and inappropriate treatment of mood disorders.

Social Distribution of Mood Disorders

The distribution of mood disorders is strongly patterned by several social factors, suggesting that the social environment may play a role in the onset of these disorders. We begin by examining some of these associations. We do not intend to be comprehensive but to provide some illustrative examples of the extent to which various social categories are associated with elevated rates of mood disorders. We draw heavily on examples from the Epidemiologic Catchment Area (ECA) study, a study of almost 20,000 institutionalized and noninstitutionalized adults, conducted between 1980 and 1983 in five communities in the United States (Robins and Regier 1991) and from the National Comorbidity Survey (NCS), the first study

Preparation of this chapter was supported by grant 1 R01 MH59575 from the National Institute of Mental Health and by the John D. and Catherine T. MacArthur Foundation Research Network on Socioeconomic Status and Health. The authors wish to thank Trisha Matelski for research assistance and preparation of the manuscript.

to use a national probability survey to assess psychiatric disorders in the United States, interviewing more than 8,000 adults between ages 15 and 54, and the NCS Replication.

Marital Status

Researchers have long noted a strong relation between marital status and the risk of depression. In the ECA study, both current marital status and marital history were strongly associated with the prevalence of mood disorders, even after sex, age, and race were controlled (Weissman et al. 1991). The widowed, and especially the separated and divorced, persons had higher adjusted odds of both major depression and bipolar disorder than did the currently married persons. Persons who were cohabiting or had a history of divorce, irrespective of current marital status, had elevated rates of bipolar disorders compared with married or widowed persons without a history of divorce. A similar relation existed for major depression. Persons who had never been married also had higher rates of bipolar disorder and major depression compared with married persons who had experienced no marital dissolution.

Data on the relation between household size and major depression (Weissman et al. 1991) may shed light on the strong relation between marital status and the prevalence of this disorder. In the ECA study, the prevalence of major depression was twice as high among persons living alone compared with those who lived with others, suggesting that social isolation may be a risk factor. However, among individuals not living alone, rates of mood disorders did not vary by household size. Further analyses suggest that it is the loss of being married (the disruption of marital status) that is the key risk factor for the elevated rates of mood disorders and not social isolation itself. For example, in the ECA study data, living alone was not related to an increased risk for mood disorders among unmarried adults. Similarly, other analyses of the ECA data found that for blacks and whites, men and women, never having been married was not significantly associated with an increased risk for major depression (Williams et al. 1992a).

Gender

One of the most consistent findings in psychiatric epidemiology is that the prevalence, incidence, and morbidity of mood disorders are higher for women than for men. These differences exist in many different cultures and countries throughout the world. In the ECA study, rates of bipolar disorder were comparable in men and women, but women had rates of major depression and dysthymia

that were more than twice as high as those in men (Weissman et al. 1991). Similarly, in the NCS, the prevalence of ever experiencing an episode of major depression and dysthymia was almost twice as high for women as for men (21.3 vs. 12.7 for major depressive episode and 8.0 vs. 4.8 for dysthymia) (Kessler and Zhao 1999). No gender difference was seen for mania; the lifetime prevalence was 1.6 for men and 1.7 for women. Piccinelli and Wilkinson's (2000) review of the determinants of gender differences in depression concluded that the gender differences in depressive disorders are not artifactual but reflect differences in the social experiences of males and females. Specifically, the available evidence suggests that gender differences in early exposures in childhood, sociocultural roles, and responses to adverse experiences play a critical role in the observed gender differences in depression. In addition, gender differences in psychological attributes and patterns of coping are likely to play a role. In contrast, fewer data indicate that genetics and biological factors play a role in the emergence of gender differences in rates of depression.

Socioeconomic Status

Low socioeconomic status (SES) is a risk factor for a broad range of health conditions, including mental illness. However, one report from the ECA study found a surprisingly weak association between SES and mood disorders. Measures of income, occupation, and education were unrelated to major depression, and only lower levels of education were associated with elevated rates of bipolar disorder (Weissman et al. 1991). However, the ECA findings differ by the indicator of SES used. When Holzer et al. (1986) used a composite measure of SES in the analyses of the ECA data, they found elevated rates of major depression at the lower levels of SES. These findings are consistent with those of the NCS. The NCS documented that the lowest levels of education and income were associated with elevated rates of any affective disorder (Kessler et al. 1994). Nonetheless, note that the association between SES and psychiatric disorders was weaker for mood disorders in both the ECA study and the NCS than for anxiety disorders or substance abuse (Holzer et al. 1986; Kessler et al. 1994).

Other data suggest that the association between SES and mood disorders varies by race/ethnicity (Dohrenwend 1990). For example, in the ECA study, major depression was inversely related to a composite measure of SES for white patients but unrelated for black patients (Williams et al. 1992b). Recent evidence also indicates that the association between SES and mood disorders is not limited to industrialized countries. A recent review documented that lower levels of income were consistently associated with elevated risk of depressive disorders in 11 community studies in six developing countries (Patel and Kleinman 2003).

Several other social status categories closely related to SES also have been associated with elevated rates of mood disorder. A study in Canada found that single motherhood was associated with an increased risk of mood disorder (Lipman et al. 1997). Both economic deprivation and social isolation may be key underlying factors. Additional analyses showed that low-income single mothers were 2.5 times more likely to meet criteria for a mood disorder in the past year compared with more economically favored mothers in two-parent families. However, single mothers who did not have low income and low-income mothers in two-parent families did not have an elevated risk for mood disorder. In the ECA study, welfare recipients (persons financially dependent on public aid) had a risk of both bipolar disorder and major depression that was three times that of persons who were financially independent (Weissman et al. 1991). Other recent studies have continued to document that rates of depression are high among welfare recipients (Lennon et al. 2002).

Some evidence also suggests that exposure to sustained economic hardship may have a cumulative adverse effect on mental health status. The Alameda County Study defined economic hardship as total household income that was less than twice the federal poverty level and examined the association between exposure to economic hardship in 1965, 1974, and 1983 and mental health status in 1994. The study found a graded association between major depression and depressive symptoms with exposure to economic hardship (Lynch et al. 1997). Persons who had experienced economic hardship at all three waves were 3.2 times more likely to be clinically depressed than were those who had never experienced economic hardship. For depressive symptoms, the odds ratio was 1.7 for those who had experienced economic hardship once but 3.8 for those who had experienced economic hardship two or three times, compared with those who had not experienced economic adversity.

Employment status also has been related to the risk for mood disorders. Among persons younger than 65 in the ECA study, the currently unemployed had a higher risk of major depression than did those who were working. Similarly, persons who had been unemployed for at least 6 months in the previous 5 years were more than three times as likely as others to meet criteria for major depression (Weissman et al. 1991). In the NCS, the currently employed subjects had lower rates of any mood disorder than did homemakers or the unemployed, retired, and disabled subjects (Kessler and Zhao 1999). Employment status also was more strongly associated with disorder risk for men than for women.

Urbanization

Increasing urbanization and exposures of larger proportions of the population to conditions linked to urban life may play a critical role in the increases observed in mood and other psychiatric disorders in the last century (Weissman et al. 1991). According to this view, large differences should be observed in the levels of psychiatric disorder in urban and rural areas.

This issue was examined at two sites of the ECA study—St. Louis, Missouri, and Durham, North Carolina—that provided variation in urbanicity. A profound pattern of urban–rural differences was observed in Durham, whereas the pattern in St. Louis was mixed. Rates of bipolar disorder were almost 4 times higher in urban than in rural areas in Durham, whereas rates of major depression were more than twice as high. In contrast, although rates of bipolar disorder were 2.2 times higher in urban St. Louis than in surrounding rural areas, the rates of major depression were significantly lower in urban St. Louis than in the adjacent rural areas.

Weissman and colleagues (1991) suggested that paying greater attention to the particular characteristics of specific geographic areas may be important in future research because they can shed light on the observed patterns. They noted, for example, that many of the rural areas in the Durham site of the ECA were substantially farther away from an urban center and less affected by urban spread than were the "rural areas" outside St. Louis. Accordingly, the greater urbanization of the St. Louis "rural areas" compared with those in Durham could account for the pattern of findings (Weissman et al. 1991). In the NCS, residents of rural areas reported slightly lower levels of mood disorders than did residents of urban areas, but the differences were not statistically significant (Kessler and Zhao 1999).

More generally, a comprehensive review of the literature on urban and rural differences in the prevalence of depressive and other psychiatric disorders also has found that the pattern of findings is mixed (Judd et al. 2002). This review concluded that a variety of sociodemographic factors are more strongly related to the prevalence of psychiatric disorders than is geographic location of residence. Judd and colleagues (2002) emphasized the need for future research that pays more attention to interactions between location of residence and other social and demographic characteristics.

Psychosocial Mechanisms: Stress, Social Roles, and Individual Vulnerability

It is very difficult to interpret the causal direction for all of the relations highlighted between the risk of mood disorders and social factors. Bidirectional influences are likely for many of the examples considered. For example, persons who are depressed may have greater challenges in both obtaining and maintaining a stable job. Similarly, someone with a history of mood disorders may be less desirable as a potential spouse, and the challenges of living with a depressed spouse could lead to marital disruption. In a similar vein, the presence of mood disorders could hinder individuals from obtaining or keeping jobs that would maintain their SES position or enhance social mobility. Thus, the presence of mood disorders or other mental illness could cause individuals to drift into lower SES groups or to fail to climb out of low SES positions at rates comparable to those of healthy adults. Nevertheless, the social distribution of mood disorders highlights the need to identify the social and psychological exposures that may lead to increased risk. We now consider the available research on key social processes and experiences that may affect the mental health risk of all people but that may systematically be differentially distributed across social groups.

Stress and Mood Disorders

A large body of research suggests that exposure to stressful life experiences may be an important link between the social environment and the risk for mood disorders. Stressful life experiences are often divided into acute life events and chronic stressors. Life events are discrete, observable stressors, whereas chronic stress refers to ongoing problems that can be divided into major role-related ones and minor irritations that are often called daily hassles. A comprehensive review of the literature on life events and depression came to four major conclusions (Kessler 1997):

1. A consistent association is seen between exposure to life events and subsequent reports of the onset of major depression.
2. The magnitude of this association varies by the assessment of life events; the association is stronger when specific features of stressful life experience are taken into account.
3. The association between life events and depression is consistently one of a dose–response relation; severe events are more strongly associated with major depression compared with events that are not severe.

4. Life events occur at a relatively high frequency in the general population, and most depressed patients experience a stressful life experience shortly before the onset of their depression. At the same time, most people who experience life events do not become depressed.

Other recent reviews provided additional evidence to support a strong association between exposure to life stress and mood disorders (Paykel 2001; Tennant 2002).

The work of George Brown and colleagues (Brown 2002; Brown and Harris 1978) illustrates both the strength of the association between stressful life events and major depression and many of the complexities in understanding and studying this association. These researchers have been studying the psychosocial factors linked to the onset of depression among working-class women in London, England. This body of research views depression as closely linked to the quality of core social roles and emphasizes the importance of understanding both the meaning that stressful life experiences has for the individual and the social context in which these experiences unfold. For example, an experience of unemployment must be understood in the light of the unemployment rate in the local community, the probability of that individual obtaining a new job, the economic resources of the individual's household, and the likely psychological and economic effects that the loss of income would have on the household unit.

The early research of Brown and Harris (1978) suggested that depression was triggered by exposure to severe events that included loss. *Loss* was broadly defined and could include the loss of a person, a social role, an important plan, or a cherished idea about one's self or a significant other. This view that loss was the key pathogenic characteristic of stressful experiences differed markedly from the prevailing view of the time, which focused on the change and adjustment caused by life events. Interestingly, Brown's work showed that severe stressful events that involved only danger were not important in predicting the risk for depression, although they played an important role in predicting the risk for anxiety disorders. However, subsequent analyses of these data suggested that the key aspects of stressful life experiences that increase the risk for major depression are those that engender feelings of entrapment and humiliation (Brown 2002). It appears that the perception of attacks on an individual's self-esteem; the undermining of a person's sense of rank, attractiveness, or value; and the experiences that seem to afford no opportunity of escape are the key factors that trigger depression. The finding that humiliation and entrapment are the key pathogenic aspects of stressful experiences was initially observed in studies of working-class women in London but has since been replicated cross-culturally in contexts as diverse as Zimbabwe, rural Spain, and the Outer Hebrides (Brown 2002).

Social Context, Social Roles, and Exposure to Stress

Exposure to stress is not randomly distributed in society. The larger social context of the individual, such as the stage of the life course and the social roles that one occupies in society, can determine exposure to stress and thus the risk for mood disorders. For example, the probability of exposure to certain stressful experiences increases with age. These include the onset or exacerbation of severe or life-threatening illness, the loss of a spouse or other loved one, disability, and a lack of social contact. In turn, all of these specific stressful experiences have been associated with the onset of depression among the elderly (Bruce 2002).

Research on gender and depression provides an illustration of how occupying certain roles in society can affect stress exposure and mental health risk. A British study of couples who had shared in the experience of a severe stressful event found that a gender difference in depression did not exist for the small number of men who had major domestic responsibilities within the household (Brown 2002). Other evidence suggests that gender differences are markedly reduced when men hold traditional women's roles. For instance, the higher prevalence of symptoms of depression among women than men is reversed when men and women are not in their traditional roles (Rosenfield 1999a). Similarly, wives who are employed have lower depression scores than do their husbands, and when women or men earn less relative to their spouses, they experience more symptoms of depression (Rosenfield 1999b). A study of teachers in Australia also found a reduction in gender differences in depression when gender roles converged (Wilhelm and Parker 1989). In addition, although women are generally better at providing emotional support than men, men who are the primary providers of child care have social support skills that are comparable to those of women (Risman 1987). Other evidence suggests that compared with men, women have lower levels of self-esteem and mastery, stronger identification with the feelings of others, and higher levels of emotional distress in response to the stressful events that happen to others (Rosenfield 1999b). All of these factors are linked to the risk of mental health problems and rooted in the socialization experiences. Thus, gender differences in socialization and social arrangements appear to play a major role in the stable pattern noted for gender differences in mood disorders.

Early Life Stressors and Adult Risk of Mood Disorders

Kendall-Tackett (2002) reviewed the literature on the relation between early childhood abuse and its behavioral, social, cognitive, and emotional sequelae. The conclusion of this review was that depression is one of the most common consequences of early childhood abuse. Some evidence suggests that the risk for depression is four times greater among adult survivors of childhood sexual abuse compared with those who do not have a history of abuse. Moreover, the evidence suggests that childhood sexual abuse makes an independent contribution to the risk for depression over and above other adverse events in childhood. Kessler (1997) also concluded that separation from a parent, family turmoil, parental psychopathology, and physical and sexual abuse are childhood adversities that have been reported more often by depressed adults.

The work of Brown (2002) and colleagues also has highlighted the importance of understanding how the social factors that determine the risk for depression unfold over the life course. Moreover, it is crucial to understand how these factors are related to one another and can create a "conveyor belt" of adversities. For example, the loss of a mother before age 11 years was associated in the initial work of Brown with an increased risk for depression once a severe event had occurred. Other childhood factors that increase the risk for depression in adulthood include marked parental neglect, physical abuse from a core social tie, or sexual abuse.

Brown's (2002) research also has identified some of the mechanisms that link exposure to early life stressors to the risk for mood disorders. For example, the early loss of a mother turned out to be important primarily because it increased the risk for neglect and abuse during childhood. In addition, the early experience of abuse and neglect could adversely affect a woman's self-esteem as well as her long-term ability to relate to others by leading to either an avoidance style that creates difficulty in establishing intimacy with others or an overdependent style in intimate relationships. That is, early childhood adversity can create psychological vulnerability that, in turn, can affect one's ability to relate to others and obtain social support, as well as increase exposure to severe events. For example, underlying social and psychological vulnerability can affect one's choice of a partner, which can determine exposure to a broad range of stressful life experiences.

Economic Change as a Macro Stressor

The stress literature identifies macro stressors as a distinct subtype of stress. Macro stressors are large-scale, systems-related stressors such as major economic changes and recessions. Aggregate indicators of such changes also have been related to rates of mental health problems. Economic change has long been suspected to have effects on mental health beyond the employees involved in the change (Weyerer and Wiedenmann 1995). Durkheim (1951) suspected that rapid economic change led to various forms of instability and suicidal behavior. Brenner (1969) studied the relation between economic change and psychological well-being. In a seminal study of mental hospitals in New York State, Brenner found that those belonging to lower socioeconomic groups experienced more psychiatric symptoms than those belonging to higher socioeconomic groups during periods of economic change. Although these results highlighted the importance of economic change for mental health, the actual causal factors to explain this link were not fully detailed. Catalano and Dooley's (1977) study of Kansas City, Missouri, residents represented an attempt to explain the link between economic change and depressive symptoms. These researchers documented that economic change was related to a significant increase in stressful events, which led to an increase in depressed mood.

Weyerer and Wiedenmann (1995) identified economic change as consisting of five broad indicators: 1) supply indicators, 2) activity indicators, 3) labor market indicators, 4) business statistics indicators, and 5) indicators of field structure change. Supply indicators include price index or income changes, whereas activity indicators include alterations in traffic, export, production, or investment volume caused by economic change. Labor market indicators include changes in unemployed and employed quotas and labor force participation, and business statistics indicators include information such as bankruptcy rates and the number of businesses in a particular area. Finally, indicators of field structure change may include changes in the distribution of the gainfully employed in a geographically defined area (Weyerer and Wiedenmann 1995).

Some research has examined the various components of these indicators. For example, Catalano and Dooley (1977) found large effects of economic change, when defined by supply indicators, on depressed mood for low-income groups. Ganzini et al. (1990) used "catastrophic financial loss" as a supply indicator and found positive associations with depressive symptoms. These two studies suggested that sudden changes in personal or household income may increase the risk for depression. Other studies have assessed the mental health correlates of activity and labor market indicators. Aneshensel and Sucoff (1996) used social disorder as an indicator of economic activity change and found positive associations with depression and anxiety in an adolescent population. Cohen and Glass

(1973) measured neighborhood noise as an activity indicator and found positive associations with anxiety.

These relations may be consistent for labor market indicators as well. For example, Tiggemann and Winefield (1984) found positive associations with depression, whereas Trovato (1986) found significant positive associations between labor market indicators and depression and suicide. Furthermore, Weyerer and Wiedenmann (1995) found positive associations between labor market indicators such as "frequency of bankruptcy" and "unemployment" and rates of depression and suicide. Similarly, Dooley et al. (2000) found higher rates of underemployment associated with increased risk of depression. Also, Beiser and Hou (2001) used "unemployment due to language fluency" as a labor market indicator and also found positive associations with depression. Other labor indicators of economic change assessed in the literature include concentration in secondary labor market and welfare system (Bennett 1987), level of managed health care (Domino et al. 1998), and transition from welfare (Dooley and Prause 2002). Bennett (1987) and Domino et al. (1998) focused on these indicators associated with depression, and Dooley and Prause (2002) considered the effect of transition to welfare on various psychiatric symptoms.

Finally, several investigators have reviewed the contributions of field structure characteristics and business statistics as indicators of economic change. Neff (1983) assessed levels of urbanization to evaluate field structure and found great usefulness in this consideration during a critique of the issue, whereas Desjarlais et al. (1995) assessed urban life as a field structure characteristic and found positive associations with depression. Heffernan and Heffernan (1986) assessed farm economic crisis as a field structure characteristic and found a positive relation with anxiety and depression, whereas Hoyt and colleagues (1997) show how rural economic stress is also a field structure that can affect psychological distress. Investigators also have used real income and frequency of bankruptcy as business statistics indicators and have found associations with depression and suicide (Weyerer and Wiedenmann 1995).

In summary, considerable empirical evidence suggests that exposure to stressful circumstances, at multiple levels of analysis, may play an important role in the onset of mood disorders. Moreover, they may importantly account for the social distribution of mood disorders. For example, Avison's (1997) research in Canada documented that stress plays a crucial role in the increased risk for major depression in single mothers. This relation is a result of the greater exposure of single mothers to acute and chronic stress but not a result of deficits in social competence or psychological resilience. Similarly, in a study of couples who had experienced the same severe event, Brown (2002) and colleagues found that the gender difference in the risk for depression could be completely accounted for by women's greater susceptibility to stressful events involving children, procreation, and housing.

Stress and Mood Disorders: Vulnerability and Protective Factors

As noted earlier, it is well documented that most individuals who are exposed to stress do not become depressed. For example, the initial work of Brown (2002) and his colleagues found that only about 20% of women who experienced a life event that was rated as severe according to their strict criteria developed depression, and only about one-third of those who had a severe event involving humiliation or entrapment developed clinical depression. There are several reasons that most persons exposed to stressful life experiences do not become depressed (Bruce 2002). First, many of the measures of stress do not adequately capture the relevant characteristics of stressors that are consequential for increasing the risk of mood disorders. Second, several stressors may work to increase the risk for mood disorders only in the context of other biological, genetic, or psychosocial variables that modify risk. Gender is an example of the latter. The risk of major depression associated with marital separation and divorce is greater for men than for women. Finally, the effect of a stressful life event may be dependent on other personality factors such as neuroticism or on the background level of chronic stressors in the individual's life.

Social status itself may also be a vulnerability factor. Persons of lower SES, as indicated by fewer years of education, low occupational status, and low income, are more vulnerable to undesirable life events, including loss of income, ill health, marital separation and divorce, other love loss, death of a loved one, and negative events within the respondents' network. Exposure to these stressors is more likely to lead to psychological distress for those of low SES than for more advantaged persons (McLeod and Kessler 1990).

The work of Brown (2002) and colleagues illustrated the central role played by vulnerability factors in affecting the strength of the association between exposure to stressful life experiences and major depression. They identified two classes of vulnerability factors: 1) psychological factors, such as low self-esteem and chronic clinical or subclinical anxiety or depression, and 2) a negative environmental factor related to the quality of social relationships in the home or the absence of a close confiding relationship with someone seen regularly. These two factors are also related to each other in complex ways. For example, the quality of core social ties in adulthood has an important influence on current self-esteem. Importantly, their work showed that a severe stressful event seldom led to the onset of major depression without the presence of at least one of these vulnerability factors. Other research confirmed that the quality of core social ties and the receipt of emotional support from family or close friends can be crucial protective factors from depression (Paykel 1994).

Social factors also shape exposure to these vulnerability factors. For instance, Brown (2002) illustrated the multiple ways in which poverty can shape exposure to the vulnerability factors for depression. Poverty can lower a sense of self-esteem and morale and adversely affect the quality of emotional support while contributing to a sense of continuing entrapment and hopelessness and increasing the individual's exposure to abuse and neglect during childhood.

Religion as a Resource

There is growing research interest in the ways in which religious involvement and participation may play a role in mental health. Religious involvement appears to be a neglected resource that can beneficially affect mental health in multiple ways (Ellison and Levin 1998; Ellison et al. 2001; Williams 1994). First, religious institutions can supply friendship networks that can provide emotional and instrumental support as well as a feeling of connectedness and belonging. Second, religious beliefs and values can provide systems of meaning that can help individuals to interpret and reinterpret stressors in ways that can reduce their negative emotional consequences. Third, religious beliefs can provide feelings of strength to cope with adversity. Fourth, by encouraging moderation in all things and discouraging negative health behaviors, religious involvement can reduce risk-taking behavior and exposure to stress. Finally, it is also recognized that there can be a dark side to religiosity. Religious beliefs and participation can generate stress, role conflicts, social conflicts, criticism, and ostracism that can adversely affect mental health.

Levels of religious involvement are very high in the United States and some other countries. A national study of prayer in the United States concluded that despite the neglect of religion by researchers, more Americans (88%) pray than have sex (Poloma and Gallup 1991). Moreover, many persons turn to religion when coping with stress. For example, a national survey that was conducted within 3–5 days of the September 11, 2001, terrorist attacks in the eastern United States found that 90% of the adults reported that they turned to prayer, religion, or spiritual feelings to cope with these events (Schuster et al. 2001). However, the relation between religiosity and prayer is complex and may vary by the indicator of religious involvement under consideration. One community survey found that in response to stress, prayer increased, but church attendance declined (Lindenthal et al. 1970).

Several studies have found that higher levels of religious attendance are associated with lower levels of depressive symptoms (e.g., Levin et al. 1996; Strawbridge et al. 1998). A review of some 80 studies concluded that individuals with high levels of general religious involvement, public participation (religious attendance), religious salience, and intrinsic religious motivation were at a reduced risk for depressive symptoms and depressive disorders (McCullough and Larson 1999). Similarly, compared with the religiously affiliated, people with no religious affiliation and from certain affiliations had an elevated risk of depressive symptoms and disorders. At the same time, private religious activity showed no reliable relation with depression, and people with extrinsic religious motivation (involved with religion for utilitarian reasons) were at increased risk for depressive symptoms. This review concluded that although the observed patterns were consistent, they were modest in size and substantially reduced in multivariate research. A more recent meta-analysis of 147 studies that examined the association between religiousness and depressive symptoms also concluded that the relation of high religious involvement to fewer symptoms of depression was strong but modest in size (Smith et al. 2003). This review also found that both an extrinsic religious orientation and negative religious coping were associated with elevated symptoms of depression.

Other evidence suggests that religious involvement can buffer or reduce the negative effects of stress on mental health (Schnittker 2001). For example, in a prospective analysis of data from New Haven, Connecticut, religious attendance did not directly reduce psychological distress, but it buffered the negative effects of undesirable life events and health problems on subsequent mental health (Williams et al. 1991). A more recent study found that a strong belief in eternal life reduced the negative effects of work-related stress on psychological distress (Ellison et al. 2001). However, cross-sectional analysis from the Alameda County Study highlights the complexity of these associations. This study found that religiosity reduced the negative effects of nonfamily stressors (financial problems, neighborhood stress, chronic illness) on depressive symptoms (Strawbridge et al. 1998). At the same time, it exacerbated the effects of child problems and family stressors on depression. The authors suggested that stressors that raise conflicts with values emphasized by religious organizations (e.g., unruly children, difficult marriages) may lead to feelings of stigmatization and low levels of active conflict resolution.

Further evidence of the potential positive and negative effects of religious involvement comes from research on religious coping. For example, a study of members of two churches coping with the 1995 bombing of the federal building in Oklahoma City, Oklahoma, found that positive religious coping (e.g., looking to God for strength, support, and guidance; trying to find a lesson from God in the crisis) was more strongly related to improved mental health status over time than was negative religious coping (e.g., felt that the bombing was God's way of punishing me; wondered whether God had abandoned us) (Pargament et al. 1998).

Investigators have much to learn about the ways in which religious involvement can enhance or impair mental health. The current literature on religion and mental health is characterized by inadequate conceptualization of religious variables and limited assessment of religion (Hill and Pargament 2003). Greater attention needs to be given to the mental health consequences of explicitly religious beliefs and behavior, such as forgiveness (Krause and Ellison 2003; Toussaint et al. 2001). The role of religious rituals and symbols has been neglected, and there are some suggestions in the literature that both the psychosocial environments of some congregations (Pargament et al. 1983) and the aspects of some religious services can facilitate the reduction of tension and the release of emotional distress (Gilkes 1980; Griffith et al. 1980). In fact, some evidence suggests that the rituals of at least some religious services provide all the key elements of a therapeutic encounter between a patient and a clinician (Griffith et al. 1980, 1984).

The extent to which spirituality as distinct from religiosity can affect mental health is another important issue to be resolved (Nelson et al. 2002). A recent national study highlighted some of the challenges in this area. More than half of Americans (52%) rated themselves as high on religiosity and spirituality, with 10% as spiritual only, 9% as religious only, and 29% as neither spiritual nor religious (Shahabi et al. 2002). Interestingly, respondents who were both spiritual and religious manifested the highest levels of public and private religious practice and the lowest levels of psychological distress. Other important issues requiring further study are the role of the clergy as gatekeepers to the mental health system (Neighbors et al. 1998; Wang et al. 2003), the counseling activities of the clergy (Young et al. 2003), and the efficacy of religiously oriented psychotherapy (Berry 2002).

Social Factors and the Course of Mood Disorders

Riso and colleagues (2002) have explored a broad range of factors that might play a role in determining the chronicity of depression. They reviewed the literature on developmental factors, personality and personality disorders, psychosocial stressors, comorbid disorders, biological factors, and cognitive factors. They concluded that at present, the strongest evidence is for the role of developmental factors in predicting the chronicity of depression. The key developmental factors are sexual or physical abuse in childhood or poor early relationships with parents. However, neuroticism, an important personality characteristic that refers to emotional instability, also seems to be a strong predictor of the chronicity of depression. Neuroticism is often used as a marker for heightened stress reactivity. Heightened stress reactivity and chronic stressors, such as ongoing medical illness or extended unemployment or marital discord, are also implicated as predictors of chronic depression (Riso et al. 2002). Other research indicates that difficulties are associated with a slower speed of recovery from a major depressive episode (Kessler 1997).

Lewis (1998) reviewed the literature suggesting that the quality of marital relationships is a strong predictor of both the severity and the course of mood disorders. This research found that high levels of emotional support from a spouse or high levels of marital conflict were among the strongest predictors of positive or negative outcome, respectively, of the treatment of major depression. Other studies found that adults who are vulnerable to depression because of the loss of a parent during childhood, for example, are protected from such risk if they receive a high level of emotional of support from their spouses. In general, this research documented that a close, confiding relationship can buffer against the onset of depression, whereas diminished marital quality can increase the severity and recurrence of depression (Lewis 1998).

Social Factors and the Treatment of Mood Disorders

Social factors are also related to both access to mental health treatment and quality of treatment for mood disorders. The organization and financing of mental health services vary across different societies, and these differences can create large inequities in the treatment of mood disorders. For example, the mental health system in the United States is fragmented organizationally and in its various sources of funding (U.S. Department of Health and Human Services 1999). These organizational characteristics combined with more generous insurance coverage for general medical care than for mental disorders have created many barriers to care. System-related barriers (e.g., inadequate funding, time pressure) often combine with patient-related (e.g., denial of psychological symptoms because of stigma) and provider-related ones (e.g., underdetection of depression and suicide risk) to adversely affect the quantity and quality of care for mood disorders.

Many individuals with mood disorders never contact a mental health care professional about their symptoms. The estimated utilization rate for individuals with depression ranges from 18.7% to 64.0% in various studies (Bland et al. 1997; Galbaud du Fort et al. 1999; Goodman and Huang 2002; Schichor et al. 1994). Some evidence suggests that help-seeking rates for major depression are increasing over time. The NCS Replication recently reported that 57% of the respondents meeting criteria for major depressive disorder in the past 12 months had received some type of treatment (Kessler et al. 2003).

Several social factors are associated with the likelihood of help seeking: being a woman, being younger than 45 years, living alone, living in a big city, and having more severe symptoms increased the likelihood of seeking treatment. Galbaud du Fort et al. (1999) reported lifetime treatment-seeking rates of 69.0% for those with major depression, 59.0% for those with a depressive illness in association with bereavement, and 57.0% for those with dysthymia. This study also found that being female and having psychomotor retardation, suicidal ideation, older age at first onset, and comorbidity with mania and panic disorder increased the likelihood of treatment seeking. In addition, comorbidity with drug abuse or dependence reduced the likelihood of professional contact (Galbaud du Fort et al. 1999). Parikh et al. (1996) found significant urban–rural differences in professional help seeking for depression. Specifically, 55% of the urban respondents compared with only 40% of the rural respondents with depression sought help. Factors found to significantly increase treatment seeking were being female, having increased associated functional impairment, and having other psychiatric disorders comorbidly. Other barriers to help seeking include difficulties in setting aside time for seeking help among working men and women (Fox et al. 2001) and the general public's attitude toward psychiatric disorders (Mojtabai et al. 2002).

Social factors also appear to affect the type of treatment received. Some research indicates that the quality of treatment for mood disorders varies by the place where it is received, with specialty mental health settings providing better overall quality than primary care settings. In particular, the rates of recognition of mood disorders and the appropriate treatment of them are low in primary care settings. Poor recognition can lead to unnecessary and expensive diagnostic procedures, and fewer than one-half of the depressed patients in primary care settings receive antidepressant medication according to recommended guidelines for dosage and duration (U.S. Department of Health and Human Services 1999). It is not surprising that 40% discontinue their medication during the first 4–6 weeks of treatment. In the United States, African American and Hispanic patients are more likely than white and Asian patients to seek treatment in the general medical sector rather than mental health specialty settings (Cooper et al. 2003; Sussman et al. 1987). Low SES is also associated with consulting a primary care physician rather than a specialist (Goodman and Huang 2002).

Mood disorders affect individuals in various ways, and people react quite differently to symptoms. Many people and their families do not recognize the symptoms of depression, are not aware that it is a medical illness, and do not know how it is treated. For example, one study found that among those individuals who met criteria for mood, anxiety, or substance use disorder, only 32% actually perceived a need for professional help. Furthermore, only 59% of those who saw a need for treatment actually sought help (Mojtabai 1999). Many in the general public think that depression is a normal part of aging. Many others, particularly men, view depression as a character flaw and as a sign of weakness. As a result, a significant amount of stigma remains attached to the idea of admitting or acknowledging symptoms of depression. The stigma against individuals with mood disorders has a major influence in determining whether an individual seeks treatment (U.S. Department of Health and Human Services 1999).

A report from the Institute of Medicine in the United States suggested that social factors also may systematically affect the quality and intensity of treatment of a broad range of health conditions, including mood disorders (Smedley et al. 2003). This review of the available research showed that across virtually every therapeutic intervention, ranging from high-tech procedures to the most elementary forms of diagnostic and treatment interventions, minorities received fewer procedures and poorer-quality medical care than did whites. Moreover, these differences persist even after differences in health insurance, SES, stage and severity of disease, comorbidity, and the type of medical facility are taken into account. Mental health was no exception to this pattern. We provide one example of the many studies of mental health treatment.

A study of 13,065 Medicaid patients diagnosed with major depressive episode found that black patients (28%) were less likely than white patients (44%) to receive antidepressant medication within 30 days of initial diagnosis (Melfi et al. 2000). This finding is important because clinical trials showed that black patients are more likely than white patients to respond to adequate antidepressant treatment. Moreover, after the investigators adjusted for demographics, provider type, and comorbidity, black patients were 55% less likely than white patients to receive any antidepressant. Of those receiving an antidepressant, black patients were 25% less likely than white patients to receive selective serotonin reuptake inhibitors compared with tricyclic antidepressants as the initial antidepressant. This difference is also instructive because other research indicated that black patients are more susceptible than white patients to side effects linked to tricyclic antidepressant use.

These racial disparities in care are striking. The ability to identify them was linked to the availability of racial identifiers in the medical records. It is likely that other social characteristics such as SES and gender also may predict variations in the quality of care provided to patients with mood (and other) disorders. Understanding the generalizability of these patterns and the factors causing them is an important priority for future research.

Needed Research

Several methodological problems need to be addressed in future research on the relation between stressful life experiences and major depression (Kessler 1997). Existing research has given inadequate attention to the role that accuracy in reporting life events may play in the observed relation between depression and stress. Given that depression can cause some life events, it is important to be able to clearly date the occurrence of stressful life experiences in relation to depression. Some research has attempted to address this issue by distinguishing the relation between dependent events and independent events with depression. Dependent events are those that could plausibly be a consequence of the individual's own action. Importantly, this research found that independent events are related to the risk for depression (see Kessler 1997).

Issues regarding the accuracy of reporting of stressful experiences are especially salient for the measurement of childhood adversities. Retrospective reports of childhood experiences have been critiqued because of the following observations: 1) the low reliability and validity of autobiographical memory, 2) memory impairment among individuals who have psychiatric disorders, and 3) mood-congruent memory biases that are also associated with psychopathology. Although some of the association between major life events and depression may be a result of events that cause depression, the condition itself may elicit difficulties or make them worse. More recent studies considering memory biases and reciprocity in the causal relation between life events and mood disorder still have detected a significant relation that is attributed in part to one or more precipitating life events.

Another important issue for future research is the need to enhance our understanding of the ways in which chronic and acute stress relate to each other and combine to affect the risk for mood disorders. Chronic stress is difficult to measure well, but chronic stress in major domains such as work and marriage likely plays an important role in exacerbating the effects of life events on episodes of major depression (Wethington et al. 1995). Other evidence suggests that chronic stress may mediate the relation between life events and depression. For example, research indicates that the adverse effects of unemployment on depression are partially mediated by chronic financial stress, and the relation between the loss of a spouse and depression is partly mediated by social isolation (Kessler 1997).

Future research must distinguish social factors that affect the first onset of mood disorders from those that affect recurrence, as well as those that affect the speed of recovery (Kessler 1997). Greater attention to the role of the history of depression also can shed important light in helping us to understand the pathways by which social factors affect depression risks. For example, Kessler (1997) showed that although the point prevalence of major depression is higher among women than among men, no sex difference is found in the recurrence of depression or in the speed of recovery from an episode of depression. He showed that in the ECA data, 91% of the respondents who reported an episode of depression in the past 12 months had a history of depression. Thus, it is important to control the history of depression in studying the short-term effects of stressors on depression. Relatedly, future work on risk factors for depressive episodes needs to look separately at the predictors of onset and the predictors of recurrence.

With the explosion of research on genetic risks for mood disorders that is likely to accompany the recent characterization of the human genome, new opportunities to understand how genetic predispositions combine with environmental triggers to affect the risks for mood disorders are probable. Variability within the gene pools of populations is unlikely to explain the large differences in rates of depression that have been observed across populations; nonetheless, genetics may play an important role in depression by determining certain temperamental aspects of personality that may increase vulnerability to environmental exposures (Brown 2002).

Conclusion

We suggest that there are pervasive ways in which social factors affect the risk for mood disorders and the course and treatment of these conditions. The evidence that the levels of these disorders and their societal costs are, at least in part, socially determined suggests that multiple opportunities exist for interventions to potentially reduce rates of mood disorders and the disability burden that they create in society. More research is needed to better delineate both pathogenic and health-enhancing psychosocial factors and the mechanisms and processes by which they operate. A central goal of such efforts should be to facilitate the identification of key intervention strategies that can improve mental health and well-being.

References

Aneshensel C, Sucoff CA: The neighborhood context of adolescent mental health. J Health Soc Behav 37:293–310, 1996

Avison WR: Single motherhood and mental health: implications for primary prevention. Can Med Assoc J 156:661–663, 1997

Beiser M, Hou F: Language acquisition, unemployment and depressive disorder among Southeast Asian refugees: a 10 year study. Soc Sci Med 53:1321–1324, 2001

Bennett M: Afro-American women, poverty and mental health: a social essay. Women Health 12:213–228, 1987

Berry D: Does religious psychotherapy improve anxiety and depression in religious adults? A review of randomized controlled studies. Int J Psychiatr Nurs Res 8:875–890, 2002

Bland RC, Newman SC, Orn H: Help-seeking for psychiatric disorders. Can J Psychiatry 42:935–942, 1997

Brenner M: Patterns of psychiatric hospitalization among different socio-economic groups in response to economic stress. J Nerv Ment Dis 148:31–38, 1969

Brown GW: Social roles, context and evolution in the origins of depression. J Health Soc Behav 43:255–276, 2002

Brown GW, Harris T: Social Origins of Depression. New York, Free Press, 1978

Bruce ML: Psychosocial risk factors for depressive disorders in late life. Biol Psychiatry 52:175–184, 2002

Catalano R, Dooley D: Economic predictors of depressed mood and stressful life events. J Health Soc Behav 18:292–307, 1977

Cohen S, Glass DC: Apartment noise, auditory discrimination, and reading ability in children. J Exp Soc Psychol 9:407–422, 1973

Cooper LA, Gonzales JJ, Gallo JJ, et al: The acceptability of treatment for depression among African-American, Hispanic, and white primary care patients. Med Care 41:479–489, 2003

Desjarlais R, Eisenberg L, Good B, et al: World Mental Health: Problems and Priorities in Low-Income Countries. New York, Oxford University Press, 1995

Dohrenwend BP: Socioeconomic status (SES) and psychiatric disorders: are the issues still compelling? Soc Psychiatry Psychiatr Epidemiol 25:41–47, 1990

Domino M, Salkever DS, Zarin DA, et al: The impact of managed care on psychiatry. Adm Policy Ment Health 26:149–157, 1998

Dooley D, Prause J: Mental health and welfare transitions: depression and alcohol abuse in AFDC women. Am J Community Psychol 30:787–813, 2002

Dooley D, Prause J, Ham-Rowbottom KA: Underemployment and depression: longitudinal relationships. J Health Soc Behav 41:421–436, 2000

Durkheim E: Suicide, a Study in Sociology. Translated by Spaulding JA, Simpson G. Glencoe, IL, Free Press, 1951

Ellison CG, Levin JS: The religion-health connection: evidence, theory, and future directions. Health Educ Behav 25:700–720, 1998

Ellison CG, Boardman JD, Williams DR, et al: Religious involvement, stress, and mental health: findings from the 1995 Detroit area study. Soc Forces 80:215–249, 2001

Fox JC, Blank M, Rovnyak VG, et al: Barriers to help seeking for mental disorders in a rural impoverished population. Community Ment Health J 37:421–436, 2001

Galbaud du Fort G, Newman SC, Boothroyd LJ, et al: Treatment seeking for depression: role of depressive symptoms and comorbid psychiatric diagnoses. J Affect Disord 52:31–40, 1999

Ganzini L, McFarland BH, Cutler D: Prevalence of mental disorders after catastrophic financial loss. J Nerv Ment Dis 178:680–685, 1990

Gilkes C: The black church as a therapeutic community: suggested areas for research into the black religious experience. Journal of the Interdenominational Theological Center 8:29–44, 1980

Goodman E, Huang B: Socioeconomic status, depressive symptoms, and adolescent substance use. Arch Pediatr Adolesc Med 156:448–453, 2002

Griffith EEH, English T, Mayfield V: Possession, prayer, and testimony: therapeutic aspects of the Wednesday night meeting in a Black church. Psychiatry 43:120–128, 1980

Griffith EEH, Young J, Smith D: An analysis of the therapeutic elements in a black church service. Hosp Community Psychiatry 35:464–469, 1984

Heffernan W, Heffernan JB: The impact of the farm crisis on families and communities. Rural Sociologist 6:160–170, 1986

Hill PC, Pargament KI: Advances in the conceptualization and measurement of religion and spirituality. Implications for physical and mental health research. Am Psychol 58:64–74, 2003

Holzer CE, Shea B, Swanson J, et al: The increased risk for specific psychiatric disorders among persons of low socioeconomic status. Am J Psychiatry 6:259–271, 1986

Hoyt D, Conger RD, Valde JG, et al: Psychological distress and help seeking in rural America. Am J Community Psychol 25:449–470, 1997

Judd FK, Jackson HJ, Komiti A, et al: High prevalence disorders in urban and rural communities. Aust N Z J Psychiatry 36:104–113, 2002

Kasen S, Cohen P, Chen H, et al: Depression in adult women: age changes and cohort effects. Am J Public Health 93:2061–2066, 2003

Kendall-Tackett K: The health effects of childhood abuse: four pathways by which abuse can influence health. Child Abuse Negl 26:715–729, 2002

Kessler RC: The effects of stressful life events on depression. Annu Rev Psychol 48:191–214, 1997

Kessler RC, Zhao S: Overview of descriptive epidemiology of mental disorders, in Handbook of the Sociology of Mental Health. Edited by Aneshensel CS, Phelan JC. New York, Kluwer Academic/Plenum, 1999, pp 127–150

Kessler RC, McGonagle KA, Zhao S, et al: Lifetime and 12-month prevalence of DSM-III-R psychiatric disorders in the United States. Arch Gen Psychiatry 51:8–19, 1994

Kessler RC, Berglund P, Demler O, et al: The epidemiology of major depressive disorder. JAMA 289:3095–3105, 2003

Krause N, Ellison CG: Forgiveness by God, forgiveness of others, and psychological well-being in late life. J Sci Study Relig 42:77–93, 2003

Lennon MC, Blome J, English K: Depression among women on welfare: a review of the literature. J Am Med Womens Assoc 57:27–31, 2002

Levin JS, Markides KS, Ray LA: Religious attendance and psychological well-being in Mexican Americans: a panel analysis of three-generations data. Gerontologist 36:454–463, 1996

Lewis JM: For better or worse: interpersonal relationships and individual outcome. Am J Psychiatry 155:582–589, 1998

Lindenthal JJ, Myers JK, Pepper M, et al: Mental status and religious behavior. J Sci Study Relig 9:143–149, 1970

Lipman EL, Offord DR, Boyle MH: Single mothers in Ontario: sociodemographic, physical and mental health characteristics. Can Med Assoc J 156:639–645, 1997

Lynch JW, Kaplan GA, Shema SJ: Cumulative impact of sustained economic hardship on physical, cognitive, psychological, and social functioning. N Engl J Med 337:1889–1995, 1997

McCullough ME, Larson DB: Religion and depression: a review of the literature. Twin Res 2:126–136, 1999

McLeod JD, Kessler RC: Socioeconomic status differences in vulnerability to undesirable life events. J Health Soc Behav 31:162–172, 1990

Melfi CA, Croghan TW, Hanna MP, et al: Racial variation in antidepressant treatment in a Medicaid population. J Clin Psychiatry 61:16–21, 2000

Mojtabai R: Datapoints: prescription patterns for mood and anxiety disorders in a community sample. Psychiatr Serv 50:1557, 1999

Mojtabai R, Olfson M, Mechanic D: Perceived need and help-seeking in adults with mood, anxiety, or substance use disorders. Arch Gen Psychiatry 59:77–84, 2002

Neff J: Urbanicity and depression reconsidered. J Nerv Ment Dis 171:546–552, 1983

Neighbors HW, Musick MA, Williams DR: The African American minister as a source of help for serious personal crises: bridge or barrier to mental health care? Health Educ Behav 25:759–777, 1998

Nelson CJ, Rosenfeld BJ, Breitbart W, et al: Spirituality, religion, and depression in the terminally ill. Psychosomatics 43:213–220, 2002

Pargament K, Silverman W, Johnson S, et al: The psychosocial climate of religious congregations. Am J Community Psychol 11:351–381, 1983

Pargament KI, Smith BW, Koenigh HG, et al: Patterns of positive and negative religious coping with major life stressors. J Sci Study Relig 37:711–725, 1998

Parikh SV, Wasylenki D, Goering P, et al: Mood disorders: rural/urban differences in prevalence, health care utilization, and disability in Ontario. J Affect Disord 38:57–65, 1996

Patel V, Kleinman A: Poverty and common mental disorders in developing countries. Bull World Health Organ 81:609–615, 2003

Paykel ES: Life events, social support and depression. Acta Psychiatr Scand Suppl 377:50–58, 1994

Paykel ES: Stress and affective disorders in humans. Semin Clin Neuropsychiatry 6:4–11, 2001

Piccinelli M, Wilkinson G: Gender differences in depression. Br J Psychiatry 177:486–492, 2000

Poloma MM, Gallup GH: Varieties of Prayer: A Survey Report. Philadelphia, PA, Trinity Press International, 1991

Risman B: Intimate relationships from a microstructural perspective: men who mother. Gender Soc 1:6–32, 1987

Riso LP, Miyatake RK, Thase ME: The search for determinants of chronic depression: a review of six factors. J Affect Disord 70:103–115, 2002

Robins LN, Regier DA: Psychiatric Disorders in America: The Epidemiologic Catchment Area Study. New York, Free Press, 1991

Rosenfield S: Gender and mental health: do women have more psychopathology, men more, or both the same (and why)?, in A Handbook for the Study of Mental Health: Social Contexts, Theories, and Systems. Edited by Horwitz A, Scheid T. New York, Cambridge University Press, 1999a, pp 348–360

Rosenfield S: Splitting the difference: gender, the self, and mental health, in Handbook of the Sociology of Mental Health. Edited by Aneshensel CS, Phelan JC. New York, Kluwer Academic/Plenum, 1999b, pp 209–224

Schichor A, Bernstein B, King S: Self-reported depressive symptoms in inner-city adolescents seeking routine health care. Adolescence 29:379–388, 1994

Schnittker J: When is faith enough? The effects of religious involvement on depression. J Sci Study Relig 40:393–411, 2001

Schuster MA, Stein BD, Jaycox LH, et al: A national survey of stress reactions after the September 11, 2001, terrorist attacks. N Engl J Med 345:1507–1512, 2001

Shahabi L, Powell LH, Musick MA, et al: Correlates of self-perceptions of spirituality in American adults. Ann Behav Med 24:59–68, 2002

Smedley BD, Stith AY, Nelson AR: Unequal Treatment: Confronting Racial and Ethnic Disparities in Health Care Washington, DC, National Academies Press, 2003

Smith T, McCullough ME, Poll J: Religiousness and depression: evidence for a main effect and the moderating influence of stressful life events. Psychol Bull 129:614–636, 2003

Strawbridge WJ, Shema SJ, Cohen RD, et al: Religiosity buffers effects of some stressors on depression but exacerbates others. J Gerontol B Psychol Sci Soc Sci 53:S118–S126, 1998

Sussman LK, Robins LN, Earls F: Treatment-seeking for depression by black and white Americans. Soc Sci Med 24:187–196, 1987

Tennant C: Life events, stress and depression: a review of recent findings. Aust N Z J Psychiatry 36:173–182, 2002

Tiggemann M, Winefield A: The effects of unemployment on the mood, self-esteem, locus of control, and depressive affect of school leavers. Journal of Occupational Psychology 57:33–42, 1984

Toussaint L, Williams DR, Musick MA, et al: Forgiveness and health: age difference in a U.S. probability sample. Journal of Adult Development 8:249–257, 2001

Trovato F: A time series analysis of international immigration and suicide mortality in Canada. Int J Soc Psychiatry 32:38–46, 1986

U.S. Department of Health and Human Services: Mental Health: A Report of the Surgeon General—Executive Summary. Rockville, MD, Center for Mental Health Services, Substance Abuse and Mental Health Services Administration, 1999

Wang PS, Berglund PA, Kessler RC: Patterns and correlates of contacting clergy for mental disorders in the United States. Health Serv Res 38:647–673, 2003

Weissman MM, Bruce ML, Leaf PJ, et al: Affective disorders, in Psychiatric Disorders in America: The Epidemiologic Catchment Area Study. Edited by Robins LN, Regier DA. New York, Free Press, 1991, pp 53–80

Wethington E, Brown GW, Kessler RC: Interview measurement of stressful life events, in Measuring Stress: A Guide for Health and Social Scientists. Edited by Cohen S, Kessler RC, Gordon L. New York, Oxford University Press, 1995, pp 59–79

Weyerer S, Wiedenmann A: Economic factors and the rates of suicide in Germany between 1881 and 1989. Psychol Rep 76:1331–1341, 1995

Wilhelm K, Parker G: Is sex necessarily a risk factor to depression? Psychol Med 19:401–413, 1989

Williams DR: The measurement of religion in epidemiologic studies, in Religious Factors in Aging and Health: Theoretical Foundations and Methodological Frontiers. Edited by Levin JS. Beverly Hills, CA, Sage, 1994, pp 125–148

Williams DR, Larson DB, Buckler RE, et al: Religion and psychological distress in a community sample. Soc Sci Med 32:1257–1262, 1991

Williams DR, Takeuchi DT, Adair R: Marital status and psychiatric disorders among blacks and whites. J Health Soc Behav 33:140–157, 1992a

Williams DR, Takeuchi D, Adair R: Socioeconomic status and psychiatric disorder among blacks and whites. Soc Forces 71:179–194, 1992b

Young JL, Griffith EE, Williams DR: The integral role of pastoral counseling by African-American clergy in community mental health. Psychiatr Serv 54:688–692, 2003

10

Evolutionary Explanations for Mood and Mood Disorders

RANDOLPH M. NESSE, M.D.

Evolution and Behavior

The evolutionary principles that have made possible major advances in the understanding of animal behavior (Alcock 1997) are just now being applied to the challenge of understanding human emotions and affects (Barkow et al. 1992; Buss 1995; Konner 2002; Plutchik 1980; E.O. Wilson 1978). In this chapter, I summarize some of those advances and some attempts to use them to better understand mood and its disorders.

Much of the opportunity, and much of the difficulty, arises because evolutionary questions about behavior and emotions are fundamentally different from proximate questions (Mayr 1983). Most medical research is about how the body's mechanisms work, how they go awry, and why some individuals become sick and others do not. Evolutionary questions, by contrast, do not ask about how the body works but instead ask why it is the way it is in all members of a species—what historical sequences, selective advantages, and other evolutionary forces account for traits being the way they are and why they fail in the ways they fail (G.W. Williams and Nesse 1991). Methods for test-

ing postulated answers can only sometimes use the familiar experimental method; they much more often use the comparative method or assessments of design features in the light of hypothesized functions (Reeve and Sherman 1993; Rose and Lauder 1996).

Although most of the recent work on mood is at the preliminary stage of attempting to formulate the correct questions and suggest possible answers, enough specific proposals have now been made and assessed to provide the rudiments of an understanding of why natural selection shaped a capacity for mood at all and why it is so likely to cause problems (Morris 1992). Before moving to those issues, a very brief overview of some recent advances in animal behavior will provide a basis for the discussion.

Two generations ago, the field of animal behavior was mostly descriptive, but it has been transformed by an evolutionary approach (Alcock 2001; Krebs and Davies 1997). The most fundamental advance is recognition that all biological traits need not only explanations of their proximate mechanisms (ranging from molecules to perceptual stimuli and cognitive and emotional mechanisms) but also evolutionary explanations of the selection forces that shaped those mechanisms. These are not alternatives

The author thanks Daniel Stein, Barbara Smuts, Norman Li, and Sean Conlan for helpful comments.

but complementary components of a complete explanation (Tinbergen 1963). For instance, previous studies of bird song were only descriptive, perhaps with some attention to development and possible functions. Now, researchers not only correlate the duration, quality, and volume of songs with characteristics of the singers but also try to determine if the singing serves to defend territories or advertise for mating partners or both.

The study of animal behavior also has been transformed by the demise of naïve group selection theories and recognition of the roles of kin selection (Hamilton 1964a, 1964b) and reciprocity (Trivers 1985) in shaping social behaviors. Behavioral traits must be explained in terms of how they increase the frequency of genes that code for them, not in terms of the benefit to the species (G.C. Williams 1966). This is not the place to provide full explanations of these advances or to describe the many other ways that considerations of evolutionary function have transformed the field of animal behavior into a theoretically based quantitative science (Alcock 1997). Recognizing this transformation is essential, however, because it has been the inspiration for attempts to use the same principles to understand human psychopathology (McGuire and Troisi 1998; McGuire et al. 1992).

These attempts to use the same principles have aroused great interest but much accompanying misunderstanding and unnecessary controversy (Buss et al. 1998; Queller 1995; Segerstråle 2000). The sociobiology wars are mostly over, and evolutionary studies of human behavior are now thriving despite their difficulties (Barrett et al. 2002). Most everyone involved recognizes that natural selection shaped human behavior-regulation mechanisms but that the human niche is distinctive and that much work remains to show how the forces of natural selection shaped the brain mechanisms that result in emergent social forces and the complexity and diversity of human behaviors (Barkow 1989; Buss 1995). Furthermore, the previous tendency to conflate behavioral genetics and evolutionary approaches to behavior is a mistake now made only rarely, and recognition is growing that a functional approach to behavior is not just not reductionistic; it is the strongest scientific antidote for reductionism. A functional approach studies the regulation of behavior at high levels of organization, relying heavily on facultative mechanisms that adjust behavior to changing circumstances. Neuroscience unravels pathways and their molecular mediators, whereas evolutionary approaches examine how those mechanisms give a selective advantage by making it possible for organisms to gather and process information that adapts their behavior to rapidly changing environments (Krebs and Davies 1984). To offer a single example, a junco given the choice to forage at a feeder that provides

three or four seeds every visit or at a feeder that provides the same mean with much more variability will choose the low-risk feeder in usual circumstances. However, if the temperature decreases from room temperature to freezing, the juncos instead prefer the more risky choice. Why? At freezing temperatures, the rate of caloric gain at the less risky feeder is too slow for them to survive the night, whereas the risky strategy offers at least some chance of survival (Caraco et al. 1990).

Evolutionary Explanations of Disorders

The other major roadblock to applying evolutionary ideas to depression has been the difficulty of seeing how selection can help to account for a disease. It seems obvious that natural selection can explain adaptive mechanisms but not defects in design. The solution to this difficulty is recognizing that although selection does not shape diseases directly, it is responsible for leaving bodies with vulnerabilities that result in diseases (Nesse and Williams 1994). From this perspective, the question becomes, for each disease, why natural selection did not design the body to be more resilient and resistant to disease. Why do we have wisdom teeth and an appendix? Why has selection not shaped better immune defenses and more effective ways of eliminating cancerous cells? Why are our bones and backs not stronger? Why do so many people experience debilitating episodes of depression?

A systematic approach to questions about the body's vulnerabilities has proved useful in the rest of medicine (Stearns 1998) and may prove even more useful in psychiatry (McGuire and Troisi 1998). In simplified outline, there are six reasons that natural selection might leave an aspect of the body vulnerable to disease (Nesse and Williams 1994). First, we live in an environment substantially different from the environment in which we evolved, and many diseases, including most chronic diseases such as addictions, obesity, and atherosclerosis, result from this mismatch (Eaton et al. 1988; Trevathan et al. 1999). Second, we remain susceptible to infection because pathogens evolve so much faster than we do (Ewald 1994). Both of these initial evolutionary explanations for disease arise because natural selection is a slow process.

The third reason for vulnerability is that no trait in the body can be perfect—all are tradeoffs. For example, if the radius and ulna were thicker, they would break less readily, but we would lose the invaluable ability to rotate our wrists. The fourth reason is that natural selection is subject to many limitations. It is subject to random happenstances that may increase the frequency of deleterious genes, and it also can never start over to correct a mistake; it works only by gradual increments. Like our poorly laid out QWERTY keyboards, our bodies are stuck with many suboptimal designs resulting from path dependence, such as our inside-out eyeballs with vessels that come between the light and the retina.

The fifth explanation is that we misunderstand what natural selection shapes. Many people imagine that it shapes bodies for health, longevity, or even happiness, but, alas, only reproductive success influences the frequency of genes in the next generation. As a result, we have many behavioral tendencies that advance the interests of our genes even as they harm our own lives, such as the notable and too often fatal bravado of young men (M. Wilson and Daly 1985). Also, the desperate goal pursuits associated with some depressions are likely ones that may benefit the individual's genes at great cost to the individual.

Finally, many responses that superficially appear to be diseases, such as fever and cough, are actually sophisticated mechanisms that help to protect us in certain circumstances. It is obvious to most people that pain can be useful, but less well known is that people born with no capacity for pain usually die by age 35 (Sternbach 1963). The utility of coughing and vomiting to clear foreign materials and toxins is obvious, but there is less recognition that the aversiveness of these experiences is a part of their design. Although the utility of anxiety is widely recognized, no one has yet systematically looked for people who have the psychiatric disorder of deficient anxiety (Marks and Nesse 1994).

Evolutionary Questions About Depression

This brief background about evolutionary approaches to behavior and to medical disorders provides a framework for formulating the evolutionary questions about depression. The global question is why depression exists at all. Each of the six evolutionary reasons for disease deserves consideration, but the last possibility is most fundamental and must be considered first. Does depression arise, like cancer and stroke, from a defect in the body's machinery; or is it, like fever and pain, a protective defensive response; or is it, like chronic pain or febrile seizures, a complication or maladaptive extreme of a useful response? The lack of agreement on an answer to this question accounts for much of the confusion that surrounds depression research. An answer, even if tentative and supported mainly by circumstantial evidence, would provide a framework for integrating our knowledge about depression and for posing new research questions.

On cursory examination, the answer seems clear. Depression is so disabling and so often fatal that it seems obvious that it must arise from a defect. As many who have had severe depression testify, the depths of melancholic depression are so physical and pervasive that any suggestion that the condition could have utility seems risible (Wolpert 1999). In my view, this is indeed sufficient evidence that severe depression is a pathological state without adaptive utility. Not all agree, however, and there are reasons for caution in accepting any conclusion on the matter too readily. Normal severe physical pain can make people completely unable to function. Even the fever, cough, fatigue, and malaise of the normal inflammatory reaction to influenza cause disability equal to all but the most severe depressions. The simple fact of intense suffering and disability is not in itself adequate evidence that depression has no useful function.

The closely related relevant question is whether the capacity for mood variation within the normal range is an adaptation or an epiphenomenon. It is certainly possible that depression has no specific function but is an epiphenomenon (Akiskal 2001). There are, however, several reasons that some believe that low mood is a useful response: it is universal, it is regulated by important and consistent aspects of the environment, it influences behavior in tangible ways, and major disruptions of the system (i.e., mood disorders) compromise function and decrease fitness (Morris 1992). Because *depression* is so often defined as a pathological state, the more generic phrase *low mood* will be used here to refer to a range of depression-like states that range from clearly normal to the possibly pathological.

Epidemiology

Several epidemiological facts about depression appear fresh in an evolutionary perspective. First, its vast prevalence, so high that it will soon be the greatest cause of disability-adjusted lost years in modern societies (Murray and Lopez 1997), argues strongly against its arising from some bodily defect, unless, like atherosclerosis, it results from living in an environment to which we are poorly suited (Eaton et al. 1988). Given the extraordinary near-perfection of most physiological systems, from renal physiology to the immune responses and our cognitive capacities, it would be most unlikely for a disorder as severe and prevalent as depression to arise simply from poor design.

Second, and even more striking, the age at onset is at the prime of life. Some cases start in childhood and some late in life, but the incidence of new onsets peaks in early adulthood when selection is the strongest (Weissman et al. 1996). This makes depression epidemiology quite different from that of almost all medical diseases. Although a few medical disorders have their peak rates of onset early in life, the incidence of most diseases rises steadily in adulthood. This is because of the good evolutionary reason that reproductive value is highest at sexual maturity, and therefore selection is strongest at this age (G.C. Williams 1957). Over the course of evolution, this has resulted in selection for modifier genes that push the expression of deleterious effects of genes and related disease onsets to later (and occasionally earlier) in the life span. The mystery of why depression tends to have its onset at just the age when everything else in the body is at its functional peak may be explained by the conflicts associated with the coincident peak of competition for mates and status.

The third epidemiological factor cast in a new light is the overwhelming influence of adverse life events on depression onset. This is often conceptualized in a model in which stressors act on mechanisms with preexisting vulnerability to cause damage and failure (Brown et al. 1986; Kessler 1997). In an alternative model, however, low mood could be, like pain, a normal and useful response to certain kinds of threats. The prevalence of mild depressive symptoms (Kessler et al. 2003), the role of certain adverse life events in precipitating or worsening these symptoms (Monroe et al. 2001), the continuous distribution of depression severity with no zone of rarity that separates pathological from more mild depression (Ruscio and Ruscio 2002), and the superior performance of models based on continua instead of categories (Angst and Merikangas 2001; Judd et al. 1998) all weigh toward considering the possibility that depression, or at least low mood, serves some defensive reaction (Morris 1992).

Evolution and Emotions

A general evolutionary framework for understanding emotions and affects is essential for considering low mood, and depression in particular. As is the case with the field of animal behavior, emotions research is now routinely based on evolutionary biology (Oatley and Jenkins 1996; Plutchik and Kellerman 1989). Work continues on just how many basic emotions there are and how they are shaped in the course of development (Ekman and Davidson 1994), but now general agreement is that the generic emotional capacities of human and animal emotions were shaped by natural selection (Oatley and Jenkins 1996). Although some approaches still try to identify the function or functions of each emotion, there is growing agreement that the organizing factor for each emotion is not its

function but the situation in which it gives a selective advantage (Nesse 1990; Tooby and Cosmides 1990). In this perspective, there is no need to argue about which aspect of an emotion is primary; cognitive, physiological, behavioral, expressive, and subjective aspects of emotions are all components of a coordinated suite of changes that helps the organism cope with the adaptive challenges of a situation that has recurred over evolutionary history. Likewise, there is no need to look for a single function; an emotion's many aspects may serve multiple functions to meet the several challenges that are associated with a situation. In panic, for instance, the physiological arousal, tendency to freeze, preoccupation with finding routes of escape, and subjective anxiety are all useful in situations that involve life-threatening danger. The positive or negative valence of emotions is expected because emotions would not be shaped for neutral situations but only for those that involve opportunities or threats. The fact that related emotional states are only partially differentiated from one another is likewise expected, and this makes it unnecessary to insist on a sharp distinction between emotions and longer-duration affects and moods (Oatley and Bolton 1985). Emotions and affects need to be understood in terms of the situations in which they are useful, the adaptive challenges of those situations, and how the characteristics of the emotion or affect help to meet those challenges (Clark 1992).

This view implies that it is a mistake to think that some emotions are inherently more useful than others. All are useful in certain circumstances and harmful in other circumstances. There is a pervasive tendency, so prevalent that it has been called "the clinician's illusion," to think of aversive states as problems instead of solutions. In medicine, this has been manifest in reflexive tendencies to prescribe drugs to block pain, fever, diarrhea, nausea, vomiting, and cough without pausing to consider their utility. This habit does little harm only because natural selection has shaped both redundant defenses and regulation mechanisms that express inexpensive defenses, such as cough and fever, according to the "smoke detector principle"—in which many false alarms are justified to be sure of responding to each actual incident of genuine threat (Nesse 2005). In psychology, a welcome turn to positive psychology has tended to seek evidence that positive feelings are generally beneficial (Seligman and Csikszentmihalyi 2000) and has attempted to understand why they are elusive (Buss 2000; Nesse 2004). Positive feelings certainly are preferable, and in the safe setting of most technological societies, they tend to be more beneficial than negative feelings. However, the core fact remains that whether an expression of an emotion is useful or harmful depends entirely on the situation.

In What Situations Is Low Mood Useful?

This background about emotions makes it possible to pose the question about low mood and depression more exactly. That is: In what situations that recurred over evolutionary history would the characteristics of low mood or depression have offered a selective advantage? Nearly a dozen partially overlapping answers have been suggested. Some were originally phrased in terms of functions, but transforming them to hypotheses about situations in which these states would be useful makes them more comparable. This is the core of current work on evolution and depression.

Situations that cause low mood are most generically associated with loss. The loss can be of property, relationships, status, health, or any other resource. Sadness caused by loss shares many features with low mood and depression, but if the loss is discrete and life can go on, then sadness is quite different from depression. It does not have the hopelessness, the global lack of motivation, or the low self-esteem and tendencies toward guilt that typify depression. Can sadness have any useful function? Certainly, losing resources is an important situation that has recurred in the lives of every one of our ancestors. Those who had a special reaction would have several possible advantages. Among the ways that sadness can be useful are

- Motivation to regain the lost resource
- Motivation to replace the lost resource
- Avoidance of situations similar to the one that resulted in the loss
- Thinking of ways to protect other resources
- Adjustment of strategies that cannot go forward in the same way without the resource
- Thinking about the situation that led to the loss to find ways to prevent future losses
- Making reparations if the loss was caused by violating a norm or a relationship partner's expectations

The exemplar of loss is the experience of infants who are separated from their mothers as studied by John Bowlby and Harry Harlow (Bowlby 1973; Harlow and Harlow 1962). Bowlby's seminal contribution was to interpret this situation in an evolutionary context in which the infant's and mother's reactions made adaptive sense. In particular, the initial protest was seen as an attempt to signal location and need to the mother, whereas the more passive "despair" phase was seen as a way to avoid predation and conserve resources if the mother was away for an

extended period. The apparently abnormal kinds of attachment he and others described (Ainsworth et al. 1978) have now been themselves reconsidered in evolutionary terms as possible facultative adaptations that infants may make to mothers with different tendencies and abilities to provide care (Belsky 1999; Chisholm 1996). The utility of passivity in situations in which resources are scarce gave rise to the phrase *conservation-withdrawal*, with emphasis again on the situation of the infant (Engel and Schmale 1972; Schmale and Engel 1975).

Loss of a relationship in adulthood usually has been interpreted in the context of attachment, with grief as the exemplar (Wortman et al. 1993). It is crucial to determine whether grief is a response shaped to cope with the loss of a loved one or an epiphenomenon of attachment. The most extensive treatment is by John Archer, who concluded that grief seems too maladaptive and too closely connected to attachment to be useful (Archer 1999). It could well be that attachments are so constrained that loss necessarily means grief or that the pain of anticipated loss is essential to the functions of attachments. However, there does not seem to be any reason that individuals could not be shaped to provide deep altruism and affection to kin who are alive and to move on without great disability after they die. Furthermore, the profound pain of grief may itself have utility to prevent future losses and to cope with the situation of having to make fundamental adjustments in life. The question is unanswered (Nesse 2000b).

A more general situation in which depression might be useful is any circumstance in which help is needed. This is consistent with crying and other low mood signals that could bring help. Aubrey Lewis (1934) emphasized this function, and it is also central in more recent treatments (Sloman et al. 1994; Watson and Andrews 2002). The general irritability of depressed patients and the wish of most people to avoid them weigh against this as a main function (Coyne et al. 1987), but data are not yet available to determine whether mild depression usually elicits help from others. The demise of extended family groups in recent decades makes the social environment fundamentally different in ways that may change the utility of pleas for help.

Perhaps the best-developed proposal is that depression is useful after loss of a status conflict. John Price (1967) originally put the hypothesis forward on the basis of animal and clinical observations that continued striving after a loss led to brutal attacks, whereas "involuntary yielding" signaled submission and ended the battle. He further developed this position in collaboration with several colleagues who have reported studies in which unwillingness to yield was associated with depression and yielding was associated with remission (Price et al. 1994;

Sloman and Price 1987; Stevens and Price 1996). This is supported by some data showing superior social judgment capacity after a low mood induction (Badcock and Allen 2003). The strength of this position is that it helps to explain the low self-esteem and lack of striving in depressed patients; exactly these traits would protect against attack, and they are the most difficult to account for otherwise. In a related vein, Hartung (1988) suggested that especially capable people often may need to conceal their abilities from their superiors to avoid attack, thus explaining some cases of depression and the self-handicapping so characteristic of neurosis.

A more general framework treats striving for status as one of many goals whose pursuit can lead to depression if there is no way to succeed but also no way to disengage (Nesse 1999, 2000a). Hamburg et al. (1975) provided an early elaborated biological model:

> A feeling of sadness and discouragement sets in [when] the subject estimates the probability of effective action is low….Depressive responses can be viewed as adaptive…in a medium range of intensity. Feelings of sadness and discouragement may be a useful stimulus to consider changing [the] situation…sadness may elicit heightened interest and sympathetic consideration on the part of significant other people. (p. 240)

In psychology, Klinger (1975) offered the most comprehensive early treatment. Since then, the model has been elaborated and further developed by many others (Brickman 1987; Diener and Fujita 1995; Emmons 1996; Higgins et al. 1997; Janoff-Bulman and Brickman 1982; Palys and Little 1983; Pyszczynski and Greenberg 1987). The importance of this work has received little recognition in psychiatry, however. Carver and Scheier's (1990, 1998) research showed that mood is influenced not by the degree of goal attainment but by the rate of approach compared with the expected rate of approach. Moving toward a goal faster than expected raises mood, whereas evidence that reaching the goal will take more time or effort than expected lowers mood. Persisting in the pursuit of a goal despite the low mood's signaling the need to disengage arouses increasingly strong and eventually pathological depression. This was at the heart of Bibring's (1953) long-admired psychoanalytic paper on depression that emphasized the central role of highly cathected desires that could not be fulfilled. A very similar focus on the role of goal pursuit is at the heart of McGuire and Troisi's (1987, 1998) recognition of the role of unrealistic wishes in depression. In a reanalysis of the best-detailed life events data available, Brown et al. (1995) found that the risk of depression is not increased equally by all severe life events; situations that involve humiliation or entrapment are much more likely to result in depression. This was interpreted as being consistent with the involuntary yielding functions of low mood, but it provides equal support for a broader view of the importance of inescapable but unreachable goals.

All of these authors recognized that there must be a mechanism for maintaining persistence in goal pursuit despite obstacles, but there also must be some mechanism for disengaging motivation from a goal when it is clear that the goal is unobtainable. Most of the research has been done on college students, but the perspective is even more powerful in the clinic. One woman's depression is precipitated by the realization that her efforts to help her daughter escape from drug addiction and likely death are futile. Another cannot stop her husband's binges but will not give up on the marriage. Some graduate students get halfway though a rigorous program, only to realize that others are doing better, no amount of work can compensate, and no other career path seems viable. In addition, millions of workers, laid off in midlife, only gradually realize that their efforts to attain comparable positions will never succeed.

This perspective also offers a possible explanation for sex differences in vulnerability to depression (Wenegrat 1995) and for why rates of depression are so high in certain modern environments (Weissman et al. 1996). Globally, media exposure and mass society increase the reference group and the range and grandeur of possible goals and possible selves to the point at which none of us can succeed, even aside from the fact that the images we see are increasingly realistic media-created fantasies (Sloman and Gilbert 2000). On a more personal level, the life goals of ordinary people are now larger and longer in duration than they were in past generations, with required investments so huge and prolonged that failure leaves few viable alternatives. This perspective also offers a framework for considering mechanisms by which personality traits may contribute to depression; intense ambition, strong attachments, fear of being alone, and a tendency to put all of life's meaning on one large goal are all traits that make it more likely that a person will find himself or herself trapped in pursuit of an unreachable goal.

Closely related is the suggestion that the capacity for mood was shaped to allocate resources and effort among various environments and strategies that vary in their propitiousness (Nesse 1999, 2000a). A situation that offers temporarily rich rewards for little effort deserves the intense effort and risk-taking made possible by high mood. Unpropitious situations, in which efforts are more expensive than gains, are best escaped or avoided. If one is stuck in such a situation, it is best to exert little effort and take few risks. If the overall life circumstance offers no current strategy in which the effort or risk is greater than the cost, the best thing to do is...nothing. The model is based on foraging theory, in which an optimally foraging animal moves to a new patch when that is worthwhile despite the time and effort of finding a new patch (Charnov 1976). When the cost of finding a new patch exceeds the overall mean rate of return, further foraging exerts a net cost and should stop until the situation becomes more propitious.

Human foraging patterns seem to follow these principles, but the resources that humans mainly strive for are not calories, but relationships, status, and the welfare of children and kin. The categories of effort used by behavioral ecologists are helpful in looking at the tradeoffs that bedevil human lives (Krebs and Davies 1997):

1. Somatic effort
   - Obtaining resources to grow and develop
   - Defending against predators, pathogens, and loss of resources

2. Reproductive effort
   - Mating
   - Parenting and helping kin

3. Social effort
   - Building relationships and alliances
   - Striving for status and power

As with every other species, humans must allocate effort among these different tasks, and every allocation to one detracts from the others (Heckhausen and Schultz 1995; Little 1999). A person who works 80 hours a week has little time or energy for taking care of children, or even taking care of self. Someone who is enmeshed in status striving will have little time and energy left for finding a mate, whereas preoccupation with making oneself an attractive mate can undermine other pursuits. However, this issue is even more complex. Different strategies in pursuit of different goals will pay off in some situations but not in others. It is essential to allocate effort to what is paying off here and now. More specifically, we should expect organisms to allocate effort according to what I call the "central Darwinian algorithm": optimal allocation of resources and effort to different enterprises requires taking whatever possible current action will give the greatest marginal gain in reproduction-limiting resources. Developmental aspects of this principle are intuitively obvious: people invest in status displays when groups are forming, they look for mates at sexual maturity, they invest enormous effort in family when they have young children, and they become generative later in life. However, from day to day and month to month, some

pursuits will be viable but others will not. A mechanism to disengage motivation from unproductive pursuits fosters reallocation to more productive strategies and enterprises (Klinger 1975; Wrosch et al. 2003). When essential investments in one area fatally deprive another area, the resulting stress should be no surprise. Most so-called life crises arise from precisely this kind of Hobson's choice. For instance, the single working mother of a chronically ill child may face the impossible choice of either keeping her job or caring for her child.

Although everyday mood variations reallocate effort among various enterprises according to what is and is not working, the same mechanism is relevant to global mood variations that reflect the productivity of efforts in all domains. When all available avenues in life appear to offer few rewards, a global pullback from habitual efforts may be warranted to avoid wasted effort and risks and to have a chance to consider possible alternative directions (Gut 1989). When such withdrawal leads to a fundamental new direction in life, depression often remits.

Situations in which efforts appear to be futile are the basis for the influential "learned helplessness" perspective on depression (Seligman 1972). Dogs that experience inescapable shock will, when a barrier is removed, stay in the shock chamber, even though they could escape. This has been used as a model for humans with depression who remain in bad situations that they could escape. The central message has been that many depressed people are far more pessimistic about their plight than is justified and far less helpless than they think they are (Seligman et al. 1979). This perspective has led to helpful interventions designed to give people a sense of increased efficacy (Peterson et al. 1993). The same perspective is found in cognitive therapy, which seeks and finds evidence of cognitive distortion and unjustified pessimism that can be corrected with systematic cognitive retraining (Beck 1976).

What has been somewhat absent from the learned helplessness literature, however, is attention to the origins of the mechanisms that result in dogs staying where they are shocked. The stimulus is so unnatural that it is difficult to tell what is actually going on. Does the pain arouse systems shaped to cope with loss of a hierarchy battle? Have dogs that persisted in the face of related natural situations fared even worse?

A clue is offered by the Porsolt test, which measures the duration of active swimming for rats dropped in a beaker of water. Drugs that prolong swimming time often have proved to be effective antidepressants in this model (Porsolt et al. 1978). A closer, ecological analysis found something different, however (Nadeau 1999). When the rats stop swimming, they do not just drown; they float quietly, with just their noses above the water. This is not a pathological helpless response but a useful adaptation for a rat swept into deep water when there is no quick way out. Rats that swim too vigorously for too long will certainly drown sooner. This makes a sobering prediction: in a natural situation, and likely even in a beaker in a laboratory, rats given antidepressants will drown sooner than those given placebo.

Attempts to bring the literature about self-esteem into an evolutionary framework have begun. Sociometry theories suggest that self-esteem is designed to indicate one's position in a group, with low self-esteem signaling the need to invest more in the group or to consider giving up on the group (Leary and Baumeister 2000). Further research suggests that people whose self-esteem is contingent on achieving goals set by others, or contingent on rising in a hierarchy, are vulnerable to depression as compared with those who pursue more "noble goals" or personal goals that do not involve social comparison (Crocker and Wolfe 2001). An explicitly evolutionary perspective recognizes competition everywhere and sees the task of adapting to it as central to life (Gilbert 1997; Gilbert et al. 1995), with depression playing an essential role in coping with status loss. In an elaboration and variation, Allen and Badcock (2003) suggested that people carefully monitor their social investment potential; when they perceive it as low and are at risk of being excluded from the group, a state of depression offers protection by inhibiting risk-taking and increasing monitoring of others' assessments. A different slant on related phenomena notes the prevalence of guilt and, especially, survivor guilt as vulnerability factors for depression and the social utility of capacity for guilt (O'Connor et al. 2002).

In situations characterized by a nonviable central life goal or strategy, it may be best to quit striving and to invest effort and time instead in mulling over the situation in preparation for possible major changes. Emmy Gut (1989) has written particularly well about these benefits of low mood when a fundamental reappraisal is needed. The benefits of pulling back and reconsidering all options without being distracted by constant pressures and striving are also central to many other presentations about the utility of depression. In particular, the social navigation hypothesis proposed by Watson and Andrews (2002) emphasizes the utility, in the face of social damage, of experiencing an emotion akin to physical pain and of sending honest signals to kin that the current situation is unworkable. They summarized evidence that depressive thinking is in some respects more realistic, but whether this is really an adaptation or simply a move toward accuracy from the usual rose-colored view (Sedikides 1993) is not certain. Neither is it clear that depression actually motivates

others to help more (Coyne et al. 1987), although Hagen (2002) provided some evidence that postpartum depression does engage helping and improves some outcomes.

Watson and Andrews (2002) have supported Hagen's (2002) suggestion that depression may have been shaped specifically to manipulate others into providing help, either after childbirth or in any social situation in which a person can influence others only by going "on strike." These ideas fit well with certain themes in behavioral ecology in which all animal communications are seen as manipulations (Krebs and Dawkins 1984) and in which the honesty of such signals is guaranteed only by high costs (Zahavi and Zahavi 1997) of the sort that are present in depression. The possibility that depression could have such a manipulation or extortion function is odious to those who are striving to remove stigma from depression, and the main evidence in favor of it is the otherwise explainable data that depression is more common in people who are in untoward circumstances. A critique of the social navigation hypothesis and adaptationist hypotheses in general suggests that wide trait variation offers a simpler explanation (Nettle 2004). The test will be whether others really do respond to these signals with predicted help that is greater than the huge costs of being depressed and with more help than they would offer to a different kind of request for aid.

Assessment of Functions of Low Mood and Depression

Despite the variety of hypotheses proposed for possible functions of low mood and depression, the main possibilities refer to just a few situations: loss of position in a hierarchy, changes in propitiousness of goal pursuit more generally, and communication with and manipulation of others by signaling a need for help or by failing to contribute to essential tasks. As noted earlier, testing evolutionary hypotheses about the selective forces that shaped a trait is quite a different and more difficult enterprise than testing proximate hypotheses about structures and mechanisms. The main differences encountered in testing evolutionary, as compared with proximate, hypotheses are that evolutionary hypotheses are not mutually exclusive, so evidence against one hypothesis is not strong evidence for alternative hypotheses. The difficulties of finding and using comparative data mean that the assessment often comes down to whether a trait's characteristics sufficiently match those expected to justify support for the hypothesis. Although such methods do not offer the strong inference that is so often available in testing proximate hypotheses (O'Donohue and Buchanan 2001; Platt

1964), the complications do not mean that the questions are impossible to answer—only that they are difficult and that hypothesis assessment requires considerable judgment in addition to relevant data.

The universal experience of low mood and its close regulation by circumstances involving unrewarded efforts or absence or loss of crucial resources or rank in a hierarchy offer support for the hypothesis that it has some adaptive function related to regulation of behavior. Nonetheless, investigators are just beginning to determine the exact circumstances that arouse normal low mood, what adaptive challenges they contain, and how some characteristics of low mood could help to meet those challenges. A closely related protective response, anxiety, seems to have been differentiated into a cluster of partially overlapping subtypes, each shaped to cope with a specific kind of danger (Marks and Nesse 1994). Thus, animal phobias, social phobias, and panic disorder show differences as well as overlapping symptoms, and people vulnerable to one kind of anxiety are often also vulnerable to others (Barlow 1988). This idea is just now being applied to depression, but preliminary studies suggest that the symptoms of depression arising from failure are different from those arising from loss or lack of a crucial resource (Keller and Nesse 2005). More detailed data allowing comparison of depression symptoms for cases with different precipitants may help to resolve the question.

Another major unanswered question is whether these findings about ordinary low mood and mild depression have anything to do with serious depression. They could be as little associated as the muscle stiffness after exercise and the muscle stiffness encountered in parkinsonism. The question is difficult, but the possibilities are clear. Depression could itself be 1) an adaptation to certain situations (akin to fever), 2) a pathological extreme of a normal response (akin to chronic pain), 3) a pathological complication (akin to the dehydration that can result from diarrhea), or 4) pathology unrelated to normal mood and its regulation (akin to Parkinson's disease). The position taken here is that answering the question about the situations in which low mood is helpful is a necessary but incomplete precursor to questions about full-fledged depression. Furthermore, there may well be subtypes of low mood, each shaped to cope with different situations.

Differences in Vulnerability to Depression

Explaining why individuals differ in their vulnerability to depression is an entirely different question from the ques-

tion of why all humans have a capacity for low mood. An evolutionary perspective does offer useful directions regarding this question, however. The high heritability of vulnerability to depression is well recognized (Wallace et al. 2002). The evolutionary question is whether the responsible genes are simply mutations not yet selected out or whether their prevalence is maintained for some reason (Houle 1998). In addition, variation in vulnerability results from differences in early experiences. In this case, the question is whether the effects are best understood as effects of facultative mechanisms that adjust the organism to its environment or as the results of experiences that damage brain mechanisms. I consider genetic differences first.

Genetic Differences

At first blush, it seems as if genes that make individuals vulnerable to depression must be defective mutations that selection has not yet been able to eliminate. Even aside from the severe selective effect of suicide, the disability and social costs associated with recurrent depression must have decreased reproductive success, even in Paleolithic times. However, extensive efforts have thus far failed to find single genes that account for more than 5% of the variation in the risk for depression. Geneticists are increasingly cautioning that depression appears to be a polygenic disease whose risk may depend on dozens of genes, in which case the force of selection becomes so tiny that mutations can persist for many generations and even drift to higher frequencies, despite some small negative effect of selection (Risch and Merikangas 1996). Furthermore, massive epigenetic effects may mean that the effects of a gene on phenotype may vary considerably from individual to individual, thus helping to explain the persistence of considerable genetic and associated phenotypic diversity. This all seems quite likely.

Trait Variation and Selection

However, considering the functions of low mood and related regulation mechanisms suggests possibilities beyond the simple notion of genetic mutation and the limited power of selection. If low mood can be a useful response in certain situations, then genetic variations will influence the threshold and intensity of the response, with maximum fitness at some intermediate level. The perils of excessive low mood are obvious, but deficits in capacity for low mood also should reduce Darwinian fitness. Furthermore, the fitness of different degrees of responsiveness may change dramatically with changes in the environment. Optimistic investors did well in the late

1990s but lost their gains and more in the early years of the new millennium, while pessimists reaped profits from bonds. Likewise, in secure environments of plenty, a deficient tendency to low mood may be optimal, but at times of famine, political unrest, and rigid hierarchies, those who lack a capacity for low mood may be at a serious disadvantage. In practical terms, it would be extremely difficult to differentiate individuals who lack a normal capacity for low mood from those who have simply been fortunate in life. However, if new antidepressants ever become both reliably effective and free from most side effects, tests of this idea will be carried out, whether wittingly or unwittingly, as we observe the lives of those who lack the normal capacity for low mood.

The optimal baseline level of mood and the optimal mood change in response to unpropitious circumstances are two distinct traits shaped by different selection forces. The optimal level of general stable mood will vary depending on the nature of the long-term environment, but if the main value of the capacity for mood is to adjust behavior so that investments and risk-taking are increased or decreased in concert with changes in propitiousness, the absolute level of mood may have relatively little influence on fitness; more will depend on the ability to change behavior in the right direction at the right time. If this is correct, then selection may act only weakly on the absolute level of baseline mood compared with its actions on the responsiveness of mood to environmental variations.

Much attention has been paid to the possibility that it may be difficult to identify genes for mental disorders because the heritable factors may differ in different lineages; less attention has been paid to the possibility that genes can lead to depression via their effects on intermediate states. The evidence that exposure to life events is heritable is striking but is obvious in retrospect, given what we know about genetic influences on sensation seeking and other personality traits that correlate with experiencing many life events (Kendler and Karkowski-Shuman 1997). Less obvious is the possibility that genes may increase vulnerability to depression by influence on temperament (Ono et al. 2002), which makes it more likely that certain people will get themselves into situations where they cannot disengage from the pursuit of unreachable goals. As already noted, several routes often lead to such situations. Extreme ambition, of the sort sometimes associated with neuroticism, makes it likely that an individual will constantly feel inadequate and unable to accomplish what seem to be essential life goals. A tendency to make very strong attachments is likely to result in continuing a relationship and trying vainly to improve it, despite abuse or lack of love. A tendency to have only a few attachments, or only one big life goal, provides fewer options when

things go badly. Extreme moral compunctions also are often associated with situations that make it difficult to escape from exploitation. General fearfulness also inhibits individuals from taking the risks necessary to get out of bad situations, as may a general lack of self-esteem. Most general of all, a tendency to see one's life in terms of one overpoweringly important central goal makes it more likely that the person will find himself or herself trapped in a nonviable overall life situation.

These ideas are somewhat theoretical but have important implications not only for the general view of genetic effects on mood but also for specific research strategies. In particular, they suggest the need to conduct phenotyping that goes beyond mere enumeration of symptoms and episodes. An ecologically based phenotyping would incorporate the relation of specific symptoms to not only the number of severe life events but also the nature of those life events; the individual's temperament, values, and life goals; and how the life events influence assessments of ability to progress toward those goals. It is conceivable that it will be possible to identify different routes to depression associated with specific genes that increase depression vulnerability—a degree of gene–environment interaction that may be essential to consider despite its complexity.

Balancing Selection

Yet another possibility is that genes that cause depression give a selective advantage either via pleiotropic effects or by benefits that accrue only in certain environments or in combination with certain other genes. This has been proposed most specifically in the case of bipolar disorder, for which the costs of illness are even more horrendous than they are for unipolar depression and in which some potential benefits are obvious (Jamison 1993; D.R. Wilson 1998). The grand creativity, sexual attractiveness, and disinhibition of people in the throes of mania give a clear route to short-term reproductive success. The more moderate but sustained productivity of those with hypomania offers another route (Akiskal 2003), but if higher mood reliably offered a fitness benefit, it already should have spread unless there were significant tradeoffs. Even aside from the advantages and disadvantages associated with clinical syndromes, close relatives of those with bipolar disorder might experience benefits without the costs associated with clinical disorders. There is ample evidence for increased creativity of people with manic depression, and some convincing evidence shows that their relatives also are more creative than average (Andreasen 1987; Richards et al. 1988). Whether they are especially sexually attractive or successful is another unanswered question.

Genes for bipolar disorder could be selected for if the creativity associated with mania benefits the group to an extent that outweighs the costs to the individual. It is certainly plausible that groups with more creative individuals tend to succeed and displace those without such inspiration. However, one of the main recent advances in evolutionary biology has been recognition that the power of selection acting at the level of the group is too weak to counteract any but the tiniest deleterious effects on individuals. While lemming groups might well do better if many of their members drown themselves when there is too little food, there will always be variation in the tendency to commit suicide for the good of the group, and genes that incline individuals against such self-sacrifice will soon take over despite the dire effects of uncontrolled population growth.

A control systems view suggests examination of mood as a trait regulated in the same way as body temperature or hemoglobin concentration. Values that are above or below a reference value initiate homeostatic mechanisms that restore the baseline value (Cziko 2000). In certain conditions, however, different levels give an advantage, and rheostatic mechanisms adjust the set point accordingly (Mrosovsky 1990). In infections, a higher body temperature helps to fight the pathogens. When individuals live at high altitude, low oxygen tension stimulates erythropoietin, which raises hemoglobin concentration to an appropriate level.

In any feedback-regulated system, cyclic oscillations are expected. If a thermostat turns on a furnace whenever the temperature drops below a set point, then the furnace will still be pouring out heat when the set point is reached, so the temperature will overshoot the optimal level. To minimize the range of these variations, most modern thermostats use anticipation mechanisms that turn on the furnace just before the set point as the temperature falls and turn it off just before the set point as the heat from the furnace raises the temperature. The cycles in cyclothymic disorder match what one would expect if there were a defect in the anticipation mechanism, with wide swings precipitated by small perturbations. The more severe extremes of manic depression are better characterized by uncontrolled positive feedback that leads to extremes of effort, energy expenditure, and lack of sleep that escalate until a shutdown mechanism sends the system crashing into depression. The characteristic sudden switch from mania to depression matches this pattern. Note that these principles do not depend on what brain mechanisms actually instantiate them, any more than it matters whether a furnace thermostat mechanism uses a bimetal strip or a digital detector.

Although these ideas about bipolar disorder are important to pursue, no concrete evidence so far indicates that bipolar genes give any selective advantage. It seems likely that they are simply defects that interfere with the evolved mechanisms that normally regulate mood. Nonetheless, epidemiological studies have not yet addressed systematically the possibility that selection maintains the frequency of the responsible genes.

Adjustment of Mood Mechanisms as a Function of Life Experience

Extensive evidence documents the effects of early life events on vulnerability to depression (Lin et al. 1986). Attachment difficulties and lack of parental love lead to problematic relationships and increased risks for depression (Beatson and Taryan 2003; Sloman et al. 2003). Other early childhood adversity, especially sexual abuse, increases the risk for depression (Harkness and Monroe 2002). Although some studies have not controlled for possible genetic mediation of the effects, it seems clear that some experiences do influence rates of depression. The question posed by an evolutionary view is whether these effects are best interpreted as damage from abnormal experiences or whether they result from properly functioning facultative mechanisms that monitor certain aspects of the environment and adjust mood mechanisms adaptively.

The exemplar is the relation between disorders of attachment and later depression. Early work treated secure attachment as normal and other kinds of attachment as pathological results of faulty parenting. Newer approaches consider the additional possibility that variation in family conditions over the course of human history made anxious and ambivalent attachment styles advantageous in certain circumstances (Belsky 1999; Chisholm 1996). This hypothesis is difficult to test but is supported by the prevalence of insecure attachment styles, their association with parental difficulty or ambivalence, and the surprising lack of heritability of attachment styles.

The best-documented and strongest risk factor for depression is previous low mood or depression (Kessler et al. 2003), and the stimulus required to set off depression seems to decrease with each subsequent episode so that the onset of depression becomes increasingly autonomous from life events (Kendler 1998). This has been interpreted as akin to the "kindling" phenomenon that makes neurons increasingly vulnerable to seizures after repeated stimulation (Post and Weiss 1998). Whether or not neural kindling is the responsible proximate mechanism, an evolutionary view asks if the change in threshold results simply from damage, or if repeated exposure to certain situations engages a mechanism that adjusts the low mood threshold accordingly and adaptively.

Certainly, other response thresholds are adjusted in light of experience, the most notable being the reduction in panic threshold after a life-threatening experience (or even after a "spontaneous" panic attack).

Population Differences in Vulnerability

Extensive evidence documents the substantial differences in rates of depression in different populations (Brown et al. 1996; Weissman et al. 1996). Some of these differences may arise from variations in reporting and cultural differences in the expression of depressive symptoms (Kleinman and Good 1985), but increasing standardization of methods allows confidence that rates do vary enormously in different groups. The simplest explanation is that differing social conditions expose people in some groups to more severe life events than others. Although differences in rates of severe life events are correlated with rates of depression, no one has examined whether systematic differences in the motivational structures of people's lives in different societies might provide an even more powerful explanation for different rates of depression. Resource allocation/goal disengagement theory predicts that depression should be more prevalent in populations where many people make enormous investments in just a few major life goals that have an uncertain payoff and no ready alternatives. Conversely, depression should be less common in groups where people pursue more limited and more relationship-related goals that offer more social support and more options if efforts to reach one particular goal fail.

The more salient population variations from an evolutionary perspective are those between ancestral and modern populations. Some studies looking for changes in depression rates in recent decades have reported positive findings (Klerman and Weissman 1989) and some have not (Murphy et al. 2000). However, the evolutionary question is whether novel aspects of the environment have increased vulnerability to depression in the same way that the ready availability of fatty and sweet foods has increased rates of atherosclerosis. Unfortunately, no reliable evidence regarding these rates is available, not even evidence on rates of depression in surviving groups of hunter-gatherers. Although methodological obstacles are high, including small group sizes and different languages, data on rates of depression in these groups may prove as crucial as the data showing that hunter-gatherers have very low rates of hypertension, obesity, and atherosclerosis. Social differences are especially salient, but many other factors could adversely influence brain mechanisms in modern environments, including artificial light, abnormal sleep patterns, dietary deficiencies of omega 3 relative to omega 6 fatty acids, and low levels of exercise.

Although gene–environment interactions in the causes of depression are now widely appreciated (Caspi et al. 2003; Kendler 1997), their implications for the effects of novel environments are still being recognized. When essentially all members of a population are exposed to evolutionarily novel environmental factors, much of the within-population variation in rates of pathology will arise from genetic differences that had no significant effects on ancestral conditions. It is thus incorrect to call these genes "defects." They are better recognized as "quirks" that become significant only when they interact with a novel environment. Many genes that predispose to atherosclerosis are examples. Variation in traits such as nearsightedness or atherosclerosis in a modern population might well be overwhelmingly genetic in origin, even though the pathogenesis requires exposure to an environmental factor, such as abnormalities in diet or early exposure to small print.

Whether genetic differences exist between groups that might influence rates of depression is unknown. Recent findings of population differences that influence the rates of other diseases offer examples, and group differences in the prevalence of the short genotype for the serotonin promoter transporter allele are interesting, but no solid evidence shows that genetic differences explain different rates of depression. The case of seasonal affective disorder offers a particularly intriguing test. If seasonal affective disorder is a defect, then populations that have lived in extreme northern or southern latitudes gradually would have been shaped to resist the syndrome as compared with populations from areas where light levels are more stable, unless it simply reflects the slowness of selection (Sher 2000). If, however, the seasonal changes in mood are useful adaptations in areas with extreme seasonal climate variations, then populations that evolved in extreme latitudes should have increased tendencies to experience winter depression.

Research Implications

An evolutionary perspective on depression has two main implications for research. The first is the need to seriously consider and test hypotheses about the evolutionary origins and functions of low mood and its possible relation to clinical depression. The second is to call attention to the possibility that we have been studying all cases of major depression as if they represent the same condition, when different individuals may get depressed by very different routes (Akiskal and McKinney 1973). Closely related is the possibility that selection has partially differentiated subtypes of depression to deal with different kinds of situations that have recurred over evolutionary history. If this is the case, then it will be essential to define depression subtypes on the basis of contributing etiological factors and to further subtype cases of depression on the basis of the nature of the precipitating life situation.

An evolutionary perspective has further implications for brain studies. Such studies seem to be moving from models based on presumed brain defects to models based on mechanisms that regulate normal and abnormal mood. However, if low mood is useful, then it seems possible that many of the brain changes associated with depression are not themselves pathological but may represent the activation of an adaptive defense mechanism. The anatomical localization of areas of increased activity in states of depression (Davidson et al. 2003) tends to support this position. If depression involves mechanisms that adaptively inhibit motivation, then effective drugs and physical treatments would not be expected to work at just one site. Instead, disruption of the low mood system at any of several points should lead to improvement, in the same way that pain can be relieved by drugs that disrupt cytokine systems at several different points or that act on opiate receptors. Furthermore, the genetic differences in vulnerability to depression may be similar to individual differences in tendency to get fever with a cold or variations in tendency to vomit in response to chemotherapy or other toxins.

Clinical Implications

Despite attempts to find ways that evolutionary views might make psychotherapy more effective (Gilbert and Bailey 2000; Weisfeld 1977), an evolutionary perspective does not specify a particular kind of treatment for depression. Its attention to the normal functions of low mood should, however, offer a useful foundation for clinical psychiatric practice in the same way that an understanding of the functions and causes of cough, fever, and vomiting provide a foundation for the practice of general medicine. Unfortunately, we are not yet in a position to offer this kind of basic science functional knowledge for the clinical practice of psychiatry. Our understanding of the proximate mechanisms involved with depression has far outstripped our understanding of what those mechanisms might be for, with much resulting confusion.

A central issue among members of the lay public is whether depression is really a disease or whether it is a normal response to certain situations. We can confidently answer the question in the case of severe, recurrent depression, but we still lack the kind of understanding that would allow us to address the question scientifically for a wide range of moods and situations. This has important implications for the psychiatric diagnosis in general and for planning for DSM-V in particular. Although the exclusion of contextual factors from diagnostic criteria fosters reliability, it makes the DSM criteria incapable of distinguishing responses that are excessive from those that are normal and useful (Nesse 2001; Wakefield 1992, 1997). An evolutionary perspective offers a solid foundation for diagnosis, one only now being appreciated (Cosmides and Tooby 1999; Wakefield 1999). If pain disorders were diagnosed in the same way, the diagnosis of chronic pain would depend on only the duration and intensity of symptoms, not on the presence or absence of a cause for the pain. The exclusion of ordinary grief already protects against some false-positive diagnoses of depression. As we develop a more confident and refined understanding of the normal functions and regulation of low mood, it should be possible to differentiate aversive but normal responses from pathological conditions with criteria more scientifically based than merely severity and duration.

The evolutionary insight with the most direct clinical utility, prefigured by many clinicians, may be the normal role of low mood in disengaging individuals from goals they cannot reach. This principle does not need to be derived from evolutionary principles; it has been developed, elaborated, and confirmed by psychologists over the past four decades. So far, however, it is little appreciated in psychiatry and has not been applied to clinical populations. From Bibring to Beck and forward, expert clinicians often have focused on what people are trying to do in their lives, why they persist in trying to please others who cannot be pleased, why they try to impress others who will not be impressed, and why they persist in unrequited love. Although it usually turns out to be difficult to help people to reassess such situations and their options, this perspective has shown enduring usefulness that could be augmented by a growing evolutionary sophistication in understanding its origins and significance and the broader framework of goals that people pursue. It could also help to unite apparently diverse therapeutic approaches, each of which intervenes at one or another point in the systems that maintain depression. As with any powerful tool, however, careless application will cause harm. There is no justification for crudely analyzing a person's main life efforts and advising him or her to change. The clinical challenge is the same as it has always been—trying to understand people and their relationships, goals, and feelings in order to understand, and help them understand, why they do what they do and why they feel what they feel. That, in combination with new diagnostic tests, genomic findings, and effective new drugs that block depression, will offer a bright future for treating depression.

References

Ainsworth MD, Blehar MC, Waters E, et al: Patterns of Attachment: A Psychological Study of the Strange Situation. Hillsdale, NJ, Lawrence Erlbaum, 1978

Akiskal HS: Dysthymia and cyclothymia in psychiatric practice a century after Kraepelin. J Affect Disord 62:17–31, 2001

Akiskal HS: The evolutionary significance of affective temperaments. CME article presented at the 156th annual meeting of the American Psychiatric Association, San Francisco, CA, May 17–22, 2003. Available at: http://www.medscape.com/viewarticle/457152.

Akiskal HS, McKinney WTJ: Depressive disorders: toward a unified hypothesis. Science 182:20–29, 1973

Alcock J: Animal Behavior: An Evolutionary Approach. Sunderland, MA, Sinauer, 1997

Alcock J: The Triumph of Sociobiology. New York, Oxford University Press, 2001

Allen NB, Badcock PBT: The social risk hypothesis of depressed mood: evolutionary, psychosocial and neurobiological perspectives. Psychol Bull 129:887–913, 2003

Andreasen NC: Creativity and mental illness: prevalence rates in writers and their first-degree relatives. Am J Psychiatry 144:1288–1292, 1987

Angst J, Merikangas KR: Multi-dimensional criteria for the diagnosis of depression. J Affect Disord 62:7–15, 2001

Archer J: The Nature of Grief. New York, Oxford University Press, 1999

Badcock PBT, Allen NB: Adaptive social reasoning in depressed mood and depressive vulnerability. Cognition and Emotion 17:647–670, 2003

Barkow JH: Darwin, Sex, and Status: Biological Approaches to Mind and Culture. Toronto, Ontario, University of Toronto Press, 1989

Barkow J, Cosmides L, Tooby J (eds): The Adapted Mind. New York, Oxford University Press, 1992

Barlow DH: Anxiety and Its Disorders. New York, Guilford, 1988

Barrett L, Dunbar RIM, Lycett J: Human Evolutionary Psychology. Basingstoke, UK, Palgrave, 2002

Beatson J, Taryan S: Predisposition to depression: the role of attachment. Aust N Z J Psychiatry 37:219–225, 2003

Beck AT: Cognitive Therapy and the Emotional Disorders. New York, International Universities Press, 1976

Belsky J: Modern evolutionary theory and patterns of attachment, in Handbook of Attachment: Theory, Research, and Clinical Applications. Edited by Cassidy J, Shaver PR. New York, Guilford, 1999, pp 141–161

Bibring E: The mechanisms of depression, in Affective Disorders. Edited by Greenacre P. New York, International Universities Press, 1953, pp 13–48

Bowlby J: Separation: Anxiety and Anger. New York, Basic Books, 1973

Brickman P: Commitment, Conflict, and Caring. Englewood Cliffs, NJ, Prentice-Hall, 1987

Brown GW, Bifulco A, Harris T, et al: Life stress, chronic subclinical symptoms and vulnerability to clinical depression. J Affect Disord 11:1–19, 1986

Brown GW, Harris TO, Hepworth C: Loss, humiliation and entrapment among women developing depression: a patient and non-patient comparison. Psychol Med 25:7–21, 1995

Brown GW, Harris TO, Eales MJ: Social factors and comorbidity of depressive and anxiety disorders. Br J Psychiatry Suppl 30:50–57, 1996

Buss DM: Evolutionary psychology: a new paradigm for psychological science. Psychological Inquiry 6:1–30, 1995

Buss DM: The evolution of happiness. Am Psychol 55:15–23, 2000

Buss DM, Haselton MG, Shackelford TK, et al: Adaptations, exaptations, and spandrels. Am Psychol 53:533–548, 1998

Caraco T, Blanckenhorn B, Gregory G, et al: Risk sensitivity: ambient temperature affects foraging choice. Anim Behav 39:338–345, 1990

Carver CS, Scheier MF: Origins and functions of positive and negative affect: a control-process view. Psychol Rev 97:19–35, 1990

Carver CS, Scheier MF: On the Self-Regulation of Behavior. New York, Cambridge University Press, 1998

Caspi A, Sugden K, Moffitt TE, et al: Influence of life stress on depression: moderation by a polymorphism in the 5-HTT gene. Science 301:386–389, 2003

Charnov EL: Optimal foraging: the marginal value theorem. Theor Popul Biol 9:129–136, 1976

Chisholm J: The evolutionary ecology of human attachment organization. Hum Nat 7:1–38, 1996

Clark MS: Emotion. Newbury Park, CA, Sage Publications, 1992

Cosmides L, Tooby J: Toward an evolutionary taxonomy of treatable conditions. J Abnorm Psychol 108:453–464, 1999

Coyne JC, Kessler RC, Tal M, et al: Living with a depressed person. J Consult Clin Psychol 55:347–352, 1987

Crocker J, Wolfe CT: Contingencies of self-worth. Psychol Rev 108:593–623, 2001

Cziko G: The Things We Do. Cambridge, MA, MIT Press, 2000

Davidson RJ, Irwin W, Anderle MJ, et al: The neural substrates of affective processing in depressed patients treated with venlafaxine. Am J Psychiatry 160:64–75, 2003

Diener E, Fujita F: Resources, personal strivings, and subjective well-being: a nomothetic ideographic approach. J Pers Soc Psychol 68:926–935, 1995

Eaton SB, Konner M, Shostak M: Stone agers in the fast lane: chronic degenerative diseases in evolutionary perspective. Am J Med 84:739–749, 1988

Ekman P, Davidson RJ (eds): The Nature of Emotion: Fundamental Questions. New York, Oxford University Press, 1994

Emmons RA: Striving and feeling: personal goals and subjective well-being, in The Psychology of Action: Linking Cognition and Motivation to Behavior. Edited by Gollwitzer PM. New York, Guilford, 1996, pp 313–337

Engel G, Schmale A: Conservation-withdrawal: a primary regulatory process for organismic homeostasis, in Physiology, Emotion, and Psychosomatic Illness, Vol 8 (N.S.). Edited by Porter R, Night J. Amsterdam, CIBA, 1972, pp 57–85

Ewald P: Evolution of Infectious Disease. New York, Oxford University Press, 1994

Gilbert P: The evolution of social attractiveness and its role in shame, humiliation, guilt and therapy. Br J Med Psychol 70:112–147, 1997

Gilbert P, Bailey KG: Genes on the Couch: Explorations in Evolutionary Psychotherapy. East Sussex, UK, Brunner/Routledge, 2000

Gilbert P, Price J, Allen S: Social comparison, social attractiveness and evolution: how might they be related? New Ideas in Psychology 13:149–165, 1995

Gut E: Productive and Unproductive Depression. New York, Basic Books, 1989

Hagen EH: Depression as bargaining: the case postpartum. Evol Hum Behav 23:323–336, 2002

Hamburg DA, Hamburg BA, Barchas JD: Anger and depression in perspective of behavioral biology, in Emotions: Their Parameters and Measurement. Edited by Levi L. New York, Raven, 1975, pp 235–278

Hamilton WD: The genetical evolution of social behaviour, I. J Theor Biol 7:1–16, 1964a

Hamilton WD: The genetical evolution of social behaviour, II. J Theor Biol 7:17–52, 1964b

Harkness KL, Monroe SM: Childhood adversity and the endogenous versus nonendogenous distinction in women with major depression. Am J Psychiatry 159:387–393, 2002

Harlow HF, Harlow MK: Social deprivation in monkeys. Sci Am 207:136–146, 1962

Hartung J: Deceiving down, in Self Deception: An Adaptive Mechanism? Edited by Lockard JS, Paulhus D. Englewood Cliffs, NJ, Prentice-Hall, 1988, pp 170–185

Heckhausen J, Schultz R: A life-span theory of control. Psychol Rev 102:284–304, 1995

Higgins ET, Shah J, Friedman R: Emotional responses to goal attainment: strength of regulatory focus as moderator. J Pers Soc Psychol 72:515–525, 1997

Houle D: How should we explain variation in the genetic variance of traits? Genetica 102/103:241–253, 1998

Jamison KR: Touched With Fire: Manic-Depressive Illness and the Artistic Temperament. New York, Free Press, 1993

Janoff-Bulman R, Brickman P: Expectations and what people learn from failure, in Expectations and Action. Edited by Feather NT. Hillsdale, NJ, Lawrence Erlbaum, 1982, pp 207–237

Judd LL, Akiskal HS, Maser JD, et al: Major depressive disorder: a prospective study of residual subthreshold depressive symptoms as predictor of rapid relapse. J Affect Disord 50:97–108, 1998

Keller MB, Nesse RM: Is low mood an adaptation? Evidence for sub-types with symptoms that match precipitants. J Affect Disord 86:27–35, 2005

Kendler KS: The genetic epidemiology of psychiatric disorders: a current perspective. Soc Psychiatry Psychiatr Epidemiol 32:5–11, 1997

Kendler KS: Major depression and the environment: a psychiatric genetic perspective. Pharmacopsychiatry 31:5–9, 1998

Kendler KS, Karkowski-Shuman L: Stressful life events and genetic liability to major depression: genetic control of exposure to the environment? Psychol Med 27:539–547, 1997

Kessler RC: The effects of stressful life events on depression. Annu Rev Psychol 48:191–214, 1997

Kessler RC, Berglund P, Demler O, et al: The epidemiology of major depressive disorder: results from the National Comorbidity Survey Replication (NCS-R). JAMA 289:3095–3105, 2003

Kleinman A, Good B: Culture and Depression: Studies in the Anthropology and Cross-Cultural Psychiatry of Affect and Disorder. Berkeley, University of California Press, 1985

Klerman G, Weissman M: Increasing rates of depression. JAMA 261:2229–2235, 1989

Klinger E: Consequences of commitment to and disengagement from incentives. Psychol Rev 82:1–25, 1975

Konner M: The Tangled Wing: Biological Constraints on the Human Spirit. New York, Times Books, 2002

Krebs JR, Davies NB (eds): Behavioral Ecology: An Evolutionary Approach. Sunderland, MA, Sinauer, 1984

Krebs JR, Davies NB: Behavioral Ecology: An Evolutionary Approach. Oxford, England, Blackwell Science, 1997

Krebs J, Dawkins R: Animal signals: mind-reading and manipulation, in Behavioral Ecology: An Evolutionary Approach. Edited by Krebs JR, Davies NB. Sunderland, MA, Sinauer, 1984, pp 380–402

Leary MR, Baumeister RF: The nature and function of self-esteem: sociometer theory, in Advances in Experimental Social Psychology, Vol 32. Edited by Zanna MP. San Diego, CA, Academic Press, 2000, pp 2–51

Lewis AJ: Melancholia: a clinical survey of depressive states. J Ment Sci 80:1–43, 1934

Lin N, Dean A, Ensel WM: Social Support, Life Events, and Depression. New York, Academic Press, 1986

Little BR: Personal projects and social ecology: themes and variation across the life span, in Action and Self Development: Theory and Research Through the Life Span. Edited by Brandtstadter J, Lerner RM. Thousand Oaks, CA, Sage Publications, 1999, pp 79–87

Marks IM, Nesse RM: Fear and fitness: an evolutionary analysis of anxiety disorders. Ethol Sociobiol 15:247–261, 1994

Mayr E: How to carry out the adaptationist program? American Naturalist 121(March):324–333, 1983

McGuire MT, Troisi A: Unrealistic wishes and physiological change: an overview. Psychother Psychosom 47:82–94, 1987

McGuire MT, Troisi A: Darwinian Psychiatry. Cambridge, MA, Harvard University Press, 1998

McGuire M, Marks I, Nesse R, et al: Evolutionary biology: a basic science for psychiatry. Acta Psychiatr Scand 86:89–96, 1992

Monroe SM, Harkness K, Simons AD, et al: Life stress and the symptoms of major depression. J Nerv Ment Dis 189:168–175, 2001

Morris WN: A functional analysis of the role of mood in affective systems. Review of Personality and Social Psychology 21:736–746, 1992

Mrosovsky N: Rheostasis. New York, Oxford University Press, 1990

Murphy JM, Laird NM, Monson RR, et al: A 40-year perspective on the prevalence of depression: the Stirling County Study. Arch Gen Psychiatry 57:209–215, 2000

Murray CJ, Lopez AD: Global mortality, disability, and the contribution of risk factors: Global Burden of Disease Study. Lancet 349(9063):1436–1442, 1997

Nadeau B: The forced swim test: an empirical and rational analysis of immobility and its reduction by antidepressants. Unpublished doctoral thesis, Department of Psychology, Simon Fraser University, Vancouver, BC, 1999

Nesse RM: Evolutionary explanations of emotions. Hum Nat 1:261–289, 1990

Nesse RM: The evolution of hope and despair. J Soc Issues 66:429–469, 1999

Nesse RM: Is depression an adaptation? Arch Gen Psychiatry 57:14–20, 2000a

Nesse RM: Is grief really maladaptive? Review of The Nature of Grief, by John Archer. Evol Hum Behav 21:59–61, 2000b

Nesse RM: On the difficulty of defining disease: a Darwinian perspective. Med Health Care Philos 4:37–46, 2001

Nesse RM: A signal detection analysis of the smoke detector principle. Evol Hum Behav 26:88–105, 2005

Nesse RM: Natural selection and the elusiveness of happiness. Philos Trans R Soc Lond B Biol Sci 359:1333–1347, 2004

Nesse RM, Williams GC: Why We Get Sick: The New Science of Darwinian Medicine. New York, Vintage, 1994

Nettle D: Evolutionary origins of depression: a review and reformulation. J Affect Disord 81:91–102, 2004

Oatley K, Bolton W: A social-cognitive theory of depression in reaction to life events. Psychol Rev 92:372–388, 1985

Oatley K, Jenkins JM: Understanding Emotions. Cambridge, MA, Blackwell, 1996

O'Connor LE, Berry JW, Weiss J, et al: Guilt, fear, submission, and empathy in depression. J Affect Disord 71:19–27, 2002

O'Donohue W, Buchanan JA: The weakness of strong inference. Behavior and Philosophy 29:1–20, 2001

Ono Y, Ando J, Onoda N, et al: Dimensions of temperament as vulnerability factors in depression. Mol Psychiatry 7:948–953, 2002

Palys TS, Little BR: Perceived life satisfaction and the organization of personal project systems. J Pers Soc Psychol 44:1221–1230, 1983

Peterson C, Maier SF, Seligman MEP: Learned Helplessness. New York, Oxford University Press, 1993

Platt JR: Strong inference. Science 146:347–353, 1964

Plutchik R: Emotion: A Psychoevolutionary Synthesis. New York, Harper & Row, 1980

Plutchik R, Kellerman H (eds): Emotion: Theory, Research, and Experience. New York, Academic Press, 1989

Porsolt RD, Anton G, Blavet N, et al: Behavioral despair in rats: a new model sensitive to antidepressant treatments. Eur J Pharmacol 47:379–391, 1978

Post RM, Weiss SR: Sensitization and kindling phenomena in mood, anxiety, and obsessive-compulsive disorders: the role of serotonergic mechanisms in illness progression. Biol Psychiatry 44:193–206, 1998

Price JS: The dominance hierarchy and the evolution of mental illness. Lancet 2:243–246, 1967

Price J, Sloman L, Gardner R, et al: The social competition hypothesis of depression. Br J Psychiatry 164:309–315, 1994

Pyszczynski T, Greenberg J: Self-regulatory perseveration and the depressive self-focusing style: a self-awareness theory of reactive depression. Psychol Bull 102:122–138, 1987

Queller DC: The spaniels of St. Marx and the Panglossian paradox: a critique of a rhetorical programme. Q Rev Biol 70:485–489, 1995

Reeve HK, Sherman PW: Adaptation and the goals of evolutionary research. Q Rev Biol 68:1–32, 1993

Richards RL, Kinner DK, Lunde I, et al: Creativity in manic-depressives, cyclothymes and their normal first-degree relatives: a preliminary report. J Abnorm Psychol 97:281–288, 1988

Risch N, Merikangas K: The future of genetic studies of complex human diseases. Science 273:1516–1517, 1996

Rose MR, Lauder GV (eds): Adaptation. San Diego, CA, Academic Press, 1996

Ruscio J, Ruscio A: A structure-based approach to psychological assessment: matching measurement models to latent structure. Assessment 9:4–16, 2002

Schmale A, Engel GL: The role of conservation-withdrawal in depressive reactions, in Depression and Human Existence. Edited by Benedek T, Anthony EJ. Boston, MA, Little, Brown, 1975, pp 83–198

Sedikides C: Assessment, enhancement, and verification determinants of the self-evaluation process. J Pers Soc Psychol 65:317–338, 1993

Segerstråle UCO: Defenders of the Truth. New York, Oxford University Press, 2000

Seligman ME: Learned helplessness. Annu Rev Med 23:407–412, 1972

Seligman ME, Csikszentmihalyi M: Positive psychology: an introduction. Am Psychol 55:5–14, 2000

Seligman ME, Abramson LY, Semmel A, et al: Depressive attributional style. J Abnorm Psychol 88:242–247, 1979

Sher L: The role of genetic factors in the etiology of seasonality and seasonal affective disorder: an evolutionary approach. Med Hypotheses 54:704–707, 2000

Sloman L, Gilbert P: Subordination and Defeat: An Evolutionary Approach to Mood Disorders. Mahwah, NJ, Lawrence Erlbaum, 2000

Sloman L, Price JS: Losing behavior (yielding subroutine) and human depression: proximate and selective mechanisms. Ethol Sociobiol 8 (3 suppl):99–109, 1987

Sloman L, Price J, Gilbert P, et al: Adaptive function of depression: psychotherapeutic implications. Am J Psychother 48:1–16, 1994

Sloman L, Gilbert P, Hasey G: Evolved mechanisms in depression: the role and interaction of attachment and social rank in depression. J Affect Disord 74:107–121, 2003

Stearns S (ed): Evolution in Health and Disease. Oxford, England, Oxford University Press, 1998

Sternbach RA: Congenital insensitivity to pain. Psychol Bull 60:252–264, 1963

Stevens A, Price J: Evolutionary Psychiatry: A New Beginning. London, Routledge, 1996

Tinbergen N: On the aims and methods of ethology. Z Tierpsychol 20:410–463, 1963

Tooby J, Cosmides L: The past explains the present: emotional adaptations and the structure of ancestral environments. Ethol Sociobiol 11:375–424, 1990

Trevathan WR, McKenna JJ, Smith EO (eds): Evolutionary Medicine. New York, Oxford University Press, 1999

Trivers RL: Social Evolution. Menlo Park, CA, Benjamin/Cummings, 1985

Wakefield JC: Disorder as harmful dysfunction: a conceptual critique of DSM-III R's definition of mental disorder. Psychol Rev 99:232–247, 1992

Wakefield JC: Diagnosing DSM-IV—part I: DSM-IV and the concept of disorder. Behav Res Ther 35:633–649, 1997

Wakefield JC: Evolutionary versus prototype analyses of the concept of disorder. J Abnorm Psychol 108:374–399, 1999

Wallace J, Schneider T, McGuffin P: Genetics of depression, in Handbook of Depression. Edited by Gotlib IH, Hammen CL. New York, Guilford, 2002, pp 169–191

Watson PJ, Andrews PW: Toward a revised evolutionary adaptationist analysis of depression: the social navigation hypothesis. J Affect Disord 72:1–14, 2002

Weisfeld GE: A Sociobiological Basis for Psychotherapy. New York, Grune & Stratton, 1977

Weissman MM, Bland RC, Canino GJ: Cross-national epidemiology of major depression and bipolar disorder. JAMA 276:293–296, 1996

Wenegrat B: Illness and Power. New York, New York University Press, 1995

Williams GC: Pleiotropy, natural selection, and the evolution of senescence. Evolution 11:398–411, 1957

Williams GC: Adaptation and Natural Selection: A Critique of Some Current Evolutionary Thought. Princeton, NJ, Princeton University Press, 1966

Williams GW, Nesse RM: The dawn of Darwinian medicine. Q Rev Biol 66:1–22, 1991

Wilson DR: Evolutionary epidemiology and manic depression. Br J Med Psychol 71:375–395, 1998

Wilson EO: On Human Nature. Cambridge, MA, Harvard University Press, 1978

Wilson M, Daly M: Competitiveness, risk taking, and violence: the young male syndrome. Ethol Sociobiol 6:59–73, 1985

Wolpert L: Malignant Sadness: The Anatomy of Depression. New York, Free Press, 1999

Wortman CB, Silver RC, Kessler RC: The meaning of loss and adjustment to bereavement, in Handbook of Bereavement. Edited by Stroebe MS, Stroebe W, Hansson RO. Cambridge, UK, Cambridge University Press, 1993, pp 349–366

Wrosch C, Scheier MF, Miller GE: Adaptive self-regulation of unattainable goals: goal disengagement, goal reengagement, and subjective well-being. Pers Soc Psychol Bull 29:1494–1508, 2003

Zahavi A, Zahavi A: The Handicap Principle: A Missing Piece of Darwin's Puzzle. New York, Oxford University Press, 1997

PART 3

Investigating Mood Disorders

SECTION EDITOR: HUSSEINI K. MANJI, M.D.

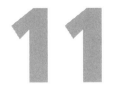

Anatomical Pathology

GRAZYNA RAJKOWSKA, PH.D.

IN VIVO NEUROIMAGING and postmortem morphological and neurochemical studies of the last two decades point to anatomical substrates associated with the neuropathology of mood disorders. Whereas neuroimaging studies have unraveled the gross morphological localization of dysfunctional brain regions in depression, postmortem studies provide further insights into the neurochemical, cellular, and molecular correlates of depression.

New and exciting histopathological studies have been conducted at the microscopic level in recent years. These studies have established that primary mood disorders, long considered to be of neurochemical origin, are also associated with morphological cell abnormalities. Postmortem cell-counting studies in recent years have reported alterations in the density and size of neuronal and glial cells in several distinct frontolimbic brain regions, including prefrontal cortex, orbitofrontal cortex, anterior cingulate cortex, amygdala, and hippocampus, in major depressive disorder (MDD) and bipolar disorder. This is in accord with findings of structural and functional neuroimaging studies showing volumetric and metabolic changes in the same frontolimbic brain regions. Co-localization of cellular changes detected postmortem at the microscopic level with in vivo neuroimaging observations

proves that postmortem studies provide an important interface between clinical and basic research in unraveling neuroanatomical substrates of depression.

The localizations of region-specific and cell type–specific alterations in neuronal and glial architecture reported in mood disorders also coincide with the hypotheses of specific monoaminergic, glutamatergic, and γ-aminobutyric acid (GABA) neurotransmitter system dysfunction in these disorders. Moreover, postmortem studies in depression suggest that although MDD and bipolar illness are clearly not neurodegenerative disorders, these disorders are associated with impaired cellular neuroplasticity and resilience. However, no specific molecular markers that may possibly be related to cell abnormalities observed postmortem have been identified in mood disorders to date.

It remains to be fully elucidated to what extent postmortem histopathological findings represent neurodevelopmental abnormalities, disease progression, or biochemical changes (e.g., in glucocorticoid levels) accompanying repeated depressive episodes. Furthermore, it has yet to be established whether the cellular changes observed postmortem in mood disorders could be reversed by antidepressant and mood-stabilizing medications. Efforts to

---

The work reviewed here was supported by grants from the National Institute of Mental Health (MH60451, MH61578, and MH63187).

identify specific groups of genes that are compromised in depression have recently been undertaken by investigators in the postmortem research field.

Neuronal Pathology

Regional Alterations in Neuronal Density and Size

Cerebral Cortex

Reductions in the neuronal density and size in some populations of cortical neurons have been reported by independent laboratories in both MDD and bipolar disorder. These abnormalities have thus far been described in the heteromodal association cortices, dorsolateral prefrontal cortex, orbitofrontal cortex, and anterior cingulate cortex (Table 11–1) but not in the primary sensory regions or somatosensory (Ongur et al. 1998) or visual cortex (Bouras et al. 2001). Thus, neuronal abnormalities at the microscopic level in mood disorders seem to be specific to frontolimbic cortical regions, and this is in agreement with in vivo neuroimaging observations on volumetric and metabolic alterations in the same cortical regions.

Neuronal abnormalities in mood disorders are not immediately evident given that no significant reduction in the overall density of neurons is detected when the entire population of Nissl-stained neurons is analyzed (Cotter et al. 2002b; Ongur et al. 1998; Rajkowska et al. 2001). Nonetheless, when neurons are analyzed in individual cortical layers or in size-dependent or immunohistochemistry-dependent separate subtypes (Figure 11–1), marked reductions are found in both MDD and bipolar disorder (Table 11–1). For example, reductions in the density of neurons with large cell body size were found in cortical layers II–VI in the dorsolateral prefrontal and rostral orbitofrontal cortex in MDD (Rajkowska et al. 1999). These reductions were accompanied by increases in the density of neurons with smaller sizes (Figure 11–2). Such parallel decreases in the density of large neurons and increases in the density of small neurons indicate that either neuronal shrinkage or a deficient development, rather than neuronal loss, underlies neuronal abnormalities in mood disorders (the "cell loss" issue is further discussed later in this chapter in section "Do Reductions in Cell Density Equal Cell Loss?").

Decreases in laminar neuronal densities also have been reported in the dorsolateral prefrontal cortex (Rajkowska et al. 2001) and anterior cingulate cortex (Benes et al. 2001; Bouras et al. 2001; Cotter et al. 2002a) in bipolar disorder but not by all studies (Cotter et al. 2001; Ongur et al. 1998; see Table 11–1). Moreover, reduced density of pyramidal neurons in cortical layers III and V (Rajkowska et al. 2001) and nonpyramidal neurons in layer II (Benes et al. 2001) has been observed in the same regions. This last observation coincides with reports on reductions in the density of layer II nonpyramidal neurons that are identified with specific antibodies against the calcium-binding protein calbindin in the anterior cingulate cortex (Cotter et al. 2002a) and dorsolateral prefrontal cortex (Reynolds et al. 2000) in bipolar disorder. Calbindin-immunoreactive neurons are known to co-localize GABA. Our recent measurements of the density and size of calbindin-immunoreactive neurons in layer II and the upper part of layer III of the dorsolateral prefrontal cortex showed a 43% reduction in the density of these neurons in MDD as compared with control subjects (Rajkowska et al. 2002). This is in agreement with emerging clinical evidence suggesting that MDD is associated with decreased levels of GABA (Sanacora et al. 2004).

Another manifestation of neuronal pathology in mood disorders is the reduced size of neuronal cell bodies (Figure 11–1F). Smaller soma sizes have been reported in the dorsolateral prefrontal cortex (Cotter et al. 2002b; Rajkowska et al. 1999), orbitofrontal cortex (Rajkowska et al. 1999), and anterior cingulate cortex (Chana et al. 2003; Cotter et al. 2001) in subjects with MDD as compared with control subjects. However, two other studies did not find significant changes in neuronal size in the anterior cingulate cortex (Bouras et al. 2001; Ongur et al. 1998). Interestingly, in the rostral orbitofrontal cortex, there was a trend for a negative correlation between the duration of depression and sizes of neuronal cell bodies (Rajkowska et al. 1999). The longer the duration of illness, the smaller the neurons were, suggesting that the progression of neuronal damage is parallel to the progression of the disease. Subtler than in MDD, reductions in neuronal soma size have been observed in bipolar disorder (Chana et al. 2003; Rajkowska et al. 2001), but not by all investigators (Bouras et al. 2001; Cotter et al. 2001; Ongur et al. 1998). In one other study, a minor increase in the size of small nonpyramidal neurons was noted in the anterior cingulate cortex in subjects with bipolar disorder (Benes et al. 2001).

The cause of reductions in neuronal size is unknown. It is possible to speculate that smaller soma size is related to smaller dendritic trees and/or abnormal morphology of synaptic contacts. However, systematic studies using the Golgi silver impregnation method, which permits visualization of neuronal dendritic trees, have not yet been conducted in cerebral cortex in mood disorders. Two studies of synaptic proteins in the anterior prefrontal cortex (Honer et al. 1999) and anterior cingulate cortex (Eastwood and Harrison 2001) described reductions (Eastwood and Harrison 2001) or no changes (Honer et al. 1999) in synaptic proteins in mood

TABLE 11–1. Morphological abnormalities in the cerebral cortex in mood disorders

Disease (No. of subjects)	Area; hemisphere	Methods	Neurons	Glia	Authors
Prefrontal cortex					
MDD (12)/ CTRL (12)	dlPFC (BA 9); left	Nissl	↓Density of large neurons (20%–60% L II, III, VI) ↑Density of small neurons ↓Size (5% L III, 7% L VI)	↓Density (20%–30% L III, V) ↑Size (6% L IIIa)	Rajkowska et al. 1999
BPD (10)/ CTRL (11)	dlPFC (BA 9); left	Nissl	↓Density of all (19% L III) and pyramidal neurons (17%–30% L III, V)	↓Density (19% L IIIc; 12% L Vb) ↑Size (9% L I, 7% L IIIc)	Rajkowska et al. 2001
MDD (15)/ BPD (15)/ CTRL (15)	dlPFC (BA 9); left+right	Nissl	↓Size (20% L VI) in MDD ↓Size (14% L V, 18% L VI) in BPD	↓Density (30% L V) in MDD =Size in MDD, BPD	Cotter et al. 2002b
MDD (14)/ CTRL (15)	dlPFC (BA 9); left	GFAP IHC	Not examined	↓Area fraction and density (L III–V) in subgroup of young MDD subjects =Area and density in young and old subjects combined	Miguel-Hidalgo et al. 2000
MDD (12)/ CTRL (12)	ORB (BA 10, 47); left ORB (BA 47); left	Nissl	↓Density of large neurons (20%–60% L II–IV) ↑Density of small neurons (L III) ↓Size (9% L II, III) ↓Density (L IIIa, Va) ↓Size (6% L II)	=Density ↓Density (15%–18% L IIIc–VI)	Rajkowska et al. 1999
Anterior cingulate cortex					
MDD (4f)/ BPD (4f)/ CTRL (5f)	Subgenual (BA 24); left+right	Nissl	=Density in MDD, BPD =Number in MDD, BPD =Size in MDD, BPD	↓Number (24% overall) in MDD ↓Number (41% overall) in BPD =Size in MDD, BPD	Ongur et al. 1998
MDD (15)/ BPD (15)/ CTRL (15)	Supragenual (BA 24); left+right	Nissl	↓Size (18% L VI) in MDD =Density in MDD, BPD	↓Density (22% L VI) in MDD =Density in BPD	Cotter et al. 2001

TABLE 11–1.   Morphological abnormalities in the cerebral cortex in mood disorders (continued)

Disease (No. of subjects)	Area; hemisphere	Methods	Neurons	Glia	Authors
MDD (20)/BPD (21)/ CTRL (55)	Supra- and subgenual (BA 24); left	Nissl	↓Density (L III, V, VI) in BPD but not in MDD =Size in MDD, BPD	Not examined	Bouras et al. 2001
BPD (10)/CTRL (12)	Pregenual (BA 24); no hemisphere specified	Nissl	↓Density (27% L II) ↑Size (L II, III) of nonpyramidal neurons	=Density	Benes et al. 2001
MDD (15)/BPD (15)/ CTRL (15)	Supragenual (BA 24); left+right	Nissl	↓Size (9% L V) in MDD and (16% L V) in BPD ↓Neuronal clustering in BPD ↑Density (L V) in MDD and (LVI) in BPD)	↑Size (13% L I, 10% L II) in MDD =Density in MDD, BPD	Chana et al. 2003
MDD (15)/BPD (15)/ CTRL (15)	Supragenual (BA 24); left+right	CB, PV, CR, IHC	↓Density of CB neurons (L II) in BPD ↑Clustering of PV neurons in BPD =Density of CB, PV, CR in MDD	Not examined	Cotter et al. 2002a

Note.   Ant=anterior; BA=Brodmann's area; BPD=bipolar disorder; CB=calbindin; CR=calretinin; CTRL=control; dlPFC=dorsolateral prefrontal cortex; f=familial; GFAP=glial fibrillary acidic protein; IHC=immunohistochemistry; L=layer; MDD=major depressive disorder; ORB=orbitofrontal cortex; PV=paravalbumin; ↓, ↑=significantly different from control; ==not significantly different from control.

disorders. Future systematic studies of dendritic trees, synaptic contacts, and their proteins in prefrontal and cingulate areas are warranted to shed some light on the possible causes of smaller neuronal somata and related synaptic transmission in mood disorders.

Hippocampus

The hippocampus constitutes the major part of the limbic archicortex (phylogenetically older than neocortex and consisting of only three layers). This structure has long been implicated in the structural neuropathology of depression and the response to stress. For example, in vivo neuroimaging studies indicate that major depression is associated with hippocampal atrophy (Bremner et al. 2000; Shah et al. 1998), which correlates with the total duration of depression (Sheline et al. 1999). Surprisingly, there have been very few postmortem studies on the hippocampal formation in mood disorders and until recently no systematic cell-counting studies in MDD in this region.

Two studies conducted on the postmortem hippocampal formation in a small sample of subjects with bipolar disorder reported decreased density and size of nonpy-

ramidal neurons in the CA2 region (Benes et al. 1998) and some disorganization in neuronal clusters in layers II and III of the entorhinal cortex (Beckmann and Jakob 1991; Bernstein et al. 1998a). Examination of apoptotic and cell stress immunocytochemical markers in hippocampal subfields in patients with mood disorders, as compared with nonpsychiatric control subjects and steroid-treated patients, did not detect significant differences between the studied groups (Lucassen et al. 2001).

In the first large study in which neuronal and glial cell packing density and soma size were estimated in the hippocampal subfields in 19 patients with MDD and 21 age-matched control subjects, prominent abnormalities in the CA regions and dentate gyrus were found in the MDD subjects (Stockmeier et al. 2004). Neuronal density in MDD was markedly increased by 30%–40% above the control level, and neuronal cell body size was significantly decreased in the CA1–CA3 subfields and dentate gyrus. An increase in packing density paralleled by smaller cell sizes in MDD suggests a decrease in neuropil, consisting of neuronal and glial processes and their synapses. This reduced neuropil hypothesis is consistent with findings from other

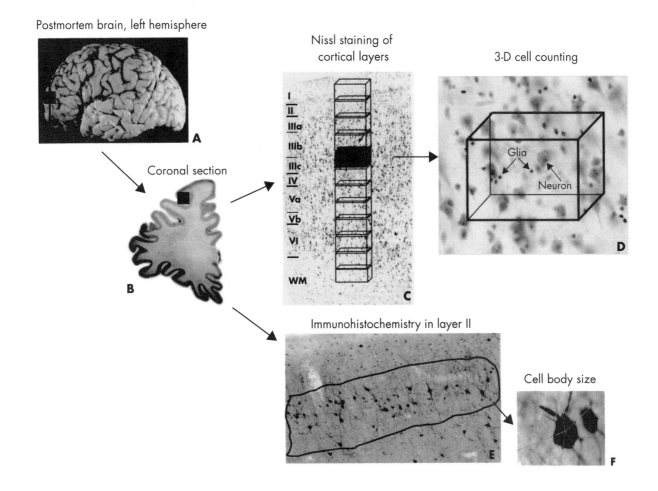

Postmortem brain, left hemisphere

A

Coronal section

B

Nissl staining of
cortical layers

C

3-D cell counting

Glia

Neuron

D

Immunohistochemistry in layer II

E

Cell body size

F

FIGURE 11–1. **Steps involved in methods used for the estimation of cell density, total cell number, and cell body size in human postmortem tissue.**

Left cerebral hemisphere **(A)** is removed at the autopsy, fixed in formalin, embedded in celloidin, and cut into 40-μm coronal sections **(B)**. Sections are stained in a given brain region (*black square, dorsolateral prefrontal cortex*) for Nissl's staining method to visualize neuronal and glial cell bodies. The packing density of cells is calculated in a stack of optically defined three-dimensional counting boxes spanning the six cortical layers **(C)**. In each counting box, the number of neuronal or glial cells is counted, under high magnification, within an optically defined volume of tissue to determine the density of specific cell types (neurons or glia) **(D)**. Additional sections adjacent to the Nissl-stained sections are immunostained with a specific antibody (in this case, against a calbindin D-28 protein) to estimate a total cell number of immunoreactive neurons in a defined cortical layer (marked by contour on **E**) with a systematic random sampling with three-dimensional counting boxes. Cell body size is estimated with a Stereological Nucleator Probe (Stereo Investigator-MicroBrightField, Inc, Williston, Vermont, USA) by marking a point at the center of the cell, extending a set of five rays from that point, and marking the intersection of the rays and the boundary of the cell **(F)**.

Source. Reprinted from Rajkowska G: "Depression: What We Can Learn From Postmortem Studies." *The Neuroscientist* 9(4):273–284, 2003. Copyright © 2003 by Sage Publications. Reprinted by permission of Sage Publications.

postmortem studies that indicated decreased dendritic length and spine density on subicular neurons (Rosoklija et al. 2000) and a decreased expression of synaptic proteins in several hippocampal regions in subjects with mood disorder (Eastwood and Harrison 2000; Webster et al. 2001). Taken together, changes in cell packing density, neuronal size, and interneuronal neuropil detected postmortem may

be the basis of decreased hippocampal volume noted by some in vivo neuroimaging studies in MDD.

The different pattern of neuronal pathology in the frontal cortex (decrease in density) and hippocampus (increase in density) suggests unique involvement of these brain regions in the neuropathology of depression. One possible rationale for varied neuronal pathology in frontal cortex compared

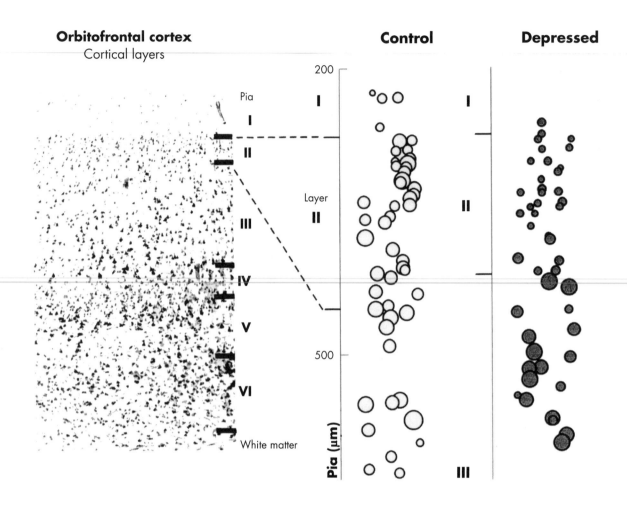

FIGURE 11–2. **Changes in neuronal size and size-dependent density in layer II of rostral orbitofrontal cortex in a subject with major depression as compared with a matched healthy control subject (Caucasian women, 73 and 71 years old, respectively; postmortem delay <17 hours; fixation time <10 months).**
Photomicrograph of the cell composition across the six cortical layers in rostral orbitofrontal cortex (*upper left*). Expanded printouts of cortical layers with neuronal cell bodies represented by equivalent-diameter circles with the area measured for the individual neuron in its equatorial plane (*right panel*). Note that in the depressed subject, neuronal sizes are smaller in layers II and III than in the control subject. Note especially dramatic increases in the density of small neurons in layer II associated with significant reductions in the density of the largest neurons of this layer.
Source.   Reprinted from Rajkowska G, Miguel-Hidalgo JJ, Wei J, et al: "Morphometric Evidence for Neuronal and Glial Prefrontal Cell Pathology in Major Depression," *Biological Psychiatry* 45:1085–1098, 1999, copyright 1999, with permission from Society of Biological Psychiatry.

with hippocampus might be the differential development of neuronal circuits in these structures (Super et al. 1998) and their involvement in cognitive dysfunction in MDD.

Subcortical Structures

The search for morphological abnormalities in subcortical structures from postmortem brains of patients with mood disorders has not been as intense as that in cortical regions.

Only a few postmortem studies have attempted to estimate the number of neurons in subcortical structures such as the hypothalamus, dorsal raphe, locus coeruleus, and amygdala, and most of these studies were conducted on a very small sample size. Results of these subcortical histopathological studies were somewhat inconsistent. Increases, decreases, or no change in the cell number or density were reported by different authors in the hypothalamus and brain stem nuclei in depressed subjects.

Stereological investigation of specific types of hypothalamic neurons found increased numbers of arginine-vasopressin (AVP)–immunoreactive neurons, oxytocin-expressing neurons, and corticotropin-releasing hormone (CRH) neurons in the paraventricular nucleus in patients with bipolar disorder and MDD, compared with control subjects without mood disorders (Purba et al. 1996; Raadsheer et al. 1994). Moreover, increases in CRH–messenger ribonucleic acid (mRNA) and in the number of CRH neurons co-localizing AVP also were found in depressed patients (Raadsheer et al. 1995; Swaab et al. 1993). These findings of increases in specific immunoreactive neurons are consistent with the evidence of activation of the hypothalamic-pituitary-adrenal (HPA) axis in some subsets of depressed patients (Holsboer et al. 1992). In contrast, a prominent reduction in the total number of Nissl-stained neurons was reported in the paraventricular hypothalamic nucleus in a mixed group of subjects with MDD and bipolar disorder (Manaye et al. 2005). Decreased number and density of nitric oxide synthase–containing neurons were also described in the paraventricular hypothalamic nucleus in a small group of subjects with MDD and bipolar disorder (Bernstein et al. 1998b).

Subtle structural abnormalities in the monoaminergic brain stem nuclei, which are the major source of serotonergic (dorsal raphe), noradrenergic (locus coeruleus), and dopaminergic (amygdala) projections to the cerebral cortex, have been reported in mood disorders, but not by all studies. Increased number and density of immunopositive serotonergic neurons were observed in the dorsal raphe of suicide victims with MDD as compared with control subjects (Underwood et al. 1999). In contrast, a decrease in the number of tyrosine hydroxylase–immunoreactive neurons was reported in the locus coeruleus of depressed subjects not dying by suicide; however, no difference in the number of these neurons was found when all depressed subjects were compared with control subjects (Baumann et al. 1999). Likewise, another morphometric study, which had a larger sample size, found no differences in the number of pigmented neurons between MDD and control subjects at several anatomical levels of locus coeruleus (Klimek et al. 1997). No changes in the neuronal densities were detected in amygdala in patients with either MDD or bipolar disorder as compared with control subjects without mood disorders (Bowley et al. 2002).

Together, these postmortem findings suggest that some rearrangement in the morphology of hypothalamic and brain stem neurons projecting to the cerebral cortex may take place in mood disorders. However, further stereological studies with a larger number of subjects are required to determine the exact pathology of hypothalamic neurons in depression and whether locus coeruleus

changes are specific to bipolar disorder and whether changes in dorsal raphe are specific to MDD and suicide.

Implication for Pathology of Neural Circuits

Morphological abnormalities detected postmortem in mood disorders are most likely related to dysfunction of neural circuits regulating emotional, cognitive, and somatic symptoms in depressed and bipolar patients. In fact, alterations in neuronal density and size have been found in the dorsolateral prefrontal, orbitofrontal, and anterior cingulate cortex, neurons of which give rise to the frontal circuits critical for higher cognitive and limbic functioning (Alexander et al. 1990). Subtle neuronal alterations are also reported in the main limbic regions, hypothalamus, and hippocampus, providing further support for the dysfunction of limbic circuits in depression.

Monoaminergic Circuits

Some of the cellular abnormalities detected postmortem in cortical and subcortical structures from patients with MDD and bipolar disorder could be related to the disruption of monoaminergic transmission reported in depression. Neurochemical postmortem studies report alterations in serotonin and norepinephrine receptors and transporters in the dorsolateral prefrontal cortex and ventrolateral or orbitofrontal cortex in brains from suicide victims with or without clinical depression (reviewed in Stockmeier and Jurjus 2002). Abnormal cell density and size are found in these same cortical regions in postmortem cell-counting studies. For example, cellular changes found in superficial layers of the prefrontal cortex in MDD may be related to alterations in serotonin type 1A ($5\text{-}HT_{1A}$) receptors that are present in significant numbers in these layers (Arango et al. 1995). Recent reexamination of $5\text{-}HT_{1A}$ receptors with agonist versus antagonist radioligands in the cortical layers of the orbitofrontal cortex in patients with MDD and matched nonpsychiatric control subjects found a significant decrease in only antagonist binding to $5\text{-}HT_{1A}$ receptors specifically in layer II in MDD (C.A. Stockmeier, G. Rajkowska, unpublished observation, July 2004). This preliminary postmortem observation coincides with findings in a neuroimaging study by Sargent et al. (2000). The authors found that the binding to $5\text{-}HT_{1A}$ receptors was decreased in nonmedicated patients with MDD across several cortical regions, including medial temporal cortex, temporal pole, orbitofrontal cortex, anterior cingulate cortex, insula, and dorsolateral prefrontal cortex. Expression of another component of serotonin neurotransmission, the serotonin transporter, also was decreased in the dorsolateral prefrontal and ventral or orbitofrontal cortex in postmortem brains from depressed suicide victims (Austin et al. 2002; Mann et al. 2000).

Detailed laminar analysis of the density of serotonin transporter–immunoreactive axons showed that this deficit was localized in cortical layer VI of the dorsolateral prefrontal cortex (Austin et al. 2002). This serotonin transporter deficit may be related to the pathology of layer VI neurons reported in the same cortical layer by postmortem cell-counting studies in depression (Table 11–1).

Moreover, subtle neuronal abnormalities in the monoaminergic brain stem nuclei reported by some studies suggest dysfunction of monoaminergic projections originating from the brain stem neurons and terminating in frontolimbic cortical regions. The functions and morphology of cortical neurons are probably affected by alterations in the functional state of noradrenergic, serotonergic, and dopaminergic neurons that project axons to prefrontal and anterior cingulate cortex. Postmortem neurochemical studies report alterations in noradrenergic receptors and transporters in the locus coeruleus (Klimek et al. 1997; Ordway et al. 1994; Zhu et al. 1999), serotonin receptors in the dorsal raphe (Stockmeier et al. 1998), and dopaminergic receptors and transporters in the amygdala (Klimek et al. 2002) in MDD.

Glutamatergic and GABAergic Circuits

Layer-specific changes in neuronal density and size, found in mood disorders, imply that reductions in both inhibitory local circuit neurons and excitatory projection types of cortical neurons could be involved in the neuropathology of mood disorders. Nonpyramidal GABAergic inhibitory neurons are localized mainly in layer II and establish local (within the frontal lobe) corticocortical connections. In contrast, pyramidal glutamatergic excitatory neurons reside predominantly in cortical layers III, V, and VI and give rise to long projections to other cortical association regions (layer III), striatum (layer V), and thalamus (layer VI).

Neuronal pathology detected in cortical layers III, V, and VI of the dorsolateral prefrontal cortex and anterior cingulate cortex in MDD (Table 11–1) may be associated with the pathology of excitatory pyramidal neurons that use glutamate as their neurotransmitter because these cells are most abundant in these cortical laminae. Moreover, the density of pyramidal neurons was selectively reduced in the dorsolateral prefrontal cortex in subjects with bipolar disorder (Rajkowska et al. 2001), further confirming the pathology of glutamatergic neurons. This coincides with reports of altered levels of glutamate in depression (Auer et al. 2000; Sanacora et al. 2004) and with

emerging evidence from postmortem studies on alterations in glutamate signaling in MDD. A study of suicide victims, some of whom were diagnosed with MDD, indicated alterations in the radioligand binding to gluamate N-methyl-D-aspartate (NMDA) receptor regulatory site in the anterior prefrontal cortex (Nowak et al. 1995). Recently, abnormally high amounts of 2C subunit of NMDA receptor have been observed in the locus coeruleus of depressed subjects (Karolewicz et al. 2005). Moreover, agents that reduce glutamatergic activity or glutamate receptor–related signal transduction may also have antidepressant effects (Berman et al. 2000; Harkin et al. 1999; Papp and Moryl 1994).

Reductions in size and density of layer II neurons in the orbitofrontal and dorsolateral prefrontal cortex and reductions in nonpyramidal neuronal density in layer II of the anterior cingulate cortex (Table 11–1) suggest deficient GABAergic neurotransmission. Most nonpyramidal neurons in cortical layer II are known to co-localize GABA, and recent clinical evidence suggests that MDD is associated with decreased levels of GABA (Sanacora et al. 2004).

In summary, localization of morphological abnormalities in mood disorders is consistent with dysfunction of prefrontolimbic circuits regulating emotional, cognitive, and somatic symptoms of depression. Layer-specific neuronal pathology further supports the involvement of monoaminergic, glutamatergic, and GABAergic neurotransmitter systems in this pathology (see Delgado and Moreno, Chapter 6, in this volume). It remains to be determined whether this structural pathology is the reason for or consequence of neurotransmitter dysfunction in depression.

Glial Pathology

Regional Alterations in Glial Number, Density, and Size

Unforeseen, but prominent, reductions in the density and number of glial cells have, to date, been the most consistent cell abnormality described in mood disorders. Glial cell reductions have been reported consistently by independent laboratories in the anterior cingulate cortex, dorsolateral prefrontal cortex, and orbitofrontal cortex in MDD and bipolar disorder subjects (Table 11–1). For example, a 24%–41% reduction in the number of general population of Nissl-stained glial cells was found in the subgenual region of the anterior cingulate cortex (ventral part of Brodmann area 24) in a small subgroup of patients with familial MDD and familial bipolar disorder, as compared with control subjects (Ongur et al. 1998). However, when familial and unfamilial subgroups of patients were combined, the reductions were not found. The estimation of glial cell number in this study was combined across all six cortical layers. Thus, no information on laminar specificity of glial loss was provided.

In contrast, in four other studies, reductions in glial cell density were reported in specific cortical layers of the anterior cingulate cortex and prefrontal cortex. These reductions were observed in layer VI of the supragenual anterior cingulate cortex (Cotter et al. 2001); layers III and V of the dorsolateral prefrontal cortex (Cotter et al. 2002b; Rajkowska et al. 1999, 2001); and layers III, IV, V, and VI of the caudal orbitofrontal cortex (Rajkowska et al. 1999) in patients with mood disorders.

Glial cell size and shape, in addition to density, appear to be affected in mood disorders. Size of glial cell bodies (corresponding to glial cell nuclei in Nissl-stained material) was estimated in five different studies. In three of these investigations, glial size was increased, whereas two other studies found that glial size was unchanged in MDD or bipolar disorder (Table 11–1). Significant increases in glial size were observed in the dorsolateral prefrontal cortex in bipolar disorder (Rajkowska et al. 2001) and to a smaller degree in MDD subjects (Rajkowska et al. 1999), as compared with control subjects. More recently, similar increases were noted in the anterior cingulate cortex in subjects with MDD (Chana et al. 2003). Furthermore, in the dorsolateral prefrontal cortex in bipolar disorder, the shape of glial nuclei changed to a less rounded conformation (Rajkowska et al. 2001). Reductions in glial density paralleled by an increase in the size of glial nuclei suggest that some compensatory mechanisms might take place. It could be speculated that decreased density of glial cells is indicative of a decrease in the number of normally functioning glial cells. At the same time, glial cells that survive and are not damaged might be forced to work harder to support the metabolic needs of the surrounding neurons. As a consequence, the nuclei of these glial cells are enlarged in size and changed in shape. Glutamate-induced swelling of astroglia reported in animal cell cultures (Hansson et al. 2000) also could account for enlarged glial cells in depression.

Evidence is accumulating to suggest that glial pathology extends beyond the frontal cortex to the hippocampus. A recent study of the hippocampus in 40 major depressive and age-matched control subjects reported marked increases in glial cell density and unchanged sizes of glial nuclei in all hippocampal CA subfields and the granule cell layer of the dentate gyrus (Stockmeier et al. 2004). Increases in glial cell packing density detected postmortem in MDD are suggestive of reduction in sur-

rounding neuropil and may be related to decreases in hippocampal volume noted by neuroimaging studies in MDD (see "Hippocampus" subsection in the "Neuronal Pathology" section earlier in this chapter).

Glial cell pathology in mood disorders may not be universally noted throughout the cerebral cortex. Changes in glial cell density or number were not found in the sensorimotor cortex in either MDD or bipolar disorder populations (Ongur et al. 1998). Recent reports suggest a lack of marked glial pathology in the supragenual part of the anterior cingulate cortex (Chana et al. 2003) and the entorhinal cortex in bipolar disorder and MDD (Bowley et al. 2002), as well as in the most rostral part of the orbitofrontal cortex corresponding to the transitional cortex between Brodmann areas 10 and 47 in subjects with MDD (Rajkowska et al. 1999).

Glial pathology in mood disorders has not been systematically studied in subcortical structures to date. Only one recent report suggested that glial pathology might extend to limbic subcortical regions because a significant reduction in glial number has been found in the amygdala in patients with MDD and unmedicated bipolar subjects (Bowley et al. 2002).

Glial Cell Type Affected in Depression: Implication for Glial Dysfunction

The glial cells analyzed in the above-mentioned studies do not represent a homogeneous population. They are composed of distinct populations of oligodendrocytes, microglia, and astrocytes. The crucial role of glial cell types in brain function is currently being reevaluated. In addition to their traditional roles in neuronal migration (radial glial), myelin formation (oligodendrocytes), and inflammatory processes (astrocytes and microglia), glia (predominantly astrocytes) are now accepted to have roles in providing trophic support to neurons, neuronal metabolism, and the formation of synapses and neurotransmission (reviewed in Cotter et al. 2002c).

Glial Cell Types in Depression

The three distinct glial cell types cannot be identified in any of the previously mentioned studies because those tissues were stained for Nissl substance and such staining does not distinguish reliably between specific glial cell types. Nissl's staining method shows only morphological features of glial cell bodies and not glial cell processes. However, recent immunohistochemical examination of an astroglial marker, glial fibrillary acidic protein (GFAP), in the dorsolateral prefrontal cortex suggested the involvement of astrocytes in overall glial pathology in

MDD (Miguel-Hidalgo et al. 2000). Although no significant group differences in GFAP-reactive astrocytes' cell packing density were present in this study, when the entire group of MDD (young and old) was compared with control subjects without MDD, a significant correlation was seen between age and GFAP immunoreactivity among subjects with MDD. Significant reductions in the population of reactive astroglia were found in a small subgroup of young (30–45 years old) MDD subjects as compared with young control subjects and older (46–86 years old) MDD subjects (Figure 11–3A, 11–3B). This subgroup of young adults with MDD also had a shorter duration of depression, and most of these subjects were suicide victims. Recent observation from our laboratory further confirms that the levels of GFAP protein are also reduced in these young adults with MDD as compared with age-matched control subjects (Figure 11–3C, 11–3D) and that GFAP levels are positively correlated with age at the time of death and age at onset of depression (Si et al. 2004). This last observation implies that the involvement of GFAP expression in early- versus late-life depression differs because the underlying pathophysiology in early-life depression is different from that in late-life depression. Increasing clinical evidence confirms that late-onset depression (first depressive episode after age 50 years) differs from early-onset depression by its etiology, phenomenology, and cerebrovascular pathology (Heun et al. 2000; Krishnan et al. 1995; Lavretsky et al. 1998).

Alterations in GFAP in both bipolar disorder and MDD were also suggested by a recent proteomic study in which different forms of GFAP proteins had disease-specific abnormalities (Johnston-Wilson et al. 2000). Another type of glial cell, oligodendroglia, also may be involved in the general glial pathology because reduced density and immunoreactivity and ultrastructural changes in oligodendrocytes were found in the dorsolateral prefrontal and anterior frontal cortex in subjects with bipolar disorder and MDD (Uranova et al. 2001, 2004). Moreover, a reduction of key oligodendrocyte-related and myelin-related gene expression was recently reported in the dorsolateral prefrontal cortex in bipolar disorder (Tkachev et al. 2003).

Although these results are intriguing, further immunohistochemical and molecular studies are needed to definitively determine which specific glial cell types are compromised in bipolar disorder and whether the same or different glial cell types are involved in the pathology reported in MDD.

Functional Significance of Glial Pathology

Reductions in glial number and density, in addition to changes in their size and shape, might be related to the dysfunction of monoaminergic and glutamatergic systems reported extensively in depression. For example, astrocytes express virtually all of the receptor systems and ion channels found in neurons, including transporter systems that regulate both the concentration of neurotransmitters at synapses and the availability of neurotransmitters for release (reviewed in Cotter et al. 2002c). Thus, glia may play a role in serotonin, norepinephrine, or dopamine neurotransmission via postsynaptic monoaminergic receptors distributed on glial cell bodies and processes. Moreover, astroglia are the primary sites of glutamate uptake by glial transporters and are important in regulating NMDA receptor activity. Astroglia regulate the levels of extracellular glutamate and have been shown in vitro to protect neurons from cell death and to provide the energy requirement for neurons. Astrocytic pathology in MDD may indirectly promote glutamate-mediated neuronal excitotoxicity, with consequences that can be detected by functional neuroimaging.

Do Reductions in Cell Density Equal Cell Loss?

Postmortem studies cannot yet clearly define whether a true loss of cells underlies prominent reductions in cell density and size detected in mood disorders. For the estimation of a total number of neurons or glia in a particular brain region, it is essential that the total volume of a studied area be calculated. To do this, the exact borders of the studied region must be established (Rajkowska and Goldman-Rakic 1995; Uylings et al. 2000) so that sampling is confined to the region within these borders. Unfortunately, in most postmortem studies on mood disorders, the true estimation of the total cell number and, consequently, the estimation of whether a cell loss occurs in depression are not possible because of technical restrictions. Limitations in tissue availability or in reliable distinction of cytoarchitectonic borders of a studied region have made the estimation of a total volume and total cell number impossible. In one study in which the total cell number was estimated in the subgenual cortex, a loss of glial but not neuronal cells was found in familial mood disorders (Ongur et al. 1998). Glial reductions reported in this study may in fact reflect a true loss of glial cells because the neuroimaging studies in the same cortical region show reduction in gray matter volume (Drevets et al. 1997).

Future studies in which a total volume of individual brain regions is estimated, and consequently the total cell number is calculated, will establish whether cell loss, in

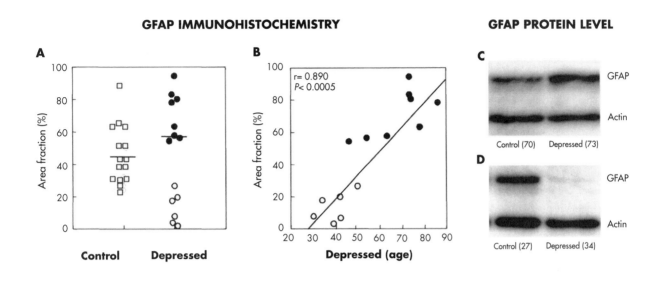

FIGURE 11–3. Pathology of glial cells found in the dorsolateral prefrontal cortex in postmortem studies on major depressive disorder

Reductions in the glial fibrillary acidic protein (GFAP)-immunoreactive astroglia were found in a subgroup of young adults with major depression as compared with age-matched control subjects and older subjects with major depression **(A),** and these reductions were correlated with age of subjects at the time of death **(B).** Recent observations from our laboratory (Si et al. 2004) indicate that the levels of GFAP in the same area of the dorsolateral prefrontal cortex are also reduced in these young **(D)** but not old **(C)** subjects with major depression as compared with age-matched control subjects. Note that the level of another protein, actin, is unchanged in a depressed subject as compared with the control subject, indicating the specificity of GFAP pathology.

Source. Miguel-Hidalgo et al. 2000; Rajkowska et al. 1999. Parts A and B reprinted from Miguel-Hidalgo JJ, Baucom C, Dilley G, et al: "Glial Fibrillary Acidic Protein Immunoreactivity in the Prefrontal Cortex Distinguishes Younger From Older Adults in Major Depressive Disorder," *Biological Psychiatry* 48:861–873, 2000, copyright 2000, with permission from Society of Biological Psychiatry.

addition to alterations in cell density and size, underlies the neuropathology of mood disorders.

Potential Confounding Variables and Medication Effect

The alterations in cell density and size in mood disorders are likely to be related to the disorder itself and not to the age of subjects at the time of death, postmortem delay, or the time of tissue fixation. Statistical analyses conducted in all of the morphometric studies mentioned earlier yielded no significant correlation between cell density or size and any of these confounding variables. It cannot be ruled out, however, that some of the cellular alterations in mood disorders are related to prior treatment with antidepressants and lithium (for further discussion, see Miguel-Hidalgo and Rajkowska 2002).

Whether cell abnormalities can be attributed to the effect of therapeutic medications remains open to debate. No systematic studies have been done on the effect of antidepressants and mood stabilizers on cell number and morphology in the postmortem human brain, most likely because of the insufficient number of treated compared with untreated subjects. However, molecular studies in human cell cultures and in the in vivo animal brain suggest that these medications have significant effects on the regulation of specific gene expression in the central nervous system. For example, both the second-messenger system (e.g., cyclic adenosine monophosphate [cAMP] cascade) and neurotrophins (e.g., brain-derived neurotrophic factor [BDNF]) are reported to be upregulated by antidepressants (Duman et al. 2000) and mood stabilizers (reviewed in Chang et al. 2002; Manji et al. 2001). Therefore, abnormalities in cell signaling pathways may be critical to the pathophysiology and treatment of depression (Coyle and Duman 2003) (see also Singh et al., Chapter 12, in this volume). Not surprisingly, several laboratories have undertaken studies on postmortem tissues to determine whether any abnormalities exist in these pathways in depression and, if so, whether the abnormalities are related to the therapeutic medication treatment. Some of these studies reported changes at multiple sites of the cAMP pathway in the cerebral cortex in patients with mood disorders (Chang et al. 2002; Dowlatshahi et al. 1999). Hippocampal BDNF immunoreactivity increased in subjects given antidepressant medications at time of death, compared with antidepressant-untreated subjects (B. Chen et al. 2001). In another postmortem study, significant reductions in mRNA and protein levels of BDNF and its tyrosine kinase B receptor were found in the dorsolateral prefrontal cortex and hippocampus in brains of suicide victims, nearly half of whom had a diagnosis of major depression. However, in this study, the comparison of suicide subjects who were taking antidepressants with those who were not receiving treatment showed no significant differences in levels of BDNF or tyrosine kinase B receptors. Although these studies are encouraging, more work is needed with a larger sample of antidepressant-treated and medication-free subjects.

A mounting body of data suggests that treatment with antidepressants or mood stabilizers not only regulates neuronal survival but also influences neurogenesis. Pharmacologically induced increases in neurogenesis in adult rodent brain have been reported recently by two independent studies (G. Chen et al. 2000; Malberg et al. 2000). Moreover, evidence indicates that treatment with lithium induces increases in the astrocytic protein GFAP in rodent hippocampus (Rocha and Rodnight 1994; Rocha et al. 1998) and the neural lobe of the pituitary (Levine et al. 2000). However, whether these increases represent a protective or compensatory effect of these medications and the mechanisms underlying the regulation of neurogenesis and glial proliferation must be further investigated. Furthermore, a precise link between cell loss and atrophy, observed in the postmortem human brain, and medication-induced production of new cells, observed in the animal brain, has yet to be established.

How Specific Are Cell Abnormalities in Depression?

Reductions in cell density, similar to those found in frontolimbic cortex in mood disorders, have been reported recently in alcohol dependence. Postmortem investigation of the dorsolateral prefrontal cortex in brains from patients with uncomplicated alcoholism found an overall pattern of glial pathology similar to that observed in depression (Miguel-Hidalgo et al. 2002). Prominent

reductions in the density of the general (Nissl-stained) population of glial cells and the density of immunospecific astroglia were found in prefrontal layers V and VI in a subgroup of alcoholic patients with depressed symptoms and to a lesser degree in alcoholic patients without depression. Glial changes in alcoholic patients with depressed symptoms were even more prominent and spread across more cortical layers than those changes in subjects with MDD who did not have alcohol addiction. The only difference in glial pathology between alcoholism and depression was opposite changes in glial nucleus size (reduction in alcoholism and increase in depression) (Miguel-Hidalgo and Rajkowska 2003).

Reduced glial nuclear size and cell density in alcoholism might be related to the cytotoxic effects of prolonged alcohol exposure; however, in MDD without alcohol abuse, other processes (e.g., stress-induced glucocorticoid neurotoxicity) might be responsible for the increase in the average size of glial nuclei and reduced cell packing density. In either case, abnormal function related to glial reduction seems to be associated with depressive symptoms. The association between alcoholism and major depression has been reevaluated recently, and prior alcohol dependence increases the risk for current MDD more than fourfold (Hasin and Grant 2002). Future molecular and genetic studies will establish whether individuals with alcohol dependence and those with depression share genetic loci for specific brain pathology.

Some reductions in glial density and atrophic changes in neurons are also reported in frontal cortical regions of postmortem brains from schizophrenic patients (reviewed in Cotter et al. 2002c and Selemon 2001). However, these changes in schizophrenia seem to be more restricted to a specific cortical region or cortical layer, and increases rather than decreases in cell densities are found in some prefrontal regions (Selemon et al. 1995, 1998).

It is interesting that the abnormalities in glial cell density found in the cerebral cortex in mood disorders (reductions) are in opposition to those described in neurological neurodegenerative disorders (increases), such as Huntington's disease and Alzheimer's disease. This suggests that depression is not characterized by classic neurodegenerative pathology, at least in younger subjects with MDD, because glial proliferation associated with degeneration and loss of neurons is not observed in young and middle-aged subjects with MDD. It cannot, however, be ignored that some neurodegeneration happens in depressed patients later in life as the disease progresses. Findings from immunohistochemical studies in which GFAP-immunoreactive astrocytes and levels of GFAP were increased in older patients with MDD as opposed to the younger patients support this hypothesis.

Cellular Abnormalities Correspond to In Vivo Neuroimaging Findings

Cellular abnormalities in mood disorders reviewed here have been observed consistently in the dorsolateral prefrontal cortex, anterior cingulate cortex, orbitofrontal cortex, hippocampus, and amygdala (Figure 11–4). In these same brain regions, neuroimaging studies report volumetric, metabolic, and neurochemical alterations in patients with mood disorders.

Structural neuroimaging studies in mood disorders provide evidence of modest but intriguing volumetric changes suggestive of cell loss and/or atrophy (reviewed in Soares and Mann 1997) (see also Singh et al., Chapter 12, and Mayberg, Chapter 13, in this volume). Some, but not all, studies report enlargement of the lateral and third ventricles (Elkis et al. 1995), which may be indicative of atrophy of surrounding cortical and subcortical regions.

Functional neuroimaging studies lend further support to physiological abnormalities in cortical and subcortical frontolimbic regions in MDD and bipolar disorder. Dysregulation of glucose metabolism, regional cerebral blood flow, and high-energy phosphate metabolism has been observed in the prefrontal and temporal cortex, basal ganglia, and amygdala in mood disorders (reviewed in Drevets 2000) (see also Mayberg, Chapter 13, this volume). Neuroimaging studies that examined neurochemical changes in the living brain provided further support for the hypothesis that mood disorders are associated with changes in cell viability and function. For example, recent studies that used high-resolution magnetic resonance spectroscopy in unmedicated patients with bipolar disorder reported decreased *N*-acetylaspartate (NAA) levels bilaterally in the hippocampus (Bertolino et al. 1999) and in the dorsolateral prefrontal cortex (Winsberg et al. 2000) as compared with healthy control subjects. In contrast, therapeutic doses of lithium increase levels of NAA in the brain of bipolar patients (Moore et al. 2000). These increases occur in several regions, including frontal cortex, and are localized almost exclusively to gray matter. NAA is regarded as a measure of neuronal viability and function; therefore, the changes in NAA levels seen in bipolar disorder strongly implicate alterations in neuronal viability, which, itself, may be related to alterations in cell number, density, and size and related volumetric changes. Interestingly, a recent magnetic resonance spectroscopic study of nonhuman primates exposed to early life stressors also indicated significant decreases in NAA as well as increases in glutamate-glutamine-GABA metabolites (changes observed 10 years later) in the adult anterior cin-gulate cortex of these animals. These NAA measures reflect neuronal integrity and metabolism, whereas changes in glutamate-glutamine-GABA metabolites may be a reflection of changes in membrane structure, glial functions, and glutamate content. Together, the above data suggest that structural and metabolic alterations observed in vivo may be related to alterations in cell viability, which, itself, may be related to alterations in cell number, density, and size observed in postmortem tissues at the microscopic level.

Conclusion: Strengths and Limitations of Human Postmortem Studies

The studies reviewed here undeniably prove the usefulness of postmortem tissue in unraveling the microanatomical substrate of depression. Postmortem cell-counting studies in mood disorders have established for the first time that MDD and bipolar illness are brain diseases with unique pathological features of neuronal and glial cells.

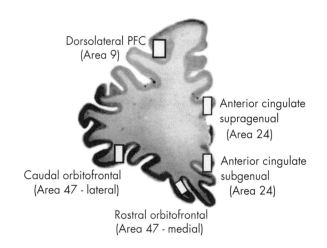

Dorsolateral PFC
(Area 9)

Anterior cingulate
supragenual
(Area 24)

Anterior cingulate
subgenual
(Area 24)

Caudal orbitofrontal
(Area 47 - lateral)

Rostral orbitofrontal
(Area 47 - medial)

FIGURE 11–4. **Localization of cortical brain regions where cell pathology (reductions in glial and/or neuronal density and soma size) is reported by postmortem morphometric studies.**

PFC=prefrontal cortex.
Source. Reprinted from Rajkowska G: "Cell Pathology in Mood Disorders." *Seminars in Clinical Neuropsychiatry* 7:281–292, 2002. Used with permission.

The precise region-specific and layer-specific alterations in neuronal and glial architecture observed in mood disorders are consistent with the hypotheses of specific monoaminergic, glutamatergic, and GABA neurotransmitter system dysfunction in these disorders. Moreover, co-localization of cellular changes detected in postmortem tissues with in vivo neuroimaging proves that postmortem studies provide an important interface between clinical and basic research in unraveling neuroanatomical substrates of depression. Both postmortem and neuroimaging studies have found changes in the same frontolimbic brain regions.

Postmortem studies in depression also indicate that MDD and bipolar disorder are clearly not neurodegenerative disorders but are associated with impaired cellular neuroplasticity and resilience. It remains to be fully elucidated to what extent these findings represent neurodevelopmental abnormalities, disease progression, biochemical changes (in levels of glucocorticoid or trophic factors) accompanying repeated affective episodes, or the results of treatment with therapeutic medications. Furthermore, it has yet to be established whether the cellular changes observed postmortem in mood disorders can be reversed by antidepressant and mood-stabilizing medications. Finally, molecular and genetic mechanisms associated with depression are yet to be unraveled. Preliminary findings from ongoing studies on gene expression in postmortem brain tissues from patients with mood disorder in which microarray technology is being used confirm that the dorsolateral prefrontal and anterior cingulate cortex are the sites of pathology in mood disorders (Evans et al. 2002; Tomita et al. 2003).

Postmortem studies also have some limitations. The small sample size, insufficient tissue or inadequate expertise in cytoarchitectonic delineation of individual brain regions, incomplete medical history, and lack of details on medication treatment are among some of the caveats of postmortem studies in depression. Ideally, longitudinal clinical studies in well-characterized patients should be linked to subsequent postmortem studies in depression, and recently a few laboratories have undertaken such efforts.

References

Alexander GE, Crutcher MD, DeLong MR: Basal ganglia-thalamocortical circuits: parallel substrates for motor, oculomotor, "prefrontal" and "limbic" functions. Prog Brain Res 85:119–146, 1990

Arango V, Underwood MD, Gubbi AV, et al: Localized alterations in pre- and postsynaptic serotonin binding sites in the ventrolateral prefrontal cortex of suicide victims. Brain Res 688:121–133, 1995

Auer DP, Putz B, Kraft E, et al: Reduced glutamate in the anterior cingulate cortex in depression: an in vivo proton magnetic resonance spectroscopy study. Biol Psychiatry 47:305–313, 2000

Austin MC, Whitehead RE, Edgar CL, et al: Localized decrease in serotonin transporter-immunoreactive axons in the prefrontal cortex of depressed subjects committing suicide. Neuroscience 114:807–815, 2002

Baumann B, Danos P, Diekmann S, et al: Tyrosine hydroxylase immunoreactivity in the locus coeruleus is reduced in depressed non-suicidal patients but normal in depressed suicide patients. Eur Arch Psychiatry Clin Neurosci 249:212–2199, 1999

Beckmann H, Jakob H: Prenatal disturbances of nerve cell migration in the entorhinal region: a common vulnerability factor in functional psychoses? J Neural Transm Gen Sect 84:155–164, 1991

Benes FM, Kwok EW, Vincent SL, et al: A reduction of nonpyramidal cells in sector CA2 of schizophrenics and manic depressives. Biol Psychiatry 44:88–97, 1998

Benes FM, Vincent SL, Todtenkopf M: The density of pyramidal and nonpyramidal neurons in anterior cingulate cortex of schizophrenic and bipolar subjects. Biol Psychiatry 50:395–406, 2001

Berman RM, Cappiello A, Anand A, et al: Antidepressant effects of ketamine in depressed patients. Biol Psychiatry 47:351–354, 2000

Bernstein HG, Krell D, Baumann B, et al: Morphometric studies of the entorhinal cortex in neuropsychiatric patients and controls: clusters of heterotopically displaced lamina II neurons are not indicative of schizophrenia. Schizophr Res 33:125–132, 1998a

Bernstein HG, Stanarius A, Baumann B, et al: Nitric oxide synthase-containing neurons in the human hypothalamus: reduced number of immunoreactive cells in the paraventricular nucleus of depressive patients and schizophrenics. Neuroscience 83:867–875, 1998b

Bertolino A, Frye M, Callicott JH, et al: Neuronal pathology in the hippocampal area of patients with bipolar disorder. Biol Psychiatry 45:135S, 1999

Bouras C, Kovari E, Hof PR, et al: Anterior cingulate cortex pathology in schizophrenia and bipolar disorder. Acta Neuropathol (Berl) 102:373–379, 2001

Bowley MP, Drevets WC, Ongur D, et al: Low glial numbers in the amygdala in major depressive disorder. Biol Psychiatry 52:404–412, 2002

Bremner JD, Narayan M, Anderson ER, et al: Hippocampal volume reduction in major depression. Am J Psychiatry 157:115–118, 2000

Chana G, Landau S, Beasley C, et al: Two-dimensional assessment of cytoarchitecture in the anterior cingulate cortex in major depressive disorder, bipolar disorder, and schizophrenia: evidence for decreased neuronal somal size and increased neuronal density. Biol Psychiatry 53:1086–1098, 2003

Chang A, Li PP, Warsh JJ: cAMP signal transduction abnormalities in the pathophysiology of mood disorders: contributions from postmortem brain studies, in The Postmortem Brain in Psychiatric Research. Edited by Agam G, Everall IP, Belmaker RH. Boston, MA, Kluwer Academic Publishers, 2002, pp 341–361

Chen B, Dowlatshahi D, MacQueen GM, et al: Increased hippocampal BDNF immunoreactivity in subjects treated with antidepressant medication. Biol Psychiatry 50:260–265, 2001

Chen G, Rajkowska G, Du F, et al: Enhancement of hippocampal neurogenesis by lithium. J Neurochem 75:1729–1734, 2000

Cotter D, Mackay D, Landau S, et al: Reduced glial cell density and neuronal size in the anterior cingulate cortex in major depressive disorder. Arch Gen Psychiatry 58:545–553, 2001

Cotter D, Landau S, Beasley C, et al: The density and spatial distribution of GABAergic neurons, labelled using calcium binding proteins, in the anterior cingulate cortex in major depressive disorder, bipolar disorder, and schizophrenia. Biol Psychiatry 51:377–386, 2002a

Cotter D, Mackay D, Chana G, et al: Reduced neuronal size and glial cell density in area 9 of the dorsolateral prefrontal cortex in subjects with major depressive disorder. Cereb Cortex 12:386–394, 2002b

Cotter DR, Pariante CM, Rajkowska G: Glial pathology in major psychiatric disorders, in The Postmortem Brain in Psychiatric Research. Edited by Agam G, Everall IP, Belmaker RH. Boston, MA, Kluwer Academic Publishers, 2002c, pp 49–73

Coyle JT, Duman RS: Finding the intracellular signaling pathways affected by mood disorder treatments. Neuron 38:157–160, 2003

Dowlatshahi D, MacQueen GM, Wang JF, et al: G Protein-coupled cyclic AMP signaling in postmortem brain of subjects with mood disorders: effects of diagnosis, suicide, and treatment at the time of death. J Neurochem 73:1121–1126, 1999

Drevets WC: Neuroimaging studies of mood disorders. Biol Psychiatry 48:813–829, 2000

Drevets WC, Price JL, Simpson JR Jr, et al: Subgenual prefrontal cortex abnormalities in mood disorders. Nature 386:824–827, 1997

Duman RS, Malberg J, Nakagawa S, et al: Neuronal plasticity and survival in mood disorders. Biol Psychiatry 48:732–739, 2000

Eastwood SL, Harrison PJ: Hippocampal synaptic pathology in schizophrenia, bipolar disorder and major depression: a study of complexin mRNAs. Mol Psychiatry 5:425–432, 2000

Eastwood SL, Harrison PJ: Synaptic pathology in the anterior cingulate cortex in schizophrenia and mood disorders: a review and a Western blot study of synaptophysin, GAP-43 and the complexins. Brain Res Bull 55:569–578, 2001

Elkis H, Friedman L, Wise A, et al: Meta-analyses of studies of ventricular enlargement and cortical sulcal prominence in mood disorders. Arch Gen Psychiatry 52:735–746, 1995

Evans S, Akil H, Choudary P, et al: Microarray studies in mood disorders: distinct patterns seen between major depression and bipolar disorder in two frontal cortical regions. Scientific Abstract 36 presented at the 41st annual meeting of the American College of Neuropsychopharmacology, San Juan, Puerto Rico, December 8–12, 2002

Hansson E, Muyderman H, Leonova J, et al: Astroglia and glutamate in physiology and pathology: aspects on glutamate transport, glutamate-induced cell swelling and gap-junction communication. Neurochem Int 37:317–329, 2000

Harkin AJ, Bruce KH, Craft B, et al: Nitric oxide synthase inhibitors have antidepressant-like properties in mice. 1: acute treatments are active in the forced swim test. Eur J Pharmacol 372:207–213, 1999

Hasin DS, Grant BF: Major depression in 6050 former drinkers: association with past alcohol dependence. Arch Gen Psychiatry 59:794–800, 2002

Heun R, Kockler M, Papassotiropoulos A: Distinction of early and late-onset depression in the elderly by their lifetime symptomatology. Int J Geriatr Psychiatry 15:1138–1142, 2000

Holsboer F, Spengler D, Heuser I: The role of corticotropin-releasing hormone in the pathogenesis of Cushing's disease, anorexia nervosa, alcoholism, affective disorders and dementia. Prog Brain Res 93:385–417, 1992

Honer WG, Falkai P, Chen C, et al: Synaptic and plasticity-associated proteins in anterior frontal cortex in severe mental illness. Neuroscience 91:1247–1255, 1999

Johnston-Wilson NL, Sims CD, Hofmann JP, et al: Disease-specific alterations in frontal cortex brain proteins in schizophrenia, bipolar disorder, and major depressive disorder. The Stanley Neuropathology Consortium. Mol Psychiatry 5:142–149, 2000

Karolewicz B, Stockmeier CA, Ordway GA: Elevated levels of the NR2C subunit of the NMDA receptor in the locus coeruleus in depression. Neuropsychopharmacology [Epub ahead of print: PMID 15920498, May 25, 2005]

Klimek V, Stockmeier C, Overholser J, et al: Reduced levels of norepinephrine transporters in the locus coeruleus in major depression. J Neurosci 17:8451–8458, 1997

Klimek V, Schenck JE, Han H, et al: Dopaminergic abnormalities in amygdaloid nuclei in major depression: a postmortem study. Biol Psychiatry 52:740–748, 2002

Krishnan K, Hays J, Tupler L, et al: Clinical and phenomenological comparisons of late-onset and early onset depression. Am J Psychiatry 152:785–788, 1995

Krystal JH, Sanacora G, Blumberg H, et al: Glutamate and GABA systems as targets for novel antidepressant and mood-stabilizing treatments. Mol Psychiatry 7:S71–S80, 2002

Lavretsky H, Lesser IM, Wohl M, et al: Relationship of age, age at onset, and sex to depression in older adults. Am J Geriatr Psychiatry 6:248–256, 1998

Levine S, Saltzman A, Klein AW: Proliferation of glial cells in vivo induced in the neural lobe of the rat pituitary by lithium. Cell Prolif 33:203–207, 2000

Lucassen PJ, Muller MB, Holsboer F, et al: Hippocampal apoptosis in major depression is a minor event and absent from subareas at risk for glucocorticoid overexposure. Am J Pathol 158:453–468, 2001

Malberg JE, Eisch AJ, Nestler EJ, et al: Chronic antidepressant treatment increases neurogenesis in adult rat hippocampus. J Neurosci 20:9104–9110, 2000

Manaye KF, Lei DL, Tizabi Y, et al: Selective neuron loss in the paraventricular nucleus of hypothalamus in patients suffering from major depression and bipolar disorder. J Neuropathol Exp Neurol 64:224–229, 2005

Manji HK, Drevets WC, Charney DS: The cellular neurobiology of depression. Nat Med 7:541–547, 2001

Mann JJ, Huang YY, Underwood MD, et al: A serotonin transporter gene promoter polymorphism (5-HTTLPR) and prefrontal cortical binding in major depression and suicide. Arch Gen Psychiatry 57:729–738, 2000

Miguel-Hidalgo JJ, Rajkowska G: Morphological brain changes in depression: can antidepressants reverse them? CNS Drugs 16:361–372, 2002

Miguel-Hidalgo JJ, Rajkowska G: Comparison of prefrontal cell pathology between depression and alcohol dependence. J Psychiatr Res 37:411–420, 2003

Miguel-Hidalgo JJ, Baucom C, Dilley G, et al: Glial fibrillary acidic protein immunoreactivity in the prefrontal cortex distinguishes younger from older adults in major depressive disorder. Biol Psychiatry 48:861–873, 2000

Miguel-Hidalgo JJ, Wei J, Overholser JC, et al: Glial pathology in the prefrontal cortex in alcohol dependence with and without depressive symptoms. Biol Psychiatry 52:1121–1133, 2002

Moore GJ, Bebchuk JM, Hasanat K, et al: Lithium increases N-acetyl-aspartate in the human brain: in vivo evidence in support of bcl-2's neurotrophic effects? Biol Psychiatry 48:1–8, 2000

Nowak G, Ordway GA, Paul IA: Alterations in the N-methyl-D-aspartate (NMDA) receptor complex in the frontal cortex of suicide victims. Brain Res 675:157–164, 1995

Ongur D, Drevets WC, Price JL: Glial reduction in the subgenual prefrontal cortex in mood disorders. Proc Natl Acad Sci U S A 95:13290–13295, 1998

Ordway GA, Widdowson PS, Smith KS, et al: Agonist binding to alpha 2-adrenoceptors is elevated in the locus coeruleus from victims of suicide. J Neurochem 63:617–624, 1994

Papp M, Moryl E: Antidepressant activity of non-competitive and competitive NMDA receptor antagonists in a chronic mild stress model of depression. Eur J Pharmacol 263:1–7, 1994

Purba JS, Hoogendijk WJ, Hofman MA, et al: Increased number of vasopressin- and oxytocin-expressing neurons in the paraventricular nucleus of the hypothalamus in depression. Arch Gen Psychiatry 53:137–143, 1996

Raadsheer FC, Hoogendijk WJ, Stam FC, et al: Increased numbers of corticotropin-releasing hormone expressing neurons in the hypothalamic paraventricular nucleus of depressed patients. Neuroendocrinology 60:436–444, 1994

Raadsheer FC, van Heerikhuize JJ, Lucassen PJ, et al: Corticotropin-releasing hormone mRNA levels in the paraventricular nucleus of patients with Alzheimer's disease and depression. Am J Psychiatry 152:1372–1376, 1995

Rajkowska G, Goldman-Rakic PS: Cytoarchitectonic definition of prefrontal areas in the normal human cortex, II: variability in locations of areas 9 and 46. Cereb Cortex 4:323–337, 1995

Rajkowska G, Miguel-Hidalgo JJ, Wei J, et al: Morphometric evidence for neuronal and glial prefrontal cell pathology in major depression. Biol Psychiatry 45:1085–1098, 1999

Rajkowska G, Halaris A, Selemon LD: Reductions in neuronal and glial density characterize the dorsolateral prefrontal cortex in bipolar disorder. Biol Psychiatry 49:741–752, 2001

Rajkowska G, O'Dwyer G, Shao Q, et al: Calbindin immunoreactive non-pyramidal neurons are reduced in the dorsolateral prefrontal cortex in major depression and schizophrenia (Program No. 497.20), in 2002 Abstract Viewer/ Itinerary Planner (CD-ROM). Washington, DC, Society for Neuroscience, 2002

Reynolds GP, Zhang ZJ, Patten I, et al: Selective deficits of frontal cortical gabaergic neuronal subtypes defined by calcium binding proteins in psychotic illness (abstract). Schizophr Res 41:255, 2000

Rocha E, Rodnight R: Chronic administration of lithium chloride increases immunodetectable glial fibrillary acidic protein in the rat hippocampus. J Neurochem 63:1582–1584, 1994

Rocha E, Achaval M, Santos P, et al: Lithium treatment causes gliosis and modifies the morphology of hippocampal astrocytes in rats. Neuroreport 9:3971–3974, 1998

Rosoklija G, Toomayan G, Ellis SP, et al: Structural abnormalities of subicular dendrites in subjects with schizophrenia and mood disorders: preliminary findings. Arch Gen Psychiatry 57:349–356, 2000

Sanacora G, Mason GF, Krystal JH: Impairment of GABAergic transmission in depression: new insights from neuroimaging studies. Crit Rev Neurobiol 14:23–45, 2000

Sanacora G, Gueorguieva R, Epperson CN, et al: Subtype-specific alterations of gamma-aminobutyric acid and glutamate in patients with major depression. Arch Gen Psychiatry 61:705–713, 2004

Sargent PA, Kjaer KH, Bench CJ, et al: Brain serotonin1A receptor binding measured by positron emission tomography with [11C]WAY-100635: effects of depression and antidepressant treatment. Arch Gen Psychiatry 57:174–180, 2000

Selemon LD: Regionally diverse cortical pathology in schizophrenia: clues to the etiology of the disease. Schizophr Bull 27:349–377, 2001

Selemon LD, Rajkowska G, Goldman-Rakic PS: Abnormally high neuronal density in the schizophrenic cortex: a morphometric analysis of prefrontal area 9 and occipital area 17. Arch Gen Psychiatry 52:805–818, 1995

Selemon LD, Rajkowska G, Goldman-Rakic PS: Elevated neuronal density in prefrontal area 46 in brains from schizophrenic patients: application of a three-dimensional, stereologic counting method. J Comp Neurol 392:402–412, 1998

Shah PJ, Ebmeier KP, Glabus MF, et al: Cortical grey matter reductions associated with treatment-resistant chronic unipolar depression: controlled magnetic resonance imaging study. Br J Psychiatry 172:527–532, 1998

Sheline YI, Sanghavi M, Mintun MA, et al: Depression duration but not age predicts hippocampal volume loss in medically healthy women with recurrent major depression. J Neurosci 19:5034–5043, 1999

Si X, Miguel-Hidalgo JJ, O'Dwyer G, et al: Age-dependent reductions in the level of glial fibrillary acidic protein in the prefrontal cortex in major depression. Neuropsychopharmacology 29:2088–2096, 2004

Soares J, Mann J: The anatomy of mood disorders—review of structural neuroimaging studies. Biol Psychiatry 41:86–106, 1997

Stockmeier CA, Jurjus G: Monoamine receptors in postmortem brain: do postmortem brain studies cloud or clarify our understanding of the affective disorders?, in The Postmortem Brain in Psychiatric Research. Edited by Agam G, Everall IP, Belmaker RH. Boston, MA, Kluwer Academic Publishers, 2002, pp 363–385

Stockmeier CA, Shapiro LA, Dilley GE, et al: Increase in serotonin-1A autoreceptors in the midbrain of suicide victims with major depression—postmortem evidence for decreased serotonin activity. J Neurosci 18:7394–7401, 1998

Stockmeier CA, Mahajan GJ, Konick L, et al: Cellular changes in the postmortem hippocampus in major depression. Biol Psychiatry 56:640–650, 2004

Super H, Soriano E, Uylings HB: The functions of the preplate in development and evolution of the neocortex and hippocampus. Brain Res Brain Res Rev 27:40–64, 1998

Swaab DF, Hofman MA, Lucassen PJ, et al: Functional neuroanatomy and neuropathology of the human hypothalamus. Anat Embryol (Berl) 187:317–330, 1993

Tkachev D, Mimmack ML, Ryan MM, et al: Oligodendrocyte dysfunction in schizophrenia and bipolar disorder. Lancet 362:798–805, 2003

Tomita H, Vawter M, Evans S, et al: Gene expression profiles in postmortem brains of mood disorder patients (Program No. 640.19.2003), in Abstract Viewer/Itinerary Planner Available at: http://apu.sfn.org/content/Meetings_Events/AnnualMeeting2004/Abstracts_Symposia/AbstractViewerandItineraryPlanner1/index.html. Washington, DC, Society for Neuroscience, 2003

Underwood MD, Khaibulina AA, Ellis SP, et al: Morphometry of the dorsal raphe nucleus serotonergic neurons in suicide victims. Biol Psychiatry 46:473–483, 1999

Uranova N, Orlovskaya D, Vikhreva O, et al: Electron microscopy of oligodendroglia in severe mental illness. Brain Res Bull 55:597–610, 2001

Uranova NA, Vostrikov VM, Orlovskaya DD, et al: Oligodendroglial density in the prefrontal cortex in schizophrenia and mood disorders: a study from the Stanley Neuropathology Consortium. Schizophr Res 67:269–275, 2004

Uylings HB, Sanz Arigita E, de Vos K, et al: The importance of a human 3D database and atlas for studies of prefrontal and thalamic functions. Prog Brain Res 126:357–368, 2000

Webster MJ, Shannon-Weickert C, Herman MM, et al: Synaptophysin and GAP-43 mRNA levels in the hippocampus of subjects with schizophrenia. Schizophr Res 49:89–98, 2001

Winsberg ME, Sachs N, Tate DL, et al: Decreased dorsolateral prefrontal N-acetyl aspartate in bipolar disorder. Biol Psychiatry 47:475–481, 2000

Zhu MY, Klimek V, Dilley GE, et al: Elevated levels of tyrosine hydroxylase in the locus coeruleus in major depression. Biol Psychiatry 46:1275–1286, 1999

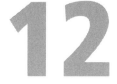

CHAPTER

12

Molecular and Cellular Neurobiology of Severe Mood Disorders

JASKARAN B. SINGH, M.D.

JORGE A. QUIROZ, M.D.

TODD D. GOULD, M.D.

CARLOS A. ZARATE JR., M.D.

HUSSEINI K. MANJI, M.D.

THERE HAS BEEN considerable progress in our understanding of the underlying molecular and cellular basis of mood disorders in recent years. Recent evidence from our laboratory and others indicates that impairments in intracellular signaling pathways that rely on enzymes such as protein kinase C (PKC), inositol monophosphatase, and glycogen synthase kinase-3 (GSK-3) may play a role in the pathophysiology of mood disorders. Mood stabilizers exert major effects on signaling pathways, which regulate neuro-plasticity and cell survival; these pathways have generated considerable excitement among the clinical neuroscience community and are reshaping views about the neurobiological underpinnings of these disorders (Duman 2002; T.D. Gould et al. 2004a; Nestler et al. 2002; Quiroz et al. 2004). In this chapter, we review these data and discuss their implications for changing existing conceptualizations about the pathophysiology of mood disorders and for the strategic development of improved therapeutics.

The authors would like to acknowledge the support of the Intramural Research Program of the National Institute of Mental Heath, the National Alliance for Research on Schizophrenia and Depression, and the Stanley Medical Research Institute. Chris Gavin provided outstanding editorial assistance.

Neuroplasticity and Cellular Resilience in Mood Disorders

The term *neuroplasticity* encompasses diverse processes of vital importance by which the brain perceives, adapts to, and responds to a variety of internal and external stimulation. At the cellular level, the term *cellular resilience* denotes the ability of cells in the brain to adapt adequately and respond to stress. Examples of neuroplasticity in the adult central nervous system (CNS) include alterations of dendritic function, synaptic remodeling, long-term potentiation (LTP), axonal sprouting, neurite extension, synaptogenesis (the birth of new synapses), and even neurogenesis (the birth of new neurons). Although the potential relevance of neuroplastic events to the pathophysiology of psychiatric disorders has been articulated for some time, recent morphometric studies (measuring the size, shape, and function) of the brain (both in vivo and postmortem) are leading to a greater appreciation of the magnitude and nature of the neuroplastic events involved in the pathophysiology of mood disorders.

Impairments of Structural Plasticity and Cellular Resilience in Mood Disorders

The evidence for impairments of structural plasticity and cellular resilience in mood disorders comes from several sources and methods of investigation. New brain imaging techniques of the structure of the brain, as well as postmortem studies of the brains of patients with mood disorders, have provided data related to the changing structural plasticity in the brain of subjects with mood disorders.

Structural Imaging

Brain imaging studies have shown reduced gray matter volumes in areas of the orbital and medial prefrontal cortex (PFC), ventral striatum, and hippocampus and subsequent enlargement of the third ventricle in subjects with mood disorders in comparison with healthy subjects (reviewed in Mayberg, Chapter 13, in this volume). Other impairments detected by structural imaging include the increase in the presence of white matter hyperintensities in the brains of elderly depressed patients and in children and adults with bipolar disorder. White matter hyperintensities may result from numerous causes, including cerebrovascular accidents, neuronal demyelination, loss of axons, dilated perivascular space, minute brain cysts, and necrosis, or they may be inherited. There is a growing awareness of the effect of white matter hyperintensities on neuropsychological functioning, and evidence suggests that white matter hyperintensities represent damage to the structure of brain tissue. Diffusion tensor imaging, which uses diffusion-weighted pulse sequences sensitive to microscopic random motion of water molecules of brain tissue, has been used to study white matter tract disruption in mood disorders. Taylor and colleagues (2001) found that white matter hyperintensities show a higher apparent diffusion quotient (a measurement of isotropic diffusion) and lower anisotropy (diffusion as influenced by tissue structure) than normal regions in both depressed subjects and control subjects. Recent evidence suggests that subcortical hyperintensities correlate with cortical gray matter changes (Lee et al. 2003; Sheline 2001). Together, these findings suggest that white matter hyperintensities damage the structure of brain tissue and likely disrupt the neuronal connectivity necessary for normal affective functioning. Although the cause of white matter hyperintensities in mood disorders is unknown, their presence—particularly in the brains of young bipolar patients—suggests importance in the pathophysiology of the disorder.

Postmortem Studies

As reviewed by Rajkowska in Chapter 11 of this volume, postmortem neuropathological studies of the brains of patients with mood disorders show changes similar to those seen in imaging studies. These postmortem studies in mood disorders show reductions in cortex volume and region- and layer-specific reductions in number, density, and size of neurons and glial cells in the subgenual PFC, orbital cortex, dorsal anterolateral PFC, amygdala, basal ganglia, and dorsal raphe nuclei.

However, it is currently unclear whether these alterations seen in functional and structural imaging or postmortem studies are developmental abnormalities conferring vulnerability to severe mood episodes, compensatory changes to other pathogenic processes, sequelae of recurrent affective episodes, or a unique phenomenon that lacks significance in the pathophysiology of mood disorders. Understanding these issues will partly depend on experiments that delineate the onset of such abnormalities within the illness course and determine whether they predate mood episodes in high-risk patients. Furthermore, there has not been complete reproducibility in other neuroimaging or postmortem studies, which may represent variations in experimental design (including medication effects), an effect of low sample size, or difficulty in clearly defining disease phenotypes within a heterogeneous group of disorders. Further studies are required to understand if more rigorously defined subtypes of mood disorders are associated with specific alterations.

Stress and Glucocorticoids Modulate Neuroplasticity

In developing hypotheses regarding the pathogenesis of these histopathological changes, the alterations in cellular morphology resulting from various stressors have been the focus of considerable recent research (McEwen 1999) and have helped increase understanding of these changes in mood disorders. Although mood disorders have a strong genetic basis, considerable evidence has shown that severe stressors are associated with a substantial increase in the risk for the onset of mood disorders in susceptible individuals and represent important gene–environment interactions (Caspi et al. 2003). Stress is primarily mediated by the hypothalamic-pituitary-adrenal (HPA) axis, and multiple lines of evidence suggest HPA axis activation in mood disorders (see Seidman, Chapter 7, in this volume).

Cushing's syndrome, a disorder resulting from increased adrenocortical secretion of cortisol, is, for example, associated with several psychiatric and psychological disturbances, regardless of its etiology. Major depression, mania, anxiety disorders, cognitive dysfunction or delirium, and hippocampal atrophy (reduction or loss) are frequently reported in Cushing's syndrome. Interestingly, treatment with antiglucocorticoid therapeutics has resulted in an improvement in mood and/or cognitive function in these patients, as well as an enlargement of hippocampal volume in proportion to the treatment-associated decrement in urinary free cortisol after corrective surgery.

Detailed studies of glucocorticoid receptors (GR) and mineralocorticoid receptors (MR) in subjects with mood disorders are ongoing. However, postmortem studies in subjects with mood disorders showed significantly lower GR and MR protein and mRNA levels in the PFC compared with control subjects. In a recent in vivo study of MR function in subjects with depression receiving spironolactone (an MR antagonist), Young and colleagues (2003) found that patients with depression had higher functional activity of the MR system and increased secretion of cortisol in response to spironolactone in comparison with matched control subjects.

Mechanisms Underlying Stress-Induced Morphometric Changes

Most studies of atrophy and survival of neurons in response to stress, as well as hormones of the HPA axis, have focused on the hippocampus. This is due, in part, to the well-defined and easily studied neuronal populations of this limbic brain region, including the dentate gyrus granule cell layer and the CA1 and CA3 pyramidal cell layers. Another major reason for studying the hippocampus is that the highest levels of GR are expressed in this brain region.

One of the most consistent effects of stress on cellular morphology in preclinical (animal) models is atrophy of hippocampal neurons (McEwen 1999; Sapolsky 2000a). This atrophy is observed in the CA3 pyramidal neurons but not in other hippocampal cell groups (i.e., CA1 pyramidal and dentate gyrus granule neurons). The stress-induced atrophy of CA3 neurons (i.e., decreased number and length of the apical dendritic branches) occurs after 2–3 weeks of exposure to restraint stress or more long-term social stress and has been observed in rodents and tree shrews. Atrophy of CA3 pyramidal neurons also occurs on exposure to high levels of glucocorticoids, suggesting that activation of the HPA axis likely plays a major role in mediating the stress-induced atrophy.

Preclinical research also has identified histopathological changes in rat PFC after corticosterone administration, although this area has not been as extensively studied as the hippocampus. Wellman (2001) investigated pyramidal neurons in layers II–III of the medial PFC and quantified dendritic morphology in three dimensions. This study found a significant redistribution of apical dendrites in corticosterone-treated animals; the amount of dendritic material proximal to the soma (the body of the nerve cell) was increased, and distal dendritic material was decreased. These findings suggest that stress may produce a significant reorganization of the apical dendritic arbor (treelike structure of the dendrite, with branches) in the medial PFC in rats (Wellman 2001).

More recently, Lyons (2002) reported that for years after a brief stressor (intermittent postnatal separations from maternal availability), young adult squirrel monkeys showed significantly larger right ventral medial prefrontal volumes; neither overall brain volumes nor left prefrontal measures were altered, suggesting selective (rather than nonspecific) effects. It is interesting to speculate that these preclinical findings are related to the clinical observations of reduced size of prefrontal cortical regions, gray matter changes, and postmortem alterations of neurons and glial cells in mood disorder subjects, as previously noted.

Mechanisms Mediating the Effects of Stress

Glutamate

Microdialysis studies have shown that stress increases extracellular levels of glutamate in the hippocampus, and N-methyl-D-aspartate (NMDA) glutamate receptor antagonists attenuate stress-induced atrophy of CA3 pyramidal

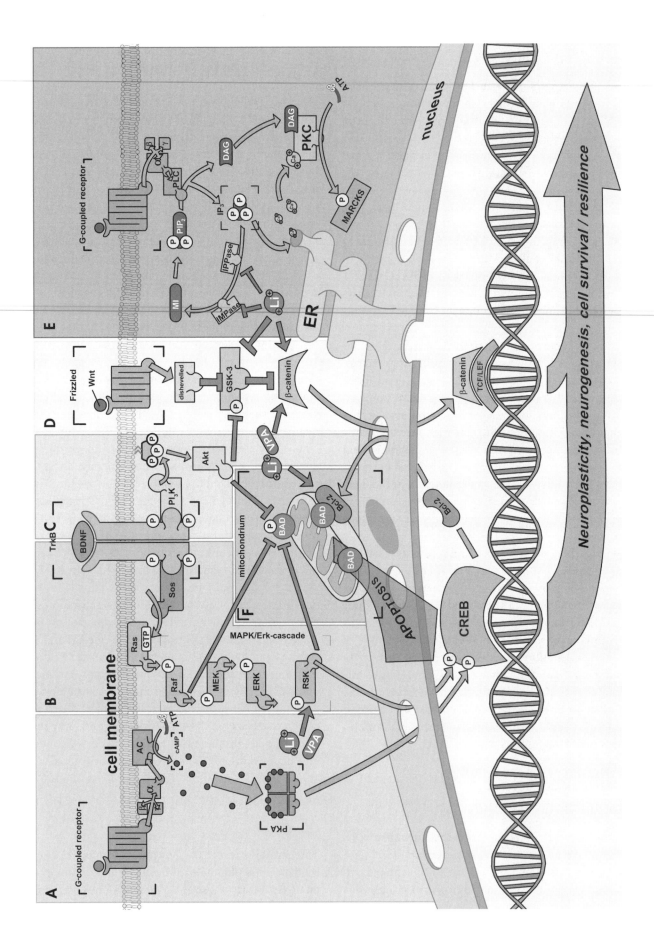

FIGURE 12–1. Signaling cascades and their involvement in neuroplasticity, neurogenesis, and cell survival/resilience.

A: Adenylate cyclase (AC) signaling pathway: This pathway is also mediated through a G protein–coupled receptor, which activates—via AC—another second messenger called cyclic adenosine monophosphate (cAMP). One of the effects of cAMP is activation of protein kinase A (PKA), an enzyme that phosphorylates many substrates including the cAMP response element binding protein (CREB). After activation, this protein binds to the cAMP response element (CRE), a gene sequence found in the promoter of certain genes. **B:** MAP/ERK pathway: The influence of neurotrophic factors on cell survival is mediated by activation of the mitogen-activated protein (MAP) kinase cascade through activation of the neurotrophic factor receptor also referred to as receptor tyrosine kinases (RTK). RTK belong to the tyrosine kinase (Trk) family of receptors. Recruitment of the guanine nucleotide exchange factor Sos results in activation of the small guanosine triphosphate binding protein Ras, which leads to the activation of a cascade of serine/threonine kinases. This includes Raf, MAP kinase kinase (MEK) and MAP kinase (also referred to as extracellular response kinase, ERK). One target of the MAP kinase cascade is ribosomal S6 kinase (RSK), which influences cell survival by phosphorylating and inactivating the pro-apoptotic factor BAD. RSK also phosphorylates CREB and thereby increases the expression of the anti-apoptotic factor bcl-2 and brain-derived neurotrophic factor (BDNF). These mechanisms underlie many of the long-term effects of neurotrophins, including neurite outgrowth, cytoskeletal remodeling and cell survival. Lithium and valproate appear to activate the ERK MAP kinase pathway. **C:** Phosphatidylinositol-3-kinase (PI_3K) pathway: This pathway can be also be activated by RTK. One way in which PI_3K signals cells to survive and grow is by indirectly activating protein kinase Akt. Akt phosphorylates a variety of target proteins. Some of them are the same that are also phosphorylated via the MAP/ERK pathway, e.g. BAD. A main substrate of Akt is glycogen synthase kinase 3 (GSK-3). **D:** GSK-3 and Wnt pathway: GSK-3 mediates a number of signaling pathways, including the Wnt pathway, neurotrophic pathways, and the insulin/PI_3 kinase pathway. In the Wnt signaling pathway Wnt glycoproteins interact with the frizzled family of receptors to stimulate the disheveled-mediated inactivation of GSK-3 and activation of the transcription factor ß-catenin. Following GSK-3 inhibition, nondegraded (nonphosphorylated) ß-catenin binds to LEF/TCF transcription factors, targeting transcription of specific genes. Disheveled inactivation of GSK-3 results via interactions with a protein complex that contains adenomatous polyposis coli (APC), axin, and FRAT1. Lithium is a direct inhibitor of GSK-3; both lithium and valproate increase ß-catenin levels. **E:** Phosphoinositol signaling pathway and protein kinase C (PKC): After ligand binding to a G-protein coupled receptor, the three subunits of the G protein dissociate from both each other and the receptor and through this activation induces phospholipase C (PLC) hydrolysis of phosphoinositide 4,5 (PIP_2) to diacylglycerol (DAG) and inositol-1, 4, 5-triphosphate (IP_3). DAG and IP_3 function as second messenger. DAG activates PKC, an enzyme that has many effects including activation of myristoylated alanine–rich C kinase substrate (MARCKS). IP_3 binds to the IP_3 receptor that also functions as a calcium channel in the cell. IP_3 is recycled back to PIP_2 by the enzymes inositol monophosphate phosphatase (IMPase) and inositol polyphosphatase phosphatase (IPPase), both of which are direct targets of lithium. **F:** Mitochondria, calcium, and bcl-2: Bcl-2 attenuates apoptosis by sequestering proforms of caspases (death-driving cysteine proteases), by preventing the release of mitochondrial apoptogenic (programed cell death) factors such as calcium, cytochrome c, and apoptosis-inducing factor (AIF) into the cytoplasm, and by enhancing mitochondrial calcium uptake. Before classic signs of apoptosis occur, mitochondria undergo major changes in membrane integrity, such as disruption of the inner transmembrane potential and the release of intermembrane proteins through the outer membrane. Bcl-2 stabilizes mitochondrial membrane integrity and prevents opening of the permeability transition pore, a key event in cell death. Lithium and valproate increase bcl-2 levels.

Source. Adapted from Yuang P, Gould TD, Graya NA, et al: "Neurotrophic Signaling Cascades Are Major Long-Term Targets for Lithium: Clinical Implications." *Clinical Neuroscience Research* 4:137–153, 2004.

neurons (McEwen 1999; Sapolsky 2000a). The preponderance of the evidence to date suggests that the atrophy, and possibly death, of CA3 pyramidal neurons arises, at least in part, from increased glutamate neurotransmission. Note, however, that although NMDA antagonists block stress-induced hippocampal atrophy, no studies have shown that they are able to block the cell death (apoptosis) induced by severe stress. Thus, the mechanisms underlying atrophy and death of neurons in the hippocampus may work on a continuum, with severe (or prolonged) stresses "recruiting" additional pathogenic pathways in addition to enhancing NMDA-mediated neurotransmission.

Overactivation of the glutamate ionotropic receptors contributes to the neurotoxic effects of a variety of insults, including repeated seizures and ischemia. Neurotoxicity is a response to overactivation of calcium-dependent enzymes and the generation of oxygen free radicals. Stress or glucocorticoid exposure also compromises the metabolic capacity of neurons, thereby increasing the vulnerability to other types of neuronal insults.

Corticotropin-Releasing Hormone and the HPA Axis

Activation of the HPA axis appears to play a critical role in mediating these effects because stress-induced neuronal atrophy is prevented by adrenalectomy (removal of adrenal glands) and duplicated by exposure to high concentrations of glucocorticoids (see Seidman, Chapter 7, in this volume). Increasingly, recent data also suggest a critical role for corticotropin-releasing hormone (CRH) in the long-term effects of early life stresses on hippocampal integrity and function. The administration of CRH to the brains of immature rats has been reported to reduce memory function throughout life; these deficits are associated with progressive loss of hippocampal CA3 neurons and chronic upregulation of hippocampal CRH expression, effects that do not require the presence of stress levels of glucocorticoids (see Seidman, Chapter 7, in this volume).

The CRH_1 receptor, which binds CRH with higher affinity than does the CRH_2 receptor, plays a major role in regulating corticotropin release and has been implicated in animal models of anxiety. The central administration of CRH_1 antisense oligodeoxynucleotides has been shown to have anxiolytic effects against both CRH and psychological stressors. Although CRH_2 receptors appear to act in an antagonistic manner (i.e., CRH_1 activates and CRH_2 attenuates the stress response), their precise role is still being characterized. Interestingly, pretreatment with a CRH antagonist also attenuates the stress-induced increases in MR levels in hippocampus, neocortex, frontal cortex, and amygdala.

Glucose Transport

Glucocorticoids are known to inhibit glucose transport, thereby diminishing the capability of energy production and augmenting the susceptibility to hypoglycemic conditions. The potential functional significance of these effects is supported by the demonstration that overexpression of the glucose transporter blocks the neurotoxic effects of neuronal insults (Manji and Duman 2001; Sapolsky 2000a).

Stress and Glucocorticoids Impair Cellular Resilience

In addition to directly causing neuronal atrophy, stress and glucocorticoids appear to reduce cellular resilience, thereby making certain neurons more vulnerable to other insults, such as ischemia, hypoglycemia, and excitatory amino acid toxicity (Sapolsky 2000a). The reduction in the resilience of discrete brain regions, including the hippocampus and potentially the PFC, also may reflect the propensity for various stressors to decrease the expression of brain-derived neurotrophic factor (BDNF) in this brain region. The mechanisms underlying the downregulation of BDNF by stress have not been fully elucidated. Adrenoglucocorticoids do not appear to account for these actions of stress because administration of a high dose of glucocorticoid is not sufficient to decrease BDNF, and adrenalectomy does not block the effect of stress (Lauterborn et al. 1998).

Thus, recurrent stress, and presumably recurrent mood disorder episodes, which are often associated with hypercortisolemia, may lower the threshold for cellular death or atrophy in response to a variety of physiological (e.g., aging) and pathological (e.g., ischemic) events. Such processes also may conceivably play a role in the relation between mood disorders and cerebrovascular events, considering that patients who develop their first depressive episode in late life have an increased likelihood of showing magnetic resonance imaging evidence of cerebrovascular disease. Furthermore, inflammatory reactions consistent with ischemia are also suggested by the finding of elevated intercellular adhesion molecule-1 (ICAM-1) in dorsolateral PFC in postmortem studies of patients with late-life depression.

Stress, Glucocorticoids, and Neurogenesis

Neurogenesis in the adult brain (see Figure 12–1) is the target of significant research on the role of stress and the HPA axis. Neurogenesis and the localization of pluripotential progenitor cells, which can differentiate into various specialized types of tissue elements, occur in restricted brain regions, with the greatest density of new cell birth observed in the subventricular zone and in the subgranular layer of the hippocampus. An enriched environment, exercise, and hippocampal-dependent learning can increase neurogenesis in the hippocampus in rodents. Upregulation of neurogenesis in response to these behavioral stimuli and the localization of this process to the hippocampus have led to the proposal that new cell birth is involved in learning and memory (E. Gould et al. 2000).

Studies have shown that decreased neurogenesis occurs in response to both acute and chronic stress (E. Gould et al. 2000). Preclinical studies in animals have shown that adrenalectomy increases neurogenesis and that treatment with high levels of glucocorticoids reproduces the downregulation of neurogenesis that occurs in response to stress. Lowering glucocorticoid levels in aged animals restores neurogenesis to levels observed in younger animals, indicating that the population of progenitor cells remains stable but is inhibited by glucocorticoids.

Treatments commonly used in mood disorders, such as antidepressants and lithium, increase neurogenesis in the hippocampus. However, the importance of neurogenesis in mood disorder treatment and pathophysiology is still a matter of important debate. Santarelli and colleagues (2003) recently conducted a series of critical experiments, suggesting that behavioral effects of chronic antidepressant use may be mediated by new neuronal growth in the hippocampus and that this neurogenesis may be necessary for its antidepressant effects.

Preclinical findings in the hippocampus in animals are consistent with clinical findings showing that patients with depression of longer duration and multiple hospitalizations (associated with prolonged hypercortisolemia) have smaller hippocampal volumes (MacQueen et al. 2003; Sheline et al. 1999). Furthermore, antidepressant treatment may offer some protection against hippocampal volume loss (Sheline et al. 2003). However, some studies suggest that smaller hippocampal volumes are at least in part an inherited characteristic of the brain (Gilbertson et al. 2002; Lyons et al. 2001), highlighting the need for caution in attributing causality in the cross-sectional human morphometric studies of the hippocampus and preclinical data on the effects of stress on the hippocampus in animals.

Neurotrophic Signaling Cascades

Neurotrophins are an important family of regulatory factors in the brain that mediate the differentiation and sur-

vival of neurons, as well as the modulation of synaptic transmission and synaptic plasticity. The neurotrophin family now includes 1) nerve growth factor (NGF), 2) BDNF, 3) neurotrophin-3 (NT-3), 4) NT-4/5, and 5) NT-6 (Patapoutian and Reichardt 2001). These various proteins are closely related in terms of sequence homology and receptor specificity. They bind to, and activate, specific receptor tyrosine kinases belonging to the Trk family of receptors, including TrkA, TrkB, TrkC, and a pan-neurotrophin receptor (p75).

Additionally, there are two isoforms (slightly different versions) of TrkB receptors: the full-length TrkB and the truncated form of TrkB, which does not contain the intracellular tyrosine kinase domain. The truncated form of TrkB can thus function as a dominant negative inhibitor for TrkB, providing another mechanism to regulate BDNF signaling in the CNS (Figure 12–2).

Neurotrophins can be secreted constitutively or transiently and often in an activity-dependent manner. Within the neurotrophin family, BDNF is a potent physiological survival factor implicated in a variety of pathophysiological conditions, including mood disorders. BDNF and other neurotrophic factors are necessary for the survival and function of neurons, implying that a sustained reduction of these factors could affect neuronal viability. However, somewhat less well appreciated is that BDNF also has some acute effects on synaptic plasticity and neurotransmitter release, including facilitating the release of glutamate, γ-aminobutyric acid (GABA), dopamine, and serotonin (5-HT). In this context, BDNF has been shown to potentiate both excitatory and inhibitory neuronal transmission, albeit via different mechanisms; BDNF strengthens excitation primarily by augmenting the amplitude of α-amino-3-hydroxy-5-methyl-4-isoxazolepropionic acid (AMPA) receptor–mediated miniature excitatory postsynaptic currents but enhances inhibition by increasing the frequency of miniature inhibitory postsynaptic currents and increasing the size of GABAergic synaptic terminals.

Furthermore, full-length TrkB receptor immunoreactivity has been found not only in glutamatergic pyramidal and granule cells but also in some interneuron axonal initial segments, in axon terminals forming inhibitory-type synapses onto somata and dendritic shafts, and in excitatory-type terminals likely to originate extrahippocampally. Together, these results suggest that TrkB is contained in some GABAergic interneurons, neuromodulatory (e.g., cholinergic, dopaminergic, and noradrenergic) afferents, and glutamatergic afferents.

Notably, although endogenous neurotrophic factors have traditionally been viewed as increasing cell survival by providing necessary trophic support, it is now clear

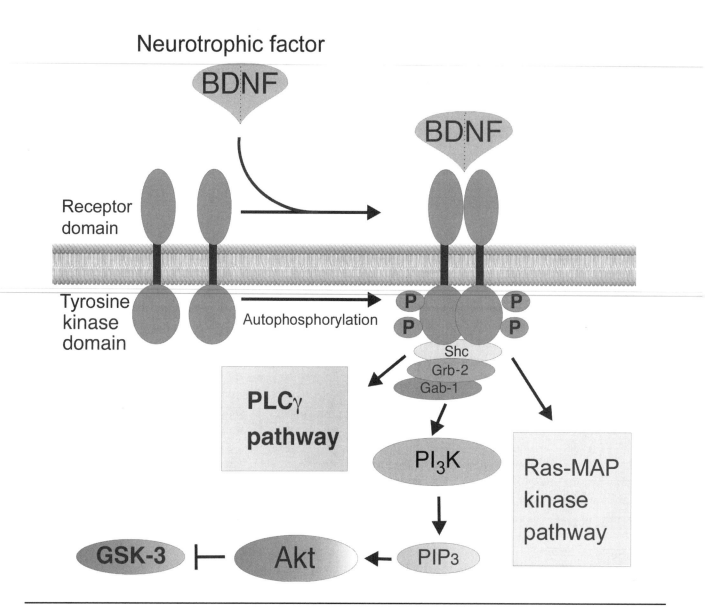

FIGURE 12–2.   **Neurotrophic cascades.**

Cell survival is dependent on neurotrophic factors, such as brain-derived neurotrophic factor (BDNF) and nerve growth factor, and the expression of these factors can be induced by synaptic activity. Phosphorylation of tyrosine receptor kinase (Trk) receptors activates a critical signaling pathway, the Ras–mitogen-activated protein (MAP) kinase pathway. Phosphorylated Trk receptors also recruit the phosphoinositide-3 kinase (PI$_3$K) pathway through at least two distinct pathways, the relative importance of which differs between neuronal subpopulations. In many neurons, Ras-dependent activation of PI$_3$K is the most important pathway through which neurotrophins promote cell survival. In some cells, however, PI$_3$K also can be activated through three adaptor proteins (Shc, Grb-2, and Gab-1). PI$_3$K directly regulates certain cytoplasmic apoptotic pathways. Akt has been proposed to act both prior to the release of cytochrome *c* by pro-apoptotic Bcl-2 family members and subsequent to the release of cytochrome *c* by regulating components of the apoptosome. Akt phosphorylates the pro-apoptotic Bcl-2 family member BAD (Bcl-xl/Bcl-2–associated death promoter), thereby inhibiting BAD's pro-apoptotic functions. Akt also may promote survival in an indirect fashion by regulating another major signaling enzyme: glycogen synthase kinase-3 (GSK-3). Phosphorylated Trk receptors also recruit phospholipase C-γ1 (PLC-γ1). Trk then phosphorylates and activates PLC-γ1, which acts to hydrolyze phosphatidylinositides to generate diacylglycerol (DAG) and inositol 1,4,5-triphosphate (IP$_3$).

Source.   Reprinted from Szabo ST, Gould TD, Manji HK: "Neurotransmitters, Receptors, Signal Transduction, and Second Messengers in Psychiatric Disorders," in *The American Psychiatric Publishing Textbook of Psychopharmacology*, 3rd Edition. Edited by Schatzberg AF, Nemeroff CB. Arlington, VA, American Psychiatric Publishing, 2004, pp. 3–52. Copyright 2004 American Psychiatric Publishing. Used with permission.

that their survival-promoting effects are mediated in large part by an inhibition of cell death cascades. Increasing evidence suggests that neurotrophic factors inhibit cell death cascades by activating the mitogen-activated protein (MAP) kinase signaling pathway and the phosphoinositide-3 (PI₃) kinase/Akt pathway (Figure 12–3). One important mechanism by which the MAP kinase signaling cascades inhibit cell death is by increasing the expression of the antiapoptotic protein Bcl-2.

Accumulating data suggest that Bcl-2 not only is neuroprotective but also exerts neurotrophic effects and promotes neurite sprouting, neurite outgrowth, and axonal regeneration. Moreover, a recent study reported that severe stress exacerbates stroke outcome by suppressing Bcl-2 expression (DeVries et al. 2001). In this study, the stressed mice expressed approximately 70% less Bcl-2 mRNA than did the unstressed mice after ischemia. Furthermore, stress greatly exacerbated infarct in control mice but not in transgenic mice that constitutively expressed increased neuronal Bcl-2. Finally, high corticosterone concentrations correlated with larger infarcts in wild-type mice but not in Bcl-2-overexpressing transgenic mice. Thus, enhanced Bcl-2 expression appears to be capable of offsetting the potentially deleterious consequences of stress-induced neuronal endangerment, suggesting that pharmacologically induced upregulation of Bcl-2 may have considerable utility in the treatment of a variety of disorders associated with endogenous or acquired impairments of cellular resilience.

Overall, it is clear that the neurotrophic factors–MAP kinase–Bcl-2 signaling cascade plays a critical role in cell survival in the CNS and that a fine balance is maintained between the levels and activities of cell survival and cell death factors. Modest changes in this signaling cascade or in the levels of the Bcl-2 family of proteins (potentially caused by genetic, illness-, or insult-related factors) may therefore profoundly affect cellular viability. We now turn to a discussion of the growing body of data suggesting that neurotrophic signaling molecules play important roles in the treatment of mood disorders.

Antidepressant Treatment and Cell Survival Pathways

Seminal studies from Duman's laboratory have investigated the possibility that the factors involved in neuronal atrophy and survival could be the target of antidepressant treatments (D'Sa and Duman 2002; Duman et al. 1999). These studies showed that one pathway involved in cell survival and plasticity—the cyclic adenosine monophosphate (cAMP)–response element binding protein (CREB)

cascade—is upregulated by antidepressant treatment (Figures 12–2 and 12–3). This group also reported that antidepressant treatment in vivo increases CREB phosphorylation and cAMP response element–mediated gene expression in mouse limbic brain regions (Thome et al. 2000). Upregulation of CREB and BDNF occurs in response to several different classes of antidepressant treatments, indicating that the cAMP CREB cascade and BDNF are common postreceptor targets of these therapeutic agents.

In addition, upregulation of CREB and BDNF is dependent on chronic treatment over weeks, consistent with the time to onset of therapeutic effects of antidepressants. In addition, induced CREB overexpression in the dentate gyrus results in an antidepressant-like effect in the learned-helplessness paradigm and the forced swim test in rats. Indirect human evidence comes from studies showing increased hippocampal BDNF expression in postmortem brains of subjects with mood disorders treated with antidepressants at the time of death compared with antidepressant-untreated subjects (Chen et al. 2001).

Cellular and Neurotrophic Actions of Antidepressant Treatments

Several studies support the hypothesis that antidepressant treatment produces neurotrophic-like effects. One study reported that antidepressant treatment induced a greater regeneration of catecholamine axon terminals in the cerebral cortex (Nakamura 1990). Chronic administration of an atypical antidepressant, tianeptine, was reported to block the stress-induced atrophy of CA3 pyramidal neurons in adult male rats (Watanabe et al. 1992). Czeh et al. (2001) recently reported results from preclinical studies, in which stress-induced changes in brain structure and neurochemistry were counteracted by treatment with tianeptine. These glucocorticoid-induced stress effects were prevented or reversed in shrews treated concomitantly with tianeptine (Czeh et al. 2001). However, the generalizability of these effects to other classes of antidepressants is unclear.

Signaling Pathway Components and Mood Stabilizers

Investigators have begun to identify components of cellular signal transduction pathways in the brain, such as PKC, that may not only play a role in the pathophysiology of mood disorders but also represent targets for the action of the most effective treatments (e.g., lithium and

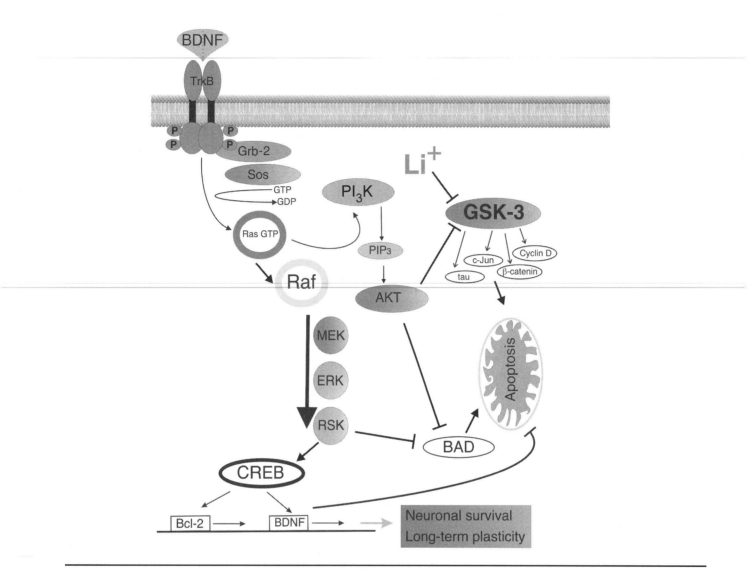

FIGURE 12–3.   **Extracellular response kinase (ERK)–mitogen-activated protein (MAP)–kinase signaling pathway.**

The influence of neurotrophic factors on cell survival is mediated by activation of the MAP kinase cascade. Activation of neurotrophic factor receptors—also referred to as tyrosine receptor kinases (Trks)—results in activation of the MAP kinase cascade via several intermediate steps, including phosphorylation of the adaptor protein Shc and recruitment of the guanine nucleotide exchange factor Sos. This results in activation of the small guanosine triphosphate (GTP)–binding protein Ras, which leads to activation of a cascade of serine/threonine kinases. This includes Raf, MAP kinase kinase (MEK), and MAP kinase (also referred to as ERK). Ras also activates the phosphoinositide-3 kinase (PI_3K) pathway, a primary target of which is the enzyme glycogen synthase kinase-3 (GSK-3). Activation of the PI_3K pathway deactivates GSK-3. GSK-3 has multiple targets in cells, including transcription factors (β-catenin and c-Jun) and cytoskeletal elements such as tau. Many of the targets of GSK-3 are pro-apoptotic when activated. Thus, deactivation of GSK-3 via activation of the PI_3K pathway results in neurotrophic effects. Lithium inhibits GSK-3, an effect that may be, at least in part, responsible for lithium's psychotropic effects. One target of the MAP kinase cascade is the ribosomal S6 kinases, known as RSK, which influences cell survival in at least two ways. RSK phosphorylates and inactivates the pro-apoptotic factor BAD (Bcl-xl/Bcl-2–associated death promoter). RSK also phosphorylates cyclic adenosine monophosphate response element binding protein (CREB) and thereby increases the expression of the antiapoptotic factor Bcl-2 and brain-derived neurotrophic factor (BDNF). These mechanisms underlie many of the long-term effects of neurotrophins, including neurite outgrowth, cytoskeletal remodeling, and cell survival.

GDP=guanosine diphosphate; PIP_3=phosphatidylinositol triphosphate.

Source.   Adapted from Gould TD, Chen G, Manji HK: "Mood Stabilizer Pharmacology." *Clinical Neuroscience Research* 2:193–212, 2003.

valproate). This experimental strategy (of investigating signal transduction pathways) may prove to be most promising because it provides data derived from the physiological response of the system in affected patients and addresses the critical dynamic interaction with pharmacological agents that effectively modify the clinical expression of the pathophysiology (T.D. Gould et al. 2004a).

What is lithium's initial target? Most of the data suggest that it is an intracellular enzyme dependent on magnesium. Lithium has a hydrated ionic radius that is very similar to that of magnesium and inhibits a few select enzymes through competition for this often-required cofactor. Lithium inhibits several enzymes to some degree, but only a few of the enzymes are significantly inhibited at therapeutic serum lithium concentrations. Lithium inhibits a group of at least four related phosphomonoesterases—a group of magnesium-dependent phosphatases in mammals. These include inositol polyphosphate 1-phosphatase (IPPase), inositol monophosphate phosphatase (IMPase), fructose 1,6-bisphosphastase, and bisphosphate nucleotidase. All members of this small group contain a conserved amino acid sequence motif and have a common core tertiary structure that binds metal ions and participates in catalytic functions of the enzyme.

Lithium also inhibits the metabolic enzymes phosphoglucomutase and a kinase that functions as an intermediary in numerous intracellular signaling pathways: GSK-3. Major research efforts have focused on IMPase and GSK-3 as possible therapeutically relevant targets of lithium inhibition predominantly on the basis of what roles these enzymes play in neurological functions (T.D. Gould et al. 2004b). Here, we describe IMPase (and secondarily IPPase) and GSK-3 in greater depth and suggest possible roles that regulation of pathways dependent on these enzymes may have in the pathophysiology of mood disorders. We follow with a discussion of PKC, reelin, and sleep deprivation regulation of signaling components, all processes that may have major relevance to mood disorder pathophysiology and treatment.

Phosphoinositol Signaling

IMPase and IPPase are enzymes involved in recycling and de novo synthesis of inositol, which is a necessary component of a primary intracellular signaling pathway, the phosphoinositol signaling pathway (Figure 12–4). Many extracellular receptors (such as serotonin type 2 [5-HT$_2$], α_1, M_1, M_3, M_5) are coupled to the G protein, $G_{q/11}$, which, through activation of phospholipase C (PLC), mediates the hydrolysis of a membrane phospholipid, phosphatidylinositol 4,5-biphosphate (PIP$_2$), to form the second messengers diacylglycerol (DAG) and inositol 1,4,5-triphosphate (IP$_3$). DAG and IP$_3$ subsequently modulate the activity of a multitude of intracellular events. Several IPPase enzymes are involved in the dephosphorylation (recycling) of IP$_3$ to inositol, which is a precursor of membrane PIP$_2$. This recycling is necessary to maintain phosphoinositol-mediated signaling in cell types in which inositol is not freely available.

The enzyme IMPase is the final (and rate limiting) IPPase prior to conversion to inositol. IPPase removes a phosphate from inositol 1,4-bisphosphate at a stage just before IMPase acts. Both appear to be critical steps in the maintenance of inositol levels and continuation of phosphoinositol-mediated signaling. IMPase is also required for the de novo synthesis of inositol. Lithium's direct effect on IMPase and secondarily on IPPase led to the inositol depletion hypothesis of lithium's action.

Heuristically, the inositol depletion hypothesis suggests that lithium, via inhibition of IMPase, decreases the availability of inositol and thus the amount of PIP$_2$ available for G protein–mediated cellular signaling that relies on this pathway. Hypothetically, the brain is especially sensitive to lithium because of inositol's relatively poor penetration across the blood-brain barrier or a reduced ability of specific neuronal populations to transport inositol across their cell membrane. Furthermore, because of the noncompetitive inhibition profile of lithium, more active cells and brain regions may be affected to a greater degree. Lithium has consistently been shown to decrease free inositol levels in brain sections and in the brains of rodents receiving lithium.

Thus, investigators have looked for dysregulation of inositol and intracellular signaling pathways regulated by inositol signaling in patients with mood disorders to explain the causes and mechanisms of the illness. In a postmortem study by Shimon and colleagues (1997), free inositol levels were lower in brains from patients with bipolar disorder compared with levels in brains from control subjects, a finding that was restricted to the PFC. There are, however, negative studies of inositol levels in patients with mood disorders. IMPase activity has been found to be decreased in lymphocyte-derived cell lines from bipolar patients (Shaltiel et al. 2001). This finding is consistent with a report of low expression of one of the human IMPase genes in lymphocytes derived from some subgroups of bipolar patients.

The levels of the G protein $G_{\alpha q/11}$ were elevated in the occipital cortex of bipolar patients. Jope and colleagues (1996) found that G protein–stimulated phosphoinositol hydrolysis was decreased in brains from patients with bipolar disorder. Further downstream in the signal transduction pathway, Rosel and colleagues (2000) reported that levels of IP$_3$ were significantly increased in the hippocampus, but not in the frontal cortex, of depressed sui-

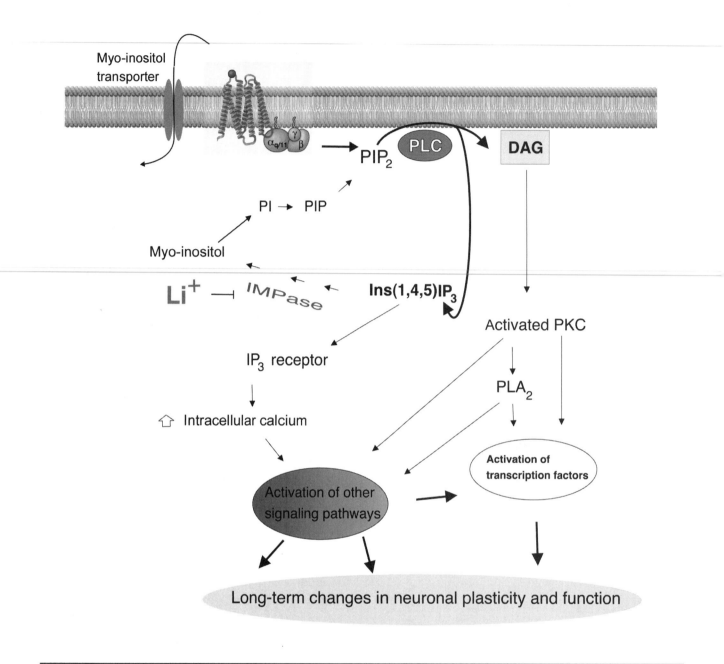

FIGURE 12–4. **Phosphoinositide (PI) signaling pathway.**

A number of receptors in the central nervous system (including M_1, M_3, M_5, $5\text{-}HT_{2C}$) are coupled, via $G_{\alpha q/11}$, to activation of PI hydrolysis. Activation of these receptors induces phospholipase C (PLC) hydrolysis of phosphatidylinositol 4,5-biphosphate (PIP_2) to diacylglycerol (DAG) and inositol 1,4,5-triphosphate (IP_3). DAG activates protein kinase C (PKC), an enzyme that has many effects, including the activation of phospholipase A_2 (PLA_2; an activator of arachidonic acid signaling pathways). IP_3 binds to the IP_3 receptor, which results in the release of intracellular calcium from intracellular stores, most notably the endoplasmic reticulum. Calcium is an important signaling molecule and initiates several downstream effects, such as activation of calmodulins and calmodulin-dependent protein kinases. IP_3 is recycled back to PIP_2 by the enzymes inositol monophosphatase (IMPase) and inositol polyphosphate 1-phosphatase (IPPase), both of which are targets of lithium. Thus, lithium may initiate many of its therapeutic effects by inhibiting these enzymes, thereby bringing about a cascade of downstream effects involving PKC and gene expression changes.

Source.   Adapted from Gould TD, Chen G, Manji HK: "Mood Stabilizer Pharmacology." *Clinical Neuroscience Research* 2:193–212, 2003.

cide victims compared with control subjects, and Wang and Friedman (1996) measured PKC-mediated phosphorylation in postmortem brains and found it to be increased in the brains of patients with bipolar disorder. Pandey et al. (2002) recently reported that PKC activity, PLC activity, and expression of their specific isozymes were decreased in the platelets of bipolar patients compared with control subjects. This investigative group also reported that expression of myristoylated alanine-rich C kinase substrate (MARCKS), a major PKC substrate, was decreased in these same samples (Pandey et al. 2002).

Thus, there is ample evidence of alterations of phosphoinositol signaling in patients with mood disorders. It remains to be seen, however, if these differences observed are relevant to the pathophysiology of mood disorders.

GSK-3

GSK-3 is a serine/threonine kinase that is normally highly active in cells and is deactivated by signals originating from numerous signaling pathways (e.g., the Wnt pathway, PI_3 kinase pathway, protein kinase A, PKC). It is found in two forms, alpha and beta, that have similar, but not always identical, biological functions. Cellular targets of GSK-3 are numerous and often depend on the signaling pathway that is acting on it (because of cellular localization and regional sequestration). For example, Wnt pathway inhibition of GSK-3 activates the transcription factor β-catenin, whereas inhibition of GSK-3 in the insulin–PI_3 kinase signaling pathway activates the enzyme glycogen synthase. Targets of GSK-3 include transcription factors (β-catenin, CREB, c-Jun), proteins bound to microtubules (tau, microtubule associate protein 1B [MAP1B], kinesin light chain), cell cycle mediators (cyclin D, human ninein), and regulators of metabolism (glycogen synthase, pyruvate dehydrogenase).

As a component of many signaling pathways, with multiple cellular targets to choose from, GSK-3 regulates a diverse array of cellular processes such as glycogen synthesis, gene transcription, events related to synaptic plasticity, apoptosis, and the circadian cycle. Although many of these functions are likely critically important to both cellular and organism functioning, GSK-3 is currently receiving the most interest as a regulator of apoptosis and cellular resilience. Generally, increased activity of GSK-3 is pro-apoptotic, whereas inhibiting GSK-3 attenuates or prevents apoptosis.

In 1996, Klein and Melton observed that lithium administration to developing *Xenopus* embryos resulted in duplication of the dorsal axis, similar to downregulation of GSK-3. This led to the discovery of GSK-3-inhibitory effects of lithium (Klein and Melton 1996). Recent studies suggest a significant inhibition of this enzyme in the rodent brain at therapeutic serum lithium levels during long-term treatment. For example, T.D. Gould and colleagues (2004a) found that 9 days of lithium treatment increased cytosolic protein levels of β-catenin (a transcription factor regulated directly by GSK-3). This protein level increase was accompanied by a small but significant decrease in β-catenin mRNA levels, further suggesting that lithium exerted its actions posttranslationally by inhibiting GSK-3 (the mRNA changes reflecting cellular compensation) (T.D. Gould et al. 2004a).

A great deal of hormonal, physiological, and behavioral evidence suggests that dysregulation of circadian rhythms occurs in both bipolar disorder and unipolar depression (Buysse et al., Chapter 43, in this volume). It has been known for quite some time that lithium treatment lengthens the circadian period in diverse species, ranging in complexity from individual cells to humans, suggesting that there is a single evolutionarily conserved target for this action. However, the cellular target for lithium's effect on circadian cycles is unknown. Recent evidence suggests that lithium also may regulate circadian cycles through inhibition of GSK-3. Of relevance may be a recent preclinical finding in *Drosophila* (fruit fly) suggesting that GSK-3 is an important mediator of the circadian cycle. It is therefore interesting to speculate that GSK-3 has a similarly general—and evolutionarily conserved—action in the function of the mammalian circadian clock (T.D. Gould and Manji 2002).

Recent evidence suggests that GSK-3 may regulate certain forms of memory in the mammalian brain. Specifically, Hernandez et al. (2002) described water maze spatial learning deficits in a transgenic mouse that conditionally overexpresses GSK-3β in the brain. Thus, the evidence cumulatively presented suggests possible roles that increased expression of GSK-3 (or increased activity of GSK-3–regulated pathways) may play in mood disorders—specifically, regulation of 1) apoptosis and cellular resiliency, 2) circadian rhythms, and 3) learning and memory, which are all impaired in mood disorders, as discussed in this chapter and elsewhere in the text.

Postmortem studies of GSK-3 levels in the brains of patients with mood disorders to date have not found decreased levels. However, as noted previously, GSK-3 is involved in a multitude of cellular signaling pathways and regulates a diverse array of targets. Thus, future studies will likely address many of these additional molecules for putative involvement.

PKC

Current animal models of mania that have been used in the study of mood disorders include kindling, behavioral or amphetamine sensitization, and glucocorticoid administration.

Kindling is an animal model for epilepsy that has been proposed to have similarities with pathophysiological aspects of bipolar disorder, in which repeated administration of electrical stimuli (that are subthreshold to produce seizures by themselves) results in an epileptic focus and a permanent state of hyperexcitability to the stimulus. Studies on rats have consistently shown the upregulatory effect of kindling on PKC activity and protein concentration in the amygdala and in the neocortex.

Studies also have implicated alterations in PKC activity as mediators of long-term alterations in neuronal excitability in the brain following chronic stimulant use. Several independent laboratories have now shown that both acute and chronic amphetamine use produces an alteration in PKC activity, its relative cytosol-to-membrane distribution, as well as the phosphorylation of a major PKC substrate, growth-associated protein (GAP)-43, which has been implicated in long-term alterations of neurotransmitter release. Furthermore, PKC inhibitors have been shown to block the acute responses (as assessed by both behavioral and in vivo microdialysis studies) to amphetamine and cocaine, as well as cocaine-induced sensitization.

Abnormalities of circulating glucocorticoids are well known to be associated with affective symptomatology, and interestingly, elevated glucocorticoids have been associated with both depressive and manic symptomatology. Repeated administration of dexamethasone for 10 days results in a significant increase in maximal binding capacity (B_{max}) of [^{3}H]phorbol 12,13-dibutyrate binding to PKC, increased PKC activity, and increased levels of PKC-α and -ϵ in the rat hippocampus. It is indeed striking that behavioral sensitization and kindling models (postulated to represent models of bipolar disorder and mania) as well as dexamethasone administration all produce alterations in the PKC signaling pathway in critical limbic structures because lithium and valproate also target the very same biochemical targets. Thus, although considerable caution obviously needs to be used when extrapolating from rodent brain and animal behavioral models, the fact that these two models and glucocorticoid administration are associated with opposite effects on PKC signaling to those observed with chronic lithium or valproate is compelling (T.D. Gould et al. 2004a).

Interestingly, evidence also suggests that chronic antidepressant administration may modulate PKC activity in limbic and limbic-associated areas of rat brain. PKC has been shown to regulate the activity of norepinephrine, dopamine, and serotonin transporters. Whether these complex effects of antidepressants on PKC activity underlie their apparent ability to trigger manic episodes, and perhaps promote rapid cycling in susceptible individuals, remains to be determined.

Reelin

Recent postmortem studies have found that an unexpected molecule may be involved in the pathophysiology of severe neuropsychiatric disorders, including bipolar disorder and schizophrenia. Reelin is a member of a growing group of diverse proteins whose absence is associated with an almost invariable phenotype—inversion of cerebral cortical layers and reduction or absence of cerebellar foliation. Costa et al. (2001) first showed that reelin protein and mRNA were reduced in several brain areas in both schizophrenia and psychotic bipolar disorder, leading to their suggestion that reelin deficiency may be a vulnerability factor for psychosis independent of diagnosis.

Subsequently, Fatemi et al. (2000) confirmed Costa and colleagues' findings but also found similar reductions in reelin protein in hippocampi of nonpsychotic bipolar and depressed patients, suggesting that reelin deficiency was not a marker of psychosis alone. Hong et al. (2000) showed that blood levels of reelin were extremely low to undetectable in children afflicted with a variant of lissencephaly (lack of the normal complex folding of the cortex in the brain). These children had various mutations involving the *RELN* gene and had severe delays in neurological and cognitive development. Later, Fatemi et al. (2002) and others found deficits in reelin protein in the brain and blood of subjects with autism, another neurodevelopmental disorder that is associated with significant cognitive dysfunction, in combination with a vulnerability toward defective reelin inheritance.

Bipolar subjects also had significant deficits in glutamic acid decarboxylase proteins of 65 and 67 kDA (GAD 65 and GAD 67) compared with nonbipolar control subjects (Fatemi et al. 2005). In contrast, reelin deficiency was limited to the 180-kDa species in the schizophrenic cerebella. All schizophrenic and depressed subjects also showed significant reductions in GAD 65 and GAD 67 proteins compared with control subjects. These results confirm a recent report by Benes and colleagues (cited in Heckers et al. 2002) showing a global deficit in levels of GAD 65 and 67 in the hippocampi of patients with bipolar disorder. Interestingly, some brain GABAergic interneurons share the synthetic machinery for production of reelin and GAD 65 and 67 proteins and appear to be dysfunctional in bipolar subjects. Finally, deficits in hippocampal and cerebellar reelin levels in bipolar subjects correlate well with decreases in levels of blood reelin in patients with bipolar disorder. Future larger studies should correlate the extent of reelin deficiency observed in the hippocampus and cerebellum of patients with bipolar disorder with blood and cerebrospinal fluid levels of the same protein to define better the role of reelin in the etiology of bipolar disorder and other neurodevelopmental disorders, such as schizophrenia and autism.

Sleep Deprivation

Sleep deprivation is the only known therapeutic maneuver that appears to alter mood in most bipolar and unipolar patients in a matter of hours. Sleep deprivation is also capable of triggering switches into mania or hypomania; therefore, the study of the potential cellular mechanisms by which sleep deprivation may bring about these rapid behavioral changes in patients with mood disorders may be particularly informative. Incontrovertible evidence now indicates that the expression of selected critical genes varies dramatically during sleep and waking events, which likely plays a major role in regulating various and long-term neuroplastic events (Cirelli and Tononi 2000). mRNA differential display, microarray, and biochemical studies have shown that short-term sleep deprivation is associated with an immediate 1) increase in levels of pCREB (the active form of this transcription factor), 2) increase in expression of BDNF, and 3) increase in expression of BDNF's receptor TrkB.

As discussed earlier, these are precisely the plasticity-related molecules whose expression is increased by chronic antidepressant treatment. In an extension of the gene expression studies, Cirelli and Tononi (2000) hypothesized that a key factor responsible for the induction of the plasticity genes might be the level of activity of the neuromodulatory noradrenergic and serotonergic systems. Both of these systems project diffusely to most of the brain, where they regulate gene expression, and are quiescent only during rapid eye movement sleep.

During normal sleep, the noradrenergic system, represented by the locus coeruleus (LC), is quiescent during rapid eye movement sleep. During sleep deprivation, the noradrenergic system is activated at a time when it is normally quiet. The activity of the noradrenergic system in a different postsynaptic environment than normal may be the key factor in inducing physiological changes that result in mood elevation in depressed patients. One possible effect of an active noradrenergic system during a time when it is normally quiescent is an effect on gene expression. For example, the *CREB* and *BDNF* genes, which are known to be involved with neuroplasticity, may increase their expression levels in response. Increases in the expression of these genes have been shown to be downstream effects of antidepressants. Thus, a more rapid increase in their expression by manipulations of the noradrenergic system may underlie the rapid antidepressant response to sleep deprivation (Payne et al. 2002).

Human Evidence of Neuroplasticity

The body of preclinical (animal) data showing neurotrophic and neuroprotective effects of mood stabilizers is striking; however, considerable caution must be exercised in extrapolating to the clinical situation with humans. In view of lithium's consistent effects on the levels of the cytoprotective protein Bcl-2 in the frontal cortex, Drevets (2000) reanalyzed data indicating approximately 40% reductions in subgenual PFC volumes in subjects with familial mood disorder. The results of this reanalysis showed that, consistent with the neurotrophic and neuroprotective effects of lithium, the patients receiving chronic lithium or valproate had subgenual PFC volumes that were significantly higher than the volumes in non-lithium-treated or non-valproate-treated patients and not significantly different from the volumes in control subjects.

N-Acetylaspartate

Although the results of the aforementioned studies suggest that mood stabilizers may have provided neuroprotective effects during naturalistic use, considerable caution is warranted in view of the small sample size and cross-sectional nature of the study. To investigate the potential neurotrophic effects of lithium in humans more definitively, a longitudinal clinical study (Moore et al. 2000a) used ^{1}H-magnetic resonance spectroscopy to quantitate *N*-acetylaspartate (NAA), a putative marker of neuronal viability levels. Four weeks of lithium treatment produced a significant increase in NAA levels, effects that were localized almost exclusively to gray matter in the brain. These findings provide intriguing indirect support for the contention that chronic lithium use increases neuronal viability and function.

Furthermore, the correlation between lithium-induced NAA increases and regional voxel gray matter content was ~0.97, providing evidence for co-localization with the regional specific Bcl-2 increases observed (e.g., gray vs. white matter) in the rodent brain cortices. These results suggest that chronic lithium use may exert not only consistent neuroprotective effects (as has been seen in a variety of preclinical paradigms) but also neurotrophic effects in humans.

Gray Matter

A follow-up volumetric magnetic resonance imaging study has reported that 4 weeks of lithium treatment also significantly increased total gray matter content in the human brain (Moore et al. 2000b), suggesting an increase in the volume of the neuropil, the mosslike layer composed of axonal and dendritic fibers that occupies much of the cortex gray matter volume. A more detailed subregional analysis of this brain imaging data is ongoing and clearly shows that lithium produces a regionally selective increase in gray matter, with prominent effects in the hippocampus and caudate. No changes in overall gray matter volume were observed in healthy volunteers treated chronically with lithium, suggesting that lithium produces a reversal of illness-related atrophy rather than nonspecific gray matter increases (Sassi et al. 2002).

Ongoing studies are attempting to determine the precise relation between the lithium-induced increases in regional NAA levels and gray matter volumes and treatment response. Michael and associates (2003) investigated the effects of a course of electroconvulsive therapy (ECT) on NAA levels in the left amygdalar region in 28 severely depressed patients. They found that a significant increase in NAA was observed only in ECT responders ($n=14$). Moreover, 5 of the 14 nonresponders to ECT monotherapy were then given adjunctive antidepressants (while ECT continued) and rescanned; these investigators found that this combination therapy group showed both clinical improvement and a significant increase in NAA. Although these clinical results are preliminary, they suggest that the neurotrophic effects of antidepressant treatments (and likely lithium) are indeed associated with treatment response (although a causal relation has yet to be established).

Neuroimmune Modulators and the Pathophysiology of Mood Disorders

Increasing evidence shows that immune modulators may play a critical role in the pathophysiology of mood disorders or the generation of specific mood symptoms. It is beyond the scope of this chapter to review this growing literature in detail. The interested reader is referred to several outstanding reviews (Kronfol and Remick 2000; Leonard 2001; Raison and Miller 2001). Here, we discuss salient aspects most pertinent to the impairments of cellular plasticity observed in mood disorders.

Cytokines and the Immune System

The immune system and the CNS form a bidirectional communication network. The association of the immune system with mood disorders comes from two directions: 1) evidence is mounting that sickness-like behavior (somnolence, reduced appetite, fatigue) seen in mood disorders may be associated with altered immune function, and

2) numerous medical disorders (e.g., hepatitis C, multiple sclerosis) and treatments that regulate immune function are associated with psychiatric symptomatology.

Nonspecific immune defenses begin rapidly after the entry of a microbial product into the body. Activated immune cells release proinflammatory cytokines, which play a critical role in recruiting additional immune cells to the site of infection, leading to a shift toward increased production of acute-phase reactants, such as C-reactive proteins and haptoglobin. Cytokines are large proteins that are not able to cross the blood-brain barrier but may be able to reach the CNS by stimulating peripheral nerves (e.g., the vagus nerve) with de novo synthesis of cytokines in the brain. Each cytokine interacts with a specific plasma membrane α receptor named for the associated cytokine. The α subunits form heterodimeric complexes with other proteins and subsequently form a tripartite receptor associated with a protein tyrosine kinase called Janus kinase (JAK).

The sequence of events leading to altered gene expression from a cytokine-bound receptor begins with activation of the receptor-associated JAK, which is critical for further signal transduction. The activated JAK phosphorylate tyrosine resides in the intracellular domains of receptor chains, creating docking sites for src homology 2 (SH2) domain–containing signaling proteins and activating signal transducers and activators of transcription (STATs), which reside latent in the cytoplasm in the absence of cytokine stimulation. JAK phosphorylates the receptor-associated STATs, which subsequently dissociate from the receptors, dimerize through their SH2 domains, and translocate to the nucleus. The STAT dimers bind to specific elements in the promoter regions of their target genes to induce transcription together with several other transcriptional coactivators.

Cytokines and Depression

Initial interest in cytokines in mood disorders came from the observations of emerging depressive symptoms in patients receiving purified or recombinant cytokines and observations of increased peripheral levels of proinflammatory cytokines in mood disorders. However, it is unclear whether the cytokine elevations contribute to the provocation of the disorder or are secondary to the illness (i.e., directly or indirectly elevated by the depression). The data showing involvement of cytokines in mood disorders are as follows:

- Animals treated with cytokines, such as interleukin (IL)-1β or tumor necrosis factor (TNF)-α, show a constellation of centrally mediated symptoms referred to as "sickness behaviors." These behaviors include reduced locomotor activity, diminished social interactions, anhedonia, and diminished consumatory behaviors.

- The above data suggest that cytokines may induce depression-like symptoms; conversely, Maes and colleagues (1993a, 1993b, 1993c) initially reported an increase in plasma concentrations of IL-1 and IL-6 in subjects with major depression. Levine et al. (1999) reported high IL-1β, low IL-6, and normal TNF-α levels in the cerebrospinal fluid of 13 hospitalized patients with untreated major depression, compared with healthy volunteers. Multiple studies have reported that depression is accompanied by increased levels of circulating cytokines or their soluble receptors, including IL-2, soluble IL-2 receptors, IL-1β, IL-1 receptor antagonist, IL-6, soluble IL-6 receptor, and λ-interferon (IFN) (Maes 1999).

  However, not all studies are consistent. One of the limitations of measuring cytokine levels is that cytokine-induced cell activation also leads to a release of soluble receptors (which inhibit the biological activity of the cytokine); therefore, circulating levels do not accurately reflect the functional state of the affected organ. Therefore, the differences in circulating levels of any specific cytokine between subject groups may not be useful.

- Administration of cytokines in humans (typically in patients with cancer, hepatitis C, and AIDS) with high doses of IL-2, IFN-α, and TNF-α have been reported to induce neuropsychiatric symptoms, including depressed mood, anhedonia, loss of appetite, fatigue, and cognitive disturbances, which are related to cytokine treatment rather than to the primary illness. The onset of these symptoms is sooner with subjects receiving IL-2 (first week); in contrast, it takes 4–8 weeks in subjects receiving IFN-α. Symptoms of hypersomnolence, decreased appetite, and decreased energy often precede a depressed mood. Furthermore, in cancer patients, treatment with the antidepressant paroxetine was useful in preventing the development of a depressed mood but not fatigue.

Vulnerability Factors for Cytokine-Induced Depression

The rate of depression in chronically medically ill patients is 5–10 times higher than in the general population. In a prospective study of neuropsychiatric effects in subjects with hepatitis C treated with IFN-α and ribavirin over 24 weeks, the treated group had a significant increase in depression, whereas the control group that did not

receive any treatment did not. Patients with depression before treatment was initiated tended to have higher scores on multiple rating scales for depression (Dieperink et al. 2003). These results suggest that preexisting depression, however mild, is a vulnerability factor. However, the specificity of this finding and biological factors involved are yet to be elucidated.

Possible Mechanisms of Cytokine-Associated Depression

Cytokines may induce or precipitate depression by several mechanisms, including impaired synthesis of serotonin with tryptophan depletion; dopamine depletion; HPA axis and plasticity effects; and disruption of neurogenesis.

Impaired Synthesis of Serotonin and Tryptophan Depletion

Immune system activation is associated with the induction of indoleamine 2,3-dioxygenase, an enzyme that switches the metabolism of tryptophan toward the synthesis of kynurenine and quinolinic acid. In a recent study of 16 subjects with renal cell carcinoma or malignant melanoma, subjects who received IFN-α or IL-2, or combined treatment, had decreased serum levels of tryptophan during the course of therapy, which correlated with the severity of depression (Capuron et al. 2002). Similarly, in another study, patients with malignant melanoma were randomized to either paroxetine or placebo treatment, 2 weeks prior to initiating IFN-α therapy. All subjects had significant increases in kynurenine, neopterin (a marker for immune activation), and the kynurenine to tryptophan ratio. Decreases in tryptophan levels in patients who were receiving placebo correlated with depressive, anxious, and cognitive symptoms but not with neurovegetative symptoms. Patients who received paroxetine had similar increases in neopterin and kynurenine as those who received placebo, but the decrease in tryptophan was not statistically significant. This finding suggests that paroxetine's antidepressant effects in subjects receiving IFN-α are likely due to its central serotonergic regulation (Capuron et al. 2003).

Maes and colleagues (2001) reported that IL-2 alone or in combination with IFN-α induced a decrease in serum dipeptidyl peptidase IV (DPP IV), a membrane-bound serine protease that acts to catalyze the cleavage of at least some cytokines and peptides, hence affecting cytokine production and immune activity. At 3–5 days after treatment, depression scores were elevated in patients receiving treatment for metastatic cancer, with increases in the kynurenine/tryptophan quotient, and were inversely related to DPP IV levels. In addition, the treatment resulted in elevated levels of IL-6 and the IL-2 receptor, which were inversely related to DPP IV levels. These data cumulatively suggest that one of the mechanisms by which cytokines may induce depression is by tryptophan depletion, which has been shown to induce depression in vulnerable subjects.

Dopamine Depletion

Chronic treatment with IFN-α has been associated with psychomotor retardation; Parkinson's disease that is responsive to levodopa; and impaired memory, cognitive, and executive functions. These effects suggest a depletion of dopamine in the basal ganglia and a relation between dopamine depletion and cytokine-associated depression.

HPA Axis and Plasticity

The seminal work of Besedovsky showed that the intraperitoneal injection of IL-1β activates the HPA axis in rats; this effect has been replicated in multiple studies (Dunn 2000). These effects occur predominantly after administration of IL-1, TNF-α, and IL-6 and are not seen as frequently with IL-2 or IFN-α. The activation of the HPA axis by IL-1, IL-6, and TNF-α is at least partly the result of an increase in secretion of corticotropin-releasing factor (CRF) because the increase in glucocorticoids is blocked by CRF antiserum. The data that an exaggerated corticotropin and cortisol response to an initial injection of IFN-α predicts subsequent development of depression further support this finding. Moreover, pretreatment with a CRF receptor antagonist (CP-154,526) and imipramine, but not naloxone or indomethacin, attenuates the depressive effects of IFN-α. The depressive effects of high proinflammatory cytokines may in part be mediated by the HPA axis. Further, Raison and Miller (2003) argued that chronically high glucocorticoids lead to desensitization of glucocorticoid receptors, resulting in insufficient glucocorticoid signaling and unrestrained immune activation.

The above review suggests that treatment with cytokines is associated in early stages with neurovegetative symptoms, which may in part be related to insufficient glucocorticoid signaling and dopamine depletion, and later with manifestation of a depressed mood, reversible by antidepressants, which may in part be induced by tryptophan depletion and reduced serotonin availability. A full understanding of the mechanisms by which the immune system is able to mediate its effects through specified signaling pathways in the CNS undoubtedly will be of increasing importance in the understanding of these complex disorders.

Disruption of Neurogenesis

In a novel theory, a failure of adult hippocampal neurogenesis has been proposed to underlie the biological and cellular basis of major depression (reviewed in Kempermann and Kronenberg 2003). Santarelli et al. (2003) reported that irradiation of the hippocampus in a mouse model blocked the effectiveness of antidepressant drugs in promoting neurogenesis and in alleviating depression and anxiety-like behavior. Monje et al. (2003) suggested that irradiation may inhibit neurogenesis through inflammation. They showed that irradiation blocked differentiation of neural stem cells in vivo. Irradiation perturbed the structural microenvironment of the "stem cell niche" in the hippocampus, disrupting close interactions between stem cells and blood vessels, leading to a decrease in adult neurogenesis. Furthermore, blocking inflammation elicited by either irradiation or injection of bacterial lipopolysaccharide with indomethacin restored hippocampal neurogenesis (Monje et al. 2003).

Evidence Suggesting That Mitochondrial Function May Play a Critical Role in the Pathophysiology and Treatment of Bipolar Disorder

Is bipolar disorder associated with impairments of mitochondrial function? Indeed, Kato and Kato (2000) had anticipated some of the recent developments in the field when they first proposed that mitochondrial dysfunction may play an important role in the pathophysiology of bipolar disorder. Since then, there have been a host of human neuroimaging and postmortem brain studies, as well as preclinical molecular and cellular biological studies, which strongly support the argument that mitochondria may play a central role in the impairments of plasticity and cellular resilience manifest in bipolar disorder. It is important to emphasize at the outset that it is not our contention that bipolar disorder is a classical mitochondrial disorder; thus, the vast majority of bipolar disorder patients do not show the symptoms of classical mitochondrial disorders, such as optic and retinal atrophy, seizures, dementia, ataxia, myopathy, exercise intolerance, cardiac conduction defects, diabetes, and lactic acidosis.

Studies of fibroblasts from patients with the syndrome of mitochondrial encephalomyopathy, lactic acidosis, and strokelike episodes (which is frequently caused by a mutation in the mitochondrial transfer RNA) have shown an elevated basal level of ionized calcium (Ca^{2+}) with impairments in normal sequestration of Ca^{2+} influxes induced by depolarization and alterations in maintaining normal mitochondrial membrane potentials. This inability to buffer intracellular Ca^{2+} may cause toxic cell injury and compromise long-term viability of neurons in patients with mitochondrial encephalomyopathies. It is thus clear that dysregulation of Ca^{2+} homeostasis is an essential component of the pathophysiology in classical mitochondriopathies. As discussed earlier, Ca^{2+} is a common signaling element and plays a critical role in the CNS by regulating the activity of diverse enzymes and facilitating neurotransmitter release. Importantly, excessively high levels of Ca^{2+} are also a critical mediator of cell death cascades within neurons, necessitating diverse homeostatic mechanisms to regulate intracellular calcium levels very precisely (Szabo et al. 2004).

Interestingly, impaired regulation of Ca^{2+} cascades has been one of the most reproducible biological abnormalities described in bipolar disorder research. For this reason, mechanisms involved in Ca^{2+} regulation have been postulated to underlie aspects of the pathophysiology of bipolar disorder (Bowden et al. 1988).

Most recently, Kato and associates (2003) investigated cytosolic and mitochondrial Ca^{2+} responses to platelet-activating factor; carbonyl cyanide *m*-chlorophenylhydrazone (CCCP), a mitochondrial uncoupler that abolishes mitochondrial Ca^{2+} uptake; and thapsigargin in lymphoblastoid cells from subjects with bipolar disorder. They found that the thapsigargin-induced cytosolic Ca^{2+} response was significantly higher in patients with bipolar disorder, effects that were not seen when the effects of Ca^{2+} influx from outside the plasma membrane was eliminated with a Ca^{2+}-free measurement buffer. By contrast, response to thapsigargin tended to be higher in patients with bipolar disorder when at the Ca^{2+}-free conditions. Furthermore, CCCP-induced Ca^{2+} responses differed significantly between mitochondrial DNA 5178/10398 haplotypes that had been reported to be associated with bipolar disorder. Together, these results clearly suggest that the mitochondrial–endoplasmic reticulum calcium regulation system contributes to the Ca^{2+} abnormalities seen in bipolar disorder (Kato et al. 2003).

Overall, these findings are of great importance in view of the growing body of evidence showing the potential toxic effects of elevated intracellular Ca^{2+} in neuronal and glial cerebral cells. In fact, studies have reported that both the subcellular compartmentalization of Ca^{2+} and the source of the Ca^{2+} may be greater determinants of neurotoxicity than the absolute intracellular Ca^{2+} levels per se (Sapolsky 2000b), and there are major relations between Ca^{2+} released from IP_3-sensitive endoplasmic reticulum stores and mitochondrial Ca^{2+} uptake (Mattson et al. 2000). Most recently, Konradi and associates (2004) have undertaken an elegant series of postmortem brain microarray studies that showed that nuclear mRNA coding for mitochondrial proteins was decreased in bipolar disorder in comparison with schizophrenia. These nuclear mRNA codings are involved in gene expression of regulating oxidative phosphorylation in the mitochondrial inner membrane and the adenosine triphosphate–dependent process of proteosome degradation (includes subunits of complexes I [the reduced form of nicotinamide-adenine dinucleotide dehydrogenase], IV [cytochrome *c* oxidase], and V [adenosine triphosphate synthase]) (Konradi et al. 2004).

Conclusion

As we have shown, a considerable body of evidence both conceptually and experimentally supports abnormalities in the regulation of signaling as integral to the underlying neurobiology of recurrent mood disorders. The pathophysiology of this illness must account for not only the profound changes in mood but also a constellation of neurovegetative features derived from dysfunction in limbic-related regions, such as the hippocampus, hypothalamus, and brain stem. The highly integrated monoamine and prominent neuropeptide pathways are known to originate and project heavily within these regions of the brain; thus, it is not surprising that abnormalities have been noted in their function across clinical studies. In fact, the contribution of these pathways to the pathophysiology of mood disorders must be reasonably consistent, given the variability that might be expected in assessing such dynamic systems under the constraints in experimental design imposed on such research. In the past, much of the research effort in the neurobiology of mood disorders focused on identifying which of these systems might be etiological in nature; we suggest that a greater understanding would be achieved if we investigated the relative contributions in the response of the system to the underlying neurobiology of the disease process. This will become particularly important as we begin to identify the susceptibility genes for bipolar disorder in the coming years.

It is also becoming increasingly clear that for many patients with refractory major depressive disorders, new drugs simply mimicking the "traditional" drugs that directly or indirectly alter neurotransmitter levels and those that bind to cell-surface receptors may be of limited benefit (Nestler 1998). This is clear because such strategies implicitly assume that the target receptor(s)—and downstream signal mediators—are functionally intact and that altered synaptic activity thus will be transduced to modify the postsynaptic "throughput" of the system. However, the possible existence of abnormalities in signal transduction pathways (noted extensively in this chapter) suggests that for patients with major depressive disorders refractory to conventional medications, improved therapeutics may be obtained only by the direct targeting of postreceptor sites. Recent discoveries of various mechanisms involved in the formation and inactivation of second messengers offer the promise for the development of novel pharmacological agents designed to target signal transduction pathways (Guo et al. 2000).

Although clearly more complex than the development of receptor-specific drugs, the design of novel agents to selectively affect second messenger systems may be possible because they are quite heterogeneous at the molecular and cellular levels, are linked to receptors in a variety of ways, and are expressed in different stoichiometries in diverse cell types (Manji and Duman 2001). Additionally, because signal transduction pathways have certain unique characteristics depending on their activity state, they offer built-in targets for relative specificity of action, depending on the set point of the substrate. It is also noteworthy that various strategies to enhance neurotrophic factor signaling are under investigation. An increasing number of strategies are being investigated to develop small molecular switches for protein-protein interactions, which have the potential to regulate the activity of growth factors, MAP kinase cascades, and interactions between homo- and heterodimers of the Bcl-2 family of proteins (Guo et al. 2000). These developments hold much promise for the advancement of novel therapeutics for the long-term treatment of mood disorders.

References

Bowden CL, Huang LG, Javors MA, et al: Calcium function in affective disorders and healthy controls. Biol Psychiatry 23:367–376, 1988

Capuron L, Ravaud A, Neveu PJ, et al: Association between decreased serum tryptophan concentrations and depressive symptoms in cancer patients undergoing cytokine therapy. Mol Psychiatry 7:468–473, 2002

Capuron L, Neurauter G, Musselman DL, et al: Interferon-alpha-induced changes in tryptophan metabolism: relationship to depression and paroxetine treatment. Biol Psychiatry 54:906–914, 2003

Caspi A, Sugden K, Moffitt TE, et al: Influence of life stress on depression: moderation by a polymorphism in the 5-HTT gene. Science 301:386–389, 2003

Chen B, Dowlatshahi D, MacQueen GM, et al: Increased hippocampal BDNF immunoreactivity in subjects treated with antidepressant medication. Biol Psychiatry 50:260–265, 2001

Cirelli C, Tononi G: Differential expression of plasticity-related genes in waking and sleep and their regulation by the noradrenergic system. J Neurosci 20:9187–9194, 2000

Costa E, Davis J, Grayson DR, et al: Dendritic spine hypoplasticity and downregulation of reelin and GABAergic tone in schizophrenia vulnerability. Neurobiol Dis 8:723–742, 2001

Czeh B, Michaelis T, Watanabe T, et al: Stress-induced changes in cerebral metabolites, hippocampal volume, and cell proliferation are prevented by antidepressant treatment with tianeptine. Proc Natl Acad Sci U S A 98:12796–12801, 2001

DeVries AC, Joh HD, Bernard O, et al: Social stress exacerbates stroke outcome by suppressing Bcl-2 expression. Proc Natl Acad Sci U S A 98:11824–11828, 2001

Dieperink E, Ho SB, Thuras P, et al: A prospective study of neuropsychiatric symptoms associated with interferon-α-2b and ribavirin therapy for patients with chronic hepatitis C. Psychosomatics 44:104–112, 2003

Drevets WC: Neuroimaging studies of mood disorders. Biol Psychiatry 48:813–829, 2000

D'Sa C, Duman RS: Antidepressants and neuroplasticity. Bipolar Disord 4:183–194, 2002

Duman R: Synaptic plasticity and mood disorders. Mol Psychiatry 7 (suppl 1):S29–S34, 2002

Duman RS, Malberg J, Thome J: Neural plasticity to stress and antidepressant treatment. Biol Psychiatry 46:1181–1191, 1999

Dunn AJ: Cytokine activation of the HPA axis. Ann N Y Acad Sci 917:608–617, 2000

Fatemi SH, Earle JA, McMenomy T: Reduction in Reelin immunoreactivity in hippocampus of subjects with schizophrenia, bipolar disorder and major depression. Mol Psychiatry 5:654–663, 571, 2000

Fatemi SH, Stary JM, Egan EA: Reduced blood levels of reelin as a vulnerability factor in pathophysiology of autistic disorder. Cell Mol Neurobiol 22:139–152, 2002

Fatemi SH, Stary JM, Earle JA, et al: GABAergic dysfunction in schizophrenia and mood disorders as reflected by decreased levels of glutamic acid decarboxylase 65 and 67 kDA and Reelin proteins in cerebellum. Schizophr Res 72:109–122, 2005

Gilbertson MW, Shenton ME, Ciszewski A, et al: Smaller hippocampal volume predicts pathologic vulnerability to psychological trauma. Nat Neurosci 5:1242–1247, 2002

Gould E, Tanapat P, Rydel T, et al: Regulation of hippocampal neurogenesis in adulthood. Biol Psychiatry 48:715–720, 2000

Gould TD, Manji HK: The Wnt signaling pathway in bipolar disorder. Neuroscientist 8:497–511, 2002

Gould TD, Quiroz JA, Singh J, et al: Emerging experimental therapeutics for bipolar disorder: insights from the molecular and cellular actions of current mood stabilizers. Mol Psychiatry 9:734–755, 2004a

Gould TD, Zarate CA, Manji HK: Glycogen synthase kinase-3: a target for novel bipolar disorder treatments. J Clin Psychiatry 65:10–21, 2004b

Guo Z, Zhou D, Schultz PG: Designing small-molecule switches for protein-protein interactions. Science 288:2042–2045, 2000

Heckers S, Stone D, Walsh J, et al: Differential hippocampal expression of glutamic acid decarboxylase 65 and 67 messenger RNA in bipolar disorder and schizophrenia. Arch Gen Psychiatry 59:521–529, 2002

Hernandez F, Borrell J, Guaza C, et al: Spatial learning deficit in transgenic mice that conditionally over-express GSK-3beta in the brain but do not form tau filaments. J Neurochem 83:1529–1533, 2003

Hong SE, Shugart YY, Huang DT, et al: Autosomal recessive lissencephaly with cerebellar hypoplasia is associated with human RELN mutations. Nat Genet 26:93–96, 2000

Jope RS, Song L, Li PP, et al: The phosphoinositide signal transduction system is impaired in bipolar affective disorder brain. J Neurochem 66:2402–2409, 1996

Kato T, Kato N: Mitochondrial dysfunction in bipolar disorder. Bipolar Disord 2 (3 pt 1):180–190, 2000

Kato T, Ishiwata M, Mori K, et al: Mechanisms of altered Ca2+ signalling in transformed lymphoblastoid cells from patients with bipolar disorder. Int J Neuropsychopharmacol 6:379–389, 2003

Kempermann G, Kronenberg G: Depressed new neurons? Adult hippocampal neurogenesis and a cellular plasticity hypothesis of major depression. Biol Psychiatry 54:499–503, 2003

Klein PS, Melton DA: A molecular mechanism for the effect of lithium on development. Proc Natl Acad Sci U S A 93:8455–8459, 1996

Konradi C, Eaton M, MacDonald ML, et al: Molecular evidence for mitochondrial dysfunction in bipolar disorder. Arch Gen Psychiatry 61:300–308, 2004

Kronfol Z, Remick DG: Cytokines and the brain: implications for clinical psychiatry. Am J Psychiatry 157:683–694, 2000

Lauterborn JC, Poulsen FR, Stinis CT, et al: Transcript-specific effects of adrenalectomy on seizure-induced BDNF expression in rat hippocampus. Brain Res Mol Brain Res 55:81–91, 1998

Lee SH, Payne ME, Steffens DC, et al: Subcortical lesion severity and orbitofrontal cortex volume in geriatric depression. Biol Psychiatry 54:529–533, 2003

Leonard BE: The immune system, depression and the action of antidepressants. Prog Neuropsychopharmacol Biol Psychiatry 25:767–780, 2001

Levine J, Barak Y, Chengappa KN, et al: Cerebrospinal cytokine levels in patients with acute depression. Neuropsychobiology 40:171–176, 1999

Lyons DM: Stress, depression, and inherited variation in primate hippocampal and prefrontal brain development. Psychopharmacol Bull 36:27–43, 2002

Lyons DM, Yang C, Sawyer-Glover AM, et al: Early life stress and inherited variation in monkey hippocampal volumes. Arch Gen Psychiatry 58:1145–1151, 2001

MacQueen GM, Campbell S, McEwen BS, et al: Course of illness, hippocampal function, and hippocampal volume in major depression. Proc Natl Acad Sci U S A 100:1387–1392, 2003

Maes M: Major depression and activation of the inflammatory response system. Adv Exp Med Biol 461:25–46, 1999

Maes M, Bosmans E, Meltzer HY, et al: Interleukin-1 beta: a putative mediator of HPA axis hyperactivity in major depression? Am J Psychiatry 150:1189–1193, 1993a

Maes M, Scharpe S, Meltzer HY, et al: Relationships between increased haptoglobin plasma levels and activation of cell-mediated immunity in depression. Biol Psychiatry 34:690–701, 1993b

Maes M, Scharpe S, Meltzer HY, et al: Relationships between interleukin-6 activity, acute phase proteins, and function of the hypothalamic-pituitary-adrenal axis in severe depression. Psychiatry Res 49:11–27, 1993c

Maes M, Capuron L, Ravaud A, et al: Lowered serum dipeptidyl peptidase IV activity is associated with depressive symptoms and cytokine production in cancer patients receiving interleukin-2-based immunotherapy. Neuropsychopharmacology 24:130–140, 2001

Manji HK, Duman RS: Impairments of neuroplasticity and cellular resilience in severe mood disorders: implications for the development of novel therapeutics. Psychopharmacol Bull 35:5–49, 2001

Mattson MP, LaFerla FM, Chan SL, et al: Calcium signaling in the ER: its role in neuronal plasticity and neurodegenerative disorders. Trends Neurosci 23:222–229, 2000

McEwen BS: Stress and hippocampal plasticity. Annu Rev Neurosci 22:105–122, 1999

Michael N, Erfurth A, Ohrman P, et al: Neurotrophic effects of electroconvulsive therapy: a proton magnetic resonance study of the left amygdalar region in patients with treatment resistant depression. Neuropsychopharmacology 28:720–725, 2003

Monje ML, Toda H, Palmer TD: Inflammatory blockade restores adult hippocampal neurogenesis. Science 302:1760–1765, 2003

Moore GJ, Bebchuk JM, Hasanat K, et al: Lithium increases N-acetyl-aspartate in the human brain: in vivo evidence in support of bcl-2's neurotrophic effects? Biol Psychiatry 48:1–8, 2000a

Moore GJ, Bebchuk JM, Wilds IB, et al: Lithium-induced increase in human brain grey matter. Lancet 356:1241–1242, 2000b

Nakamura S: Antidepressants induce regeneration of catecholaminergic axon terminals in the rat cerebral cortex. Neurosci Lett 111:64–68, 1990

Nestler EJ: Antidepressant treatments in the 21st century. Biol Psychiatry 44:526–533, 1998

Nestler EJ, Barrot M, DiLeone RJ, et al: Neurobiology of depression. Neuron 34:13–25, 2002

Pandey GN, Dwivedi Y, SridharaRao J, et al: Protein kinase C and phospholipase C activity and expression of their specific isozymes is decreased and expression of MARCKS is increased in platelets of bipolar but not in unipolar patients. Neuropsychopharmacology 26:216–228, 2002

Patapoutian A, Reichardt LF: Trk receptors: mediators of neurotrophin action. Curr Opin Neurobiol 11:272–280, 2001

Payne JL, Quiroz JA, Zarate CA Jr, et al: Timing is everything: does the robust upregulation of noradrenergically regulated plasticity genes underlie the rapid antidepressant effects of sleep deprivation? Biol Psychiatry 52:921–926, 2002

Quiroz JA, Singh J, Gould TD, et al: Emerging experimental therapeutics for bipolar disorder: clues from the molecular pathophysiology. Mol Psychiatry 9:756–776, 2004

Raison CL, Miller AH: The neuroimmunology of stress and depression. Semin Clin Neuropsychiatry 6:277–294, 2001

Rosel P, Arranz B, San L, et al: Altered 5-HT(2A) binding sites and second messenger inositol trisphosphate (IP(3)) levels in hippocampus but not in frontal cortex from depressed suicide victims. Psychiatry Res 99:173–181, 2000

Santarelli L, Saxe M, Gross C, et al: Requirement of hippocampal neurogenesis for the behavioral effects of antidepressants. Science 301:805–809, 2003

Sapolsky RM: Glucocorticoids and hippocampal atrophy in neuropsychiatric disorders. Arch Gen Psychiatry 57:925–935, 2000a

Sapolsky RM: The possibility of neurotoxicity in the hippocampus in major depression: a primer on neuron death. Biol Psychiatry 48:755–765, 2000b

Sassi RB, Nicoletti M, Brambilla P, et al: Increased gray matter volume in lithium-treated bipolar disorder patients. Neurosci Lett 329:243–245, 2002

Shaltiel G, Shamir A, Nemanov L, et al: Inositol monophosphatase activity in brain and lymphocyte-derived cell lines of bipolar patients. World J Biol Psychiatry 2:95–98, 2001

Sheline YI: 3D MRI studies of neuroanatomic changes in unipolar major depression: the role of stress and medical comorbidity. Biol Psychiatry 48:791–800, 2000

Sheline YI, Sanghavi M, Mintun MA, et al: Depression duration but not age predicts hippocampal volume loss in medically healthy women with recurrent major depression. J Neurosci 19:5034–5043, 1999

Sheline YI, Gado MH, Kraemer HC: Untreated depression and hippocampal volume loss. Am J Psychiatry 160:1516–1518, 2003

Shimon H, Agam G, Belmaker RH, et al: Reduced frontal cortex inositol levels in postmortem brain of suicide victims and patients with bipolar disorder. Am J Psychiatry 154:1148–1150, 1997

Szabo ST, Gould TD, Manji HK: Neurotransmitters, receptors, signal transduction, and second messengers in psychiatric disorders, in The American Psychiatric Publishing Textbook of Psychopharmacology, 3rd Edition. Edited by Schatzberg AF, Nemeroff CB. Washington, DC, American Psychiatric Publishing, 2004, pp 3–52

Taylor WD, Payne ME, Krishnan KR, et al: Evidence of white matter tract disruption in MRI hyperintensities. Biol Psychiatry 50:179–183, 2001

Thome J, Sakai N, Shin K, et al: cAMP response element-mediated gene transcription is upregulated by chronic antidepressant treatment. J Neurosci 20:4030–4036, 2000

Wang HY, Friedman E: Enhanced protein kinase C activity and translocation in bipolar affective disorder brains. Biol Psychiatry 40:568–575, 1996

Watanabe Y, Gould E, Daniels DC, et al: Tianeptine attenuates stress-induced morphological changes in the hippocampus. Eur J Pharmacol 222:157–162, 1992

Wellman CL: Dendritic reorganization in pyramidal neurons in medial prefrontal cortex after chronic corticosterone administration. J Neurobiol 49:245–253, 2001

Young EA, Lopez JF, Murphy-Weinberg V, et al: Mineralocorticoid receptor function in major depression. Arch Gen Psychiatry 60:24–28, 2003

13

Brain Imaging

HELEN S. MAYBERG, M.D.

LINKING BRAIN STRUCTURE and brain function is one of the principal strategies used in the study of neurobehavioral syndromes. Historically, localization of specific behaviors used lesion–deficit correlations inferred from patient symptoms and later confirmed by postmortem pathological examinations. Now, X-ray computed tomography (CT) and magnetic resonance imaging (MRI) provide an in vivo means to investigate these same structure–function relations. Physiological mapping also can be performed with methods ranging from direct brain stimulation with measures of single unit electrical activity to noninvasive recordings that use evoked potentials and magnetoencephalography. Positron emission tomography (PET) and single-photon emission computed tomography (SPECT), functional magnetic resonance imaging (fMRI), and magnetic resonance spectroscopy (MRS) offer additional methods to assess many neurophysiological and neurochemical variables, including regional brain blood flow, oxygen and glucose metabolism, blood-brain barrier permeability, tissue pH, amino acid transport, neurotransmitter synthesis, degradation enzyme concentrations, presynaptic transporter sites, and postsynaptic neuroreceptor density and affinity (Toga and Mazziotta 2002). The diversity of the available imaging methods provides a versatile platform for investigating the neurobiology of mood disorders, in which relations between genetics, biochemistry, anatomy, functional neurocircuitry, and systems levels behaviors are strongly implicated but not yet fully characterized. These methods also provide potential

strategies for future development of clinically relevant biomarkers that may improve diagnostic accuracy, guide treatment selection, and identify vulnerable individuals at risk for both illness onset and relapse.

Brain Localization: Historical Perspective

Since Broca's first descriptions of the great limbic lobe, the cingulate (Broca 1878), limbic structures have been a primary focus of studies of emotion. An equally critical role for the frontal lobes, however, has emerged in the characterization of brain regions mediating pathological disturbances of mood. Modern theories regarding the neural localization of depressive illness date back to the 1930s. Kleist's early observations of specific mood and emotional sensations following direct stimulation of the ventral frontal lobes (Brodmann areas 47 and 11) and anterior cingulate highlighted primary limbic as well as frontal and paralimbic regions (Kleist 1937). These experimental studies were paralleled by early neurosurgical procedures targeting the frontal lobes to treat refractory melancholia (Moniz 1937). Studies by Papez (1937), Fulton (1951), and MacLean (1949), among others, further characterized the anatomical pathways linking these limbic and paralimbic regions, thus providing the first anatomical templates for putative "emotional circuits."

Comparative cytoarchitectural, connectivity, and neuro-chemical studies have since delineated reciprocal path-ways linking various limbic structures with widely distrib-uted brain stem, striatal, paralimbic, and neocortical sites (Alexander et al. 1990; Carmichael and Price 1996; Haber et al. 2000; Nauta 1986; Ongur and Price 2000; Vogt and Pandya 1987). Physiological associations between specific pathways and various aspects of motivational, affective, and emotional behaviors in animals are now increasingly well defined (Barbas 1995; Rolls 2000; Tremblay and Schultz 1999).

Building on this preclinical foundation, disruption of pathways mediating normal emotional responses can be seen as the likely pathological substrate for a range of neuropsychiatric syndromes, including major depression. This hypothesis is supported by numerous neuroimaging studies of depressed patient populations and comple-mented by parallel experiments of specific affective be-haviors mapped in healthy volunteers. Together, these converging studies suggest that depression is best charac-terized as a systems level disorder, affecting discrete but functionally linked pathways involving specific cortical, subcortical, and limbic sites and their associated neu-rotransmitter and peptide mediators critical for the nor-mal regulation of mood, motivation, reinforcement, and circadian functioning (Mayberg 1997, 2003). Structural and functional neuroimaging have assumed a unique po-sition in characterizing these pathways.

Structural Imaging Studies

Depression in Neurological Disease

Lesion–deficit correlation studies indicate that certain disorders are more likely to be associated with major de-pression than are others: 1) discrete brain lesions, as seen with trauma, surgery, stroke, tumors, and certain types of ep-ilepsy; 2) neurodegenerative diseases with regionally con-fined pathologies, such as Parkinson's disease, Hunting-ton's disease, and Alzheimer's disease; 3) disorders affecting diffuse or multiple random locations, such as multiple sclerosis; and 4) system illness with known central ner-vous system effects, such as thyroid disease, cancer, and acquired immunodeficiency syndrome (AIDS) (Starkstein and Robinson 1993).

CT and MRI studies in stroke patients have shown a high association of mood changes with infarctions of the frontal lobe and basal ganglia, particularly those occur-ring in close proximity to the frontal pole or involving the caudate nucleus (Robinson et al. 1984; Starkstein et al. 1987). Studies of patients with head trauma, brain tumors,

and surgical resections (Stuss and Benson 1986) further suggest that dorsolateral rather than ventral-frontal le-sions are more commonly associated with depression and depressive-like symptoms such as apathy and psycho-motor slowing. As might be expected, more precise local-ization of "depression-specific regions" is hampered by the heterogeneity of these types of lesions.

These limitations shifted the focus to those diseases in which the neurochemical or neurodegenerative changes are reasonably well localized, as in many of the basal gan-glia disorders. Notable is the high association of depres-sion with Parkinson's disease and Huntington's disease, for example (reviewed in Mayberg 1994; Starkstein and Robinson 1993). These observations directly comple-ment the findings described in studies of discrete brain le-sions and further suggest the potential importance of functional circuits linking these regions (Alexander et al. 1990; Haber et al. 2000).

Despite these apparent patterns, certain paradoxes re-main. First, despite comparable underlying pathologies, not all patients with a given disorder develop depressive symptoms. For instance, in Parkinson's disease and Hun-tington's disease, the reported rate is about 50%. As pos-tulated for primary mood disorders, mechanisms for this discordance focus on genetic and temperament markers. The second issue concerns the actual type of affective dis-turbance. For several neurological conditions, depression and mania are both recognized. With the exception of stroke, no localizing or regional differences can be offered to explain this phenomenon. There is also no consensus as to whether the left or the right hemisphere is dominant in the expression of depressive symptoms in any neuro-logical disorder.

Reports of patients with traumatic frontal lobe injury indicate a high correlation between affective disturbances and right-hemisphere pathology (Grafman et al. 1986). Secondary mania, although rare, is most consistently seen with right-sided basal frontotemporal or subcortical dam-age (Starkstein et al. 1990). However, studies of stroke pa-tients suggest that left-sided lesions of both the frontal cortex and the basal ganglia are more likely to result in de-pressive symptoms than are right-sided lesions, for which euphoria or indifference predominates (Robinson et al. 1984). There is, however, considerable debate on this is-sue (Carson et al. 2000). Similar contradictions are seen in studies of patients with temporal lobe epilepsy and multi-ple sclerosis, in which an association between affective symptoms (both mania and depression) and left- and right-sided lesions has been described (Altshuler et al. 1990; Honer et al. 1987). Anatomical studies have yet to define the critical sites within the temporal lobe most closely associated with mood changes.

Last, and in some ways counterintuitive, is the absence of depressive symptoms reported with primary injury to limbic structures such as the amygdala, hippocampus, and hypothalamus, despite their fundamental involvement in critical aspects of motivational and emotional processes. This contradiction would suggest that these key regions have a much more complex role than is apparent with classic lesion–deficit correlation methods.

Primary Unipolar Depression

Macroscopic anatomical findings in patients with primary mood disorders have been less consistent than those in depressed patients with neurological disorders (reviewed in Sheline 2003 and in Rajkowska, Chapter 11, in this volume). Brain anatomy is grossly normal, and focal neocortical abnormalities are not visible on standard clinical structural scans. Volume loss has been described in various subdivisions of the orbital frontal cortex with quantitative MRI measures (Ballmaier et al. 2004; Drevets et al. 1997; Lee et al. 2003) and is most consistently seen in geriatric depressed subgroups. Amygdala abnormalities are also described, but both increases and decreases are reported, as well as clear differences between bipolar and unipolar patients (Altshuler et al. 2000; Blumberg et al. 2003). Hippocampal changes are a major focus of research, with reduced hippocampal volumes consistently seen across studies (Campbell et al. 2004; Frodl et al. 2004; Sheline et al. 1999) (Figure 13–1). Postulated mechanisms for these changes include glucocorticoid neurotoxicity and stress-induced changes in structural plasticity consistent with both animal models (Mirescu et al. 2004; Sapolsky 2000) and studies of patients with posttraumatic stress disorder. More recent studies suggest a more critical role of chronicity and reversibility with atrophy best correlated with both number of lifetime depressed days and lack of treatment (Sheline et al. 1999, 2004).

Nonspecific changes in ventricular size and T_2-weighted MRI changes in subcortical gray and periventricular white matter have been reported in some patient subgroups, most notably, elderly depressed patients (Hickie et al. 1997; Lee et al. 2003). Newer studies are examining more subtle white matter abnormalities with microstructural measures such as fractional anisotropic and magnetization transfer MRI techniques (Alexopoulos et al. 2002; Kumar et al. 2004; Taylor et al. 2004). Parallels between these observations and regional abnormalities described in lesion and neurological patients with depression are tantalizing but not yet fully characterized. Further studies of new-onset patients or preclinical at-risk subjects are needed to clarify whether these changes reflect disease pathophysiology or are the consequence of chronic illness or treatment.

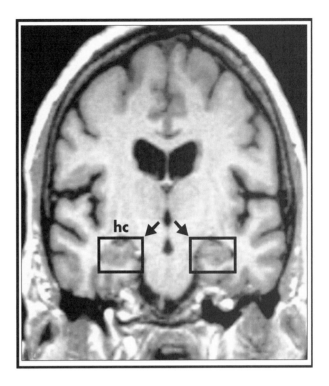

FIGURE 13–1. **Decreased hippocampal volume in depression.**
Depressed patients have smaller hippocampi (hc) than do nondepressed control subjects. Antidepressant use is associated with less atrophy.
Source. Courtesy of Yvette Sheline, Washington University.

Neuropathological Correlates

In vivo structural abnormalities identified with X-ray CT and MRI have provided a foundation for the systematic examination of histological and cellular correlates in postmortem brain (Harrison 2002). To this end, morphometric and immunocytochemical changes in neurons and glia as well as synaptic and dendritic markers have been reported, with studies targeting some subdivisions of the frontal cortex (Rajkowska 2000), anterior cingulate (Cotter et al. 2001; Ongur et al. 1998), hippocampus, and brain stem (Harrison 2002). A loss of glia is the best-replicated and most consistent finding, affecting orbital-frontal (ventral-prefrontal) and prefrontal cortex as well as the cingulate (subgenual, pregenual). Glial abnormalities are seen in both bipolar and unipolar disorders and are most consistent in patients with a positive family history of mood disorder (Ongur et al. 1998). Neuronal abnormalities are less consistently identified and generally involve a decrease in size, not number, of prefrontal neurons (Rajkowska 2000). Synaptic terminal and dendritic abnormalities, in support of aberrant cellular plasticity or impaired neurodevelopment, are also reported but appear to be a more selective marker of bipolar disorder. Preclinical correlates of hippocampal atrophy seen on MRI have been pursued, with new links identified between stress-induced alterations in structural plasticity as indexed by neurogenesis (Gould et al. 1998; Mirescu et al. 2004). These changes appear sensitive to antidepressants, suggesting a target for new treatment development (Malberg and Duman 2003; Santarelli et al. 2003). Direct links to depression pathogenesis have not yet been established (Henn and Bollmayr 2004; Lucassen et al. 2001).

Functional Imaging Studies

Functional imaging further complements structural imaging findings in that the consequences of lesions on global and regional brain function in putative functional neurocircuits also can be assessed. In addition, one can test how similar mood symptoms occur with anatomically or neurochemically distinct disease states as well as determine why comparable lesions do not always result in comparable behavioral phenomena. Specific cohorts such as healthy family members or sib-pairs and presence or absence of specific risk factors (e.g., high and low neuroticism, specific genetic polymorphisms, family history, early abuse) can be systematically targeted. Parallel studies of primary mood disorders and patients with neurological depression similarly provide complementary perspectives.

Syndromal Markers

Metabolic and Blood Flow Studies

Resting state, PET, and SPECT studies of both primary depression (unipolar, bipolar) and depression associated with specific neurological conditions (focal lesions, degenerative diseases, epilepsy, multiple sclerosis) have identified many common regional abnormalities (reviewed in Ketter et al. 1996; Mayberg 1994; Videbech 2000).

Studies of depressed neurological patients with well-characterized basal ganglia disorders (Parkinson's disease, Huntington's disease, and caudate stroke) report frontal, cingulate, and temporal hypometabolism (Mayberg 1994), consistent with disruption of specific frontostriatal and basotemporal limbic pathways characterized in primates. These findings are also seen in other neurological disorders, including epilepsy and Alzheimer's disease (Bromfield et al. 1992; Hirono et al. 1998), further suggesting the common involvement of a distributed limbic-cortical-

subcortical network in the pathogenesis of depressive symptoms across neurological diagnoses. These observations in neurological patients with depression further provide perspective for interpreting studies of primary mood disorders.

Across the many studies of primary depression, frontal and cingulate abnormalities are most commonly reported, in general agreement with the pattern seen in neurological depression (Baxter et al. 1989; Bench et al. 1992; Buchsbaum et al. 1986; Ebert et al. 1996; George et al. 1994; Ketter et al. 1996; Mayberg et al. 1994, 1997; Post et al. 1987; Videbech 2000). Other limbic-paralimbic (amygdala, anterior temporal, insula) and subcortical (basal ganglia, thalamus) abnormalities also have been identified (Buchsbaum et al. 1986; Mayberg et al. 1994, 1997; Post et al. 1987), but the findings are more variable. Across studies, the most consistent finding is decreased frontal lobe function, although normal frontal and hyperfrontal activity also has been reported (Baxter et al. 1989; Brody et al. 2001a; Drevets et al. 1992; Goldapple et al. 2004) (Figure 13–2). Localization of abnormalities within the frontal lobe includes dorsolateral and ventral-lateral prefrontal cortex (Brodmann areas 9, 46, 10, 47) as well as orbitofrontal cortices (Brodmann areas 10, 11). Findings are generally bilateral, although asymmetries are described. Cingulate changes are also commonly seen and consistently involve anterior dorsal sectors (Bench et al. 1992; Ebert and Ebmeier 1996; Mayberg et al. 1994, 1997).

Biochemical Studies

Several neurochemical markers also have been examined in depressed patients via PET and SPECT. Decreases in serotonin transporter (SERT) binding have been reported in the brain stem (Malison et al. 1998) but not in any of the other regions identified in postmortem studies of depressed patients who committed suicide, such as ventral prefrontal cortex or anterior cingulate (Meyer et al. 2004). Serotonin type 1A ($5-HT_{1A}$) and $5-HT_{2A}$ receptor densities also have been examined, but with inconsistent findings in the drug-free state (Drevetz et al. 1999, 2001; Meltzer et al. 1999; Messa et al. 2003; Meyer et al. 1999; Mintun et al. 2004; Sargent et al. 2000). Dopamine markers have been less informative, with no significant change in D_2 receptors found with either PET or SPECT (Klimke et al. 1999; Parsey et al. 2001). Relations between receptor and transporter markers or between neurochemical and regional metabolic changes have not yet been systematically explored, as is a growing trend in many postmortem studies. Studies of other targets of interest are limited by the lack of suitable radioligands.

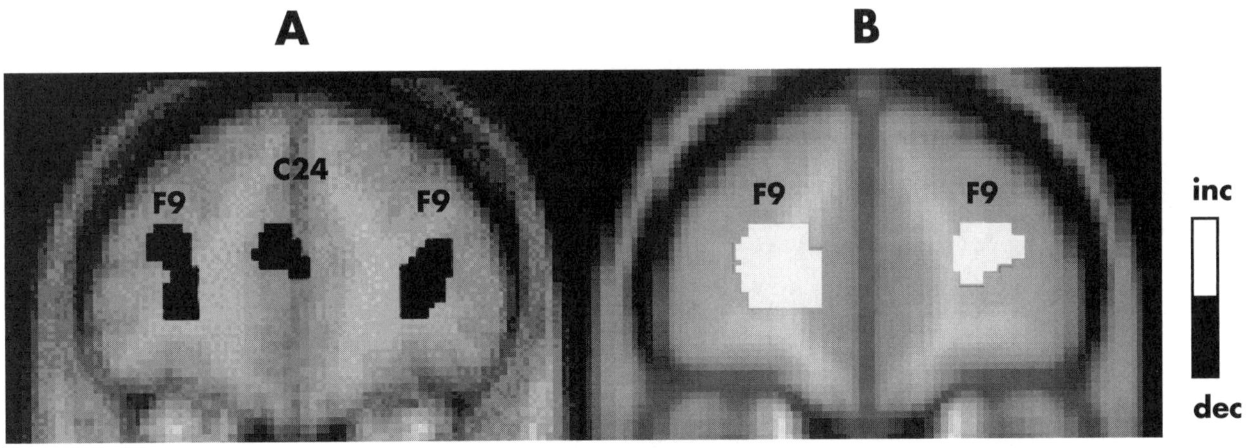

FIGURE 13–2. **Frontal metabolic abnormalities in depression.**

Symmetric prefrontal (F9) hypometabolism (A) and hypermetabolism (B) are both reported in studies of untreated depression of comparable severity. C24=anterior cingulate; inc=increased; dec=decreased (metabolic activity). Numbers designate Brodmann areas.

Behavioral Correlates

Clinical Correlations

The best-replicated behavioral correlate of a resting state abnormality in depression is that of an inverse relation between prefrontal activity and depression severity (reviewed in Ketter et al. 1996). Prefrontal activity also has been linked to psychomotor speed and executive functions (Bench et al. 1993; Mayberg et al. 1994); parietal and parahippocampus have been linked with anxiety (Bench et al. 1993; Osuch et al. 2000); mediofrontal and cingulate have been linked with cognitive performance (Bench et al. 1993; Dunn et al. 2002); and amygdala has been linked with cortisol status (Drevets et al. 2002). A more complex ventrodorsal segregation of frontal lobe functions also has been described, with anxiety and tension positively correlated with ventral prefrontal activity and psychomotor and cognitive slowing negatively correlated with dorsolateral activity (Brody et al. 2001a). The prefrontal cortex overactivity seen in patients with a more ruminative or anxious clinical presentation is also consistent with findings described in primary anxiety and obsessional disorders (Saxena and Rauch 2000), memory-evoked anxiety and fear in healthy subjects (Liotti et al. 2000), and even normal variations in individual response to the testing environment caused by novelty or state anxiety (Gur et al. 1987). Decreased caudate fluorodopa uptake has been reported in depressed patients with pronounced psychomotor slowing, suggesting biochemical subtype differences as well (Martinot et al. 2001).

An alternative to the more classic behavioral localization or correlational approach is to consider further that a given metabolic pattern is a combination of a functional lesion and an ongoing process of attempted self-correction or adaptation (Figure 13–3) (Mayberg 2003; McEwen 2003). From this perspective, the net regional activity or sum total of various synergistic and competing inputs (likely influenced by factors such as heredity, temperament, early life experiences, and previous depressive episodes) is what accounts for the observed clinical symptoms. For instance, frontal hyperactivity would now be viewed as an exaggerated or a maladaptive compensatory process resulting in psychomotor agitation and rumination, serving to override a persistent negative mood generated by abnormal chronic activity of limbic-subcortical structures.

In contrast, frontal hypometabolism seen with increasing depression severity would be interpreted as failure to initiate or maintain such a compensatory state, with resulting apathy, psychomotor slowness, and impaired executive functioning. From this perspective, one might postulate that a specific metabolic signature may ultimately provide a therapeutic road map for optimal treatment selection based on known patterns of differential change with different treatment interventions, if the contribution of these adaptive and maladaptive compensatory responses can be fully defined. Toward this goal, strategies to characterize such treatment-specific effects are discussed below.

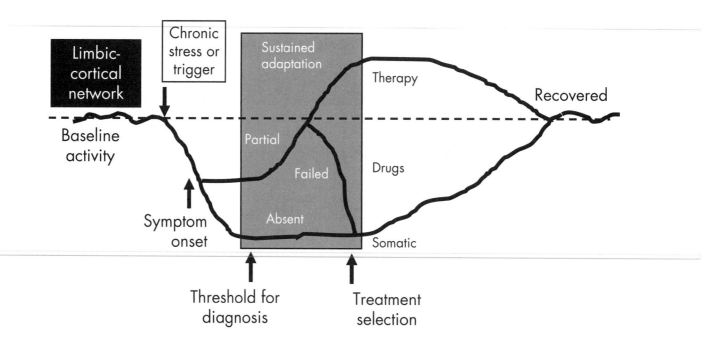

FIGURE 13–3.   Postulated mechanism of frontal variability.

Positron emission tomography abnormalities are viewed as the net effect of a triggering "insult" and subsequent adaptive neural processes, providing a framework for developing brain-based algorithms to guide treatment selection.

Mapping Studies

Correlational studies of resting state patterns with syndromal features are complemented by parallel functional activation experiments examining specific cognitive, motor, circadian, and affective behaviors mapped in healthy volunteers. With respect to specific deficits, not only can the neural correlates of performance decrements observed in depressed patients be quantified, but also the compensatory reorganization of brain regions involved in performing specific tasks can be identified. For example, blunting of an expected anterior cingulate increase during performance of a Stroop task has been demonstrated in depressed patients, with a shift to the left dorsolateral prefrontal cortex (George et al. 1997), a region not normally recruited for this task in healthy subjects. In the Tower of London test, a similar attenuation in depressed patients of an expected increase in dorsolateral prefrontal cortex is described, with failure to activate anterior cingulate and caudate seen in nondepressed control subjects (Elliott et al. 1997).

More subtle variations in cognitive processing, such as the well-recognized negative bias of depressed patients, also can be examined. Elliott et al. (2002) identified depression-specific patterns of medial and orbital prefrontal

activations in mediating this mood-congruent processing bias. Others have used complementary strategies, showing that depressed patients evaluate positive and negative emotional stimuli without the expected activation of dorsomedial prefrontal cortex seen in never-depressed healthy control subjects (Mitterschiffthaler et al. 2003). Siegle et al. (2002) have reported that depressed patients show abnormally sustained amygdala responses to negative words in comparison to control subjects. This sustained amygdala response, in the context of negative information processing, is postulated to be an important neural correlate of sustained self-rumination—a common feature of a major depressive episode.

These complementary studies provide important insights into neural correlates of the dysfunctional mood and emotional-processing strategies characteristic of depressed patients. They also emphasize the need for experimental approaches that can effectively evaluate the effect of treatments on such reorganized behavioral systems. To this end, normalization by venlafaxine of aberrant amygdala responses to aversive picture viewing in patients with major depression studied before and after treatment has been recently reported (Davidson et al. 2003; Sheline et al. 2001). Effects of nonpharmacological interventions on these neural pathways would be of additional interest.

Treatment Studies

Theoretical Considerations

Imaging studies to date have focused primarily on neural mechanisms mediating pharmacological and somatic treatments, although a small but growing number have examined nonpharmacological interventions. In general, pharmacotherapy studies tend to emphasize a bottom-up cascade; brain stem, limbic, and subcortical sites are viewed as the primary sites of drug action, with secondary cortical changes seen as secondary effects of chronic treatment (Blier 2001; Freo et al. 2000; Santarelli et al. 2003; Vaidya and Duman 2001). In contrast, nonpharmacological antidepressant treatments such as cognitive-behavioral therapy (CBT) work to facilitate alteration of depression-relevant cognitions, affective bias, and maladaptive information processing that also may modify specific but alternative neural processes (Beck et al. 1979; Teasdale et al. 2002). Surgical ablation provides additional evidence for involvement of specific neural pathways. Three standard approaches—anterior capsulotomy, cingulotomy, and subcaudate tractotomy—all show comparable clinical efficacy but disrupt different white matter targets (Cosgrove and Rauch 1995). Both top-down (corticothalamic, corticolimbic) and bottom-up (thalamocortical, limbic-cortical) mechanisms can be postulated, though the precise limbic, subcortical, and cortical targets or pathways necessary for amelioration of depressive symptoms are not well characterized. Towards testing one such theory, explicit targeting of overactive subgenual cingulate activity using deep brain stimulation has been piloted in treatment-resistant patients (Mayberg et al. 2005).

Regional Activity Changes

Changes in regional metabolism and blood flow with recovery from a major depressive episode consistently include normalization of many regional abnormalities identified in the pretreatment state. Changes in cortical (prefrontal, parietal), limbic-paralimbic (cingulate, amygdala, insula), and subcortical (caudate/pallidum, thalamus, brain stem) areas have been described following various treatments, including medication, psychotherapy, sleep deprivation, electroconvulsive therapy (ECT), repetitive transcranial magnetic stimulation (rTMS), vagal nerve stimulation (VNS), and ablative surgery (Bench et al. 1995; Brody et al. 2001b; Buchsbaum et al. 1997; Chae et al. 2003; Malizia 1997; Mayberg et al. 2000; Nobler et al. 2001; Teneback et al. 1999) (see Nobler and Sackeim, Chapter 20, and George et al., Chapter 21, in this volume). Normalization of frontal hypometabolism is the best-replicated finding, seen mainly with all classes of medication, although normalization of frontal hypermetabolism is also reported, including changes seen with CBT and interpersonal psychotherapy (Brody et al. 2001b; Goldapple et al. 2004). Changes in limbic-paralimbic and subcortical regions are also seen, often involving changes in previously "normally" functioning regions. Requisite changes mediating clinical recovery have not been determined, although differences between responders and nonresponders on comparable treatment have been shown for certain interventions such as selective serotonin reuptake inhibitor (SSRI) pharmacotherapy (Klimke et al. 1999; Mayberg et al. 2000).

Several studies of SSRI pharmacotherapy (Goldapple et al. 2004; Kennedy et al. 2001; Mayberg et al. 2000) found a correlation between improvement in depressive symptoms and increases in prefrontal cortex (F9/46) and decreases in subgenual cingulate (Cg25), suggesting that these changes may be important for illness remission with this class of medications. In further support of the critical role of reciprocal dorsocortical and ventrolimbic changes are reports of fluoxetine treatment in depressed patients with Parkinson's disease (Stefurak and Mayberg 2003) as well as with inactive fluoxetine as part of a placebo-controlled experiment (Mayberg et al. 2002). Cg25 hypometabolism in fully recovered patients receiving maintenance SSRI treatment is also reported (Liotti et al. 2002), suggesting that persistent limbic changes in remitted patients are the adaptive homeostatic response necessary to maintain a recovered state. Complementary preclinical studies of treatment mechanisms lend further support for these hypotheses; a cascade of adaptive neurochemical and molecular changes in brain stem, limbic, and neocortical regions is reported with chronic antidepressant treatment (Freo et al. 2000; Vaidya and Duman 2001). Interestingly, placebo response was not associated with changes in brain stem, hippocampus, or striatum, as seen with active medication, lending further support that changes in these regions may be medication specific.

Receptor Changes

Treatment studies with SSRIs or tricyclic antidepressants report downregulation of 5-HT$_{2A}$ receptors consistent with pharmacological studies in animals (Klimke et al. 1999; Meyer et al. 2001; Yatham et al. 1999). Like abnormalities in the pretreatment state, reported changes are global rather than focal. 5-HT$_{1A}$ receptors show no change with treatment, suggesting that the pretreatment abnormalities may be a compensatory rather than a primary etiological finding (Sargent et al. 2000), as postulated in recent postmortem studies of these markers. Although no direct comparisons of SSRI and norepinephrine reuptake inhibitor action on serotonin binding have been done, the areas with the greatest magnitude of change with desipramine treatment were ventromedial frontal regions—overlapping sites of the most consistent metabolic decreases with more selective SSRIs such as fluoxetine and areas of highest concentration of the SERT (Mann et al. 2000). Striatal dopamine D_2 changes also have been reported (Ebert et al. 1996), with upregulation of receptors associated with clinical improvement (Klimke et al. 1999). Extrastriatal measurements are not yet reliable with currently available tracers.

Medication Versus Psychotherapy

Despite the apparent convergence of regional metabolic changes with pharmacotherapy, the final common pathway hypothesis requires the definitive demonstration of comparable changes with a formal nonpharmacological intervention. The few published studies of interpersonal psychotherapy thus far showed no common pattern to support or refute this hypothesis (Brody et al. 2001b; Martin et al. 2001).

More recent studies of CBT identified a different set of regional changes than those seen with pharmacotherapy, supporting an alternative hypothesis of treatment-specific rather than common response effects (Goldapple et al. 2004) (Figure 13–4). Changes with CBT include lateral prefrontal decreases and hippocampal increases in a pattern exactly opposite to that seen with pharmacotherapy. Orbital and medial frontal decreases and cingulate increases occur uniquely in the CBT group. It is also notable that subgenual cingulate changes, characteristic of SSRIs, do not occur with CBT. The pattern of changes across treatments suggests that pharmacotherapy and cognitive interventions both target a unique set of brain regions but also affect changes in certain common sites within an integrative neural systems framework. The overall modulation of this complex system rather than any one focal regional change may be most critical for disease remission. Additional support for this hypothesis will require additional studies of non-SSRI antidepressants as well as other available somatic treatments, as has been most recently demonstrated using deep brain stimulation (Mayberg et al. 2005).

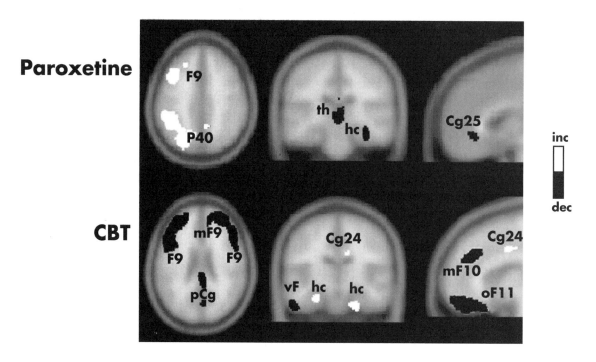

FIGURE 13–4. **Metabolic change patterns with cognitive-behavioral therapy (CBT) and medication.**
A pattern of prefrontal (F9) decreases and hippocampal (hc) increases is seen with CBT. The reverse pattern is seen with paroxetine. Additional unique changes are seen with each treatment: increases in anterior cingulate (Cg24) and decreases in medial (mF9/mF10) and orbitofrontal (oF11) cortex with CBT; decreases in subgenual cingulate (Cg25) and thalamus (th) with paroxetine. pCg=posterior cingulate; vF=ventral frontal; inc=increased; dec=decreased (metabolic activity).

Response Predictors

Baseline Markers

In light of the described differences between responders and nonresponders to a given treatment as well as variable brain changes with response to disparate treatments, an obvious related question is whether baseline scan patterns might effectively predict treatment outcome or potentially even guide treatment selection. To these future goals, several studies have found that pretreatment metabolic activity in the rostral (pregenual) cingulate uniquely distinguishes medication responders from nonresponders (Mayberg et al. 1997) (Figure 13–5), a pattern replicated in Parkinson's disease and other unipolar depressed cohorts (Davidson et al. 2003; Kennedy et al. 2001; Pizzagalli et al. 2001; Stefurak and Mayberg 2003). A similar pattern also predicts good response to one night of sleep deprivation (Smith et al. 2002; Wu et al. 1999). Additional evidence of persistent hypermetabolism in patients in full remission receiving maintenance SSRI treatment for more than a year further suggests a critical compensatory or adaptive role for the rostral cingulate in facilitating and maintaining clinical response long term (Liotti et al. 2002). Taken together, these data would suggest not just focal differences but also network differences among patient subgroups relevant to mechanisms mediating brain plasticity and adaptation to illness with potential future implications for clinical management of individual patients.

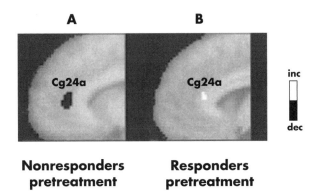

A   **B**

Cg24a   Cg24a

inc

dec

Nonresponders pretreatment   **Responders pretreatment**

FIGURE 13–5. **Scan pattern predicting treatment response.**

Metabolic activity in rostral anterior cingulate (Cg24a) identified prior to treatment predicts response to pharmacotherapy. Nonresponders are hypometabolic (A), and responders are hypermetabolic (B) relative to control subjects. inc=increased; dec=decreased (metabolic activity).

Early Treatment Effects

Examination of time course of changes and differences between responders and nonresponders to a given treatment provides additional localizing clues to brain changes critical for clinical remission (Mayberg et al. 2000) (Figure 13–6). Responders and nonresponders to 6 weeks of fluoxetine, for example, showed similar regional metabolic changes after 1 week of treatment (brain stem, hippocampus increases; posterior cingulate, striatal, thalamic decreases) concordant with absence of clinical change in both groups. In contrast, the 6-week metabolic change pattern discriminated them, with clinical improvement uniquely associated with limbic-paralimbic and striatal decreases (subgenual cingulate, hippocampus, pallidum, insula) and brain stem and dorsocortical increases (prefrontal, anterior cingulate, posterior cingulate, parietal). Failed response to fluoxetine was associated with a persistent 1-week pattern (hippocampal increases; striatal, posterior cingulate decreases) and absence of either subgenual cingulate or prefrontal changes. This reversal of the week 1 pattern at 6 weeks in only those patients showing a clinical response might suggest a requisite process of neural adaptation in specific brain regions over time with chronic treatment (Freo et al. 2000; Vaidya and Duman 2001). The presence of an inverse pattern in responders and nonresponders at the 6-week time point further suggests that failure to induce these adaptive changes underlies treatment nonresponse. Needed are careful time course experiments to identify the point of regional metabolic "switching" that may actually predict SSRI or other treatment response down the line. This type of approach may be useful in evaluating new antidepressant agents with purported earlier onset of clinical effects.

Relapse Risk and Illness Vulnerability

A further need concerns identification of patients at risk for illness onset as well as those vulnerable to illness relapse. Challenge or stress tests might be seen as a possible avenue toward this goal. Along these lines, mood induction experiments initially studied in healthy subjects to define brain regions mediating modulation of acute changes in mood states relevant to the depressive dysphoria have been similarly performed in acutely depressed and remitted depressed subjects and have identified disease-specific modifications of these pathways. Specifically, with acute sad mood induction in healthy volunteers, ventral and subgenual cingulate increases are consistently described (Damasio et al. 2000; Liotti et al. 2000; Mayberg et al. 1999). These cingulate increases are not found

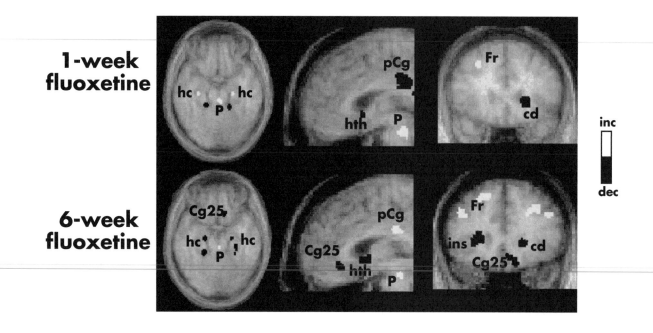

FIGURE 13-6.   Time course of treatment changes.

Metabolic changes are seen after 1 week of treatment in caudate (cd), brain stem, hippocampus (hc), hypothalamus (hth), and posterior cingulate (pCg). At 6 weeks, striatal, hypothalamic, and brain stem changes persist but are now accompanied by widespread cortical increases (frontal [Fr], parietal [P]) and by subgenual cingulate (Cg25) and insula (ins) decreases. Activity in hc and pCg shows a switch in activity over time.

in depressed patients comparably provoked, in whom unique dorsal cingulate increases and medial and orbital frontal decreases are seen instead. Similar findings in both euthymic-remitted and acutely depressed patients suggest that these differences may be depression trait markers (Kruger et al. 2003; Liotti et al. 2002). In addition, the pattern seen with memory-provoked sadness shows striking similarities to resting state studies of refractory unipolar and neurologically depressed patients, as well as to the changes seen following acute tryptophan depletion during the early phase of SSRI treatment (Bremner et al. 1997). This pattern also has been described when fMRI was used in a recent case of iatrogenic mood symptoms induced by high-frequency deep-brain stimulation of the right subthalamic nucleus for treatment of intractable Parkinson's disease in a patient with a remote history of major depression (Stefurak and Mayberg 2003). Consistent with recent clinical studies reporting increased relapse risk in those remitted depressed patients with persistent hypersensitivity to negative emotional stimuli (Teasdale et al. 2002), the converging imaging evidence suggests strategies for future studies of potential neural mechanisms of relapse vulnerability.

Challenge experiments of this type may additionally identify presyndromal subjects with high illness risk as suggested by preliminary studies indicating differential rest-

and mood-stress-induced patterns of change in healthy control subjects selected for high and low neurotic temperaments (Keightley et al. 2003; Zald et al. 2002). For example, the activation pattern in the high neuroticism groups is similar but not identical to that seen in remitted depressed patients, which suggests a potential vulnerability marker, unmasked only with emotional stress. This is of interest because high neuroticism not only is highly associated with the presence of a mood disorder but also appears to be a major depression risk factor (Kendler et al. 2001). Further development of these types of paradigms has future potential for preclinical testing of unaffected family members of genetically defined cohorts (Caspi et al. 2003; Hariri and Weinberger 2003; Neumeister et al. 2002).

Limbic-Cortical Dysregulation Model of Depression

To synthesize the findings described in the previous sections, regions with known anatomical interconnections that also show consistent changes across studies are summarized in a simplified schematic model illustrated in Figure 13–7. Regions within the model are clustered into working compartments based on consistent patterns of

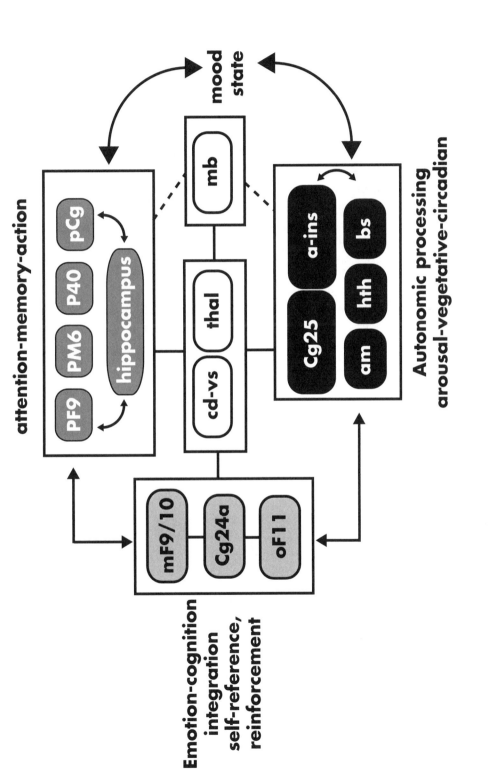

FIGURE 13–7. Limbic-cortical dysregulation model.

Regions with known anatomical interconnections that show consistent changes across converging imaging experiments form the basis of this model. Regions are grouped into three main compartments reflecting general behavioral dimensions of depression and regional targets of various antidepressant treatments. mF=medial prefrontal; Cg24a=rostral anterior cingulate; oF=orbital frontal; cd–vs=caudate–ventral striatum; thal=thalamus; mb=midbrain; Cg25=subgenual cingulate; a-ins=anterior insula; am=amygdala; hth=hypothalamus; bs=brain stem; PF=dorsolateral prefrontal; PM=premotor; P=parietal; pCg=posterior cingulate; numbers=Brodmann's area designations.

behavior across different experiments. These functional groupings further attempt to accommodate the major defining symptom clusters of major depression (mood, motor, cognitive, circadian) as well as brain regions associated with specific cognitive, motivational, and autonomic functions of obvious relevance. A consistent reciprocal relation between dorsocortical (regions in black) and ventrolimbic (in dark gray) regions is seen across studies examining both depression and transient negative mood states. Variations in mediofrontal regions (in light gray), including the anterior cingulate, account most consistently for depression-specific deviations observed with both affective and cognitive challenges (Fossati et al. 2003; Kruger et al. 2003; Liotti et al. 2002). Earlier versions of this model emphasized a central role for the rostral anterior cingulate (Cg24a) (Mayberg 1997), given its known connections to regions in both the dorsocortical and the ventral compartments and its unique behavior in predicting antidepressant treatment response (Mayberg et al. 1997), but more recent studies suggested that the subgenual cingulate (Cg25) may be more critical to the core features of a major depressive episode—namely, dysregulated motivational, circadian, and cognitive responses to sustained negative mood (Mayberg 2003; Mayberg et al. 2005; Seminowicz et al. 2004). Last, it is postulated that the initial modulation of unique targets by specific treatments facilitates adaptive changes in particular pathways necessary for network homeostasis and resulting clinical recovery.

This type of network or neural systems approach is a deliberate oversimplification. It nonetheless provides a flexible platform to systematically test future hypotheses regarding the contribution of additional genetic, environmental, and subtype variables to disease pathogenesis and treatment response. Advances in imaging methods and analytic strategies that optimally integrate these factors will be a critical next step in fully characterizing the depression phenotype at the neural systems level and in the development of strategies leading to brain-based algorithms that optimize care of individual depressed patients.

References

Alexander GE, Crutcher MD, De Long MR: Basal ganglia-thalamocortical circuits: parallel substrates for motor, oculomotor, "prefrontal" and "limbic" functions. Prog Brain Res 85:119–146, 1990

Alexopoulos GS, Kiosses DN, Choi SJ, et al: Frontal white matter microstructure and treatment response of late-life depression: a preliminary study. Am J Psychiatry 159:1929–1932, 2002

Altshuler LL, Devinsky O, Post RM, et al: Depression, anxiety, and temporal lobe epilepsy: laterality of focus and symptoms. Arch Neurol 47:284–288, 1990

Altshuler LL, Bartzokis G, Grieder T, et al: An MRI study of temporal lobe structures in men with bipolar disorder or schizophrenia. Biol Psychiatry 48:147–162, 2000

Ballmaier M, Toga AW, Blanton RE: Anterior cingulate, gyrus rectus, and orbitofrontal abnormalities in elderly depressed patients: an MRI-based parcellation of the prefrontal cortex. Am J Psychiatry 161:99–108, 2004

Barbas H: Anatomical basis of cognitive-emotional interactions in the primate prefrontal cortex. Neurosci Biobehav Rev 19:499–510, 1995

Baxter LR Jr, Schwartz JM, Phelps ME, et al: Reduction of prefrontal cortex glucose metabolism common to three types of depression. Arch Gen Psychiatry 46:243–250, 1989

Beck AT, Rush AJ, Shaw BF: Cognitive Therapy of Depression. New York, Guilford, 1979

Bench CJ, Friston KJ, Brown RG, et al: Anatomy of melancholia—focal abnormalities of cerebral blood flow in major depression. Psychol Med 22:607–615, 1992

Bench CJ, Friston KJ, Brown RG: Regional cerebral blood flow in depression measured by positron emission tomography: the relationship with clinical dimensions. Psychol Med 23:579–590, 1993

Bench CJ, Frackowiak RSJ, Dolan RJ: Changes in regional cerebral blood flow on recovery from depression. Psychol Med 25:247–251, 1995

Blier P: Crosstalk between the norepinephrine and serotonin systems and its role in the antidepressant response. J Psychiatry Neurosci 26 (suppl):S3–10, 2001

Blumberg HP, Kaufman J, Martin A, et al: Amygdala and hippocampal volumes in adolescents and adults with bipolar disorder. Arch Gen Psychiatry 60:1201–1208, 2003

Bremner JD, Innis RB, Salomon RM, et al: Positron emission tomography measurement of cerebral metabolic correlates of tryptophan depletion-induced depressive relapse. Arch Gen Psychiatry 54:364–374, 1997

Broca P: Anatomie comparée des circonvolutions cérébrales: le grant lobe limbique et la scissure limbique dans la série des mammifères. Revue Anthropologia 1:385–498, 1878

Brody AL, Saxena S, Mandelkern MA, et al: Brain metabolic changes associated with symptom factor improvement in major depressive disorder. Biol Psychiatry 50:171–178, 2001a

Brody AL, Saxena S, Stoessel P, et al: Regional brain metabolic changes in patients with major depression treated with either paroxetine or interpersonal therapy. Arch Gen Psychiatry 58:631–640, 2001b

Bromfield EB, Altshuler L, Leiderman DB, et al: Cerebral metabolism and depression in patients with complex partial seizures. Arch Neurol 49:617–623, 1992

Buchsbaum MS, Wu J, DeLisi LE, et al: Frontal cortex and basal ganglia metabolic rates assessed by positron emission tomography with [18F]2-deoxyglucose in affective illness. J Affect Disord 10:137–152, 1986

Buchsbaum MS, Wu J, Siegel BV, et al: Effect of sertraline on regional metabolic rate in patients with affective disorder. Biol Psychiatry 41:15–22, 1997

Campbell S, Marriott M, Nahmias C, et al: Lower hippocampal volume in patients suffering from depression: a meta-analysis. Am J Psychiatry 161:598–607, 2004

Carmichael ST, Price JL: Connectional networks within the orbital and medial prefrontal cortex of macaque monkeys. J Comp Neurol 371:179–207, 1996

Carson AJ, MacHale S, Allen K, et al: Depression after stroke and lesion location: a systematic review. Lancet 356:122–126, 2000

Caspi A, Sugden K, Moffitt TE, et al: Influence of life stress on depression: moderation by a polymorphism in the 5-HTT gene. Science 301:386–389, 2003

Chae JH, Nahas Z, Lomarev M, et al: A review of functional neuroimaging studies of vagus nerve stimulation (VNS). J Psychiatr Res 37:443–455, 2003

Cosgrove GR, Rauch SL: Psychosurgery. Neurosurg Clin N Am 6:167–176, 1995

Cotter D, MacKay D, Landau S, et al: Reduced glial cell density and neural size in the anterior cingulate cortex in major depressive disorder. Arch Gen Psychiatry 58:545–553, 2001

Damasio AR, Grabowsky TJ, Bechara A, et al: Subcortical and cortical brain activity during the feeling of self-generated emotions. Nat Neurosci 3:1049–1056, 2000

Davidson RJ, Irwin W, Anderle MJ, et al: The neural substrates of affective processing in depressed patients treated with venlafaxine. Am J Psychiatry 160:64–75, 2003

Drevets WC, Videen TO, Price JL: A functional anatomical study of unipolar depression. J Neurosci 12:3628–3641, 1992

Drevets WC, Price JL, Simpson JR Jr, et al: Subgenual prefrontal cortex abnormalities in mood disorders. Nature 386:824–827, 1997

Drevets WC, Frank E, Price JC: PET imaging of serotonin 1A receptor binding in depression. Biol Psychiatry 46:1375–1387, 1999

Drevets WC, Price JL, Bardgett ME: Glucose metabolism in the amygdala in depression: relationship to diagnostic subtype and plasma cortisol levels. Pharmacol Biochem Behav 71:431–447, 2002

Dunn RT, Kimbrell TA, Ketter TA, et al: Principal components of the Beck Depression Inventory and regional cerebral metabolism in unipolar and bipolar depression. Biol Psychiatry 51:387–399, 2002

Ebert D, Ebmeier K: Role of the cingulate gyrus in depression: from functional anatomy to depression. Biol Psychiatry 39:1044–1050, 1996

Ebert D, Feistel H, Loew T, et al: Dopamine and depression—striatal dopamine D2 receptor SPECT before and after antidepressant therapy. Psychopharmacology (Berl) 126:91–94, 1996

Elliott R, Baker SC, Roger RD, et al: Prefrontal dysfunction in depressed patients performing a complex planning task: a study using PET. Psychol Med 27:931–942, 1997

Elliott R, Rubinsztein JS, Sahakian BJ, et al: The neural basis of mood-congruent processing biases in depression. Arch Gen Psychiatry 59:597–604, 2002

Fossati P, Hevenor SJ, Graham SJ, et al: In search of the emotional self: a fMRI study using positive and negative emotional words. Am J Psychiatry 160:1938–1945, 2003

Freo U, Ori C, Dam M, et al: Effects of acute and chronic treatment with fluoxetine on regional glucose cerebral metabolism in rats: implications for clinical therapies. Brain Res 854:35–41, 2000

Frodl T, Meisenzahl EM, Zetzsche T: Hippocampal and amygdala changes in patients with major depressive disorder and healthy controls during a 1-year follow-up. J Clin Psychiatry 65:492–499, 2004

Fulton JF: Frontal Lobotomy and Affective Behavior: A Neurophysiological Analysis. London, England, Chapman & Hall, 1951

George MS, Ketter TA, Post RM: Prefrontal cortex dysfunction in clinical depression. Depression 2:9–72, 1994

George MS, Ketter TA, Parekh PI, et al: Blunted left cingulate activation in mood disorder subjects during a response interference task (the Stroop). J Neuropsychiatry Clin Neurosci 9:55–63, 1997

Goldapple K, Segal Z, Garson C, et al: Modulation of cortical-limbic pathways in major depression: treatment specific effects of cognitive behavioral therapy. Arch Gen Psychiatry 61:34–41, 2004

Gould E, Tanapat P, McEwen BS, et al: Proliferation of granule cell precursors in the dentate gyrus of adult monkeys is diminished by stress. Proc Natl Acad Sci U S A 95:3168–3171, 1998

Grafman J, Vance SC, Weingartner H, et al: The effects of lateralized frontal lesions on mood regulation. Brain 109 (pt 6):1127–1148, 1986

Gur RC, Gur RE, Resnick SM, et al: The effect of anxiety on cortical cerebral blood flow and metabolism. J Cereb Blood Flow Metab 7:173–177, 1987

Haber SN, Fudge JL, McFarland NR: Striato-nigro-striatal pathways in primates form an ascending spiral from the shell to the dorsolateral striatum. J Neurosci 20:2369–2382, 2000

Hariri AR, Weinberger DR: Functional neuroimaging of genetic variation in serotonergic neurotransmission. Genes Brain Behav 2:341–349, 2003

Harrison P: The neuropathology of primary mood disorder. Brain 125:1428–1449, 2002

Henn FA, Bollmayr B: Neurogenesis and depression: etiology or epiphenomenon? Biol Psychiatry 56:146–150, 2004

Hickie I, Scott E, Wilhelm K, et al: Subcortical hyperintensities on magnetic resonance imaging in patients with severe depression—a longitudinal evaluation. Biol Psychiatry 42:367–374, 1997

Hirono N, Mori E, Ishii K, et al: Frontal lobe hypometabolism and depression in Alzheimer's disease. Neurology 50:380–383, 1998

Honer WG, Hurwitz T, Li DKB, et al: Temporal lobe involvement in multiple sclerosis patients with psychiatric disorders. Arch Neurol 44:187–190, 1987

Keightley ML, Seminowicz DA, Bagby RM, et al: Personality influences limbic-cortical interactions during sad mood induction. Neuroimage 41:585–596, 2003

Kendler KS, Thornton LM, Gardner CO: Genetic risk, number of previous depressive episodes, and stressful life events in predicting onset of major depression. Am J Psychiatry 158:582–586, 2001

Kennedy SH, Evans K, Kruger S, et al: Changes in regional glucose metabolism with PET following paroxetine: treatment for major depression. Am J Psychiatry 158:899–905, 2001

Ketter TA, George MS, Kimbrell TA: Functional brain imaging, limbic function, and affective disorders. Neuroscientist 2:55–65, 1996

Kleist K: Bericht über die Gehirnpathologie in ihrer Bedeutung für Neurologie und Psychiatrie. Zeitschrift für des gesamte Neurologie und Psychiatrie 158:159–193, 1937

Klimke A, Larisch R, Janz A, et al: Dopamine D2 receptor binding before and after treatment of major depression measured by [123I]IBZM SPECT. Psychiatry Res 90:91–101, 1999

Kruger S, Seminowicz D, Goldapple K, et al: Regional cerebral blood flow in bipolar disorder: differences between remitted and depressed patients identified with an acute mood challenge. Biol Psychiatry 54:1274–1283, 2003

Kumar A, Gupta RC, Albert M: Biophysical changes in normal-appearing white matter and subcortical nuclei in late-life major depression detected using magnetization transfer. Psychiatry Res 130:131–140, 2004

Lee SH, Payne ME, Steffens DC, et al: Subcortical lesion severity and orbitofrontal cortex volume in geriatric depression. Biol Psychiatry 54:529–533, 2003

Liotti M, Mayberg HS, Brannan SK, et al: Differential neural correlates of sadness and fear in healthy subjects: implications for affective disorders. Biol Psychiatry 48:30–42, 2000

Liotti M, Mayberg HS, McGinnis S, et al: Mood challenge in remitted unipolar depression unmasks disease-specific cerebral blood flow abnormalities. Am J Psychiatry 159:1830–1840, 2002

Lucassen PJ, Muller MB, Holsboer F, et al: Hippocampal apoptosis in major depression is a minor event and absent from sub-areas at risk for glucocorticoid overexposure. Am J Pathol 158:453–468, 2001

MacLean PD: Psychosomatic disease and the visceral brain: recent developments bearing on the Papez theory of emotion. Psychosom Med 11:338–353, 1949

Malberg JE, Duman RS: Cell proliferation in adult hippocampus is decreased by inescapable stress: reversal by fluoxetine treatment. Neuropsychopharmacology 28:1562–1571, 2003

Malison RT, Price LH, Berman RM, et al: Reduced midbrain serotonin transporter binding in depressed vs healthy subjects as measured by 123b-CIT SPECT. Biol Psychiatry 44:1090–1098, 1998

Malizia A: Frontal lobes and neurosurgery for psychiatric disorders. J Psychopharmacol 11:179–187, 1997

Mann JJ, Huang Y, Underwood MD, et al: A serotonin transporter gene promoter polymorphism (5-HTTLPR) and prefrontal cortical binding in major depression and suicide. Arch Gen Psychiatry 57:729–738, 2000

Martin SD, Martin E, Rai SS, et al: Brain blood flow changes in depressed patients treated with interpersonal psychotherapy or venlafaxine hydrochloride. Arch Gen Psychiatry 58:641–664, 2001

Martinot M, Bragulat V, Artiges E, et al: Decreased presynaptic dopamine function in the left caudate of depressed patients with affective flattening and psychomotor retardation. Am J Psychiatry 158:314–316, 2001

Mayberg HS: Frontal lobe dysfunction in secondary depression. J Neuropsychiatry Clin Neurosci 6:428–442, 1994

Mayberg HS: Limbic-cortical dysregulation: a proposed model of depression. J Neuropsychiatry Clin Neurosci 9:471–481, 1997

Mayberg HS: Modulating dysfunctional limbic-cortical circuits in depression: towards development of brain-based algorithms for diagnosis and optimised treatment. Br Med Bull 65:193–207, 2003

Mayberg HS, Lewis PJ, Regenold W, et al: Paralimbic hypoperfusion in unipolar depression. J Nucl Med 35:929–934, 1994

Mayberg HS, Brannan SK, Mahurin RK, et al: Cingulate function in depression: a potential predictor of treatment response. Neuroreport 8:1057–1061, 1997

Mayberg H, Liotti M, Brannan S, et al: Reciprocal limbic-cortical function and negative mood: converging PET findings in depression and normal sadness. Am J Psychiatry 156:675–682, 1999

Mayberg HS, Brannan SK, Tekell JL, et al: Regional metabolic effects of fluoxetine in major depression: serial changes and relationship to clinical response. Biol Psychiatry 48:830–843, 2000

Mayberg HS, Silva JA, Brannan SK, et al: The functional neuroanatomy of the placebo effect. Am J Psychiatry 159:728–737, 2002

Mayberg HS, Lozano AM, Voon V, et al: Deep brain stimulation for treatment-resistant depression. Neuron 45:651–660, 2005

McEwen BS: Mood disorders and allostatic load. Biol Psychiatry 54:200–207, 2003

Meltzer CC, Price JC, Mathis CA: PET imaging of serotonin type 2A receptors in late-life neuropsychiatric disorders. Am J Psychiatry 156:1871–1878, 1999

Messa C, Colombo C, Moresco RM, et al: 5-HT(2A) receptor binding is reduced in drug-naive and unchanged in SSRI-responder depressed patients compared to healthy controls: a PET study. Psychopharmacology (Berl) 167:72–78, 2003

Meyer J, Kapur S, Houle S, et al: Prefrontal cortex 5-HT2 receptors in depression: a [18F] setoperone PET imaging study. Am J Psychiatry 156:1029–1034, 1999

Meyer JH, Kapur S, Eisfeld B, et al: The effect of paroxetine upon 5-HT$_{2a}$ receptors in depression: an [^{18}F] setoperone PET imaging study. Am J Psychiatry 158:78–85, 2001

Meyer JH, Houle S, Sagrati S, et al: Brain serotonin transporter binding potential measured with carbon 11–labeled DASB PET: effects of major depressive episodes and severity of dysfunctional attitudes. Arch Gen Psychiatry 61:1271–1279, 2004

Mintun MA, Sheline YI, Moerlein SM, et al: Decreased hippocampal 5-HT2A receptor binding in major depressive disorder: in vivo measurement with [18F]-altanserin positron emission tomography. Biol Psychiatry 55:217–224, 2004

Mirescu C, Peters JD, Gould E: Early life experience alters response of adult neurogenesis to stress. Nat Neurosci 7:841–846, 2004

Mitterschiffthaler MT, Kumari V, Malhi GS, et al: Neural response to pleasant stimuli in anhedonia: an fMRI study. Neuroreport 14:177–182, 2003

Moniz E: Prefrontal leucotomy in the treatment of mental disorders. Am J Psychiatry 93:1379–1385, 1937

Nauta WJH: Circuitous connections linking cerebral cortex, limbic system, and corpus striatum, in The Limbic System: Functional Organization and Clinical Disorders. Edited by Doane BK, Livingston KE. New York, Raven, 1986, pp 43–54

Neumeister A, Konstantinidis A, Stastny J, et al: Association between serotonin transporter gene promoter polymorphism (5HTTLPR) and behavioral responses to tryptophan depletion in healthy women with and without family history of depression. Arch Gen Psychiatry 59:613–620, 2002

Nobler MS, Oquendo MA, Kegeles LS, et al: Decreased regional brain metabolism after ECT. Am J Psychiatry 158:305–308, 2001

Ongur D, Price JL: The organization of networks within the orbital and medial prefrontal cortex of rats, monkeys and humans. Cereb Cortex 10:206–219, 2000

Ongur D, Drevet WC, Price JL: Glial reduction in the subgenual prefrontal cortex in mood disorders. Proc Natl Acad Sci U S A 95:13290–13295, 1998

Osuch EA, Ketter TA, Kimbrell TA, et al: Regional cerebral metabolism associated with anxiety symptoms in affective disorder patients. Biol Psychiatry 48:1020–1030, 2000

Papez JW: A proposed mechanism of emotion. Arch Neurol Psychiatry 38:725–743, 1937

Parsey RV, Oquendo M, Zea-Ponce Y, et al: Dopamine D2 receptor availability and amphetamine-induced dopamine release in unipolar depression. Biol Psychiatry 50:313–322, 2001

Pizzagalli D, Pascual-Marqui RD, Nitschke JB, et al: Anterior cingulate activity as a predictor of degree of treatment response in major depression: evidence from brain electrical tomography analysis. Am J Psychiatry 158:405–415, 2001

Post RM, DeLisi LE, Holcomb HH, et al: Glucose utilization in the temporal cortex of affectively ill patients: PET. Biol Psychiatry 22:545–553, 1987

Rajkowska G: Postmortem studies in mood disorders indicate altered number of neurons and glial cells. Biol Psychiatry 48:766–777, 2000

Robinson RG, Kubos KL, Starr LB, et al: Mood disorders in stroke patients: importance of location of lesion. Brain 107:81–93, 1984

Rolls ET: The orbitofrontal cortex and reward. Cereb Cortex 10:284–294, 2000

Santarelli L, Saxe M, Gross C, et al: Requirement of hippocampal neurogenesis for the behavioral effects of antidepressants. Science 301:805–809, 2003

Sapolsky RM: The possibility of neurotoxicity in the hippocampus in major depression: a primer on neuron death. Biol Psychiatry 48:755–765, 2000

Sargent PA, Kjaer KH, Bench CJ, et al: Brain serotonin-1A receptor binding measured by PET with 11C-Way-100635. Arch Gen Psychiatry 57:174–180, 2000

Saxena S, Rauch SL: Functional neuroimaging and the neuroanatomy of obsessive-compulsive disorder. Psychiatr Clin North Am 23:563–586, 2000

Seminowicz DA, Mayberg HS, McIntosh AR, et al: Limbic-frontal circuitry in major depression: a path modeling met-analysis. Neuroimage 22:409–418, 2004

Sheline YI: Neuroimaging studies of mood disorder effects on the brain. Biol Psychiatry 54:338–352, 2003

Sheline YI, Sanghavi M, Mintun MA, et al: Depression duration but not age predicts hippocampal volume loss in medically healthy women with recurrent major depression. J Neurosci 19:5034–5043, 1999

Sheline YI, Barch DM, Donnelly JM, et al: Increased amygdala response to masked emotional faces in depressed subjects resolves with antidepressant treatment: an fMRI study. Biol Psychiatry 50:651–658, 2001

Sheline YI, Gado MH, Kraemer HC: Untreated depression and hippocampal volume loss. Am J Psychiatry 161:1309–1310, 2003

Siegle GJ, Steinhauer SR, Thase ME, et al: Can't shake that feeling: event-related fMRI assessment of sustained amygdala activity in response to emotional information in depressed individuals. Biol Psychiatry 51:693–707, 2002

Smith GS, Reynolds CF, Houck PR, et al: Glucose metabolic response to total sleep deprivation, recovery sleep, and acute antidepressant treatment as functional neuroanatomic correlates of treatment outcome in geriatric depression. Am J Geriatr Psychiatry 10:561–567, 2002

Starkstein SE, Robinson RG (eds): Depression in Neurologic Diseases. Baltimore, MD, Hopkins University Press, 1993

Starkstein SE, Robinson RG, Price TR: Comparison of cortical and subcortical lesions in the production of post-stroke mood disorders. Brain 110:1045–1059, 1987

Starkstein SE, Mayberg HS, Berthier ML, et al: Mania after brain injury: neuroradiological and metabolic findings. Ann Neurol 27:652–659, 1990

Stefurak T, Mayberg HS: Cortico-limbic-striatal dysfunction in depression: converging findings in basal ganglia disease and primary affective disorders, in Mental and Behavioral Dysfunction in Movement Disorders. Edited by Bedard MA. Totowa, NJ, Humana, 2003, pp 321–338

Stuss DT, Benson DF: The Frontal Lobes. New York, Raven, 1986

Taylor WD, MacFall JR, Payne ME, et al: Late-life depression and microstructural abnormalities in dorsolateral prefrontal cortex white matter. Am J Psychiatry 161:1293–1296, 2004

Teasdale JD, Moore RG, Hayhurst H, et al: Metacognitive awareness and prevention of relapse in depression: empirical evidence. J Consult Clin Psychol 70:275–287, 2002

Teneback CC, Nahas Z, Speer AM, et al: Changes in prefrontal cortex and paralimbic activity in depression following two weeks of daily left prefrontal TMS. J Neuropsychiatry Clin Neurosci 11:426–435, 1999

Toga AW, Mazziotta JC (eds): Brain Mapping: The Methods, 2nd Edition. San Diego, CA, Academic Press, 2002

Tremblay L, Schultz W: Relative reward preference in primate orbitofrontal cortex. Nature 398:704–708, 1999

Vaidya VA, Duman RS: Depression—emerging insights from neurobiology. Br Med Bull 57:61–79, 2001

Videbech P: PET measurements of brain glucose metabolism and blood flow in major depressive disorder: a critical review. Acta Psychiatr Scand 101:11–20, 2000

Vogt BA, Pandya DN: Cingulate cortex of the rhesus monkey, II: cortical afferents. J Comp Neurol 262:271–289, 1987

Wu J, Buchsbaum MS, Gillin JC, et al: Prediction of antidepressant effects of sleep deprivation on metabolic rates in ventral anterior cingulate and medial prefrontal cortex. Am J Psychiatry 156:1149–1158, 1999

Yatham LN, Liddle PF, Dennis J, et al: Decrease in brain serotonin 2 receptor binding in patients with major depression following desipramine treatment. Arch Gen Psychiatry 56:705–711, 1999

Zald DH, Mattson DL, Pardo JV: Brain activity in ventromedial prefrontal cortex correlates with individual differences in negative affect. Proc Natl Acad Sci U S A 99:2450–2454, 2002

14

Genetics of Bipolar and Unipolar Disorders

WADE BERRETTINI, M.D., PH.D.

IN THIS CHAPTER, I review some aspects of the genetic epidemiology and molecular genetic research on bipolar disorders and recurrent unipolar disorders. I also review the genetic concepts of linkage and linkage disequilibrium. Given that the inherited susceptibilities for bipolar disorder and recurrent unipolar disorder are explained by multiple genes of small effect, simulations indicate that *universal* confirmation of vulnerability genes cannot be expected because of power issues, sampling variation, and genetic heterogeneity. With this background, I review several valid linkages of bipolar disorder to genomic regions, including some that may be shared with schizophrenia. These results suggest that nosology must be changed to reflect the genetic origins of the multiple disorders that are collectively described by the term *bipolar disorders*. The briefer history of recurrent unipolar disorder molecular linkage and linkage disequilibrium studies is reviewed as well.

Bipolar Disorders

Genetic Epidemiology

Family Studies

The optimal design for a bipolar disorder family study is one in which relatives of control subjects and relatives of bipolar disorder probands are directly interviewed, and diagnoses are made by individuals who are blind to the identity and family origin of the individual under scrutiny. Family studies of bipolar disorders show that a spectrum of mood disorders is found among the first-degree relatives of bipolar disorder probands: bipolar I disorder, bipolar II disorder (hypomania and recurrent major depressive episodes in the same person), schizoaffective disorders, and recurrent unipolar disorder (Angst et al. 1980; Baron et al. 1983; Gershon et al. 1982; Helzer and Winokur 1974; James and Chapman 1975; Johnson and Leeman 1977; Maier et al. 1993; Taylor et al. 1993; Tsuang et al. 1980; Weissman et al. 1984; Winokur et al. 1982, 1995). The family studies suggest shared liability for bipolar disorder and recurrent unipolar disorder.

No bipolar disorder family study, conducted in an optimal manner, reports increased risk for schizophrenia among relatives of bipolar disorder probands. Similarly, no schizophrenia family study reports increased risk for bipolar disorder among relatives of schizophrenia probands. However, several schizophrenia family studies reported increased risk for recurrent unipolar disorder and schizoaffective disorder among relatives of schizophrenia probands (Gershon et al. 1988; Kendler et al. 1993; Maier et al. 1993; Taylor et al. 1993). These family studies are consistent with some degree of overlap in susceptibility to recurrent unipolar disorder and schizoaffec-

TABLE 14–1. Concordance rates for mood disorders in monozygotic and dizygotic twins[a]

Study	Monozygotic twins		Dizygotic twins	
	Concordant pairs/ total pairs	Concordance (%)	Concordant pairs/ total pairs	Concordance (%)
Luxemberger 1930	3/4	75.0	0/13	0.0
Rosanoff et al. 1935	16/23	69.6	11/67	16.4
Slater 1953	4/7	57.1	4/17	23.5
Kallman 1954	25/27	92.6	13/55	23.6
Harvald and Hauge 1975	10/15	66.7	2/40	5.0
Allen et al. 1974	5/15	33.3	0/34	0.0
Bertelsen et al. 1977	32/55	58.2	9/52	17.3
Totals	95/146	65.1	39/278	14.0

[a]Data not corrected for age. Diagnoses include both bipolar and unipolar illness.

tive disorder for relatives of bipolar disorder probands and relatives of schizophrenia probands. Kendler et al. (1993) specifically noted an increase in risk for psychotic affective disorders among the relatives of schizophrenia probands.

Potash et al. (2001, 2003) reported that psychotic mood disorders cluster in families. Risk for psychotic mood disorders was significantly higher among the relatives of psychotic bipolar disorder probands, compared with the risk for relatives of nonpsychotic bipolar disorder probands. This raises the possibility that the partial overlap in risk for bipolar disorder and schizophrenia nosological categories is due to a subset of bipolar disorders characterized by psychotic symptoms. This subset of bipolar disorders is probably quite common because most of the bipolar disorder probands from the Potash et al. (2003) study were psychotic.

Twin Studies

Twin studies of bipolar disorder have been conducted over the past 70 years. In nearly all these reports, recurrent unipolar disorder in the co-twin of a bipolar disorder index case was grounds for categorizing the twin pair as concordant. Bertelsen et al. (1977) and Allen et al. (1974) reported that approximately 20% of concordant monozygotic twin pairs were composed of a bipolar disorder index twin and a recurrent unipolar disorder co-twin. These older studies (see Table 14–1) were conducted before the introduction of operationalized diagnostic criteria and semistructured interviews. However, the older results are quite consistent with the more recent studies (Kendler et al. 1993; McGuffin et al. 2003), which reported significantly higher monozygotic twins' concor-

dance rates, compared with those for dizygotic twins (see Figure 14–1). Recent estimates of heritability are about 85%, and about 30% of this is shared liability with recurrent unipolar disorder (McGuffin et al. 2003).

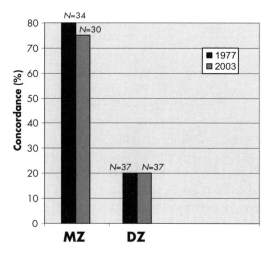

FIGURE 14–1. Heritability estimates: bipolar disorder twin studies.

Two bipolar disorder twin studies, conducted 25 years apart, are compared for concordance rates in monozygotic (MZ) and dizygotic (DZ) twins. Twins were clinically ascertained through a bipolar disorder proband. Co-twins were concordant if bipolar disorder or recurrent unipolar disorder was present. These studies yielded very similar results, including estimates of heritability of approximately 80%.

Source. Bertelsen et al. 1977; McGuffin et al. 2003.

Adoption Studies

Mendlewicz and Rainer (1977) reported a controlled adoption study of bipolar disorder probands, including a control group of probands with poliomyelitis. The biological relatives of the bipolar disorder probands had a 31% risk for bipolar disorder or unipolar disorders, as opposed to 2% in the relatives of the control probands. The risk for affective disorder in the biological relatives of adopted bipolar disorder patients was similar to the risk in the relatives of bipolar disorder patients who were not adopted away (26%). Adoptive relatives do not show increased risk compared with relatives of control probands.

Wender et al. (1986) and Cadoret (1978) studied unipolar and bipolar disorder probands. Although evidence for genetic susceptibility was found, adoptive relatives of affective probands had a tendency to excess affective illness themselves, compared with the adoptive relatives of control subjects. Von Knorring et al. (1983) did not find concordance in psychopathology between adoptees and biological relatives when examining the records of 56 adoptees with unipolar disorders.

Molecular Linkage Studies

Linkage refers to the observation that two DNA sequences, found near each other on the same chromosome, tend to be inherited together more often than expected by chance within families. Such DNA sequences are said to be *linked*. *Lod score* refers to the probability that observed cosegregation of alleles at distinct DNA sequences within a family has occurred because the two DNA sequences are linked. A lod score greater than 3 is evidence (not proof) that two DNA sequences are linked. The numerical value of the lod score is dependent on the proposed mode of inheritance (dominant, recessive, sex-linked) and penetrance. Because the lod score is dependent on these parameters (mode of inheritance and penetrance), it is sometimes termed a *parametric* statistic. This dependence on mode of inheritance and penetrance distinguishes the lod score from *nonparametric* statistics (including affected sibling pair and affected pedigree member methods) because such statistics are not dependent on mode of inheritance or penetrance. These nonparametric statistics use kinship coefficients to estimate the randomly expected degree of DNA sharing among affected members of the same family. For example, siblings share 50% of DNA sequences randomly because they have the same parents. If one has DNA samples from 1,000 pairs of ill siblings, one could search through the genomes of those 2,000 persons to find regions where DNA sequences are shared significantly greater than the baseline 50% rate. Regions of increased

DNA sharing may harbor genes that may explain (in part) why both members of each sibling pair are affected.

What level of statistical significance should be required for declaring linkage? A recommended level of statistical significance for an initial report ($P \leq \sim 0.00002$) is a stringent criterion according to simulations indicating that this level of significance would occur less than 5 times randomly in 100 genome scans for linkage (Lander and Kruglyak 1995). This statistical criterion assumes that all the genetic information within the pedigrees studied would be extracted, an assumption that is not true in practice. Typically, no more than about 80% of the genetic information in a pedigree series is extracted through genotyping. As in any other area of science, however, no single report of linkage should be accepted as valid without independent confirmation. The requirement for independent confirmations (at $P \leq 0.01$) is not waived, regardless of what level of statistical significance has been achieved in a single report. This confirmation requirement should be viewed within the context that valid linkages will not be confirmed in some studies. Indeed, nonconfirmations should be expected, intuitively, because of population (ethnic) differences, sampling procedures, and genetic heterogeneity.

Suarez et al. (1994) examined the probability of confirmation in simulations. They simulated a disorder caused by any one of six loci and determined that a large sample size and substantial time would be required for an initial linkage to be confirmed in a second sample. From their simulations, it is clear that consistent detection of a locus of moderate effect cannot be expected. Nonconfirmatory studies always will occur when an initially detected linkage is valid.

One of the most critical issues in confirmation of reported linkages is power. Attempts at confirmation of a reported susceptibility locus should state what power has been achieved to detect the locus initially described. For example, if a locus increases risk for bipolar disorder by a factor of two, it may be necessary to study approximately 200 affected sibling pairs to have adequate (90%) power to detect such a locus (Hauser et al. 1996). Unfortunately, few studies address this key issue. If 200 affected sibling pairs are required to achieve adequate (90%) power to detect a previously described locus, then a publication with fewer than 150 sibling pairs does not address the central issue of confirmation. However, such power-limited publications may have an important role in meta-analyses, in that they identify invaluable sources of additional data.

Comprehensive scans of the human genome have been completed with sufficient numbers (e.g., >100) of bipolar disorder individuals (Bennett et al. 2002; Cichon et al. 2001; Detera-Wadleigh et al. 1999; Dick et al. 2003; Ekholm et al. 2003; Kelsoe et al. 2001; Liu et al. 2003;

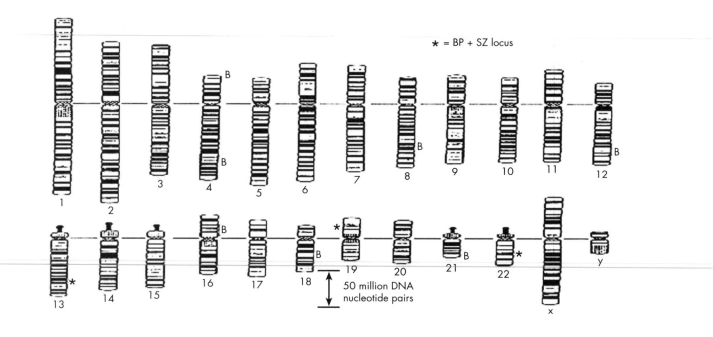

FIGURE 14–2.   **Loci with confirmed linkages for bipolar disorder (BP) and reported linkages for schizo-phrenia (SZ) mapped onto an ideogram of the human genome.**

To the right of the indicated chromosome, a B is placed for a confirmed bipolar disorder susceptibility locus; an asterisk is placed to the right of the indicated chromosome for a confirmed bipolar disorder + schizophrenia susceptibility locus.

McInnis et al. 2003; Rice et al. 1997). If a major locus (explaining more than 50% of the risk in more than 50% of the patients with bipolar disorder) existed, it would have been detected in many of these studies. Thus, no such major locus exists for bipolar disorder. Several reports of loci of smaller effect have been confirmed, which can be termed *susceptibility loci*. These loci are neither necessary nor sufficient for disease but increase risk for the disorder in a non-Mendelian manner.

From these genome scans and from additional, smaller studies, a picture has emerged in which approximately 10 bipolar disorder linkage regions have been confirmed across the genome. It is highly probable that additional confirmed bipolar disorder linkages will be identified through future linkage studies. These bipolar disorder linkage regions are confirmed by virtue of at least one study with strong statistical significance ($P<0.0001$) and at least two confirmatory studies ($P<0.01$). As noted elsewhere (Berrettini 2003), in some cases, these confirmed bipolar disorder linkage regions overlap with schizophrenia linkage reports, suggesting that the same loci may be involved in some aspects of both disorders. In Figure 14–2, these loci are mapped onto an ideogram of the human genome. The studies that support these findings are listed in

Table 14–2, with the identified primary report cited as the first study with genomewide statistical significance.

Two methodological approaches have been used to conduct meta-analyses of bipolar disorder linkage studies (Badner and Gershon 2002; Levinson et al. 2003). Badner and Gershon (2002) analyzed linkage results with a multiple-scan probability approach in which P values are combined across studies, after they adjusted for the size of the linkage region. These authors concluded that two genomic regions, 13q32 and 22q11–13, were the most promising loci for bipolar disorder. Segurado et al. (2003) used the method of Levinson et al. (2003), which ranks the P values across the genome of each study and then sums the rankings for each genomic "bin." In this approach, no genomic region reached genomewide significance, although the region that seemed most promising was the pericentromeric region of 18 (Segurado et al. 2003).

Linkage Disequilibrium Studies

The human genome consists of about 3 billion base pairs of DNA (Venter et al. 2001). The completion of draft genomic sequences of the human genome (Venter et al.

TABLE 14–2. Linkage studies of bipolar disorder

Location	Primary report	Independent confirmations	Comments
18p11.2	Berrettini et al. 1997	Bennett et al. 2002; Nothen et al. 1999; Stine et al. 1995; Turecki et al. 1999a	Paternal parent-of-origin effect; see Lin and Bale 1997; Schwab et al. 1998
21q22	Straub et al. 1994	Aita et al. 1999; Detera-Wadleigh et al. 1996; Kwok et al. 1999; Morissette et al. 1999; Smyth et al. 1996	
22q11–13	Kelsoe et al. 2001	Detera-Wadleigh et al. 1994, 1999; Lachman et al. 1996	Velocardiofacial syndrome region; overlap with a schizophrenia locus: Gill et al. 1996
18q22	Stine et al. 1995	De Bruyn et al. 1996; McInnes et al. 1996; McInnis et al. 2003; McMahon et al. 1997	See Freimer et al. 1996
12q23	Morissette et al. 1999	Curtis et al. 2003; Dawson et al. 1995; Ekholm et al. 2003; Ewald et al. 2002; Maziade et al. 2005	Morissette et al. (1999) studied a Canadian isolate; Abkevich et al. 2003
8q24	Cichon et al. 2001	Dick et al. 2003; McInnis et al. 2003	
13q32	Detera-Wadleigh et al. 1999	Badenhop et al. 2001; Kelsoe et al. 2001; Liu et al. 2003; Potash et al. 2003	See Blouin et al. 1998; Brzustowicz et al. 1999; Chumakov et al. 2002
16p12	Ewald et al. 2002	Dick et al. 2003; Ekholm et al. 2003	
4q32	Ekholm et al. 2003	Adams et al. 1998; Liu et al. 2003; McInnis et al. 2003	
4p15	Blackwood et al. 1996	Cichon et al. 2001; Detera-Wadleigh et al. 1999; Ewald et al. 2002; Morissette et al. 1999	See Ginns et al. 1998

2001) is consistent with about 35,000–40,000 genes. Physical distance along the linear sequence of DNA can be expressed in terms of base pairs of DNA. The most common sequence variation in the human genome is a single nucleotide polymorphism, in which two different nucleotides from the possible four (adenine [A], guanine [G], thymine [T], and cytosine [C]) are found among humans at the same position on different chromosomes. Single nucleotide polymorphisms with a common minor allele (frequency of ~20%) occur approximately every 1,000 base pairs of DNA (Venter et al. 2001). Analysis of closely spaced single nucleotide polymorphisms in outbred populations suggests a complex pattern of inheritance, in which recombination is inhibited in a small region of DNA, such that blocks of DNA (containing multiple single nucleotide polymorphisms) tend to be inherited intact over many generations (Gabriel et al. 2002). Thus, blocks of DNA are shared among present-day individuals who may have had a common ancestor 10,000 generations ago. These blocks are variable in length and often contain multiple single nucleotide polymorphisms, but among outbred human populations, the block length rarely exceeds around 100,000 base pairs. Alleles of single nucleotide polymorphisms within a block form a *haplotype* (a set of alleles) that usually is inherited across many generations. Such single nucleotide poly-

morphisms are said to be in strong linkage disequilibrium with one another. Linkage disequilibrium refers to the fact that two (or more) alleles can be found together in *unrelated* individuals more often than predicted by chance. The interested reader is referred to primary reports concerning linkage disequilibrium (e.g., Gabriel et al. 2002). Figure 14–3 presents an example of a haplotype block that contains two single nucleotide polymorphisms.

Linkage disequilibrium is a useful tool to investigate the relatively small genomic regions that have been implicated in the genetic origins of bipolar disorder through linkage studies (see Table 14–2). In this process, single nucleotide polymorphisms spaced across genes in the linkage region are assessed in large groups (ideally several hundred at least) of ethnically matched patients and control subjects. Investigators compare allele and genotype frequencies among groups of patients and control subjects.

A multitude of linkage disequilibrium studies in bipolar disorder have been done over the past decade. In a typical report, allele and genotype frequencies in the bipolar disorder patients and control subjects are examined at a single candidate gene variant. If nominally significant differences in allele or genotype frequencies are found between groups, the authors might conclude that the variant influences risk for bipolar disorder. Most often, these studies have assembled a small group of bipolar disorder

LINKAGE DISEQUILIBRIUM

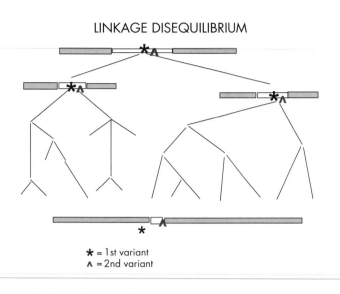

★ = 1st variant
∧ = 2nd variant

FIGURE 14–3. **Linkage disequilibrium.**

The first variant and the second variant represent two single nucleotide polymorphisms located in the same small region of an ancestral chromosome. Across thousands of generations, recombination between the two single nucleotide polymorphisms tends to be rare because they are located so close to each other. About 10,000 generations later, only about 5,000 base pairs are shared. Individuals who share the common ancestor shown here will retain that ancestor's alleles at both single nucleotide polymorphisms.

patients and unaffected control subjects from a population. These studies typically have used one variant in a single candidate gene, which is selected on the basis of presumed central nervous system (CNS) function, in relation to bipolar disorder pathophysiological theories. Unfortunately, the nearly complete absence of pathophysiological data on bipolar disorder makes the process of rational candidate gene selection difficult. Additionally, these studies have typically involved smaller numbers of bipolar disorder patients than is optimal, given that the effect size of individual alleles on risk must be small. Last, these studies often have used gene variants that are not known to confer functional differences in the gene. Despite these difficulties, several candidate genes deserve mention.

One promising candidate gene is the *G72* locus on 13q32, the site of a confirmed linkage in bipolar disorder and schizophrenia (see Table 14–2). *G72* is a primate-specific brain-expressed gene that activates D-amino acid oxidase (Chumakov et al. 2002). D-Amino acid oxidase may control levels of D-serine, which regulates glutamatergic receptors (Stevens et al. 2003). Chumakov et al. (2002) identified a haplotype from *G72* single nucleotide polymorphisms (without obvious functional significance)

that were in linkage disequilibrium with schizophrenia in a French-Canadian sample. This has been confirmed in distinct schizophrenia populations, including Russian (Chumakov et al. 2002) and German (Schumacher et al. 2004), although different haplotypes have been associated in different ethnic populations. Similarly, in bipolar disorder, there have been several positive findings with distinct haplotypes in different populations, including American (Chen et al. 2004; Hattori et al. 2003) and German (Schumacher et al. 2004) bipolar disorder samples. Although the data are promising, no clear functional variants have been defined at this locus.

A second promising candidate gene is brain-derived neurotrophic factor (BDNF), for which there are several positive reports of a functional missense variant (Neves-Pereira et al. 2002; Sklar et al. 2002). In the several European origin populations studied, at a G/A single nucleotide polymorphism (valine/methionine), the G (valine) allele was overtransmitted. Egan et al. (2001) reported that this single nucleotide polymorphism confers functional difference. These reports are promising because they consistently identify a functional variant contributing to genetic risk for bipolar disorder. However, small studies of Japanese and Chinese bipolar disorder patients did not show any evidence of this variant influencing risk for bipolar disorder (Hong et al. 2003; Nakata et al. 2003). The effect may be limited to populations of European origin. Alternatively, the negative studies may have been underpowered. It must be remembered that some variants will be relatively specific to particular ethnic groups. Consider that the protective effect of aldehyde dehydrogenase deficiency on risk for alcoholism is easily shown in Chinese, Korean, and Japanese populations because the deficiency allele has a frequency of approximately 30% (Harada et al. 1982; Thomasson et al. 1991). Much larger sample sizes are required to detect this influence in European populations because the deficiency allele frequency is lower by an order of magnitude.

There have been numerous independent association studies of bipolar disorder and recurrent unipolar disorder and a monoamine oxidase–A (MAO-A) $(CA)_n$ repeat polymorphism in European (Craddock et al. 1995; Furlong et al. 1999; Lim et al. 1995; Nothen et al. 1995; Parsian and Todd 1997; Preisig et al. 2000; Turecki et al. 1999b) and Asian (Kawada et al. 1995; Muramatsu et al. 1997) populations. Those studies reporting a positive association (Furlong et al. 1999; Kawada et al. 1995; Lim et al. 1995; Preisig et al. 2000) generally detected an overrepresentation of allele 5 or 6 of the MAO-A $(CA)_n$ repeat among bipolar disorder patients, compared with control subjects, an observation that may be particularly evident among women. The effect size was small (odds ratio=

1.49) (Preisig et al. 2000), and the sample size required for adequate power to detect was larger than in most of the negative studies (Craddock et al. 1995; Muramatsu et al. 1997; Nothen et al. 1995; Parsian and Todd 1997; Turecki et al. 1999b). An MAO-A promoter polymorphism is also found (Kunugi et al. 1999). These studies involved multiple ethnic groups, case–control methods, and family-based designs, with some studies having limited power to detect a small effect size. Thus, it is understandable that conflicting studies are reported.

Another intensively studied candidate gene is the serotonin transporter (*5HTT*), a functional candidate gene for which multiple bipolar disorder linkage disequilibrium studies have been published. The *5HTT* represents a logical candidate gene because many antidepressants act through binding to the 5-HTT protein (Ramammorthy et al. 1993). Two variants of the *5HTT* gene have been studied in bipolar disorder, and both have functional significance, according to in vitro analysis of these noncoding polymorphisms. The first variant is an insertion/deletion polymorphism in the 5-HTT promoter region. The shorter allele has much less transcriptional activity than the longer allele (Collier et al. 1996a; Heils et al. 1996). Moreover, the shorter allele has been associated with anxiety-related personality traits in humans (Lesch et al. 1996). The second variant is a variable number of tandem repeats (VNTR) polymorphism in intron 2.

The two most common alleles are the 10 and 12 repeats, which confer differential transcriptional activity in an embryonic stem cell line (Fiskerstrand et al. 1999). Collier et al. (1996a) first reported that the *5HTT* intron 2 VNTR allele 12 was in linkage disequilibrium with bipolar disorder among patients from the United Kingdom. Collier et al. (1996b) also reported that the short allele of the *5HTT* promoter variant was more common among 454 European bipolar disorder and recurrent unipolar patients, compared with 570 European control subjects, although the statistical significance was marginal (*P*=0.03), emphasizing the small effect size involved. Analysis by genotype suggested that homozygosity for the short allele was associated with bipolar disorder (*P*<0.05) and recurrent unipolar disorder (*P*<0.01). Rees et al. (1997) confirmed the observation of Collier et al. (1996a) in that allele 12 of the intron 2 VNTR was in linkage disequilibrium with bipolar disorder among 171 bipolar disorder probands, compared with 121 control subjects (*P*=0.031). Similarly, Rees et al. (1998) studied bipolar disorder patients and control subjects and reported an excess of bipolar disorder patients among individuals homozygous for the shorter promoter allele, implying a recessive mode of inheritance. Note that the sample sizes for Rees et al. (1997) and for Collier et al. (1996b) were in the hundreds.

Vincent et al. (1999) studied an initial sample of about 100 bipolar disorder probands from Canada and confirmed the observation that the promoter short allele was in linkage disequilibrium with bipolar disorder, compared with about 100 control subjects, but then failed to confirm this observation in a second set of about 100 bipolar disorder probands. Sampling variation and the small effect size, coupled with limited power of this sample size, are probable explanations for these results.

Gutierrez et al. (1998) studied bipolar disorder probands and control subjects of Spanish origin. They reported no evidence for linkage disequilibrium with *5HTT* alleles. This may be secondary to the ethnic background of patients or to small sample size. Bocchetta et al. (1999) studied approximately 55 Sardinian parent–child bipolar disorder trios and found no evidence for transmission disequilibrium in the *5HTT* gene, although sample size was a limiting factor in their conclusions. In a study of 123 bipolar disorder parent–child trios of European origin, Mundo et al. (2000) reported no evidence for linkage disequilibrium with the *5HTT* promoter alleles. Mynett-Johnson et al. (2000) studied approximately 100 Irish bipolar disorder parent–child trios from multiplex families and reported that a haplotype including the shorter promoter allele and a 3′ untranslated-region single nucleotide polymorphism conferred risk for bipolar disorder. Kirov et al. (1999) studied 122 parent–child trios of British ethnic background, with no nominally significant results at either polymorphism. In a study of 50 Indian bipolar disorder patients and control subjects, no evidence for linkage disequilibrium was reported with the VNTR variant (Saleem et al. 2000); this result was limited by the small sample size. From another ethnic perspective, Mendes de Oliveira et al. (1998) studied a small number of Brazilian bipolar disorder patients and found no evidence for linkage disequilibrium with the 5-HTT promoter polymorphism. Kunugi et al. (1997) studied these two polymorphisms in a Japanese sample of 191 patients with mood disorders (142 bipolar and 49 unipolar) and 212 control subjects. They reported nominally significant linkage disequilibrium between the VNTR and bipolar disorder, with no evidence for linkage disequilibrium with the promoter variant.

Furlong et al. (1999) reported results of a meta-analysis for approximately 1,400 individuals of European origin, including 772 control subjects, 375 bipolar patients, and 299 unipolar patients. Although no evidence was seen for linkage disequilibrium with mood disorders for the VNTR, a marginally significant result was found for the short allele of the 5-HTT promoter polymorphism. This result is important because it suggests that samples in the thousands will be necessary to draw firm conclusions because of the small effect sizes involved.

What clinical characteristics might describe those bipolar disorder probands with illness secondary to *5HTT* alleles? One preliminary answer was derived from two studies on independent populations. Coyle et al. (2000) studied bipolar women with postpartum psychotic episodes and found a large effect size for the *5HTT* promoter short allele, with an attributable risk of 69%. Ospina-Duque et al. (2000) studied 100 bipolar disorder patients from a Colombian population isolate and approximately 100 control subjects; those patients with psychosis as part of the phenotype showed linkage disequilibrium with the shorter *5HTT* promoter allele. Their conclusions may be similar to those of Coyle et al. (2000) and suggest that this allele deserves further study.

In another large European study, Mendlewicz et al. (2004) examined the genetic contribution of the 5-HTT promoter polymorphism in a case–control sample, including 539 recurrent unipolar disorder patients, 572 bipolar disorder patients, and 821 control subjects. No evidence of linkage disequilibrium was found for recurrent unipolar disorder or bipolar disorder, and subdividing the sample according to family history, suicidal attempts, and psychotic features did not show any role of the promoter variant in the genetic susceptibilities to these disorders.

In a recent population-based study, Caspi et al. (2003) noted that individuals with one or more copies of the short allele of the 5-HTT promoter variants were at increased risk for depression depending on the occurrence of adverse life events. This article described a plausible gene-by-environment interaction that may help explain the conflicting results for the 5-HTT promoter variant noted earlier in this section.

Recurrent Unipolar Disorders

Genetic Epidemiology

Family Studies

In considering optimally designed family studies of recurrent unipolar disorder (with blinded interviews and simultaneous examination of control relatives), there are five reports in the literature (Gershon et al. 1982; Maier et al. 1993; Tsuang et al. 1980; Weissman et al. 1984, 1993). These five reports had remarkably similar results; each study concluded that the first-degree relatives of recurrent unipolar disorder probands were at increased risk for recurrent unipolar disorders, compared with the first-degree relatives of control probands. Across the five studies, a two- to fourfold increased risk for recurrent unipolar disorder was found among the first-degree relatives of recurrent unipolar disorder probands.

Characteristics of recurrent unipolar disorders that yield a more heritable phenotype include early onset (i.e., before age 30) (Bland et al. 1986; Cadoret et al. 1977; Kupfer et al. 1989; Mendlewicz and Baron 1981; Stancer et al. 1987; Weissman et al. 1986, 1993) and a high degree of recurrence (Bland et al. 1986; Gershon et al. 1986; Kendler et al. 1994, 1999; Reich et al. 1987). A third characteristic that may identify a separate group of disorders is the presence of psychosis (Kendler et al. 1993). Additional genetic subtypes of recurrent unipolar disorder may be identified through examination of comorbidities with panic disorder and other anxiety disorders and with alcoholism (e.g., Merikangas et al. 1994; Nurnberger et al. 2001; Winokur et al. 1971).

Twin Studies

A review of twin studies in recurrent unipolar disorder estimated heritability at 37%, with a substantial component of unique individual environmental risk but little shared environmental risk (Sullivan and Kendler 2001). These twin studies included four community-ascertained samples (Bierut et al. 1999; Kendler and Prescott 1999; Kendler et al. 1995; Lyons et al. 1998) and two clinically ascertained samples, one from the United Kingdom (McGuffin et al. 1996) and one from Sweden (Kendler et al. 1995). The results were quite consistent in concluding that genetic influence is a significant factor in risk for recurrent unipolar disorder, independent of ascertainment and country of origin.

Molecular Linkage Studies

Only a few recurrent unipolar disorder genome scans have been done with more than 100 affected individuals, in contrast to the numbers for bipolar disorder. Holmans et al. (2004) reported on the first phase of a multisite collaborative effort. The sample consisted of 297 informative multiplex families (containing 685 informative affected relative pairs, 555 sibling pairs, and 130 other pair types). Affected patients had recurrent unipolar disorder, with onset before age 31 for probands or before age 41 for other affected relatives; the mean age at onset was 18.5, and the mean number of depressive episodes was 7.3, indicating a highly recurrent form of illness. Families were excluded if a first- or second-degree relative had bipolar disorder. Linkage was observed on chromosome 15q25.3–26.2 (empirical genomewide $P=0.023$). The linkage was not sex specific. This was the sole significant linkage peak observed by this group.

Abkevich et al. (2003) reported a genome scan on 110 Utah pedigrees (each with at least 4 affected individuals), which consisted of 784 individuals with recurrent unipolar disorder, 161 persons with single-episode major depressive disorder, and 162 individuals with bipolar disorder, who also were considered affected. They observed a highly significant linkage signal at 12q23 ($P=0.0000007$), confirming a previously identified bipolar disorder locus (see Table 14–2). No other linkage peaks approached statistical significance. It is probable that this study has detected the same bipolar disorder 12q23 locus, even though their families were ascertained from a recurrent unipolar disorder proband, because most kindreds probably did have at least one individual with bipolar disorder. These results confirm family and twin studies, suggesting genetic overlap between bipolar disorder and recurrent unipolar disorders, and this study identified the 12q23 region as a locus that increases risk for both bipolar disorder and recurrent unipolar disorders.

Zubenko et al. (2003b) reported on a genome scan of 81 families ascertained through a proband with early-onset nonpsychotic recurrent unipolar disorder. They described a highly significant linkage ($P<0.0001$) of this phenotype to 2q35 near marker *D2321*, which is near a candidate gene, *CREB1* (cyclic adenosine monophosphate response element–binding protein 1). Sequence variants in the *CREB* gene were found to segregate with recurrent unipolar disorder among women in 2 of these 81 extended kindreds (Zubenko et al. 2003a), thus nominating *CREB* as a recurrent unipolar disorder susceptibility gene. These intriguing results await independent confirmation.

Conclusion

Family, twin, and adoption studies of bipolar disorders and recurrent unipolar disorders, in general, show substantial heritable components to risk, with the bipolar disorders having higher heritability than the recurrent unipolar disorders. Multiple regions of the genome (including 18p11, 18q22, 12q24, 21q21, 13q32, 4p15, 4q32, 16p12, 8q24, and 22q11) have been implicated in the genetic origins of bipolar disorder by several independent groups. Most of these regions will likely yield susceptibility genes within the next 5 years, through the application of linkage disequilibrium mapping methods to large sample sizes. Linkage disequilibrium approaches to candidate genes have yielded several promising candidate genes, including *G72* and *BDNF* for bipolar disorder. For each of these candidate genes, several independent bipolar disorder populations have yielded data consistent with the existence of one or more haplotypes as susceptibility sequences. Only several genome scans for recurrent unipolar disorders have been published, and confirmations are required.

References

Abkevich V, Camp NJ, Hensel CH, et al: Predisposition locus for major depression at chromosome 12q22–12q23.2. Am J Hum Genet 73:1271–1281, 2003

Adams LJ, Mitchell PB, Fielder SL, et al: A susceptibility locus for bipolar affective disorder on chromosome 4q35. Am J Hum Genet 62:1084–1091, 1998

Aita VM, Liu J, Knowles JA, et al: A comprehensive linkage analysis of chromosome 21q22 supports prior evidence for a putative bipolar affective disorder locus. Am J Hum Genet 64:210–217, 1999

Allen MG, Cohen S, Pollin W, et al: Affective illness in veteran twins: a diagnostic review. Am J Psychiatry 131:1234–1239, 1974

Angst J, Frey R, Lohmeyer R, et al: Bipolar manic depressive psychoses: results of a genetic investigation. Hum Genet 55:237–254, 1980

Badenhop RF, Moses MJ, Scimone A, et al: A genome screen of a large bipolar affective disorder pedigree supports evidence for a susceptibility locus on chromosome 13q. Mol Psychiatry 6:396–403, 2001

Badner JA, Gershon ES: Meta-analysis of whole-genome linkage scans of bipolar disorder and schizophrenia. Mol Psychiatry 7:405–411, 2002

Baron M, Gruen R, Anis L, et al: Schizoaffective illness, schizophrenia and affective disorders: morbidity risk and genetic transmission. Acta Psychiatr Scand 65:253–262, 1983

Bennett P, Segurado R, Jones I, et al: The Wellcome trust UK-Irish bipolar affective disorder sibling pair genome screen: first stage report. Mol Psychiatry 7:189–200, 2002

Berrettini WH: Evidence for shared susceptibility in bipolar disorder and schizophrenia. Am J Med Genet 123C:59–64, 2003

Berrettini W, Ferraro T, Choi H, et al: Linkage studies of bipolar illness. Arch Gen Psychiatry 54:32–39, 1997

Bertelsen A, Harvald B, Hauge M: A Danish twin study of manic-depressive disorders. Br J Psychiatry 130:330–351, 1977

Bierut LJ, Heath AC, Bucholz KK, et al: Major depressive disorder in a community-based twin sample: are there different genetic and environmental contributions for men and women? Arch Gen Psychiatry 56:557–563, 1999

Blackwood DHR, He L, Morris SW, et al: A locus for bipolar affective disorder on chromosome 4p. Nat Genet 12:427–430, 1996

Bland RC, Newman SC, Orn H: Recurrent and nonrecurrent depression. Arch Gen Psychiatry 43:1085–1089, 1986

Blouin JL, Dombroski BA, Nath SK, et al: Schizophrenia susceptibility loci on chromosomes 13q32 and 8p21. Nat Genet 20:70–73, 1998

Bocchetta A, Piccardi MP, Palmas MA, et al: Family based association study between bipolar disorder and DRD2, DRD4, DAT, and SERT in Sardinia. Am J Med Genet 88:522–526, 1999

Brzustowicz LM, Honer WG, Chow EWC, et al: Linkage of familial schizophrenia to chromosome 13q32. Am J Hum Genet 65:1096–1103, 1999

Cadoret RJ: Evidence for genetic inheritance of primary affective disorder in adoptees. Am J Psychiatry 135:463–466, 1978

Cadoret RJ, Woolson R, Winokur G: The relationship of age of onset in unipolar affective illness to risk of alcoholism and depression in parents. J Psychiatr Res 13:137–142, 1977

Caspi A, Sugden K, Moffitt TE, et al: Influence of life stress on depression: moderation by a polymorphism in the 5-HTT gene. Science 301:386–389, 2003

Chen YS, Akula N, Detera-Wadleigh SD, et al: Findings in an independent sample support an association between bipolar affective disorder and the G72/G30 locus on chromosome 13q33. Mol Psychiatry 9:87–92, 2004

Chumakov I, Blumenfeld M, Guerassimenko O, et al: Genetic and physiological data implicating the new human gene G72 and the gene for D-amino acid oxidase in schizophrenia. Proc Natl Acad Sci U S A 99:13675–13680, 2002 [published erratum appears in 99:17221, 2002]

Cichon S, Schumacher J, Muller DJ, et al: A genome screen for genes predisposing to bipolar affective disorder detects a new susceptibility locus on 8q. Hum Mol Genet 10:2933–2944, 2001

Collier DA, Arranz MJ, Sham P, et al: The serotonin transporter is a potential susceptibility factor for bipolar affective disorder. Neuroreport 7:1675–1679, 1996a

Collier DA, Stober G, Li T, et al: A novel functional polymorphism within the promoter of the serotonin transporter gene: possible role in susceptibility to affective disorders. Mol Psychiatry 1:453–460, 1996b

Coyle N, Jones I, Robertson E, et al: Variation at the serotonin transporter gene influences susceptibility to bipolar affective puerperal psychosis. Lancet 356:1490–1491, 2000

Craddock N, Daniels J, Roberts E, et al: No evidence for allelic association between bipolar disorder and MAOA gene polymorphisms. Am J Med Genet 60:322–324, 1995

Curtis D, Kalsi G, Brynjolfsson J, et al: Genome scan of pedigrees multiply affected with bipolar disorder provides further support for the presence of a susceptibility locus on chromosome 12q23-q24, and suggests the presence of additional loci on 1p and 1q. Psychiatr Genet 13:77–84, 2003

Dawson E, Parfitt E, Roberts Q, et al: Linkage studies of bipolar disorder in the region of the Darier's disease gene on chromosome 12q23–24.1. Am J Med Genet 60:94–102, 1995

De Bruyn A, Souery D, Mendelbaum K, et al: Linkage analysis of families with bipolar illness and chromosome 18 markers. Biol Psychiatry 39:679–688, 1996

Detera-Wadleigh SD, Hsieh WT, Berrettini WH, et al: Genetic linkage mapping for a susceptibility locus to bipolar illness: chromosomes 2, 3, 4, 7, 9, 10p, 11p, 22, and Xpter. Am J Med Genet 54:206–218, 1994

Detera-Wadleigh SD, Badner JA, Berrettini WH, et al: A high-density genome scan detects evidence for a bipolar-disorder susceptibility locus on 13q32 and other potential loci on 1q32 and 18p11.2. Proc Natl Acad Sci U S A 96:5604–5609, 1999

Dick DM, Foroud T, Flury L, et al: Genome-wide linkage analyses of bipolar disorder: a new sample of 250 NIMH Genetics Initiative pedigrees. Am J Hum Genet 73:107–114, 2003

Egan MF, Goldberg TE, Kolachana BS, et al: Effect of COMT Val108/158 Met genotype on frontal lobe function and risk for schizophrenia. Proc Natl Acad Sci U S A 98:6917–6922, 2001

Ekholm JM, Kieseppa T, Hiekkalinna T, et al: Evidence of susceptibility loci on 4q32 and 16p12 for bipolar disorder. Hum Mol Genet 12:1907–1915, 2003

Ewald H, Flint T, Kruse TA, et al: A genome-wide scan shows significant linkage between bipolar disorder and chromosome 12q24.3 and suggestive linkage to chromosomes 1p22–21, 4p16, 6q14–22, 10q26 and 16p13.3. Mol Psychiatry 7:734–744, 2002

Fiskerstrand CE, Lovejoy EA, Quinn JP: An intronic polymorphic domain often associated with susceptibility to affective disorders has allele-dependent differential enhancer activity in embryonic stem cells. FEBS Lett 458:171–174, 1999

Freimer NB, Reus VI, Escamilla MA, et al: Genetic mapping using haplotype, association and linkage methods suggests a locus for severe bipolar disorder (BPI) at 18q22-q23. Nat Genet 12:436–441, 1996

Furlong RA, Ho L, Rubinszstein JS, et al: Analysis of the MAOA gene in bipolar affective disorder by association studies, meta-analyses and sequencing of the promoter. Am J Med Genet 88:398–406, 1999

Gabriel SB, Schaffner SF, Nguyen H, et al: The structure of haplotype blocks in the human genome. Science 296:2225–2227, 2002

Gershon ES, Hamovit J, Guroff JJ, et al: A family study of schizoaffective, bipolar I, bipolar II, unipolar, and normal control probands. Arch Gen Psychiatry 39:1157–1167, 1982

Gershon ES, Weissman MM, Guroff JJ, et al: Validation of criteria for major depression through controlled family study. J Affect Disord 11:125–131, 1986

Gershon ES, DeLisi LE, Hamovit J, et al: A controlled family study of chronic psychoses. Arch Gen Psychiatry 45:328–336, 1988

Gill M, Vallada H, Collier D, et al: A combined analysis of D22S278 marker alleles in affected sib-pairs: support for a susceptibility locus for schizophrenia at chromosome 22q12. Am J Med Genet 67:40–45, 1996

Ginns EI, St Jean P, Philibert RA, et al: A genome-wide search for chromosomal loci linked to mental health wellness in relatives at high risk for bipolar affective disorder among the Old Order Amish. Proc Natl Acad Sci U S A 95:15531–15536, 1998

Gutierrez B, Arranz MJ, Collier DA, et al: Serotonin transporter gene and risk for bipolar affective disorder: an association study in Spanish population. Biol Psychiatry 43:843–847, 1998

Harada S, Agarwal DP, Goedde HW: Aldehyde dehydrogenase deficiency as cause of the flushing reaction to alcohol in Japanese. Lancet ii(8253):982, 1982

Harvald B, Hauge M: Manic-depression, in Genetics and the Epidemiology of Chronic Diseases (PHS Publ No 1163). Edited by Neal JV, Shaw MW, Shull WJ. Washington, DC, U.S. Department of Health, Education and Welfare, 1975, pp 61–76

Hattori E, Liu C, Badner JA, et al: Polymorphisms at the G72/G30 gene locus on 13q33 are associated with bipolar disorder in two independent pedigree series. Am J Hum Genet 72:1131–1140, 2003

Hauser ER, Boehnke M, Guo S-W, et al: Affected sib pair interval mapping and exclusion for complex genetic traits. Genet Epidemiol 13:117–137, 1996

Heils A, Teufel A, Petri S, et al: Allelic variation of human serotonin transporter gene expression. J Neurochem 66:2621–2624, 1996

Helzer JE, Winokur G: A family interview study of male manic-depressives. Arch Gen Psychiatry 31:73–77, 1974

Holmans P, Zubenko GS, Crowe RR, et al: Genomewide significant linkage to recurrent, early-onset major depressive disorder on chromosome 15q. Am J Hum Genet 74:1154–1167, 2004

Hong CJ, Huo SJ, Yen FC, et al: Association study of a brain-derived neurotrophic factor genetic polymorphism and mood disorders, age of onset and suicidal behavior. Neuropsychobiology 48:186–189, 2003

James NM, Chapman CJ: A genetic study of bipolar affective disorder. Br J Psychiatry 126:449–456, 1975

Johnson GFS, Leeman MM: Analysis of familial factors in bipolar affective illness. Arch Gen Psychiatry 34:1074–1083, 1977

Kallman F: Genetics of depression, in Depression. Edited by Hoch PH, Zubin J. New York, Grune & Stratton, 1954, pp 1–24

Kawada Y, Hattori M, Dai XY: Possible association between MAOA gene and bipolar affective disorder. Am J Hum Genet 56:335–336, 1995

Kelsoe JR, Spence MA, Loetscher E, et al: A genome survey indicates a possible susceptibility locus for bipolar disorder on chromosome 22. Proc Natl Acad Sci U S A 98:585–590, 2001

Kendler KS, Prescott CA: A population-based twin study of lifetime major depression in men and women. Arch Gen Psychiatry 56:39–44, 1999

Kendler KS, McGuire M, Gruenberg AM, et al: The Roscommon family study. Arch Gen Psychiatry 50:527–540, 1993

Kendler KS, Neale MC, Kessler RC, et al: The clinical characteristics of major depression as indices of the familial risk to illness. Br J Psychiatry 165:66–72, 1994

Kendler KS, Pedersen N, Johnson L, et al: A pilot Swedish twin study of affective illness, including hospital- and population-ascertained subsamples. Behav Genet 25:217–232, 1995

Kendler KS, Gardner CO, Prescott CA: Clinical characteristics of major depression that predict risk of depression in relatives. Arch Gen Psychiatry 56:322–327, 1999

Kirov G, Rees M, Jones I, et al: Bipolar disorder and the serotonin transporter gene: a family based association study. Psychol Med 29:1249–1254, 1999

Kunugi H, Hattori M, Kato T, et al: Serotonin transporter gene polymorphisms: ethnic difference and possible association with bipolar affective disorder. Mol Psychiatry 2:457–462, 1997

Kunugi H, Ishida S, Kato T, et al: A functional polymorphism in the promoter region of MAOA gene and mood disorders. Mol Psychiatry 4:393–395, 1999

Kupfer DJ, Frank E, Carpenter LL, et al: Family history in recurrent depression. J Affect Disord 17:113–119, 1989

Kwok JB, Adams LJ, Salmon JA, et al: Non-parametric simulation-based statistical analyses for bipolar affective disorder locus on chromosome 21q22.3 Am J Med Genet 88:99–102, 1999

Lachman HM, Kelsoe JR, Remick RA, et al: Linkage studies support a possible locus for bipolar disorder in the velocardiofacial syndrome region on chromosome 22. Am J Med Genet 74:121–128, 1996

Lander E, Kruglyak L: Genetic dissection of complex traits: guidelines for interpreting and reporting linkage results. Nat Genet 11:241–247, 1995

Lesch K-P, Bengel D, Heils A, et al: Association of anxiety related traits with a polymorphism in the serotonin transporter gene regulatory region. Science 274:1527–1531, 1996

Levinson DF, Levinson MD, Sequardo R, et al: Genome scan meta-analysis of schizophrenia and bipolar disorder, part I: methods and power analysis. Am J Hum Genet 73:17–33, 2003

Lim LC, Powell J, Sham P, et al: Evidence for a genetic association between alleles of MAOA gene and bipolar affective disorder. Am J Med Genet 60:325–331, 1995

Lin JP, Bale SJ: Parental transmission and D18S37 allele sharing in bipolar affective disorder. Genet Epidemiol 14:665–668, 1997

Liu J, Juo SH, Dewan A, et al: Evidence for a putative bipolar disorder locus on 2p13–16 and other potential loci on 4q31, 7q34, 8q13, 9q31, 10q21–24, 13q32, 14q21 and 17q11–12. Mol Psychiatry 8:333–342, 2003

Luxemberger H: Psychiatrisch-neurologische Zwillings pathologie [Psychiatric-neurological twin pathology]. Zentralblatt fur diagesamte Neurologie und Psychiatrie 14:56–57, 145–180, 1930

Lyons MJ, Eisen SA, Goldberg J, et al: A registry-based twin study of depression in men. Arch Gen Psychiatry 55:468–472, 1998

Maier W, Lichtermann D, Minges J, et al: Continuity and discontinuity of affective disorders and schizophrenia: results of a controlled family study. Arch Gen Psychiatry 50:871–883, 1993

Maziade M, Roy MA, Chagnon YC, et al: Shared and specific susceptibility loci for schizophrenia and bipolar disorder: a dense genome scan in Eastern Quebec families. Mol Psychiatry 10:486–499, 2005

McGuffin P, Katz R, Watkins S, et al: A hospital-based twin register of the heritability of DSM-IV unipolar depression. Arch Gen Psychiatry 53:129–136, 1996

McGuffin P, Rijsdijk S, Andrew M, et al: The heritability of bipolar affective disorder and the genetic relationship to unipolar depression. Arch Gen Psychiatry 60:497–502, 2003

McInnes LA, Escamilla MA, Service SK, et al: A complete genome screen for genes predisposing to severe bipolar disorder in two Costa Rican pedigrees. Proc Natl Acad Sci U S A 93:13060–13065, 1996

McInnis MG, Lan TH, Willour VL, et al: Genome-wide scan of bipolar disorder in 65 pedigrees: supportive evidence for linkage at 8q24, 18q22, 4q32, 2p12, and 13q12. Mol Psychiatry 8:288–298, 2003

McMahon FJ, Hopkins PJ, Xu J, et al: Linkage of bipolar affective disorder to chromosome 18 markers in a new pedigree series. Am J Hum Genet 61:1397–1404, 1997

Mendes de Oliveira JR, Otto PA, Vallada H, et al: Analysis of a novel functional polymorphism within the promoter region of the serotonin transporter gene (5-HTT) in Brazilian patients affected by bipolar disorder and schizophrenia. Am J Med Genet 81:225–227, 1998

Mendlewicz J, Baron M: Morbidity risks in subtypes of unipolar depressive illness: differences between early and late onset forms. Br J Psychiatry 139:463–466, 1981

Mendlewicz J, Rainer JD: Adoption study supporting genetic transmission in manic-depressive illness. Nature 368 (5618):327–329, 1977

Mendlewicz J, Massat I, Souery D, et al: Serotonin transporter 5HTTLPR polymorphism and affective disorders: no evidence of association in a large European multicenter study. Eur J Hum Genet 12:377–382, 2004

Merikangas KR, Risch NJ, Weissman MM: Co-morbidity and co-transmission of alcoholism, anxiety and depression. Psychol Med 24:69–80, 1994

Morissette J, Villeneuve A, Bordeleau L, et al: Genome-wide search for linkage of bipolar affective disorders in a very large pedigree derived from a homogeneous population in Quebec points to a locus of major effect on chromosome 12q23-q24. Am J Med Genet 88:567–587, 1999

Mundo E, Walker M, Tims H, et al: Lack of linkage disequilibrium between serotonin transporter protein gene (SLC6A4) and bipolar disorder. Am J Med Genet 96:379–383, 2000

Muramatsu T, Matsushita S, Kanba S, et al: MAO genes polymorphisms and mood disorder. Am J Med Genet 19:494–496, 1997

Mynett-Johnson L, Kealey C, Claffey E, et al: Multimarker haplotypes within the serotonin transporter gene suggest evidence of an association with bipolar disorder. Am J Med Genet 96:845–849, 2000

Nakata K, Ujike H, Sakai A, et al: Association study of the BDNF gene with bipolar disorder. Neurosci Lett 337:17–20, 2003

Neves-Pereira M, Mundo E, Muglia P, et al: The brain-derived neurotrophic factor gene confers susceptibility to bipolar disorder: evidence from a family based association study. Am J Hum Genet 71:651–655, 2002

Nothen MM, Eggermann K, Albus M, et al: Association analyses of the MAOA gene in bipolar affective disorder by using family based controls. Am J Hum Genet 57:975–977, 1995

Nothen MM, Cichon S, Rohleder H, et al: Evaluation of linkage of bipolar affective disorder to chromosome 18 in a sample of 57 German families. Mol Psychiatry 4:76–84, 1999

Nurnberger JI, Foroud T, Flury L, et al: Evidence for a locus on chromosome 1 that influences vulnerability to alcoholism and affective disorder. Am J Psychiatry 158:718–724, 2001

Ospina-Duque J, Duque C, Carvajal-Carmona L, et al: An association study of bipolar mood disorder (type I) with the 5-HTTLPR serotonin transporter polymorphism in a human population isolate from Colombia. Neurosci Lett 292:199–202, 2000

Parsian A, Todd RD: Genetic association between monoamine oxidase and manic-depressive illness: comparison of relative risk and haplotype relative risk data. Am J Med Genet 74:475–479, 1997

Potash JB, Willour VL, Chiu Y-F, et al: The familial aggregation of psychotic symptoms in bipolar disorder pedigrees. Am J Psychiatry 158:1258–1264, 2001

Potash JB, Chiu Y-F, MacKinnon DF, et al: Familial aggregation of psychosis in a replication set of 69 bipolar pedigrees: Am J Med Genet 116B:90–97, 2003

Preisig M, Bellivier F, Fenton BT, et al: Association between bipolar disorder and MAOA gene polymorphisms: results of a multicenter study. Am J Psychiatry 157:948–959, 2000

Ramammorthy S, Bauman AL, Moore KR, et al: Antidepressant and cocaine sensitive human transporter: molecular cloning, expression and chromosomal localization. Proc Natl Acad Sci U S A 90:2542–2546, 1993

Reich T, Van Eerdewegh P, Rice J, et al: The familial transmission of primary major depressive disorder. J Psychiatr Res 21:613–624, 1987

Rice JP, Goate A, Williams JT, et al: Initial genome scan of the NIMH Genetics Initiative bipolar pedigrees: chromosomes 1, 6, 8, 10, and 12. Am J Med Genet 74:247–253, 1997

Rosanoff AJ, Handy L, Plesset IR: The etiology of manic-depressive syndromes with special reference to their occurrence in twins. Am J Psychiatry 91:725–762, 1935

Saleem Q, Ganesh S, Vijaykumar M, et al: Association analysis of 5HT transporter gene in bipolar disorder in the Indian population. Am J Med Genet 96:170–172, 2000

Schumacher J, Jamra RA, Freudenberg J, et al: Examination of G72 and D-amino acid oxidase as genetic risk factors for schizophrenia and bipolar affective disorder. Mol Psychiatry 9:203–207, 2004

Schwab SG, Hallmayer J, Lerer B, et al: Support for a chromosome 18p locus conferring susceptibility to functional psychoses in families with schizophrenia, by association and linkage analysis. Am J Hum Genet 63:1139–1152, 1998

Segurado R, Detera-Wadleigh SD, Levinson DF, et al: Genome scan meta-analysis of schizophrenia and bipolar disorder, part III: bipolar disorder. Am J Hum Genet 73:49–62, 2003

Sklar P, Gabriel SP, McInnis MG, et al: Family based association study of 76 candidate genes in bipolar disorder: BDNF is a susceptibility locus. Mol Psychiatry 7:579–593, 2002

Slater E: Psychotic and neurotic illness in twins. Medical Research Council Special Report Series no. 278. London, Her Majesty's Stationery Office, 1953

Smyth C, Kalsi G, Brynjolfsson J, et al: Further tests for linkage of bipolar affective disorder to the tyrosine hydroxylase gene locus on chromosome 11p15 in a new series of multiplex British affective disorder pedigrees. Am J Psychiatry 153:271–274, 1996 [Erratum: 154:1396, 1997]

Stancer HC, Persad E, Wagener DK, et al: Evidence for homogeneity of major depression and bipolar affective disorder. J Psychiatr Res 21:37–53, 1987

Stevens ER, Esguerra M, Kim PM, et al: D-Serine and serine racemase are present in the vertebrate retina and contribute to the physiological activation of NMDA receptors. Proc Natl Acad Sci U S A 100:6789–6794, 2003

Stine OC, Xu J, Koskela R, et al: Evidence for linkage of bipolar disorder to chromosome 18 with a parent-of-origin effect. Am J Hum Genet 57:1384–1394, 1995

Straub RE, Lehner T, Luo Y, et al: A possible vulnerability locus for bipolar affective disorder on chromosome 21q22.3. Nat Genet 8:291–296, 1994

Suarez B, Harpe CL, Van Eerdewegh P: Problems of replicating linkage claims in psychiatry, in Genetic Approaches to Mental Disorders. Edited by Gershon ES, Cloninger CR. Washington, DC, American Psychiatric Press, 1994, pp 23–46

Sullivan P, Kendler K: Genetic case-control studies in neuropsychiatry. Arch Gen Psychiatry 58:1015–1024, 2001

Taylor MA, Berenbaum SA, Jampala VC, et al: Are schizophrenia and affective disorder related? preliminary data from a family study. Am J Psychiatry 150:278–285, 1993

Thomasson HR, Edenberg HJ, Crabb DW, et al: Alcohol and aldehyde dehydrogenase genotypes and alcoholism in Chinese men. Am J Hum Genet 48:677–681, 1991

Tsuang MT, Winokur G, Crowe RR: Morbidity risks of schizophrenia and affective disorders among first degree relatives of patients with schizophrenia, mania, depression and surgical conditions. Br J Psychiatry 137:497–504, 1980

Turecki G, Grof P, Cavazzoni P, et al: Lithium responsive bipolar disorder, unilineality and chromosome 18: a linkage study. Am J Med Genet 88:411–415, 1999a

Turecki G, Grof P, Cavazzoni P, et al: MAOA: association and linkage studies with lithium responsive bipolar disorder. Psychiatr Genet 9:13–16, 1999b

Venter JC, Adams MD, Myers EW, et al: The sequence of the human genome. Science 291:1304–1351, 2001

Vincent JB, Masellis M, Lawrence J, et al: Genetic association analysis of serotonin system genes in bipolar affective disorder. Am J Psychiatry 156:136–138, 1999

Von Knorring AL, Cloninger CR, Bohman M, et al: An adoption study of depressive disorders and substance abuse. Arch Gen Psychiatry 40:943–950, 1983

Weissman MM, Gershon ES, Kidd KK, et al: Psychiatric disorders in the relatives of probands with affective disorder. Arch Gen Psychiatry 41:13–21, 1984

Weissman MM, Merikangas KR, Wickramaratne P, et al: Understanding the clinical heterogeneity of major depression using family data. Arch Gen Psychiatry 43:430–434, 1986

Weissman MM, Wickramaratne P, Adams PB, et al: The relationship between panic disorder and major depression: a new family study. Arch Gen Psychiatry 50:767–780, 1993

Wender H, Kety SS, Rosenthal D, et al: Psychiatric disorders in the biological and adoptive families of adopted individuals with affective disorders. Arch Gen Psychiatry 43:923–929, 1986

Winokur G, Cadoret R, Dorsab J, et al: Depressive disease: a genetic study. Arch Gen Psychiatry 24:135–144, 1971

Winokur G, Tsuang MT, Crowe RR: The Iowa 500: affective disorder in relatives of manic and depressed patients. Am J Psychiatry 139:209–212, 1982

Winokur G, Coryell W, Keller M, et al: A family study of manic-depressive (bipolar I) disease. is it a distinct illness separable from primary unipolar depression? Arch Gen Psychiatry 52:367–373, 1995

Zubenko GS, Hughes HG, Stiffler JS, et al: Sequence variations in CREB1 co-segregate with depressive disorders in women. Mol Psychiatry 8:611–618, 2003a

Zubenko GS, Maher B, Hughes HB, et al: Genome-wide linkage survey for genetic loci that influence the development of depressive disorders in families with recurrent early onset major depression. Am J Med Genet 123B:1–18, 2003b

PART 4

Somatic Interventions for Mood Disorders

SECTION EDITOR: MARK S. GEORGE, M.D.

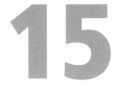

CHAPTER

15

Tricyclics, Tetracyclics, and Monoamine Oxidase Inhibitors

WILLIAM ZEIGLER POTTER, M.D., PH.D.

ROBERT A. PADICH, PH.D.

MATTHEW V. RUDORFER, M.D.

K. RANGA RAMA KRISHNAN, M.B., CH.B.

IN THIS CHAPTER, we focus on the first generation of antidepressants: tricyclic and tetracyclic antidepressants (TCAs meaning either type) and monoamine oxidase inhibitors (MAOIs). They share a common heritage in that their usefulness in treating depression was recognized through incidental observation rather than planned, theoretically based research. These drugs are no longer first-line therapies, not because of poor efficacy but because of potentially serious side effects. For example, amitriptyline, one of the earliest TCAs to become available, produces disturbances of cardiac conduction at therapeutic doses (Ray et al. 2004), and there have been reports of sudden death among children taking desipramine and other TCAs (Varley 2001). Despite their inherently low toxicity, MAOIs produce serious interactions with other drugs and some common foods.

Antidepressants are still among the top prescription drugs of choice used in suicide attempts, although the completion rate for suicide by drug overdose is declining, probably because of the lower toxicity of selective serotonin reuptake inhibitors (SSRIs) (Frey et al. 2000; Ohberg et al. 1998). Amitriptyline (along with other TCAs) is still a leading vehicle for completed suicide attempts. It accounts for up to 82% of deaths by antidepressant poisoning, leading some to seriously question the continued use of these antidepressants (Montgomery 1997).

Nevertheless, because of their broad spectrum of efficacy, TCAs and MAOIs continue to be prescribed. Moreover, expectations of differential efficacy compared with other classes of antidepressants continue to fuel work on new forms of MAOIs (Youdim and Weinstock 2004).

History and Discovery

Monoamine Oxidase Inhibitors

Bloch and colleagues (1954) reported that tubercular patients receiving iproniazid experienced improved mood. Subsequently, Zeller (1963) reported that iproniazid was a potent inhibitor of monoamine oxidase enzymes both in vitro and in vivo and could reverse the effects of reserpine, which was long known to produce depression as a side effect.

Other MAOIs soon replaced iproniazid, which had significant hepatotoxicity risks. Although these drugs were far less hepatotoxic, their use became limited by the discovery of a risk for serious hypertensive crisis precipitated through interaction with tyramine in common foods such as cheese (Blackwell et al. 1967). The TCAs quickly replaced the MAOIs, although new MAOIs with better safety profiles have been, and continue to be, developed.

Tricyclic and Tetracyclic Antidepressants

The antidepressant effects of imipramine were first reported by the Swiss psychiatrist Roland Kuhn (1958, 1970), who tested the compound to determine whether it might be useful in calming agitated patients. It was not; however, symptoms improved in a subset of patients with depression. Numerous structurally similar antidepressant drugs were developed. They had the same core of three contiguous rings—hence, the name *tricyclic antidepressants*. The tricyclic and closely related tetracyclic antidepressants dominated the pharmacological treatment of depression for the next 30 years, although compliance problems developed because of unpleasant side effects and many fatalities following intentional overdoses.

Classification and Mechanisms of Action

Tricyclic and Tetracyclic Antidepressants

The TCAs affect norepinephrine (NE) and serotonin (5-HT) function in both preclinical models and humans through a direct primary action as inhibitors of the respec-

tive transporter proteins for NE and serotonin. These transporter proteins, also called reuptake sites, are located mainly on the presynaptic nerve ending and serve at least two major functions: 1) deactivation of released NE or serotonin and 2) recycling of neurotransmitters into intraneuronal storage vesicles in the nerve endings, which can be released again on stimulation. The latter is not often emphasized because the functional importance of such recycling of NE and serotonin has not been fully elucidated. Rather, research to understand how these drugs work has focused on the many "downstream" effects of increasing intrasynaptic NE or serotonin above basal pretreatment levels.

Because of their relative potency as inhibitors of NE or serotonin transporter antagonism in various preclinical models (including cloned human transporters in vitro), TCAs traditionally have been categorized as preferentially acting on NE or serotonin, as summarized in Table 15–1.

In humans, however, the tertiary amine TCAs (which are initially more potent on serotonin) are sufficiently metabolized to secondary amines (more potent on NE) such that they are all likely to act as mixed reuptake inhibitors at therapeutic doses.

Interestingly, positron emission tomography (PET) imaging with ligands for the serotonin transporter shows that all SSRIs (see Shelton and Lester, Chapter 16, in this volume) have a similar high occupancy (approximately 80%) at effective doses. Initial results with a newly described ligand for NE transporters suggest that a similar high occupancy will prevail for effective selective norepinephrine reuptake inhibitors (Andree et al., in press). Therefore, we predict that doses of tertiary amine TCAs associated with efficacy will show high occupancy of both serotonin and NE transporters. Secondary amine TCAs, particularly desipramine, may show higher occupancy of the NE transporter than the serotonin transporter and thus have a narrower spectrum of activity.

Antagonism of multiple neurotransmitter receptors produces many of the side effects of TCAs—dry mouth, orthostatic hypotension, and excessive somnolence—which are poorly tolerated by many patients, thus making TCAs second-line drugs despite their efficacy and low cost. In populations such as the elderly, TCAs may be contraindicated because of potent antagonism of cholinergic receptors (worsening of memory impairments) and α_1-noradrenergic receptors (orthostatic hypotension with falls). Importantly, these receptor interactions, per se, cannot explain the lethality of TCAs that can occur after ingestion of 2,500 mg or more, a rather narrow multiple when average efficacy doses range between 100 and 300 mg/day. One suggested mechanism is based on the fact that TCAs can modestly affect cardiac conduction time at therapeu-

TABLE 15–1.   Acute biochemical activity of tricyclic and tetracyclic antidepressants in vitro

Antidepressant	Reuptake inhibition			Receptor affinity				
	NE	5-HT	DA	α_1	α_2	H_1	M	D_2
Imipramine	+	+	0	++	0	+	++	0
Desipramine	+++	0	0	+	0	0	+	0
Amitriptyline	±	++	0	+++	±	++++	++++	0
Nortriptyline	++	±	0	+	0	+	++	0
Clomipramine	+	+++	0	++	0	+	++	0
Trimipramine	+	0	0	++	±	+++	++	+
Doxepin	++	+	0	++	0	+++	++	0
Protriptyline	++	0	0	+	0	+	++	0
Amoxapine	++	0	0	++	±	±	0	++
Maprotiline	++	0	0	+	0	++	+	0

Note.   NE=norepinephrine; 5-HT=serotonin; DA=dopamine; α= α-adrenergic receptor; H=histamine receptor; M=muscarinic acetylcholine receptor; D=dopaminergic receptor; + through ++++=active to strongly active; 0=lacking; ±=weakly active.
Source.   Reprinted from Potter WZ, Manji HK, Rudorfer MV: "Tricyclics and Tetracyclics," in *The American Psychiatric Press Textbook of Psychopharmacology*, 2nd Edition. Edited by Schatzberg AF, Nemeroff CB. Washington, DC, American Psychiatric Press, 1998. Used with permission.

tic doses (Ray et al. 2004), which can be especially dangerous if the patient has preexisting ischemic heart disease (for a review, see Glassman 1998).

In summary, the *acute* biochemical effects of TCAs include those related to immediate side effects (antagonism of multiple receptors) and those initiating a cascade of events leading to efficacy (reuptake inhibition).

Monoamine Oxidase Inhibitors

Like TCAs, MAOIs increase the amount of NE and serotonin in the synapse but through a different primary mechanism than that used by TCAs. Because dopamine (DA) is also a substrate for monoamine oxidase (MAO), its intrasynaptic concentration is also increased. Altered DA function may be relevant to antidepressant effects, given that in some brain regions DA is transported by the NE transporter into the presynaptic neuron (Wong and Bymaster 2002). Therefore, in those brain regions rich in NE nerve terminals, TCAs may act like a DA uptake inhibitor but indirectly through inhibition of NE uptake.

The MAOIs act by inhibiting the target function of MAO in the central nervous system. Oxidative monoamine neurotransmitter metabolism depends on two isozymes: monoamine oxidase A (MAO-A) and monoamine oxidase B (MAO-B) (Cesura and Pletscher 1992). The relative distribution of these isozymes across different types of neurons and glia is relevant to the actions of selective inhibitors.

Because MAO is bound to the outer surface of the plasma membrane of the mitochondria, it is unable to deaminate those amines that are stored in vesicles within the neuron and only metabolizes those amines that are present in the cytoplasm. As a result, MAO activity maintains a low cytoplasmic concentration of amines. MAOIs therefore increase the amine content within the cytoplasm. This, in turn, increases the amount available for storage in vesicles such that more amine neurotransmitter is released into the synapse per vesicle that is mobilized to the cell surface during activation of release mechanisms (Finberg and Youdim 1984; Murphy et al. 1987). MAOIs can be subdivided according to not only the particular isoenzyme that is inhibited but also the *type* of inhibition: reversible or irreversible. Irreversible inhibitors bind so tightly to the MAO that it is permanently inactivated such that new MAO must be synthesized to regain activity, a process that requires weeks to fully restore the pretreatment state. Reversible inhibitors act like the general class of competitive inhibitors whereby the degree of inhibition is related to the concentration of inhibitor present at any moment. Thus, MAO activity can be regained simply by reducing the concentration over the few hours that it takes to eliminate this class of MAOIs from the body.

Because both TCAs and MAOIs are effective antidepressants, their common property of increasing intrasynaptic NE and serotonin appears to be core to their mechanism of action. The MAOIs' additional property of increasing DA in multiple brain regions may be relevant to their efficacy in patients whose symptoms do not respond to TCAs (Rush and Ryan 2002). As noted in Table 15–1, at least for the TCAs, mechanisms related to side effects from antagonism of receptors (e.g., cholinergic) will produce immediate side effects (e.g., dry mouth). Therapeutic effects do not become manifest until 1 or 2 weeks and in many patients require 3–6 weeks. Research over the last two decades has focused on trying to understand the cascade of events that occurs over time following acute treatment. In experimental animals, TCAs and MAOIs, as well as SSRIs and the newer serotonin-norepinephrine reuptake inhibitors (SNRIs), reduce one or more NE (β, α_1, and α_2 adrenoceptors) or serotonin (1A and 2) receptor subtypes (Hyman and Nestler 1996; Lenox and Fraser 2002). Recent studies suggest that 5-HT$_{2A}$ antagonism may play a useful role in antidepressant action (Marek et al. 2003). Whether the reduction of the number of receptors is necessary for antidepressant action or is only a normal compensatory reaction to increasing intrasynaptic concentrations of neurotransmitter is not known.

One case in which receptor downregulation has been argued to play a substantial role is that of 5-HT$_{1A}$ receptors, which mediate an acute negative feedback of serotonin on firing of serotonergic neurons (Artigas et al. 1996). Another is downregulation of noradrenergic α_2 receptors, which mediate a negative feedback of NE on its own release (Svensson and Usdin 1978). Thus, when synaptic serotonin or NE concentrations are increased after TCA or MAOI administration, these feedback mechanisms tend to counteract the acute drug effect by inhibiting neurotransmitter release. The downregulation of 5-HT$_{1A}$ and α_2 receptors after chronic drug administration results in greater extraneuronal concentrations of serotonin and NE, a time-dependent effect that may be related to the onset of antidepressant efficacy. Such findings led to the hypothesis that adding either a 5-HT$_{1A}$ antagonist or an α_2 antagonist to a standard antidepressant can accelerate the onset of antidepressant effects (Artigas et al. 1996; Crews et al. 1981). This hypothesis remains to be tested because no generally accepted, safe, and selective antagonists have been available.

The most current hypotheses on the critical biochemical intermediaries of antidepressant effects focus on a wide range of intracellular targets. Detailed reviews describing the effects of antidepressants on cyclic adenosine monophosphate (cAMP), protein kinase A, calcium- or calmodulin-dependent protein kinase, cAMP response element–binding protein (CREB), and brain-derived neurotrophic factor (BDNF) highlight the possibility that these drugs produce long-term changes that might even increase neuron growth and function (Duman et al. 2000) (see Delgado and Moreno, Chapter 6, in this volume). Indeed, some degree of neurogenesis in the hippocampus might be necessary for some of the behavioral effects of antidepressants in animal models (Santarelli et al. 2003). Other preclinical research, however, shows that potentially more relevant behavioral effects can occur without alterations of neurotrophic factors such as BDNF (Conti et al. 2002). Furthermore, longer-term changes in presynaptic regulation of transporters also may be relevant to antidepressant action (Benmansour et al. 2004). Which of these diverse preclinical effects are truly relevant to antidepressant action cannot be determined until methods are available that show which of these actions also result in clinical benefit in humans.

Indications

A plethora of head-to-head studies have compared the efficacy of the different classes of antidepressants (MAOIs, TCAs, SSRIs, and SNRIs). Comparisons have been made between and within classes, among various subtypes of depression, and by subgroups such as age, sex, and comorbidity. No class of antidepressant consistently stands out in large controlled or naturalistic outpatient trials as having unique efficacy (for reviews, see Anderson 2001; Silverstone 2001). Importantly, antidepressants can work in the presence of comorbidities that may discourage drug treatment. For example, antidepressants were effective in the short-term treatment of comorbid alcohol dependence and depression in the few well-controlled studies that have been performed (Mason et al. 1996; McGrath et al. 1996).

Depression (Broadly Defined)

Currently, TCAs are second-line treatments for depression. Initially, it appeared that major depressive disorder, with melancholic features, responded better to TCAs than did depression without melancholic features (Paykel 1972; Raskin and Crook 1976). Cumulative data from the field have not supported such selectivity of response, perhaps reflecting the changing population of patients available for such studies (Paykel 1989). Among the best predictors of positive response to both TCAs and MAOIs are severity (Stewart et al. 1989), good premorbid personality (as with most psychiatric disorders), and whether depression is primary (i.e., depression not preceded by other psychiatric diagnoses or medical illness) (Coryell and Turner 1985; Fairchild et al. 1986).

Overall, the response rate for TCAs is 80% in nonpsychotic patients who have a primary diagnosis of major depressive disorder, with melancholic features, and an illness duration of less than 1 year, if plasma levels are maintained in therapeutic ranges for 4–6 weeks. Lower response rates reported in this type of patient are most likely a result of inadequate dosage over too short a time. In some series, about half of the tricyclic partial or nonresponders showed augmented antidepressant effect with the addition of a second drug—most commonly, lithium (Heit and Nemeroff 1998) or, less consistently, thyroid hormone, generally in the form of triiodothyronine (T_3).

The two major MAOIs approved for the treatment of depression in the United States are phenelzine and tranylcypromine. Isocarboxazid, a third effective member of this class, a hydrazine compound like phenelzine, was returned to the market in the late 1990s, several years after its license was acquired by a new company. Tranylcypromine, a nonhydrazine, bears a structural relationship to amphetamine, and there is some evidence for amphetamine-like active metabolites of this drug and phenelzine (Rudorfer and Potter 1997). Another marketed MAOI, selegiline (formerly called deprenyl), has been shown to be effective in the treatment of early Parkinson's disease at doses selective for MAO-B (e.g., 10 mg/day), which obviate the need for a tyramine-free diet. At higher dosages (e.g., 30 mg/day), selegiline may have antidepressant effects. However, at such doses, it becomes a nonselective MAOI, making dietary precautions necessary. A transdermal (skin patch) formulation is under development for the treatment of depression that has received an approval letter from the FDA. The development of selective reversible inhibitors of MAO-A (RIMAs) had appeared to offer the possibility of MAOI efficacy with an improved safety profile (Rudorfer 1992). However, although such compounds (e.g., moclobemide) are marketed in many countries, their efficacy appears less than that of the older agents for both mood and anxiety disorders. It is not clear whether their approval will be sought in the United States.

Because MAOIs have an even higher propensity than TCAs for producing adverse events and serious interactions with foods and other drugs, MAOIs are often the final somatic treatment before initiating electroconvulsive therapy (ECT). Many studies have reported the efficacy of MAOIs in the treatment of different types of depression, including major depressive disorder, with melancholic features, and atypical depression (Davidson et al. 1987; McGrath et al. 1986; Vallejo et al. 1987; White et al. 1984). Other studies have documented the efficacy of high doses of tranylcypromine in treating so-called *anergic depression* and the more thoroughly defined treatment-resistant depression (Himmelhoch et al. 1982, 1991; McGrath et al. 1993; O'Reardon and Amsterdam 2000; Thase et al. 1992; White and White 1986).

Atypical Depression

Atypical forms of depression have been formally recognized only recently. Previously, *atypical depression* referred simply to the absence of melancholic features. Atypical depression is now listed as a major depressive disorder characterized by a combination of mood reactivity (i.e., inability to experience a positive response to favorable events), overeating, oversleeping, and chronic sensitivity to rejection (DSM-IV-TR; American Psychiatric Association 2000). The best predictors of poor response to TCAs among patients with atypical depression are early age at onset and chronicity (Stewart et al. 2002). Patients with atypical depression often have a better response to MAOIs than to TCAs (see Stewart et al., Chapter 33, in this volume). Bipolar depression, which shares with atypical depression a pattern of reversed vegetative symptoms, also responds well to MAOIs.

Delusional Depression (With Psychotic Features)

Patients with major depression who have delusions (DSM-IV-TR [American Psychiatric Association 2000] major depressive disorder, severe with psychotic features) show a very poor response to TCA monotherapy but often respond to the combination of an antipsychotic and a TCA (see Flores and Schatzberg, Chapter 34, in this volume). Alternatively, the response rates to ECT among patients with delusional depression are excellent, with an 86% response rate in the aggregate from a dozen studies (Kroessler 1985). There have been no studies of MAOIs marketed in the United States to support their use in delusional depression for the last 30 years.

Depression in the Very Old and Very Young

Adjustments are often required in dealing with mood disorders at the extremes of the life cycle. For example, given the sensitivity of older adults to cognitive impairment and falls, TCAs with strong anticholinergic effects or propensity to cause orthostatic hypotension should be avoided. Reduced renal function with age may dictate downward dosage adjustments. Conversely, children often require proportionally larger doses of antidepressants because of the enhanced hepatic metabolizing capacity of young people.

Considerations for Treating Depression in Elderly Patients

Contemporary treatment of geriatric depression is safe and effective (see Roose and Devanand, Chapter 36, in this volume). The combination of nortriptyline and interpersonal psychotherapy produced a 69% remission rate in older adults with *bereavement-related* major depression and had the lowest recurrence rate (Reynolds et al. 1999a).

Medication alone was second best, but the relapse rate doubled to 43%. Nearly two-thirds of the patients receiving maintenance psychotherapy only relapsed, as did 90% of the pill placebo group. There appears to be a plasma level–response relation. In long-term treatment of depression in the elderly with nortriptyline, borderline-low plasma concentrations maintained for 3 years were associated with less stable mood, a tradeoff in that fewer side effects occurred than with full-strength dosing (Reynolds et al. 1999b).

On a cautionary note, TCA use in elderly nursing home residents has been associated with increases in falls and hip fractures (Liu et al. 1998; Ruthazer and Lipsitz 1993; Thapa et al. 1998). The milder side-effect profile of the newer antidepressants should confer a better quality of life during treatment, although overall response and remission rates in older people appear lower than with TCAs.

Considerations for Treating Depression in the Very Young

Research on treatment of mood disorders in children and adolescents has lagged behind that directed at older individuals (see Emslie et al., Chapter 35, in this volume). Essentially all well-designed double-blind studies of TCAs have failed to show superiority of tricyclics over placebo in this age group (Hazell et al. 2002). Moreover, in addition to the risk of fatality by overdose, a concern has been raised that TCAs might increase the risk of cardiac tachyarrhythmias (Mezzacappa et al. 1998) and even sudden death in vulnerable young patients (Biederman et al. 1995), although there is no definitive proof.

Other Uses

The first-generation antidepressants have been found to be useful for many conditions not directly related to depression, which are not covered here. These antidepressants are effective in some psychiatric conditions, such as obsessive-compulsive disorder, for which clomipramine remains an effective treatment (Ackerman and Greenland 2002); panic and other anxiety disorders, for which MAOIs such as phenelzine have proved to be most efficacious (Heimberg et al. 1998; Liebowitz et al. 1992); and attention-deficit/hyperactivity disorder, for which TCAs were shown to be effective (Biederman et al. 1989; Wilens et al. 1996) but which may be too risky for use in young children (Riddle et al. 1993). Other uses range from low-

dose imipramine for enuresis (Rapoport et al. 1980) to TCAs for neuropathic pain (McCleane 2003).

Adverse Events

Tricyclic and Tetracyclic Antidepressants

The TCAs are associated with various unpleasant adverse events that reflect their relative lack of specificity of action at the receptor level (see Table 15–1). The most potentially serious adverse event is disruption of cardiac conduction, with possible sudden death (Glassman 1998). The most common side effects of TCAs include drowsiness, dizziness, headache, blurred vision, dry mouth, urinary retention, postural hypotension, photosensitivity, increased appetite, and weight gain. In elderly patients, cognitive impairment may be exacerbated by the anticholinergic activity of many TCAs.

Monoamine Oxidase Inhibitors

The major liability associated with MAOI therapy has been the frequency of adverse events ranging from severe headaches to serious hypertensive crisis by interaction with certain common foods, such as cheese. This drug–food interaction has been classically attributed to increased levels of tyramine, which is present in many foods and has a pressor action. An alternative explanation is that NE levels are increased, which is prompted by the occurrence of spontaneous hypertensive crises in some patients (O'Brien et al. 1992; Zajecka and Fawcett 1991). Headaches also can be caused by increased levels of histamine during MAOI treatment. Histamine headaches are usually accompanied by hypotension, colic, loose stools, salivation, and lacrimation (Cooper 1967).

The most common adverse events with MAOIs include dizziness, headache, dry mouth, insomnia, constipation, blurred vision, nausea, peripheral edema, forgetfulness, orthostatic hypotension, urinary hesitancy, weakness, and myoclonic jerks. Hepatotoxicity is less common with the newer MAOIs, but transaminase levels are elevated in 3%–5% of patients. Liver function must be monitored if patients have or develop symptoms such as malaise, jaundice, and excessive fatigue.

Adverse events that may develop with extended treatment (maintenance) include weight gain, edema, muscle cramps, carbohydrate craving, sexual dysfunction, pyridoxine (vitamin B_6) deficiency, hypoglycemia, hypomania, urinary retention, and disorientation. For a more in-depth review of adverse events that may accompany treatment with MAOIs and tips for their management, see Krishnan (2004). Adverse events are more frequent with the MAOIs than with the TCAs and newer classes of antidepressants, relegating MAOIs to the third tier of somatic treatment choices and possibly the last resort before ECT.

Drug Interactions

Tricyclic and Tetracyclic Antidepressants

TCAs interact, pharmacodynamically and pharmacokinetically, with a variety of other compounds. Most pharmacodynamic adverse interactions with other medications result in additive sedative or anticholinergic effects (e.g., with hypnotics or neuroleptics). The TCAs are heavily dependent on hepatic metabolism, and most adverse pharmacokinetic interactions are with drugs that induce or impair cytochrome P450 (CYP) hepatic microsomal enzyme system activity (Rudorfer and Potter 1997, 1999). For example, barbiturates and carbamazepine induce hepatic enzymes, resulting in accelerated tricyclic metabolism and reduced steady-state blood levels. The competitive inhibition of CYP2D6-mediated drug metabolism by some currently marketed SSRIs is of particular clinical relevance. The interactions of TCAs and SSRIs can produce dramatic elevations of steady-state TCA plasma concentrations, although such combinations may be used safely and effectively provided the TCA dosages are adjusted downward (Rudorfer et al. 1994).

Potentially serious interactions with TCAs include those with

- *MAOIs.* Although combinations of TCAs and MAOIs have been used successfully in refractory depression, convulsions, stroke, hyperpyrexia, and death are possible.
- *Norepinephrine and epinephrine.* There may be unexpectedly large increases in blood pressure and a greater incidence of arrhythmias when given for other medical indications.
- *Phenothiazines.* Although combinations of TCAs and phenothiazines are useful in delusional (psychotic) depression, the additive anticholinergic effects may increase psychosis and agitation in elderly patients.

Monoamine Oxidase Inhibitors

Because of their broad spectrum of enzyme inhibition, the MAOIs are open to many interactions, not only with prescription psychotropic medications but also with common over-the-counter medications. For example, many cough medicines and allergy or cold medicines sold without a prescription contain sympathomimetic agents that can precipitate hypertensive crises in patients taking MAOIs. The prospect of surgery poses added hazard for patients taking MAOIs. In addition to the expected potentiation of sympathomimetics, a rare but potentially fatal interaction with narcotic analgesics, especially meperidine, is possible; this interaction can produce a reaction characterized by coma, hyperpyrexia, and hypertension (Stack et al. 1988).

Other potentially serious interactions with MAOIs include those with

- *TCAs.* Severe adverse effects are possible, as discussed in the previous subsection.
- *SSRIs, L-tryptophan, fenfluramine.* Serotonin syndrome may result.
- *Dextromethorphan.* Brief psychosis may occur.
- *Oral hypoglycemics and insulin.* Hypoglycemia may worsen.
- *Recreational drugs.* The interaction may cause further increases in blood pressure (cocaine, amphetamines) and possible serotonin syndrome (lysergic acid diethylamide, methylenedioxyethylamphetamine, methylenedioxymethamphetamine [MDMA; Ecstasy]). For instance, MDMA is a serotonin-releasing analogue of amphetamine that is heavily dependent on the CYP2D6 metabolic pathway (Oesterheld et al. 2004), and some reported deaths have been attributed to MDMA and MAOI in combination (Vuori et al. 2003).

Given the higher incidence of physical complaints in patients with depression, the high rate of depression in the patients with chronic illnesses, and the increasing age of the world population in general, it is not unusual for patients to take more than one medication. Thorough drug histories and careful risk-benefit evaluations are always necessary in light of the potentially serious drug interactions that can occur with ever more powerful medications.

Role of Plasma Concentrations

Tricyclic and Tetracyclic Antidepressants

The most important clinical advance to emerge from studies of the pharmacology of the TCAs over the past 40 years is an appreciation of their complex pharmacokinetics (Amsterdam et al. 1980; Rudorfer and Potter 1987). TCAs undergo side-chain demethylation, aromatic ring hydroxylation, and glucuronide conjugation of the hydroxy metabolites, with less than 5% of a dose being excreted unchanged. The demethylated metabolites of the tertiary amines (amitriptyline, imipramine, and clomipramine) are pharmacologically active, as are all unconjugated hydroxy metabolites (Bertilsson et al. 1979; Potter et al. 1979). The clinical relevance of active metabolites includes both efficacy and side effects (Rudorfer and Potter 1987). Metabolism is determined by individual genetics; 7%–9% of the Caucasian population are classified as "slow hydroxylators" and have 30-fold or higher concentrations in blood than expected for the average patient (Brosen et al. 1985; Evans et al. 1980).

Functional polymorphisms of the CYP2D6 gene explain variations in the rate of hydroxylation of TCAs. Population differences in this polymorphism can guide dosing; for instance, patients of Asian background may need lower than usual doses. A greater percentage of slow metabolizers is also seen among African Americans compared with those of European background (Gaedigk et al. 2002). An allele associated with ultrarapid drug metabolism by CYP2D6 also exists, making it difficult for therapeutic medication levels to be achieved. The clinician also must consider the influence of exogenous substances, including other drugs, alcohol, and smoking, on cytochrome oxidative enzymes (Rudorfer and Potter 1997, 1999).

Clearance of TCAs varies considerably across the life span. The known decline of renal clearance with age predictably reduces the urinary excretion of unconjugated hydroxy metabolites, resulting in substantially increased steady-state concentrations of active metabolites in elderly patients (Kitanaka et al. 1982; Pollock and Perel 1989). In prepubescent children, TCA clearance is higher than in adults, often resulting in a lower plasma concentration at the same mg/kg dose (Geller 1991; Rapoport and Potter 1981).

Definitive concentrations are not well established for all TCAs, despite current appreciation for the great variability in metabolism of tricyclic drugs and the consequent need to individualize treatment. Therapeutic levels have been defined only for nortriptyline, imipramine, and desipramine (American Psychiatric Association Task Force 1985; Perry et al. 1987; Rudorfer and Potter 1987). Nonetheless, estimates of reasonable therapeutic ranges for all marketed TCAs are based on cumulative experience with therapeutic monitoring rather than on prospective controlled studies (Orsulak 1989; Stewart et al. 2002). Indications for measuring plasma drug levels include a lack of response, toxicity, a desire to minimize adverse effects by using the minimal effective dose, and a need to monitor suspected pharmacokinetic interactions (e.g., neuroleptics or SSRIs). For example, nortriptyline requires monitoring because plasma levels greater than 150 ng/mL are as ineffective as doses that yield a subtherapeutic level (<50 ng/mL). Tricyclic antidepressants have a narrow

therapeutic index, with considerable risk of significant toxicity when blood concentrations are two to six times therapeutic levels. Thus, a 1-week supply may be fatal if taken all at once (Gram 1990; Rudorfer and Robins 1982).

In general, concentrations greater than 1,000 ng/mL are associated with prolongation of the QRS interval, an effect that may be seen even at 500 ng/mL (Preskorn and Irwin 1982; Spiker et al. 1985). This relatively narrow therapeutic index is of special concern for depressed patients with suicide potential who may intentionally take an overdose. TCA blood concentrations may remain elevated for several days after overdose, presenting cardiac risk even after apparent clinical improvement (Jarvis 1991). Furthermore, central nervous system toxicity of TCAs with resulting coma, shock, respiratory depression, delirium, seizures, and hyperpyrexia may contribute as much to fatalities as the quinidine-like effects on cardiac conduction.

Monoamine Oxidase Inhibitors

Inhibition of MAO activity persists well after these drugs are no longer detectable in plasma; therefore, conventional pharmacokinetic measures such as plasma half-life are not useful. Although MAOIs are easily absorbed via the gastrointestinal system, the rate of elimination varies. For example, phenelzine metabolism is heavily dependent on hepatic acetylation, which can result in higher than expected levels in those individuals who are phenotypically "slow acetylators." In general, MAO inhibition persists for about 7 days after stopping tranylcypromine and up to 3 weeks after stopping phenelzine. See Lenox and Fraser (2002) for a more complete discussion.

References

Ackerman DL, Greenland S: Multivariate meta-analysis of controlled drug studies for obsessive-compulsive disorder. J Clin Psychopharmacol 22:309–317, 2002

American Psychiatric Association: Diagnostic and Statistical Manual of Mental Disorders, 4th Edition, Text Revision. Washington, DC, American Psychiatric Association, 2000

American Psychiatric Association Task Force: Task Force on the Use of Laboratory Tests in Psychiatry: tricyclic antidepressants—blood level measurements and clinical outcome. Am J Psychiatry 142:155–162, 1985

Amsterdam J, Brunswick D, Mendels J: The clinical application of tricyclic antidepressant pharmacokinetics and plasma levels. Am J Psychiatry 137:653–662, 1980

Anderson IM: Meta-analytical studies on new antidepressants. Br Med Bull 57:161–178, 2001

Andree B, Seneca N, Schou M, et al: [11C]MeNER human PET study: high occupancy of the central norepinephrine transporter induced by reboxetine at clinical doses (abstract). J Nucl Med 45 (suppl 1):191–192, 2004

Artigas F, Bel N, Casanovas JM, et al: Adaptive changes of the serotonergic system after antidepressant treatments. Adv Exp Med Biol 398:51–59, 1996

Benmansour S, Altamirano AV, Jones DJ, et al: Regulation of the norepinephrine transporter by chronic administration of antidepressants. Biol Psychiatry 55:313–316, 2004

Bertilsson L, Mellstrom B, Sjoqvist F: Pronounced inhibition of noradrenaline uptake by 10-hydroxymetabolites of nortriptyline: Life Sci 25:1285–1292, 1979

Biederman J, Baldessarini RJ, Wright V, et al: A double-blind placebo controlled study of desipramine in the treatment of ADD, I: efficacy. J Am Acad Child Adolesc Psychiatry 28:777–784, 1989

Biederman J, Thisted RA, Greenhill LL, et al: Estimation of the association between desipramine and the risk for sudden death in 5- to 14-year-old children. J Clin Psychiatry 56:87–93, 1995

Blackwell B, Marley E, Price J, et al: Hypertensive interactions between monoamine oxidase inhibitors and foodstuffs. Br J Psychiatry 113:349–365, 1967

Bloch RG, Doonief AS, Buchberg AS, et al: The clinical effect of isoniazid and iproniazid in the treatment of pulmonary tuberculosis. Ann Intern Med 40:881–900, 1954

Brosen K, Otton SV, Gram LF: Sparteine oxidation polymorphism in Denmark. Acta Pharmacol Toxicol (Copenh) 57:357–360, 1985

Cesura AM, Pletscher A: The new generation of monoamine oxidase inhibitors. Prog Drug Res 38:171–297, 1992

Conti AC, Cryan JF, Dalvi A, et al: cAMP response element binding is essential for the upregulation of brain-derived neurotrophic factor transcription but not the behavioral or endocrine responses to antidepressant drugs. J Neurosci 22:3262–3268, 2002

Cooper AJ: M.A.O. inhibitors and headache. Br Med J 4(516):420, 1967

Coryell W, Turner R: Outcome with desipramine therapy in subtypes of nonpsychotic major depression. J Affect Disord 9:149–154, 1985

Crews FT, Paul SM, Goodwin FK: Acceleration of beta-receptor desensitization in combined administration of antidepressants and phenoxybenzamine. Nature 209:787–789, 1981

Davidson J, Raft D, Pelton S: An outpatient evaluation of phenelzine and imipramine. J Clin Psychiatry 48:143–146, 1987

Duman RS, Malberg J, Nakagawa S, et al: Neuronal plasticity and survival in mood disorders. Biol Psychiatry 48:732–739, 2000

Evans DA, Mahgoub A, Sloan TP, et al: A family and population study of the genetic polymorphism of debrisoquine oxidation in a white British population. J Med Genet 17:102–105, 1980

Fairchild CJ, Rush AJ, Vasavada N, et al: Which depressions respond to placebo? Psychiatry Res 18:217–226, 1986

Finberg JPM, Youdim MBH: Reversible monoamine oxidase inhibitors and the cheese effect, in Monoamine Oxidase and Disease: Prospects for Therapy With Reversible Inhibitors. Edited by Tipton KF, Dostert P, Strolin-Benedetti M. New York, Academic Press, 1984, pp 479–485

Frey R, Schreinzer D, Stimpfl T, et al: Suicide by antidepressant intoxication identified at autopsy in Vienna from 1991–1997: the favourable consequences of the increasing use of SSRIs. Eur Neuropsychopharmacol 10:133–142, 2000

Gaedigk A, Bradford LD, Marcucci KA, et al: Unique CYP2D6 activity distribution and genotype-phenotype discordance in black Americans. Clin Pharmacol Ther 72:76–89, 2002

Geller B: Psychopharmacology of children and adolescents: pharmacokinetics and relationships of plasma/serum levels to response. Psychopharmacol Bull 27:401–409, 1991

Glassman AH: Cardiovascular effects of antidepressant drugs. J Clin Psychiatry 50 (suppl 15):13–18, 1998

Gram LF: Inadequate dosing and pharmacokinetic variability as confounding factors in assessment of efficacy of antidepressants. Clin Neuropharmacol 13 (suppl 1):S35–S44, 1990

Hazell P, O'Connell D, Heathcote D, et al: Tricyclic drugs for depression in children and adolescents. Cochrane Database Syst Rev (2):CD002317, 2002

Heimberg RG, Liebowitz MR, Hope DA, et al: Cognitive behavioral group therapy vs phenelzine therapy for social phobia: 12-week outcome. Arch Gen Psychiatry 55:1133–1141, 1998

Heit S, Nemeroff CB: Lithium augmentation of antidepressants in treatment-refractory depression. J Clin Psychiatry 59 (suppl 6):28–33, 1998

Himmelhoch JM, Fuchs CZ, Symons BJ: A double-blind study of tranylcypromine treatment of major anergic depression. J Nerv Ment Dis 170:628–634, 1982

Himmelhoch JM, Thase ME, Mallinger AG, et al: Tranylcypromine versus imipramine in anergic bipolar depression. Am J Psychiatry 148:910–916, 1991

Hyman SE, Nestler EJ: Initiation and adaptation: a paradigm for understanding psychotropic drug action. Am J Psychiatry 153:151–162, 1996

Jarvis MR: Clinical pharmacokinetics of tricyclic antidepressant overdose. Psychopharmacol Bull 27:541–550, 1991

Kitanaka I, Ross RJ, Cutler NR, et al: Altered hydroxydesipramine concentrations in elderly depressed patients. Clin Pharmacol Ther 31:51–55, 1982

Krishnan KRR: Monoamine oxidase inhibitors, in The American Psychiatric Publishing Textbook of Psychopharmacology, 3rd Edition. Edited by Schatzberg AF, Nemeroff CB. Arlington, VA, American Psychiatric Publishing, 2004, pp 303–314

Kroessler D: Relative efficacy rates for therapies of delusional depression. Convuls Ther 1:173–182, 1985

Kuhn R: The treatment of depressive states with G 22355 (imipramine hydrochloride). Am J Psychiatry 115:459–464, 1958

Kuhn R: The imipramine story, in Discoveries in Biological Psychiatry. Edited by Ayd FJ, Blackwell B. Philadelphia, PA, JB Lippincott, 1970, pp 205–217

Lenox RH, Frazer A: Mechanisms of action of antidepressants and mood stabilizers, in Neuropsychopharmacology: The Fifth Generation of Progress. Edited by Davis KL, Charney D, Coyle JT, et al. Philadelphia, PA, Lippincott Williams & Wilkins, 2002, pp 1139–1163

Liebowitz MR, Schneier F, Campeas R, et al: Phenelzine vs atenolol in social phobia: a placebo-controlled comparison. Arch Gen Psychiatry 49:290–300, 1992

Liu B, Anderson G, Mittmann N, et al: Use of selective serotonin-reuptake inhibitors of tricyclic antidepressants and risk of hip fractures in elderly people. Lancet 351(9112):1303–1307, 1998

Marek GJ, Carpenter LL, McDougle CJ, et al: Synergistic action of 5-HT2A antagonists and selective serotonin reuptake inhibitors in neuropsychiatric disorders. Neuropsychopharmacology 28:402–412, 2003

Mason BJ, Kocsis JH, Ritvo EC, et al: A double-blind, placebo-controlled trial of desipramine for primary alcohol dependence stratified on the presence or absence of major depression. JAMA 275:761–767, 1996

McCleane G: Pharmacological management of neuropathic pain. CNS Drugs 17:1031–1043, 2003

McGrath PJ, Stewart JW, Harrison W, et al: Phenelzine treatment of melancholia. J Clin Psychiatry 47:420–422, 1986

McGrath PJ, Stewart JW, Nunes EV, et al: A double-blind crossover trial of imipramine and phenelzine for outpatients with treatment-refractory depression. Am J Psychiatry 150:118–123, 1993

McGrath PJ, Nunes EV, Stewart JW, et al: Imipramine treatment of alcoholics with primary depression: a placebo-controlled clinical trial. Arch Gen Psychiatry 53:232–240, 1996

Mezzacappa E, Steingard R, Kindlon D, et al: Tricyclic antidepressants and cardiac autonomic control in children and adolescents. J Am Acad Child Adolesc Psychiatry 37:52–59, 1998

Montgomery SA: Suicide and antidepressants. Ann N Y Acad Sci 836:329–338, 1997

Murphy DL, Sunderland T, Garrick NA, et al: Selective amine oxidase inhibitors: basic to clinical studies and back, in Clinical Pharmacology in Psychiatry. Edited by Dahl SG, Gram A, Potter W. Berlin, Germany, Springer, 1987, pp 35–146

O'Brien S, McKeon P, O'Regan M, et al: Blood pressure effects of tranylcypromine when prescribed singly and in combination with amitriptyline. J Clin Psychopharmacol 12:104–109, 1992

Oesterheld JR, Armstrong SC, Cozza KL: Ecstasy: pharmacodynamic and pharmacokinetic interactions. Psychosomatics 45:84–87, 2004

Ohberg A, Klaukka T, Lonnqvist J: Antidepressants and suicide mortality. J Affect Disord 50:225–233, 1998

O'Reardon JP, Amsterdam JD: Mechanisms and management of treatment-resistant depression, in Pharmacotherapy for Mood, Anxiety, and Cognitive Disorders. Edited by Halbreich U, Montgomery SA. Washington, DC, American Psychiatric Press, 2000, pp 285–304

Orsulak PJ: Therapeutic monitoring of antidepressant drugs: guidelines updated. Ther Drug Monit 11:497–507, 1989

Paykel ES: Correlates of a depressive typology. Arch Gen Psychiatry 27:203–210, 1972

Paykel ES: Treatment of depression: the relevance of research for clinical practice. Br J Psychiatry 155:754–763, 1989

Perry PJ, Pfohl BM, Holstad SG: The relationship between antidepressant response and tricyclic antidepressant plasma concentrations: a retrospective analysis of the literature using logistic regression analysis. Clin Pharmacokinet 13:381–392, 1987

Pollock BG, Perel JM: Tricyclic antidepressants: contemporary issues for therapeutic practice. Can J Psychiatry 34:609–617, 1989

Potter WZ, Calil HM, Manian AA, et al: Hydroxylated metabolites of tricyclic antidepressants: preclinical assessment of activity. Biol Psychiatry 14:601–613, 1979

Potter WZ, Manji HK, Rudorfer MV: Tricyclics and tetracyclics, in The American Psychiatric Press Textbook of Psychopharmacology, 2nd Edition. Edited by Schatzberg AF, Nemeroff CB. Washington, DC, American Psychiatric Press, 1998, pp 199–218

Preskorn SH, Irwin HA: Toxicity of tricyclic antidepressants—kinetics, mechanism, intervention: a review. J Clin Psychiatry 43:151–156, 1982

Rapoport JL, Potter WZ: Tricyclic antidepressants: use in pediatric psychopharmacology, in Pharmacokinetics: Youth and Age. Edited by Raskin A, Robinson D. Amsterdam, The Netherlands, Elsevier, 1981, pp 105–123

Rapoport JL, Mikkelsen EJ, Zavadil A, et al: Childhood enuresis, II: psychopathology, tricyclic concentration in plasma, and antienuretic effect. Arch Gen Psychiatry 37:1146–1152, 1980

Raskin A, Crook TH: The endogenous–neurotic distinction as a predictor of response to antidepressant drugs. Psychol Med 6:59–70, 1976

Ray WA, Meredith S, Thapa PB, et al: Cyclic antidepressants and the risk of sudden cardiac death. Clin Pharmacol Ther 75:234–241, 2004

Reynolds CF 3rd, Miller MD, Pasternak RE, et al: Treatment of bereavement-related major depressive episodes in later life: a controlled study of acute and continuation treatment with nortriptyline and interpersonal psychotherapy. Am J Psychiatry 156:202–208, 1999a

Reynolds CF 3rd, Perel JM, Frank E, et al: Three-year outcomes of maintenance nortriptyline treatment in late-life depression: a study of two fixed plasma levels. Am J Psychiatry 156:1177–1181, 1999b

Riddle MA, Geller B, Ryan N: Another sudden death in a child treated with desipramine. J Am Acad Child Adolesc Psychiatry 32:792–797, 1993

Rudorfer MV: Monoamine oxidase inhibitors: reversible and irreversible. Psychopharmacol Bull 28:45–57, 1992

Rudorfer MV, Potter WZ: Pharmacokinetics of antidepressants, in Psychopharmacology: The Third Generation of Progress. Edited by Meltzer HY. New York, Raven, 1987, pp 1353–1364

Rudorfer MV, Potter WZ: The role of metabolites of antidepressants in the treatment of depression. CNS Drugs 7:273–312, 1997

Rudorfer MV, Potter WZ: Metabolism of tricyclic antidepressants. Cell Mol Neurobiol 19:373–409, 1999

Rudorfer MV, Robins E: Amitriptyline overdose: clinical effects on tricyclic antidepressant plasma levels. J Clin Psychiatry 43:457ñ460, 1982

Rudorfer MV, Manji HK, Potter WZ: Comparative tolerability profiles of the newer versus older antidepressants. Drug Saf 10:18–46, 1994

Rush AJ, Ryan ND: Current therapeutics for depression, in Neuropsychopharmacology: The Fifth Generation of Progress. Edited by Davis KL, Harney D, Coyle JT, et al. Philadelphia, PA, Lippincott Williams & Williams, 2002, pp 1081–1095

Ruthazer R, Lipsitz LA: Antidepressants and falls among elderly people in long-term care. Am J Public Health 83:746–749, 1993

Santarelli L, Saxe M, Gross C, et al: Requirement of hippocampal neurogenesis for the behavioral effects of antidepressants. Science 301(5634):805–809, 2003

Silverstone T: Moclobemide vs imipramine in bipolar depression: a multicenter double-blind clinical trial. Acta Psychiatr Scand 104:104–109, 2001

Spiker DG, Weiss JC, Dealy RS, et al: The pharmacological treatment of delusional depression. Am J Psychiatry 142:430–436, 1985

Stack CG, Rogers P, Linter SP: Monoamine oxidase inhibitors and anaesthesia. Br J Anaesth 60:222–227, 1988

Stewart JW, McGrath PJ, Quitkin FM, et al: Relevance of DSM-III depressive subtype and chronicity of antidepressant efficacy in atypical depression: differential response to phenelzine, imipramine, and placebo. Arch Gen Psychiatry 46:1080–1087, 1989

Stewart JW, McGrath PJ, Quitkin FM: Do age of onset and course of illness predict different treatment outcome among DSM IV depressive disorders with atypical features? Neuropsychopharmacology 26:237–245, 2002

Svensson TH, Usdin T: Feedback inhibition of brain noradrenaline neurons by tricyclic antidepressants: α-receptor mediation. Science 202:1089–1091, 1978

Thapa PB, Gideon P, Cost TW, et al: Antidepressants and the risk of falls among nursing home residents. N Engl J Med 339:875–882, 1998

Thase ME, Mallinger AG, McKnight D, et al: Treatment of imipramine-resistant recurrent depression, IV: a double-blind crossover study of tranylcypromine for anergic bipolar depression. Am J Psychiatry 149:195–198, 1992

Vallejo J, Gasto C, Catalan R, et al: Double-blind study of imipramine versus phenelzine in melancholias and dysthymic disorders. Br J Psychiatry 151:639–642, 1987

Varley CK: Sudden death related to selected tricyclic antidepressants in children: epidemiology, mechanisms and clinical implications. Paediatr Drugs 3:613–627, 2001

Vuori E, Henry JA, Ojanpera I, et al: Death following ingestion of MDMA (ecstasy) and moclobemide. Addiction 98:365–368, 2003

White K, White J: Tranylcypromine: patterns and predictors of response. J Clin Psychiatry 47:380–382, 1986

White K, Razani J, Cadow B, et al: Tranylcypromine vs nortriptyline vs placebo in depressed outpatients: a controlled trial. Psychopharmacology (Berl) 82:258–262, 1984

Wilens TE, Biederman J, Prince J, et al: Six-week, double-blind, placebo-controlled study of desipramine for adult attention deficit hyperactivity disorder. Am J Psychiatry 153:1147–1153, 1996

Wong DT, Bymaster FP: Dual serotonin and noradrenaline uptake inhibitor class of antidepressants potential for greater efficacy or just hype? Prog Drug Res 58:169–222, 2002

Youdim MBH, Weinstock M: Therapeutic applications of selective and non-selective inhibitors of monoamine oxidase A and B that do not cause significant tyramine potentiation. Neurotoxicology 25:243–250, 2004

Zajecka J, Fawcett J: Susceptibility to spontaneous MAOI hypertensive episodes. J Clin Psychiatry 52:513–514, 1991

Zeller EA: Diamine oxidase, in The Enzymes, Vol 8, 2nd Edition. Edited by Boyer PD, Lardy H, Myrback K. London, Academic Press, 1963, pp 313–335

16

Selective Serotonin Reuptake Inhibitors and Newer Antidepressants

RICHARD C. SHELTON, M.D.

NATALIE LESTER, B.S.

THE INTRODUCTION of the selective serotonin reuptake inhibitors (SSRIs) has had an enormous effect on the practice of medicine in general and the practice of psychiatry in particular. Before the introduction of fluoxetine to the United States market in late 1998, antidepressants were used infrequently in the primary care setting and often at subtherapeutic doses. Since then, antidepressants have become among the most widely prescribed drugs worldwide, with a market representing billions of dollars per year. The SSRIs and later medications have changed the face of the treatment of depression. In this chapter, we review antidepressant medications approved by the U.S. Food and Drug Administration (FDA) since 1997.

Background and History

Tricyclic and monoamine oxidase inhibitor (MAOI) antidepressants have a high side-effect burden, cardiotoxicity, risk in overdosage, and drug interactions that limit their usefulness in practice. By the late 1960s, it was clear that newer treatments with improved risk and tolerability profiles were needed. Because both the MAOIs and the tricyclics appeared to work by enhancement of monoaminergic synaptic transmission, including that of norepinephrine (NE), serotonin (5-HT), and, to a lesser degree, dopamine (DA), investigators pursued the hypothesis that the therapeutic effects of these drugs resulted from increased levels of these neurotransmitters, culminating in the monoamine hypothesis of depression (Schildkraut 1965). Initially, this hypothesis largely focused on noradrenergic mechanisms, but later work by investigators such as Arvid Carlsson and James Maas began to shift the focus toward serotonin as an important target of antidepressant action (Nemeroff and Owens 2003). Pharmaceutical research in Europe and the United States focused on developing drugs that blocked the serotonin reuptake site, referred to as the serotonin transporter (SERT), without the concomitant receptor-binding profile of the tricyclics. This led to the synthesis of zimelidine, the first marketed SSRI, and fluoxetine, the first SSRI marketed in the United States (Fuller et al. 1991; Huitfeldt and Montgomery 1983; Montgomery et al. 1981a, 1981b).

Following the remarkable success of fluoxetine, various companies introduced compounds that were relatively potent and selective antagonists of the SERT. The "modern" era of antidepressant treatment had begun in earnest. In parallel with this development, many companies continued to focus considerable efforts on the synthesis of drugs that were similar to tricyclics in action but not serotonin selective. Much of the development of antidepressants over the last 30 years or more has focused on the goal of the development of "cleaned-up" tricyclics—drugs that inhibit the reuptake of NE or serotonin, or both, but that have low affinity for other receptors. The result was a new generation of antidepressants, including the SSRIs, selective NE reuptake inhibitors (NRIs), and dual serotonin-NE reuptake inhibitors (SNRIs).

Monoamine Transporters

Most antidepressant compounds, both old and newer, act by the blockade of the transporter proteins for either serotonin or NE or both. The SERT and the NE transporter are chemically related structures with distinct genetic loci. They are part of a larger family of transporters powered by Na^+/ K^+ adenosine triphosphatases (ATPases). The function of a transporter is to remove neurotransmitter from the synapse, thus terminating stimulation of the postsynaptic neuron. In addition, it serves as a recycling agent, allowing the presynaptic cell to reuse the serotonin that it collects (Blakely et al. 1994; Qian et al. 1995).

Like other members of the transporter family, the SERT is a glycoprotein complex embedded in a plasma membrane by 12 transmembrane domains. Its glycosylation plays an important role in protein folding and protection against degradation (Blakely et al. 1994). These transporters are located on the axon terminals and cell bodies of serotonergic neurons. Each transporter contains binding sites for serotonin, Na^+, Cl^-, K^+, and pharmacological agents (such as SSRIs, cocaine, and amphetamines). To initiate serotonin reuptake, the SERT binds extracellular serotonin, Na^+, and Cl^-. This induces a conformational change in the SERT that moves these ions and serotonin into the cell, where they are released. Intracellular K^+ then binds to the complex, another conformational change ensues, and the complex returns to its initial configuration. SSRIs inhibit the SERT by binding to a site on the SERT protein at a location other than the active uptake site for serotonin (allosteric inhibition). Thus, SSRIs do not completely prevent the SERT from functioning because they do not prevent the binding of serotonin. However, therapeutic doses of SSRIs decrease SERT functioning by 60%–80%.

The NE transporter is structurally and functionally very similar to SERT, and many antidepressants inhibit both of these transporters. In addition, the NE transporter has a moderate affinity for DA; therefore, antidepressants that act on the NE transporter enhance transmission of both NE and DA (Pacholczyk et al. 1991). Finally, at least one antidepressant, sertraline, has a modest effect on the transporter for DA directly, although the clinical implications of this are unknown (Owens et al. 1997). Binding affinities for the NE transporter and SERT (expressed as the inhibition constant [K_i]) are listed in Table 16–1.

Desensitization of specific serotonin and NE receptors, which occurs after uptake blockade, has been postulated to be the principal mechanism of action of antidepressants (Sulser et al. 1978). Hyman and Nestler (1996) suggested that this desensitization serves as a marker of adaptation rather than as the mechanism through which therapeutic actions are mediated. Enhanced transsynaptic signaling by NE and serotonin leads to downstream effects of gene expression that may, ultimately, result in therapeutic effects. Thus, rather than being directly associated with the antidepressant effects, receptor desensitization could co-occur with the amelioration of side effects.

Therapeutic Implications of Serotonin and Norepinephrine Reuptake Blockade

Antidepressants, including the SSRIs, SNRIs, and NRIs, are indicated for the treatment of not only depression but also a variety of other psychiatric conditions, particularly anxiety disorders. Table 16–2 lists the trade names, FDA-approved dosage ranges and indications, and "extreme" doses (i.e., dosing minima and maxima used in clinical practice) of these newer antidepressants.

A natural question that arises is whether the full therapeutic effect of antidepressants can be realized by enhancement of either NE or serotonin alone or, alternatively, whether some meaningful differences in therapeutic action exist between the two principal mechanisms of action. Note that although all of the marketed antidepressants have at least some evidence of benefit in depression, this does not mean that most patients recover with treatment. The existing data, both from clinical trials and from more naturalistic outcomes studies, suggest that most patients do not experience a therapeutic remission with any single antidepressant (Simon et al. 1999).

Over the last 20 years, data have emerged to suggest that mood is not a simple "good" versus "bad" or "high" versus "low" construct. Rather, several component features have come forth. For example, L.A. Clark and Watson (1991) conceptualized the mood–anxiety spectrum as composed of three dominant bimodal (i.e., high vs. low) factors. These

TABLE 16–1. Pharmacodynamics and pharmacokinetics of selected newer antidepressants

Drug	K_i^a (SERT) (nmol)	K_i^a (NET) (nmol)	K_i (NET)/ K_i (SERT)	Protein binding (%)	Half-life
Citalopram	8.9	30,285	3,403	80	20 h (Fredricson 1982)
Duloxetine	0.8 (Bymaster et al. 2001)	7.5 (Bymaster et al. 2001)	9	95 (Chalon et al. 2003)	12.5 h (Sharma et al. 2000)
Fluoxetine[b]	20	2,186	109	98	4–6 d
Fluvoxamine	14	4,743	339	80	15 h (van Harten 1995)
Nefazodone	549	713	1.3	99 (DeVane et al. 2002)	4–8 h (DeVane et al. 2002)
Paroxetine	0.83	328	395	95	21 h
Sertraline[c]	3.3	1,716	520	98	26 h
Venlafaxine[d]	102	1,644	16	27	5–7 h

Note. SERT=serotonin transporter; NET=norepinephrine transporter.

[a]Uptake binding site binding affinity is expressed as the inhibition constant (K_i), which is an inverse scale (i.e., lower values are more potent) and is expressed as nanomolar (nmol).

[b]The half-life of the principal metabolite norfluoxetine is >200 hours.

[c]The half-life of the principal metabolite desmethylsertraline is 66 hours.

[d]O-desmethylvenlafaxine half-life is 11 hours.

Source. Adapted from Owens et al. (1997) and the *Physicians' Desk Reference* (2002), except as noted.

emanated from factor analytic studies of mood descriptors in large nonsymptomatic control and symptomatic populations and comprise *somatic anxiety*, *positive affect*, and *general distress* (also termed *negative affect*) (D.A. Clark et al. 1994; L.A. Clark and Watson 1991; Watson et al. 1995a, 1995b). Somatic anxiety involves physiological arousal, with features such as tachycardia, tachypnea, tremor, diaphoresis, and other evidence of acute fear, and is found in conditions such as panic attacks. Positive affect suggests a bimodal dimension with a positive emotional state involving enthusiasm, motivation, optimism, and so forth at the one end and anhedonia, which is fairly specific to depression, at the other end. General distress refers to a range of negative emotions (e.g., sadness, anxiety, worry, rumination, tension) and general dissatisfaction and is common to both anxiety and mood disorders. The focusing on these components may contribute to misdiagnosis or multiple diagnostic assignment (i.e., comorbidity).

A question arises as to whether therapeutic response maps to any of these dimensions of mood. Enhancement of serotonin transmission appears to improve elements of somatic anxiety (e.g., panic, social phobia) and general distress (e.g., generalized anxiety disorder), which seem to be class effects and are not specific to a limited set of compounds (Shelton and Tomarken 2001). This would distinguish the difference between therapeutic *effect*, based on some under-

lying neurochemical mechanism of action, and therapeutic *indication*, based on submission of research data to the FDA or other regulatory agencies. By contrast, serotonin uptake inhibitors seem to produce a more mixed effect with regard to positive affect. Although some patients clearly experience a broad effect on mood symptoms with SSRIs, only about one-third experience remission in a typical 8- to 12-week therapeutic trial. Moreover, some patients describe a mood "flattening" effect with SSRIs. In fact, persisting symptoms in depression are often in the "positive" rather than the "negative" affective domains.

By contrast, the effects of NE (including the indirect effects on dopaminergic mechanisms) appear to be significant mediators of arousal and activation. Antidepressants that act on catecholamines have been shown to have a beneficial effect in the positive affect domain. Bupropion, a drug acting predominantly via a catecholaminergic mechanism, has been shown to have a more consistent effect in the positive affective than in the general distress domains (Tomarken et al. 2004).

Clearly, some depressed patients achieve full therapeutic remission with SSRIs, and noradrenergically active drugs have been shown to produce benefit in anxiety. However, the therapeutic effect of imipramine has been shown to be inversely proportional to the plasma level of the desipramine metabolite in both panic disorder (Mavissakalian and Perel

TABLE 16–2. Newer antidepressants and related compounds approved for the treatment of depressive or anxiety disorders by the U.S. Food and Drug Administration (FDA)

Drug	U.S. trade name	Dosing range (mg/day) FDA approved	"Clinical"[a]	FDA–approved indications
Atomoxetine	Strattera	10–60	10–100	Attention-deficit disorder
Bupropion	Wellbutrin Wellbutrin SR Wellbutrin XL Zyban	SR: 150–400 XL: 150–450	100–400	Depression Smoking cessation (Zyban)
Citalopram	Celexa	20–60	10–80	Depression
Duloxetine	Cymbalta	60–120	—	Depression
Escitalopram	Lexapro	10–20	5–40	Depression
Fluoxetine	Prozac Prozac Weekly Serafem	20–80 Weekly: 90–180	10–120	Depression Bulimia nervosa Obsessive-compulsive disorder Panic disorder Premenstrual dysphoric disorder (Serafem)
Fluvoxamine	Luvox	50–300	25–400	Obsessive-compulsive disorder (adults, children)
Mirtazapine	Remeron Remeron Soltab	15–45	7.5–75	Depression
Nefazodone	Serzone	200–600	50–750	Depression
Paroxetine	Paxil Paxil CR	Paxil: 20–50 Paxil CR: 25–62.5	Paxil: 5–70 Paxil CR: 25–75	Depression Generalized anxiety disorder Panic disorder Posttraumatic stress disorder Premenstrual dysphoric disorder Social phobia (social anxiety disorder)
Sertraline	Zoloft	50–200	12.5–250	Depression Obsessive-compulsive disorder Panic disorder Posttraumatic stress disorder Premenstrual dysphoric disorder Social phobia (social anxiety disorder)
Venlafaxine	Effexor Effexor XR	75–375 XR: 75–225	37.5–450	Depression Generalized anxiety disorder

[a]Dosing minima and maxima typically used in clinical practice. Dash indicates no data available.

1996) and generalized anxiety disorder (McLeod et al. 2000), which led the investigators to conclude that the antianxiety benefits of imipramine derived primarily from the serotonergic rather than the noradrenergic effects. Thus, the therapeutic specificity of antidepressant mechanisms of action remains somewhat controversial, but at least some evidence indicates that the effects of serotonergic agents shade toward reduction in anxiety, whereas catecholaminergic drugs shade toward reduction in anhedonia.

Selective Serotonin Reuptake Inhibitors

As a class of drugs, SSRIs share many characteristics. In addition to their specificity for the SERT and relatively low affinity for other neurotransmitter receptors, they have low side-effect profiles relative to tricyclics and MAOIs, are relatively safe in overdose, and are readily absorbed from the gastrointestinal tract. Most circulate in a form that is highly bound to protein and that is in equilibrium with the unbound, biologically active form. Metabolized in the liver, these antidepressants are broken down by hepatic microsomal enzymes and conjugated, usually with glucuronic acid, allowing clearance in the urine. Thus, hepatic or renal dysfunction reduces clearance of the drug. Despite these similarities, these drugs are unique in terms of their receptor affinity and pharmacokinetic properties.

Today, five SSRIs are approved by the FDA for treatment of depression (fluoxetine, sertraline, paroxetine, citalopram, and escitalopram), and another (fluvoxamine) is marketed for obsessive-compulsive disorder (OCD) but has been prescribed for depression in Europe and other parts of the world. Table 16–2 lists the available SSRIs, their typical dosing ranges, and FDA-approved indications.

Clinical Use of Selective Serotonin Reuptake Inhibitors

Because newer antidepressants are safer and better tolerated by patients, there has been an increased willingness among clinicians to prescribe them and among patients to take them. The popularity of the SSRIs has stemmed largely from their increased tolerability and not from an increase in drug efficacy (i.e., response or remission). Although overall outcomes of treatment may not have improved, SSRIs and later drugs appear to have increased the proportion of patients receiving antidepressant drugs, which is likely to have a favorable effect that is independent of the benefits of any single agent.

Increase in antidepressant tolerability has resulted in a substantial shift in the physicians who treat depression; depression was once treated mainly by mental health professionals, but nearly three-quarters of all patients seeking treatment for depression now visit a primary care physician (Montano 1994). Between 1987 and 1997, the rate of people seeking treatment increased from 0.73 to 2.33 per 100 people per year (Olfson et al. 2002), about a threefold increase. The percentage of depressed individuals in treatment who are given antidepressants has doubled, from 37.3% in 1987 to 74.5% in 1997. Use is increasing in children as well: between 1988 and 1994, use of antidepressants in children increased three- to fivefold (Zito 2002).

Specific Selective Serotonin Reuptake Inhibitors

Fluoxetine

In late 1987, fluoxetine became the first SSRI approved for use in the United States. Once ingested, it is con-
verted to its active metabolite, norfluoxetine. Both parent compound and metabolite are relatively selective for the SERT: the K_i for fluoxetine and norfluoxetine is 0.9 and 2.3 nmol, respectively, versus tritium-labeled ($[^3H]$) citalopram in human transfected cells (SERT affinity), as opposed to 777 and 3,947 nmol, respectively, versus $[^3H]$nesoxetine binding (NE transporter affinity) (Owens et al. 1997). Typical fluoxetine dosing starts at 20 mg, once daily, and dosage can be increased in increments of 10–20 mg in a dosing range of up to 80 mg/day. Because of the relatively long half-life (4–6 days for fluoxetine, 7–15 days for norfluoxetine), a weekly dosing schedule and formulation has been approved, with a dose of 90 mg once or twice per week. Its long half-life also makes it less likely than other SSRIs to produce a discontinuation syndrome in patients stopping treatment (Haddad 2001). It is very highly protein bound (98%) and is an inhibitor of cytochrome P450 (CYP) 2D6 and 2C and somewhat less so for 1A2 and 3A4 (Table 16–3).

Fluoxetine has been studied for a variety of conditions and is currently approved in the United States for depression, bulimia nervosa, OCD, panic disorder, and premenstrual dysphoric disorder (Table 16–2). For the latter, it is marketed under the trade name Serafem.

Sertraline

Sertraline, which was approved in 1992, has been among the most widely used antidepressants. Like fluoxetine, sertraline has been studied for a wide group of disorders and has been approved by the FDA for depression, OCD, panic disorder, posttraumatic stress disorder, premenstrual dysphoric disorder, and social phobia (Table 16–2). It is highly protein bound (Table 16–1), and it inhibits metabolism of other drugs via CYP2C, CYP2D6, and CYP3A4 (Table 16–3). A typical starting dose is 50 mg (although lower doses are sometimes used in anxiety disorders such as panic disorder), and it can be prescribed up to 200 mg. Sertraline is a very potent serotonin uptake inhibitor: sertraline and its primary metabolite, desmethylsertraline, potently block the SERT, as measured by displacement of $[^3H]$citalopram (K_i=0.15 and 3.7 nmol, respectively) or $[^3H]$serotonin (K_i=3.3 and 187 nmol, respectively) (Owens et al. 1997). Both are weak NE uptake inhibitors (K_i vs. $[^3H]$citalopram or $[^3H]$serotonin in the range of 85 or 328 nmol for sertraline and 811 or 2,365 nmol for desmethylsertraline).

Sertraline is sometimes touted as a DA uptake inhibitor, although the binding affinity for the DA transporter is modest. Tatsumi et al. (1997) found the affinity (K_D) for sertraline and desmethylsertraline to be 25 and 129 nmol, respectively. However, this is much more potent than

TABLE 16–3. Estimated relative inhibition of selected cytochrome P450 enzymes by newer antidepressants

Drug	Cytochrome P450 enzyme inhibited	Relative inhibition
Bupropion	2D6	+
Citalopram/ escitalopram	1A2	+
	2C	+
Duloxetine (Skinner et al. 2003)	2D6	++
Fluoxetine	1A2	+
	2D6	++
	2C	++
	3A4	+
Fluvoxamine	1A2	++
	2C	++
	2D6	+
	3A4	++
Mirtazapine	2D6	+
Nefazodone	3A4	+++
Paroxetine	2C	+
	2D6	+++
	3A4	+
Sertraline	2D6	+
	2C	++
	3A4	++
Venlafaxine	None	–

Note.   +=low but significant; ++=moderate; +++=high.
Source.   Adapted from Nemeroff et al. (1996) and Greenblatt et al. (1998).

other antidepressant drugs (e.g., citalopram K_D=28,100 nmol). To our knowledge, it has not been tested via putative dopaminergic markers in humans (e.g., frontally mediated eye blink rates), and the effect of sertraline at the DA transporter in humans is unknown.

Paroxetine

Paroxetine was released soon after sertraline and was initially touted as a highly selective serotonin uptake inhibitor as a result of its high potency of SERT binding and its high ratio of serotonin to NE transporter binding affinity (Boyer and Feighner 1992). Like other SSRIs, it has been widely studied, and it is approved for the treatment of depression, generalized anxiety disorder, panic disorder, posttraumatic stress disorder, premenstrual dysphoric disorder, and social phobia (Table 16–2). The usual dosage

is 20 mg, once daily, and this can be increased to 60 mg/day or more. Paroxetine has a mild affinity to muscarinic receptors, leading some patients to experience anticholinergic side effects, such as dry mouth and constipation (Owens et al. 1997). In addition, it is a moderately potent histamine-1 antagonist, which can result in drowsiness (Owens et al. 1997). An enteric-coated, controlled-release form of paroxetine also has recently been released and appears to be associated with a somewhat lower profile of initial gastrointestinal side effects than the immediate-release version.

Paroxetine truly is a potent blocker of SERT: K_i=0.65 nmol ([^{3}H]citalopram displacement) or 0.83 nmol ([^{3}H]serotonin displacement) (Owens et al. 1997). However, although the ratio of SERT to NE transporter inhibition is high, binding at the NE transporter is not inconsequential: in vitro K_i=85 and 328 nmol versus [^{3}H]nisoxetine and [^{3}H]NE, respectively (Owens et al. 1997), which is mirrored by in vivo effects in rats (Owens et al. 2000). An important question, then, is whether this is reflected in human pharmacology.

Prior tests of NE transporter blockade by paroxetine in humans, such as the tyramine pressor test, have had negative results, although the dosage of paroxetine was low in those studies (20 mg/day). However, Gilmor and colleagues (2002) found that paroxetine inhibited NE uptake by 27% at an average serum concentration of 100 ng/mL and by 43% at 200 ng/mL, suggesting that paroxetine could be a meaningful NE uptake inhibitor in humans, at least at higher doses. However, the relation between the in vitro effects measured in this study and the in vivo effects in the brains of humans is unclear.

Citalopram and Escitalopram

Citalopram and its *S*-isomer, *S*-citalopram (escitalopram), have been approved for treatment of depression in the United States. These drugs are potent and selective serotonin uptake inhibitors (K_i=approximately 1–10 nmol) with negligible effects on the NE or DA transporters (K_i>3,000 nmol) (Owens et al. 1997). They also have very low binding affinity at other receptor sites (e.g., receptors for NE, serotonin, DA, histamine, or acetylcholine) (Baumann 1996). Citalopram is prescribed at a dose of 20 mg, which can be increased to 60 mg/day or more. Escitalopram typically is dosed in a range of 10–30 mg/day. Only the *S*-isomer is the active form of the compound (Burke 2002); when citalopram is administered, only about 35% of the circulating plasma level in humans is in the escitalopram form (Rochat et al. 1995). Comparative clinical trials usually have contrasted absolute doses of escitalopram at half the dose of citalopram (e.g., 10 mg vs. 20 mg)

(Montgomery et al. 2001), which, therefore, may not be therapeutically equivalent.

Citalopram and escitalopram are substrates for CYP3A4, CYP2C19, and CYP2D6 (Olesen and Linnet 1999; von Moltke et al. 1999). Neither citalopram nor the *S*-isomer substantially inhibits cytochrome P450 metabolism, although modest inhibition of CYP1A2 and CYP2C has been reported (Greenblatt et al. 1998; Nemeroff et al. 1996). Escitalopram appears to have somewhat lower plasma protein binding affinity (56%) in contrast to racemic citalopram (~80%) (DeVane 1998). This suggests that protein binding of the *R*-isomer is higher still, a potential therapeutic advantage for escitalopram when plasma protein displacement is of concern.

Fluvoxamine

Fluvoxamine is an SSRI approved in the United States only for the treatment of OCD, although it has been used as an antidepressant in Europe since 1984 (Rapaport et al. 1996). Placebo-controlled depression registration trials were conducted in the United States, but the findings were not sufficient to gain approval by the FDA (Ware 1997). Trials in OCD in both adults and children have suggested a strong effect (Goodman et al. 1997; Grados and Riddle 2001; Riddle et al. 2001).

The effects in depression, OCD, and other anxiety disorders are predictable according to the primary mechanism of action: fluvoxamine is a highly potent serotonin uptake inhibitor (K_i=1.6 nmol vs. [^{3}H]citalopram and =14 nmol vs. [^{3}H]serotonin) with minimal effects on the NE transporter (K_i=4,743 nmol) (Owens et al. 1997). Like other SSRIs, it inhibits a variety of cytochrome P450 enzymes, including CYP1A2, CYP2C, CYP2D6, and CYP3A4 Table 16–3). Protein binding is relatively high at 80%, although this is lower than for other SSRIs (Table 16–1). It is metabolized into various relatively inactive compounds, primarily via oxidative deamination and demethylation. The half-life of fluvoxamine is about 15 hours initially, although this is increased with continued exposure as a result of autoinhibition of metabolism (van Harten 1995). The starting dose usually is 50 mg/day; however, fluvoxamine tends to be effective at a dose of 150–200 mg.

Comparative Effectiveness

Drug responsiveness generally refers to a significant decrease in symptomatology—for example, as measured by a 50% or greater decrease in score on a scale for depression, such as the Hamilton Rating Scale for Depression (Ham-D). In contrast, a patient is considered to be "in

remission" if his or her level of symptoms is brought within the normal range, typically defined as a 17-item Ham-D score of 7 or less. Although response rather than remission has long been the primary measure of efficacy, many investigators are advocating the use of remission rates with the suggestion that remission is a better indicator for long-term outcome (Thase 2003). In general, rates of response do not vary significantly among antidepressant drugs (Kroenke et al. 2001). Most effective antidepressants produce response rates of 60%–75% in the typical 8- to 12-week clinical trial. By contrast, remission rates in those same trials can be quite low—ranging from 30% to 50%. It is important not to consider these rates as somehow representing what would happen in clinical practice; trials are artificially truncated, and data usually are reported as last observation carried forward. Therefore, reports of remission may be valid for comparing effectiveness but may not reflect the realities of treatment.

However, some data indicate that SSRIs may induce remission at a rate that is less than that for alternative treatments, at least among certain subpopulations. Specifically, evidence suggests that tricyclic compounds may be more effective than SSRIs in treating the melancholic subtype of depression (Perry 1996). It has been speculated that the reason for this more favorable response characteristic is that tricyclics generally block the uptake of both NE and serotonin. The Danish University Antidepressant Group ("Citalopram: Clinical Effect Profile in Comparison With Clomipramine: A Controlled Multicenter Study" 1986; "Paroxetine: A Selective Serotonin Reuptake Inhibitor Showing Better Tolerance, But Weaker Antidepressant Effect Than Clomipramine in a Controlled Multicenter Study" 1990) found that clomipramine, a potent NE and serotonin uptake inhibitor, produced a higher proportion of remission in contrast to either citalopram or paroxetine. In addition, a meta-analysis of registration trials with venlafaxine, a putative serotonin-NE uptake inhibitor, suggested that a small but statistically significantly higher proportion of patients achieve therapeutic remission with this drug in contrast to the SSRIs, at least in their "SERT-selective doses" (Thase et al. 2001). Alternatively, however, some recent data suggested that the overall therapeutic effect of venlafaxine may not be greater than that of comparably dosed SSRIs (Montgomery et al. 2004). Therefore, whether SNRIs exert a greater effect than SSRIs or a heightened effect in a subgroup of depressed patients is unknown.

The concept of "subgroup specificity" of response was initially supported by findings in the atypical subtype of depression, suggesting that SSRIs were preferentially effective. Atypical depression is characterized by so-called reversed vegetative features, including increased appetite and sleep along with heightened mood reactivity (Stewart et al., Chapter 33, in this volume). The boundaries of this condition were described in the past with regard to differential responsiveness to treatment—specifically, a preferential effect with MAOIs relative to tricyclics. Earlier open and small-scale controlled treatment research suggested that SSRIs might be preferentially effective over tricyclics in this subtype. However, at least two subsequent controlled trials did not support this contention, and another report suggested that atypical features predicted earlier relapse in continuation and maintenance treatment after initial response.

Despite this recent debate over the efficacy of SSRIs, these newer antidepressants have clearly had a positive effect on patient care because they have made pharmacological treatment much more accessible to many patients with depression. Their relatively long half-lives (most are approximately 24 hours) have made once-daily dosing possible with most SSRIs, a factor that promotes drug adherence.

Clinically Relevant Mechanisms of Action

When is an SSRI truly selective? Early in the evolution of SSRIs, serotonin selectivity was touted as a therapeutic advantage, playing off of the idea that the broader receptor-binding profiles of tricyclics produced considerable side effects; theoretically, then, selectivity would be expected to reduce the side-effect burden. However, given the more recent data suggesting a modestly improved effect with SNRIs, several studies have tested the relative selectivity of antidepressant drugs. Most of the newer antidepressants are more potent serotonin than NE uptake inhibitors, and determining when a drug has a dual or a single mechanism has been the focus of fierce debate. Much discussion has focused on the relative binding affinities of drugs for SERT and NE transporters in vitro (expressed as SERT–to–NE transporter ratio), which is essentially a meaningless concept. The potency of a given drug at a site of action is the product of both binding affinity and concentration. Therefore, a drug with very low affinity but a high concentration in brain may ultimately produce an equivalent effect to another drug with the opposite properties.

Paroxetine did not show evidence of effect on the tyramine pressor test as compared with amitriptyline (Hassan et al. 1985). Given the very high ratio of SERT to NE transporter binding affinity, this has been taken as evidence of relative selectivity of paroxetine for the SERT. However, although paroxetine binds to the SERT much more potently, its affinity for the NE transporter may not be trivial relative to other antidepressants. The

in vitro binding affinity of [^{3}H]NE for the human NE transporter is 328 compared with that of venlafaxine (1,644 nmol). We have used the term *serotonin-selective dose* to describe doses of antidepressants in which the serotonergic effects predominate over the noradrenergic; for example, doses such as paroxetine 20 mg, sertraline 50 mg, or venlafaxine 75 mg/day. However, on the basis of relative affinity, certain compounds exert alternative binding affinity (e.g., for NE transporter) as the dose is increased. However, exactly where these effects occur can be obscure. Gilmor et al. (2002), as noted earlier, found that higher plasma levels of paroxetine produced moderate blockade of NE transporter; low concentrations of paroxetine produced relatively modest NE transporter blockade (27%), but this increased somewhat at 200 ng/mL (43%), leading the investigators to conclude that paroxetine at higher doses and plasma concentrations could have a clinically meaningful noradrenergic effect. Again, the actual effect in brain is unclear.

Serotonin-Norepinephrine Reuptake Inhibitors

Venlafaxine

Venlafaxine is a structurally unique antidepressant that was introduced into the United States in 1994. It is a weak inhibitor of serotonin and NE reuptake (Table 16–1) and a very weak inhibitor of DA uptake. Nonetheless, as noted earlier, in human studies it shows significant effects in measurements of both SERT and NE transporter blockade. This is partly a result of the relatively high plasma and cerebrospinal levels of the parent compound and the primary metabolite, *O*-desmethylvenlafaxine, and very low protein binding. The low protein binding, and the fact that venlafaxine does not significantly interact with cytochrome P450 enzymes, suggests that drug–drug interactions typically would not be expected to occur (Ereshefsky and Dugan 2000). It is approved in a dosing range of 75–225 mg/day (375 mg/day for the immediate-release form). The dosing range in practice is between 37.5 and 450 mg/day (Table 16–2). Because of its short half-life, twice-daily dosing is required for the immediate-release form; however, the extended-release form of venlafaxine can be dosed once a day.

Venlafaxine has been approved by the FDA for the treatment of both major depression and generalized anxiety disorder (Gutierrez et al. 2003). Montgomery and colleagues (2002) conducted a survival analysis with data from two longer-term studies in this population, which suggested that patients tended to do well with venlafaxine overall and that, as a rule, higher doses (up to 150 mg/day) were better. That is, an overall better response and fewer dropouts occurred at 150 mg/day relative to the 75- and 37.5-mg doses (Montgomery et al. 2002).

As discussed earlier in this subsection, venlafaxine has a short half-life, and therefore discontinuation reactions can be observed, even after only brief interruptions (Haddad 2001). Like other sustained-release preparations (e.g., Paxil CR), extended-release venlafaxine is not less prone to inducing such reactions. Therefore, patients should be warned about interruptions in dosing. Venlafaxine is also associated with mild elevations in blood pressure; the immediate-release form at higher doses is somewhat more liable in this regard. It should be emphasized that these are not severe hypertensive events as seen with MAOIs, and hypertensive responses are not more common in patients with a history of hypertension. However, monitoring blood pressure is recommended (Feighner 1995).

Duloxetine

Duloxetine is another dual uptake inhibitor, recently approved for marketing for major depressive disorder in the United States. Dosing in clinical trials has ranged up to 40 mg twice per day, and the drug has shown good tolerability (Nemeroff et al. 2002; Schatzberg 2003; Sharma et al. 2000). In contrast to venlafaxine, duloxetine appears to induce low rates of spontaneous hypertension (<2%) (Schatzberg 2003).

Because mild hypertensive reactions occur with other NE uptake inhibitors such as tricyclics and venlafaxine, the question that arises is whether duloxetine causes a clinically meaningful blockade of NE reuptake. Duloxetine binds to the SERT and NE transporter at K_i=0.8 and 7.5 nmol, respectively, yielding a SERT–to–NE transporter ratio of 9 (Bymaster et al. 2001) as opposed to 16 for venlafaxine (Owens et al. 1997; see Table 16–1). Work by Turcotte et al. (2001) and Chalon and colleagues (2003) has called into question the in vivo potency of the drug at blocking the uptake of NE.

Two properties of duloxetine should be mentioned. The drug has been shown to reduce subjective ratings of pain in depressed patients as measured by a visual analog scale. Other antidepressants, including tricyclics and SSRIs, have been shown to produce benefit in pain syndromes, and the relative effect of duloxetine in this regard is unknown. In addition, duloxetine has been shown to be effective in reducing stress incontinence in women (Moore 2004).

Other Antidepressants

Bupropion

Bupropion is a moderately potent NE and DA uptake inhibitor (EC_{50} [effective concentration 50%]=5.0 and 2.0 μmol, respectively), with minimal effects on serotonin uptake (EC_{50}=58 μmol) (Horst and Preskorn 1998). Furthermore, it has at least two active metabolites with NE and DA uptake inhibiting effects: hydroxybupropion (EC_{50}=7.0 and 23 μmol, respectively) and threohydrobupropion (EC_{50}=16 and 47 μmol, respectively) (Horst and Preskorn 1998). However, more recent data suggest that bupropion may enhance presynaptic release of these catecholamines (Dong and Blier 2001; Gobbi et al. 2003). The drug increases synaptic availability of these transmitters, according to a variety of animal models of action, in concentration ranges that are associated with positive effects on animal models of antidepressant actions. Therefore, the principal mechanisms of action of bupropion seem to be enhanced synaptic transmission of the catecholamines, with minimal or no direct effects on the serotonin system.

This mechanism of action has yielded some unique properties to the compound. For example, bupropion is now widely used to target symptoms that are putatively related to these catecholamines: anergia, anhedonia, fatigue, and hypersomnia. In fact, clinicians have come to use bupropion more as an augmenting agent, typically added to SSRIs, than as a primary antidepressant. Furthermore, the relative lack of effects on the serotonin system tends to produce a reduced sexual side-effect burden. Bupropion has been used to treat SSRI-induced sexual side effects directly and as an alternative antidepressant when sexual side effects are intractable.

Bupropion may be somewhat less prone to inducing rapid cycling in bipolar depression. In an early open trial of adding bupropion to lithium or levothyroxine, bupropion was reported not to induce an increased frequency of cycles. In a very small study, Stoll et al. (1994) found that bupropion and MAOIs were somewhat less likely to induce cycles than other antidepressants. Although bupropion often is recommended for bipolar depression, the contention that it has less propensity to induce cycling has limited empirical support (Compton and Nemeroff 2000).

Bupropion is registered (FDA approved) for smoking cessation (Hays and Ebbert 2003). The effect of bupropion on mesolimbic catecholamines has suggested that it also has an effect in attention-deficit/hyperactivity disorder (ADHD). Clinical trials in both children and adults support this view. However, the effectiveness as compared with stimulants (e.g., methylphenidate) is not clear. More research is needed before any claim for equivalence can be supported.

The side-effect profile of bupropion is relatively benign; adverse events can include anxiety, agitation, insomnia, palpitations, dry mouth, dizziness, and nausea ("Wellbutrin SR package insert" 2002). Although headache is common, it was not reported more frequently than placebo in clinical trials ("Wellbutrin SR package insert" 2002). However, the seizure risk appears to be somewhat greater for bupropion than for other marketed antidepressants: 0.4% (4 of 1,000 exposures) in the dosing range of 300–450 mg/day for the immediate-release form; the risk with the sustained-release form was 0.1% at 100–300 mg/day and 0.4% at 400 mg/day ("Wellbutrin SR package insert" 2002). Thus, the manufacturer recommends avoiding bupropion in people with increased risks of seizures. Such risk factors include 1) history of seizures, 2) prior severe head trauma, 3) central nervous system tumor, 4) severe hepatic compromise (which would be expected to result in increased plasma levels), 5) use of other drugs that lower seizure threshold, 6) bulimia (i.e., bingeing and purging), and 7) use in situations involving concomitant use of stimulants (e.g., cocaine) or the potential withdrawal of sedative-hypnotics (including excessive alcohol or benzodiazepine use) ("Wellbutrin SR package insert" 2002). Doses higher than 400 mg/day for the sustained-release preparation and 450 mg/day for the immediate-release or extended-release formulation seem to increase the incidence of seizures further.

Nefazodone

Nefazodone is a phenylpiperazine derivative structurally similar to trazodone but with a somewhat improved side-effect profile (Owens et al. 1997). It has a weak potency for the human SERT and NE transporter ($K_i = 549$ and 713 nmol, respectively) (Owens et al. 1997). By contrast, binding of nefazodone and its principal metabolite, hydroxynefazodone, to the 5-HT_{2A} receptor is considerably greater than its binding to the serotonin or the norepinephrine transporter (ketanserin binding, $K_i = 7.1$ and 7.2 nmol, respectively) (Owens et al. 1997). Therefore, blockade of this receptor seems to be the basis of the therapeutic effect of nefazodone, much as it is with trazodone. 5-HT_{2A} blockade shows considerable antidepressant and antianxiety effects in animal behavioral models. Nefazodone is a relatively potent NE α_1 receptor antagonist ($K_i = 5.5$ nmol) (Owens et al. 1997) and modestly potent histamine-1 blocker ($K_i = 30$ nmol), which may account for some of the side-effect profile associated with nefaz-

odone, including orthostatic hypotension and sedation. The drug has a very short half-life (4–8 hours) (DeVane et al. 2002), requiring it to be dosed at least twice per day. Nefazodone usually is initiated at 200 mg/day, and it is typically advanced to the 300–600 mg/day range, divided into two doses. Rates of sexual dysfunction are relatively low. However, some significant concerns are associated with this drug. For example, it is a potent inhibitor of CYP3A4, an enzyme that is responsible for the metabolism of many drugs (Table 16–3) (Nemeroff et al. 1996). In addition, it has been reported to induce severe hepatotoxicity, resulting in liver failure. The rate of serious hepatotoxicity is low (about 1 in 250,000–300,000 exposures) ("Serzone package insert" 2002), but the outcome is potentially catastrophic. Routine monitoring of hepatic function has not been shown to be effective in preventing toxicity and is not required by the FDA, although early detection may improve outcome. Alternatively, counseling patients with regard to this adverse outcome and the symptoms of hepatic dysfunction (e.g., nausea, jaundice, anorexia, malaise) is essential. Furthermore, nefazodone should be avoided in people with baseline elevated transaminase levels, not because of an established increased risk in these patients but because of difficulties in prospective monitoring ("Serzone package insert" 2002).

Mirtazapine

Mirtazapine was introduced in the United States in 1997. It has a tetracyclic structure, reminiscent of tricyclics and, like those drugs, has histamine-1-blocking properties, which contribute to its side-effect profile. The primary mechanism of action appears to be antagonism of the NE α_2 receptor (de Boer et al. 1996). A significant function of this receptor is presynaptic inhibition of the release of both NE and serotonin. Blockade, therefore, enhances the availability of both neurotransmitters and is likely to be the main action for the therapeutic effect. However, mirtazapine also is an antagonist at 5-HT_2 and 5-HT_3 receptors, which may contribute to its anxiolytic effects and to the relative lack of sexual side effects. In addition, the histamine-1-blocking effects of the drug are similar to those of traditional antihistamines and tricyclic antidepressants. These effects account for not only the common side effects of sedation, increased appetite, and weight gain that occur at lower doses but also the positive effects on insomnia.

In a meta-analysis of eight double-blind, randomized, controlled trials of mirtazapine in major depression, Fawcett and Barkin (1998a) concluded that mirtazapine was consistently superior to placebo and comparable to tricyclics, particularly amitriptyline, which was the most common comparator agent. In particular, the data suggested that the drug was especially effective for symptoms of anxiety, including agitation and somatization. If valid, this efficacy is likely to be related to the 5-HT_2- and 5-HT_3-receptor-blocking effects. 5-HT_2 antagonists such as nefazodone and trazodone have been shown to have beneficial effects on anxiety, and 5-HT_3-blocking drugs such as ondansetron have been shown to reduce both physical and psychic symptoms of anxiety. The typical dosing range is between 15 and 45 mg/day.

Mirtazapine is metabolized by CYP1A2, CYP2D6, and CYP3A4 (Fawcett and Barkin 1998b). Although it appears not to have significant inhibiting effects at those enzymes, coadministration with other drugs that do inhibit them should be done with caution. The desmethyl metabolite is weakly active relative to the parent compound. The side-effect profile of mirtazapine appears to be bimodal, with histamine-1-blockade–associated sedation, increased appetite, and weight gain predominating at lower doses (i.e., <30 mg/day) and activation occurring at higher dosages. Thus, mirtazapine dosing involves a type of "balancing act" between those extremes. Finally, the drug appears to be relatively free of significant cardiotoxicity, including hyper- or hypotension.

Studies in special populations have been limited. Halikas (2003) compared mirtazapine with trazodone and placebo and found mirtazapine to be safe, effective, and well tolerated in elderly patients. It could be considered a good choice for elderly patients with decreased appetite and weight loss. Mirtazapine has received a limited amount of human study for both anxiety and insomnia.

Reboxetine and Atomoxetine

Both reboxetine (Brunello et al. 2002; Kasper et al. 2000) and atomoxetine (Kratochvil et al. 2003) are potent and relatively selective NRIs. Therefore, these drugs are similar in their therapeutic potential to tricyclics such as desipramine. Although reboxetine seems to be effective in depression and is available outside of the United States, FDA-regulated controlled registration trials have not been positive to date. In May 2001, the FDA declined the license application for reboxetine. This may be the result of failed rather than negative trials; that is, failure caused by a relatively high placebo response rate. The FDA cited no specific safety concerns, but its decision might have been influenced by the fact that no positive clinical trials have been reported in the United States. On the other hand, atomoxetine has received approval in the United States for ADHD as a result of significant controlled trials. Also, although atomoxetine has not been approved for treatment of depressive disorders, it was shown in at least

one published Phase II clinical trial to be effective in depression. Although atomoxetine is not widely used for the treatment of depression, the similarity to bupropion or tricyclics suggests potential benefit as a combination strategy with serotonergic agents.

Special Considerations

Serotonin Reuptake Inhibitor Discontinuation Syndrome

Abrupt termination of treatment with serotonin uptake inhibitors can result in a rapid onset of one or more characteristic symptoms now associated with the discontinuation syndrome: anxiety, crying, dizziness, "electrical sensations," headache, increased dreaming, insomnia, irritability, myoclonus, nausea (with occasional vomiting), paresthesias (including "electrical sensations"), and tremor. This phenomenon appears to be linked to three significant factors: 1) serotonin uptake blockade, 2) short half-life, and 3) a relatively rapid decrease in dose or termination of the medication. The anticholinergic effects of tricyclics also have been often mentioned as contributing to the problems associated with these drugs, especially in the face of symptoms that are more consistent with cholinergic rebound (including gastrointestinal hypermotility, movement disorders such as akathisia, and arrhythmias). However, it is a consistent property of serotonin reuptake inhibitors, although half-life is key: long half-life drugs such as fluoxetine seldom if ever produce the discontinuation syndrome, whereas short half-life drugs such as paroxetine or venlafaxine produce the discontinuation syndrome very often.

Serotonin reuptake inhibitor discontinuation syndrome is not peculiar to the newer generation of agents such as venlafaxine. In fact, the phenomenon has been reported with tricyclics such as imipramine and clomipramine and MAOIs as well (Lejoyeux and Ades 1997). In fact, the highest relative rates of discontinuation symptoms have been with tricyclic antidepressants (21.5%–100%) (Lejoyeux and Ades 1997), although this has not been confirmed in head-to-head comparisons.

Prevention is the ideal approach to the management of the syndrome. When patients are receiving shorter half-life serotonin reuptake inhibitors, slow tapering typically prevents significant symptoms. Furthermore, patients taking any serotonin reuptake inhibitor should be warned about the incidence of discontinuation symptoms after abrupt withdrawal. However, even with very slow tapering, some patients will experience intolerable symptoms. Slowing the tapering process sometimes helps, but at times, the substitution of another serotonin reuptake inhibitor with a longer half-life is needed.

Sexual Dysfunction

Sexual dysfunction is a side-effect property common to all serotonin reuptake inhibitors; although other chemical properties such as α-adrenergic and muscarinic cholinergic receptor blockade may contribute, the most consistent theme is the blockade of serotonin reuptake. Sexual side effects were reported with serotonergic tricyclics in the past. Common side effects of serotonin reuptake inhibitors include decreased libido, impairment in erection (in men) or labial engorgement (in women), and inhibition of orgasm. Therefore, patients taking these medications must be monitored carefully for persisting sexual side effects because this class of adverse reactions contributes significantly to premature discontinuation. Reported rates of sexual dysfunction with serotonin reuptake inhibitors have varied widely, depending more on the ascertainment method than on the type of drug. Conservatively, about half of the patients taking serotonin reuptake inhibitors will experience significant dysfunction, with 15% or more experiencing persisting symptoms. For a comprehensive review, see Ferguson (2001).

However, caution needs to be exercised when evaluating sexual dysfunction associated with serotonin reuptake inhibitors. Decreased sexual drive and arousal are common in depression; about half of depressed patients report significantly decreased sexual interest. Therefore, a baseline sexual history is an important part of information gathering in the evaluation of depression. Persistent sexual dysfunction may be a side effect of antidepressant therapy but also may be a residual symptom of depression and, if so, should be addressed accordingly.

Management of sexual dysfunction can involve several approaches. As noted, many patients will experience some improvement with time. However, it is often an intolerable side effect and should be managed aggressively to prevent premature termination of treatment. Decreasing or discontinuing the dose for a short period has been recommended, although this typically is ineffective and risks a return of depressive symptoms or the discontinuation syndrome. One alternative is switching to a drug with fewer side effects; for example, from the serotonin reuptake inhibitor to bupropion, nefazodone, or mirtazapine, all of which have been reported to be effective. However, some patients experience a significant return of depressive symptoms on tapering of the serotonin reuptake inhibitor and, therefore, must be restarted on the original drug. The addition of bupropion to the serotonin reuptake inhibitor is one management strategy; the addition of bupropion in the dose range of 100–300 mg/day has been reported to be somewhat effective. The addition of cyproheptadine, yohimbine, or sildenafil may be effective.

Suicide Risk

In 1990, Teicher et al. reported on a series of six inpatients who, at baseline, had reported no suicidal ideation but who developed intense and violent suicidal preoccupation after initiating treatment with fluoxetine. According to the investigators, this state persisted for 3 days to 3 months after discontinuation. This set off a firestorm of controversy about the potential that SSRIs could induce suicidal ideation in patients who did not previously have self-destructive thoughts. Furthermore, allegations have arisen that the risk of suicidal ideation with SSRIs has been downplayed by researchers because of compelling economic interests, which are the product of the financial relationships between pharmaceutical companies and universities (Healy 2003).

On the one side of the equation are case series that suggest that SSRIs do, in fact, enhance suicidal ideation in some patients. For example, Donovan et al. (2000) retrospectively evaluated 2,776 patients with deliberate self-harm presenting to the emergency department of the Derbyshire Royal Infirmary in the United Kingdom. The incidence of self-harm by drug was estimated from the number of prescriptions written for either a tricyclic or an SSRI in the Southern Derbyshire District for the same time interval. They found a higher incidence of deliberate self-harm in the SSRI-treated patients than in the tricyclic-treated patients. The relative risk of overdosage (setting imipramine at 1.0) was highest for fluoxetine at 2.8, followed closely by flupentixol (an antipsychotic) at 2.6. The mean relative risk for SSRIs was 2.3 and for tricyclics was 1.7. However, as the authors noted, the SSRI-related risk was skewed by the risk for fluoxetine; for example, the risk with sertraline was 1.4 and with paroxetine was 1.9, whereas the risk for the tricyclic clomipramine was 2.0 and lofepramine was 2.5. These kinds of data have led some to conclude that the risk of self-harm is increased with SSRIs, especially fluoxetine (Healy 2002). However, Donovan et al. (2000) stated:

> Equally relevant, however, is the pragmatic consideration that prescribers are heeding advice to prescribe safer-in-overdose antidepressants to patients who are perceived to be at greater risk of DSH [deliberate self-harm]. This effectively "loads the dice" against antidepressants such as the SSRIs, so that this manifests as an apparent excess of self-harm behaviour in patients who had been prescribed these antidepressants. (p. 556)

On the other side of the debate, data from controlled clinical trials generally have not indicated that SSRIs enhance risk relative to non-SSRI antidepressants or placebo. Khan et al. (2000) assessed frequency of suicides, suicide attempts, and symptom reduction derived from clinical trials information on seven drugs in the FDA database: fluoxetine, sertraline, paroxetine, venlafaxine, nefazodone, mirtazapine, and bupropion. A total of 19,639 participants were included. The investigators found no differences among the three groups compared collectively or within any given drug data set. However, fluoxetine information was not available via that avenue, and therefore no comment could be made with regard to fluoxetine risk per se. However, suicide risk with fluoxetine has been assessed by other studies.

Beasley et al. (1991) conducted a meta-analysis of 17 controlled clinical trials comparing fluoxetine ($n=1,765$ exposures) with tricyclics ($n=731$), placebo ($n=569$), or both. The pooled incidence of suicidal behavior did not differ among groups (suicidal acts: fluoxetine, 0.3%; tricyclics, 0.4%; placebo, 0.2%; and suicidal ideation: fluoxetine, 1.2%; tricyclics, 3.6%; placebo, 2.5%). Together, these data make a compelling case for a lack of association between SSRIs and an increase in suicidal potential.

Alternatively, clinical trial databases may not be the best place to evaluate risk for increased suicidal potential. For example, patients with active suicidal ideation typically are excluded from outpatient trials. Furthermore, subsets of patients who may be at greater risk, such as those with borderline personality disorder, are routinely excluded as well. However, data from nonrandomized populations run the risk cited by Donovan et al. (2000)—that patients with greater suicidal risk may be given drugs with less potential for fatality, hence inflating apparent liability.

More recently, marginal differences in rates of suicidal ideation or suicide attempts from individual clinical trials have led the FDA and other regulatory authorities to issue warnings about the potential for certain SSRIs to enhance suicide risk in adolescents. As reviewed by Wooltorton (2003), the FDA issued a warning based on a meta-analysis of three unpublished controlled trials in depressed adolescents that failed to show differences between paroxetine and placebo. In these studies, suicidal thoughts, suicide attempts, and episodes of self-harm were more frequent among adolescents taking paroxetine (5.3% of 378) compared with those taking placebo (2.8% of 285). A similar result was reported in studies of adolescents with social anxiety disorder (paroxetine: 2.4% of 165; placebo: 0% of 157). In this review, Wooltorton (2003) stated that "Paroxetine is contraindicated for patients under the age of 18...any pediatric patient currently taking

paroxetine should be screened for suicidal thoughts, suicide attempts or episodes of self-harm" (p. 446).

On the basis of similar data, clinicians have been warned about the risk of suicidal behavior in adolescents receiving extended-release venlafaxine. This FDA warning came from an analysis of children and adolescents between ages 6 and 17 years treated in both open and controlled clinical trials. Wyeth, Inc., the manufacturer of venlafaxine, outlined adverse event information from trials in depression and generalized anxiety disorder conducted in children and adolescents in a "Dear Healthcare Professional" letter. The company noted an excess of discontinuations for adverse events in three categories—hostility (venlafaxine, 2%; placebo, <1%), suicidal ideation (2% vs. 0%), and abnormal or changed behavior (1% vs. 0%)—and concluded: "Effexor and Effexor XR have not been and are not now recommended for use in pediatric patients."

A careful look at the numbers leads, perhaps, to an alternative conclusion. Taking the paroxetine data as a launching point, the excesses in each category of adverse experiences are relatively small. For example, as noted, suicidal ideation and behavior occurred in 5.3% of 378 patients taking paroxetine compared with 2.8% of 285 children and adolescents taking placebo. However, this translates into 20 versus 8 actual incidences. Because there were fewer individuals in the placebo group, normalizing the data yields a relative incidence rate of 20 in the paroxetine group versus 11 in the placebo group (results for χ^2 not significant). On the basis of these kinds of data, clinicians have been prohibited from using either paroxetine or venlafaxine in children or adolescents.

A key question, then, is why there is an apparent excess of suicidal ideation and behavior at all. The first and most compelling answer can be derived from the venlafaxine findings; specifically, the increases in suicidal ideation and behavior are due to the induction of a manic or mixed state (evidenced by hostility). The presence of an occult bipolar disorder could have resulted in the induction of a mixed state by the active drug that could have led to an increase in agitation, anxiety, irritability, hostility, and suicidal preoccupation. Second, antidepressants can induce anxiety and agitation in depressed patients, even in the absence of a bipolar diathesis, but with a similar outcome. Third, both paroxetine and venlafaxine have short half-lives and are known to induce withdrawal reactions. Missing one or more doses could result in an abrupt return of depressive, anxious, and other symptoms, leading to suicidal ideation. Finally, suicidal preoccupation may be induced by SSRIs in a fraction of patients. However, according to the data presented to date, it is impossible to determine whether a vulnerable subgroup of this type exists or whether the explanation is related to one or more of the more conventional answers. These kinds of factors together could contribute to an excess of suicidal ideation, suicide attempts, or hostility described in the two data sets.

So, what is the concern? Often, risk is appraised in a vacuum—that is, risk is assessed in a way that is independent of other relevant factors. In the particular case of the increased incidence of suicidal ideation with paroxetine or venlafaxine, clinicians have been advised to avoid using these medications in children and adolescents. However, the risk of a choice is more properly appraised against alternative choices, such as a different antidepressant or no treatment at all. Clearly, the major risk in a depressed child or adolescent is that of the illness itself; the use of antidepressants seems to have reduced that risk. For example, Olfson et al. (2003) used a large pharmacy database to evaluate the relation between the changes in regional antidepressant medication treatment and suicide in adolescents from 1990 to 2000. They found that a 1% increase in frequency of prescription of antidepressant drugs resulted in a decrease in suicide frequency by 0.23 per 100,000. In addition, for the period of 1991–2001 in the United States, the suicide rate for children ages 10–14 years declined approximately 14%, whereas the rate for 15- to 19-year-olds decreased 31.5% (Centers for Disease Control and Prevention 2004). The increase in frequency of antidepressant prescriptions over the same period suggests that these medications contributed to this decline.

A major concern is that clinicians, patients, and their family members will shy away from using an antidepressant or discontinue an effective medication in a vulnerable child. Given the high propensity for suicide, especially among adolescents, this could be catastrophic.

Drug–Drug Interactions

The newer antidepressants are generally safe, but they do confer risks for serious drug–drug interactions in certain circumstances. Perhaps the most serious is the combination of SSRIs and MAOIs, which can lead to the development of a potentially fatal "serotonin syndrome." These drugs should never be taken in combination, and patients should not begin taking an MAOI for at least 2 weeks after discontinuing an SSRI (for fluoxetine, 4 or more weeks). The serotonin syndrome presents within 24 hours of initiating or increasing the dose of a serotonergic agent and results from overstimulation of 5-HT$_{1A}$ and possibly 5-HT$_2$ receptors. It consists of a constellation of mental, autonomic, and neurological symptoms. The full-blown syndrome is diagnosed when a patient presents with at

least four major symptoms or at least three major and two minor symptoms. Major symptoms include confusion, elevated mood, coma, fever, tremors, chills, and rigidity (among others), and minor symptoms include agitation, insomnia, tachycardia, tachypnea, and impaired coordination. Treatment always involves the discontinuation of the serotonergic agent and replacement of fluids.

A second way in which dangerous drug–drug interactions can occur is through competitive protein binding. Antidepressants circulate in a state highly bound to proteins such as albumin, and other drugs that circulate in a highly bound state can displace the antidepressants, resulting in an increase in the fraction of the drug that is unbound. This may amplify the drug's effects, particularly the side effects (Table 16–2).

A third way in which antidepressants may confer risk for drug–drug interactions is that they inhibit cytochrome P450 enzymes, the microsomal enzymes of the liver that metabolize many drugs before they are cleared from the body (Tables 16–3 and 16–4). The antidepressants themselves are broken down by these enzymes, and some even inhibit their own metabolism. CYP2D6 is strongly inhibited by fluoxetine and paroxetine and weakly inhibited by sertraline and citalopram (Nemeroff et al. 1996). Drugs that are normally metabolized by this isoform include antipsychotics, antiseizure medication, β-blockers, and angiotensin-converting enzyme inhibitors. CYP3A4 is inhibited by nefazodone, norfluoxetine, and fluvoxamine; thus, they can cause increased plasma levels of cyclosporine and other drugs metabolized by CYP3A4 (Nemeroff et al. 1996). Venlafaxine and mirtazapine may have lower potential for drug–drug interactions than other antidepressants.

Conclusion

The introduction of SSRIs and newer antidepressants has dramatically changed the treatment of depression over the past two decades. Earlier antidepressants such as the tricyclics were effective but had significant side effects because they interacted with a variety of neurotransmitter receptors. SSRIs rapidly became the most widely prescribed class of antidepressants, indeed one of the most widely prescribed classes of drugs, and have been used in the treatment of depression in millions of people worldwide. Although questions remain about their comparative effectiveness, they continue to be widely used. More research is needed to create pharmacological agents that treat depression more quickly and effectively.

TABLE 16–4. Representative drugs metabolized by specific cytochrome P450 enzymes

1A2	2C	2D6	3A4
Caffeine	Amitriptyline	Brofaromine	Alprazolam
Clomipramine	Citalopram	Citalopram	Astemizole
Clozapine	Clomipramine	Codeine	Calcium channel inhibitors
Fluvoxamine	Diazepam	Dextromethorphan	Carbamazepine
Haloperidol	Hexobarbital	Encainide	Clomipramine
Imipramine	Imipramine	Fluoxetine	Cyclosporine
Mirtazapine	Mephobarbital	Haloperidol	Dexamethasone
Phenacetin	Moclobemide	Maprotiline	Dextromethorphan
Tacrine	NSAIDs	Metoprolol	Erythromycin
Tertiary amine tricyclics	Omeprazole	Mianserin	Imipramine
Theophylline	Phenytoin	Mirtazapine	Lidocaine
Verapamil	Proguanil	Paroxetine	Midazolam
	Tolbutamide	Perphenazine	Mirtazapine
	Tricyclic antidepressants	Propafenone	Nefazodone
	Warfarin	Propranolol	Quinidine
		Remoxipride	Sertraline
		Risperidone	Steroids
		Thioridazine	Terfenadine
		Trazodone	Triazolam
		Tricyclic antidepressants	Tricyclic antidepressants
		Venlafaxine	Verapamil
			Vinblastine

Note. NSAIDs=nonsteroidal anti-inflammatory drugs.
Source. Adapted from Nemeroff et al. (1996).

References

Baumann P: Pharmacokinetic-pharmacodynamic relationship of the selective serotonin reuptake inhibitors. Clin Pharmacokinet 31:444–469, 1996

Beasley CM Jr, Dornseif BE, Bosomworth JC, et al: Fluoxetine and suicide: a meta-analysis of controlled trials of treatment for depression. BMJ 303:685–692, 1991

Blakely RD, De Felice LJ, Hartzell HC: Molecular physiology of norepinephrine and serotonin transporters. J Exp Biol 196:263–281, 1994

Boyer WF, Feighner JP: An overview of paroxetine. J Clin Psychiatry 53 (suppl):3–6, 1992

Brunello N, Mendlewicz J, Kasper S, et al: The role of noradrenaline and selective noradrenaline reuptake inhibition in depression. Eur Neuropsychopharmacol 12:461–475, 2002

Burke WJ: Escitalopram. Expert Opin Investig Drugs 11:1477–1486, 2002

Bymaster FP, Dreshfield-Ahmad LJ, Threlkeld PG, et al: Comparative affinity of duloxetine and venlafaxine for serotonin and norepinephrine transporters in vitro and in vivo, human serotonin receptor subtypes, and other neuronal receptors. Neuropsychopharmacology 25:871–880, 2001

Centers for Disease Control and Prevention: Methods of suicide among persons aged 10–19 years—United States, 1992–2001. MMWR Morb Mortal Wkly Rep 53:471–474, 2004

Chalon SA, Granier LA, Vandenhende FR, et al: Duloxetine increases serotonin and norepinephrine availability in healthy subjects: a double-blind, controlled study. Neuropsychopharmacology 28:1685–1693, 2003

Citalopram: clinical effect profile in comparison with clomipramine: a controlled multicenter study. Danish University Antidepressant Group. Psychopharmacology (Berl) 90:131–138, 1986

Clark DA, Steer RA, Beck AT: Common and specific dimensions of self-reported anxiety and depression: implications for the cognitive and tripartite models. J Abnorm Psychol 103:645–654, 1994

Clark LA, Watson D: Tripartite model of anxiety and depression: psychometric evidence and taxonomic implications. J Abnorm Psychol 100:316–336, 1991

Compton MT, Nemeroff CB: The treatment of bipolar depression. J Clin Psychiatry 61 (suppl 9):57–67, 2000

de Boer TH, Nefkens F, van Helvoirt A, et al: Differences in modulation of noradrenergic and serotonergic transmission by the alpha-2 adrenoceptor antagonists, mirtazapine, mianserin and idazoxan. J Pharmacol Exp Ther 277:852–860, 1996

DeVane CL: Differential pharmacology of newer antidepressants. J Clin Psychiatry 59 (suppl 20):85–93, 1998

DeVane CL, Grothe DR, Smith SL: Pharmacology of antidepressants: focus on nefazodone. J Clin Psychiatry 63:10–17, 2002

Dong J, Blier P: Modification of norepinephrine and serotonin, but not dopamine, neuron firing by sustained bupropion treatment. Psychopharmacology (Berl) 155:52–57, 2001

Donovan S, Clayton A, Beeharry M, et al: Deliberate self-harm and antidepressant drugs: investigation of a possible link. Br J Psychiatry 177:551–556, 2000

Ereshefsky L, Dugan D: Review of the pharmacokinetics, pharmacogenetics, and drug interaction potential of antidepressants: focus on venlafaxine. Depress Anxiety 12 (suppl 1):30–44, 2000

Fawcett J, Barkin RL: A meta-analysis of eight randomized, double-blind, controlled clinical trials of mirtazapine for the treatment of patients with major depression and symptoms of anxiety. J Clin Psychiatry 59:123–127, 1998a

Fawcett J, Barkin RL: Review of the results from clinical studies on the efficacy, safety and tolerability of mirtazapine for the treatment of patients with major depression. J Affect Disord 51:267–285, 1998b

Feighner JP: Cardiovascular safety in depressed patients: focus on venlafaxine. J Clin Psychiatry 56:574–579, 1995

Ferguson JM: The effects of antidepressants on sexual functioning in depressed patients: a review. J Clin Psychiatry 62 (suppl 3):22–34, 2001

Fredricson OK: Kinetics of citalopram in man; plasma levels in patients. Prog Neuropsychopharmacol Biol Psychiatry 6:311–318, 1982

Fuller RW, Wong DT, Robertson DW: Fluoxetine, a selective inhibitor of serotonin uptake. Med Res Rev 11:17–34, 1991

Gilmor ML, Owens MJ, Nemeroff CB: Inhibition of norepinephrine uptake in patients with major depression treated with paroxetine. Am J Psychiatry 159:1702–1710, 2002

Gobbi G, Slater S, Boucher N, et al: Neurochemical and psychotropic effects of bupropion in healthy male subjects. J Clin Psychopharmacol 23:233–239, 2003

Goodman WK, Ward H, Kablinger A, et al: Fluvoxamine in the treatment of obsessive-compulsive disorder and related conditions. J Clin Psychiatry 58 (suppl 5):32–49, 1997

Grados MA, Riddle MA: Pharmacological treatment of childhood obsessive-compulsive disorder: from theory to practice. J Clin Child Psychol 30:67–79, 2001

Greenblatt DJ, von Moltke LL, Harmatz JS, et al: Drug interactions with newer antidepressants: role of human cytochromes P450. J Clin Psychiatry 59 (suppl 15):19–27, 1998

Gutierrez MA, Stimmel GL, Aiso JY: Venlafaxine: a 2003 update. Clin Ther 25:2138–2154, 2003

Haddad PM: Antidepressant discontinuation syndromes. Drug Saf 24:183–197, 2001

Halikas JA: Org 3770 (mirtazapine) versus trazodone: a placebo controlled trial in depressed elderly patients. Hum Psychopharmacol 10:125S–133S, 2003

Hassan SM, Wainscott G, Turner P: A comparison of the effect of paroxetine and amitriptyline on the tyramine pressor response test. Br J Clin Pharmacol 19:705–706, 1985

Hays JT, Ebbert JO: Bupropion for the treatment of tobacco dependence: guidelines for balancing risks and benefits. CNS Drugs 17:71–83, 2003

Healy D: SSRIs and deliberate self-harm. Br J Psychiatry 180:547–548, 2002

Healy D: In the grip of the python: conflicts at the university-industry interface. Sci Eng Ethics 9:59–71, 2003

Horst WD, Preskorn SH: Mechanisms of action and clinical characteristics of three atypical antidepressants: venlafaxine, nefazodone, bupropion. J Affect Disord 51:237–254, 1998

Huitfeldt B, Montgomery SA: Comparison between zimeldine and amitriptyline of efficacy and adverse symptoms—a combined analysis of four British clinical trials in depression. Acta Psychiatr Scand Suppl 308:55–69, 1983

Hyman SE, Nestler EJ: Initiation and adaptation: a paradigm for understanding psychotropic drug action. Am J Psychiatry 153:151–162, 1996

Kasper S, el Giamal N, Hilger E: Reboxetine: the first selective noradrenaline re-uptake inhibitor. Expert Opin Pharmacother 1:771–782, 2000

Khan A, Warner HA, Brown WA: Symptom reduction and suicide risk in patients treated with placebo in antidepressant clinical trials: an analysis of the Food and Drug Administration database. Arch Gen Psychiatry 57:311–317, 2000

Kratochvil CJ, Vaughan BS, Harrington MJ, et al: Atomoxetine: a selective noradrenaline reuptake inhibitor for the treatment of attention-deficit/hyperactivity disorder. Expert Opin Pharmacother 4:1165–1174, 2003

Kroenke K, West SL, Swindle R, et al: Similar effectiveness of paroxetine, fluoxetine, and sertraline in primary care: a randomized trial. JAMA 286:2947–2955, 2001

Lejoyeux M, Ades J. Antidepressant discontinuation: a review of the literature. J Clin Psychiatry 58 (suppl 7):11–15, 1997

Mavissakalian MR, Perel JM: The relationship of plasma imipramine and N-desmethylimipramine to response in panic disorder. Psychopharmacol Bull 32:143–147, 1996

McLeod DR, Hoehn-Saric R, Porges SW, et al: Therapeutic effects of imipramine are counteracted by its metabolite, desipramine, in patients with generalized anxiety disorder. J Clin Psychopharmacol 20:615–621, 2000

Montano CB: Recognition and treatment of depression in a primary care setting. J Clin Psychiatry 55 (suppl):18–34, 1994

Montgomery SA, McAuley R, Rani SJ, et al: A double blind comparison of zimelidine and amitriptyline in endogenous depression. Acta Psychiatr Scand Suppl 290:314–327, 1981a

Montgomery SA, Rani SJ, McAuley R, et al: The antidepressant efficacy of zimelidine and maprotiline. Acta Psychiatr Scand Suppl 290:219–224, 1981b

Montgomery SA, Loft H, Sanchez C, et al: Escitalopram (S-enantiomer of citalopram): clinical efficacy and onset of action predicted from a rat model. Pharmacol Toxicol 88:282–286, 2001

Montgomery SA, Mahe V, Haudiquet V, et al: Effectiveness of venlafaxine, extended release formulation, in the short-term and long-term treatment of generalized anxiety disorder: results of a survival analysis. J Clin Psychopharmacol 22:561–567, 2002

Montgomery SA, Huusom AK, Bothmer J: A randomised study comparing escitalopram with venlafaxine XR in primary care patients with major depressive disorder. Neuropsychobiology 50:57–64, 2004

Moore K: Duloxetine: a new approach for treating stress urinary incontinence. Int J Gynaecol Obstet 86 (suppl 1):S53–S62, 2004

Nemeroff CB, Owens MJ: Neuropharmacology of paroxetine. Psychopharmacol Bull 37 (suppl 1):8–18, 2003

Nemeroff CB, DeVane CL, Pollock BG: Newer antidepressants and the cytochrome P450 system. Am J Psychiatry 153:311–320, 1996

Nemeroff CB, Schatzberg AF, Goldstein DJ, et al: Duloxetine for the treatment of major depressive disorder. Psychopharmacol Bull 36:106–132, 2002

Olesen OV, Linnet K: Studies on the stereoselective metabolism of citalopram by human liver microsomes and cDNA-expressed cytochrome P450 enzymes. Pharmacology 59:298–309, 1999

Olfson M, Marcus SC, Druss B, et al: National trends in the outpatient treatment of depression. JAMA 287:203–209, 2002

Olfson M, Shaffer D, Marcus SC, et al: Relationship between antidepressant medication treatment and suicide in adolescents. Arch Gen Psychiatry 60:978–982, 2003

Owens MJ, Morgan WN, Plott SJ, et al: Neurotransmitter receptor and transporter binding profile of antidepressants and their metabolites. J Pharmacol Exp Ther 283:1305–1322, 1997

Owens MJ, Knight DL, Nemeroff CB: Paroxetine binding to the rat norepinephrine transporter in vivo. Biol Psychiatry 47:842–845, 2000

Pacholczyk T, Blakely RD, Amara SG: Expression cloning of a cocaine- and antidepressant-sensitive human noradrenaline transporter. Nature 350:350–354, 1991

Paroxetine: a selective serotonin reuptake inhibitor showing better tolerance, but weaker antidepressant effect than clomipramine in a controlled multicenter study. Danish University Antidepressant Group. J Affect Disord 18:289–299, 1990

Perry PJ: Pharmacotherapy for major depression with melancholic features: relative efficacy of tricyclic versus selective serotonin reuptake inhibitor antidepressants. J Affect Disord 39:1–6, 1996

Physicians' Desk Reference, 52nd Edition. Montvale, NJ, Medical Economics, 2002

Qian Y, Melikian HE, Rye DB, et al: Identification and characterization of antidepressant-sensitive serotonin transporter proteins using site-specific antibodies. J Neurosci 15:1261–1274, 1995

Rapaport M, Coccaro E, Sheline Y, et al: A comparison of fluvoxamine and fluoxetine in the treatment of major depression. J Clin Psychopharmacol 16:373–378, 1996

Riddle MA, Reeve EA, Yaryura-Tobias JA, et al: Fluvoxamine for children and adolescents with obsessive-compulsive disorder: a randomized, controlled, multicenter trial. J Am Acad Child Adolesc Psychiatry 40:222–229, 2001

Rochat B, Amey M, Baumann P: Analysis of enantiomers of citalopram and its demethylated metabolites in plasma of depressive patients using chiral reverse-phase liquid chromatography. Ther Drug Monit 17:273–279, 1995

Schatzberg AF: Efficacy and tolerability of duloxetine, a novel dual reuptake inhibitor, in the treatment of major depressive disorder. J Clin Psychiatry 64 (suppl 13):30–37, 2003

Schildkraut JJ: The catecholamine hypothesis of affective disorders: a review of supporting evidence. Am J Psychiatry 122:509–522, 1965

Serzone package insert. Princeton, NJ, Bristol-Myers Squibb Company, 2002

Sharma A, Goldberg MJ, Cerimele BJ: Pharmacokinetics and safety of duloxetine, a dual-serotonin and norepinephrine reuptake inhibitor. J Clin Pharmacol 40:161–167, 2000

Shelton RC, Tomarken AJ: Can recovery from depression be achieved? Psychiatr Serv 52:1469–1478, 2001

Simon GE, Heiligenstein J, Revicki D, et al: Long-term outcomes of initial antidepressant drug choice in a "real world" randomized trial. Arch Fam Med 8:319–325, 1999

Skinner MH, Kuan HY, Pan A, et al: Duloxetine is both an inhibitor and a substrate of cytochrome P4502D6 in healthy volunteers. Clin Pharmacol Ther 73:170–177, 2003

Stoll AL, Mayer PV, Kolbrener M, et al: Antidepressant-associated mania: a controlled comparison with spontaneous mania. Am J Psychiatry 151:1642–1645, 1994

Sulser F, Vetulani J, Mobley PL: Mode of action of antidepressant drugs. Biochem Pharmacol 27:257–261, 1978

Tatsumi M, Groshan K, Blakely RD, et al: Pharmacological profile of antidepressants and related compounds at human monoamine transporters. Eur J Pharmacol 340:249–258, 1997

Teicher MH, Glod C, Cole JO: Emergence of intense suicidal preoccupation during fluoxetine treatment. Am J Psychiatry 147:207–210, 1990

Thase ME: Effectiveness of antidepressants: comparative remission rates. J Clin Psychiatry 64 (suppl 2):3–7, 2003

Thase ME, Entsuah AR, Rudolph RL: Remission rates during treatment with venlafaxine or selective serotonin reuptake inhibitors. Br J Psychiatry 178:234–241, 2001

Tomarken AJ, Dichter GS, Freid C, et al: Assessing the effects of bupropion SR on mood dimensions of depression. J Affect Disord 78:235–241, 2004

Turcotte JE, Debonnel G, de Montigny C, et al: Assessment of the serotonin and norepinephrine reuptake blocking properties of duloxetine in healthy subjects. Neuropsychopharmacology 24:511–521, 2001

van Harten J: Overview of the pharmacokinetics of fluvoxamine. Clin Pharmacokinet 29 (suppl 1):1–9, 1995

von Moltke LL, Greenblatt DJ, Grassi JM, et al: Citalopram and desmethylcitalopram in vitro: human cytochromes mediating transformation, and cytochrome inhibitory effects. Biol Psychiatry 46:839–849, 1999

Ware MR: Fluvoxamine: a review of the controlled trials in depression. J Clin Psychiatry 58 (suppl 5):15–23, 1997

Watson D, Clark LA, Weber K, et al: Testing a tripartite model, II: exploring the symptom structure of anxiety and depression in student, adult, and patient samples. J Abnorm Psychol 104:15–25, 1995a

Watson D, Weber K, Assenheimer JS, et al: Testing a tripartite model, I: evaluating the convergent and discriminant validity of anxiety and depression symptom scales. J Abnorm Psychol 104:3–14, 1995b

Wellbutrin SR package insert. Research Triangle Park, NC, GlaxoSmithKline, 2002

Wooltorton E: Paroxetine (Paxil, Seroxat): increased risk of suicide in pediatric patients. CMAJ 169:446, 2003

Zito JM: Five burning questions. J Dev Behav Pediatr 23:S23–S30, 2002

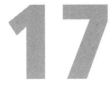

CHAPTER 17

Lithium and Mood Stabilizers

PAUL E. KECK JR., M.D.
SUSAN L. McELROY, M.D.

LITHIUM HERALDED the modern era of biological treatments for mental illnesses more than 50 years ago and was the first mood stabilizer. In the last 10 years, several new agents have been investigated in randomized, controlled trials as potential treatments for various phases of bipolar disorder. In this chapter, we review the psychopharmacology of lithium and the anticonvulsants, focusing on data from randomized, controlled trials of lithium and other medications in the treatment of acute manic, mixed, and depressive episodes and in the prevention of further symptoms and episodes. Evidence is growing for the efficacy of new-generation antipsychotics in bipolar disorder, but this subject is covered elsewhere in this volume (see Strakowski and Shelton, Chapter 18).

Lithium

Acute Manic and Mixed Episodes

Lithium, the oldest medication in the pharmacological armamentarium for bipolar disorder, remains a first-line treatment for all phases of the illness (Hirschfeld et al. 2002). Lithium's efficacy in the treatment of acute mania

was initially established in placebo-controlled trials in the 1950s and 1960s (Goodwin et al. 1969; Maggs 1963; Schou et al. 1954; Stokes et al. 1971). Several more recent placebo-controlled trials of different agents in which lithium was used as an active comparator continue to confirm the results of these earlier studies (Bowden et al. 1994; Paulsson 2003). In head-to-head comparison trials, lithium had efficacy comparable to that of divalproex (Bowden et al. 1994), carbamazepine (Lerer et al. 1987; Small et al. 1991), risperidone (J. Segal et al. 1998), olanzapine (Berk et al. 1999), quetiapine (Paulsson 2003), and first-generation antipsychotics (neuroleptics) (Garfinkel et al. 1980; Johnson et al. 1976; Platman 1970; Prien et al. 1972; Shopsin et al. 1975; Spring et al. 1970; Takahashi et al. 1975). Although most of these studies were not powered to detect significant differences among active agents, the uniformity of lithium response in these studies in aggregate is striking. Lithium exerted therapeutic effects in all manic symptom domains in these trials, including improvement in psychosis in patients with psychotic mania. The time course of response ranged between 5 and 14 days after treatment initiation (Keck and McElroy 2001), which often began at a subtherapeutic dose with subsequent upward titration.

Persuasive predictors of lithium response are lacking in acute mania. However, post hoc analysis of the Bowden et al. (1994) trial suggested that the patients with classic or euphoric mania (Bowden 1995), hyperactivity (Swann et al. 2002), and few lifetime mood episodes (Swann et al. 1999) had better responses to lithium compared with patients with mixed episodes and numerous (>10) lifetime mood episodes.

Lithium's antimanic efficacy appears to be positively correlated with plasma concentrations within the therapeutic range (0.6–1.2 mEq/L) (Stokes et al. 1971). The rate of lithium titration to mid- to high therapeutic plasma concentrations also may affect response. Goldberg et al. (1998) found a strong correlation between the rapidity with which therapeutic concentrations of antimanic mood-stabilizing agents (e.g., lithium, divalproex, carbamazepine) were achieved and onset of antimanic effect. In a pilot trial consistent with this observation, Keck et al. (2001) reported significant reduction in manic symptoms in 5 days when manic patients achieved therapeutic lithium concentrations within 24 hours, via administration of 20 mg/kg/day dosing. Side effects associated with acute lithium treatment include nausea, vomiting, diarrhea, tremor, somnolence, weight gain, and cognitive slowing (Dunner 2003).

Acute Bipolar Depressive Episodes

In eight of nine placebo-controlled trials, lithium was superior to placebo in the acute treatment of bipolar depression (reviewed in Zornberg and Pope 1993). Zornberg and Pope (1993) analyzed the magnitude of lithium response in five placebo-controlled studies, which quantified improvement sufficiently to distinguish partial from full antidepressant response. They found that 36% of the patients had an "unequivocal" response, whereas 79% had at least partial improvement. Because approximately two-thirds of the patients taking lithium for bipolar depression do not have a full antidepressant response, adjunctive use of antidepressants in bipolar depression is common.

Two studies examined the antidepressant efficacy of lithium in placebo-controlled trials of adjunctive treatment with paroxetine (Nemeroff et al. 2001; Young et al. 2000). Nemeroff et al. (2001) found no significant difference in antidepressant efficacy among patients receiving paroxetine, imipramine, and placebo who also had lithium concentrations greater than 0.8 mEq/L. However, paroxetine was superior to placebo in patients with lithium concentrations of 0.8 mEq/L or less. These findings have been interpreted to suggest that higher lithium concentrations were associated with better antidepressant response. In the second trial, Young et al. (2000) found comparable efficacy between the addition of paroxetine and the alternative mood stabilizer (lithium or divalproex) in patients with bipolar I disorder experiencing breakthrough depressive episodes while taking lithium or divalproex. This study was not adequately powered to detect significant differences in efficacy between treatment groups, however.

Maintenance Treatment

Lithium remains the most well-studied agent in the long-term prevention of mood episodes in patients with bipolar I disorder. Pooled data from randomized, placebo-controlled trials conducted primarily in the 1960s and 1970s showed that lithium reduced the risk of relapse fourfold compared with placebo at 6 months and 1 year (Keck et al. 2000). The recent Cochrane analysis (Burgess et al. 2003) of nine studies that included 825 patients randomized to lithium or placebo found lithium to be more effective than placebo in preventing overall bipolar relapse. Two recent 18-month placebo-controlled studies of lamotrigine maintenance treatment in bipolar type I patients that used lithium as an active comparator found that lithium was superior to placebo in preventing manic relapse (Bowden et al. 2001, 2003). However, only a small proportion of the patients were taking lithium alone by the end of the study. These findings are consistent with those of naturalistic studies that found that only about one-third of the patients maintained on lithium had sustained responses (Harrow et al. 1990; Maj et al. 1991; O'Connell et al. 1991; Tondo et al. 2001a). This limitation is not restricted to lithium because most patients with bipolar I and II disorders require combination therapy to prevent syndromal relapse and symptom, especially depressive symptom, recurrence (Grof 2003; Judd et al. 2003).

Unfortunately, very few studies have compared the maintenance efficacy of lithium in combination with other agents. Solomon et al. (1997) compared the efficacy of lithium monotherapy with the combination of lithium and divalproex over 1 year in 12 patients. Despite the small sample size in this pilot trial, the combination therapy group had significantly fewer relapses compared with the monotherapy group, although at the cost of more side effects.

In addition to its efficacy as a long-term mood stabilizer, lithium appears to reduce significantly the risk of suicide in patients with bipolar disorder apart from its palliative effects on mood symptoms (Baldessarini et al. 2003; Goodwin et al. 2003; Muller-Oerlinghausen 2001; Tondo et al. 2001b). In a naturalistic study, Goodwin et al. (2003) found significantly lower suicide attempts and deaths from suicide in patients receiving lithium compared with divalproex. Although an order effect may have contributed to these findings (patients not responsive to lithium subsequently were given divalproex), they are nevertheless consistent with results of large meta-analyses (Baldessarini et al. 2003; Tondo et al. 2001b) and post hoc analyses of large multicenter trials (Muller-Oerlinghausen 2001).

Because of its heritage as a long-term treatment of bipolar disorder in controlled and naturalistic studies, some predictors of response to lithium maintenance treatment have been identified. Rapid cycling; multiple prior mood episodes; negative family history of mood disorder; co-occurring anxiety, alcohol, or substance use disorders; and episode sequence of depression-mania-euthymia have negative prognostic significance to lithium treatment (Bowden 1995; Henry et al. 2003; Maj 2000; Sasson et al. 2003). In contrast, Grof et al. (2002) recently reported a strong association between unequivocal lithium response among family members with bipolar disorder.

Hopkins and Gelenberg (2000) reviewed studies that compared different serum lithium concentrations and long-term outcome in bipolar disorder and concluded that therapeutic maintenance concentrations normally should range from 0.6 to 1.0 mEq/L. Although some individuals may benefit from concentrations less than 0.6 mEq/L, most studies found that lower concentrations were associated with higher relapse rates. In a reanalysis of data from the pivotal Gelenberg et al. (1989) study that compared the efficacy of high (0.8–2.0 mEq/L) and low (0.4–0.6 mEq/L) therapeutic plasma concentration ranges, Perlis et al. (2002) found that abrupt decreases in lithium concentrations, even within the therapeutic range, were a more powerful predictor of relapse than assignment to the high or low concentration. Within the therapeutic range of 0.6–1.0 mEq/L, side effects are more likely at the higher end and may lead to poorer treatment adherence (Hopkins and Gelenberg 2000).

Valproate

Acute Manic and Mixed Episodes

Divalproex was the second agent (after lithium) to receive U.S. Food and Drug Administration (FDA) approval for the treatment of acute bipolar mania, based on its superior efficacy as monotherapy in two placebo-controlled, randomized trials (Bowden et al. 1994; Pope et al. 1991). These pivotal trials confirmed the promising findings of two earlier small, placebo-controlled studies (Brennan et al. 1984; Emrich et al. 1981). In other randomized, controlled trials in acute bipolar mania, divalproex or related formulations of valproic acid were comparable in efficacy

to lithium (Bowden et al. 1994; T.W. Freeman et al. 1992), haloperidol (McElroy et al. 1996), and olanzapine (Zajecka et al. 2002). As with most lithium-comparator studies, these trials were not powered to find significant differences in efficacy between agents but nevertheless showed consistent antimanic efficacy across studies. One active comparator trial of adequate power found olanzapine superior to divalproex in mean reduction of manic symptoms and in the proportion of patients in remission at the end of the 3-week trial (Tohen et al. 2002). Muller-Oerlinghausen et al. (2000) compared the combination of valproate and first-generation antipsychotics with placebo plus antipsychotic and found that patients receiving combination treatment needed significantly lower antipsychotic doses and had higher overall response rates.

As with lithium, preliminary data identify putative predictors of response to valproate in acute bipolar mania. The presence of prominent depressive symptoms during mania (T.W. Freeman et al. 1992; Swann et al. 1997), impulsivity and hyperactivity (Swann et al. 2002), and multiple prior mood episodes (>10) was more predictive of response to valproate compared with lithium in studies involving both agents. When divalproex was compared with first- (McElroy et al. 1996) and second-generation antipsychotics (Tohen et al. 2002; Zajecka et al. 2002), no significant differences in efficacy were found among the treatment groups in reduction of psychotic symptoms.

The therapeutic plasma concentrations for antimanic response to valproate range from 50 to 125 mg/L, with higher concentrations associated with greater degrees of improvement (Bowden et al. 1999; Hirschfeld et al. 2003; Zajecka et al. 2002). Plasma concentrations greater than 125 mg/L may be necessary for response in some patients but are associated with more frequent dose-related side effects (somnolence, nausea, vomiting, tremor). Several studies have reported that divalproex can be safely administered at a therapeutic starting dose of 20–30 mg/kg/day (Hirschfeld et al. 1999; Keck et al. 1993; Martinez et al. 1998; McElroy et al. 1993, 1996; Zajecka et al. 2002) and that this strategy may produce a more rapid onset of action (Hirschfeld et al. 2003). In addition to the dose-related side effects described earlier, other common side effects include weight gain and cognitive slowing. The enteric-coated and extended-release formulations of divalproex appear to be better tolerated than the valproic acid or sodium valproate formulations. However, the extended-release formulation requires a 20% dose adjustment upward to achieve plasma concentrations comparable to those of immediate-release agents. Rare adverse events associated with valproate formulations include hepatic failure, pancreatitis, and hyperammonemic encephalopathy in individuals with urea cycle disorders.

Acute Bipolar Depressive Episodes

The efficacy of divalproex in the treatment of acute bipolar depression has been examined in only one randomized, controlled trial (Sachs and Collins 2001). Although there were significant differences in favor of divalproex over placebo at several time points in this 8-week trial, there were no significant differences in reduction of depressive symptoms between divalproex and placebo at study end point. Clearly, further research needs to be done to determine whether divalproex has efficacy in acute bipolar depression.

Maintenance Treatment

A recent Cochrane review of studies of valproate maintenance treatment concluded that "the efficacy [in maintenance treatment of bipolar disorder] and acceptability of valproate compared with placebo and lithium cannot be made with any degree of confidence" (Macritchie et al. 2003, p. 1). This review was based primarily on the only randomized, placebo-controlled maintenance trial of divalproex in bipolar I disorder, a 1-year study that found no significant difference in the time to relapse into any mood episode among patients receiving divalproex, lithium, or placebo (Bowden et al. 2000). However, some unanticipated design problems influenced the results of this trial. Among patients who received divalproex during an open-label period prior to randomization, divalproex was superior to placebo in rate of early termination (29% vs. 50%) during the subsequent year due to any mood episode. These post hoc findings have clinical relevance in that they suggest that in patients who are stabilized on divalproex acutely, long-term maintenance treatment has greater efficacy than placebo.

The only other randomized, controlled trial of divalproex maintenance therapy in bipolar I disorder was a 47-week comparison with olanzapine (Tohen et al. 2003). Patients were randomly assigned to receive either agent as inpatients for the treatment of acute mania for an initial 3-week trial (Tohen et al. 2002). Patients who responded to either agent were then asked to continue taking the medication blind to its identity for an additional 44 weeks to determine the maintenance of antimanic efficacy following acute treatment. Patients receiving olanzapine had significantly greater improvement in manic symptoms compared with patients receiving divalproex for the first 15 weeks; thereafter, there were no significant differences in mean reduction of manic symptoms or in relapse rates (olanzapine, 45%; divalproex, 52%). At the end of the 47-week study period, only 15% of the patients in each treatment group remained in the trial, emphasizing the difficulty of monotherapy maintenance treatment. Patients receiving olanzapine experienced significantly greater weight gain (mean=3.4 kg) compared with patients receiving divalproex (mean=1.7 kg).

Two other open-label, randomized trials compared the effectiveness of valproate with lithium. Lambert and Venaud (1992) reported that the valpromide formulation (available in Europe) of valproate produced a 20% lower relapse rate compared with lithium over 18 months. Revicki et al. (1999) found comparable effectiveness and health care resource costs between lithium and divalproex over 1 year in patients initially treated with either agent for acute mania.

Analysis of plasma concentration data from the Bowden et al. (2000) 1-year maintenance trial suggested that the optimal therapeutic range was 75–100 mg/L (Keck et al. 2002) for most patients. However, interindividual differences in tolerability and efficacy indicate that titration to doses with minimal side effects that ameliorate subsyndromal symptoms is a useful clinical approach (Hirschfeld et al. 2002).

Carbamazepine and Oxcarbazepine

Acute Manic and Mixed Episodes

Although carbamazepine has been studied in several randomized, controlled trials in acute bipolar mania, most of the early studies of this agent were limited by small sample sizes or other design complications (Keck et al. 1992). Two recent placebo-controlled, parallel-group, monotherapy trials of the Equetro formulation of carbamazepine found significant efficacy for this agent over placebo (Weisler et al. 2004, 2005). These findings were consistent with those of the only other placebo-controlled study, a crossover trial by Ballenger and Post (1978). In other trials, carbamazepine was comparable to lithium (Lerer et al. 1987; Small et al. 1991) and chlorpromazine (Grossi et al. 1984; Okuma et al. 1979) but not valproate (Vasudev et al. 2000). Common side effects of carbamazepine reported in these trials included diplopia, blurred vision, ataxia, somnolence, fatigue, and nausea. Rash, hyponatremia, and mild leukopenia and thrombocytopenia are less common side effects associated with carbamazepine. Rare but serious adverse effects include agranulocytosis, aplastic anemia, thrombocytopenia, hepatic failure, pancreatitis, and exfoliative dermatitis.

Oxcarbazepine has some putative advantages over carbamazepine, including a lower rate of side effects and less hepatic enzyme induction (Emrich 1991). However, no well-designed studies of oxcarbazepine in the treatment of acute bipolar mania have been done. Two small active comparator trials were limited by the use of adjunctive antimanic agents (Emrich 1991; Muller and Stoll 1984). Thus, the use of oxcarbazepine in acute bipolar mania is based on assumptions of similarities in mechanism of action and efficacy with carbamazepine.

Acute Bipolar Depressive Episodes

Three small controlled trials examined the efficacy of carbamazepine in the treatment of acute bipolar and unipolar treatment-refractory depression (Kramlinger and Post 1989; Post et al. 1986; Small 1990). The response rates to carbamazepine in these trials ranged from 32% to 35%. Although these response rates are comparatively low, they may have clinical relevance given the treatment refractoriness of depressive symptoms in the patients involved. No randomized, controlled trials of oxcarbazepine in the treatment of acute bipolar depression have been done.

Maintenance Treatment

Many studies examined the efficacy of carbamazepine in the maintenance treatment of bipolar disorder but were limited by methodological drawbacks (Dardennes et al. 1995). Three recently reported trials compared carbamazepine with lithium. Denicoff et al. (1997) found no significant differences in relapse rates after 1 year between carbamazepine (37%) and lithium (31%). Greil et al. (1997) conducted an open-label, randomized 2.5-year study and found that lithium was superior to carbamazepine on several outcome measures. Patients with atypical symptoms responded better to carbamazepine than to lithium. Hartong et al. (2003) randomly assigned 94 patients with bipolar I disorder, who had not received lithium for more than 6 months of their lifetime, to carbamazepine or lithium and monitored relapse rates for up to 2 years. Significantly fewer patients receiving lithium relapsed (27%) compared with patients receiving carbamazepine (42%). However, significantly more patients receiving lithium dropped out of the study before 2 years. No data are available regarding serum concentration–treatment response relations for carbamazepine maintenance treatment.

No randomized, controlled trials of oxcarbazepine in the maintenance treatment of bipolar disorder have been done.

Other Antiepileptic Agents

Acute Manic and Mixed Episodes

Three novel antiepileptic agents—gabapentin, lamotrigine, and topiramate—have been studied in randomized, controlled trials of acute bipolar mania. Gabapentin did not provide significantly greater efficacy than placebo in two controlled trials (Frye et al. 2000; Pande et al. 2000). Similarly, topiramate was not superior to placebo in five controlled trials (Calabrese 2000). In three small studies, all with significant methodological limitations, lamotrigine was not superior to placebo in reduction of manic symptoms in two studies (Anand et al. 1999; Frye et al. 2000) but was comparable to lithium in an underpowered trial (Ichim et al. 2000).

Acute Bipolar Depressive Episodes

Among the new antiepileptic agents, only lamotrigine has been examined in randomized, controlled trials of acute bipolar depression (Bowden 2001; Calabrese et al. 1999; Frye et al. 2000). In the first study (Calabrese et al. 1999), 195 patients with bipolar I depression were randomized to 50 mg/day of lamotrigine, 200 mg/day of lamotrigine, or placebo for 7 weeks. The two lamotrigine groups had significantly greater reductions in depressive symptoms, as measured by the Montgomery-Åsberg Depression Rating Scale, compared with the placebo group. Mood-switching rates (3%–8%) were not significantly different among the three groups. In the second study, Bowden (2001) did not find significantly greater efficacy for lamotrigine over placebo in patients with bipolar I or bipolar II depression. However, lamotrigine was superior to placebo in patients with bipolar I depression in post hoc analysis. Frye et al. (2000) reported significantly greater efficacy for lamotrigine compared with placebo in improvement of depressive symptoms in a series of 6-week crossover trials in patients with treatment-refractory rapid-cycling bipolar I disorder.

Common side effects of lamotrigine in these studies included headache, nausea, infection, and xerostomia. The risk of rare but serious rash can be minimized by adhering to *Physicians' Desk Reference*–recommended lamotrigine titration rates, but patients should be warned of this risk and the need to report rash immediately.

Maintenance Treatment

Among the recent novel antiepileptic agents, only lamotrigine has been studied in the maintenance treatment of bipolar disorder. Two large placebo-controlled 18-month trials comparing lamotrigine (200–400 mg/day) with lithium (0.8–1.1 mEq/L) found lamotrigine, but not lithium, superior to placebo in preventing depressive relapse (Bowden et al. 2001, 2003). However, lithium, but not lamotrigine, was superior to placebo in preventing manic relapses. One obvious implication of these trials is that the combination of lithium and lamotrigine might be especially useful in preventing both types of mood episodes, although this has not yet been proven in prospective studies.

Calabrese et al. (2000) conducted one of the only maintenance studies specifically for patients with rapid-cycling bipolar I or II disorder; lamotrigine (mean dose=288 mg/day) was compared with placebo over 6 months. Overall, no significant difference in relapse prevention was seen between lamotrigine and placebo. However, a trend in favor of lamotrigine emerged in patients with bipolar II disorder.

Role of Lithium and Anticonvulsants in Other Areas

Major Depressive Disorder

Lithium

Lithium augmentation of unimodal antidepressants in the treatment of partially responsive major depressive disorder (MDD) has been one of the better-studied augmentation strategies in randomized, controlled trials (M.P. Freeman et al. 2004). M.P. Freeman et al. (2004) reviewed five placebo-controlled trials of lithium augmentation of tricyclics, monoamine oxidase inhibitors, trazodone, and serotonin reuptake inhibitors and found significant improvement in 56%–96% of the patients receiving lithium. The time course of onset of lithium augmentation, duration of subsequent maintenance treatment, and optimal serum lithium concentration for antidepressant augmentation remain unclear from these trials (Heit and Nemeroff 1998).

Valproate

No randomized, controlled trials of valproate in the treatment of MDD have been done.

Carbamazepine and Oxcarbazepine

Carbamazepine was examined in the treatment of MDD in three small randomized, controlled trials (Neumann et al. 1984; Post et al. 1986; Small 1990) that also included patients with bipolar depression. Pooled response rates in these trials were 35%, but many patients were refractory to treatment with unimodal antidepressants. No randomized, controlled trials of oxcarbazepine in the treatment of major depressive disorder have been reported.

Conclusion

Lithium, valproate, carbamazepine, and first- and second-generation antipsychotics all have established efficacy in the treatment of acute bipolar manic episodes. Lithium and olanzapine have demonstrated efficacy in the treatment of bipolar depressive episodes. More lim-ited data suggest that lamotrigine and carbamazepine also have efficacy in the treatment of acute bipolar depression. Lithium, olanzapine, and lamotrigine had efficacy in the maintenance treatment of bipolar disorder in at least two randomized, controlled trials. Data regarding the efficacy of valproate and carbamazepine in maintenance treatment are suggestive but limited. Thus, the data to date indicate that lithium and olanzapine have established efficacy in the treatment of acute manic and depressive episodes and in maintenance therapy and meet the most comprehensive definition of a mood stabilizer.

In practice and as studies have shown, many patients with bipolar disorder require combination therapy for all phases of the illness. All studies comparing combination antimanic agents with monotherapy found that combination therapy produced better overall acute response rates in mania. Combining antidepressants with mood stabilizers is often necessary in acute bipolar depression to bring about symptom remission, but with a risk of mood switching. Long-term maintenance treatment with mood stabilizer combinations is very common but not well studied. In the two studies available, combination therapy was superior to mood stabilizer monotherapy in relapse prevention but, not surprisingly, at the expense of more side effects.

Several clinical trials are under way or near completion to examine the efficacy of second-generation antipsychotics other than olanzapine in the treatment of acute bipolar depression and as maintenance therapy. The results of these studies should provide important evidence about how well these agents may fit the comprehensive definition of a mood stabilizer.

References

Anand A, Oren DA, Berman RM: Lamotrigine treatment of lithium failure in outpatient mania: a double-blind, placebo-controlled trial. Paper presented at the Third International Conference on Bipolar Disorder, Pittsburgh, PA, June 14, 1999

Baldessarini RJ, Tondo L, Hennen J: Lithium treatment and suicide risk in major affective disorders: update and new findings. J Clin Psychiatry 64 (suppl 5):44–52, 2003

Ballenger JC, Post RM: Therapeutic effects of carbamazepine in affective illness: a preliminary report. Commun Psychopharmacol 2:159–175, 1978

Berk M, Ichim L, Brook S: Olanzapine compared to lithium in mania: a double-blind randomized controlled trial. Int Clin Psychopharmacol 14:339–343, 1999

Bowden CL: Predictors of response to divalproex and lithium. J Clin Psychiatry 56 (suppl 2):25–30, 1995

Bowden CL: Novel treatments for bipolar disorder. Expert Opin Investig Drugs 10:661–671, 2001 [published erratum appears in 10:following 1205, 2001]

Bowden CL, Brugger AM, Swann AC, et al: Efficacy of divalproex versus lithium and placebo in the treatment of mania. JAMA 271:918–924, 1994

Bowden CL, Janicak PG, Orsulak P: Relation of serum valproate concentration to response in mania. Am J Psychiatry 153:765–770, 1999

Bowden CL, Calabrese JR, McElroy SL, et al: Efficacy of divalproex versus lithium and placebo in maintenance treatment of bipolar disorder. Arch Gen Psychiatry 57:481–489, 2000

Bowden CL, Calabrese JR, Sachs GS, for the Lamictal 605 Study Group: A placebo-controlled 18-month trial of lamotrigine and lithium maintenance treatment in recently depressed patients with bipolar I disorder. Paper presented at the 40th annual meeting of the American College of Neuropsychopharmacology, San Juan, PR, December 11, 2001

Bowden CL, Calabrese JR, Sachs GS, et al: A placebo-controlled 18-month trial of lamotrigine and lithium maintenance treatment in recently manic or hypomanic patients with bipolar I disorder. Arch Gen Psychiatry 60:392–400, 2003

Brennan MJW, Sandyk R, Borsook D: Use of sodium valproate in the management of affective disorders: basic and clinical aspects, in Anticonvulsants in Affective Disorders. Edited by Emrich HM, Okuma T, Muller AA. Amsterdam, The Netherlands, Excerpta Medica, 1984, pp 56–65

Burgess S, Geddes J, Hawton K, et al: Lithium for maintenance treatment of mood disorders (Cochrane Review), in The Cochrane Library, Issue 4. Chichester, UK, Wiley, 2003

Calabrese JR: A placebo-controlled trial of topiramate in acute mania. Paper presented at the European College of Neuropsychopharmacology Annual Meeting, Munich, Germany, September 22, 2000

Calabrese JR, Bowden CL, Sachs GS, et al: A double-blind placebo-controlled study of lamotrigine monotherapy in outpatients with bipolar I disorder. J Clin Psychiatry 60:79–88, 1999

Calabrese JR, Suppes T, Bowden CL, et al: A double-blind, placebo-controlled prophylaxis study of lamotrigine in rapid-cycling bipolar disorder. J Clin Psychiatry 61:841–850, 2000

Dardennes R, Even C, Bange F: Comparison of carbamazepine and lithium in the prophylaxis of bipolar disorders: a meta-analysis. Br J Psychiatry 166:375–381, 1995

Denicoff KC, Smith-Jackson EE, Disney ER, et al: Comparative prophylactic efficacy of lithium, carbamazepine, and the combination in bipolar disorder. J Clin Psychiatry 58:470–478, 1997

Dunner DL: Drug interactions of lithium and other antimanic/mood-stabilizing medications. J Clin Psychiatry 64 (suppl 5):38–43, 2003

Emrich HM: Studies of oxcarbazepine (Trileptal®) in acute mania. Int J Clin Psychopharmacol 5:83–88, 1991

Emrich HM, von Zerssen D, Kissling W: On a possible role of GABA in mania: therapeutic efficacy of sodium valproate, in GABA and Benzodiazepine Receptors. Edited by Costa E, Dicharia G, Gessa GL. New York, Raven, 1981, pp 287–296

Freeman MP, Wiegand C, Gelenberg AJ: Lithium, in The American Psychiatric Publishing Textbook of Psychopharmacology, 3rd Edition. Edited by Schatzberg AF, Nemeroff CB. Washington, DC, American Psychiatric Publishing, 2004, pp 547–565

Freeman TW, Clothier JL, Pazzaglia P, et al: A double-blind comparison of valproate and lithium in the treatment of acute mania. Am J Psychiatry 149:108–111, 1992

Frye MA, Ketter TA, Kimbrell TA, et al: A placebo-controlled study of lamotrigine and gabapentin monotherapy in refractory mood disorders. J Clin Psychopharmacol 20:607–614, 2000

Garfinkel PE, Stancer HC, Persad E: A comparison of haloperidol, lithium and their combination in the treatment of mania. J Affect Disord 2:279–288, 1980

Gelenberg AJ, Kane JM, Keller MB, et al: Comparison of standard and low serum lithium levels of lithium maintenance treatment of bipolar disorder. N Engl J Med 321:1489–1493, 1989

Goldberg JF, Garno JL, Leon AC, et al: Rapid titration of mood stabilizers predicts remission from mixed and pure mania in bipolar patients. J Clin Psychiatry 59:151–158, 1998

Goodwin FK, Murphy DL, Bunney WE Jr: Lithium carbonate treatment of depression and mania: a longitudinal double-blind study. Arch Gen Psychiatry 21:486–496, 1969

Goodwin FK, Fireman B, Simon GE, et al: Suicide risk in bipolar disorder during treatment with lithium and divalproex. JAMA 290:1467–1473, 2003

Greil W, Ludwig-Mayerhofer W, Erazo N: Lithium versus carbamazepine in the maintenance treatment of bipolar disorders—a randomised study. J Affect Disord 43:151–161, 1997

Grof P: Selecting effective long-term treatment for bipolar patients: monotherapy and combinations. J Clin Psychiatry 64 (suppl 5):53–61, 2003

Grof P, Duffy A, Cavazzoni P, et al: Is response to prophylactic lithium a familial trait? J Clin Psychiatry 63:942–947, 2002

Grossi E, Sacchetti E, Vita A: Carbamazepine versus chlorpromazine in mania: a double-blind trial, in Anticonvulsants in Affective Disorders. Edited by Emrich HM, Okuma T, Muller AA. Amsterdam, the Netherlands, Excerpta Medica, 1984, pp 177–187

Harrow M, Goldberg JF, Grossman LS, et al: Outcome in manic disorders: a naturalistic follow-up study. Arch Gen Psychiatry 47:665–671, 1990

Hartong EGTM, Moleman P, Hoogduin CAL, et al: Prophylactic efficacy of lithium versus carbamazepine in treatment-naïve bipolar patients. J Clin Psychiatry 64:144–151, 2003

Heit S, Nemeroff CG: Lithium augmentation of antidepressants in treatment-refractory depression. J Clin Psychiatry 59 (suppl 6):28–33, 1998

Henry C, Van den Bulke D, Bellivier F, et al: Anxiety disorders in 318 bipolar patients: prevalence and impact on illness severity and response to mood stabilizer. J Clin Psychiatry 64:331–335, 2003

Hirschfeld RMA, Allen MH, McEvoy JP, et al: Safety and tolerability of oral loading divalproex sodium in acutely manic bipolar patients. J Clin Psychiatry 60:815–818, 1999

Hirschfeld RMA, Bowden CL, Gitlin MJ, et al: Practice guideline for the treatment of patients with bipolar disorder (revision). Am J Psychiatry 159 (suppl):1–50, 2002

Hirschfeld RMA, Baker JD, Wozniak P, et al: The safety and early efficacy of oral-loaded divalproex versus standard titration divalproex, lithium, olanzapine, and placebo in the treatment of acute mania associated with bipolar disorder. J Clin Psychiatry 64:841–846, 2003

Hopkins HS, Gelenberg AJ: Serum lithium levels and the outcome of maintenance therapy of bipolar disorder. Bipolar Disord 2(3 pt 1):174–179, 2000

Ichim L, Berk M, Brook S: Lamotrigine compared with lithium in mania: a double-blind randomized controlled trial. Ann Clin Psychiatry 12:5–10, 2000

Johnson G, Gershon S, Burdock EI, et al: Comparative effects of lithium and chlorpromazine in the treatment of acute manic states. Br J Psychiatry 119:267–276, 1976

Judd LL, Schettler PJ, Akiskal HS, et al: Long-term symptomatic status of bipolar I vs. bipolar II disorder. Int J Neuropsychopharmacol 6:127–137, 2003

Keck PE Jr, McElroy SL: Definition, evaluation, and management of treatment refractory mania. Psychopharmacol Bull 35:130–148, 2001

Keck PE Jr, McElroy SL, Nemeroff CB: Anticonvulsants in the treatment of bipolar disorder. J Neuropsychiatry Clin Neurosci 4:395–405, 1992

Keck PE Jr, McElroy SL, Tugrul KC, et al: Valproate oral loading in the treatment of acute mania. J Clin Psychiatry 54:305–308, 1993

Keck PE Jr, Welge JA, Strakowski SM, et al: Placebo effect in randomized, controlled maintenance studies of patients with bipolar disorder. Biol Psychiatry 47:756–765, 2000

Keck PE Jr, Strakowski SM, Hawkins JM, et al: A pilot study of rapid lithium administration in the treatment of acute mania. Bipolar Disord 3:68–72, 2001

Keck PE Jr, Meinhold JM, Prihoda T, et al: Relation of serum valproate and lithium concentrations to efficacy and tolerability in maintenance therapy for bipolar disorder. Paper presented at the 41st annual meeting of the American College of Neuropsychopharmacology, San Juan, PR, December 8–12, 2002

Kramlinger KG, Post RM: The addition of lithium to carbamazepine. Arch Gen Psychiatry 46:794–800, 1989

Lambert PA, Venaud G: Comparative study of valpromide versus lithium as prophylactic treatment of affective disorders. Nervure J Psychiatrie 4:1–9, 1992

Lerer B, Moore N, Meyendorff E, et al: Carbamazepine versus lithium in mania: a double-blind study. J Clin Psychiatry 48:89–93, 1987

Macritchie KAN, Geddes JR, Scott J, et al: Valproic acid, valproate, and divalproex in the maintenance treatment of bipolar disorder (Cochrane Review), in The Cochrane Library, Issue 4. Chichester, UK, Wiley, 2003

Maggs R: Treatment of manic-depressive illness with lithium carbonate. Br J Psychiatry 109:56–65, 1963

Maj M: The impact of lithium prophylaxis on the course of bipolar disorder: a review of the research evidence. Bipolar Disord 2:93–101, 2000

Maj M, Pirozzi R, Kemali D: Long-term outcome of lithium prophylaxis in bipolar patients. Arch Gen Psychiatry 48:772–773, 1991

Martinez JM, Russell JM, Hirschfeld RMA: Tolerability of oral loading of divalproex in the treatment of acute mania. Depress Anxiety 7:83–86, 1998

McElroy SL, Keck PE Jr, Tugrul KC, et al: Valproate as a loading treatment in acute mania. Neuropsychobiology 27:146–149, 1993

McElroy SL, Keck PE Jr, Stanton SP, et al: A randomized comparison of divalproex oral loading versus haloperidol in the initial treatment of acute psychotic mania. J Clin Psychiatry 57:142–146, 1996

Muller AA, Stoll KD: Carbamazepine and oxcarbazepine in the treatment of manic episodes: studies in Germany, in Anticonvulsants in Affective Disorders. Edited by Emrich HM, Okuma T, Muller AA. Amsterdam, the Netherlands, Excerpta Medica, 1984, pp 134–147

Muller-Oerlinghausen B: Arguments for the specificity of the antisuicidal effect of lithium. Eur Arch Psychiatry Clin Neurosci 251 (suppl 2):72–75, 2001

Muller-Oerlinghausen B, Retzow A, Henn FA, et al: Valproate as an adjunct to neuroleptic medication for the treatment of acute episodes of mania: a prospective, randomized, double-blind, placebo-controlled, multicenter study. J Clin Psychopharmacol 20:195–203, 2000

Nemeroff CB, Evans DL, Gyulai L, et al: Double-blind, placebo-controlled comparison of imipramine and paroxetine in the treatment of bipolar depression. Am J Psychiatry 62:195–203, 2001

Neumann J, Seidel K, Wunderlich HP: Comparative studies of the effect of carbamazepine and trimipramine in depression, in Anticonvulsants in Affective Disorders. Edited by Emrich HM, Okuma T, Muller AA. Amsterdam, The Netherlands, Excerpta Medica, 1984, pp 160–166

O'Connell RA, Mayo JA, Flatow L: Outcome in bipolar disorder on long-term treatment with lithium. Br J Psychiatry 159:123–129, 1991

Okuma T, Inanaga K, Otsuki S, et al: Comparison of the antimanic efficacy of carbamazepine and chlorpromazine: a double-blind controlled study. Psychopharmacology 66:211–217, 1979

Pande AC, Crockatt JG, Janney CA, et al: Gabapentin in bipolar disorder: a placebo-controlled trial of adjunctive therapy. Bipolar Disord 2:249–255, 2000

Paulsson B: Quetiapine monotherapy for the treatment of bipolar mania. Paper presented at the Fifth International Conference on Bipolar Disorder, Pittsburgh, PA, June 12–14, 2003

Perlis RH, Sachs GS, Lafer B, et al: Effect of abrupt change from standard to low serum levels of lithium: a re-analysis of double-blind lithium maintenance data. Am J Psychiatry 159:1155–1159, 2002

Platman SR: A comparison of lithium carbonate and chlorpromazine in mania. Am J Psychiatry 127:351–353, 1970

Pope HG Jr, McElroy SL, Keck PE Jr, et al: Valproate in the treatment of acute mania: a placebo-controlled study. Arch Gen Psychiatry 48:62–68, 1991

Post RM, Uhde TW, Roy-Byrne PP: Antidepressant effects of carbamazepine. Am J Psychiatry 43:29–34, 1986

Prien RF, Caffey EM Jr, Klett CJ: Comparison of lithium carbonate and chlorpromazine in the treatment of mania: report of the Veterans Administration and National Institute of Mental Health Collaborative Study Group. Arch Gen Psychiatry 26:146–153, 1972

Revicki D, Hirschfeld RMA, Keck PE Jr: Cost-effectiveness of divalproex sodium vs. lithium in long-term therapy for bipolar disorder. Paper presented at the 43rd annual meeting of the American College of Neuropsychopharmacology, Waikoloa, HI, December 15, 1999

Sachs GS, Collins MC: A placebo-controlled trial of divalproex sodium in acute bipolar depression. Paper presented at the 40th annual meeting of the American College of Neuropsychopharmacology, San Juan, PR, December 12, 2001

Sasson Y, Chopra M, Harrari E, et al: Bipolar comorbidity: from diagnostic dilemmas to therapeutic challenge. Int J Neuropsychopharmacol 6:139–144, 2003

Schou M, Juel-Nielson M, Stromgren E, et al: The treatment of manic psychoses by administration of lithium salts. J Neurol Neurosurg Psychiatry 17:250–260, 1954

Segal J, Berk M, Brook S: Risperidone compared with both lithium and haloperidol in mania: a double-blind randomized, controlled trial. Clin Neuropharmacol 21:176–180, 1998

Shopsin B, Gershon S, Thompson H, et al: Psychoactive drugs in mania: a controlled comparison of lithium carbonate, chlorpromazine, and haloperidol. Arch Gen Psychiatry 32:34–42, 1975

Small JG: Anticonvulsants in affective disorders. Psychopharmacol Bull 26:25–36, 1990

Small JG, Klapper MH, Milstein V, et al: Carbamazepine compared with lithium in the treatment of mania. Arch Gen Psychiatry 48:915–921, 1991

Solomon DA, Ryan CE, Keitner GI: A pilot study of lithium carbonate plus divalproex sodium for the continuation and maintenance treatment of patients with bipolar I disorder. J Clin Psychiatry 58:95–99, 1997

Spring G, Schweid D, Gray C, et al: A double-blind comparison of lithium and chlorpromazine in the treatment of manic states. Am J Psychiatry 126:1306–1310, 1970

Stokes PE, Shamoian CA, Stoll PM, et al: Efficacy of lithium as acute treatment of manic-depressive illness. Lancet 1:1319–1325, 1971

Swann AC, Bowden CL, Morris D, et al: Depression during mania: treatment response to lithium or divalproex. Arch Gen Psychiatry 54:37–42, 1997

Swann AC, Bowden CL, Calabrese JR, et al: Differential effect of number of previous episodes of affective disorder on response to lithium or divalproex in mania. Am J Psychiatry 156:1264–1266, 1999

Swann AC, Bowden CL, Calabrese JR, et al: Pattern of response to divalproex, lithium, or placebo in four naturalistic subtypes of mania. Neuropsychopharmacology 26:530–536, 2002

Takahashi R, Sakuma A, Itoh K, et al: Comparison of efficacy of lithium carbonate and chlorpromazine in mania: report of collaborative study group on treatment of mania in Japan. Arch Gen Psychiatry 32:1310–1318, 1975

Tohen M, Baker RW, Altshuler LL, et al: Olanzapine versus divalproex in the treatment of acute mania. Am J Psychiatry 159:1011–1017, 2002 [published erratum appears in 162:102, 2005]

Tohen M, Ketter TA, Zarate CA Jr, et al: Olanzapine versus divalproex sodium for the treatment of acute mania and maintenance of remission: a 47-week study. Am J Psychiatry 160:1263–1271, 2003

Tondo L, Baldessarini RJ, Floris G: Long-term clinical effectiveness of lithium maintenance treatment in types I and II bipolar disorders. Br J Psychiatry 178 (suppl 41):184–190, 2001a

Tondo L, Hennen J, Baldessarini RJ: Lower suicide risk with long-term lithium treatment in major affective illness: a meta-analysis. Acta Psychiatr Scand 104:163–172, 2001b

Vasudev K, Goswami U, Kohli K: Carbamazepine and valproate monotherapy: feasibility, relative safety and efficacy, and therapeutic drug monitoring in manic disorders. Psychopharmacology 150:15–20, 2000

Weisler RH, Kalali AH, Ketter TA, et al: A multicenter, randomized, double-blind, placebo-controlled trial of extended-release carbamazepine capsules as monotherapy for bipolar disorder patients with manic or mixed episodes. J Clin Psychiatry 65:478–484, 2004

Weisler RH, Keck PE, Swann AC, et al: Extended-release carbamazepine capsules as monotherapy for acute mania in bipolar disorder: a multicenter, randomized, double-blind, placebo-controlled trial. J Clin Psychiatry 66:323–330, 2005

Young LT, Joffe RT, Robb JC, et al: Double-blind comparison of addition of a second mood stabilizer versus an antidepressant to an initial mood stabilizer for treatment of patients with bipolar depression. Am J Psychiatry 157:124–127, 2000

Zajecka JM, Weisler R, Sachs GS, et al: A comparison of the efficacy, safety, and tolerability of divalproex sodium and olanzapine in the treatment of bipolar disorder. J Clin Psychiatry 63:1148–1155, 2002

Zornberg GL, Pope HG Jr: Treatment of depression in bipolar disorder: new directions for research. J Clin Psychopharmacol 13:397–408, 1993

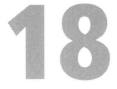

Antipsychotic Medications

STEPHEN M. STRAKOWSKI, M.D.
RICHARD C. SHELTON, M.D.

ALTHOUGH MOST ANTIPSYCHOTIC medications entered United States practice through U.S. Food and Drug Administration (FDA) approval for the treatment of schizophrenia (Table 18–1), these drugs are widely used in the management of other psychiatric disorders. In particular, antipsychotic medications are often prescribed as adjunctive therapies to treat psychotic symptoms in patients with mood disorders, although they are also widely administered to nonpsychotic patients with mood disorders. Moreover, newer antipsychotics are rapidly becoming first-line interventions in bipolar disorder. In this chapter, we review the role of antipsychotic medications in patients with mood disorders.

History and Discovery

The first antipsychotic, chlorpromazine, was identified essentially by chance. Chlorpromazine was synthesized as an antihistamine, but because of its sedating and anticholinergic properties, in 1952, the French physician Henri Laborit experimented with chlorpromazine as a preanesthetic (Laborit et al. 1952). He noticed that the drug

appeared to be calming in his surgical patients, an effect that was likened to a "chemical lobotomy," so he encouraged its use in psychiatric contexts (Lehmann and Ban 1997). Subsequently, the French physicians Delay and Deniker (1952) reported that chlorpromazine appeared to have efficacy for acute psychosis in schizophrenic and bipolar patients. These reports rapidly spread, and the drug became widely prescribed within 5 years after its discovery (Janicak et al. 2001). The efficacy of chlorpromazine for schizophrenia was firmly established by the U.S. Veterans Administration Study Group (J.F. Casey et al. 1960a, 1960b). Chlorpromazine provided a treatment for a group of patients who otherwise would have been simply chronically institutionalized with little hope of recovery; it therefore revolutionized the practice of psychiatry.

Because chlorpromazine is a phenothiazine, pharmaceutical companies began the search for chemically related drugs, which, by trial and error, also were identified as antipsychotics. In fact, clozapine, the first atypical antipsychotic, was identified in this way in 1959 (Baldessarini and Frankenburg 1991). This process of human trial-and-error testing is inefficient, so animal models were developed to identify antipsychotic compounds. Potential antipsychotics

TABLE 18–1. Commonly prescribed antipsychotic medications approved by the Food and Drug Administration for use in the United States

Classification and generic name	Brand name	Typical daily dose range (mg)
First-generation antipsychotics		
Low-potency agents		
Chlorpromazine	Thorazine	100–1,000
Thioridazine	Mellaril	50–800
Mesoridazine	Serentil	20–200
Moderate-potency agents		
Loxapine	Loxitane	20–100
Trifluoperazine	Stelazine	10–60
Perphenazine	Trilafon	8–60
High-potency agents		
Fluphenazine	Prolixin	5–30
Thiothixene	Navane	6–60
Haloperidol	Haldol	2–20
Pimozide	Orap	1–10
Second-generation antipsychotics		
Clozapine	Clozaril	100–900
Risperidone	Risperdal	1–8
Olanzapine	Zyprexa	5–30
Quetiapine	Seroquel	50–800
Ziprasidone	Geodon	40–160
Aripiprazole	Abilify	5–30

were identified if they caused specific motor responses (e.g., catalepsy) in animal models. These motor responses arise from the dopamine antagonist properties of antipsychotics in the basal ganglia. Consequently, the development of antipsychotic drugs was, for many years, specifically linked to the ability of the compounds to cause neuromotor effects in animals—namely, to act as neuroleptics. During the next 10 years, more than 20 antipsychotic compounds were identified, primarily phenothiazine derivatives (Lehmann and Ban 1997). Haloperidol also was serendipitously identified in 1958 as a by-product of research with meperidine (Lehmann and Ban 1997), and this expanded the search for new antipsychotic medications to include butyrophenone derivatives. Importantly, as a direct

result of the manner in which these drugs were identified, all of the antipsychotics developed before the mid-1980s (except clozapine) have neuromotor (extrapyramidal) side-effect liability.

Clozapine was the only pre-1985-developed compound that was observed to be an effective antipsychotic but not to produce the typical neuromotor effects in animal models. In fact, this lack of neuromotor effects probably contributed to the low use of clozapine after initially promising reports in the mid-1960s because clinicians were skeptical of its efficacy (Lehmann and Ban 1997). Additionally, the risk of clozapine's side effects, including hypotension, decreased seizure threshold, and agranulocytosis, further limited its use until the landmark study by Kane et al. (1988), which reported that clozapine was more efficacious in treatment-resistant schizophrenia than was chlorpromazine. Clozapine was subsequently made available for use in the United States (as Clozaril) and received FDA approval in 1990. Its success launched a widespread effort to identify similar nonneuroleptic antipsychotic compounds. This wave of investigation led to the development of the second-generation antipsychotic risperidone. The success of risperidone, which offered an effective antipsychotic with lower extrapyramidal symptoms (EPS) liability than conventional antipsychotics and which also lacked the risk of agranulocytosis of clozapine, encouraged the development of several other second-generation antipsychotic medications (Table 18–1). During the last decade, the advantages of these newer medications, particularly with regard to their low neuromotor side-effect liability, have resulted in their supplanting the older antipsychotics.

Classification and Mechanisms of Action

Antipsychotic medications have been loosely classified into two general categories. As noted, the older medications (except clozapine) are called *conventional* or *first-generation antipsychotics* and are the so-called neuroleptic agents. *Neuroleptic* literally means "to grab the neuron" and specifically refers to the propensity of first-generation antipsychotics to produce neurological side effects—namely, EPS and tardive dyskinesia (TD). These drugs are all dopamine type 2 (D_2) receptor antagonists with a relatively narrow therapeutic window between antipsychotic and neuroleptic effects. Newer antipsychotics are characterized by having fewer extrapyramidal effects at therapeutic doses and, thus, have consequently been called *atypical* or *second-generation antipsychotics*. Second- and first-generation antipsychotic medications also may be separated by different pharmacological properties, which produce differences in receptor binding and, potentially, efficacy and tolerability.

First-Generation Antipsychotics

The specific mechanisms of action of first-generation antipsychotics that produce clinical efficacy in mood disorders are not known. However, as noted, all of these drugs are potent dopamine D_2 receptor antagonists, and this property is thought to underlie the ability of these medications to alleviate psychosis. This dopamine hypothesis of antipsychotic action was first proposed by Carlsson and Lindqvist (1963) and verified by X-ray crystallography (Lehmann and Ban 1997). It is generally believed that the antipsychotic (and, likely, antimanic) effects of these drugs occur by blocking the action of dopamine originating from dopaminergic neurons in the ventral tegmentum that project into mesolimbic and frontal cortical areas (A10 system). In contrast, blocking postsynaptic dopamine D_2 receptors in the basal ganglia, released from neurons in the substantia nigra (the A9 system), produces EPS. Historically, the first-generation antipsychotics were further classified by their relative affinity for dopamine receptors into low-, moderate-, and high-potency agents (Table 18–1).

In general, the first-generation antipsychotics with high potency are relatively specific dopamine antagonists, whereas those with lower potency are less specific and show activity at other receptors, particularly muscarinic cholinergic receptors. Consequently, the dopaminergic potency of first-generation antipsychotics is, in general, inversely related to anticholinergic activity. Therefore, high-potency agents tend to have minimal anticholinergic risk, whereas low-potency agents commonly cause anticholinergic side effects. Because cholinergic activity is inversely related to dopaminergic activity in the basal ganglia, low-potency agents may be less likely to produce EPS. Additionally, cholinergic mechanisms have been suggested to underlie the expression of mood symptoms, although this has not been specifically confirmed, and anticholinergic medications have not proven to be effective antidepressant or mood-stabilizing agents. Some of the first-generation antipsychotics also show antagonist properties in noradrenergic and serotonergic neurotransmitter systems. Increasing synaptic serotonin and norepinephrine has been indirectly associated with antidepressants. Moreover, these neurotransmitter systems may be involved in the expression of mania (Goodwin and Jamison 1990). Therefore, noradrenergic and serotonergic actions of antipsychotic agents may have relevance for the treatment of mood disorders; this is discussed in more detail in the next subsection.

Second-Generation Antipsychotics

As with the first-generation antipsychotics, the specific mechanisms of action that contribute to the effects of second-generation antipsychotics on mood disorders are unknown. All of the second-generation antipsychotics, except aripiprazole, are also dopamine D_2 antagonists, which likely underlies their antipsychotic effects. However, what may truly separate first- and second-generation antipsychotics is a wider margin between medication doses that bind sufficient numbers of dopamine D_2 receptors to treat psychosis and doses that lead to EPS (Kapur and Seeman 2001; Kapur et al. 2000). Specifically, positron emission tomography (PET) studies suggest that psychosis improves when a drug blocks approximately 65% of striatal dopamine D_2 receptors. However, when approximately 80% of the receptors are blocked, the risk of EPS increases substantially (Strakowski 2003). This explains the neuroleptic side effects of conventional antipsychotics because the dosing margin between 65% and 80% dopamine blockade tends to be narrow (Kapur and Seeman 2001; Kapur et al. 2000). For example, for haloperidol, 65% occupancy occurs with doses as low as 2 mg, and 80% occupancy occurs at doses around 3 mg (Kapur et al. 2000). In contrast, second-generation antipsychotics appear to have a much wider dosing margin, between 65% and 80% dopamine receptor occupancy. For example, for risperidone, 65% occupancy occurs at approximately 2 mg, whereas 80% occupancy does not occur until doses higher than 8 mg. For some of the second-generation antipsychotics, such as quetiapine and clozapine, 80% occupancy does not occur with even very high therapeutic doses. Consequently, the EPS risk of these latter agents is at the level of placebo. This wider therapeutic dopamine D_2 binding window appears to most clearly separate first- and second-generation antipsychotics.

Aripiprazole has a novel mechanism of action that is unlike any other antipsychotic, leading some investigators to consider it a "third-generation" antipsychotic. Specifically, as noted, all other antipsychotics are dopamine D_2 receptor antagonists, whereas aripiprazole shows dopamine D_2 partial agonist properties (Strakowski et al. 2003). Therefore, in situations with high dopamine release, aripiprazole appears to function as an antagonist, whereas with low dopamine levels, it acts as an agonist. In addition to animal and cellular studies that support this mechanism of action, aripiprazole is a potent binder to the dopamine D_2 receptor, achieving more than 90% occupancy in PET studies, even with low therapeutic doses (e.g., 10 mg) (Yokoi et al. 2002). Nonetheless, it has a low propensity for EPS, consistent with its partial agonist effects.

Other pharmacological effects of second-generation antipsychotics also have been hypothesized to be associated with the lower propensity of these drugs to produce neuro-leptic side effects. Namely, these compounds are serotonin type 2 (5-HT$_2$) receptor antagonists, which has been hypothesized to decrease the risk for EPS in the presence of dopamine D$_2$ receptor blockade. However, the specific mechanism underlying this putative effect is not established.

Importantly, 5-HT$_2$ receptor antagonists have antidepressant properties, suggesting that second-generation antipsychotics may be antidepressant. Additionally, several of these agents show other pharmacological properties associated with antidepressants. Specifically, ziprasidone is a partial agonist at 5-HT$_{1A}$ and an antagonist at 5-HT$_{1D}$ receptors and is both a serotonin and a norepinephrine transporter inhibitor. Risperidone has α_2 antagonist properties, and aripiprazole is a partial agonist at the 5-HT$_{1A}$ receptor and a serotonin reuptake inhibitor. Therefore, the dopamine D$_2$ effects of second-generation antipsychotics may underlie their demonstrated antimanic effects (discussed later in this chapter under "Acute Mania and Mixed States"), whereas their 5-HT$_2$ and other serotonergic and noradrenergic effects may lead to antidepressant properties. Potentially, the combination of pharmacological properties present in these drugs may provide mood stabilization in bipolar patients, as well as new treatments for depressive disorders. Clinical studies supporting these hypothetical possibilities are reviewed later in this chapter (in the section "Acute Bipolar Depression").

Indications

Several antipsychotic medications are FDA approved for use in mood disorders. Olanzapine, risperidone, quetiapine, ziprasidone, aripiprazole, and chlorpromazine are approved for use in bipolar mania, and olanzapine and aripiprazole are approved for relapse prevention; olanzapine is also approved for bipolar depression (as a fluoxetine-olanzapine combination). Thioridazine was previously approved for the treatment of agitated depression, but recent changes in labeling, related to an increased appreciation of cardiotoxic side effects, now restrict thioridazine's use to treatment-resistant schizophrenia. Nonetheless, antipsychotics have been widely used outside specific FDA labeling in the treatment of mood disorders, both as adjunctive treatments and as monotherapies.

Bipolar Disorder

Acute Mania and Mixed States

Virtually every antipsychotic medication that has been systematically studied in manic and mixed bipolar patients has been shown to be an effective antimanic agent. Among the first-generation antipsychotics, chlorpromazine has been most widely studied in controlled clinical trials (Keck et al. 1998). In fact, Prien et al. (1972), in a large multisite study, reported that chlorpromazine was more effective than lithium for mania, particularly in highly agitated patients. However, in a meta-analysis of these studies, Janicak et al. (1988) found superior efficacy overall for lithium compared with first-generation antipsychotics. Nonetheless, it is likely that first-generation antipsychotic medications as a class are effective antimanic agents, and, in fact, they have been used for this purpose worldwide for more than 50 years.

Concerted research efforts in recent years into the efficacy of second-generation antipsychotics in bipolar disorder have established all of these compounds as effective antimanic agents. Each of the second-generation antipsychotics has been studied in large double-blind, placebo-controlled clinical trials that support their efficacy in acute mania (Table 18–2; Strakowski 2003). Additionally, olanzapine monotherapy was found to be significantly more efficacious than divalproex for the treatment of acute mania in one study (Tohen et al. 2002a). However, in a second study, although the numerical difference between the compounds' response was similar to that in the first study, a statistically significant difference was not observed (Zajecka et al. 2002). Several of these drugs, including risperidone, olanzapine, quetiapine, and ziprasidone, also have been shown to be effective augmentation agents or co-therapies when administered with classic mood stabilizers (i.e., lithium and divalproex; Table 18–2). Typically, these studies have suggested increased rapidity of response, and possibly greater overall response, with the combination of an antipsychotic and a mood stabilizer compared with lithium or divalproex alone. There is little doubt, then, that second-generation antipsychotics are effective acute antimanic agents. The combination of a second-generation mood stabilizer with lithium or divalproex appears to be associated with a faster and possibly greater clinical response (Strakowski 2003).

Second-generation antipsychotics, along with lithium and divalproex, are all reasonable first-line treatments of acute mania. Patients with acute mania often require medication doses at the higher end of the therapeutic ranges listed in Table 18–1. Specifically, olanzapine can be initiated at 15 mg/day. Risperidone can be initiated at 2 mg/day but then can be rapidly increased to 4–6 mg/day as needed over a couple of days. Quetiapine can be initiated at 100 mg/day and titrated by 100 mg/day to a target dosage of 400–600 mg/day. Similarly, ziprasidone should be initiated at 80 mg/day and then increased to 160 mg on day 2. Finally, aripiprazole can be initiated at 10–15 mg on the first day and then can be increased to 30 mg/day if necessary, although because of the partial agonist properties of this compound, the addi-

TABLE 18-2.   **Studies of the newer second-generation antipsychotics in the treatment of bipolar disorder**

Medication	Acute mania monotherapy	Acute mania add-on therapy	Acute depression	Relapse prevention
Risperidone	++	++	ND	ND
Olanzapine	++	+	+	++
Quetiapine	++	++	+	ND
Ziprasidone	++	+	ND	ND
Aripiprazole	++	ND	ND	++

Note. +=one double-blind, controlled study; ++=two or more double-blind, controlled studies; ND=not done or not yet reported.

Sources.   Bourin et al. 2003; Delbello et al. 2002; Hirschfeld et al. 2002; M.W. Jones and Huizar 2003; Keck et al. 2003b, 2003c; Khanna et al. 2003; Marcus et al. 2003; Price et al. 2003; Sachs et al. 2002a, 2002b; Tohen et al. 1999, 2000, 2002a, 2002b, 2003a, 2003b, 2003c, 2003d, 2003e; Yatham et al. 2003; Zajecka et al. 2002.

tional efficacy of increasing doses above 15 mg is unclear. In clinical trials of patients with schizophrenia, for example, little additional benefit was gained by increasing the aripiprazole dose from 15 to 30 mg/day. With all of the compounds, doses and titration schedules should be adjusted according to tolerability and clinical factors (e.g., age) that might affect tolerability (Strakowski 2003).

As noted, the combination of a second-generation antipsychotic plus lithium or divalproex appears to lead to a faster response. However, combining medications leads to different, and typically increased, side-effect risks than with either agent alone. Therefore, in a given patient, clinicians must balance the need for a more rapid treatment response with the likely increased risk of side effects. With our current state of knowledge, it is reasonable to treat acute mania with second-generation antipsychotics, lithium, or divalproex as monotherapy; to initiate a mood stabilizer or an antipsychotic and then to add the other class of medication (i.e., antipsychotic or mood stabilizer, respectively) if response to monotherapy is insufficient; or to start a second-generation antipsychotic and mood stabilizer simultaneously. This choice typically will be an individualized risk versus benefit decision based on specific patient factors (e.g., severity of symptoms or sensitivity to side effects). Regardless, the advent of second-generation antipsychotics has significantly enhanced treatment alternatives for acute mania and expanded possibilities for improving the lives of affected people.

Acute Bipolar Depression

Several outcome studies have found that bipolar patients will spend more time throughout their lives struggling with depressive than manic symptoms, yet treatments for bipolar depression are underdeveloped (Judd et al. 2002; Strakowski 2003; Strakowski et al. 2002, 2003). No controlled studies support the efficacy of first-generation antipsychotics in the

treatment of the depressed phase of bipolar disorder. Nonetheless, they were often used in this role, particularly to manage psychotic symptoms during bipolar depression (Keck et al. 1998). However, previous studies, albeit with significant limitations, have suggested that first-generation antipsychotics are ineffective in the treatment and prevention of bipolar depression and, potentially, may worsen the depressive course of bipolar disorder (Ahlfors et al. 1981; McElroy et al. 1996). Therefore, first-generation antipsychotics have a limited role in the treatment of bipolar depression.

The role of second-generation antipsychotics in the treatment of bipolar depression is also not as well defined as in bipolar mania. However, these compounds possess pharmacological properties that suggest that they may have antidepressant effects and have been found to improve depressive symptoms in schizophrenia better than first-generation agents (Keck et al. 2000b). Therefore, investigators have hypothesized for several years that second-generation antipsychotics may have thymoleptic properties in bipolar disorder. Although this remains speculative, recent investigations with olanzapine, quetiapine, and risperidone support the role of these medications in bipolar depression (Calabrese et al. 2004; Shelton et al. 2001; Tohen et al. 2003e).

These studies provide direct support for the efficacy of certain second-generation antipsychotics in the treatment of bipolar depression and also suggest that antipsychotic-antidepressant combinations may be of use in some patients. Given the pharmacology of the other second-generation antipsychotics, and their common efficacy for reducing depressive symptoms in schizophrenia, it seems likely that several, if not all, will prove to have antidepressant effects in bipolar disorder (Strakowski 2003).

Currently, then, second-generation antipsychotics appear to have a secondary role (to lithium and lamotrigine) in the treatment of acute bipolar depression. Nonetheless, the recent studies are promising and suggest that the role of second-generation antipsychotics may expand in the management of bipolar depression. Therefore, they represent a reasonable treatment alternative in patients who have failed to improve with first-line agents. Additionally, unlike antidepressants, second-generation antipsychotics would be unlikely to precipitate mania (because they are antimanic agents), so they may be safer than antidepressants in this regard.

Relapse Prevention

Bipolar disorder is a recurrent or chronic condition that requires extended therapy. Consequently, much of the treatment focus is to identify medications that prevent affective relapses. To date, only lithium, aripiprazole, olanzapine, and lamotrigine are FDA approved for relapse prevention, although other anticonvulsants (carbamazepine and divalproex) likely possess these properties as well (Strakowski et al. 2002, 2003). Conventional antipsychotics have been widely prescribed in the long-term maintenance therapy for bipolar disorder (Keck et al. 1998). However, first-generation antipsychotics have not been shown to be effective maintenance treatments (Keck et al. 2000a). In fact, as noted in the previous subsection, these drugs do not appear to prevent depressive relapses (Ahlfors et al. 1981), which are the most common affective symptoms during the course of bipolar illness in most patients. Given the long-term side-effect risks of first-generation antipsychotics (namely, TD and hyperprolactinemia) in the absence of demonstrated benefit, the role of first-generation antipsychotics in the long-term maintenance treatment of bipolar disorder is limited.

With their different pharmacological profiles and possible antidepressant effects, second-generation antipsychotics hold promise as bipolar maintenance therapies. This promise has been realized recently in several longer-term relapse prevention studies, primarily with olanzapine, but also with aripiprazole (Marcus et al. 2003; Tohen et al. 2003a, 2003d). Relapse prevention studies with other second-generation antipsychotics are currently under way but have not been completed. Again, it is likely that several of these other drugs will show relapse prevention properties. Therefore, long-term maintenance therapy with these other second-generation antipsychotics is a reasonable alternative to consider in patients who fail to respond to or cannot tolerate the first-line agents.

Major (Unipolar) Depression

Acute Depression

In general, the role of first-generation antipsychotics in the acute management of unipolar depression is rela-

tively limited. At times, conventional antipsychotics have been used as adjunctive therapy for patients with treatment-resistant depression, but this practice is not well supported by research and puts patients at risk for side effects such as EPS or TD (Thase 2002). In contrast, conventional antipsychotics do have an established role in the treatment of unipolar major depression with psychotic features. It has been shown that treatment response in psychotic depression is much better with the combination of a standard antidepressant and antipsychotic than with either the antidepressant or the antipsychotic alone (see Flores and Schatzberg, Chapter 34, in this volume).

In general, second-generation antipsychotics have replaced conventional antipsychotics as the treatments of choice in combination with an antidepressant (typically a selective serotonin reuptake inhibitor) for managing unipolar depression with psychotic features. Because the second-generation agents appear to have antidepressant properties, as noted earlier, investigators have studied whether these drugs are effective as monotherapy in psychotic depression. However, the data suggest that the combination of a second-generation antipsychotic and an antidepressant appears to be indicated over monotherapy with either agent for managing psychotic depression.

One question has been essentially unanswered: How long should antipsychotic therapy be maintained in the treatment of psychotic depression? Work by Rothschild and Duval (2003) suggests that most patients do not require long-term antipsychotic treatment past 4 months, which serves as a good benchmark for clinical practice. Additional studies of this area are needed to identify patients who require even shorter antipsychotic exposure, as well as those who may require longer-term combination treatment.

Because of the antidepressant effects of the second-generation antipsychotics in schizophrenia, several studies have also investigated the use of these agents in non-psychotic (particularly treatment-resistant) depression (Thase 2002). *Treatment-resistant depression* can be defined as failure to respond to at least two 6-week trials of antidepressant therapy at adequate doses with medications from two separate classes (Thase 2002). These studies suggest a potential role for atypical antipsychotics in this patient population (Ostroff and Nelson 1999; Shelton et al. 2001; Viner et al. 2003). Nonetheless, at this time, lithium is the best-established augmentation strategy in cases of antidepressant nonresponse or partial response, although second-generation antipsychotics also may begin to fill this role (Thase 2002). Additional studies are needed to clarify the value of second-generation antipsychotics in the management of acute unipolar depression.

Relapse Prevention

Long-term conventional antipsychotic therapy is generally not indicated in the relapse prevention of recurrent depression. The risk of adverse effects exceeds any putative benefit, which has not been seen with these agents, for most patients. Similarly, although second-generation antipsychotics have shown potential as long-term mood stabilizers in bipolar disorder, whether they are effective for preventing relapse in unipolar depression is not yet known. The potential benefits of these drugs in the long-term management of recurrent unipolar depression have not yet been shown to justify the known risks of long-term side effects (e.g., weight gain). However, in one 76-week open-label study of 560 patients with treatment-resistant depression, the combination of olanzapine plus fluoxetine was found to sustain a "robust" improvement in depressive symptoms with a relatively safe side-effect profile, similar to that of the individual drugs (Corya et al. 2003). Given the current thymoleptic properties of second-generation antipsychotics, these agents do have promise for relapse prevention of recurrent unipolar depression in at least some patients.

Adverse Effects

Antipsychotics are associated with numerous adverse effects, both as a class and for individual compounds. Although adverse effects are relatively common with most of these agents, these side effects tend to be mild, and most patients are able to tolerate one or more medications with minimal problems. In this section, we review the more common side effects associated with antipsychotic medications.

Extrapyramidal Symptoms

EPS appear to arise from the activity of dopamine antagonists in the basal ganglia of treated patients. Three major categories of EPS have been identified: parkinsonism, acute dystonias, and akathisia. Antipsychotic-induced parkinsonism resembles that produced by idiopathic Parkinson's disease and is characterized by pill-rolling resting tremor, masklike facies, psychomotor retardation, shuffling gait, and cogwheeling. A more subtle form also has been reported, which consists of emotional blunting and an inability to engage in social activity, which can be confused with depression (Janicak et al. 2001). Acute dystonias are sudden, involuntary muscular contractions that occur throughout the body, such as torticollis (contraction of neck muscles). Less common but potentially life-threatening dystonias involve contraction of multiple large muscle groups that produce posturing (oculogyric crisis and opisthotonos).

Laryngeal dystonias also can be life-threatening, leading to suffocation. Finally, akathisia is a sensation of internal restlessness accompanied by the inability to sit still. All of these EPS are uncomfortable, and the dystonias, specifically, can be quite dramatic and frightening.

EPS are a relatively common side effect of the first-generation antipsychotics, and EPS are more common as the potency of the agent increases. In contrast, the second-generation antipsychotics appear to be much less likely to induce EPS, secondary to the wider therapeutic margin between the antipsychotic and the neuroleptic properties of these drugs. In particular, both clozapine and quetiapine appear to have a very low risk for EPS. Risperidone, olanzapine, and ziprasidone have a dose-related risk of EPS, although in the typical therapeutic dose ranges listed in Table 18–1, this risk is relatively low. The newest antipsychotic, aripiprazole, also appears to have a relatively low risk of EPS, although its use has been associated with akathisia. However, because aripiprazole may have dopamine agonist properties, it is not entirely clear whether the restlessness reported in some patients is akathisia or a mild activation syndrome from the potential stimulant effects of this compound. Regardless, all of the second-generation antipsychotics are less likely to cause EPS than are the first-generation medications.

The most effective treatment for EPS is to lower the antipsychotic dose or to switch to an antipsychotic with a lower propensity for causing EPS. When this is not possible, pharmacological interventions can often manage these symptoms. Acute dystonias usually occur early in treatment and will typically improve rapidly with an antiparkinsonian agent, such as benztropin, procyclidine, or diphenhydramine. Parkinsonian side effects typically will respond to similar interventions. Akathisia tends to be more difficult to treat, but adding a β-blocker, a benzodiazepine, or an antiparkinsonian agent may help. Again, the best treatment for EPS is to attempt to lower the medication dose or switch to an alternative agent; adding a second medication to manage side effects introduces the risk of additional adverse effects.

Tardive Dyskinesia

TD is characterized by the development of abnormal, involuntary, repetitive movements that typically involve lip smacking, choreiform movements of the tongue, lateral jaw movements, or choreiform or athetoid movement of the limbs and trunk (Janicak et al. 2001). TD is usually mild, nonprogressive, and reversible, although in some patients, it can become disfiguring and uncomfortable. It generally occurs after long-term exposure to antipsychotic medications, although spontaneous dyskinetic movements have been observed in first-episode patients and were reported prior to the pharmacological era. Therefore, these spontaneous cases account for a small fraction of cases of TD. Studies with predominantly schizophrenic patients suggest that the risk for TD while taking first-generation antipsychotics is about 4% per year (Kane et al. 1992). However, this risk may be increased in patients with mood disorders.

The rate of TD with the second-generation antipsychotics is not known because there is a dearth of long-term studies. Nonetheless, it appears to be significantly lower than with the first-generation agents. For example, Beasley et al. (1999) followed up more than 600 patients with schizophrenia and found a 1-year incidence of TD in 0.5% of the patients receiving olanzapine compared with 7.5% of the patients receiving haloperidol.

The specific mechanism underlying the development of TD is not known; however, it is assumed to arise from a denervation hypersensitivity that occurs in the basal ganglia with long-term neuroleptic exposure (D.E. Casey 1996). Therefore, it is reasonable to assume that drugs that produce EPS (as a sign of significant basal ganglia dopamine D_2 receptor blockade) have a potential risk for producing TD. Consequently, the second-generation antipsychotics that carry a dose-dependent liability for EPS (risperidone, ziprasidone, and olanzapine) are likely to possess a risk for TD, even if given at lower rates than conventional agents. Drugs without this EPS risk (i.e., quetiapine and clozapine) may consequently have little or no risk for this adverse event. The risk of TD for a dopamine partial agonist such as aripiprazole is not known, but as noted earlier, its EPS liability appears to be low, suggesting a similarly low risk for TD.

The only known effective treatment for TD is to discontinue the neuroleptic agent thought to be responsible for its development. Importantly, TD may transiently worsen after discontinuing the causative neuroleptic because the continued dopamine receptor blockade, present when receiving the drug, masks some of the symptoms. With the offending agent gone, TD usually remits over time (often weeks). In some cases, TD may remit spontaneously even with continued antipsychotic treatment (Janicak et al. 2001); therefore, when discontinuing medication, a careful risk (continued TD) versus benefit (alleviation of psychosis) discussion with the patient should occur. An alternative to discontinuing the antipsychotic altogether is, of course, switching to another antipsychotic with a potentially lower risk for TD, such as clozapine or quetiapine, or another class of medication (e.g., lithium).

Neuroleptic Malignant Syndrome

Neuroleptic malignant syndrome (NMS) is a rare but potentially fatal adverse effect of neuroleptics. The symptoms of NMS include fever (often >104°F), muscle rigidity, autonomic instability (e.g., tachycardia, hypotension), and altered sensorium (Janicak et al. 2001). Creatine kinase levels are typically elevated and may be accompanied by an elevated white blood cell count. The risk of developing NMS from antipsychotics appears to be low (0.2%) and usually occurs early in treatment. Risk factors may include dehydration, agitation, and a mood disorder diagnosis, although with rare syndromes such as NMS, definitively establishing risk factors is difficult. Both first- and second-generation agents appear to impart a risk for NMS, although whether some are less likely to produce this condition is unknown.

The effective treatment of NMS involves rapid diagnosis, discontinuation of the offending antipsychotic, and aggressive supportive care. The syndrome appears to be related to the dopaminergic antagonist properties of antipsychotics, so that a dopaminergic agonist (e.g., bromocriptine) may be helpful. Additionally, dantrolene sodium, which inhibits contraction of skeletal muscles, also may be useful in reducing mortality (Caroff et al. 1998).

Subsequent treatment of a mood disorder in a patient who has developed NMS should focus on using medications other than antipsychotics whenever possible (e.g., lithium or anticonvulsants). However, if an antipsychotic is deemed necessary, switching to a different chemical family might be useful, and then the medication should be reintroduced very slowly (i.e., low dose, slow titration) with a high index of suspicion for recurrence and careful monitoring for symptoms of NMS. Some experts also recommend prescribing bromocriptine concomitantly for several weeks, with gradual tapering after that while watching closely for signs of NMS (Janicak et al. 2001), although the efficacy of this practice is not fully established.

Prolactin Effects

All of the first-generation antipsychotics increase serum prolactin levels. In contrast, with the second-generation medications, this problem occurs only with risperidone. Hyperprolactinemia is a consequence of antipsychotic antagonism of dopamine receptors in the tuberoinfundibular system. Although acute increases in serum prolactin levels are benign, longer-term (weeks to months) elevation is associated with sexual dysfunction (decreased libido, anorgasmia), infertility (amenorrhea, decreased sperm motility), galactorrhea, increased risk of breast cancer, and osteoporosis (Strakowski et al. 2003). In patients receiving a long-term first-generation antipsychotic or risperidone, it is probably prudent to monitor for these adverse effects.

Anticholinergic Effects

Several antipsychotic medications are likely to produce anticholinergic side effects. These result from blockade of muscarinic cholinergic receptors and include symptoms such as dry mouth, blurred vision, constipation, and urinary retention. The low-potency first-generation antipsychotics are the most likely to produce these side effects, and in these older medications, anticholinergic side-effect risk occurs approximately inversely to the dopaminergic potency of the drug. Of the second-generation antipsychotics, clozapine has significant anticholinergic effects. Of the newer antipsychotics, only olanzapine has any significant muscarinic receptor activity; nonetheless, the risk for anticholinergic side effects with this drug is relatively low. The best treatment for anticholinergic side effects is either to lower the dose of the offending antipsychotic or to switch to an alternative antipsychotic that lacks this risk.

Sedation

All antipsychotics can cause sedation. In some cases, sedation is a desired effect in patients who have insomnia or are agitated. The relative risk of sedation with the first-generation antipsychotics tends to be inversely related to the dopaminergic potency of the drug. Clozapine is the most sedating of the second-generation agents, followed by olanzapine and quetiapine (Strakowski et al. 2003). Aripiprazole is relatively nonsedating. Sedation is best managed by prescribing medications at bedtime, although some patients may need to switch to a less-sedating agent if this adverse effect does not resolve.

Cardiovascular Effects

Orthostatic hypotension is the most common cardiovascular adverse effect associated with antipsychotics (Janicak et al. 2001). Again, low-potency first-generation agents and clozapine are the most likely to produce this problem, which is primarily mediated through α-adrenergic blockade. Orthostatic hypotension also has been reported for the second-generation antipsychotics, particularly risperidone and quetiapine. In vulnerable populations, such as the elderly, slowing the dose titration and checking postural blood pressure can manage this side effect. Orthostatic hypotension is dose dependent, and most patients will rapidly accommodate. Treatment involves slowing the dose titration or switching to another antipsychotic agent.

Antipsychotics have been associated with sudden death, presumably from ventricular dysrhythmias. The meaning of this association has been difficult to determine; it is unclear whether this is a coincidental association; a real but very rare risk; or a risk secondary to the primary psychiatric conditions for which antipsychotics are prescribed (e.g., schizophrenia, bipolar disorder). As noted by Janicak et al. (2001): "Medical examiners should refrain from attributing sudden death to these drugs… until research clearly establishes a causal rather than coincidental link" (p. 167).

However, some antipsychotics have been linked with prolonged QTc intervals. Specifically, as noted earlier, thioridazine had its FDA-approved indication restricted to treatment-resistant schizophrenia because of its association with lengthening the QTc interval. The risk of an elongated QTc interval that exceeds 500 ms is the development of ventricular dysrhythmias, specifically torsades de pointes, which can be fatal. A similar risk may exist for mesoridazine, the active metabolite of thioridazine (Janicak et al. 2001). Thioridazine and mesoridazine are therefore contraindicated in patients with a history of cardiac dysrhythmias, in combination with other drugs that lengthen the QTc interval, or in combination with drugs that inhibit the antipsychotic's metabolism.

Ziprasidone use also has been associated with QTc elongation in some patients, although this risk is less than with thioridazine (Taylor 2003). To date, in clinical practice, ziprasidone has not been associated with an increased risk of cardiac dysrhythmias or sudden death. However, it is probably prudent to obtain a baseline and serial electrocardiograms when initiating this medication in patients with a history of cardiac conditions or electrolyte disturbances (Taylor 2003). Additionally, prescribing ziprasidone with other drugs that lengthen the QTc interval should be avoided (Taylor 2003).

Weight Gain

Most antipsychotic medications are associated with weight gain with extended use. For the first-generation agents, the risk of weight gain roughly inversely correlates with dopaminergic potency, so that, for example, chlorpromazine is much more likely to be associated with weight gain than is haloperidol. Weight gain has been among the most commonly expressed concerns with the second-generation agents. Clozapine appears to have the highest propensity for inducing weight gain (6–10 kg), although it is followed fairly closely by olanzapine (B. Jones et al. 2001; Kinon et al. 2001; Nasrallah 2003; Strakowski et al. 2002, 2003). Recent longer-term studies in patients with schizophrenia suggested that olanzapine is associated with mean weight increases of more than 6 kg, with increases of more than 12 kg in some studies during a single year (Strakowski et al. 2003). Similarly, in studies of patients with bipolar disorder, olanzapine showed weight gain risks similar to those reported in schizophrenia, suggesting that this is not a diagnostically specific effect. Significant weight gain with olanzapine (e.g., >7%) occurs in as many as 40% of the patients in studies, yet treatment discontinuation for weight gain is relatively uncommon. Quetiapine and risperidone are associated with modest risks of weight gain, averaging 2–3 kg over 12 months. Ziprasidone and aripiprazole appear to be relatively "weight neutral," even with longer-term treatment.

Overweight and obesity are significant health concerns in the United States in general because they are associated with metabolic and cardiovascular conditions (Nasrallah 2003). Moreover, because many mood disorders are often treated with a second-generation antipsychotic in combination with other drugs (e.g., divalproex, lithium), which also contribute significant weight gain liability, the likelihood of significant weight gain is magnified. The risks associated with overweight and obesity are significant enough to suggest that weight should be regularly monitored in patients receiving antipsychotics. With even relatively modest gains (e.g., 2–4 kg), it is prudent to introduce dietary, exercise, and other interventions to minimize this adverse effect.

Metabolic Disturbances

Several case reports have been filed linking antipsychotics, particularly second-generation agents, to metabolic disturbances. In particular, type 2 diabetes mellitus and hyperlipidemia have been reported. Most cases reported have involved clozapine, followed by olanzapine, risperidone, and quetiapine. However, these uncontrolled case series did not establish causality and were difficult to interpret. Studies from the prepharmacological era suggested that the prevalence of type 2 diabetes is greater in patients with psychotic and mood disorders at baseline than in the general population (Keck et al. 2003a). In a study of drug-naïve patients with first-episode schizophrenia, Ryan et al. (2003) found that 15% of the patients had abnormal glucose metabolism, which correlated with intra-abdominal obesity. Results from studies to determine the effects of antipsychotics on metabolic disorders have been mixed (Gianfrancesco et al. 2002; Koro et al. 2002a, 2002b; Lindenmayer et al. 2003; Sernyak et al. 2002); the specific liability of the second-generation antipsychotics for causing type 2 diabetes has not been fully defined.

As noted, whether the association between antipsychotics and metabolic disturbances is a direct medication effect on glucose metabolism or an indirect association with weight gain or other risk factors is not known. One approach for clarifying this problem is to examine prospectively the effects of antipsychotics on metabolic indicators. Additionally, the risk for metabolic abnormalities associated with antipsychotic use seems to be directly correlated with the relative weight gain propensity associated with each of the various antipsychotics. However, metabolic disturbances have been reported with a variety of antipsychotics and thus do not yet appear to be specific for any given drug. Nonetheless, these reports suggest that it is prudent to check baseline glucose, lipid, and cholesterol levels before prescribing antipsychotics. These levels should rechecked periodically, especially in patients who have gained weight or who present with any other symptoms of diabetes.

Idiosyncratic Effects

In addition to the side effects commonly associated with antipsychotics as a drug class, several of the medications have idiosyncratic side effects that warrant mention. Clozapine has a well-known risk for inducing agranulocytosis. In the United States, the risk of agranulocytosis after 1 year of treatment is slightly less than 1% (Alvir et al. 1993). Because of the clozapine monitoring system, the death rate associated with clozapine-induced agranulocytosis has decreased, but careful clinical monitoring, even with regular blood cell counts, is still necessary. Clozapine also has a greater risk for producing seizures than other antipsychotics, particularly at doses greater than 900 mg. Finally, paradoxically (given its anticholinergic effects), clozapine may produce a hypersalivation syndrome. This can be bothersome for patients but is otherwise benign.

Chlorpromazine can produce dermatological side effects. This medication increases the sensitivity of skin to sunlight, increasing the risk of sunburn as well as discoloration. Patients taking this medication should wear sunscreen when they are exposed to sun. Chlopromazine and thioridazine both have been associated with ocular side effects. Chlorpromazine use has been associated with developing lenticular and corneal opacities. Thioridazine at high doses (e.g., 800 mg/day) may cause retinitis pigmentosa. Both of these conditions require a high index of suspicion by the treating psychiatrist to identify and then refer to an ophthalmologist for verification. The best treatment in both cases is to switch to alternative therapies.

Drug Interactions

In general, antipsychotic medications do not affect the pharmacokinetics of other compounds. Antipsychotics are typically metabolized through the hepatic cytochrome

P450 enzyme system (especially 2D6 and 3A4), so other medications that affect these enzymes can alter antipsychotic medication serum levels. Consequently, selective serotonin reuptake inhibitors, which inhibit these enzymes, may increase antipsychotic levels, increasing the risk of antipsychotic-induced side effects. Drugs such as carbamazepine that induce these enzymes may decrease antipsychotic levels, with loss of clinical response.

In addition to pharmacokinetic interactions, antipsychotics may have pharmacodynamic interactions with other drugs. Typical pharmacodynamic drug interactions occur when the concomitant drug shares a side-effect liability similar to that of the antipsychotic. For example, combining a sedative with antipsychotics may lead to excessive drowsiness. Combining a second drug with weight gain liability with an antipsychotic may produce even greater weight gain than with either drug alone (Tohen et al. 2002b). Antipsychotics with potentially dangerous side effects (e.g., the agranulocytosis of clozapine or the QTc interval lengthening of thioridazine) should not be combined with other drugs that share these same risks. Monotherapy should be used whenever possible. However, in many patients, combination therapy is necessary and common. Combinations should therefore be based not only on careful efficacy considerations but also on tolerability profiles and potential shared adverse-effect risks (Strakowski et al. 2002, 2003).

Role of Plasma Concentrations

The utility of serum blood levels with antipsychotic therapy remains controversial (Janicak et al. 2001). To date, convincing evidence is lacking for the utility of blood levels for anything more than to verify treatment adherence. Titrating antipsychotic doses by therapeutic response balanced with tolerability remains the mainstay of administering antipsychotic medications.

Conclusion

Antipsychotic medications are commonly used in the treatment of mood disorders. Recent studies have suggested that the newer second-generation antipsychotics are first-line agents for the treatment of bipolar mania and may become first-line interventions for other phases of bipolar disorder as well (Strakowski 2003). These newer drugs also have promise in the treatment of depression, particularly when psychotic features are present. Antipsychotic use is associated with numerous adverse effects, which must be

carefully considered when adding these drugs to the treatment regimen of patients with mood disorders. Nonetheless, given the efficacy of these drugs for many patients, these adverse-effect risks can typically be balanced against the benefit these compounds provide. As research continues to refine the role of antipsychotic medication in patients with mood disorders, and as new antipsychotic compounds become available, these drugs likely will continue to gain a growing role in the management of mood disorders. Regardless, advances in antipsychotics in the past decade have significantly enhanced treatment options for patients with mood disorders.

References

Ahlfors UG, Baastrup PC, Dencker SJ, et al: Flupenthixol decanoate in recurrent manic-depressive illness: a comparison with lithium. Acta Psychiatr Scand 64:226–237, 1981

Alvir JM, Lieberman JA, Safferman AZ, et al: Clozapine-induced agranulocytosis: incidence and risk factors in the United States. N Engl J Med 329:162–167, 1993

Baldessarini RJ, Frankenburg FR: Clozapine: a novel antipsychotic agent. N Engl J Med 324:736–754, 1991

Beasley CM, Dellva MA, Tamura RN, et al: Randomised double-blind comparison of the incidence of tardive dyskinesia in patients with schizophrenia during long-term treatment with olanzapine or haloperidol. Br J Psychiatry 174:23–30, 1999

Bourin M, Auby P, Marcus RN, et al: Aripiprazole versus haloperidol for maintained treatment effect of acute mania. Paper presented at the 156th annual meeting of the American Psychiatric Association, San Francisco, CA, May 17–22, 2003

Calabrese J, McFadden W, McCoy R, et al: Double-blind placebo controlled study of quetiapine in bipolar depression. Paper presented at the 157th annual meeting of the American Psychiatric Association, New York, NY, May 1–6, 2004

Carlsson A, Lindqvist M: Effect of chlorpromazine or haloperidol on formation of 3-methoxytyramine and normetanephrine in mouse brain. Acta Pharmacol Toxicol (Copenh) 20:140–144, 1963

Caroff SN, Mann SC, Keck PE Jr: Specific treatment of the neuroleptic malignant syndrome. Biol Psychiatry 44:378–381, 1998

Casey DE: Extrapyramidal syndromes and new antipsychotic drugs: findings in patients and non-human primate models. Br J Psychiatry 168 (suppl 29):32–39, 1996

Casey JF, Bennet IF, Lindley CJ, et al: Drug therapy in schizophrenia: a controlled study of the relative effectiveness of chlorpromazine, promazine, phenobarbital and placebo. Arch Gen Psychiatry 2:210–220, 1960a

Casey JF, Lasky JJ, Klett CJ, et al: Treatment of schizophrenic reactions with phenothiazine derivatives. Am J Psychiatry 117:97–105, 1960b

Corya SA, Andersen SW, Detke HC, et al: Long-term antidepressant efficacy and safety of olanzapine/fluoxetine combination: a 76-week open label study. J Clin Psychiatry 64:1349–1356, 2003

Delay J, Deniker P: Le traitement des psychoses par une methode neurolytique derive de l'hibernotherapie. Congres des médecins alienists et neurologists de France, Luxembourg, July 1952, pp 497–502

Delbello MP, Schwiers ML, Rosenberg HL, et al: A double-blind, randomized, placebo-controlled study of quetiapine as adjunctive treatment for adolescent mania. J Am Acad Child Adolesc Psychiatry 41:1216–1223, 2002

Gianfrancesco FD, Grogg AL, Mahmoud RA, et al: Differential effects of risperidone, olanzapine, clozapine, and conventional antipsychotics on type 2 diabetes: findings from a large health plan database. J Clin Psychiatry 63:920–930, 2002

Goodwin FK, Jamison KR: Manic-Depressive Illness. London, Oxford University Press, 1990

Hirschfeld R, Keck PE, Karcher K, et al: Rapid antimanic effect of risperidone monotherapy: a 3-week multicenter, double-blind, placebo-controlled trial. Paper presented at the 41st annual meeting of the American College of Neuropsychopharmacology, San Juan, PR, December 8–12, 2002

Janicak PG, Bresnahan DB, Sharma R, et al: A comparison of thiothixene with chlorpromazine in the treatment of mania. Clin Psychopharmacol 8:33–37, 1988

Janicak PG, Davis JM, Preskorn SH, et al: Principles and Practice of Psychopharmacotherapy, 3rd Edition. Philadelphia, PA, Lippincott Williams & Wilkins, 2001, pp 73–192

Jones B, Basson BR, Walker DJ, et al: Weight change and atypical antipsychotic treatment in patients with schizophrenia. J Clin Psychiatry 62 (suppl 2):41–44, 2001

Jones MW, Huizar K: Quetiapine monotherapy for acute mania associated with bipolar disorder. Poster presented at the 156th annual meeting of the American Psychiatric Association, San Francisco, CA, May 17–22, 2003

Judd LL, Akiskal HS, Schettler PJ, et al: The long-term natural history of the weekly symptomatic status of bipolar I disorder. Arch Gen Psychiatry 59:530–537, 2002

Kane J, Honigfeld G, Singer J, et al: Clozapine for the treatment-resistant schizophrenic: a double-blind comparison with chlorpromazine. Arch Gen Psychiatry 45:789–796, 1988

Kane JM, Jeste DV, Barnes TRE, et al: Tardive Dyskinesia: A Task Force Report of the American Psychiatric Association. Washington, DC, American Psychiatric Press, 1992

Kapur S, Seeman P: Does fast dissociation from the dopamine d(2) receptor explain the action of atypical antipsychotics? A new hypothesis. Am J Psychiatry 158:360–369, 2001

Kapur S, Zipursky R, Jones C, et al: A positron emission tomography study of quetiapine in schizophrenia: a preliminary finding of an antipsychotic effect with only transiently high dopamine D2 receptor occupancy. Arch Gen Psychiatry 57:553–559, 2000

Keck PE Jr, McElroy SL, Strakowski SM: Anticonvulsants and antipsychotics in the treatment of bipolar disorder. J Clin Psychiatry 59:74–81, 1998

Keck PE Jr, McElroy SL, Strakowski SM, et al: Antipsychotics in the treatment of mood disorders and risk of tardive dyskinesia. J Clin Psychiatry 61 (suppl 4):33–38, 2000a

Keck PE Jr, Strakowski SM, McElroy SL: The efficacy of atypical antipsychotics in the treatment of depressive symptoms, hostility and suicidality in patients with schizophrenia. J Clin Psychiatry 61 (suppl 3):4–9, 2000b

Keck PE Jr, Buse JB, Dagogo-Jack S, et al: Managing metabolic concerns in patients with severe mental illness: a special report. Postgrad Med, Minneapolis, MN, McGraw-Hill, 2003a, pp 1–85

Keck PE Jr, Marcus R, Tourkodimitris S, et al: A placebo-controlled, double-blind study of the efficacy and safety of aripiprazole in patients with acute bipolar mania. Am J Psychiatry 160:1651–1658, 2003b

Keck PE Jr, Versiani M, Potkin S, et al: Ziprasidone in the treatment of acute bipolar mania: a three-week, placebo-controlled, double-blind, randomized trial. Am J Psychiatry 160:741–748, 2003c

Khanna S, Hirschfeld RMA, Karcher K, et al: Risperidone monotherapy in acute bipolar mania. Paper presented at the 156th annual meeting of the American Psychiatric Association, San Francisco, CA, May 17–22, 2003

Kinon BJ, Basson BR, Gilmore JA, et al: Long-term olanzapine treatment: weight change and weight-related health factors in schizophrenia. J Clin Psychiatry 62:92–100, 2001

Koro CE, Fedder DO, L'Italien GJ, et al: An assessment of the independent effects of olanzapine and risperidone exposure on the risk of hyperlipidemia in schizophrenic patients. Arch Gen Psychiatry 59:1021–1026, 2002a

Koro CE, Fedder DO, L'Italien GJ, et al: Assessment of independent effects of olanzapine and risperidone on risk of diabetes among patients with schizophrenia: population based nested case-control study. BMJ 325:243–247, 2002b

Laborit H, Huguenard P, Alluaume R: Un nouveau stabilisateur végétatif, le 4560 RP [A new vegetative stabilizer; 4560 RP]. Presse Med 60:206–208, 1952

Lehmann HE, Ban TA: The history of the psychopharmacology of schizophrenia. Can J Psychiatry 42:152–162, 1997

Lindenmayer JP, Czobor P, Volavka J, et al: Changes in glucose and cholesterol levels in patients with schizophrenia treated with typical or atypical antipsychotics. Am J Psychiatry 160:290–296, 2003

Marcus R, Carson W, McQuada R, et al: Long-term efficacy of aripiprazole in the maintenance treatment of bipolar disorder. Paper presented at the 42nd annual meeting of the American College of Neuropsychopharmacology, San Juan, PR, December 7–11, 2003

McElroy SL, Keck PE Jr, Strakowski SM: Mania, psychosis and antipsychotics. J Clin Psychiatry 57 (suppl 3):14–26, 1996

Nasrallah H: A review of the effect of atypical antipsychotics on weight. Psychoneuroendocrinology 28:83–96, 2003

Ostroff RB, Nelson CJ: Risperidone augmentation of selective serotonin reuptake inhibitors in major depression. J Clin Psychiatry 60:256–259, 1999

Price LH, Weisler RS, Loebel A, et al: Ziprasidone in adjunctive treatment of acute bipolar mania: randomized, double-blind, placebo-controlled trial. Paper presented at the 42nd annual meeting of the American College of Neuropsychopharmacology, San Juan, PR, December 7–11, 2003

Prien RF, Caffey EM, Klett CJ: Comparison of lithium carbonate and chlorpromazine in the treatment of mania: report of the Veterans Administration and National Institute of Mental Health Collaborative Study Group. Arch Gen Psychiatry 26:146–153, 1972

Rothschild AJ, Duval SE: How long should patients with psychotic depression stay on the antipsychotic medication? J Clin Psychiatry 64:390–396, 2003

Ryan MC, Collins P, Thakore JH: Impaired fasting glucose tolerance in first-episode, drug-naive patients with schizophrenia. Am J Psychiatry 160:284–289, 2003

Sachs GS, Grossman F, Ghaemi SN, et al: Combination of a mood stabilizer with risperidone or haloperidol for treatment of acute mania: a double-blind, placebo-controlled comparison of efficacy and safety. Am J Psychiatry 159:1146–1154, 2002a

Sachs G, Mullen J, Devine N, et al: Quetiapine versus placebo as an adjunct to mood stabilizer for the treatment of acute bipolar mania. Paper presented at the 3rd European Stanley Foundation Conference on Bipolar Disorder, Freiburg, Germany, September 12–14, 2002b

Sernyak MJ, Leslie DL, Alarcon RD, et al: Association of diabetes mellitus with use of atypical neuroleptics in the treatment of schizophrenia. Am J Psychiatry 159:561–566, 2002

Shelton RC, Addington S, Augenstein E, et al: Risperidone and paroxetine in bipolar disorder. Paper presented at the 154th annual meeting of the American Psychiatric Association, New Orleans, LA, May 5–10, 2001

Strakowski SM: Clinical update in bipolar disorders: second-generation antipsychotics in the maintenance therapy of bipolar disorder. Available at http://www.medscape.com/viewprogram/2496. Release date June 26, 2003

Strakowski SM, DelBello MP, Adler CM: Comparative efficacy and tolerability of drug treatments for bipolar disorder. CNS Drugs 15:701–708, 2002

Strakowski SM, Del Bello MP, Adler CM, et al: Atypical antipsychotics in the treatment of bipolar disorder. Expert Opin Pharmacother 4:751–760, 2003

Taylor D: Ziprasidone in the management of schizophrenia: the QT interval issue in context. CNS Drugs 17:423–430, 2003

Thase ME: What role do atypical antipsychotic drugs have in treatment-resistant depression? J Clin Psychiatry 63:95–103, 2002

Tohen M, Sanger TM, McElroy SL, et al: Olanzapine versus placebo in the treatment of acute mania. Olanzapine HGEH Study Group. Am J Psychiatry 156:702–709, 1999

Tohen M, Jacobs TG, Grundy SL, et al: Efficacy of olanzapine in acute bipolar mania: a double-blind, placebo-controlled study. Olanzapine HGGW Study Group. Arch Gen Psychiatry 57:841–849, 2000

Tohen M, Baker RW, Altshuler LL, et al: Olanzapine versus divalproex in the treatment of acute mania. Am J Psychiatry 159:1011–1017, 2002a

Tohen M, Chengappa KN, Suppes T, et al: Efficacy of olanzapine in combination with valproate or lithium in the treatment of mania in patients partially nonresponsive to valproate or lithium monotherapy. Arch Gen Psychiatry 59:62–69, 2002b

Tohen M, Bowden CL, Calabrese JR, et al: Olanzapine versus placebo for relapse prevention in bipolar disorder. Paper presented at the 156th annual meeting of the American Psychiatric Association, San Francisco, CA, May 17–22, 2003a

Tohen M, Goldberg JF, Gonzalez-Pinto Arrillaga AM, et al: A 12-week, double-blind comparison of olanzapine vs haloperidol in the treatment of acute mania. Arch Gen Psychiatry 60:1218–1226, 2003b

Tohen M, Ketter TA, Zarate CA, et al: Olanzapine versus divalproex sodium for the treatment of acute mania and maintenance of remission: a 47-week study. Am J Psychiatry 160:1263–1271, 2003c

Tohen M, Marnernos A, Bowden C, et al: Olanzapine versus lithium in relapse prevention in bipolar disorder. Paper presented at the 156th annual meeting of the American Psychiatric Association, San Francisco, CA, May 17–22, 2003d

Tohen M, Vieta E, Calabrese J, et al: Efficacy of olanzapine and olanzapine-fluoxetine combination in the treatment of bipolar I depression. Arch Gen Psychiatry 60:1079–1088, 2003e

Viner MW, Chen Y, Bakshi I, et al: Low-dose risperidone augmentation of antidepressants in nonpsychotic depressive disorders with suicidal ideation. J Clin Psychopharmacol 23:104–106, 2003

Yatham LN, Grossman F, Augustyns I, et al: Mood stabilizers plus risperidone or placebo in the treatment of acute mania: international, double-blind, randomized controlled trial. Br J Psychiatry 182:141–147, 2003

Yokoi F, Grunder G, Biziere K, et al: Dopamine D2 and D3 receptor occupancy in normal humans treated with the antipsychotic drug aripiprazole (OPC 14597): a study using positron emission tomography and [11C]raclopride. Neuropsychopharmacology 27:248–259, 2002

Zajecka JM, Weisler R, Sachs G, et al: A comparison of the efficacy, safety, and tolerability of divalproex sodium and olanzapine in the treatment of bipolar disorder. J Clin Psychiatry 63:1148–1155, 2002

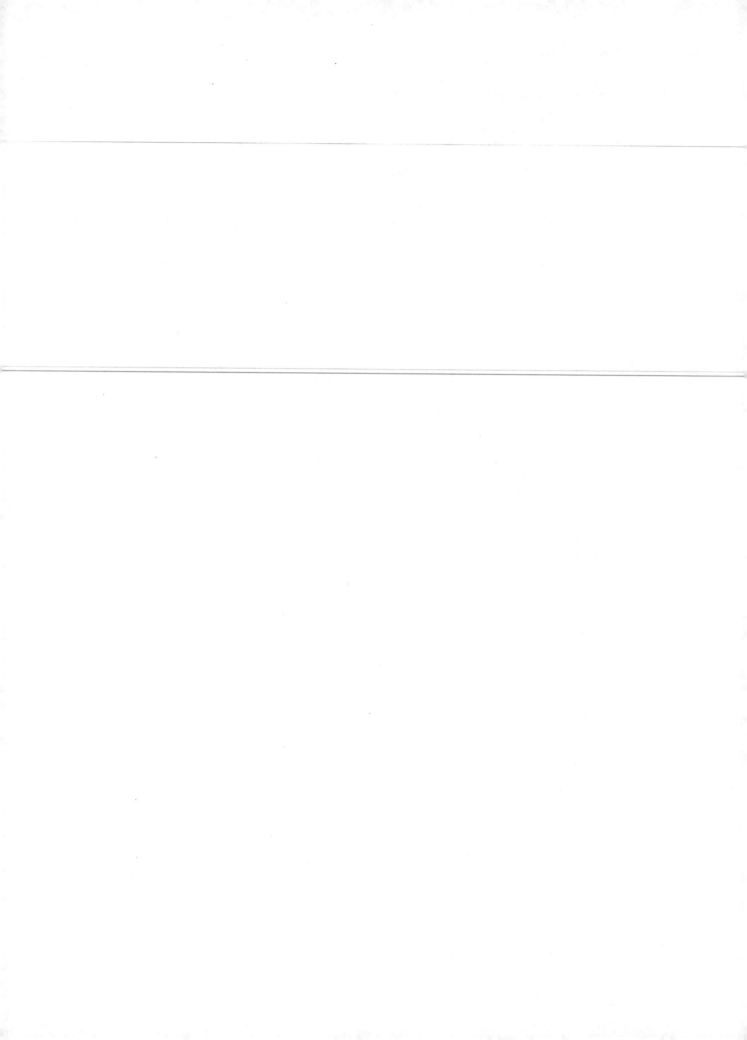

19

Targeting Peptide and Hormonal Systems

STUART N. SEIDMAN, M.D.

IN RECENT YEARS, psychotropic effects of gonadal steroids, corticosteroids, thyroid hormones, brain-secreted hormones (neurosteroids), and neuroregulatory peptides have been characterized. However, little systematic research has been done to study the application of these agents as therapeutic interventions. Although there is unequivocal support for the use of exogenous hormones in the setting of primary hormonal dysregulations (e.g., thyroid hormone replacement for hypothyroidism and testosterone replacement for male hypogonadism), hormones are not approved by the U.S. Food and Drug Administration (FDA) for any psychiatric conditions. Nonetheless, because hormones are psychotropic and because hormone-axis dysregulation is a frequent concomitant of mood disorders, it is reasonable to consider the therapeutic potential of these agents.

Accumulating evidence suggests the following: Antiglucocorticoids have psychotropic actions that have shown some therapeutic promise as antidepressant treatments; thyroid hormone may be an effective adjunct to antidepressant medication and, further, may accelerate the rate of antidepressant response; and gonadal steroids (i.e., testosterone in men and estrogen in women) may be

effective for some elderly depressed individuals. Taken together, these data suggest that exogenous hormone treatments may offer novel therapeutic opportunities in the treatment of mood disorders.

In this chapter, we explore the therapeutic promise of exogenous hormones. As an organizational and theoretical model, we approach hormonal interventions primarily with reference to the associated hormone axes and functional changes associated with mood disorders—in most cases, major depressive disorder (MDD). Although this organizational scheme uses the normally functioning hormone axes for context, this perspective does not exclude the possibility that hormones—which are undoubtedly psychotropic—can be effective pharmacological agents without reference to the normal or dysregulated functioning of their corresponding hormone axis.

History and Discovery

The recognition that hormones exert potent behavioral and emotional effects has a long history. For example,

The author thanks Donald F. Klein, M.D., and Anne Davis, M.D., for their comments on an earlier version of this manuscript and the Partnership for Gender-Specific Medicine and the National Institute of Mental Health for salary support.

castration has been a time-honored way of controlling the sexual and aggressive behavior of animals. In the now classic studies performed by Berthold in the mid-nineteenth century, implantation of testes into the abdominal cavity of castrated roosters was shown to restore the sexual, aggressive, and vocal behaviors that had disappeared following castration. He postulated that a blood-borne substance, acting on the brain, must be responsible. Modern endocrinological investigations have confirmed the role of hormones in the coordination of behavior with other physiological events in the body (e.g., sexual behavior with fertility, food seeking with the appropriate metabolic state). Recent research has explored the mechanism of hormonal influence on central nervous system (CNS) processes, such as cerebral blood flow, receptors, enzymes, cell membranes, and signal transduction. Increased interest in the application of hormones as psychotropic vehicles is primarily a result of the following observations: 1) in addition to being the regulator of hormonal systems, the brain is also a *target organ* of such agents—and activation leads to emotional and behavioral outcomes; 2) endocrinopathies commonly affect mood and behavior; and 3) mood disorders are associated with reversible hormonal dysregulations.

Mechanism of Action

The hypothalamus is situated in a critical location at the base of the brain: from this "primitive" region, it readily influences all signals that flow out into the periphery. The hypothalamus integrates disparate information about the internal and external milieu and, in turn, is the primary coordinator of mass-sustained organismic functions (e.g., osmolality, body temperature, circadian rhythms, appetite, libido, and motivational state, which may be experienced as mood) (Kasckow et al. 2003). The hormone axes are a critical component of hypothalamic-regulated homeostatic adaptations to the challenges of survival (e.g., response to life-threatening stimuli, reproduction). As such, hormones have potent and wide-ranging behavioral effects that are complemented by metabolic effects in the promotion of an adaptive response.

The accumulated evidence has shown a striking *context dependency* of the hormonal signal at the cellular level, in the historical environment (e.g., during critical periods of development), and in the present milieu (Rubinow et al. 2002). Much current research is directed toward the cellular level, such as the differential tissue response resulting from tissue-specific co-regulator proteins with which the hormone interacts, and the genetic polymor-

phisms that affect response. It is likely that the context dependency of the CNS response to hormones allows for a subtle influence of hormones on behavior, emotion, and cognition.

The two general classes of hormones are 1) proteins (including polypeptides and glycoproteins) and 2) steroids (including steroidlike compounds) (see Table 19–1). Highly differentiated glandular cells secrete hormones into the bloodstream, and these messengers then travel to adjacent or distant targets. Secretion is stimulated by the action of a neurohormone, which is a secretory product of a hypothalamic neuroendocrine transducer cell. The concentration of hormones is typically very small, and discrete mechanisms have developed to facilitate their actions. Hormones act via activation of specific membrane-bound, intracellular, or nuclear receptors, which trigger tissue-specific changes in functional activity of the target cell.

The same hormone can have different effects by acting at different sites (i.e., they are pleiotropic). This makes hormones especially well suited for modulating complex behaviors and for integrating such behaviors with a metabolic state. To do this, they must interact with the CNS in ways separate from those that serve merely a self-regulatory function (i.e., negative feedback). In addition, it should be remembered that hormonal effects are generally tonic and diffuse, setting the "gain" on a system, and they have a much longer duration of action than do neurotransmitters. This allows for more subtle influence on integrated behavioral responses. It is in this context, with the brain as an organ that is *targeted* by hormones to promote adaptive behavior, that exogenous hormone treatment derives its greatest therapeutic potential.

Hormones directly affect the CNS through at least three mechanisms:

1. *Hormones as direct neurotransmitters.* This is the likely mechanism of action of hypothalamic peptides, which bind to membrane receptors and modulate the production of second messengers such as inositol triphosphate, diacylglycerol, and cyclic adenosine monophosphate (cAMP). Second messengers activate protein kinase enzymes, which play a central role in protein phosphorylation.

2. *Hormones as neuromodulators.* Through intranuclear receptor binding, hormones modulate genomic expression and thereby regulate protein synthesis of synthetic and metabolic enzymes for neurotransmitters, neuropeptides, neurotransmitter transporters, receptors, growth factors, and signal transduction proteins. Neurotransmission can be influenced by hormones at multiple levels: neurotransmitter synthesis and stor-

age, presynaptic receptor activation, enzymatic neurotransmitter inactivation and reuptake, postsynaptic receptor concentration and binding, and membrane microviscosity.

3. *Hormones as neurotrophic factors.* Peptides such as thyrotropin-releasing hormone (TRH) and corticotropin influence cerebral cortex neuronal maturation and axon growth in vitro. Sex steroids and thyroid hormone influence the axoplasmic transport mechanisms that maintain neuronal structure and function. These are particularly important during critical developmental periods that involve structural changes of neurons and their connections, so-called organizational effects.

Classification and Physiology

The relation between hormone-axis physiology and psychiatric symptoms and syndromes is complex and bidirectional. Endocrinopathies are frequently associated with state-dependent psychiatric symptoms: male hypogonadism with loss of libido, low mood, and low energy; hypothyroidism with depression and cognitive dysfunction; hyperthyroidism with anxiety, irritability, and psychomotor agitation; acromegaly with hypersomnia and loss of libido; Cushing's syndrome and Addison's disease with dysphoric mood; hypercortisolemia with euphoria and psychosis; and hyperprolactinemia with low libido. Psychoendocrine investigators have found hormonal dysregulations associated with psychiatric conditions, particularly the hypothalamic-pituitary-adrenal (HPA) and hypothalamic-pituitary-thyroid (HPT) axes in mood disorders. A comprehensive review of the relation between endocrine physiology and mood disorders is beyond the scope of this chapter (see Seidman, Chapter 7, in this volume). In this chapter, we focus on hormonal interventions with therapeutic promise.

Hypothalamic-Pituitary-Adrenal Axis Antidepressants

Antiglucocorticoids

The antiglucocorticoid agents studied in the treatment of depression include both cortisol synthesis inhibitors (aminoglutethimide, ketoconazole, and metyrapone) and corticosteroid receptor antagonists (mifepristone and ketoconazole). Aminoglutethimide is used to reduce the hypercortisolism of Cushing's syndrome and in the treatment of estrogen-dependent breast cancers. Ketoconazole at low doses is primarily used as an antifungal drug, but at higher doses, it is a potent antiglucocorticoid and has been shown to be safe and effective for treating Cushing's syndrome and prostate cancer. Metyrapone has been frequently used in augmentation for nonresponsive Cushing's syndrome cases treated with aminoglutethimide and as a diagnostic challenge test for adrenal insufficiency. Mifepristone, a potent glucocorticoid receptor antagonist and progesterone receptor antagonist, is used primarily as an abortifacient but has some efficacy in the treatment of hormone-dependent tumors and disorders of the female reproductive system.

Multiple case reports have suggested an association between the administration of antiglucocorticoid medication and depressive remission, particularly in the setting of medication-resistant psychosis and atypical features. Murphy (1997) treated 20 treatment-resistant patients who had MDD with hypercortisolism and no history of Cushing's syndrome. A 50% reduction in Hamilton Rating Scale for Depression (Ham-D) score was used to define response; a 65% intent-to-treat response rate was seen in an 8-week trial of antiglucocorticoid treatment (together with hydrocortisone replacement throughout to avoid hypoadrenalism). Thakore and Dinan (1995) administered ketoconazole for 4 weeks to eight patients with MDD; five (63%) met response criteria. Finally, Brown et al. (2001) administered ketoconazole (up to 800 mg/day) as an add-on therapy to six depressed patients who had a diagnosis of treatment-resistant bipolar disorder. The three patients who received a dose of at least 400 mg/day had substantial reductions in depressive symptoms and no development of manic symptoms; cortisol levels were not lowered in any of the subjects.

Few placebo-controlled studies of antiglucocorticoids for MDD have been performed. Wolkowitz et al. (1999a) administered ketoconazole or placebo to 20 patients with MDD in a 4-week double-blind clinical trial. Thirteen of the 20 patients had been resistant to antidepressant treatment, and 8 had hypercortisolemia. Overall, responses were similar in the ketoconazole and the placebo groups, but in the 3 hypercortisolemic patients who had received ketoconazole, significant improvement in depressive symptoms was evident compared with the 5 hypercortisolemic patients who had received placebo (Wolkowitz et al. 1999a). Study limitations were the short trial duration and that only 3 of the 8 patients who were hypercortisolemic had received ketoconazole. Malison et al. (1999) administered ketoconazole (600–1,200 mg/day) or placebo to 16 patients with treatment-refractory MDD in a 6-week double-blind, placebo-controlled trial. None of the 8 patients assigned to placebo and 2 of the 8 patients

TABLE 19–1. Classification of hormones

Structure	Storage	Lipid soluble	Primary mechanism
Protein	Vesicles	No	Binding to membrane-bound receptors
Steroids	Diffusion after synthesis	Yes	Binding to intracellular receptor, leading to changes in DNA transcription

assigned to ketoconazole met response criteria, and the mean change in Ham-D scores did not differ between the groups. Finally, data collected by Jahn and colleagues (2004) suggest that metyrapone administered along with a serotonergic antidepressant can accelerate antidepressant response.

Overall, in a review of 11 trials (including both open and controlled studies) of antiglucocorticoid treatments for MDD, Wolkowitz and Reus (1999) reported "some degree of antidepressant response" in 67%–77% of the patients. However, because of the small sample sizes, lack of placebo controls, and heterogeneity of the populations studied, such data must be interpreted cautiously. Further, even though these studies reported few clinically significant side effects (e.g., transient light-headedness, headache, nausea or stomach cramps, and metabolic changes in 15%–20% of the patients), antiglucocorticoid treatments can cause serious hepatotoxicity and hypoadrenalism and require careful monitoring. Currently, this treatment should be considered experimental.

Corticotropin-Releasing Hormone Receptor Antagonists

The corticotropin-releasing hormone (CRH) receptor is a seven-transmembrane protein that is coupled to G proteins and linked to cAMP production. Type 1 and 2 receptors differ in structure, pharmacology, and regulatory responses. Primarily on the basis of the work of three research groups (led by Gold [1995], Holsboer [2003], and Nemeroff [2002]) that have intensively tested the hypothesis that HPA axis hyperactivity of MDD is driven by CRH hypersecretion, there has been a major effort to develop CRH receptor antagonist therapy. The most progress has been made with the CRH_1 receptor antagonist R121919, which penetrates the blood-brain barrier and occupies the CRH_1 receptor in a dose-dependent manner. In the largest published trial to date, escalating doses of R121919 (5–40 mg and 40–80 mg) were given to 27 patients with MDD. No serious side effects were noted, normal HPA axis function was not impaired, and anxiety and depression were reduced according to both patient and clinician ratings (Held et al. 2004; Kunzel et

al. 2003; Zobel et al. 2000). Nonetheless, lack of a placebo control limits interpretation of these data.

Dehydroepiandrosterone

Determining the effect of DHEA on mood has been hampered by methodological difficulties (Cameron and Braunstein 2005). In nondepressed patients, some data support a mood-enhancing effect of DHEA replacement in women with adrenal insufficiency and in HIV-positive men (Arlt et al. 1999), but placebo-controlled data are limited. Similarly, systematically collected data assessing the effects of DHEA in patients with MDD are scarce. Wolkowitz et al. (1997) administered physiologic doses of DHEA to six elderly men and women with MDD and low levels of the DHEA metabolite DHEA sulfate (DHEA[S]). Mood and aspects of memory improved significantly, and, moreover, such improvements were correlated with DHEA(S) and DHEA(S):cortisol ratio. In a follow-up study, 12 men and 10 women with MDD (all but 7 on antidepressant medication) were randomly assigned to receive DHEA or placebo for 6 weeks. Mean Ham-D score decreased 30.5% in the DHEA-treated subjects and 5.3% in the placebo-treated subjects; 5 of 11 DHEA-treated subjects were considered treatment responders, compared with none of 11 placebo-treated subjects (Wolkowitz et al. 1999b). Finally, in the largest such study, Schmidt et al. (2005) randomly assigned 23 men and 23 women with midlife-onset major or minor depression to receive 6 weeks of DHEA (3 weeks low dose and 3 weeks high dose) or placebo followed by 6 weeks of the alternative intervention. Depression scores (Ham-D and Center for Epidemiologic Studies Depression Scale) were significantly improved during DHEA treatment compared with both baseline and placebo conditions ($P<0.01$). Overall, these data provide tentative support for the antidepressant efficacy of DHEA, but more systematically collected data are needed before this treatment can be recommended.

DHEA replacement is generally well tolerated and not associated with significant changes on physical examination or in hepatic, thyroid, hematological, or prostatic function. Relatively common side effects include acne, oily skin, nasal congestion, and headache. Less commonly reported side effects include insomnia, overactivation (including disinhibition, aggression, and mania), hirsutism, increased body odor, itching, irregular menstrual cycles, and voice deepening.

Hypothalamic-Pituitary-Thyroid Axis Antidepressants and Mood Stabilizers

Thyroid supplementation as an adjunct to antidepressant medication appears to 1) improve response rate if given at the time of antidepressant medication initiation (Altshuler et al. 2001), 2) convert about 25% of treatment-resistant patients to responders (Joffe 1997), and 3) help stabilize rapid-cycling or refractory bipolar patients (Whybrow et al. 1992). The mechanism underlying these therapeutic effects is unknown, but it has been proposed that they may be due to the development of CNS hypothyroidism in the context of systemic euthyroidism or to thyroid-mediated changes in the net activity of neurotransmitters involved in the pathophysiology of depression (Halbreich 1997). Furthermore, it has been proposed that triiodothyronine (T_3) may be particularly effective because elevated cortisol levels in depressed patients could impair the intracerebral conversion of thyroxine (T_4) to T_3; exogenous T_3 would then restore CNS thyroid hormone homeostasis (Rubin 1989).

Augmentation of Inadequate Response to Antidepressant Therapy

The use of thyroid hormones in the treatment of depression was first reported in 1958 (Wilson et al. 1970). Thyroid hormones do not appear to be adequate antidepressants on their own and can cause intolerable thyrotoxicity. The accumulated literature suggests that T_3 (25–50 µg) is an effective augmentation agent in one-fourth of the depressed patients who have a suboptimal response to a tricyclic antidepressant (TCA).

Two reports have been particularly influential in guiding thyroid augmentation strategies. In the first, Joffe et al. (1993) compared augmentation with a 2-week course of T_3, lithium, or placebo in 50 patients who had TCA-resistant unipolar MDD. Response (defined as >50% Ham-D score reduction and final Ham-D score <10) rates to T_3 (10 of 17; 59%) and lithium (9 of 17; 53%) were indistinguishable from each other, and both treatments were superior to placebo (3 of 16; 19%). The second study was a meta-analysis that included eight placebo-controlled clinical trials (N=292) of T_3 augmentation to TCA nonresponders published from 1966

through mid-1995 (Aronson et al. 1996). Patients who received T_3 augmentation were twice as likely to respond as were those who received placebo (relative response=2.09; 95% confidence interval [CI]=1.31–3.32; P=0.002), and improvements in Ham-D scores were moderately large (standardized effect size=0.62; P<0.001).

Joffe and Singer (1990) compared 3-week TCA augmentation with T_3 versus T_4 in treatment-resistant depression and found a significantly higher response rate with T_3 (53%) compared with T_4 (19%). The clinical consensus became that T_3 should be the augmentation hormone of choice. Yet in more recent open studies that used high-dose T_4, response rates were greater than those expected for T_3. In a review of eight supraphysiological T_4 augmentation studies (total N=78), Baumgartner (2000) reported an antidepressant response rate of approximately 50% in patients completely resistant to multiple other antidepressant therapies. In one of these studies, Bauer et al. (1998) treated 17 treatment-resistant, euthyroid, severely depressed patients (12 bipolar, 5 unipolar) with high-dose T_4 (mean dose=482±72 µg/day). The mean Ham-D scores declined from 26.6 (±4.7) to 11.6 (±6.8) at the end of week 8; 8 of 17 (47%) met remission criteria. Remarkably, side effects were mild. This surprisingly benign safety profile was supported by a follow-up study comparing such doses in depressed and nondepressed patients (Bauer et al. 2002a).

Overall, the thyroid augmentation literature is hampered by uneven study quality: Many trials have been uncontrolled and included small and heterogeneous samples; therapeutic doses of TCAs generally were not laboratory confirmed; and thyroid abnormalities in patients at baseline were not always diagnosed (with subsequent exclusion of such subjects). Therefore, additional studies are necessary, especially placebo-controlled augmentation trials that are generalizable to modern clinical practice, such as augmentations to selective serotonin reuptake inhibitors and/or antidepressant combinations. In this regard, in an open clinical trial in which T_3 was added to a selective serotonin reuptake inhibitor (primarily fluoxetine, 40 mg) in nonresponders, 10 of 16 women (63%) and 0 of 9 men remitted (Agid and Lerer 2003).

Acceleration of Response to an Antidepressant Therapy

The delayed onset of therapeutic response to antidepressants has been a major problem in the treatment of depression. Prange et al. (1969) reported that the early addition of T_3 to TCAs appeared to hasten treatment response in women. In a meta-analysis of this literature, Altshuler et al.

(2001) identified six double-blind, placebo-controlled studies assessing the concomitant administration of T_3 and a TCA to accelerate clinical response in patients with non-refractory depression. Five of the six studies found T_3 to be significantly more effective than placebo in accelerating clinical response (weighted effect size index=0.58). Notably, the effects of T_3 acceleration were greater as the percentage of women participating in the study increased, suggesting that women might be more likely than men to benefit from this intervention (Altshuler et al. 2001). Hendrick et al. (1998) proposed that the greater prevalence of thyroid disease in women leads to a delay, on average compared with men, of their antidepressant response and that thyroid supplementation leads to an equalization of response times. Even so, such an accelerating effect of T_3 on the SSRI paroxetine was not demonstrable in a large (N=109) placebo-controlled clinical trial that was stopped before completion because of the unequivocal lack of effect (Appelhof et al. 2004).

Thyroid Hormone and Bipolar Disorder

Several case studies and an open trial indicate that two to three times the normal replacement doses of T_4 (i.e., sufficient to induce hyperthyroidism) may decrease both the frequency and the severity of cycling in bipolar patients, particularly those with rapid cycling and poor response to standard pharmacotherapy. This therapy appears to be useful for both depression and mania when added to standard mood stabilizer therapy (Bauer et al. 2002b; Post et al. 2000). Yet few controlled clinical trials of thyroid hormones in bipolar cycling have been done.

In short-term safety studies, use of supraphysiological T_4 was associated with a small increase in heart rate (5–8 beats/minute) and slight weight loss but no electrocardiogram changes or differences in bone mineral density compared with matched control subjects (Gyulai et al. 2001). However, because of the potential risks of long-term use—particularly at supraphysiological doses—treatment of rapid cycling with thyroid hormone should be considered experimental. Even so, given the limited number of effective treatment interventions for this condition, this strategy should be considered on a case-by-case basis after more traditional strategies have failed.

Hypothalamic-Pituitary-Thyroid Axis Therapies: Clinical Considerations

Patients presenting with a depressive or manic episode should have their thyroid function evaluated because of the considerable symptom overlap and comorbidity with thyroid dysfunction. Ideally, if thyroid dysfunction is present, specific treatment of the mood disorder should be undertaken, if necessary, after euthyroidism is maintained for 6 weeks. Even so, in many instances, pharmacotherapy (e.g., anxiolytic treatments in hyperthyroidism, antidepressant treatment for a severe depressive episode in hypothyroidism) is appropriately started concomitantly with HPT axis treatment. Clinical judgment should guide such treatment rather than rigid adherence to the concept of thyroid normalization as antidepressant treatment.

Considering the relatively extensive data on thyroid hormone augmentation in medication-resistant (or partially responsive) depressed patients, thyroid hormone should be an early consideration for this condition. Except for lithium augmentation, there have been far fewer clinical trials of alternative augmentation strategies, such as with second-generation antipsychotics and combinations of antidepressants. The available evidence indicates that T_3 should be the first choice, although T_4 and even T_3/T_4 combinations may be viable alternatives.

Dosing, Interactions, and Contraindications

T_3 can be started at 25 µg/day. Once-a-day dosing is common; although twice-a-day dosing would result in smoother blood levels, this does not appear to be of clinical relevance. After 1 week, the dosage can be increased to 37.5 µg/day or 50 µg/day. Thyrotoxicosis, which can occur at higher doses, presents with nervousness, mild tachycardia, sweating, flushing, and headache. When used to augment an inadequate antidepressant response, improvement is often observed within 2 weeks, although treatment should be continued at least 4 weeks to appreciate the maximum benefit.

The metabolic potency of T_4 at 100 µg is approximately equivalent to 25 µg of T_3. When treating rapid-cycling bipolar disorder, T_4 can be started at 50 µg/day. Once-a-day dosing is sufficient because of its long half-life. It is reasonable to increase the dose by 50 µg/week until 150 µg is reached; that dose may be maintained for 2–4 weeks while waiting for a clinical response and then increased again by 50 µg/week provided no symptoms of thyrotoxicosis emerge. Some experts have suggested a standard upper limit of 500 µg/day of T_4, although it has been noted that rapid-cycling bipolar patients seem relatively resistant to the metabolic effects of T_4. Serum thyrotropin should be monitored when treating rapid cycling because doses that have shown benefit in clinical trials have been at levels that suppress thyrotropin below the normal range. Serum free T_4 (or for more accuracy, free T_4 by dialysis) also can be followed up, aiming for a value approximately 150% of the upper limit of the normal range. When discontinuing therapy with thyroid hormone, it is recommended that T_3 be tapered by 12.5 µg and T_4 by 50 µg every 3 days.

Thyroid hormone may increase catabolism of vitamin K–dependent clotting factors; therefore, oral anticoagulants need to be closely monitored after initiation of thyroid hormone therapy. Thyroid hormones may increase insulin and oral hypoglycemic agent requirements. Cholestyramine binds T_3 and T_4 in the intestine, so administration of thyroid hormone within 4–5 hours of cholestyramine administration should be avoided. Estrogen can induce an increase in thyroglobulin, thereby reducing the serum free T_3 and T_4. Thyroid hormones may increase the metabolism of digitalis and also may potentiate the toxic effects of digitalis. Finally, thyroid hormones may increase the adrenergic effects of catecholamines such as epinephrine and norepinephrine, resulting in enhanced cardiovascular response. Exogenous thyroid hormone is contraindicated in pregnancy and in patients with frank cardiovascular disease, such as coronary artery disease, pathological arrhythmia, or heart failure.

Investigators have been concerned about the effect of chronic thyroid administration on bone mineral density (BMD) because of the known association between hyperthyroidism and osteoporosis. In a cross-sectional comparative study of mostly premenopausal women with rapid-cycling bipolar disorder, thyrotropin-suppressive doses of T_4 were not associated with a decreased BMD compared with a reference population (Gyulai et al. 2001). In a prospective study, BMD assessed with dual-energy X-ray absorptiometry at the femoral neck, Ward's triangle, trochanter, and lumbar vertebrae, was measured after approximately 1 and 3 years in 21 patients with mood disorders who were receiving supraphysiological doses of T_4 (mean dose=413 µg/day) (Bauer et al. 2004). In all bone regions assessed, there was no difference between the actual and age-expected group-mean decline in BMD. However, although age was identified as the primary predictor of percentage change in BMD, T_4 dose was also positively correlated with the decline of BMD at lumbar spines L1 and L4. This was primarily accounted for by one 57-year-old postmenopausal woman with bipolar disorder who was taking 600 µg/day of T_4 (and who had the highest free T_4 levels in the study group, 57 ng/l). The percentage change after 1.5 years in her lumbar spine BMD ranged from 12% (L3, L4) to 20% (L4), and the authors thought it likely that the thyroid played a role in this clinically significant bone loss. Overall, although thyroid supplementation may be recommended in certain clinical settings, the potential detrimental effects on bone should be considered, particularly in postmenopausal women and patients with known osteopenia or risk factors for its development. Regular assessment of BMD during longer-term supraphysiological thyroid hormone treatment should be standard.

Exogenous Testosterone Administration

Nondepressed Men

Testosterone has variable effects on mood. In most clinical trials in which exogenous testosterone was administered to nondepressed eugonadal men at physiological doses, significant effects on mood were not detected. For example, Tricker et al. (1996) randomly assigned 43 eugonadal men ages 19–40 to double-blind treatment with either testosterone or placebo injections weekly for 10 weeks; they found no change in self- or observer-reported measures of hostility, anger, or mood during testosterone treatment.

Administration of supraphysiological doses of testosterone to eugonadal men has been associated with mania in a small proportion of men. For example, Yates et al. (1999) administered testosterone (100, 250, or 500 mg/week) for 14 weeks to 18 men; 1 (6%) became manic. Pope et al. (2000) randomly assigned 66 men (age range=20–50) who did not have psychiatric histories to receive testosterone in doses rising to 600 mg/week or placebo for 6 weeks, followed by a 6-week no-treatment period, and then crossover to the alternate treatment. They found that testosterone administration significantly increased the mean manic score on the Young Mania Rating Scale (YMRS) (P=0.003) and on daily diaries (P=0.004), the "like the way I feel" score on daily diaries (P=0.01), and aggressive responses on the Point Subtraction Aggression Paradigm (P=0.04). Notably, two men became markedly hypomanic (YMRS score>20) after testosterone administration.

There are also well-controlled studies of testosterone administration to eugonadal men with sexual dysfunction. In general, they have found that administration of physiological doses of testosterone 1) is no more effective than placebo for erectile dysfunction, 2) leads to a modest increase in sexual interest, and 3) does not lead to a change on self-report measures of mood. For example, Schiavi et al. (1997) enrolled 18 eugonadal men (ages 46–67) who presented with the chief complaint of erectile dysfunction in a double-blind, placebo-controlled, crossover study of testosterone, 200 mg, or placebo every 2 weeks for 6 weeks. They found that during the testosterone compared with placebo phase ejaculatory frequency doubled; other measures of sexual arousal increased, but this was not statistically significant; erectile function and sexual satisfaction were unaffected; and mood, assessed by self-report instruments, was unaffected. Most subjects could not correctly identify the phase in which they had received testosterone and felt that it was not helpful. Notably, the authors were unable to show that this schedule of testosterone administration led to an increase in circulating levels 2 weeks after each intramuscular injection; thus, this dose may have been too low to override the compensatory feedback mechanisms operating in eugonadal men.

In hypogonadal men, androgen replacement clearly improves desire and some aspects of erectile functioning. It is not known whether mild, age-related hypothalamic-pituitary-gonadal hypofunctioning is associated with any sexual dysfunction and, if it is, whether androgen replacement is effective.

Depressed Men

Reports from the older psychiatric literature (1935–1960) on the "antidepressant" effects of testosterone suggested that a substantial number of "depressed" men responded immediately and dramatically to hormone replacement therapy and subsequently relapsed when treatment was discontinued (Seidman and Walsh 1999). However, standardized, syndromal psychiatric diagnoses were not used in these studies, and baseline testosterone levels were not assessed. Moreover, the lack of a control group prevents considering such results as any more than promising.

More recent anecdotal reports have suggested that in some hypogonadal men, comorbid MDD remits with testosterone replacement (Ehrenreich et al. 1999; Heuser et al. 1999) or augmentation to partially effective antidepressant medication (Seidman and Rabkin 1998) and that in hypogonadal HIV-infected men, testosterone replacement is associated with improved mood, libido, and energy (Grinspoon et al. 2000; Rabkin et al. 2000). On the basis of such reports, it had been assumed that testosterone replacement in hypogonadal men with MDD would conform to the "hypothyroid" model (i.e., hormone axis normalization as an effective antidepressant). Systematic study suggests that this is not the case.

In the past two decades, there have been at least 10 published studies of androgen treatment for men with depression in which investigators used DSM criteria for MDD and systematically followed up depressive symptoms. In a double-blind, randomized clinical trial of testosterone replacement versus placebo in 30 men with MDD and hypogonadism, Seidman et al. (2001) found testosterone replacement indistinguishable from placebo in antidepressant efficacy: 38% responded to testosterone, and 41% responded to placebo. However, more recent studies of testosterone replacement as an augmentation to antidepres-

sant partial response suggested that this strategy might be more promising (Orengo et al. 2005; Pope et al. 2003), although our unpublished findings do not support this. Overall, although initial anecdotal reports have been favorable, systematic trials of androgen replacement for depression have provided little support for its efficacy. Currently, treatment of depression with testosterone, either as replacement (i.e., in hypogonadism) or as an antidepressant supplement, should be considered experimental.

Exogenous Testosterone: Clinical Considerations

Exogenous testosterone, even at supraphysiological doses, rarely produces side effects, although there is a remote risk of developing gynecomastia (i.e., breast tenderness and breast enlargement), truncal acne (particularly for those with a history of acne), hair loss or hair growth, and weight gain. Because a modest increase in hematocrit always occurs, complete blood count should be checked pretreatment and monitored (Rolf and Nieschlag 1998; Seidman and Roose 2000). Via the negative feedback mechanism, exogenous testosterone suppresses luteinizing hormone and follicle-stimulating hormone, which leads to reduced testicular sperm production and, consequently, reduced testicular volume. Because mania and hypomania have been precipitated by testosterone administration (Pope et al. 2000; Yates et al. 1999), bipolar disorder should be considered a relative contraindication.

The primary concern regarding potential adverse effects of testosterone treatment is related to the prostate gland. Androgens play a permissive role in the growth of prostate cancer and benign prostatic hyperplasia (BPH); however, no data indicate that testosterone administration can lead to the progression of preclinical prostate cancer or to worsening BPH. Prostate cancer is an absolute contraindication to treatment with exogenous testosterone and should be excluded in all men older than 50 years (or in men older than 40 years if they have a positive family history of prostate cancer) via pretreatment prostate-specific antigen test and digital rectal examination of the prostate (Rolf and Nieschlag 1998).

Gonadal Hormones for Female Mood Disorders

Estrogen enhances mood, and its effects on the CNS (e.g., increasing monoaminergic transmission and particularly sensitivity to serotonin) have suggested to some investigators that it might be an effective antidepressant or an augmentation agent to antidepressants in treatment-resistant patients. However, clinical trials of estrogen for MDD have had consistently negative results (with a few unimpressive exceptions). This literature has serious methodological problems—most notably, the lack of structured psychiatric diagnoses and therefore heterogeneity of "depressive" samples. There is some interest, but limited data, regarding its use in treatment-resistant patients; this proposed use also requires more systematic study.

Hormonal treatments for premenstrual dysphoric disorder include gonadotropin-releasing hormone agonists, danazol, and estradiol (Kornstein and Sloan, Chapter 41, in this volume). Medical or surgical ovarian suppression has been shown to lead to an improvement in premenstrual dysphoric disorder, and this improvement is reversed by replacement with either estrogen or progesterone. In an elegant study, Schmidt et al. (1998) described the context-dependent nature of the specific interaction between hormonal milieu and this mood disorder. They used a double-blind, placebo-controlled design and first confirmed the symptomatic improvement resulting from ovarian suppression in 20 women with premenstrual syndrome and that replacement with gonadal steroids led to worsening. Then they performed the identical hormonal manipulations (with comparable hormone levels achieved) in women without premenstrual syndrome and observed no perturbations of mood. This finding supports the conclusion that the apparently "depressogenic" hormonal milieu activates this condition only in vulnerable individuals.

Hormonal treatments of postpartum depression have focused on the hypothesis that the typical postpartum "estrogen withdrawal state" (and possibly this state's effect on monoaminergic transmission) provokes MDD in vulnerable individuals. As a way to ameliorate such a state, investigators have studied high-dose estrogen treatment. In a placebo-controlled trial, Gregoire et al. (1996) randomly assigned 61 women with postpartum depression (half of whom were taking an antidepressant) to estradiol or placebo. During the first month of therapy, the women receiving estrogen improved rapidly and to a significantly greater extent than did control subjects; by 3 months, 80% of the patients receiving estrogen and 31% of the control subjects achieved remission. The estimated overall treatment effect of estrogen on the Edinburgh Postnatal Depression Scale was 4.38 points (95% CI=1.89–6.87). Progesterone has been considered for postpartum depression, but clinical trials have been methodologically flawed and generally negative.

Hormone replacement therapy in peri- and postmenopausal women is discussed elsewhere in this volume (Kornstein and Sloan, Chapter 41). Briefly, there are no conclusive data on the effects of estrogen for preventive or therapeutic effects on mood in postmenopausal women. Current data support a role for estrogen replacement therapy in improving mood, well-being, energy, and libido in surgically menopausal, depressed perimenopausal, and nondepressed postmenopausal women. These effects may be reversed by progesterone (Rubinow et al. 2002) and enhanced by androgens (Montgomery et al. 1987). Investigators have proposed that the subgroup of women who are particularly likely to respond to estrogen replacement therapy are those who have significant hypothalamic-pituitary-gonadal dysregulation (e.g., higher basal gonadotropins and exaggerated responses to luteinizing hormone–releasing hormone stimulation) (O'Toole and Rubin 1995; Rubin et al. 2002). Overall, limited data support the use of estrogen alone in postmenopausal MDD, and given the potential risks of this treatment, it should not be considered a first-line therapy.

Conclusion

In this chapter, we considered the role of hormonal interventions in the treatment of mood disorders. Such treatments are vulnerable to premature claims because exogenous hormones are clearly psychotropic and, moreover, because a vast anecdotal history supports efficacy but limited systematic data are available (and placebo response rates are high).

We focused in this chapter on the three primary hormone axes and MDD. Bipolar disorder was given little attention and other mood disorders none at all. This is because of a shortage of systematic data on the effects of hormones in mood disorders other than MDD. It is worth noting, also, that the study of hormonal interventions for mood disorders may require better refinement of the anchor points of psychiatric diagnosis against which hormonal therapies can be studied. Finally, because of space limitations we were unable to discuss a variety of novel potential interventions, such as melatonin, cholecystokinin antagonists, substance P antagonists, and leptin (see Table 19–2). This should not be interpreted as a negative assessment of their potential.

Although no hormonal treatments are FDA approved for mood disorders, accumulated evidence and clinical consensus support the following. First, in the setting of comorbid hormone axis dysfunction and MDD, hormone axis normalization (e.g., thyroid replacement) should be a treatment priority, and many would suggest that comorbid MDD is enough to justify treatment of subclinical endocrinopathies (e.g., grade II or III hypothyroidism) that

TABLE 19–2. Hormonal interventions with psychotropic activity

Hypothalamic-pituitary-adrenal axis

Cortisol antagonists

Corticotropin-releasing hormone receptor antagonists

Dehydroepiandrosterone

Hypothalamic-pituitary-thyroid axis

Thyroid hormones

Hypothalamic-pituitary-gonadal axis

Gonadal hormones (androgens, estrogens, progestins)

Ovulation suppressors

Other hormones

Neurosteroids

Melatonin

Arginine vasopressin

Oxytocin

Cholecystokinin antagonists

Prolactin inhibitors

Opioids

Substance P antagonists

Leptin

might otherwise have been watched. Second, considerable evidence supports the use of thyroid hormones to augment a poor response to antidepressants and estrogen replacement therapy alone for perimenopausal MDD. Third, evidence is accumulating that CRH antagonists may be effective for MDD. Fourth, only limited evidence supports the use of thyroid hormones in rapid-cycling bipolar patients, antiglucocorticoids for MDD, or testosterone for MDD, although these treatments may be effective in subpopulations (e.g., testosterone in HIV-infected depressed men).

In summary, the consistently equivocal evidence regarding the role of hormones in antidepressant therapies supports the notion that mood effects of these agents are idiosyncratic and context dependent. For example, about 15% of men experience profound mood effects following administration of moderately supraphysiological doses of exogenous testosterone (Pope et al. 2000; Yates et al. 1999). Again, the model we would suggest that best fits the literature is context dependence. Determination of the specific context that optimizes the antidepressant potential of these agents may require better-defined target conditions or target populations (e.g., based on androgen receptor isotype). In general, evidence is sufficient to predict a role for exogenous hormones in the treatment of mood disorders, but full delineation of such a role is left to future research.

References

Agid O, Lerer B: Algorithm-based treatment of major depression in an outpatient clinic: clinical correlates of response to a specific serotonin reuptake inhibitor and to triiodothyronine augmentation. Int J Neuropsychopharmacol 6:41–49, 2003

Altshuler LL, Bauer M, Frye MA, et al: Does thyroid supplementation accelerate tricyclic antidepressant response? A review and meta-analysis of the literature. Am J Psychiatry 158:1617–1622, 2001

Appelhof BC, Brouwer JP, van Dyck R, et al: Triiodothyronine addition to paroxetine in the treatment of major depressive disorder. J Clin Endocrinol Metab 89:6271–6276, 2004

Arlt W, Callies F, Van Vlijmen JC, et al: Dehydroepiandrosterone replacement in women with adrenal insufficiency. N Engl J Med 341:1013–1020, 1999

Arlt W, Callies F, Koehler I, et al: Dehydroepiandrosterone supplementation in healthy men with an age-related decline of dehydroepiandrosterone secretion. J Clin Endocrinol Metab 86:4686–4692, 2001

Aronson R, Offman HJ, Joffe RT, et al: Triiodothyronine augmentation in the treatment of refractory depression: a meta-analysis. Arch Gen Psychiatry 53:842–848, 1996

Bauer M, Hellweg R, Graf KJ, et al: Treatment of refractory depression with high-dose thyroxine. Neuropsychopharmacology 18:444–455, 1998

Bauer M, Baur H, Berghofer A, et al: Effects of supraphysiological thyroxine administration in healthy controls and patients with depressive disorders. J Affect Disord 68:285–294, 2002a

Bauer M, Berghofer A, Bschor T, et al: Supraphysiological doses of L-thyroxine in the maintenance treatment of prophylaxis-resistant affective disorders. Neuropsychopharmacology 27:620–628, 2002b

Bauer M, Fairbanks L, Berghofer A, et al: Bone mineral density during maintenance treatment with supraphysiological doses of levothyroxine in affective disorders: a longitudinal study. J Affect Disord 83:183–190, 2004

Baumgartner A: Thyroxine and the treatment of affective disorders: an overview of the results of basic and clinical research. Int J Neuropsychopharmacol 3:149–165, 2000

Brown ES, Bobadilla L, Rush AJ: Ketoconazole in bipolar patients with depressive symptoms: a case series and literature review. Bipolar Disord 3:23–29, 2001

Cameron DR, Braunstein GD: The use of dehydroepiandrosterone therapy in clinical practice. Treat Endocrinol 4:95–114, 2005

Ehrenreich H, Halaris A, Ruether E, et al: Psychoendocrine sequelae of chronic testosterone deficiency. J Psychiatr Res 33:379–387, 1999

Gold PW, Licinio J, Wong ML, et al: Corticotropin releasing hormone in the pathophysiology of melancholic and atypical depression and in the mechanism of action of antidepressant drugs. Ann N Y Acad Sci 771:716–729, 1995

Gregoire AJ, Kumar R, Everitt B, et al: Transdermal oestrogen for treatment of severe postnatal depression. Lancet 347:930–933, 1996

Grinspoon S, Corcoran C, Stanley T, et al: Effects of hypogonadism and testosterone administration on depression indices in HIV-infected men. J Clin Endocrinol Metab 85:60–65, 2000

Gyulai L, Bauer M, Garcia-Espana F, et al: Bone mineral density in pre- and post-menopausal women with affective disorder treated with long-term L-thyroxine augmentation. J Affect Disord 66:185–191, 2001

Halbreich U: Hormonal interventions with psychopharmacological potential: an overview. Psychopharmacol Bull 33:281–286, 1997

Held K, Kunzel H, Ising M, et al: Treatment with the CRH1-receptor-antagonist R121919 improves sleep-EEG in patients with depression. J Psychiatr Res 38:129–136, 2004

Heuser I, Hartmann A, Oertel H: Androgen replacement in a 48, XXYY-male patient (letter). Arch Gen Psychiatry 56:194–195, 1999

Holsboer F: Corticotropin-releasing hormone modulators and depression. Curr Opin Investig Drugs 4:46–50, 2003

Jahn H, Schick M, Kiefer F, et al: Metyrapone as additive treatment in major depression: a double-blind and placebo-controlled trial. Arch Gen Psychiatry 61:1235–1244, 2004

Joffe RT: Refractory depression: treatment strategies, with particular reference to the thyroid axis. J Psychiatry Neurosci 22:327–331, 1997

Joffe RT, Singer W: A comparison of triiodothyronine and thyroxine in the potentiation of tricyclic antidepressants. Psychiatry Res 32:241–251, 1990

Joffe RT, Singer W, Levitt AJ, et al: A placebo-controlled comparison of lithium and triiodothyronine augmentation of tricyclic antidepressants in unipolar refractory depression. Arch Gen Psychiatry 50:387–393, 1993

Kasckow JW, Aguilera G, Mulchahey JJ, et al: In vitro regulation of corticotropin-releasing hormone. Life Sci 73:769–781, 2003

Kunzel HE, Zobel AW, Nickel T, et al: Treatment of depression with the CRH-1-receptor antagonist R121919: endocrine changes and side effects. J Psychiatr Res 37:525–533, 2003

Malison RT, Anand A, Pelton GH, et al: Limited efficacy of ketoconazole in treatment-refractory major depression. J Clin Psychopharmacol 19:466–470, 1999

Montgomery JC, Appleby L, Brincat M, et al: Effect of oestrogen and testosterone implants on psychological disorders of the climacteric. Lancet 339:297–299, 1987

Murphy BE: Antiglucocorticoid therapies in major depression: a review. Psychoneuroendocrinology 22 (suppl 1):S125–S132, 1997

Nemeroff CB: New directions in the development of antidepressants: the interface of neurobiology and psychiatry. Hum Psychopharmacol 17 (suppl 1):S13–S16, 2002

Orengo CA, Fullerton L, Kunik ME: Safety and efficacy of testosterone gel 1% augmentation in depressed men with partial response to antidepressant therapy. J Geriatr Psychiatry Neurol 18:20–24, 2005

O'Toole SM, Rubin RT: Neuroendocrine aspects of primary endogenous depression, XIV: gonadotropin secretion in female patients and their matched controls. Psychoneuroendocrinology 20:603–612, 1995

Pope HGJ, Kouri EM, Hudson JI: Effects of supraphysiologic doses of testosterone on mood and aggression in normal men: a randomized controlled trial. Arch Gen Psychiatry 57:133–140, 2000

Pope HGJ, Cohane GH, Kanayama G, et al: Testosterone gel supplementation for men with refractory depression: a randomized, placebo-controlled trial. Am J Psychiatry 160:105–111, 2003

Post RM, Frye MA, Denicoff KD, et al: Emerging trends in the treatment of rapid cycling bipolar disorder: a selected review. Bipolar Disord 2:305–315, 2000

Prange AJ Jr, Wilson IC, Rabon AM, et al: Enhancement of imipramine antidepressant activity by thyroid hormone. Am J Psychiatry 126:457–469, 1969

Rabkin JG, Wagner G, Rabkin R: A double-blind, placebo-controlled trial of testosterone therapy for HIV-positive men with hypogonadal symptoms. Arch Gen Psychiatry 57:141–147, 2000

Rolf C, Nieschlag E: Potential adverse effects of long-term testosterone therapy. Baillieres Clin Endocrinol Metab 12:521–534, 1998

Rubin RT: Pharmacoendocrinology of major depression. Eur Arch Psychiatry Neurol Sci 238:259–267, 1989

Rubin RT, Dinan TG, Scott LV: The neuroendocrinology of affective disorders, in Hormones, Brain and Behavior. Edited by Pfaff D, Arnold AP, Etgen AM, et al. New York, Academic Press, 2002, p 467

Rubinow DR, Schmidt PJ, Roca CA, et al: Gonadal hormones and behavior in women: concentrations versus context, in Hormones, Brain and Behavior. Edited by Pfaff D, Arnold AP, Etgen AM, et al. New York, Academic Press, 2002, p 37

Schiavi RC, White D, Mandeli J, et al: Effect of testosterone administration on sexual behavior and mood in men with erectile dysfunction. Arch Sex Behav 26:231–241, 1997

Schmidt PJ, Nieman LK, Danaceau MA, et al: Differential behavioral effects of gonadal steroids in women with and in those without premenstrual syndrome. N Engl J Med 338:209–216, 1998

Schmidt PJ, Daly RC, Bloch M, et al: Dehydroepiandrosterone monotherapy in midlife-onset major and minor depression. Arch Gen Psychiatry 62:154–162, 2005

Seidman SN, Rabkin JG: Testosterone replacement therapy for hypogonadal men with SSRI-refractory depression. J Affect Disord 48:157–161, 1998

Seidman SN, Roose SP: The male hypothalamic-pituitary-gonadal axis: pathogenic and therapeutic implications in psychiatry. Psychiatr Ann 30:102–112, 2000

Seidman SN, Walsh BT: Testosterone and depression in aging men. Am J Geriatr Psychiatry 7:18–33, 1999

Seidman SN, Spatz E, Rizzo C, et al: Testosterone replacement therapy for hypogonadal men with major depressive disorder: a randomized, placebo-controlled clinical trial. J Clin Psychiatry 62:406–412, 2001

Thakore JH, Dinan TG: Cortisol synthesis inhibition: a new treatment strategy for the clinical and endocrine manifestations of depression. Biol Psychiatry 37:364–368, 1995

Tricker R, Casaburi R, Storer TW, et al: The effects of supraphysiological doses of testosterone on angry behavior in healthy eugonadal men—a clinical research center study. J Clin Endocrinol Metab 81:3754–3758, 1996

Whybrow PC, Bauer MS, Gyulai L: Thyroid axis considerations in patients with rapid cycling affective disorder. Clin Neuropharmacol 15 (suppl 1, pt A):391A–392A, 1992

Wilson IC, Prange AJ Jr, McClane TK, et al: Thyroid-hormone enhancement of imipramine in nonretarded depressions. N Engl J Med 282:1063–1067, 1970

Wolkowitz OM, Reus VI: Treatment of depression with antiglucocorticoid drugs. Psychosom Med 61:698–711, 1999

Wolkowitz OM, Reus VI, Roberts E, et al: Dehydroepiandrosterone (DHEA) treatment of depression. Biol Psychiatry 41:311–318, 1997

Wolkowitz OM, Reus VI, Chan T, et al: Antiglucocorticoid treatment of depression: double-blind ketoconazole. Biol Psychiatry 45:1070–1074, 1999a

Wolkowitz OM, Reus VI, Keebler A, et al: Double-blind treatment of major depression with dehydroepiandrosterone (DHEA). Am J Psychiatry 156:646–649, 1999b

Wolkowitz OM, Brizendine L, Reus VI: The role of dehydroepiandrosterone (DHEA) in psychiatry. Psychiatr Ann 30:123–128, 2000

Yates WR, Perry PJ, Macindoe J, et al: Psychosexual effects of three doses of testosterone cycling in normal men. Biol Psychiatry 45:254–260, 1999

Zobel AW, Nickel T, Kunzel HE, et al: Effects of the high-affinity corticotropin-releasing hormone receptor 1 antagonist R121919 in major depression: the first 20 patients treated. J Psychiatr Res 34:171–181, 2000

20

Electroconvulsive Therapy and Transcranial Magnetic Stimulation

MITCHELL S. NOBLER, M.D.

HAROLD A. SACKEIM, PH.D.

ELECTROCONVULSIVE THERAPY (ECT) has a long history within the field of psychiatry. Despite repeated demonstrations of remarkable efficacy in the short-term treatment of mood disorders and other specific conditions, ECT remains controversial in the public eye. This is partly because of misconceptions about the treatment but also because of the unfortunate presence of potentially severe cognitive side effects. There have been major advances in the past two decades in research aimed at optimizing efficacy while minimizing adverse effects (Abrams 2002; American Psychiatric Association 2001). However, there is considerable variability in the extent to which this new knowledge has been adopted in clinical practice. In addition to reviewing such fundamental information, we highlight important recent advances, including new developments in a related treatment—repetitive transcranial magnetic stimulation (rTMS). Finally, we underscore current challenges for ECT and rTMS research.

History and Discovery

Use of ECT in psychiatry began in the prepharmacological era and before the development of the methodologies used to establish the efficacy and safety of treatments. An understanding of the role of ECT as a somatic treatment in psychiatry today requires an appreciation of the historical context in which it was first introduced (Kalinowsky 1986).

Prior to World War II, definitive treatments were essentially nonexistent for severe mental illnesses, and multitudes of patients were consigned to large public psychiatric institutions, with little hope of symptomatic relief, let alone remission. Thus, from both public health and humanitarian standpoints, the need for an effective intervention was inestimable. Unfortunately, neuroscience was in its infancy, and there was little scientific rationale to guide treatment development. Indeed, the predominant belief in biological psychiatry was that the major forms of mental illness reflected either congenital or degenerative brain disease that could not be effectively treated. In other words, therapeutic nihilism was rampant. In addition, modern scientific methods, such as randomized, controlled trials, had yet to be developed. It was against this backdrop that several early somatic treatments emerged, the most important being prefrontal lobotomy, insulin coma therapy, and convulsive therapy. The latter, as it turns out, did have a theoretical basis (which was later discredited), postulating that there was a biological antagonism between generalized seizures of epilepsy and schizophrenia.

ECT was not the first form of convulsive therapy (Meduna 1935). Chemical convulsants, such as camphor oil and pentylenetetrazol, predated the first electrically induced convulsions in humans by Cerlitti and Bini in 1938. The main reason that ECT eclipsed other forms of convulsive therapy was that electrical seizure elicitation was far more controllable and predictable than were chemically induced convulsions. In fact, there was no special belief that electrical stimulation would confer additional efficacy; it was only a means to an end. This conceptualization, however, influenced several subsequent decades of ECT research and therapeutics. In essence, the field held that as long as a generalized seizure was elicited with ECT, the degree of electrical stimulation was irrelevant to efficacy, whereas increasing the intensity of the electrical stimulus would only lead to greater cognitive side effects. Only within the past 20 years has this view been successfully challenged.

In the 1940s and 1950s, as the initial enthusiasm surrounding prefrontal lobotomy and insulin coma waned, ECT, despite its sketchy scientific basis and crude methods of delivery, quickly ascended to prominence as the most important somatic treatment in psychiatry. Early experience indicated that ECT was more useful in the treatment of severe mood disorders and catatonic stupor than in chronic psychoses. The introduction of barbiturate anesthesia, muscle relaxation, and oxygenation in the 1950s and 1960s made the treatment somewhat more palatable and reduced the rate of spinal injury. Early researchers in ECT began to examine the relative advantages of unilateral electrode placement (Lancaster et al. 1958) and of modifications to the electrical waveform to provide more efficient stimulation (Kaplan et al. 1956).

However, in the United States by the early 1960s, there was a major change in the attention given to somatic treatments in psychiatry. The psychopharmacological revolution had begun, and research in ECT waned. Randomized, controlled trials of antidepressant and antipsychotic medications (which initially used ECT as the gold standard comparator condition) shifted to studies of pharmacological agents alone and soon began to eclipse ECT research. Simultaneously, along with the push toward deinstitutionalization and the documentation of short-term efficacy of antidepressant medications in major depressive episodes (MDEs), ECT was increasingly reserved for patients with treatment-resistant depression, often as the option of last resort. Throughout the 1970s and early 1980s, rates of ECT use declined (disproportionately so in public vs. private hospitals), and aside from

a core group of academic psychiatrists, there was slow progress in preclinical and clinical research, de-emphasis of the practice of ECT in residency training programs, and little initiative from the National Institute of Mental Health (NIMH). During this time, public sentiment mirrored the view of the mental health establishment (and perhaps vice versa) in its enthusiasm for psychopharmacological approaches and neglect of ECT. The popular media often depicted ECT as cruel and barbaric, frequently ignoring the improvements that had been made prior to 1980. Others contended that ECT was an abusive procedure typically inflicted on the destitute or helpless as a method of behavior control. Often, these critics contended that severe mental illness reflected societal dysfunction and was not a biological disturbance in need of a somatic intervention (Breggin 1979). Thus, ECT was the "straw man" in societal debate about mind-body issues and the role of somatic treatments in psychiatry. Because of the vehemence of this debate, use of ECT in public municipal, state, and federal facilities largely disappeared.

By the mid-1980s, this situation began to reverse. Despite the introduction of selective serotonin reuptake inhibitors (SSRIs), dual-acting antidepressants (e.g., venlafaxine), and atypical antipsychotic medications, the strengths and limitations of psychopharmacological treatment of mood disorders became apparent. It is now recognized that only about one-third of patients achieve remission of the MDE with their first pharmacological treatment. Furthermore, a large percentage of patients do not achieve remission with multiple adequate trials. The large numbers of treatment-resistant patients, coupled with the growing costs of health care (and psychiatric hospital stays in particular), spurred interest in the cost-effectiveness of ECT. At the same time, renewed scientific interest resulted in long-overdue advances in ECT treatment technique, showing that ECT could be delivered in both a highly effective and a less toxic manner (Potter and Rudorfer 1993). The American Psychiatric Association and the NIMH incorporated these advances into specific guidelines for the delivery of ECT (American Psychiatric Association 1990; American Psychiatric Association Task Force on ECT 1978; Blaine and Clark 1986). Utilization rates stabilized and began to increase. Perhaps even public opinion softened, with media reports becoming more evenhanded and important autobiographical accounts by patients appearing in bookstores (Endler 1990; Manning 1995).

However, even as we are writing this chapter, ECT remains a treatment that generates intense debate among patients, extremist organizations, the media, and politicians. Curiously, mental health professionals remain divided about ECT. Various state legislatures have passed, or are considering, bills that impose special reporting requirements for ECT or that limit patient access to care. ECT is perhaps the medical procedure with the greatest legislative restrictions and oversight in the United States. Undoubtedly, part of this stems from its unique history. Yet ignorance on the part of both the medical establishment and the general public of advances in the field also perpetuates unjustified fear of ECT. The end result is that ECT continually becomes the focal point of any debate over potential abuse of vulnerable psychiatric patients. Many ECT practitioners welcome opportunities to further enhance the safe delivery of the treatment while fully including patients and their families in the informed consent process. However, the variability clearly documented in the quality of ECT practice potentially reinforces those who would restrict or abolish access to this treatment.

Mechanisms of Action

General Considerations

A definitive explanation of "how ECT works" would represent a great advance for the field and perhaps quiet some of its opponents. This explanation does not exist. Nor does it exist for antidepressant medications (or for psychotherapy, for that matter). Complicating matters further, many early researchers believed that mechanisms of action could never be identified because the elicitation of the seizure at ECT caused such a multitude of biochemical and physiological changes that it would be improbable that any single mechanism could be found (a "needle in a haystack" effect). Of course, research into mechanisms of action has progressed and has yielded several well-replicated findings and useful avenues of investigation. It has also spurred advances in related areas of neuroscience research, such as neuroimaging of mood disorders (Coffey et al. 1991; Nobler et al. 1994) and neurogenesis (Madsen et al. 2000).

Yet several important challenges and limitations remain in this area. Although animal research into electroconvulsive shock (ECS) has been fruitful (especially in terms of neurotransmitter and receptor studies), there are still no clear animal models for the major psychiatric syndromes, which limits the interpretation of findings. Also, much of this work has not taken the time course of ECS into consideration. For example, certain biochemical effects may be quite pronounced following a single ECS session, but evaluating the effects of repeated ECS likely has greater relevance to the clinical use of ECT.

The foremost challenge in clinical research into ECT mechanisms stems from the irony that because ECT is so

highly effective, it is difficult to identify biological differences between responders and nonresponders. In other words, from a statistical standpoint, the restricted range in clinical outcomes reduces the power to test hypotheses about which specific changes are critical to efficacy. While sham-controlled trials in ECT are no longer a viable option from an ethical standpoint (although such studies did help provide critical evidence regarding efficacy), studies that used ECT modalities that differ in efficacy have provided useful data on the relations of neurobiological variables to treatment outcome (Lisanby et al. 1998; Luber et al. 2000; Nobler et al. 2000a; Sackeim et al. 1996).

Perhaps a subtler caveat is an appreciation of exactly which elements of the treatment are therapeutic. Is the elicitation of a generalized seizure both necessary and sufficient for clinical response? What role, if any, does the site of stimulation (i.e., electrode placement) or the degree of electrical stimulus intensity play? In other words, do the settings on the ECT device really matter? Clearly, as discussed earlier, effective forms of convulsive therapy have existed that did not involve electrical stimulation. Thus, it would seem that any generalized seizure elicited by ECT should be therapeutic. However, it is now established that fully generalized seizures that are of adequate duration yet lack therapeutic properties can be elicited with low-dosage, right-unilateral ECT. On the whole, studies are beginning to indicate that the interaction of electrode placement and electrical stimulus intensity is more useful in conceptualizing therapeutic mechanisms than considering each component as a separate entity. In other words, the efficacy of ECT is determined, in part, by the current paths of the ECT stimulus and the current density within those paths.

Effects on Neurotransmission

Much of the traditional research into the mechanisms of action of ECT has relied on preclinical studies that examined the similarities and differences between ECS and antidepressant medications (tricyclics, monoamine oxidase inhibitors, and SSRIs) in modulating neurotransmitter and peptide systems (Fochtmann 1994; Green et al. 1986; Kellar 1987; Kellar et al. 1981b; Lerer et al. 1986; Mann 1998). A consistent finding is that, similar to antidepressant medications, ECS leads to a downregulation of β-adrenergic receptors (Kellar et al. 1981a; Lerer et al. 1986). This finding often has been cited as evidence that the antidepressant effects of ECT share a common mechanism with that of standard medications. However, human studies of alterations in noradrenergic function have yielded inconsistent results (Rudorfer et al. 1988; Sackeim et al. 1995). Furthermore, in contrast to the downregulation of the 5-hydroxytryptamine (serotonin) type 2 (5-HT$_2$) receptor usually seen with antidepressants, ECS leads to an increased density of 5-HT$_2$ receptors (Kellar et al. 1981b; Mann 1998; Nutt et al. 1989). Thus, ECS may lead to enhanced serotonergic transmission, but this mechanism appears to be different from those of antidepressant medications.

Although human studies have reported an increase of serotonin metabolites in the cerebrospinal fluid following a course of ECT (Mann and Kapur 1994; Rudorfer et al. 1991), other probes of serotonergic function have yielded inconsistent results (Mann 1998). Animal studies have consistently found profound increases in dopaminergic tone following ECS (Fochtmann 1994; Glue et al. 1990; Zis et al. 1991). Clinical studies, although less consistent, similarly point in the direction of enhanced dopaminergic functioning with ECT (Mann and Kapur 1994). Theoretically, this may underlie the antiparkinsonian effect of ECT, but these findings are paradoxical with respect to ECT's antipsychotic effects.

Other preclinical work has focused on a variety of neurotransmitters such as γ-aminobutyric acid (GABA), adenosine, and the endogenous opioids. These systems may be particularly important in understanding the biochemical basis of the anticonvulsant effects of ECT. Overall, little evidence indicates that alterations in any specific transmitter system co-vary with ECT efficacy (Mann 1998; Newman et al. 1998), nor is there agreement on whether similarities to or differences from antidepressant medication should be the main theoretical focus.

Effects on Neuroendocrine Parameters

Another theory regarding mechanisms of action, the diencephalic hypothesis (Abrams and Taylor 1976; Fink and Ottosson 1980), has focused on the role of stimulation of deep brain structures by ECT. This theory postulates that the therapeutic properties of ECT are related to stimulation of the hypothalamic-pituitary-adrenal axis, presumably correcting a neuroendocrine dysfunction associated with major depression. The diencephalic hypothesis also recognizes that generalized seizures result in the release of numerous compounds, including prolactin, vasopressin, neurophysin, oxytocin, cortisol, and corticotropin (Apëria et al. 1985; Kronfol et al. 1991; Whalley et al. 1982). Of these, prolactin has received the most attention. For instance, it has been observed that the rise in serum prolactin levels following an ECT treatment is influenced by both electrode placement and stimulus intensity (McCall et al. 1996). Thus, the prolactin surge may reflect the "strength" of the seizure at ECT and is a potential marker for what constitutes a maximally therapeutic treatment modality. However, a direct association between the magnitude of the prolactin surge and efficacy has not been reliably established despite numerous attempts (Lisanby et al. 1998).

Effects on Neurophysiology and Functional Neuroanatomy

Another approach to mechanisms of action that is not mutually exclusive with other theories draws on preclinical and clinical observations regarding the anticonvulsant properties of ECT (Post et al. 1986; Sackeim 1999; Sackeim et al. 1983). A basic premise of this theory is that seizures do not terminate via passive mechanisms, but rather that the ictus has both excitatory and inhibitory components and that inhibition eventually overcomes excitation, resulting in termination. Moreover, sites of seizure initiation (as opposed to sites of the regional distribution of seizure propagation) may be critical because they putatively represent the areas of greatest functional inhibition. The anticonvulsant theory postulates that such inhibitory processes are the basis of therapeutic effects. It should be emphasized that inhibition within the central nervous system is an active metabolic process, presumably mediated via neurotransmitters and likely reflected in alterations of electroencephalographic patterns as well as changes in regional cerebral blood flow (rCBF) and regional cerebral metabolic rate (rCMR).

Research into the effects of ECT on both ictal and interictal electroencephalographic characteristics has been active for several decades (d'Elia and Perris 1970; Fink and Kahn 1957; Krystal et al. 1993, 2000; Luber et al. 2000; Nobler et al. 1993, 2000a; Ottosson 1962; Pacella et al. 1942; Perera et al. 2004; Sackeim et al. 1996; Small et al. 1970; Staton et al. 1981; Weiner et al. 1986a). There have been three major lines of investigation: 1) relations of changes in resting (i.e., interictal) electroencephalogram (EEG) with clinical outcome during and following a course of ECT, 2) relations of ictal EEG characteristics with clinical outcome, and 3) the practicality of using ictal EEG measures to distinguish among various ECT modalities and potentially guide treatment. The latter has less immediate relevance to mechanisms of action per se but has been useful in showing that less therapeutic forms of ECT result in EEG-measured seizures that are lower in peak slow-wave amplitudes, are less stereotyped and less coherent, and have less postictal suppression. However, the utility of electroencephalographic measures to more finely distinguish among effective and ineffective forms of ECT has limitations, and it is doubtful that electroencephalographic measures should be used in isolation to guide treatment delivery (Perera et al. 2004).

In terms of therapeutic mechanisms, very early studies noted that EEG "slowing" (increased power in the delta and theta frequency bands) develops during a course of ECT and lasts several weeks. Although this effect was not consistently noted, evidence showed that more pronounced EEG slowing, either globally or regionally, was associated with superior outcomes (Fink and Kahn 1957). More recently, power spectral analyses were used to show that short-term increases in delta activity in prefrontal cortex were associated with the magnitude of symptomatic improvement with ECT (Sackeim et al. 1996). This finding can be interpreted to indicate that effective ECT results in greater functional inhibition in prefrontal brain regions.

As noted, the ictal EEG has been observed to vary with ECT treatment modality and, consequently, might serve as a marker of maximally therapeutic ECT. There are indications that greater peak slow-wave amplitudes (especially in prefrontal cortex) and greater immediate postictal suppression are both positively correlated with treatment response, but it is still unclear if these statistical associations have clinical significance (Nobler et al. 1993; Perera et al. 2004). Nonetheless, both of these seizure characteristics reflect inhibitory processes, similar to the development of increased slow-wave activity in the interictal EEG.

Neuroimaging of patients receiving ECT represented some of the earliest studies to assess in vivo brain function (Kety et al. 1948). Over the past six decades, various imaging techniques have been used in ECT research, including xenon inhalation rCBF, single-photon emission computed tomography (SPECT), and positron emission tomography (PET). This body of work has contributed both to the understanding of mechanisms of action (Nobler et al. 2000b) and to the pathophysiology of mood disorders (Soares and Mann 1997). Preclinical studies have reported profound increases in rCBF and rCMR during generalized seizures, with reductions below baseline in the postictal period (Ackermann et al. 1986; Ingvar 1986). For technical and practical reasons, it has been difficult to capture the ictal and immediate postictal ECT response with conventional techniques, but there is at least the suggestion that the same pattern is present in humans (Saito et al. 1995). In the early postictal period (i.e., up to an hour post-ECT), rCBF values decline to levels below baseline (Nobler et al. 1994). Most studies that used xenon rCBF, SPECT, and PET have noted that postictal decreases in rCBF and rCMR persist up to several days following a course of ECT, although they become less pronounced as time from treatment progresses (Nobler et al. 2000b). There have been discrepant findings (Bonne et al. 1996), but this may be partly because of differences in imaging techniques and in whether global shifts in cerebral perfusion were taken into consideration. In terms of topography, many studies have indicated that postictal and interictal decreases in functional activity occur primarily in prefrontal regions, mirroring those brain areas that show increases in slow activity on EEG (Henry et al. 2001; Nobler et al. 1994, 2001). Most critically, evidence also indicates that the magnitude of rCBF reductions in a specific pattern of prefrontal regions is related to clinical response (Nobler et al. 1994).

Thus, convergent lines of electroencephalographic and brain imaging data support the notion that increased inhibitory activity (or decreased excitatory input) is a consequence of ECT, particularly in prefrontal cortex. Moreover, this functional change in cerebral activity may be linked to efficacy.

Other Effects

A more recent approach to mechanisms of action has focused on the effects of ECT on the potential of neurons to develop new interconnections, and possibly increase in number, especially within the hippocampus. Increased neurogenesis may be dependent on changes in neurotrophic factors in response to induced seizures (Madsen et al. 2000). All known antidepressants (ECS and medications) result in an increase in neurogenesis, and the magnitude of this effect is greatest for ECS (Scott et al. 2000). Some evidence suggests that blocking the development of neurogenesis in a knockout mouse model of mood disorder also blocks reversal of the behavioral deficits that usually follow chronic treatment with fluoxetine. This finding has led to the claim that increased neurogenesis is a precondition or is necessary for antidepressant effects. Whether such a pattern applies to ECS has yet to be determined.

Indications

Recommending ECT is a critical decision. Inappropriately administered ECT exposes the patient to unnecessary (and potentially irreversible) side effects. Unsuccessful treatment may further demoralize a patient with chronic illness and thus should not be held out as a viable option in the wrong circumstances. However, to withhold the appropriate use of ECT may lead to undue suffering (or even death) and can be viewed as unethical. This duality serves to emphasize that at least as much attention should be given to patient selection for ECT as is given to the technical considerations of the treatment. From the patient's perspective, this recommendation is often emotionally loaded and should be raised as early as possible and reinforced with clear and open discussions. Patient attitudes about ECT can be influenced by a well-balanced informed consent process that involves close family members and includes frank disclosures about the likelihood of response, the potential for medical and cognitive side effects, the necessity of strict compliance with post-ECT pharmacotherapy or continuation ECT, and the possibility of relapse.

Diagnostic Considerations

The starting point for the recommendation of ECT is careful diagnostic assessment. Current American Psychiatric Association (2001) guidelines recognize three main diagnostic categories in which ECT is indicated: major depression, mania, and schizophrenia.

Major Depression

Nearly 85% of the individuals who receive ECT in the United States have mood disorders (primarily major depression) (Thompson et al. 1994). The evidence for efficacy of ECT in major depression is extensive (Sackeim et al. 1995) and has included uncontrolled case series, controlled comparisons of ECT and medications, trials comparing active ECT with placebo or "sham ECT" (i.e., general anesthesia without the actual passage of current), and trials contrasting different forms of ECT.

In addition to the presence of major depression, diagnostic subtype partially influences the decision to refer a patient for ECT. Specifically, ECT is often considered relatively early in the treatment of melancholic or delusional major depression. There has been some empirical evidence bearing on this practice. However, the uniformly high rates of remission reduce the statistical power to detect clinically meaningful differences. Thus, in terms of melancholic depression, studies have been inconsistent—the presence of melancholic features may or may not confer a greater likelihood of responding to ECT. The data on delusional depression, however, are more consistent. Several early studies indicated that patients with psychotic features were more likely to respond to ECT (Nobler and Sackeim 1996). A multicenter trial has replicated this observation (Petrides et al. 2001). The interpretation of this finding remains open. It may simply be that delusional depression is uniquely responsive to ECT, and at a rate that exceeds that in nondelusional depression. An alternative explanation derives from the finding that patients with documented medication resistance are less likely to respond to ECT than are patients without documented treatment resistance (Prudic et al. 1990). Particularly because antidepressant pharmacotherapy alone is not sufficient treatment for delusional depression (Spiker et al. 1985), many patients with this illness are referred for ECT without ever being shown to be medication resistant. Thus, such patients would be predicted to fare better with ECT than would the nondelusional patients, who have had higher rates of not benefiting sufficiently from adequate medication trials.

Mania

Clinical practice over six decades has indicated that ECT can produce dramatic remission in acute mania and is lifesaving in cases of manic delirium (American Psychiatric Association 2001). However, in contrast to major depression, far less research has been conducted on the efficacy of ECT in acute manic episodes. This is largely because the immediate pharmacological management of mania is generally effective for most patients and because enrolling manic patients in controlled trials is difficult. Nevertheless, retrospective chart reviews and controlled studies of both ECT as first-line treatment and ECT following failure of lithium or neuroleptics have been strikingly positive (Mukherjee et al. 1994). Taken together with the experience of most ECT practitioners, the limited research data support the idea that ECT is extremely useful in the treatment of mania, either as a first-line treatment or in the setting of medication resistance.

Schizophrenia and Related Disorders

ECT was initially introduced as a treatment for psychosis. However, because of early recognition of its antidepressant effects, poor findings in patients with chronic schizophrenia, and then the enthusiastic introduction of antipsychotic medications, ECT use shifted away from primary diagnoses of schizophrenia toward mood disorders. Controlled trials indicated some advantages of ECT, but in general terms, efficacy of monotherapy with ECT was inferior to monotherapy with neuroleptic medications (Fink and Sackeim 1996).

Some clinical features help determine whether a course of ECT is indicated in a patient with schizophrenia. Perhaps most critical is the setting of "first-break" psychosis. Thus, in a young patient in whom the provisional diagnosis may be a schizophreniform disorder but in whom there has been poor response to psychotropic medications, a successful trial of ECT may forestall a lengthy illness (with the attendant possibility of institutionalization). In patients with more definite diagnoses of schizophrenia or schizoaffective disorder, certain clinical features have been associated with a higher likelihood of ECT response, including predominance of positive rather than negative symptoms, clear-cut exacerbation of psychosis, and short duration of episode. Finally, analogous to mood disorders, many patients have treatment-resistant schizophrenia. Although clozapine and the newer atypical antipsychotic medications have offered hope to many patients, some do not respond. ECT is appropriate in this setting as an adjunctive treatment (Hirose et al. 2001). However, the synergistic mechanism between ECT and neuroleptics remains unclear.

Other Diagnostic Indications

In addition to mood disorders and schizophrenia, ECT is useful in the treatment of several syndromes that bridge the gap between psychiatry and neurology. One such illness is catatonia, which for decades has been recognized as uniquely responsive to ECT. Interestingly, catatonia was once viewed primarily as a subtype of schizophrenia but is now considered a syndrome that may segregate with mood disorders or be a manifestation of a variety of medical illnesses. Although the current treatment of choice for catatonia is a benzodiazepine trial, ECT should be strongly considered as the second-line treatment because these patients are at risk for severe medical complications. Perhaps related on a pathophysiological level to catatonia ("malignant catatonia") is neuroleptic malignant syndrome, for which ECT has been reported to be of substantial benefit (Davis et al. 1991).

Among neurological illnesses, Parkinson's disease has received considerable attention as an indication for ECT (Moellentine et al. 1998). Many patients with Parkinson's disease are prone to develop severe depression. In addition, some patients become increasingly resistant to antiparkinsonian medications, leading to psychomotor stupor, whereas others develop psychosis secondary to pharmacological treatment. ECT is often dramatically effective in these clinical situations. Independent of its antidepressant and antipsychotic mechanisms in Parkinson's disease, ECT also benefits the primary motor symptoms of Parkinson's disease (Wengel et al. 1998), presumably via dopaminergic actions. Unfortunately, such benefit can be short-lived.

Aside from Parkinson's disease, other primary neurological indications for ECT are intractable epilepsy and status epilepticus (Lisanby et al. 2001a). The presumptive mechanism of action in this setting is the anticonvulsant properties of ECT, which in several models often exceeded those of anticonvulsant medications. There have been no controlled studies in this area.

Potential Diagnostic Contraindications

To date, there is no convincing evidence that ECT is useful in the treatment of dysthymic disorder, posttraumatic stress disorder (PTSD), generalized anxiety disorder, dissociative disorders, or obsessive-compulsive disorder. Of course, such conditions may be complicated by the presence of an MDE. In this circumstance, judicious use of ECT may be entertained, but patients should clearly understand at the outset that the comorbid Axis I diagnosis is not likely to remit (although some symptoms may improve) and can, in fact, temporarily worsen (especially with PTSD and the dissociative disorders).

Similarly, no evidence indicates that ECT is useful in the treatment of severe personality disorders. However, the field is faced with the dilemma that comorbid Axis II pathology is often diagnosed in many patients with chronic mood disorders. Until recently (Prudic et al. 2004), scant empirical evidence has been available in this area (DeBattista and Mueller 2001). The clinical wisdom has been that a patient with borderline personality disorder may achieve remission from a comorbid MDE, but his or her underlying interpersonal difficulties were likely to remain after the ECT course. In a more conservative scenario, depressive symptoms might remain (as a result of either misdiagnosis of major depression or failure of ECT), and the patient would be left with cognitive side effects. Given the findings of Prudic et al. (2004) suggesting that patients with Axis II disorders are less likely to respond to an acute ECT course, there is an even greater burden on both the referring psychiatrist and the ECT practitioner to consider the benefit to be gained against the risks of potential adverse medical and cognitive consequences.

Other Clinical and Demographic Considerations

In addition to psychiatric diagnosis as a consideration, ECT should be strongly considered in certain clinical situations. Current American Psychiatric Association (2001) guidelines recognize several situations in which ECT should be an initial (primary) form of treatment, including 1) when rapid response is necessary because of the severity of the psychiatric or medical condition; 2) when the risks of ECT are less than those of alternative treatments; 3) when the patient has a history of poor medication response or good ECT response in a prior episode of illness; and 4) when the patient has a preference for ECT. Situations in which ECT should be considered as a secondary treatment (i.e., after medication trials) include 1) medication resistance, 2) intolerance of medications, and 3) deterioration of the patient's condition necessitating rapid response (American Psychiatric Association 2001).

Two of these considerations have been evaluated from a research standpoint. First is the idea that severity of illness should prompt earlier use of ECT. Technically, severity of depression can be distinguished from diagnostic subtype, although, in actuality, patients with melancholic or delusional depression will have higher ratings on depression scales than will nonmelancholic and nondelusional patients. To date, there is no consensus on this topic because there has been evidence of greater initial symptom severity associated with better ECT outcome (Roberts 1959), no difference (Sackeim et al. 1987a), or even poorer outcome (Kindler et al. 1991; Pande et al. 1990). The other clinical indication that has been critically examined is a history of medication resistance. Early retrospective case series had generally supported the advantages of ECT in the setting of failure of antidepressant medication trials, but subsequent reports have indicated that patients with medication resistance are less likely to respond to ECT than are patients who have not received adequate pharmacotherapy prior to ECT (Prudic et al. 1990, 1996). It should be stressed that these findings do not imply that medication-resistant patients should not be referred for ECT. Rather, they can be interpreted to mean that more-difficult-to-treat episodes of depression are just more difficult to treat, regardless of the intervention. Moreover, given the reality that medication resistance is a rapidly growing justification for ECT referral, newer strategies involving longer trials of ECT and use of concurrent medication during and after the ECT course may be required.

Apart from published guidelines, other considerations are duration of illness and age. A well-replicated finding is that a longer index episode of major depression is associated with a poorer ECT outcome (Kindler et al. 1991; Nobler and Sackeim 1996). Indeed, this association may contribute to the relation between medication resistance and poorer ECT outcome (longer duration will necessarily accompany failed medication trials). In terms of patient age, surveys have clearly indicated that use of ECT is greater among the elderly than in any younger age group. Earlier retrospective reports of high rates of efficacy in the elderly have now been confirmed by prospective studies (O'Connor et al. 2001; Tew et al. 1999). Interpretation of this finding may be confounded by higher rates of delusional features in older patients (Petrides et al. 2001); nonetheless, it adds to growing evidence that the neurobiology of major depression in the elderly differs from that in younger patients.

Adverse Events

Medical Considerations: Alterations in the Risk-Benefit Ratio

ECT is a medically safe procedure. This is primarily because of the routine use of general anesthesia, supplemental oxygen, and muscle paralysis. However, more careful health prescreening also has added to the safety of ECT. All patients must undergo an evaluation by an internist prior to treatment, which consists of (at a minimum) a thorough physical examination, laboratory work, chest radiograph, and electrocardiogram. If there is evidence of

poor dentition, a dental consult should be obtained. If there is suspicion of focal neurological findings on examination or a history of neurological disease or symptoms, a screening neuroimaging scan (computed tomography or magnetic resonance imaging) should be considered. All medications should be reviewed, and some classes of compounds, such as anticonvulsants and theophylline preparations, should be discontinued before ECT. Both during the procedure and in the postictal recovery period, blood pressure, pulse, electrocardiogram, and oxygen saturation should be continuously monitored. If all of these guidelines are followed and patients are in good physical health, serious medical complications from ECT are rare, and mortality rates are statistically equivalent to the risks imposed by general anesthesia (Abrams 2002; American Psychiatric Association 2001).

Of course, the above description is the ideal situation. Many patients are referred for ECT precisely because they are frail, have considerable medical comorbidity, and are intolerant of psychotropic medications. Yet even though it is customary to speak of medical contraindications to ECT, it is more appropriate to consider medical conditions that alter the risk-benefit ratio of ECT. Most commonly, these include ischemic heart disease, congestive heart failure, unstable arrhythmia, vascular aneurysm, and intracranial mass lesions (particularly those associated with increased intracranial pressure). If any of these conditions are present, consultation with the appropriate medical specialist should be considered and further tests (e.g., cardiac stress test) may be advised before initiating ECT. Oral medication regimens should be optimized to control hypertension and stabilize cardiac rate and rhythm. In addition, ECT itself may be further modified to reduce risk. For example, it is now fairly routine to pretreat certain patients with intravenous β-blockers to reduce hemodynamic stress. Taken together, strategies to reduce cardiac complications have been generally successful, even in the highest-risk patients (Rice et al. 1994; Welch and Lambertus 1989; Zielinski et al. 1993). Still, on an individualized basis, the potential benefits of ECT must be weighed against the possibility of deleterious side effects. Any discussion of such alterations in the usual risk-benefit ratio should be documented as part of the informed consent process.

Cognitive Side Effects of Electroconvulsive Therapy

General Considerations

Although adverse medical events with ECT are potentially life-threatening, they are fortunately quite rare.

Furthermore, the ECT team usually is aware ahead of time of situations that pose increased medical risk and therefore can be prepared to anticipate such possibilities. The situation with adverse cognitive side effects is opposite on both accounts. First, adverse cognitive outcomes are not rare. In fact, by definition, every patient that undergoes ECT has some cognitive side effect, even if this consists of transient postictal disorientation. Second, other than when a patient has a documented cognitive disorder at baseline (e.g., dementia), we lack any objective sense of which patients are most likely to have worse cognitive outcomes.

Many myths and irrational fears surround this topic. Perhaps the most insidious is the claim that the extent of adverse cognitive effects is related to the efficacy of ECT. In fact, there is no scientific credence to this assertion because there is clearly a double dissociation between cognitive and therapeutic outcomes—patients may achieve remission without substantial memory side effects, and patients may have severe cognitive sequelae without clinical improvement. Another misconception is that ECT reduces intelligence or executive functions. In fact, evidence indicates that measures of intelligence, psychomotor performance, attention, concentration, receptive and expressive language, spatial skills, short-term memory, immediate learning, and other neuropsychological functions either are unchanged by ECT or may even improve. Nonetheless, the cognitive side effects of ECT are a real issue and represent the major factor limiting its use.

Nature of the Adverse Cognitive Effects

The most common and stereotypical cognitive effects of ECT are transient postictal disorientation, retrograde amnesia, and anterograde amnesia. In general, rapid recovery of cognitive function occurs just after the ECT course, with return to baseline by several weeks after treatment. The anterograde amnesia is time limited, and no study contrasting ECT patients and control subjects or forms of ECT has observed anterograde amnesia to persist more than 2–4 weeks (Sackeim 1992). In contrast, the retrograde amnesia may persist for months, and some degree of retrograde amnesia is permanent (McElhiney et al. 1995; Sackeim et al. 2000b; Weiner et al. 1986b). The retrograde amnesia is temporally graded and most dense for events that occurred closest in time to the treatment (Lisanby et al. 2000). These findings are congruent with patient reports long after ECT (Squire and Slater 1983). In rare cases, the retrograde amnesia may be extensive, with gaps in memory extending back years before ECT (American Psychiatric Association 2001). Such patients have been difficult to study in a systematic fashion. Without question, retrograde amnesia is the most

important adverse effect of ECT and the most bothersome to patients (Freeman and Kendell 1986; Prudic et al. 2000).

Factors Influencing Adverse Cognitive Effects

How ECT is performed has a dramatic effect on the severity and persistence of amnestic effects. Relevant factors are electrode placement, electrical waveform (sine wave vs. brief pulse vs. ultrabrief pulse), electrical dose relative to seizure threshold, and spacing of treatments. Sine wave devices are quite toxic, and their use is no longer sanctioned. Otherwise, generally speaking, bilateral ECT, higher stimulus dose, and closely spaced treatments are each associated with more profound cognitive side effects. The effect of such treatment factors is not transitory. For instance, persistent, long-term retrograde amnesia is principally seen only among patients treated with bilateral ECT.

Shortening of pulse width (i.e., moving from brief pulse to ultrabrief pulse) may confer additional safety with respect to adverse cognitive effects. In our work, we have found remarkable effect sizes in several measures of anterograde amnesia and retrograde amnesia when comparing ultrabrief pulse (<0.6 ms) with standard brief-pulse ECT. Moreover, the cognitive savings attributable to ultrabrief ECT were larger than those associated with electrode placement.

Mechanisms of Adverse Cognitive Effects

Despite the extensive neuropsychological literature on the cognitive side effects of ECT, a paucity of research exists on the neurobiological mechanisms of postictal disorientation and amnestic syndromes. Preclinical research has implicated changes in cholinergic neurotransmission as contributory to amnestic side effects (Lerer 1985), but we lack convincing human biochemical data. Our group has documented that increased interictal EEG theta activity in left frontotemporal regions was associated with longer recovery of orientation, and the magnitude of retrograde amnesia for autobiographical events correlated with increased theta activity in left frontotemporal regions (Sackeim et al. 2000a). In part, such preliminary findings challenge the long-held view that disruption in mediotemporal regions exclusively underlies the cognitive side effects of ECT.

Given the possibility of extensive retrograde amnesia following ECT, there is a pressing clinical need to identify predictors of which patients are more likely to develop severe cognitive problems. To our knowledge, the only report that has examined this issue found that both poorer baseline global cognitive function and longer times to reorient immediately following ECT predicted more severe retrograde amnesia for autobiographical information (Sobin et al. 1995).

Strategies to Minimize Adverse Cognitive Effects

There are a few reasonable strategies to minimize cognitive side effects from the outset of ECT. First, during the medical and psychiatric evaluation, special attention should be given to identifying any preexisting cognitive disturbance. Also, careful evaluation of concurrent medications should screen for compounds that might increase side effects, such as lithium or psychotropic medications with excessive anticholinergic activity. Unless there are compelling reasons to the contrary, right-unilateral ECT should be used as the initial treatment modality. If bilateral ECT is used, particular care should be given to the stimulus dose. Finally, if the clinician has an a priori concern about the development of side effects, twice-weekly treatment should be considered.

If cognitive side effects appear to be developing precipitously during the ECT course, strategies similar to those discussed previously may be instituted. For example, slowing down the frequency from three times per week to two times per week is usually helpful. If a patient is responding well to bilateral ECT, either decreasing the stimulus dose or switching to right-unilateral ECT might be considered.

There have also been experimental approaches toward reducing cognitive side effects. For instance, there has been research into the possibility of blocking the cognitive side effects of ECT by pharmacological means (Prudic et al. 1999), although much of this work has not been highly encouraging (Nobler and Sackeim 1993). Another strategy has been to alter the standard bilateral electrode placement to avoid stimulation over temporal lobes (Blumenfeld et al. 2003). Such bifrontal electrode placement has shown some statistical advantages with respect to cognitive side effects (Bailine et al. 2000; Letemendia et al. 1993), but the clinical significance of these findings awaits further study. Finally, it may be possible to target seizures focally with magnetic stimulation, thereby optimizing therapeutic effects and potentially sparing brain regions that mediate side effects. The feasibility of this novel form of convulsive treatment has already been shown (Kosel et al. 2003; Lisanby et al. 2003).

Use With Concurrent Medications

Safety

Patients referred for ECT are likely taking one or more psychotropic medications. Many are also on medication regimens for comorbid medical conditions. It is ultimately the responsibility of the ECT practitioner to review all of these medications and advise the referring clinician as to their

safety. Potentially deleterious medication interactions can be roughly conceptualized as those that might hinder the effectiveness of ECT, such as anticonvulsants (including high-dose benzodiazepines), or those that might cause complications at discrete ECT treatments or during a course of ECT. Examples of the latter include status epilepticus in the setting of theophylline (Devanand et al. 1988) and prolonged seizures or confusional states in the presence of lithium (Penney et al. 1990; Weiner et al. 1980).

Most commonly, patients referred for ECT will be taking one or more antidepressant medications. Aside from monoamine oxidase inhibitors, which are discontinued because of current anesthesia guidelines, most antidepressants are probably safe in combination with ECT (Nobler and Sackeim 1993). Nonetheless, clinicians should remain abreast of the case report literature for potential adverse interactions (Gonzalez-Pinto et al. 2002).

Augmentation

The possibility of optimizing ECT by the use of adjunctive medications dates back almost to its introduction (Bailey 1943) and generally has consisted of strategies to either synergistically enhance the antidepressant effect of ECT (Nobler and Sackeim 1993) or elicit adequate seizures in seizure-resistant patients (Datto et al. 2002). The former category has not yielded any consistently positive findings; however, the proconvulsant effects of caffeine have been successfully exploited at ECT to sustain the length of otherwise inadequate seizures, particularly in elderly male patients (Coffey et al. 1990). Current research is revisiting the feasibility of antidepressant medication concurrent with the ECT course. Such a strategy may possibly enhance ECT, resulting in the need for fewer treatments. More important, perhaps, it may forestall early relapse following response to ECT.

Treatment Considerations

Stimulus Dosing and Electrode Placement

For many clinicians outside of ECT, the technical aspects of treatment remain somewhat mysterious, and even basic variables such as electrode placement and stimulus intensity are considered irrelevant to either efficacy or side effects. For others, there has been a growing awareness of some key concepts, such as the fact that bilateral electrode placement is more likely to result in amnesia. In reality, details about electrical parameters (pulse width, frequency, and stimulus duration) are probably only relevant to ECT practitioners. The following discussion is intended to highlight key concepts that are relevant to all clinicians.

One basic concept is stimulus dose, also referred to as *electrical stimulus intensity*. Each ECT device provides an electrical output. Early devices did not modify the basic continuous sine wave pattern of electricity (sine wave devices) and were inefficient and toxic, exposing patients to far too much electrical stimulation and resulting in severe cognitive side effects (Weiner et al. 1986b). Current devices modify ordinary electrical current, breaking it down into individual pulses in the millisecond range (brief-pulse devices). These devices can deliver a broad range of stimulus dose (generally with 576 millicoulombs [mC] as the upper limit in the United States). But how much is enough, and how much is too much? The answers to these questions remain a subject of debate.

Another basic consideration is electrode placement. Bilateral ECT has consisted of a standard bifrontotemporal electrode placement for several decades, whereas right-unilateral ECT has had several manifestations, with the two electrodes being closely or widely spaced. The generally accepted standard for right-unilateral ECT has become the d'Elia placement, in which one electrode is in the right frontotemporal position and the other is placed just to the right of the vertex. Although it has long been recognized that bilateral ECT results in more cognitive side effects than right-unilateral electrode placement, many practitioners thought that bilateral ECT was more effective than right-unilateral ECT. Some studies supported this belief, but others found right-unilateral ECT to be as effective as bilateral ECT (Sackeim et al. 1995). As research has progressed, we are appreciating a critical interaction between right-unilateral electrode placement and stimulus dose (Abrams et al. 1991; McCall et al. 2000; Sackeim et al. 2000b), which may explain discrepancies in the earlier findings.

A key concept for a fuller understanding of stimulus dose is the seizure threshold, which is the minimum amount of electrical stimulus intensity required to elicit a generalized seizure. Seizure threshold is a biological variable with perhaps a 50-fold range and is dependent on factors such as age and gender (Sackeim et al. 1987b). Given this broad range, when a fixed stimulus dose is used on the ECT device, there is clearly the potential to 1) expose a patient to a stimulus dose far exceeding his or her seizure threshold; or 2) use an insufficient stimulus dose, which may lack efficacy or fail to elicit a seizure in a patient with a high seizure threshold. As mentioned previously, early researchers embraced the notion that as long as a generalized seizure of adequate duration (i.e., lasting at least 20–30 seconds) was elicited at ECT, treatment should be successful, and any increase in stimulus dose (i.e., suprathreshold stimulation) would only cause greater side effects. The latter concept is not without merit, but the former idea has been successfully challenged since

the 1980s. In England, Robin and De Tissera (1982) reported on a comparison of three fixed energy doses of bilateral ECT in a double-blind, random-assignment design. The authors found that patients receiving low-energy pulses continued receiving more ECT treatments until clinical recovery than did patients receiving either of two high-energy modalities. Furthermore, depression scores decreased significantly more slowly in the low-energy pulse group. Taken together, these findings suggested that high-energy ECT was more efficient than low-energy ECT. The authors concluded that because they could produce adequate seizures with low-energy treatments that were also weakly therapeutic and that because seizures produced with higher-energy stimuli were more efficacious than those produced with low-energy stimuli, the electrical stimulus dose was an important factor in determining therapeutic outcome.

A series of studies at Columbia University also has examined the issue of stimulus dose (and electrode placement) in relation to the efficacy of ECT (Sackeim et al. 1987a, 1993, 2000b). In contrast to studies that used fixed energy doses, this research pioneered the use of stimulus dose titration to determine each patient's seizure threshold. The protocols also involved random assignment of patients to stimulus doses at specific increases over the threshold. The first study assumed that right-unilateral ECT at a dose just above seizure threshold would be as effective as bilateral ECT given at a stimulus dose similarly just above threshold but with far fewer cognitive side effects. Although the latter was confirmed, the efficacy data were quite surprising and disappointing—only 28% of the patients receiving low-dose, right-unilateral ECT met criteria for clinical response, compared with a 70% response rate for patients receiving low-dose, bilateral ECT. Thus, adequate generalized seizures were elicited with right-unilateral ECT, but they clearly lacked efficacy. This line of inquiry was replicated and extended, with an indication that a dose–response relation exists for right-unilateral ECT whereby doses must be at least six times the seizure threshold for efficacy to match that of bilateral ECT, while still retaining advantages with respect to cognitive side effects (Sackeim et al. 2000b). Other work has suggested that the dose–response relation for right-unilateral ECT may extend up to 8–12 times the seizure threshold but that cognitive side effects may increase to unwanted levels at the high end of stimulus dosing (McCall et al. 2000).

The role of stimulus intensity in affecting the speed of response to ECT is still not completely clear. We have found that a higher stimulus dose led to more rapid recovery (i.e., fewer treatments were required) regardless of electrode placement (Sackeim et al. 1993). However, a detailed examination of pooled data indicated that the choice of statistical method used in the analysis of speed of improvement strongly influenced whether treatment differences were obtained as well as the nature of the observed effects (Nobler et al. 1997).

Frequency of Treatment

A third variable in treatment is the weekly frequency. The two most common regimens are two or three times per week. The available evidence is that slowing the frequency to two times per week may delay speed of improvement, but the same end point will be reached. The potential advantage of twice-weekly ECT is decreased cognitive side effects.

Number of Treatments: How Much Electroconvulsive Therapy Is Enough?

The typical range of treatments to achieve remission of an MDE is 6–12 treatments. However, there is no way to predict how many treatments an individual will need. In fact, among patients who are beginning to show symptomatic improvement, premature termination of the treatment course may undermine sustained clinical response and ultimately contribute to early relapse. At the same time, this must be balanced against administering "extra" ECT (i.e., treating beyond the point at which full remission has been achieved), a practice for which no empirical support exists.

Determining what constitutes an adequate trial of ECT for the patient who is not responding is a matter of some debate. Most practitioners will consider switching a patient from right-unilateral to bilateral ECT if there has been only minimal improvement by 6 to 8 treatments. This may not be long enough because with moderate-dose, right-unilateral ECT, full remission may not be achieved until 12 or more treatments. However, clinical urgency may justify a prompt modality switch. A more conservative approach would be to increase the stimulus dose of right-unilateral ECT before switching to bilateral placement. An adequate trial of bilateral ECT probably consists of 10 treatments. For some patients with treatment-resistant depression, that may not even be enough (Sackeim et al. 2000b).

Ending a Course of Electroconvulsive Therapy

A central irony in the field of ECT is that it is probably the only treatment in psychiatry that is stopped just as the patient has shown maximal benefit. Of course, there are numerous reasons for this fact. However, from a mechanisms point of view, it poses a difficult scenario. Even if post-ECT pharmacotherapy is begun during the acute course, common clinical experience is that many patients will relapse during the first 2 weeks after their final ECT treatment. In addition, there are theoretical reasons that ECT should not be stopped abruptly (analogous to abrupt discontinuation of effective psychotropic or anticonvulsant medications). Thus, in our clinical practice, we have instituted the notion of an ECT taper period. This allows both for consolidation of maximal ECT benefits and for further time for antidepressant medications to achieve steady-state plasma levels. Such a practice has not yet received research attention.

Maintenance and Continuation

Most patients are started on antidepressant medications following a successful course of ECT. Relapse rates are otherwise not acceptable. For many decades, few empirical data were available to inform the choice of post-ECT pharmacotherapy. Indeed, it was common practice to readminister the same medication that was ineffective during the index episode. This area was reexamined by Sackeim and colleagues (2001). In a multicenter, double-blind, placebo-controlled trial, 84 patients with unipolar major depression who fully remitted with ECT were randomly assigned to receive continuation treatment for 24 weeks with placebo, nortriptyline (target steady-state level=75–125 ng/mL), or combination nortriptyline and lithium (target steady-state level=0.5–0.9 mEq/L). With relapse of MDE as the main outcome measure, nortriptyline-lithium combination therapy had a marked advantage, superior both to placebo and to nortriptyline alone. The relapse rate was 84% for placebo, 60% for nortriptyline, and 39% for nortriptyline-lithium. All but one instance of relapse with nortriptyline-lithium occurred within 5 weeks of ECT termination, whereas relapse continued throughout treatment with placebo or nortriptyline alone. Patients with medication-resistant depression, female patients, and those with more severe depressive symptoms following ECT had more rapid relapse. The findings indicated that without active treatment, virtually all remitted patients relapsed within 6 months of stopping ECT and that monotherapy with nortriptyline had limited efficacy. The combination of nortriptyline and lithium was more effective, but the relapse rate was still high, particularly during the first month of continuation therapy.

A double-blind, placebo-controlled, multicenter trial is currently under way in which antidepressant medication (nortriptyline or venlafaxine) is begun at the outset of the ECT course, with the addition of lithium (or placebo) following clinical response. This study will address issues of augmenting ECT as well as optimal pharmacological strategies to prevent relapse.

Some patients either cannot tolerate medications or relapse after ECT despite adequate continuation pharmacotherapy. For these select patients, continuation ECT and maintenance ECT, respectively, represent viable short- or longer-term treatment options to forestall relapse (American Psychiatric Association 2001). In theory, maintenance ECT also may be prophylactic against recurrent episodes of major depression. There has been a long clinical tradition incorporating this practice, even though most of the supporting evidence has been anecdotal or from retrospective case series (Monroe 1991). The feasibility of randomly assigning patients to either continuation pharmacotherapy or continuation ECT via informed consent in research is difficult, and comparing continuation ECT with an inactive treatment condition (e.g., placebo) raises ethical concerns. Also, an inevitable confound is that patients would not be blinded as to whether they had received continuation ECT. Nonetheless, the clinical practice of both continuation ECT and maintenance ECT is likely increasing, so solid empirical data as to the relative superiority of further ECT compared with pharmacotherapy are sorely needed. A multicenter, NIMH-supported trial (see O'Connor et al. 2001) was recently completed in which ECT responders were randomly assigned to receive either continuation ECT or a nortriptyline-lithium combination. We hope that studies of this nature will also provide insights into which patients are more likely to benefit from continuation ECT than from medications alone, as well as explore the longer-term cognitive consequences of continuation ECT.

Transcranial Magnetic Stimulation

History and Discovery

It has been 20 years since the demonstration that a strong, pulsed magnetic field delivered adjacent to the head can induce an electrical current in the underlying tissue and thereby depolarize neurons (Barker et al. 1985). This procedure, known as *transcranial magnetic stimulation* (TMS), was originally used as a diagnostic tool within clinical neurophysiology. Subsequently, the technique was modified with increased pulse frequency and was referred to as rTMS. Early on, interest grew in the potential therapeutic applications of rTMS in neuropsychiatry, including major depression (George et al. 1995). In part, this interest derived from early observations that even single-pulse magnetic stimulation transiently elevated mood in healthy control subjects (Bickford et al. 1987) and later findings that higher-frequency rTMS led to sustained excitation of cortical neurons (Pascual-Leone et al. 1993).

At the same time, it was recognized that rTMS provides a subconvulsive form of stimulation, but at higher frequencies, it could (unintentionally) provoke generalized seizures in susceptible individuals (Pascual-Leone et al. 1993). This discovery led to an early theoretical debate over the ultimate usefulness of rTMS as a subconvulsive antidepressant therapy compared with the eventual development of magnetic stimulation as a convulsive treatment and potential alternative to ECT (George and Wassermann 1994; Sackeim 1994). Since then, both lines of investigation have proceeded.

Mechanisms of Action

For the most part, the recognition that rTMS has antidepressant effects has followed a long tradition of serendipity in clinical medicine. However, there has been a multifaceted effort to explicate how cortical excitation (or inhibition) with rTMS might be therapeutic in major depression. This effort has encompassed animal studies of neurotransmitter function (Ben-Shachar et al. 1997), immediate early gene induction (Ji et al. 1998), neuronal inhibitory effects (Chen et al. 1997), neuronal excitatory effects (Wu et al. 2000), and possible anticonvulsant effects (Ebert and Ziemann 1999).

Some studies in human volunteers indicated that rTMS could produce alterations in mood (George et al. 1996), which lent further credence to its potential role as an antidepressant treatment. However, this work has not always been replicated (Mosimann et al. 2000). Other work in both nondepressed volunteers and patients with depression has used neuroimaging to understand both local (i.e., regions under the coil) and more distant effects of rTMS on cerebral functioning (Kimbrell et al. 2002; Loo et al. 2003; Nahas et al. 2001; Speer et al. 2003; Teneback et al. 1999). It is too early to draw definitive conclusions from these studies; however, effects on rCBF and rCMR appear to be dependent on both the frequency and the intensity of rTMS, and reciprocal changes have been detected, even at remote ipsilateral and contralateral brain regions. As with ECT neuroimaging research, studies of this type should help shed light on treatment mechanisms, as well as further clarify the pathophysiological disturbances in major depression. Ultimately, they also may help identify important similarities and differences between the actions of rTMS and ECT.

Coil Placement and Stimulus Intensity

Because rTMS is a relatively new and rapidly evolving form of treatment, certain fundamental variables are still being actively investigated. Central among these are coil geometry, optimal sites of coil placement, and stimulation parameters (including intensity, frequency, train duration, and intertrain interval). The two leading sites for coil placement are left and right dorsolateral prefrontal cortex. To some extent, these locations correspond to brain regions implicated in the pathophysiology of major depression. However, physical limitations have constrained the choice of sites for coil placement. Stimulus intensity is usually expressed as a percentage relative to the motor threshold, which is the lowest amount of energy required to elicit movement in a distal hand muscle. Aside from the repeated observation that high-frequency (5–20 Hz) rTMS appears to be necessary with left prefrontal stimulation and low-frequency (1 Hz) rTMS with right prefrontal stimulation, optimal frequencies have not been identified, and there are safety limitations (Wassermann and Lisanby 2001). Similarly, many of the other treatment parameters have not yet been studied in a systematic fashion. Moreover, in addition to these technical factors, little is known as to what constitutes an optimal treatment regimen with rTMS. Is once daily the most appropriate spacing of treatment sessions, and, if so, for how many days or weeks?

Ultimately, a consensus needs to be reached as to definitions of an adequate trial of rTMS and what constitutes rTMS resistance. From a research perspective, it is important to agree on the minimal and maximal number of rTMS sessions a patient may have had in the past and still be eligible to participate in an rTMS trial. In addition, from an ethical standpoint, stringent guidelines are needed for the maximal number of treatment sessions before considering a patient as a nonresponder to rTMS. Such definitions of rTMS resistance should protect patients from being reexposed to a treatment that has been ineffective for them.

Efficacy and Indications

Major Depressive Disorder

At the time of this writing, rTMS is not a U.S. Food and Drug Administration–approved treatment in the United States. Most of the research evidence has been in populations of patients with major depression (Fitzgerald et al. 2003; George et al. 1995; Klein et al. 1999; Pascual-Leone et al. 1996). Several meta-analyses of the published trials have been done (Burt et al. 2002; Gershon et al. 2003; Martin et al. 2003; Schlaepfer et al. 2003; Wassermann and Lisanby 2001), with varying conclusions as to the strength of the findings and whether statistical significance can be equated with clinical significance. With respect to diagnostic subtype, investigators have suggested that patients with psychotic features are less likely to respond to rTMS. Overall, a moderate position at this time is that some antidepressant efficacy of rTMS has been reported but that

consistent findings across studies have been hampered by issues common to many clinical trials, such as adequate randomization, sufficient sample sizes, variability in outcome measures, and length of follow-up.

Some difficulties unique to rTMS clinical trials research also have been a source of discrepant findings. Perhaps most fundamental is the question of a controlled trial. In some ways, sham-controlled ECT studies are easier to carry out than sham-controlled rTMS studies because ECT requires general anesthesia, and patients are therefore unaware of whether they receive active ECT or sham. With rTMS, patients are fully awake, and, ideally, sham treatment consists of delivering pulses that do not stimulate the cortex. It turns out that this is a difficult task, partly dependent on factors such as the angle at which the coil is held away from the head (Lisanby et al. 2001b; Loo et al. 2000). Thus, some studies that were designed as sham-controlled likely had some activity within sham condition, potentially confounding the results. Even if a sham coil placement can be perfected, there may always be a potential confound of an enhanced placebo response to rTMS, given the drama of the treatment setting (Kaptchuk et al. 2000). Thus, it may be difficult, but not impossible, to keep patients blinded to treatment condition. However, the physician who administers rTMS cannot be blinded. To maintain blinding for research, clinical raters are kept unaware of real versus sham condition. This situation is even more difficult if rTMS is compared with another form of treatment, such as ECT or medications, in which side effects may be obvious to external raters.

A second fundamental issue in rTMS research is the accuracy of coil placement in the active treatment conditions because variability may affect efficacy. Thus, although a rule-based algorithm has commonly been used to stimulate over the left dorsolateral prefrontal cortex, magnetic resonance imaging studies of coil position indicate considerable variability. In addition, differences in patients' head size and shape affect coil position, and advancing patient age with associated cortical atrophy also may mitigate accurate placement. New methods are under way to develop more precise positioning based on functional neuroimaging.

Other Psychiatric Disorders

Aside from mood disorders, there have been some preliminary reports that right prefrontal rTMS may reduce compulsions in patients with obsessive-compulsive disorder. Also of interest are both case reports and initial controlled studies that used 1-Hz rTMS stimulation over the left temporoparietal cortex to reduce successfully the frequency and intensity of auditory hallucinations in patients with treatment-resistant schizophrenia.

Adverse Events and Drug Interactions

The most common side effects of rTMS are minor and consist of discomfort resulting from stimulation of scalp and facial muscles and headache. The most potentially serious adverse event is elicitation of generalized seizures, but this risk is minimal if appropriate screening is used. Unlike ECT, rTMS does not appear to result in amnestic syndromes (Martis et al. 2003). Thus, rTMS has major advantages compared with ECT in terms of adverse effects. It also may have side-effect advantages with respect to antidepressant medications. However, these must be weighed against the uniqueness of the treatment delivery because rTMS cannot be self-administered, requires frequent visits to a hospital or clinic, and has an unknown long-term cost burden. Finally, very little is known about potential drug interactions. In theory, analogous to ECT, there may be issues of both safety and efficacy in patients taking medications with either proconvulsant or anticonvulsant activity.

Magnetic Seizure Therapy

The recognition that rTMS can elicit seizures, either unintentionally or intentionally, raises the question as to the feasibility and potential therapeutic efficacy of deliberate seizure induction in patients under general anesthesia (magnetic seizure therapy). In many ways, the ability to spatially target the magnetic field with rTMS provides greater control over current paths and current density in the brain, overcoming some of the physical limitations of ECT and possibly minimizing adverse cognitive effects. A preliminary within-subjects trial already has shown the feasibility of magnetic seizure therapy and has found that many fewer cognitive side effects occurred compared with those caused by ECT (Lisanby et al. 2003). Further studies are well under way and will begin to address issues of efficacy more closely.

References

Abrams R: Electroconvulsive Therapy. New York, Oxford University Press, 2002

Abrams R, Taylor MA: Diencephalic stimulation and the effects of ECT in endogenous depression. Br J Psychiatry 129:482–485, 1976

Abrams R, Swartz CM, Vedak C: Antidepressant effects of high-dose right unilateral electroconvulsive therapy. Arch Gen Psychiatry 48:746–748, 1991

Ackermann R, Engel JJ, Baxter L: Positron emission tomography and autoradiographic studies of glucose utilization following electroconvulsive seizures in humans and rats. Ann N Y Acad Sci 462:263–269, 1986

American Psychiatric Association: The Practice of ECT: Recommendations for Treatment, Training and Privileging. Washington, DC, American Psychiatric Press, 1990

American Psychiatric Association: The Practice of ECT: Recommendations for Treatment, Training and Privileging, 2nd Edition. Washington, DC, American Psychiatric Publishing, 2001

American Psychiatric Association Task Force on ECT: Electroconvulsive Therapy, Task Force Report #14. Washington, DC, American Psychiatric Association, 1978

Apëria B, Bergman H, Engelbrektson K, et al: Effects of electroconvulsive therapy on neuropsychological function and circulating levels of ACTH, cortisol, prolactin, and TSH in patients with major depressive illness. Acta Psychiatr Scand 72:536–541, 1985

Bailey KC: Use of amphetamine sulphas in facilitating electrically induced convulsions. BMJ 1:250–252, 1943

Bailine SH, Rifkin A, Kayne E, et al: Comparison of bifrontal and bitemporal ECT for major depression. Am J Psychiatry 157:121–123, 2000

Barker AT, Jalinous R, Freeston IL: Non-invasive magnetic stimulation of human motor cortex. Lancet 1:1106–1107, 1985

Ben-Shachar D, Belmaker RH, Grisaru N, et al: Transcranial magnetic stimulation induces alterations in brain monoamines. J Neural Transm 104:191–197, 1997

Bickford RG, Guidi M, Fortesque P, et al: Magnetic stimulation of human peripheral nerve and brain: response enhancement by combined magnetoelectrical technique. Neurosurgery 20:110–116, 1987

Blaine J, Clark S: Report of the NIMH-NIH Consensus Development Conference on Electroconvulsive Therapy—statement of the Consensus Development Panel. Psychopharmacol Bull 22:445–454, 1986

Blumenfeld H, McNally KA, Ostroff RB, et al: Targeted prefrontal cortical activation with bifrontal ECT. Psychiatry Res 123:165–170, 2003

Bonne O, Krausz Y, Shapira B, et al: Increased cerebral blood flow in depressed patients responding to electroconvulsive therapy. J Nucl Med 37:1075–1080, 1996

Breggin PR: Electroshock: Its Brain-Disabling Effects. New York, Springer, 1979

Burt T, Lisanby SH, Sackeim HA: Neuropsychiatric applications of transcranial magnetic stimulation: a meta analysis. Int J Neuropsychopharmacol 5:73–103, 2002

Chen R, Classen J, Gerloff C, et al: Depression of motor cortex excitability by low-frequency transcranial magnetic stimulation. Neurology 48:1398–1403, 1997

Coffey CE, Figiel GS, Weiner RD, et al: Caffeine augmentation of ECT. Am J Psychiatry 147:579–585, 1990

Coffey CE, Weiner RD, Djang WT, et al: Brain anatomic effects of electroconvulsive therapy: a prospective magnetic resonance imaging study. Arch Gen Psychiatry 48:1013–1021, 1991

d'Elia G, Perris C: Seizure and post-seizure electroencephalographic pattern. Acta Psychiatr Scand 215:9–29, 1970

Datto C, Rai AK, Ilivicky HJ, et al: Augmentation of seizure induction in electroconvulsive therapy: a clinical reappraisal. J ECT 18:118–125, 2002

Davis JM, Janicak PG, Sakkas P, et al: Electroconvulsive therapy in the treatment of the neuroleptic malignant syndrome. Convuls Ther 7:111–120, 1991

DeBattista C, Mueller K: Is electroconvulsive therapy effective for the depressed patient with comorbid borderline personality disorder? J ECT 17:91–98, 2001

Devanand DP, Decina P, Sackeim HA, et al: Status epilepticus following ECT in a patient receiving theophylline (letter). J Clin Psychopharmacol 8:153, 1988

Ebert U, Ziemann U: Altered seizure susceptibility after high-frequency transcranial magnetic stimulation in rats. Neurosci Lett 273:155–158, 1999

Endler N: Holiday of Darkness: A Psychologist's Journey out of His Depression, Revised Edition. Toronto, Ontario, Wall & Thompson, 1990

Fink M, Kahn RL: Relation of electroencephalographic delta activity to behavioral response in electroshock: quantitative serial studies. Arch Neurol Psychiatry 78:516–525, 1957

Fink M, Ottosson JO: A theory of convulsive therapy in endogenous depression: significance of hypothalamic functions. Psychiatry Res 2:49–61, 1980

Fink M, Sackeim HA: Convulsive therapy in schizophrenia? Schizophr Bull 22:27–39, 1996

Fitzgerald PB, Brown TL, Marston NA, et al: Transcranial magnetic stimulation in the treatment of depression: a double-blind, placebo-controlled trial. Arch Gen Psychiatry 60:1002–1008, 2003

Fochtmann LJ: Animal studies of electroconvulsive therapy: foundations for future research. Psychopharmacol Bull 30:321–444, 1994

Freeman C, Kendell R: Patients' experiences of and attitudes to electroconvulsive therapy. Ann N Y Acad Sci 462:341–352, 1986

George MS, Wassermann EM: Rapid-rate transcranial magnetic stimulation and ECT. Convuls Ther 10:251–254, 1994

George MS, Wassermann EM, Williams WA, et al: Daily repetitive transcranial magnetic stimulation (rTMS) improves mood in depression. Neuroreport 6:1853–1856, 1995

George MS, Wassermann EM, Williams WA, et al: Changes in mood and hormone levels after rapid-rate transcranial magnetic stimulation (rTMS) of the prefrontal cortex. J Neuropsychiatry Clin Neurosci 8:172–180, 1996

Gershon AA, Dannon PN, Grunhaus L: Transcranial magnetic stimulation in the treatment of depression. Am J Psychiatry 160:835–845, 2003

Glue P, Costello MJ, Pert A, et al: Regional neurotransmitter responses after acute and chronic electroconvulsive shock. Psychopharmacology (Berl) 100:60–65, 1990

Gonzalez-Pinto A, Gutierrez M, Gonzalez N, et al: Efficacy and safety of venlafaxine-ECT combination in treatment-resistant depression. J Neuropsychiatry Clin Neurosci 14:206–209, 2002

Green AR, Heal DJ, Goodwin GM: The effects of electroconvulsive therapy and antidepressant drugs on monoamine receptors in rodent brain—similarities and differences. Ciba Found Symp 123:246–267, 1986

Henry ME, Schmidt ME, Matochik JA, et al: The effects of ECT on brain glucose: a pilot FDG PET study. J ECT 17:33–40, 2001

Hirose S, Ashby CRJ, Mills MJ: Effectiveness of ECT combined with risperidone against aggression in schizophrenia. J ECT 17:22–26, 2001

Ingvar M: Cerebral blood flow and metabolic rate during seizures: relationship to epileptic brain damage. Ann N Y Acad Sci 462:194–206, 1986

Ji RR, Schlaepfer TE, Aizenman CD, et al: Repetitive transcranial magnetic stimulation activates specific regions in rat brain. Proc Natl Acad Sci U S A 95:15635–15640, 1998

Kalinowsky L: History of convulsive therapy. Ann N Y Acad Sci 462:1–4, 1986

Kaplan JA, Liberson WT, Sherer IW, et al: Correlations of EEG and psychological findings during intensive brief stimulus therapy. Confin Neurol 16:116–125, 1956

Kaptchuk TJ, Goldman P, Stone DA, et al: Do medical devices have enhanced placebo effects? J Clin Epidemiol 53:786–792, 2000

Kellar K: Effects of electroconvulsive shock on noradrenergic and serotonergic receptors in rat brain. Pharmacopsychiatry 20:30–34, 1987

Kellar K, Cascio C, Bergstrom D, et al: Electroconvulsive shock and reserpine: effects on beta-adrenergic receptors in rat brain. J Neurochem 37:830–836, 1981a

Kellar K, Cascio C, Butler J, et al: Differential effects of electroconvulsive shock and antidepressant drugs on serotonin-2 receptors in rat brain. Eur J Pharmacol 69:515–518, 1981b

Kety SS, Woodford RB, Harmel MH, et al: Cerebral blood flow and metabolism in schizophrenia. Am J Psychiatry 104:765–770, 1948

Kimbrell TA, Dunn RT, George MS, et al: Left prefrontal-repetitive transcranial magnetic stimulation (rTMS) and regional cerebral glucose metabolism in normal volunteers. Psychiatry Res 115:101–113, 2002

Kindler S, Shapira B, Hadjez J, et al: Factors influencing response to bilateral electroconvulsive therapy in major depression. Convuls Ther 7:245–254, 1991

Klein E, Kreinin I, Chistyakov A, et al: Therapeutic efficacy of right prefrontal slow repetitive transcranial magnetic stimulation in major depression: a double-blind controlled study. Arch Gen Psychiatry 56:315–320, 1999

Kosel M, Frick C, Lisanby SH, et al: Magnetic seizure therapy improves mood in refractory major depression. Neuropsychopharmacology 28:2045–2048, 2003

Kronfol Z, Hamdan-Allen G, Goel K, et al: Effects of single and repeated electroconvulsive therapy sessions on plasma ACTH, prolactin, growth hormone and cortisol concentrations. Psychoneuroendocrinology 16:345–352, 1991

Krystal AD, Weiner RD, McCall WV, et al: The effect of ECT stimulus dose and electrode placement on the ictal electroencephalogram: an intraindividual crossover study. Biol Psychiatry 34:759–767, 1993

Krystal AD, Holsinger T, Weiner RD, et al: Prediction of the utility of a switch from unilateral to bilateral ECT in the elderly using treatment 2 ictal EEG indices. J ECT 16:327–337, 2000

Lancaster NP, Steinert RR, Frost I: Unilateral electroconvulsive therapy. J Ment Sci 104:221–227, 1958

Lerer B: Studies on the role of brain cholinergic systems in the therapeutic mechanisms and adverse effects of ECT and lithium. Biol Psychiatry 20:20–40, 1985

Lerer B, Weiner RD, Belmaker RH: ECT: Basic Mechanisms. Washington, DC, American Psychiatric Press, 1986

Letemendia FJ, Delva NJ, Rodenburg M, et al: Therapeutic advantage of bifrontal electrode placement in ECT. Psychol Med 23:349–360, 1993

Lisanby SH, Devanand DP, Prudic J, et al: Prolactin response to electroconvulsive therapy: effects of electrode placement and stimulus dosage. Biol Psychiatry 43:146–155, 1998

Lisanby SH, Maddox JH, Prudic J, et al: The effects of electroconvulsive therapy on memory of autobiographical and public events Arch Gen Psychiatry 57:581–590, 2000

Lisanby SH, Bazil CW, Resor SR, et al: ECT in the treatment of status epilepticus. J ECT 17:210–215, 2001a

Lisanby SH, Gutman D, Luber B, et al: Sham TMS: intracerebral measurement of the induced electrical field and the induction of motor-evoked potentials. Biol Psychiatry 49:460–463, 2001b

Lisanby SH, Luber B, Schlaepfer TE, et al: Safety and feasibility of magnetic seizure therapy (MST) in major depression: randomized within-subject comparison with electroconvulsive therapy. Neuropsychopharmacology 28:1852–1865, 2003

Loo CK, Taylor JL, Gandevia SC, et al: Transcranial magnetic stimulation (TMS) in controlled treatment studies: are some "sham" forms active? Biol Psychiatry 47:325–331, 2000

Loo CK, Sachdev PS, Haindl W, et al: High (15 Hz) and low (1 Hz) frequency transcranial magnetic stimulation have different acute effects on regional cerebral blood flow in depressed patients. Psychol Med 33:997–1006, 2003

Luber B, Nobler MS, Moeller JR, et al: Quantitative EEG during seizures induced by electroconvulsive therapy: relations to treatment modality and clinical features, II: topographic analyses. J ECT 16:229–243, 2000

Madsen TM, Treschow A, Bengzon J, et al: Increased neurogenesis in a model of electroconvulsive therapy. Biol Psychiatry 47:1043–1049, 2000

Mann JJ: Neurobiological correlates of the antidepressant action of electroconvulsive therapy. J ECT 14:172–180, 1998

Mann JJ, Kapur S: Elucidation of biochemical basis of the antidepressant action of electroconvulsive therapy by human studies. Psychopharmacol Bull 30:445–453, 1994

Manning M: Undercurrents: A Therapist's Reckoning with Depression. San Francisco, CA, Harper, 1995

Martin JL, Barbanoj MJ, Schlaepfer TE, et al: Repetitive transcranial magnetic stimulation for the treatment of depression: systematic review and meta-analysis. Br J Psychiatry 182:480–491, 2003

Martis B, Alam D, Dowd SM, et al: Neurocognitive effects of repetitive transcranial magnetic stimulation in severe major depression. Clin Neurophysiol 114:1125–1132, 2003

McCall WV, Weiner RD, Carroll BJ, et al: Serum prolactin, electrode placement, and the convulsive threshold during ECT. Convuls Ther 12:81–85, 1996

McCall WV, Reboussin DM, Weiner RD, et al: Titrated moderately suprathreshold vs fixed high-dose right unilateral electroconvulsive therapy: acute antidepressant and cognitive effects. Arch Gen Psychiatry 57:438–444, 2000

McElhiney MC, Moody BJ, Steif BL, et al: Autobiographical memory and mood: effects of electroconvulsive therapy. Neuropsychology 9:501–517, 1995

Meduna LJ: Versuche über die biologische Beeinflussung des Abaufes der Schizophrenie, I: Campher und Cardiozolkrämpfe [Experiments regarding the biological influences on the progression of schizophrenia, I: camphor and cardiazol]. Z Neurol Psychr 152:235–262, 1935

Moellentine C, Rummans T, Ahlskog JE, et al: Effectiveness of ECT in patients with parkinsonism. J Neuropsychiatry Clin Neurosci 10:187–193, 1998

Monroe RRJ: Maintenance electroconvulsive therapy. Psychiatr Clin North Am 14:947–960, 1991

Mosimann UP, Rihs TA, Engeler J, et al: Mood effects of repetitive transcranial magnetic stimulation of left prefrontal cortex in healthy volunteers. Psychiatry Res 94:251–256, 2000

Mukherjee S, Sackeim HA, Schnur DB: Electroconvulsive therapy of acute manic episodes: a review of 50 years' experience. Am J Psychiatry 151:169–176, 1994

Nahas Z, Lomarev M, Roberts DR, et al: Unilateral left prefrontal transcranial magnetic stimulation (TMS) produces intensity-dependent bilateral effects as measured by interleaved BOLD fMRI. Biol Psychiatry 50:712–720, 2001

Newman ME, Gur E, Shapira B, et al: Neurochemical mechanisms of action of ECS: evidence from in vivo studies. J ECT 14:153–171, 1998

Nobler MS, Sackeim HA: Augmentation strategies in electroconvulsive therapy: a synthesis. Convuls Ther 9:331–351, 1993

Nobler MS, Sackeim HA: Electroconvulsive therapy: clinical and biological aspects, in Predictors of Response in Mood Disorders. Edited by Goodnick PJ. Washington, DC, American Psychiatric Press, 1996, pp 177–198

Nobler MS, Sackeim HA, Solomou M, et al: EEG manifestations during ECT: effects of electrode placement and stimulus intensity. Biol Psychiatry 34:321–330, 1993

Nobler MS, Sackeim HA, Prohovnik I, et al: Regional cerebral blood flow in mood disorders, III: treatment and clinical response. Arch Gen Psychiatry 51:884–897, 1994

Nobler MS, Sackeim HA, Moeller JR, et al: Quantifying the speed of symptomatic improvement with electroconvulsive therapy: comparison of alternative statistical methods. Convuls Ther 13:208–221, 1997

Nobler MS, Luber B, Moeller JR, et al: Quantitative EEG during seizures induced by electroconvulsive therapy: relations to treatment modality and clinical features, I: global analyses. J ECT 16:211–228, 2000a

Nobler MS, Teneback CC, Nahas Z, et al: Structural and functional neuroimaging of electroconvulsive therapy and transcranial magnetic stimulation. Depress Anxiety 12:144–156, 2000b

Nobler MS, Oquendo MA, Kegeles LS, et al: Decreased regional brain metabolism after ECT. Am J Psychiatry 158:305–308, 2001

Nutt DJ, Gleiter CH, Glue P: Neuropharmacological aspects of ECT: in search of the primary mechanism of action. Convuls Ther 5:250–260, 1989

O'Connor MK, Knapp R, Husain M, et al: The influence of age on the response of major depression to electroconvulsive therapy: a C.O.R.E. report. Am J Geriatr Psychiatry 9:382–390, 2001

Ottosson J-O: Seizure characteristics and therapeutic efficiency in electroconvulsive therapy: an analysis of the antidepressive efficiency of grand mal and lidocaine-modified seizures. J Nerv Ment Dis 135:239–251, 1962

Pacella BL, Barrera SE, Kalinowsky L: Variations in electroencephalogram associated with electric shock therapy of patients with mental disorders. Arch Neurol Psychiatry 47:367–384, 1942

Pande AC, Grunhaus LJ, Haskett RF, et al: Electroconvulsive therapy in delusional and non-delusional depressive disorder. J Affect Disord 19:215–219, 1990

Pascual-Leone A, Houser CM, Reese K, et al: Safety of rapid-rate transcranial magnetic stimulation in normal volunteers. Electroencephalogr Clin Neurophysiol 89:120–130, 1993

Pascual-Leone A, Rubio B, Pallardo F, et al: Rapid-rate transcranial magnetic stimulation of left dorsolateral prefrontal cortex in drug-resistant depression. Lancet 348:233–237, 1996

Penney JF, Dinwiddie SH, Zorumski CF, et al: Concurrent and close temporal administration of lithium and ECT. Convuls Ther 6:139–145, 1990

Perera TD, Luber B, Nobler MS, et al: Seizure expression during electroconvulsive therapy: relationships with clinical outcome and cognitive side effects. Neuropsychopharmacology 29:813–825, 2004

Petrides G, Fink M, Husain MM, et al: ECT remission rates in psychotic versus nonpsychotic depressed patients: a report from CORE. J ECT 17:244–253, 2001

Post RM, Putnam F, Uhde TW, et al: Electroconvulsive therapy as an anticonvulsant: implications for its mechanism of action in affective illness. Ann N Y Acad Sci 462:376–388, 1986

Potter WZ, Rudorfer MV: Electroconvulsive therapy—a modern medical procedure. N Engl J Med 328:882–883, 1993

Prudic J, Sackeim HA, Devanand DP: Medication resistance and clinical response to electroconvulsive therapy. Psychiatry Res 31:287–296, 1990

Prudic J, Haskett RF, Mulsant B, et al: Resistance to antidepressant medications and short-term clinical response to ECT. Am J Psychiatry 153:985–992, 1996

Prudic J, Fitzsimons L, Nobler MS, et al: Naloxone in the prevention of the adverse cognitive effects of ECT: a within-subject, placebo controlled study. Neuropsychopharmacology 21:285–293, 1999

Prudic J, Peyser S, Sackeim HA: Subjective memory complaints: a review of patient self-assessment of memory after electroconvulsive therapy. J ECT 16:121–132, 2000

Prudic J, Olfson M, Marcus SC, et al: Effectiveness of electroconvulsive therapy in community settings. Biol Psychiatry 55:301–312, 2004

Rice EH, Sombrotto LB, Markowitz JC, et al: Cardiovascular morbidity in high-risk patients during ECT. Am J Psychiatry 151:1637–1641, 1994

Roberts JM: Prognostic factors in the electroshock treatment of depressive states: (1) clinical features from testing and examination. J Ment Sci 105:693–702, 1959

Robin A, De Tissera S: A double-blind controlled comparison of the therapeutic effects of low and high energy electroconvulsive therapies. Br J Psychiatry 141:357–366, 1982

Rudorfer MV, Risby ED, Hsiao JK, et al: Disparate biochemical actions of electroconvulsive therapy and antidepressant drugs. Convuls Ther 4:133–140, 1988

Rudorfer MV, Risby ED, Osman OT, et al: Hypothalamic-pituitary-adrenal axis and monoamine transmitter activity in depression: a pilot study of central and peripheral effects of electroconvulsive therapy. Biol Psychiatry 29:253–264, 1991

Sackeim HA: The cognitive effects of electroconvulsive therapy, in Cognitive Disorders: Pathophysiology and Treatment. Edited by Moos WH, Gamzu ER, Thal LJ. New York, Marcel Dekker, 1992, pp 183–228

Sackeim HA: Magnetic stimulation therapy and ECT. Convuls Ther 10:255–258, 1994

Sackeim HA: The anticonvulsant hypothesis of the mechanisms of action of ECT: current status. J ECT 15:5–26, 1999

Sackeim HA, Decina P, Prohovnik I, et al: Anticonvulsant and antidepressant properties of electroconvulsive therapy: a proposed mechanism of action. Biol Psychiatry 18:1301–1310, 1983

Sackeim HA, Decina P, Kanzler M, et al: Effects of electrode placement on the efficacy of titrated, low-dose ECT. Am J Psychiatry 144:1449–1455, 1987a

Sackeim HA, Decina P, Prohovnik I, et al: Seizure threshold in electroconvulsive therapy: effects of sex, age, electrode placement, and number of treatments. Arch Gen Psychiatry 44:355–360, 1987b

Sackeim HA, Prudic J, Devanand DP, et al: Effects of stimulus intensity and electrode placement on the efficacy and cognitive effects of electroconvulsive therapy. N Engl J Med 328:839–846, 1993

Sackeim HA, Devanand DP, Nobler MS: Electroconvulsive therapy, in Psychopharmacology: The Fourth Generation of Progress. Edited by Bloom F, Kupfer D. New York, Raven, 1995, pp 1123–1142

Sackeim HA, Luber B, Katzman GP, et al: The effects of electroconvulsive therapy on quantitative electroencephalograms: relationship to clinical outcome. Arch Gen Psychiatry 53:814–824, 1996

Sackeim HA, Luber B, Moeller JR, et al: Electrophysiological correlates of the adverse cognitive effects of electroconvulsive therapy. J ECT 16:110–120, 2000a

Sackeim HA, Prudic J, Devanand DP, et al: A prospective, randomized, double-blind comparison of bilateral and right unilateral electroconvulsive therapy at different stimulus intensities. Arch Gen Psychiatry 57:425–434, 2000b

Sackeim HA, Haskett RF, Mulsant BH, et al: Continuation pharmacotherapy in the prevention of relapse following electroconvulsive therapy: a randomized controlled trial. JAMA 285:1299–1307, 2001

Saito S, Yoshikawa D, Nishihara F, et al: The cerebral hemodynamic response to electrically induced seizures in man. Brain Res 673:93–100, 1995

Schlaepfer TE, Kosel M, Nemeroff CB: Efficacy of repetitive transcranial magnetic stimulation (rTMS) in the treatment of affective disorders. Neuropsychopharmacology 28:201–205, 2003

Scott BW, Wojtowicz JM, Burnham WM: Neurogenesis in the dentate gyrus of the rat following electroconvulsive shock seizures. Exp Neurol 165:231–236, 2000

Small JG, Small IF, Perez HC, et al: Electroencephalographic and neurophysiological studies of electrically induced seizures. J Nerv Ment Dis 150:479–489, 1970

Soares JC, Mann JJ: The functional neuroanatomy of mood disorders. J Psychiatr Res 31:393–432, 1997

Sobin C, Sackeim HA, Prudic J, et al: Predictors of retrograde amnesia following ECT. Am J Psychiatry 152:995–1001, 1995

Speer AM, Willis MW, Herscovitch P, et al: Intensity-dependent regional cerebral blood flow during 1-Hz repetitive transcranial magnetic stimulation (rTMS) in healthy volunteers studied with H215O positron emission tomography, II: effects of prefrontal cortex rTMS. Biol Psychiatry 54:826–832, 2003

Spiker DG, Weiss JC, Dealy RS, et al: The pharmacological treatment of delusional depression. Am J Psychiatry 142:430–436, 1985

Squire L, Slater P: Electroconvulsive therapy and complaints of memory dysfunction: a prospective three-year follow-up study. Br J Psychiatry 142:1–8, 1983

Staton RD, Hass PJ, Brumback RA: Electroencephalographic recording during bitemporal and unilateral non-dominant hemisphere (Lancaster Position) electroconvulsive therapy. J Clin Psychiatry 42:264–269, 1981

Teneback CC, Nahas Z, Speer AM, et al: Changes in prefrontal cortex and paralimbic activity in depression following two weeks of daily left prefrontal TMS. J Neuropsychiatry Clin Neurosci 11:426–435, 1999

Tew JDJ, Mulsant BH, Haskett RF, et al: Acute efficacy of ECT in the treatment of major depression in the old-old. Am J Psychiatry 156:1865–1870, 1999

Thompson JW, Weiner RD, Myers CP: Use of ECT in the United States in 1975, 1980, and 1986. Am J Psychiatry 151:1657–1661, 1994

Wassermann EM, Lisanby SH: Therapeutic application of repetitive transcranial magnetic stimulation: a review. Clin Neurophysiol 112:1367–1377, 2001

Weiner RD, Whanger AD, Erwin CW, et al: Prolonged confusional state and EEG seizure activity following concurrent ECT and lithium use. Am J Psychiatry 137:1452–1453, 1980

Weiner RD, Rogers HJ, Davidson JR, et al: Effects of electroconvulsive therapy upon brain electrical activity. Ann N Y Acad Sci 462:270–281, 1986a

Weiner RD, Rogers HJ, Davidson JR, et al: Effects of stimulus parameters on cognitive side effects. Ann N Y Acad Sci 462:315–325, 1986b

Welch CA, Lambertus LJ: Cardiovascular effects of ECT. Convuls Ther 5:35–43, 1989

Wengel SP, Burke WJ, Pfeiffer RF, et al: Maintenance electroconvulsive therapy for intractable Parkinson's disease. Am J Geriatr Psychiatry 6:263–269, 1998

Whalley L, Rosie R, Dick H, et al: Immediate increases in plasma prolactin and neurophysin but not other hormones after electroconvulsive therapy. Lancet 2:1064–1068, 1982

Wu T, Sommer M, Tergau F, et al: Lasting influence of repetitive transcranial magnetic stimulation on intracortical excitability in human subjects. Neurosci Lett 287:37–40, 2000

Zielinski RJ, Roose SP, Devanand DP, et al: Cardiovascular complications of ECT in depressed patients with cardiac disease. Am J Psychiatry 150:904–909, 1993

Zis AP, Nomikos GG, Damsma G, et al: In vivo neurochemical effects of electroconvulsive shock studied by microdialysis in the rat striatum. Psychopharmacology (Berl) 103:343–350, 1991

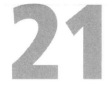

Vagus Nerve Stimulation and Deep Brain Stimulation

MARK S. GEORGE, M.D.

ZIAD NAHAS, M.D.

DARYL E. BOHNING, PH.D.

F. ANDREW KOZEL, M.D., M.S.

BERRY ANDERSON, R.N.

CHIWEN MU, M.D., PH.D.

JEFFREY BORCKARDT, PH.D.

XIANGBAO LI, M.D.

The authors are supported in part by research grants from the National Alliance for Research on Schizophrenia and Depression and the Stanley Foundation, by a National Institute of Neurological Disorders and Stroke grant (R01-AG40956), by a National Institute of Mental Health grant (Z.N.), and by a grant from the Defense Advanced Research Projects Agency. The Brain Stimulation Laboratory also has received grant support from Cyberonics (vagus nerve stimulation [VNS]) and Neotonus (transcranial magnetic stimulation) for clinical trials. None of the authors has equity or financial conflicts. Drs. George and Bohning hold a patent for interleaving transcranial magnetic stimulation with functional magnetic resonance imaging (fMRI) as a neuroscience tool and an invention disclosure (with Drs. Bohning and Nahas) to use fMRI to determine the optimum treatment settings for VNS. The authors would like to thank Minnie Dobbins for administrative help. Dr. George would like to acknowledge helpful past discussions about VNS research advances with Burke Barrett, formerly of Cyberonics, and Dr. Jake Zabara.

Vagus Nerve Stimulation

Two somatic treatments the brain routinely used as therapies in neurology offer promise as antidepressant treatments—vagus nerve stimulation (VNS) and deep brain stimulation (DBS). Recent studies in epilepsy patients, as well as those in primary depressed patients, suggest that VNS has significant antidepressant effects. In this chapter, we describe the VNS method, the clinical studies to date in depression, and potential antidepressant mechanisms of action interpreted in light of current theories concerning the antidepressant mechanisms of medications and electroconvulsive therapy (ECT). Stimulation of cranial nerves can alter brain function. In fact, throughout the past century, researchers have investigated how stimulation of the cranial nerves, especially the vagus nerve, produces observable brain effects.

The vagus nerve is actually a cable of nerve fibers that regulates the body's autonomic functions, which are important in a variety of emotional tasks. Most students are familiar with the vagus nerve's efferent functions, when it serves as the messenger for signals *from the brain* to the viscera. Traditionally, the vagus nerve has been considered a parasympathetic efferent nerve (controlling and regulating autonomic functions such as heart rate and gastric tone). The afferent role of the vagus (fibers carrying signals originating in the periphery to the brain) has been underemphasized in the traditional literature. The vagus is actually a mixed nerve composed of about 80% afferent sensory fibers carrying information *to the brain* from the head, neck, thorax, and abdomen (Foley and DuBois 1937).

Researchers have convincingly documented extensive projections of the vagus nerve via its sensory afferent connections in the nucleus tractus solitarius to diverse brain regions (MacLean 1990). For example, as early as 1938, Bailey and Bremer found that VNS in the cat elicited synchronized electroencephalogram (EEG) activity in the orbital cortex. In 1949, MacLean and Pribram stimulated the vagus nerve and recorded EEG activity from the cortical surface of anesthetized monkeys. They found that VNS caused inconsistent slow waves to be generated from the lateral frontal cortex (Maclean 1990). Shortly after that, Dell and Olson (1951) studied the effects of VNS in awake cats with high cervical spinal lesions. They found that VNS evoked a slow-wave response in the anterior rhinal sulcus, as well as in the amygdala.

Reasoning from this body of literature, as well as evidence that deep breathing (e.g., Lamaze or yoga) can calm the brain (Sovik 2000), presumably through activation of vagus afferents, Zabara (1985a, 1985b, 1992) reported an anticonvulsant action of VNS on experimental seizures in dogs. Zabara hypothesized that VNS could prevent or control the motor and autonomic components of epilepsy. Penry and others then ushered in the modern clinical application of VNS in 1988 by using an implanted device to treat epilepsy in human patients (Penry and Dean 1990).

Although the route of entry into the brain is constrained, VNS offers the potential for modulating and modifying function in several important brain regions through transsynaptic connections. (For a detailed discussion of vagus circuitry, see George et al. 2000; Henry 2002; Ter Horst and Streetland 1994.) These brainstem and limbic anatomical connections can be shown in nonhuman animals and, with functional neuroimaging, in humans.

The oncogene c-*fos* is a general marker for cellular activity. In rats, c-*fos* studies showed increased activity in the amygdala, cingulate, locus coeruleus, and hypothalamus while the vagus was being stimulated (Naritoku et al. 1995). Furthermore, the signal into the brain from VNS can be amplified or reduced by modifying the activity in several of these key relay nuclei.

In an important study that established the potential for combining VNS with general or local pharmacology, Walker and colleagues (1999) outlined a possible role of the nucleus tractus solitarius in how VNS reduces seizures. By microinjecting the nucleus tractus solitarius with either γ-aminobutyric acid (GABA) agonists or glutamate antagonists while seizing animals also were receiving VNS, they found that increased GABA or decreased glutamate in the nucleus tractus solitarius blocked seizures. Indirectly, these findings suggest that VNS may change nucleus tractus solitarius GABA and glutamate concentrations, with secondary changes in the function of specific limbic structures noted earlier (e.g., amygdala, cingulate, insula, and hippocampus).

In summary, incoming sensory (afferent) connections of the vagus nerve provide direct projections to many of the brain regions implicated in neuropsychiatric disorders. These connections provide a basis for understanding how VNS might be a portal to the brain stem and connected limbic and cortical regions. These pathways likely account for the neuropsychiatric effects of VNS, and they invite additional theoretical considerations for potential research and clinical applications. Functional imaging studies in humans have largely confirmed this important neuroanatomy of the vagus (Henry 2002; Henry et al. 1998, 1999).

Methods

The broad term *vagus nerve stimulation* generally refers to several different techniques used to stimulate the vagus nerve, including studies in animals in which the vagus was accessed through the abdomen and diaphragm. However, for virtually all human studies, VNS refers to stimulation of the left cervical vagus nerve with a commercial device: the VNS Therapy System (Cyberonics, Houston, TX) (see Figure 21–1). (An important exception to this rule was the recent work that used a modified VNS Therapy System to stimulate both subdiaphragmatic vagus nerves for the treatment of obesity [Roslin and Kurian 2001].)

VNS has been commercially available for the treatment of resistant partial-onset seizures in Europe since 1994 and in the United States since 1997. More than 22,000 people with epilepsy worldwide have been treated with the VNS Therapy System. Typically, although not always, epilepsy patients considering VNS have had unsatisfactory seizure control despite treatment with multiple medications. In many ways, VNS resembles implanting a cardiac pacemaker. With VNS, the electrical stimulation is delivered through a pulse generator—an implantable, multiprogrammable, bipolar pulse generator (about the size of a pocket watch)—that is implanted in the left chest wall to deliver electrical signals to the left vagus nerve through a bipolar lead. Thus, VNS resembles in some ways DBS (Limousin et al. 1995, 1998), with the main differences being the location of the end wire (left cervical vagus nerve with VNS, deep brain nuclei with DBS); the need for breaching the skull, with consequent risks in DBS but not VNS; and the nature of the electrical pulse (intermittent and relatively low frequency with VNS, constant and high-frequency stimulation [<100 Hz] with DBS). In VNS, the electrode is wrapped around the vagus nerve in the neck and is connected to the generator subcutaneously. The VNS implantation surgery is typically an outpatient procedure most commonly, but not exclusively, performed by neurosurgeons.

A personal computer or handheld personal digital assistant (PDA) and an infrared wand control the VNS generator. As a safety feature, the VNS Therapy System is designed to shut off in the presence of a constant magnetic field. Each patient is given a small handheld magnet that, when held over the pulse generator, turns off stimulation. When the magnet is removed, normal programmed stimulation resumes. This allows patients to control and temporarily eliminate stimulation-related side effects during key behaviors such as public speaking (voice tremor) and heavy exercising (mild shortness of breath).

Use in Epilepsy

VNS has been most extensively studied as a treatment for epilepsy. Two double-blind studies (Ben-Menachem et al. 1994) have been conducted in patients with epilepsy, with a total of 313 treatment-resistant completers. In this diffi-

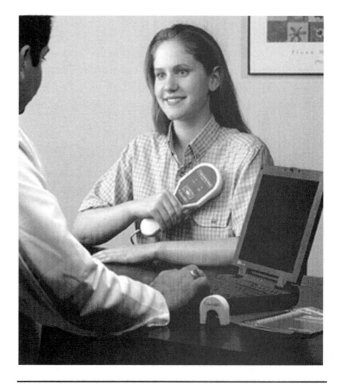

FIGURE 21–1. Vagus nerve stimulation (VNS) therapy system.
VNS therapy is coordinated by a generator and battery implanted under the skin of the left chest (similar in design to a cardiac pacemaker). The generator sends intermittent signals to the left vagus nerve through a subcutaneous wire. The physician can modify the generator settings by communicating with it through a handheld wand placed over the chest. The wand is controlled by a laptop computer. Because it is implanted, there are no issues of noncompliance or uncontrolled variations in dosing.

cult-to-treat group, the average decline acutely in seizure frequency was about 25%–30% compared with baseline.

VNS, as now delivered, generally has not been shown to be a substitute for anticonvulsant medications. In some patients, the dosage levels or numbers of antiepileptic medications have been decreased with the addition of VNS. VNS is increasingly being used in children with epilepsy, in part because VNS does not have negative cognitive effects, which are common with other anticonvulsants (Heck et al. 2002; Helmers et al. 2001).

In patients with epilepsy, the long-term efficacy of VNS is either maintained or improved, while the frequency of adverse events generally decreases as patients accommodate to stimulation (Salinsky et al. 1996). Data from uncontrolled observations suggest that, contrary to a tolerance effect, improvement in seizure control is maintained or may increase over time. It appears that little or no tolerance develops over time to the anticonvulsant actions of VNS. The patient with the longest exposure to VNS has had the system operating for 13 years.

Several different programmable variables are involved in determining how to deliver VNS. (These are also an issue with other forms of electrical brain stimulation—DBS and transcranial magnetic stimulation [TMS].) These "use parameters" include the pulse width of the electrical signal (130, 250, 500, 750, 1,000 μs), the stimulation intensity (0.25–4.00 mA is clinically tolerated), the frequency of stimulation (1–145 Hz), the length or duration of uninterrupted stimulation (7–270 seconds), and the length of time between trains of stimuli (0.2 second to 180 minutes). In general, the initial epilepsy use parameter settings were derived from the animal studies in which acute anticonvulsant effects were found. The initial epilepsy studies compared efficacy in two groups, on the basis of different use parameters: a high-stimulation group (500-μs pulse width, 30 Hz, 30 seconds on, 5 minutes off) and a low-stimulation group (130-μs pulse width, 1 Hz, 30 seconds on, 90–180 minutes off). Most of the VNS epilepsy efficacy and safety data come from trials with use parameters similar to those used in the high-stimulation group in the initial epilepsy studies. Similarly, most of the data concerning VNS effects in other neuropsychiatric disorders (depression, anxiety) involve VNS at use parameters similar to those used in the high-stimulation group in the initial epilepsy studies. These use parameters are not likely the maximally effective choices for different diseases or even individuals. It is also unlikely that the same parameters work equally well in all conditions. Epilepsy physicians commonly switch nonresponding patients to use parameters different from their current settings. However, there has been no clear proof that changing settings improves efficacy. Further work to understand the translational neurobiology of these use parameter choices, and how they relate to clinical symptoms, is an important area for future growth of the field.

Effects in Depression

The increasing literature in psychiatry indicates that anticonvulsant medications (e.g., carbamazepine) or devices (e.g., ECT) have mood-stabilizing or antidepressant effects. In early 1998, several lines of evidence suggested that VNS might have antidepressant effects. (For a full discussion of this reasoning, see George et al. 2000.) In the initial decision to perform a clinical trial of VNS in depression, the knowledge of vagus connections in the brain stem, particularly the role of the locus coeruleus, was crucial. Additional supporting information came from 1) mood effects of VNS observed in patients with epilepsy (Elger et al. 2000), 2) evidence from positron emission tomographic (PET) imaging that VNS affects

the function of important limbic structures, 3) the long history of anticonvulsant medications being useful in treating mood disorders (Ballenger and Post 1978), and 4) neurochemical studies in both animals and humans that reported that VNS alters concentrations of monoamines within the central nervous system (transmission of serotonin, norepinephrine [Krahl et al. 1998, 2000, 2001], GABA, and glutamate) (Walker et al. 1999). The initial open-label VNS depression study involved four sites (Medical University of South Carolina, Charleston; Columbia–New York State Psychiatric Institute, New York; University of Texas Southwestern Medical Center–Dallas; Baylor–Houston) and initially involved 30 subjects (Rush et al. 2000), with a later extension of 30 more subjects to clarify the effect size and look for response predictors (Sackeim et al. 2001b). The study design involved selecting patients with treatment-resistant, chronic, or recurrent major depressive episode (MDE) (unipolar or non-rapid-cycling bipolar) and then adding VNS to a stable regimen of antidepressant medications or no antidepressant medications. No stimulation was given for the first 2 weeks following implantation, creating a single-blind placebo phase and allowing for surgical recovery. All patients met eligibility criteria by failing at least two adequate treatment trials in the current MDE according to the Antidepressant Treatment History Form (Prudic et al. 1996; Sackeim et al. 1990).

Of the 59 subjects who completed the study (1 patient improved during the recovery period before the device was turned on permanently and was not included), the response rates after 3 months of treatment were 30.5% for the primary 28-item Hamilton Rating Scale for Depression measure, 34.0% for the Montgomery-Åsberg Rating Scale for Depression, and 37.3% for the Clinical Global Impression–Improvement Scale score (1 or 2). Interestingly and perhaps importantly, 2 patients developed hypomania. VNS was well tolerated in this group; side effects were similar to those encountered by epilepsy patients. The most common side effect was voice alteration or hoarseness, 60.0% (36/60), which was generally mild and related to the intensity of the output current. No adverse cognitive effects occurred (Sackeim et al. 2001a), and subjects actually improved on several cognitive measures after 8 weeks of therapy, likely because their depression had lifted. Prior antidepressant treatment resistance correlated with a poor VNS response. For example, none of the 13 patients who had not responded adequately to more than seven research-defined adequate antidepressant trials in the current episode responded to VNS, whereas 39% of the remaining 46 patients did respond (P=0.0057).

This cohort has now been followed up regularly for

more than 2 years. Changes in psychotropic medications and in VNS stimulus parameters were allowed during this long-term follow-up. Results seen at the end of the 10-week acute phase largely appear to have continued and even improved over 9 months of long-term maintenance VNS treatment (Marangell et al. 2002). According to the last observation carried forward, response rates were 30.5% (18/59) after 3 months, 42.4% (25/59) after 1 year, and 42.4% (25/59) after 2 years of VNS. Remission rates were 15.3% (9/59) at 3 months, 27.1% (16/59) at 1 year, and 22.0% (13/59) at 2 years. By 2 years, two deaths, unrelated to VNS, had occurred, and four patients had withdrawn for other reasons. At 24 months, 48/59 (81.4%) were still receiving active VNS therapy. These naturalistic open results suggest, but do not prove, that long-term beneficial effects are associated with VNS therapy for patients with chronic or recurrent treatment-resistant depression. Longer-term VNS therapy was generally well tolerated (Nahas et al., in press).

These encouraging initial open-label results led to market approval for VNS in the treatment of chronic or recurrent depression in Canada and served as the basis for a recent United States multisite double-blind trial of VNS for chronic or recurrent, low to moderate treatment-resistant depression. In this trial, VNS failed to show a statistically significant difference in acute response from the sham group. The sham response was 10%, and the active response was 15% (Rush et al., in press). There are several possible explanations for the differences between the 30% response rate in the open study and the 15% active acute response rate in the double-blind study. Some placebo response was likely in the open study. Additionally, the dose of VNS delivered in the double-blind study was markedly less than in the open study, likely because of the complex nature of the double-blind trial. However, a VNS antidepressant dose–response relation was not evident, although this does exist for epilepsy and was the basis for the initial double-blind epilepsy trials. Finally, an attempt at screening out highly treatment-resistant individuals was not fully successful.

As in the initial open study, at the end of the acute phase, subjects continued to receive VNS. Subjects were free to change or add medications or treatments. After 12 months of VNS therapy, the response rate in this cohort approached that seen in the open study (35%). The long-term outcome of a highly treatment-resistant group like this is unknown. To assess whether the presence of the VNS therapy influenced the long-term course, these D-02 data were compared with those of a control group with similar entry criteria that simply received treatment as usual (George et al., in press). The 205 depressed subjects who received VNS (D-02) were compared with 124 subjects who received treatment as usual (D-04) over the

course of 1 year. The two groups had similar baseline demographic, psychiatric, and mood disorder treatment histories. VNS (D-02) subjects had a statistically significant greater improvement per month when compared with treatment-as-usual (D-04) subjects across 12 months of therapy ($P<0.001$), by repeated-measures linear regression on the Inventory of Depressive Symptomatology–Self-Rated (Rush et al. 1986). These results suggest that, when compared in a nonrandomized fashion with usual standard of care (D-04) for 1 year, VNS therapy (D-02) provides a statistically significant benefit for depression symptoms in a chronic or recurrent treatment-resistant depression population. The company is continuing to gather long-term data on these subjects and is organizing further studies. These results have been presented to the U.S. Food and Drug Administration (FDA) for potential approval of VNS as a therapy for treatment-resistant depression. Thus, no double-blind, prospective, randomized, controlled evidence exists for VNS as an antidepressant in patients with primary depression. However, open (Harden et al. 2000) and double-blind (Elger et al. 2000) studies showed that VNS has antidepressant effects in epilepsy patients with comorbid depression.

Acute Changes in Pain Perception in Depressed Patients

Previous research suggested that VNS affects pain perception in epilepsy patients, with acute VNS decreasing pain thresholds (pronociceptive) (Ness et al. 2000) and chronic treatment increasing pain thresholds (antinociceptive) (Kirchner et al. 2000). These studies did not address whether different VNS device parameter settings had varying effects on pain perception. Divergent studies, as discussed in more detail later, suggested that different device parameters are associated with unique fiber activation and different regional brain activation. Borckardt and colleagues at the Medical University of South Carolina thus examined the effects of different VNS device parameters on pain perception in depressed adults with a thermal pain paradigm (Borckardt et al. 2005). Pronociceptive effects (pain enhancing) were found with eight depressed subjects during acute VNS device activation, and main effects were found for VNS output current, frequency, and interaction of current and frequency. The effects of VNS on pain perception were most pronounced during the first 3 seconds of the thermal pain procedures. Subjects' levels of depression did not predict VNS-induced changes in pain threshold. However, large individual differences were seen with the specific device settings associated with the largest changes in pain threshold. Further work with VNS as a potential treatment for chronic pain appears warranted.

Clinical Summary and Conclusion

Although VNS is highly promising as a potential long-term treatment for recurrent mood disorders, no prospective, randomized, double-blind data currently exist for use of VNS to treat primary depression. The double-blind data showing efficacy in treating depression within the context of epilepsy, and the long-term positive open results in treatment-resistant primary depression, suggest that VNS is an area with future promise. More research is needed.

Mechanisms of Action

What are the potential mechanisms by which VNS relieves symptoms of depression? A lack of consensus exists about the underlying pathophysiology of the depressions, and many different mechanisms of action are proposed for the currently effective and approved antidepressant treatments. Any potential VNS antidepressant mechanism of action must account for the known route of entry of VNS into the brain and also must be able to explain the relatively slow onset of antidepressant action of VNS, with continued improvement over long time frames such as 1 year. What might be happening at a neurobiological level, starting at the vagus nerve and entering the brain, over slow periods in the depressed patients who respond to VNS?

Neurotransmitters and Cerebrospinal Fluid

Both clinical and animal studies indicate that VNS likely results in changes in serotonin, norepinephrine, GABA, and glutamate, which are all neurotransmitters implicated in the pathogenesis of major depression. VNS in animals activates the locus coeruleus, the main source of central nervous system (CNS) norepinephrine-containing neuronal cell bodies (Krahl et al. 1998, 2000). In patients with epilepsy, VNS appears to increase 5-hydroxyindoleacetic acid—a metabolite of serotonin. Because many of the currently available therapies are believed to work through changes in the same neurotransmitters (serotonin or norepinephrine), VNS might be acting through mechanisms similar to antidepressant medications. It was thus surprising that a recent study of effects of VNS on cerebrospinal fluid (CSF) changes in depressed patients over time failed to confirm the finding of serotonin metabolite changes in CSF and instead found significant increases in CSF homovanillic acid, a dopamine metabolite (Carpenter et al. 2004). The two studies differed in their study subjects (epilepsy and depression), VNS use parameters, and concomitant medications, which might explain the discrepancy. Further studies are needed, but enough data have accumulated to date to conclude that VNS acts on

norepinephrine and serotonin systems and that this may be an important mechanism in explaining VNS antidepressant actions.

Antidepressant Effects Secondary to Anticonvulsant Action

A popular theory about ECT is that it invokes natural anticonvulsant cascades that then reregulate a system and improve depression. Several other anticonvulsant medications, including carbamazepine and lamotrigine, also have antidepressant effects, and the anticonvulsant effects of VNS are well established. VNS may improve depression by manipulating anticonvulsant systems in the brain. Recent work by Dean and colleagues (2002) in epilepsy patients with VNS implanted for 6–12 months showed the powerful and persistent anticonvulsant effects of VNS. These researchers used TMS to study the effects of acute VNS on motor threshold and the cortical silent period following a TMS pulse. Motor threshold and cortical silent period are TMS measures of cortical excitability. The most interesting finding was that in epilepsy patients who had been receiving VNS for more than 6 months, a significant decrease in motor cortex excitability occurred while VNS was on, compared with 30 minutes after VNS was turned off. However, not all anticonvulsants have antidepressant effects. Further work is needed to understand the mechanisms by which VNS stops seizures and whether these are the same or similar mechanisms as those working to improve mood in depression.

Changing Regional Functional Anatomy

Structural and functional imaging studies over the past 20 years in emotion regulation and depression have drawn attention to a "functional neuroanatomy of depression." One of the current main concepts is that clinical depression arises through an imbalance in prefrontal-limbic circuits. Several imaging studies over the past 10 years have examined antidepressant treatments and how they cause changes in these circuits. Through the known projections of the vagus nerve, VNS could theoretically cause changes in these limbic and orbitofrontal regions. Functional imaging studies with VNS have now shown that VNS, repeatedly and over time, causes changes in these key brain regions (Bohning et al. 2001; Henry et al. 1998, 1999; Lomarev et al. 2002; Mu et al. 2003).

Studies combining functional brain imaging with VNS offer the promise of elucidating the an0tidepressant mechanisms of action of VNS. Fast imaging methods such as functional magnetic resonance imaging (fMRI) can show the immediate effects of VNS, whereas slower imaging methods such as single-photon emission computed tomography

(SPECT) and PET can show the longer-term changes associated with constant VNS over time as a therapy (Chae et al. 2003). We have recently succeeded in performing blood oxygen level–dependent fMRI studies in depressed patients implanted with VNS as part of the initial pilot clinical study and a more recent larger double-blind trial. An initial study that used the interleaved VNS/fMRI technique showed that VNS immediately activates many anterior paralimbic regions, including the orbitofrontal cortex, insula, and medial temporal lobe (Bohning et al. 2001). A follow-up study that used the same technique showed that VNS at 5 Hz had a smaller brain effect than did VNS at 20 Hz (Lomarev et al. 2002). Most recently, we have serially scanned 17 depressed patients in the D-02 study with the VNS/fMRI interleaved technique (Mu et al. 2003). Patients were scanned at the first moments when VNS was turned on and again 2 weeks later after a ramp-up phase, when the VNS intensity was increased. Finally, subjects were scanned again with the same technique after 10 weeks of VNS therapy. These imaging data are consistent with the notion that repeated daily VNS causes immediate cortical increases and limbic (cingulate and orbitofrontal) decreases and that, over time, these immediate effects change as the system changes its dynamic homeostasis.

This prefrontal-limbic neuroanatomical theory of VNS antidepressant mechanisms of action accounts for the known projections and role of the vagus afferents, as well as the very slow and gradual time frame involved in resetting a dynamic system. As a corollary, the antidepressant effects of gamma-knife surgery and other surgical lesion treatments for depression also take 6 months to a year before reaching peak effect.

Perhaps the most important information for the entire field of VNS as therapy is improved understanding of the different effects of use parameters on VNS brain effects. This information can be partially gathered in animal studies, although it is difficult to implant VNS in small animals, and they then are immobile for most of the day. Interleaving VNS with fMRI can help solve the riddles of how different VNS use parameters differentially affect the brain. Future work with this methodology holds promise for rapidly and efficiently refining the more than 500,000 different combinations of VNS pulse width, frequency, intensity, train length, and length of time turned off.

Stress Sensitization

Another important concept in depression pathogenesis is *stress sensitization*. This term applies to the phenomenon in which repeated mild stresses, over time, build up to a point at which an animal is sensitized to developing depression (Antelman 1988; Antelman et al. 1991; Kalivas et al. 1988;

Post 1980; Post et al. 1986). Thus, a single stressful event would not produce depression, but repeated daily stresses will. Reasoning within this stress sensitization paradigm, one wonders whether VNS might be constantly and repeatedly diminishing the abnormal brain reaction to stress inherent in depression. Thus, theoretically, with each new stress that a depressed patient encounters, VNS might be blunting an otherwise amplified pathological reaction. Then the brain gradually is able to return to homeostasis without the pathological feedback from repeated stresses.

Patients taking selective serotonin reuptake inhibitors (SSRIs) commonly report that a stressful life event is no longer as stressful to them as it was before they were taking medications. Our group has similarly observed patients in VNS depression trials tolerate stressful events much better than they did before they were receiving VNS. Learning whether and to what degree VNS might "stress inoculate" or reduce anxiety and the pathological overreaction of a depressed individual to a stressful event is important. VNS may improve depression by gradually reducing the downstream effects of stressful life events, thus enabling corrective brain responses over time. This mechanism of action would account for the slow onset of antidepressant action, the continued improvement over time, and the relatively low rates of relapse (because stressful events that precipitate relapse are less neurobiologically potent during VNS regulation). To date, there is no information about whether and to what degree VNS affects serum or urinary cortisol, thyroid function, or other hypothalamic-pituitary-adrenal axis measures, such as the dexamethasone suppression test. Further research is needed.

Overall Vagus Nerve Stimulation Summary

In summary, more work is needed to establish whether VNS is an effective antidepressant and, if so, to determine what mechanisms are responsible for causing these changes. From the relatively few studies to date, it appears that VNS could improve depression through several of the current antidepressant mechanism models. Strong data support the anticonvulsant properties of VNS, as well as the changes VNS causes in regional brain activity, both acutely and gradually over time. Because of its unique method of delivery, VNS may produce brain changes through mechanisms not shared by other medications or devices.

Deep Brain Stimulation

The most anatomically discrete, and invasive, method of stimulating deep brain structures is called DBS (Ashby

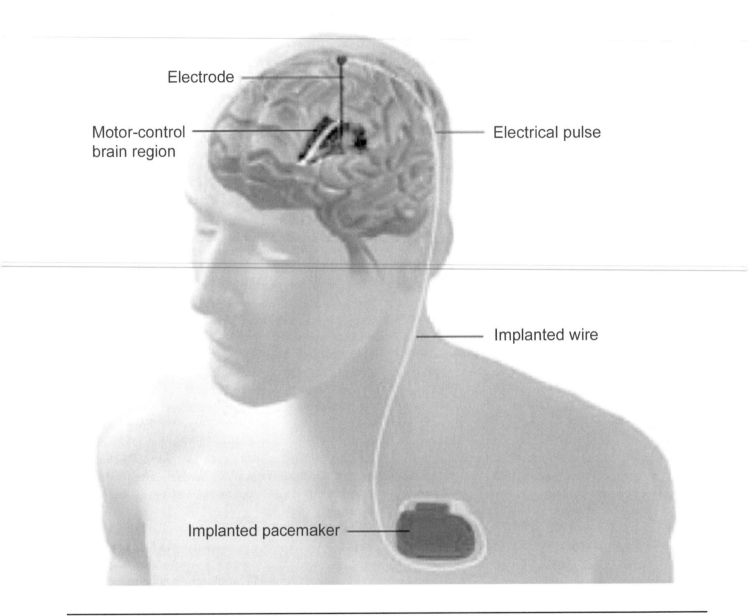

Electrode

Motor-control
brain region

Electrical pulse

Implanted wire

Implanted pacemaker

FIGURE 21–2.   Deep brain stimulation (DBS).

A neurosurgeon passes a small electrode, about the width of a human hair, directly into the brain after making a small hole in the skull. The electrode is then connected to generators implanted under the skin in the chest, connected through a wire tunneled under the skin. The DBS electrode is positioned by the surgeon using stereotactic image guidance. As with vagus nerve stimulation, the DBS generator can be programmed to deliver the electrical stimulation in any number of ways. Typically, for Parkinson's disease, the generator is constantly on, stimulating at about 120 Hz.

Source.   Reprinted from George MS: "Stimulating the Brain." *Scientific American* 289(3):66–93, September 2003, p. 70. Image created by and used with permission from Bryan Christie.

and Rothwell 2000; Bekhtereva et al. 1972; Kumar et al. 1998; Olanow et al. 2000) (see Figure 21–2). DBS of the thalamus, globus pallidus interna, or subthalamic nucleus is a new treatment for essential tremor and bradykinesia in Parkinson's disease (PD) (Kumar et al. 1998; Olanow et al. 2000; Tarsy 2001).

Use in Parkinson's Disease

In DBS, a thin electrode is inserted directly into the brain. Then different currents are applied at varying depths until the desired effects are achieved. High-frequency (>80 Hz) electrical stimulation of the middle thalamus or subthalamic nucleus has been found effective in PD (Damier 1998; Limousin et al. 1995, 1998). Stimulation can be performed at high frequencies (>50 Hz), which are thought to create a transient functional lesion and inhibit a brain region from normal participation in brain activity. Alternatively, low-frequency stimulation may intermittently activate a region (Grill 1999; Grill and McIntyre 2001).

Mood Effects

Although DBS has not been used to treat major depression, mood effects of the stimulation have been reported. In one patient with PD who had never had depression, the testing of the stimulation caused the acute onset of tearfulness, sadness, and despair. These symptoms remitted immediately when the surgeon moved the stimulator away from the substantia nigra, directly below the subthalamic nucleus. Transient acute depression was evoked 5 seconds after 130-Hz DBS of the left substantia nigra and ceased 90 seconds after DBS was stopped. Others also have reported that unilateral or bilateral DBS of the subthalamic nucleus resulted in involuntary laughter, humorous triggered imaginative associations, and feelings of well-being that lasted for several minutes until the stimulation intensity was lowered or discontinued (Kumar et al. 1998). This emotional reaction was accompanied by improved parkinsonian symptoms.

Other studies during diagnostic DBS prior to neurosurgical ablations also have reported emotional reactions. Microstimulation of the nucleus ventralis caudalis (somatosensory) was accompanied by a strong affective component of visceral pain similar to that previously observed in the patient during a comorbid PD panic attack (Lenz et al. 1995). Weeping, anxiety, and depression were reported to be elicited during neurosurgery in unanesthetized PD patients with 32-Hz stimulation for several seconds of ventral arterionucleus, ventral lateral pars oralis, and other thalamic nuclei as well as pallidum septum and hypothalamus (Schaltenbrand et al. 1973). Different emotional reactions occurred while stimulating nucleus ventralis lateralis with the floating electrode (Il'inskii 1970).

Bondarchuk and Smirnov (1969) summarized the effects of diagnostic and therapeutic DBS via long-term implanted electrodes in a large sample of patients with PD: positive emotional states occurred after stimulation of the centrum medianum area of the thalamus. Interestingly, high-frequency (ablative) DBS and also stereotaxic destruction of the anterior thalamic nuclei resulted in relief from intractable agitated depression (Mark et al. 1970). Finally, the thalamus was one of the brain structures in which Heath and colleagues recorded EEG correlates of pleasure during orgasm (Heath 1964; Heath and Guerrero-Figueroa 1968).

Thus, recent and older case report data indicate that DBS has the potential for short-term alteration of mood. However, this area has not been systematically studied in a controlled setting, and only recently have investigators been able to use powerful concurrent functional neuroimaging to trace the circuits that are activated during stimulation.

Data in Obsessive-Compulsive Disorder

Obsessive-compulsive disorder (OCD) is perhaps the major psychiatric disorder for which the most is known about regional brain pathology (Baxter 1990). Briefly, many functional and structural imaging studies have implicated the orbitofrontal cortex and the caudate nucleus in OCD pathogenesis (Breiter et al. 1996; Rauch et al. 1994). Additionally, treatment responses to medications and behavior therapy are modest at best for most OCD patients (Goodman 1999; McDougle et al. 1991). Over the past 20 years, neurosurgical ablation of the cingulate gyrus has continued to be offered as an option for treatment-resistant patients (Ballantine et al. 1987; Cosgrove and Rauch 1995; Kurlan et al. 1990; Spangler et al. 1996). This surgery likely interrupts fibers connecting the orbitofrontal cortex to the cingulate gyrus and other limbic regions. Reasoning from this literature, Nuttin and colleagues (1999) reported the first series of patients with OCD treated with DBS of the anterior limb of the internal capsule. These initial reports have been followed by continued positive reports (Greenberg et al. 2000, 2003; Nuttin et al. 2003). Double-blind studies are now under way.

Use in Depression

As discussed earlier, one of the more common, but likely incomplete, theories concerning DBS and the brain is that high-frequency DBS results in a functional ablation, or the switching off and inhibition of ongoing neuronal activity, although this theory needs more informed research (Grill 1999). Use of DBS of the subthalamic nucleus or globus pallidus is increasing in patients with PD whose symptoms have not responded to medications.

Major depression occurs in up to 40% of patients with PD (Cummings 1993; Tom and Cummings 1998). Mood changes with DBS treatment in patients with PD are now being studied. Many neurologists and neurosurgeons have commented that there may be a post-DBS hypomania in the month following surgery. Thus, clinicians are interested in whether DBS might be used for treatment-resistant depression. Although the functional neuroanatomy of normal mood regulation in health and the pathological changes in major depression are becoming

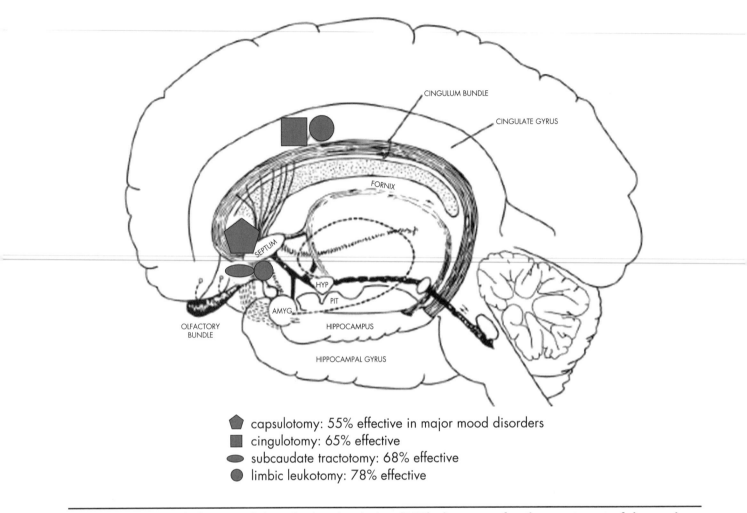

FIGURE 21–3.   Likely sites of deep brain stimulation (DBS) placement for the treatment of depression.
It is unclear exactly where the best locations might be for using DBS to treat depression that has not responded to medications or electroconvulsive therapy. Possible clues come from the neurosurgical literature illustrated here. These include capsulotomy, cingulotomy, and subcaudate tractotomy. A limbic leukotomy is the combination of a cingulotomy and a subcaudate tractotomy and has the highest reported success rate. DBS has the advantage over ablative neurosurgery that if the surgery is ineffective, the electrodes can be removed without permanent alterations in brain connections and structure. DBS targets in this proposal are in red (two sites in each hemisphere), which may equal a "virtual limbic leukotomy." AMYG=amygdala; HYP=hypothalamus; PIT=pituitary.
Source.   Courtesy of Dr. Ziad Nahas.

better understood, knowledge in this area lags drastically behind the neuroanatomical knowledge of motor dysfunction in PD or the circuitry of OCD. A key recent concept is that mood is regulated through changes in activity in the anterior paralimbic circuit (amygdala, septum, anterior cingulate cortex, anterior temporal poles, and orbitofrontal cortex) and that this system functions abnormally in major depression. Neurosurgical ablation of the anterior cingulate gyrus or the anterior limb of the internal capsule has been used for many years for treatment-resistant depression. Additionally, some researchers

have indicated that the DBS-related improvements in patients with OCD are actually more mood related than pure OCD symptoms.

With these theories in mind, several researchers in the United States are beginning small series of DBS studies in patients with treatment-resistant depression. Extreme caution is needed in these studies, particularly given the checkered history with respect to brain surgery (frontal lobotomies) for psychiatric diseases in the early 1900s. It is important to proceed cautiously in patients who have failed almost all available treatments and to integrate knowledge gained from these pilot studies with information from brain imaging and animal models of depression. Figure 21–3 shows the likely sites of DBS placement for the treatment of depression.

In addition to the incomplete knowledge about where to place the DBS leads, this area lacks complete knowledge of the mechanisms of action of DBS and how these are affected by the different use parameters.

Conclusion

In summary, VNS and DBS represent important new technologies that may rapidly develop into established treatments for depression. Both are approved and commonly used for other neuropsychiatric disorders. The initial pilot and later randomized studies of VNS for the treatment of depression are encouraging, but further studies are needed to provide prospective randomized, controlled data on efficacy. Few published data are available on the use of DBS for depression, although case reports from patients with PD and OCD hint that this may be an emerging treatment option in the years to come. Both of these treatments, along with TMS, represent a new class of brain treatments that build on knowledge of regional brain activity in disease pathogenesis. Much more information is needed, however, about the neurobiological basis of depression and the translational effects initiated by brain stimulation with VNS, DBS, or TMS.

References

Antelman SM: Stressor-induced sensitization to subsequent stress: implications for the development and treatment of clinical disorders, in Sensitization in the Nervous System. Edited by Kalivas PW, Barnes CD. Caldwell, NJ, Telford Press, 1988, pp 227–254

Antelman SM, Kocan D, Knopf S, et al: One brief exposure to a psychological stressor induces long-lasting, time-dependent sensitization of both the cataleptic and neurochemical responses to haloperidol. Life Sci 51:261–266, 1991

Ashby P, Rothwell J: Neurophysiologic aspects of deep brain stimulation. Neurology 55 (12, suppl 6):S17–S20, 2000

Bailey P, Bremer F: A sensory cortical representation of the vagus nerve. J Neurophysiol 2:405–412, 1938

Ballantine HT Jr, Bouckoms AJ, Thomas EK, et al: Treatment of psychiatric illness by stereotactic cingulotomy. Biol Psychiatry 22:807–819, 1987

Ballenger JC, Post RM: Therapeutic effects of carbamazepine in affective illness: a preliminary report. Commun Psychopharmacol 2:159–175, 1978

Baxter LR: Brain imaging as a tool in establishing a theory of brain pathology in obsessive compulsive disorder. J Clin Psychiatry 51(suppl):22–25, 1990

Bekhtereva NP, Bondarchuk AN, Smirnov VM, et al: [Therapeutic electric stimulation of deep brain structures]. Vopr Neirokhir 36:7–12, 1972

Ben-Menachem E, Manon-Espaillat R, Ristanovic R, et al: Vagus nerve stimulation for treatment of partial seizures, 1: a controlled study of effect on seizures. First International Vagus Nerve Stimulation Study Group. Epilepsia 35:616–626, 1994

Bohning DE, Lomarev MP, Denslow S, et al: Feasibility of vagus nerve stimulation-synchronized blood oxygenation level-dependent functional MRI. Invest Radiol 36:470–479, 2001

Bondarchuk AN, Smirnov VM: [Effects of electric stimulation on the thalamic median center in man.] Fiziol Zh SSSR Im I M Sechenova 55:408–413, 1969

Borckardt JJ, Kozel FA, Anderson B, et al: Vagus nerve stimulation affects perception in depressed adults. Pain Res Manag 10:9–15, 2005

Breiter HC, Rauch SL, Kwong KK, et al: Functional magnetic resonance imaging of symptom provocation in obsessive-compulsive disorder. Arch Gen Psychiatry 53:595–606, 1996

Carpenter LL, Moreno F, Kling MA, et al: Effects of vagus nerve stimulation on cerebrospinal fluid monoamine metabolites, norepinephrine, and gamma-aminobutyric acid concentrations in depressed patients. Biol Psychiatry 51:418–426, 2004

Chae JH, Nahas Z, Lomarev M, et al: A review of functional neuroimaging studies of vagus nerve stimulation (VNS). J Psychiatr Res 37:443–455, 2003

Cosgrove GR, Rauch SL: Psychosurgery. Neurosurg Clin N Am 6:167–176, 1995

Cummings JL: The neuroanatomy of depression. J Clin Psychiatry 54(suppl):14–20, 1993

Damier P: The stimulation of deep cerebral structures in the treatment of Parkinson's disease. Eur Neuropsychopharmacol 8:S89–S13.04, 1998

Dean AC, Wu AT, et al: Motor cortex excitability in epilepsy patients treated with vagus nerve stimulation. American Epilepsy Society Meeting, 2002

Dell P, Olson R: [Secondary mesencephalic, diencephalic and amygdalian projections of vagal visceral afferences.] C R Seances Soc Biol Fil 145:1088–1091, 1951

Elger G, Hoppe C, Falkai P, et al: Vagus nerve stimulation is associated with mood improvements in epilepsy patients. Epilepsy Res 42:203–210, 2000

Foley JO, DuBois F: Quantitative studies of the vagus nerve in the cat, I: the ratio of sensory and motor studies. J Comp Neurol 67:49–67, 1937

George MS, Sackeim HA, Rush AJ, et al: Vagus nerve stimulation: a new tool for brain research and therapy. Biol Psychiatry 47:287–295, 2000

George MS, Rush AJ, Sackeim H, et al: A one-year comparison of vagus nerve stimulation (VNS) with treatment as usual for treatment-resistant depression. Biol Psychiatry (in press)

Goodman WK: Obsessive-compulsive disorder: diagnosis and treatment. J Clin Psychiatry 60 (suppl 18):27–32, 1999

Greenberg BD, Murphy DL, Rasmussen SA: Neuroanatomically based approaches to obsessive-compulsive disorder: neurosurgery and transcranial magnetic stimulation. Psychiatr Clin North Am 23:671–686, 2000

Greenberg BD, Price LH, Rauch SL, et al: Neurosurgery for intractable obsessive-compulsive disorder and depression: critical issues. Neurosurg Clin N Am 14:199–212, 2003

Grill WM Jr: Modeling the effects of electric fields on nerve fibers: influence of tissue electrical properties. IEEE Trans Biomed Eng 46:918–928, 1999

Grill WM, McIntyre CC: Extracellular excitation of central neurons: implications for the mechanisms of deep brain stimulation. Thalamus Relat Syst 1:269–277, 2001

Harden CL, Pulver MC, Ravdin LD, et al: A pilot study of mood in epilepsy patients treated with vagus nerve stimulation. Epilepsy Behav 1:93–99, 2000

Heath RG: Pleasure response of human subjects to direct stimulation of the brain: physiologic and psychodynamic considerations, in The Role of Pleasure in Behavior. Edited by Heath RG. New York, Hoeber, 1964, pp 219–243

Heath RG, Guerrero-Figueroa R: Stimulation of the human brain: spontaneous and evoked electroencephalographic responses. Acta Neurol Latinoam 14:116–124, 1968

Heck CN, Helmers SL, DeGiorgio CM, et al: Vagus nerve stimulation therapy, epilepsy, and device parameters: scientific basis and recommendations for use. Neurology 59 (suppl 4):S31–S37, 2002

Helmers SL, Wheless JW, Frost M, et al: Vagus nerve stimulation therapy in pediatric patients with refractory epilepsy: retrospective study. J Child Neurol 16:843–848, 2001

Henry TR: Therapeutic mechanisms of vagus nerve stimulation. Neurology 59 (suppl 4):S15–S20, 2002

Henry TR, Bakay RA, Votaw JR, et al: Brain blood flow alterations induced by therapeutic vagus nerve stimulation in partial epilepsy, I: acute effects at high and low levels of stimulation. Epilepsia 39:983–990, 1998

Henry TR, Votaw JR, Pennell PB, et al: Acute blood flow changes and efficacy of vagus nerve stimulation in partial epilepsy. Neurology 52:1166–1173, 1999

Il'inskii IA: [Emotional-affective reactions evoked by electrostimulation of the ventrolateral nucleus of the optic thalamus]. Vopr Neirokhir 34:26–29, 1970

Kalivas PW, Duffy P, Abhold R, et al: Sensitization of mesolimbic dopamine neurons by neuropeptides and stress, in Sensitization in the Nervous System. Edited by Kalivas PW, Barnes CD. Caldwell, NJ, Telford Press, 1988, pp 119–143

Kirchner A, Birklein F, Stefan H, et al: Left vagus nerve stimulation suppresses experimentally induced pain. Neurology 55:1167–1171, 2000

Krahl SE, Clark KB, Smith DC, et al: Locus coeruleus lesions suppress the seizure attenuating effects of vagus nerve stimulation. Epilepsia 39:709–714, 1998

Krahl SE, Senanayake SS, Handforth A: Seizure suppression by systemic epinephrine is mediated by the vagus nerve. Epilepsy Res 38:171–175, 2000

Krahl SE, Senanayake SS, Handforth A: Destruction of peripheral C-fibers does not alter subsequent vagus nerve stimulation-induced seizure suppression. Epilepsia 42:586–589, 2001

Kumar R, Lozano AM, Kim YJ, et al: Double-blind evaluation of subthalamic nucleus deep brain stimulation in advanced Parkinson's disease. Neurology 51:850–855, 1998

Kurlan R, Kersun J, Ballantine HT Jr, et al: Neurosurgical treatment of severe obsessive-compulsive disorder associated with Tourette's syndrome. Mov Disord 5:152–155, 1990

Lenz FA, Gracely RH, Romanoski AJ, et al: Stimulation in the human somatosensory thalamus can reproduce both the affective and sensory dimensions of previously experienced pain. Nat Med 1:910–913, 1995

Limousin P, Pollak P, Benazzouz A, et al: Effect of parkinsonian signs and symptoms of bilateral subthalamic nucleus stimulation. Lancet 345(8942):91–95, 1995

Limousin P, Krack P, Pollak P, et al: Electrical stimulation of the subthalamic nucleus in advanced Parkinson's disease. N Engl J Med 339:1105–1111, 1998

Lomarev M, Denslow S, Nahas Z, et al: Vagus nerve stimulation (VNS) synchronized BOLD fMRI suggests that VNS in depressed adults has frequency/dose dependent effects. J Psychiatr Res 36:219–227, 2002

MacLean PD: The Triune Brain in Evolution: Role in Paleocerebral Functions. New York, Plenum, 1990

Marangell LB, Rush AJ, George MS, et al: Vagus nerve stimulation (VNS) for major depressive episodes: longer-term outcome. Biol Psychiatry 51:280–287, 2002

Mark VA, Barry H, McLardy T, et al: The destruction of both anterior thalamic nuclei in a patient with intractable agitated depression. J Nerv Ment Dis 150:266–272, 1970

McDougle CJ, Price LH, Goodman WK, et al: A controlled trial of lithium augmentation in fluvoxamine-refractory obsessive-compulsive disorder: lack of efficacy. J Clin Psychopharmacol 11:175–184, 1991

Mu Q, Bohning DE, Nahas Z, et al: Acute VNS using different pulse widths produces varying brain effects. Biol Psychiatry 55:816–825, 2004

Nahas Z, Marangell LB, et al: Two-year outcome of vagus nerve stimulation (VNS) therapy for major depressive episodes. J Clin Psychiatry (in press)

Naritoku DK, Terry WJ, Helfert RH, et al: Regional induction of Fos immunoreactivity in the brain by anticonvulsant stimulation of the vagus nerve. Epilepsy Res 22:53–62, 1995

Ness TJ, Fillingim RB, Randich A, et al: Low intensity vagal nerve stimulation lowers human thermal pain thresholds. Pain 86:81–85, 2000

Nuttin B, Cosyns P, Demeulemeester H, et al: Electrical stimulation in anterior limbs of internal capsules in patients with obsessive-compulsive disorder. Lancet 354(9189):1526, 1999

Nuttin BJ, Gabriels LA, Cosyns PR, et al: Long-term electrical capsular stimulation in patients with obsessive-compulsive disorder. Neurosurgery 52:1263–1272, 2003

Olanow CW, Brin MF, Obeso JA: The role of deep brain stimulation as a surgical treatment for Parkinson's disease. Neurology 55 (12, suppl 6):S60–S66, 2000

Penry JK, Dean JC: Prevention of intractable partial seizures by intermittent vagal nerve stimulation in humans: preliminary results. Epilepsy 31:S40–S43, 1990

Post RM: Behavioral sensitization and kindling: implications for affective illness and its treatment with carbamazepine. Rivista de Psichiatria 1:71–79, 1980

Post RM, Rubinow DR, Ballenger JC: Conditioning and sensitization in the longitudinal course of affective illness. Br J Psychiatry 149:191–201, 1986

Prudic J, Haskett RF, Mulsant B, et al: Resistance to antidepressant medications and short-term clinical response to ECT. Am J Psychiatry 153:985–992, 1996

Rauch SL, Jenike MA, Alpert NM, et al: Regional cerebral blood flow measured during symptom provocation in obsessive-compulsive disorder using oxygen 15-labeled carbon dioxide and positron emission tomography. Arch Gen Psychiatry 51:62–70, 1994

Roslin M, Kurian M: The use of electrical stimulation of the vagus nerve to treat morbid obesity. Epilepsy Behav 2:S11–S16, 2001

Rush AJ, Giles DE, Schlesser MA, et al: The Inventory of Depressive Symptomatology (IDS): preliminary findings. Psychiatry Res 18:65–87, 1986

Rush AJ, George MS, Sackeim HA, et al: Vagus nerve stimulation (VNS) for treatment-resistant depressions: a multicenter study. Biol Psychiatry 47:276–286, 2000

Rush AJ, Marangell LB, George MS, et al: Vagus nerve stimulation (VNS) therapy for treatment-resistant depression: a randomized, controlled acute phase trial. Biol Psychiatry (in press)

Sackeim HA, Prudic J, Devanand DP, et al: The impact of medication resistance and continuation pharmacotherapy on relapse following response to electroconvulsive therapy in major depression. J Clin Psychopharmacol 10:96–104, 1990

Sackeim HA, Keilp JG, Rush AJ, et al: The effects of vagus nerve stimulation on cognitive performance in patients with treatment-resistant depression. Neuropsychiatry Neuropsychol Behav Neurol 14:53–62, 2001a

Sackeim HA, Rush AJ, George MS, et al: Vagus nerve stimulation (VNS) for treatment-resistant depression: efficacy, side effects, and predictors of outcome. Neuropsychopharmacology 25:713–728, 2001b

Salinsky MC, Uthman BM, Ristanovic RK, et al: Vagus nerve stimulation for the treatment of medically intractable seizures: results of a 1-year open-extension trial. Arch Neurol 53:1176–1180, 1996

Schaltenbrand G, Spuler H, Wahren W, et al: Vegetative and emotional reactions during electrical stimulation of deep structures of the brain during stereotactic procedures. Z Neurol 205:91–113, 1973

Sovik R: The science of breathing—the yogic view. Prog Brain Res 122:491–505, 2000

Spangler WJ, Cosgrove GR, Ballantine HT Jr, et al: Magnetic resonance image-guided stereotactic cingulotomy for intractable psychiatric disease. Neurosurgery 38:1071–1076, 1996

Tarsy D: Deep brain stimulation and movement disorders. Epilepsy Behav 2 (suppl):S45–S54, 2001

Ter Horst GJ, Streetland C: Ascending projections of the solitary tract nucleus, in Nucleus of the Solitary Tract. Edited by Robin I, Barraco A. London, CRC Press, 1994

Tom T, Cummings JL: Depression in Parkinson's disease: pharmacological characteristics and treatment. Drugs Aging 12:55–74, 1998

Walker BR, Easton A, Gale K: Regulation of limbic motor seizures by GABA and glutamate transmission in nucleus tractus solitarius. Epilepsia 40:1051–1057, 1999

Zabara J: Peripheral control of hypersynchronous discharge in epilepsy. Electroencephalogr Clin Neurophysiol 61S:S162, 1985a

Zabara J: Time course of seizure control to brief, repetitive stimuli. Epilepsia 26:518, 1985b

Zabara J: Inhibition of experimental seizures in canines by repetitive vagal stimulation. Epilepsia 33:1005–1012, 1992

PART 5

Psychotherapy of Mood Disorders

SECTION EDITOR: ELLEN FRANK, PH.D.

22

Cognitive-Behavioral Therapy for Depression and Dysthymia

EDWARD S. FRIEDMAN, M.D.

MICHAEL E. THASE, M.D.

THE PAST 40 YEARS have witnessed the ascendance of cognitive-behavioral therapy (CBT) as both the most influential and the most widely studied form of psychotherapy for depression (Gloaguen et al. 1998; Thase 2001). The term *cognitive-behavioral therapy* refers to a broader class of therapies, whereas *cognitive therapy* describes a specific model of treatment that was formulated between the late 1950s and 1970s by Aaron T. Beck and colleagues (A. T. Beck 1963, 1964, 1976; A. T. Beck et al. 1979). In this chapter, we focus initially on Beck's model of therapy and then report on some recent modifications of Beckian cognitive therapy that address the issues of relapse, recurrence, and chronicity.

Cognitive therapy evolved over several decades in response to Beck's observations of stereotypical patterns of hopelessness, pessimism, and self-criticism in depressed patients. The central thesis of cognitive therapy is that cognition is the primary determinant of emotion and behavior. Cognition is linked to depressive psychopathology in terms of dysfunctional attitudes and negative automatic thoughts about self, world, and future, as well as habitual errors of information processing (A. T. Beck 1976; Dob-

son and Block 1988) (see Christensen et al., Chapter 8, in this volume). (For a detailed review of the historical basis of CBT, see Dobson and Block 1988.) In addition, Clark and colleagues (1999) provide a comprehensive and thorough review of the philosophical and theoretical assumptions behind the cognitive theory of depression.

The foundation of cognitive therapy is built on several pragmatic and theoretical assumptions. First, therapy has a psychoeducational orientation. Cognitive therapy assumes that people are capable of learning new ways of perceiving themselves, others, and their futures. They are taught to examine their reactions and learn about their vulnerabilities. Cognitive therapy also helps the patient learn about the nature of his or her depressive disorder, his or her perceptions and reactions to stressors in his or her life, and the rationale for trying out new coping strategies and problem-solving methods. Second, between-session assignments, or homework, are an integral part of the therapy and provide an opportunity for patients to practice newly learned skills outside of the therapy session, thereby enhancing and generalizing the learning of new ways of coping. Third, an objective assessment of the depressive symptomatology at each session fosters objectivity and provides a rational basis for evaluating the utility of the therapy. Fourth, therapy is directive and requires a high level of therapist activity. Each session follows an orderly sequence or agenda, and the therapist is responsible for ensuring that sessions adhere to this structure. Fifth, for most patients, the therapy is time limited, generally consisting of 12–20 weekly sessions. Sixth, cognitive therapy is based on empirical evidence that validates its theoretical orientation and guides the therapist's choice of therapeutic techniques. Seventh, the therapist uses a style of engagement known as *collaborative empiricism*, which reflects both the use of specific techniques (guided discovery, Socratic questioning, and elicitation of feedback) and the willingness to modify therapeutic tactics in response to patient feedback.

The Cognitive Model

Beck's cognitive model of psychopathology is based on the theoretical assumption that environmental stimuli are filtered through the individual's perception (orienting scheme), thereby triggering cognitive structures and products that define the personal meaning of the event for that person. The perception also elicits physiological and affective arousal. Emotions, subsequently, have a potent reciprocal effect on cognitive content and information processing, resulting in depressive ideation characterized by cascades of dysfunctional thoughts that are reinforced by undesired behavioral outcomes. The individual's behavioral responses to stimuli and negative thoughts are interpreted to be both the product and the cause of his or her depression. Cognitive therapy identifies treatment interventions that can target any or all of the components of the model.

This classic model of cognitive therapy has been expanded to consider other factors that are involved in the etiology of depression, including genetic predisposition, state-dependent neurobiological changes, and comorbidity with other psychiatric disorders. An expanded cognitive-behavioral model (Figure 22–1) synthesizes (Clark et al. 1999; Wright and Thase 1992) cognitive and neurobiological/pharmacological factors in a combined treatment model. In light of this expanded model, contemporary researchers are trying to understand how best to combine or sequence cognitive therapy and pharmacotherapy and how to relate cognitive therapy techniques to new advances in cognitive neuroscience.

The cognitive model assumes that behaviors represent the learned responses an individual has formed in response to his or her early childhood environment. These learned responses manifest as patterns of thinking, emotional reactivity, and behavior. The patterns of thinking that the individual uses to deal with environmental challenges compose the "rules" that characterize his or her cognitive processing and reveal deep-rooted beliefs about himself or herself. Maladaptive beliefs are continuously reinforced by unconscious, automatic negative thoughts and undesirable behavioral outcomes. Over the course of a trial of cognitive therapy, these factors are analyzed in a graded and increasingly comprehensive manner so that the patient comes to recognize and ultimately reframe his or her maladaptive cognitions and replace his or her maladaptive behaviors with more satisfying and healthy ones. Tables 22–1 to 22–3 summarize the evidence from randomized clinical trials of the effectiveness of cognitive therapy in the treatment of major depression.

Dysfunctional Information Processing

In the first treatment manual for cognitive therapy, A. T. Beck and colleagues (1979) described how systematic errors maintain depressed patients' beliefs in the validity of their automatic negative thoughts despite the presence of evidence to the contrary. The identification, assessment, and modification of dysfunctional thinking are the core techniques of cognitive therapy (A. T. Beck 1976; Dobson and Shaw 1986; Segal 1988; Teasdale 1983). At the more superficial level are the automatic negative thoughts, which are stream-of-consciousness cognitions (e.g., thoughts, memories, or images) that may either arise spontaneously or occur in response to an environmental stimulus. Automatic negative thoughts may be provoked by affective arousal (e.g., anger, anxiety, or sadness), or, conversely, affective arousal may trigger familiar automatic negative thoughts (Teasdale 1983). They are called *automatic* to reflect their rapid speed of entry into awareness. Furthermore, because automatic negative thoughts are implicitly believed to be true, they are said to have emotional validity (Thase and Beck 1993). Before patients learn cognitive therapy, most are unaware of their automatic negative thoughts or do not examine them with any rigor or in any detail. Errors in interpretation of events thus go unquestioned. Consider an example from everyday life: it is common to have the thought "This always happens to me" when one has selected the wrong (i.e., slow-moving) line at the grocery store or bank, when in actuality, the speed of a particular line is, more likely than not, a random event that is outside the individual's control. Although all people experience auto-

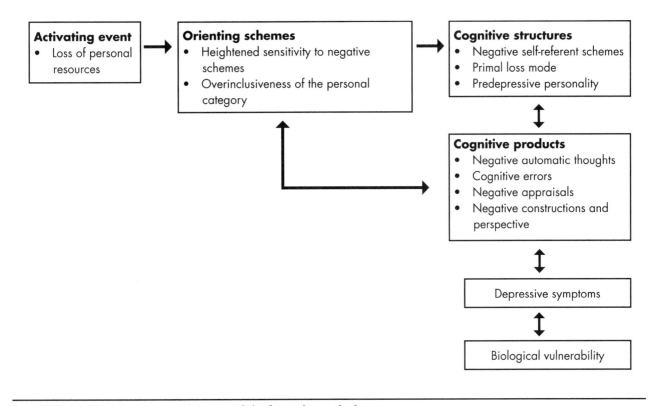

FIGURE 22–1. **Beck's cognitive model of psychopathology.**

Source. Modified from Clark DA, Beck AT, Alford BA: *Scientific Foundations of Cognitive Theory and Therapy of Depression.* New York, Wiley, 1999, pp 76–112. Copyright © 1999 by John Wiley & Sons, Inc. Used with permission of John Wiley & Sons, Inc.

matic negative thoughts at times of emotional activation, in depression, these thoughts are distinguished by their greater intensity and frequency (LeFebvre 1981).

A.T. Beck (1967) proposed the concept of the *cognitive triad* to describe the stereotypical content of automatic negative thinking. He observed that patients' automatic negative thoughts fall into three major groups: 1) negative thoughts about oneself, 2) negative thoughts about the world (i.e., their interpersonal interactions with other people in their lives), and 3) negative thoughts about the future. In psychopathological states, a collection of these thoughts can be used to point to one or more patterns or themes, which can be organized to infer a "deeper" type of cognition—core beliefs. In cognitive therapy, patients are taught to examine these beliefs, to evaluate their utility in attaining goals, and to consider whether alternative beliefs might increase the likelihood of desired outcomes. In a modification of cognitive therapy described in more detail later, McCullough (2000) increased the therapeutic focus on helping the patient to identify desired and obtained outcomes in everyday life, as well as practicing alternative methods of social problem solving. This more specific focus may be particularly useful for more chronically de-

pressed patients, who tend to have more global (and less specific) recollections of problematic interactions.

Beck and associates (A.T. Beck and Emery 1985; A.T. Beck et al. 1979; Wright and Beck 1983) have described stereotypical errors in logic in the thinking of depressed patients. These errors are termed *cognitive errors* or *cognitive distortions* and are characterized by a selective distortion of information processing that shapes the content of the automatic negative thoughts. Examples of cognitive distortions include all-or-none thinking, magnification or minimization, overgeneralization, personalization, emotional reasoning, jumping to conclusions, and selective abstraction. Definitions of several common cognitive distortions are included in Table 22–4.

Effective cognitive therapists look for examples of automatic negative thoughts that are associated with heightened affective states (i.e., "hot cognitions"). During times of affective arousal, one's focus is narrowed, information processing is simplified, and more basic or "overlearned" behavioral responses are intensified. Thase and Beck (1993) suggested that such changes in thinking might have had evolutionary benefit by priming the individual to respond decisively in a crisis situation. This view is consistent

TABLE 22–1. Randomized clinical trials comparing cognitive therapy (CT) and nonpharmacological control conditions as acute-phase treatments of major depressive disorder

Study	N	Duration (weeks)	Comparison of efficacy
Shaw 1977	32	4	CT (group)>attentional control CT (group) >waiting list CT (group)=BT (group)
Fleming and Thornton 1980	35	4	CT (group)[a]≤BT (group) CT (group)[a]=dynamic psychotherapy (group)
Comas-Diaz 1981	26	4	CT (group)[a]>waiting-list assessment
Gallagher and Thompson 1982 (geriatric patients)	37	12	CT=BT CT≥dynamic psychotherapy
Wilson et al. 1983	25	8	CT[a]>waiting list CT[a]=BT
Steuer et al. 1984 (geriatric patients)	33	36	CT (group)≥dynamic therapy (group)
Ross and Scott 1985	51	12	CT>waiting list CT (group)=CT (individual)
Rude 1986	48	5	CT[a]>waiting list CT[a]=BT
Beutler et al. 1987	56	20	CT (group)+placebo>supportive care+placebo
Covi and Lipman 1987	70	14	CT (group)>"traditional" process group
Thompson et al. 1987 (geriatric patients)	91	16	CT>waiting list CT=dynamic psychotherapy CT=BT
Hogg and Deffenbacher 1988 (college students)	37	8	CT (group)[a]=waiting list[b] CT (group)[a]=dynamic psychotherapy (group)
Elkin et al. 1989	239	16	CT≥placebo+clinical management[c] CT=IPT
M.J. Scott and Stradling 1990 (study 1: primary care setting)	67	12	CT>waiting list CT (group)=CT (individual)
(study 2: employee assistance setting)	36	12	CT (group)=CT (individual)
Selmi et al. 1990	36	6	CT=computerized CT CT>waiting list
N.S. Jacobson et al. 1991	72	16	CT[d]≥BT (marital)
Beach and O'Leary 1992	45	15	CT>waiting list CT=BT (marital)
Propst et al. 1992[e] (devoutly religious patients)	59	12	CT ("conventional")>waiting list CT ("conventional")=pastoral counseling CT (religious)>pastoral counseling CT (religious)≥CT (nonreligious)
Shapiro et al. 1994		16	CT≥psychodynamic IPT
N.S. Jacobson et al. 1996	149	16	CT=AT=BA

Note. BT=behavior therapy; IPT=interpersonal psychotherapy; AT=automatic thoughts; ">" indicates more efficacy; "≥" indicates at least as much efficacy and sometimes more; "=" indicates equal efficacy.
[a]CT condition is not fully representative of A.T. Beck's (1976) model of treatment.
[b]Waiting-list group was not randomly assigned. Waiting-list subjects' treatment was delayed by the Christmas holiday break in classes.
[c]General pattern of results favored active treatments over control, especially for IPT (relative to placebo) in more severely depressed patients.
[d]CT was more effective in couples whose marriages were not distressed.
[e]This study included two forms of CT: "conventional" and a specially modified form integrating religious beliefs and metaphors.
Source. Adapted and updated from Thase 2001.

TABLE 22–2. Randomized, controlled clinical trials comparing depression-focused cognitive therapy (CT) and pharmacotherapy as acute-phase treatments of major depressive disorder

Study	N	Duration (weeks)	Comparison of efficacy
Rush et al. 1977	41	12	CT>imipramine
Rush and Watkins 1981	39	12	Combined (tricyclic)[a]>CT
Blackburn et al. 1981	64	12	Combined=CT>tricyclic[a] (general practice clinic setting) Combined[b]≥CT=tricyclic[a] (psychiatric clinic setting)
Teasdale et al. 1984	34	15	CT+TAU>TAU[c]
Murphy et al. 1984	70	12	Combined=CT=nortriptyline
Beck et al. 1985	33	12	Combined (amitriptyline)=CT
Beutler et al. 1987	56	20	CT (group)+alprazolam>alprazolam alone
Covi and Lipman 1987	70	14	Combined (imipramine)=CT (group)
Elkin et al. 1989	239	16	CT≤imipramine[e]
Hollon et al. 1992	106	12	Combined[b]≥CT=imipramine
McKnight et al. 1992	43	8	CT=amitriptyline[c]
Murphy et al. 1995	37	16	CT=RT>desipramine
Blackburn and Moore 1997	75	16	CT=antidepressants[a]
Jarrett et al. 1999	108	10	CT=phenelzine>placebo
Keller et al. 2000	681	12	Combined>CT=nefazodone

Note. TAU=treatment as usual; RT=relaxation therapy; ">" indicates more efficacy; "≥" indicates at least as much efficacy and sometimes more; "=" indicates equal efficacy.
[a]This indicates physician's choice of medication.
[b]Advantage of combined treatment was limited to selected measures.
[c]TAU was provided by primary care physician.
[d]Imipramine was more rapidly effective than either form of psychotherapy. Also, imipramine was more effective than CT in patients with Hamilton Rating Scale for Depression scores>2.
[e]Melancholic and hypercortisolemic patients in both cells had significantly poorer outcomes.
Source. Adapted from Thase 2001.

with recent findings that elucidated the distinct affective and cognitive pathways composing the neurocircuitry of brain fear pathways. LeDoux (1988) reported that activation of the fear pathway causes a sequential activation of affective (limbic-amygdala branch) and cognitive (hippocampal-cortical branch) pathways. Because the affective pathway is shorter, it activates milliseconds before the cognitive pathway. Thus, environmental situations that elicit fear trigger this sequential affective and cognitive response. Similarly, environmental situations that elicit thoughts of worthlessness, hopelessness, and futility trigger depressive affective and cognitive responses.

Core beliefs or schemas represent the learned templates that guide perception, organize experience, and shape the probability of certain behavioral responses. A schema is composed of the basic assumptions about oneself and attitudes and expectations about others and is operationalized by the individual's rules of conduct that translated beliefs into actions (Segal 1988; Wright and Beck 1983; Young and Lindermann 1992). Some of the easiest schemas to conceptualize are the ones that permit us to tie our shoes or ride a bicycle. More pertinent to the vulnerability to depression are schemas relating to one's intimate relationships and competence. Schemas that pertain to safety, vulnerability to threat, and the trustworthiness of caregivers are common in related and often comorbid psychopathologies (A.T. Beck et al. 1990; Blackburn et al. 1986a; Segal 1988; Young and Lindermann 1992).

Although schemas certainly can be understood as the product of a lifetime of experience (and, thus, are subject

TABLE 22–3.   Effect sizes of cognitive therapy

Source	Comparison group	Outcome/ end point	Estimated effect size (Cohen's *d* or *w*)	NNT
Depression Guideline Panel 1993	Waiting list	Response rate	>1.0	>2
Depression Guideline Panel 1993; Thase 2001	Placebo	Response rate	0.2	10
Depression Guideline Panel 1993; Thase 2001	Other psychotherapies	Response rate	0	Undefined
Depression Guideline Panel 1993; Thase 2001	Pharmacotherapy	Response rate	0	Undefined
Fava et al. 1994	No-treatment control group	Relapse rate	>1.0	>2
Fava et al. 1998	No-treatment control group	Recurrence risk	>1.0	2
Paykel et al. 1999	No-treatment control group	Relapse rate	0.4	5
Jarrett et al. 2001	No-treatment control group	Relapse rate	0.6	4

Note.   NNT=number needed to treat.

to change or revision), it is also true that many events that shape our core beliefs take place in childhood and adolescence. Maladaptive early childhood experiences that teach the person to see himself or herself as vulnerable to the demands of others, as not valuable or loved by others, or as incompetent in endeavors are incorporated into his or her adult schema. Bowlby (1985) noted that most psychopathologically relevant schemas are developed early in life when the individual is relatively powerless and dependent on caregivers.

Some of the psychopathological implications of schemas can be dormant or "silent" for decades. For example, the schematic dictum that "I must succeed in order to be worthwhile" may not have harsh emotional consequences unless one encounters vocational setbacks. Schemas become activated when a person is confronted with new environmental stimuli that are relevant to a particular type of vulnerability (Clark et al. 1999). Being fired from a job is generally experienced as a stressful life event, but it is only depressogenic for the subset of individuals whose well-being is contingent on success. In this manner, the cognitive model of depression emphasizes a diathesis-stress model (Metalasky et al. 1987; Thase and Beck 1993). A considerable amount of evidence confirms the role of dysfunctional information processing in depression. Negative automatic thoughts have been found to be more common in depressed patients than in control subjects (Blackburn et al. 1986b; Dobson and Shaw 1986; LeFebvre 1981; Watkins and Rush 1983). Patients with

high levels of anxiety were found to have automatic thoughts about uncontrollability, threat, or danger (Ingram and Kendall 1987; Kendall and Hollon 1989). In some clinical studies, depressed patients have had higher levels of dysfunctional attitudes (Blackburn et al. 1986b; DeRubeis et al. 1990; Simons et al. 1984), distorted attributions to life events (Abramson et al. 1978; Deutscher and Cimbolic 1990; Peterson et al. 1985; Sweeney et al. 1986; Zautra et al. 1985), and negatively biased responses to feedback (DeMonbreun and Craighead 1977; Rizley 1978; Wenzloff and Grozier 1988). Miranda and colleagues (Miranda and Persons 1999; Miranda et al. 1990) have found that dysfunctional attitudes are mood-state dependent and that the endorsement of dysfunctional beliefs depends on a formerly depressed person's current mood state. Segal and Gemar (Gemar et al. 2001; Segal et al. 1999) have shown that previously depressed individuals had an increase in dysfunctional attitudes and a more negative evaluative bias for self-relevant information after the induction of a negative mood when compared with healthy control subjects.

Basic Strategies and Techniques Used in Cognitive Therapy

Cognitive therapy uses several specific techniques to effect therapeutic change. These techniques are derived from a body of empirical research that has accumulated

TABLE 22–4. Common patterns of irrational thinking in anxiety and depression

Overgeneralization	Evidence drawn from one experience or a small set of experiences that reaches an unwarranted conclusion with far-reaching implications
Catastrophic thinking	An extreme example of overgeneralization in which the effect of a clearly negative event or experience is amplified to extreme proportions (e.g., "If I have a panic attack, I will lose all control and go crazy [or die].")
Maximizing and minimizing	The tendency to exaggerate negative experiences and minimize positive experiences in one's activities and interpersonal relationships
All-or-none (black-or-white, absolutistic) thinking	An unnecessary division of complex or continuous outcomes into polarized extremes (e.g., "Either I am a success at this or I am a total failure.")
Jumping to conclusions	Use of pessimism or earlier experiences of failure to predict failure prematurely or inappropriately in a new situation (also known as fortune telling)
Personalization	Interpretation of an event, situation, or behavior as salient or personally indicative of a negative aspect of self
Selective negative focus—"ignoring the evidence" or "mental filter"	Undesirable or negative events, memories, or implications that are focused on at the expense of recalling or identifying other, more neutral or positive information (In fact, positive information may be ignored or disqualified as irrelevant, atypical, or trivial.)

over the past 40 years (Clark et al. 1999; Dobson and Block 1988). Although these basic techniques may be viewed as the cornerstones of cognitive therapy, there is considerable leeway for flexibility and creativity on the part of individual therapists in developing a case formulation and implementing a course of therapy. Ultimately, theory and technique must be adapted to fit the needs of the patient and to maximize the likelihood of a successful outcome.

As in all psychotherapies, the therapist must develop a productive therapeutic alliance with the patient. From the onset of therapy, the therapist begins formulating an individualized case conceptualization with the information learned from patterns of the patient's automatic negative thoughts, rules, and beliefs. The most important treat-ment strategies used to help depressed patients are summarized here, and the interested reader may find more detailed accounts elsewhere (A.T. Beck et al. 1979; J.S. Beck 1995; Freeman et al. 1989; Greenberger and Padesky 1995; Persons 1989; Persons et al. 2001).

Structure and Pacing of Sessions

Cognitive therapy sessions follow a standard format. The initial segment, which typically lasts 5–10 minutes, includes a review of symptomatic status (typically with the Beck Depression Inventory or a similar self-report scale), a review of homework activities (described in the "Homework" subsection later in this chapter), and the creation of an agenda for the remainder of the session. The second segment consists of the "work" of the sessions, which usually consists of one or two focused interventions. The third segment is used to summarize the work that was accomplished in the session and to develop a new homework assignment. Effective therapists are able to maintain an appropriate pace throughout the session and facilitate smooth transitions by seeking feedback from the patient before moving on to the next segment.

Collaborative Empiricism

One distinguishing characteristic of the therapeutic relationship in cognitive therapy is based on the notion of collaborative empiricism. Unlike more traditional psychotherapies, cognitive therapy sessions follow a particular structure, and the therapist's explicit task is to manage each session actively within that structure. Collaborative empiricism can be thought of as the stylistic fulcrum that permits the helping alliance to thrive within the artificial constraints of structured sessions. This is accomplished through two principles: 1) the patient must perceive that his or her feedback and understanding of therapeutic interchanges are essential to the success of therapy; and 2) together, therapist and patient adopt a scientific approach based on testing the validity of dysfunctional cognitions and the utility of maladaptive behaviors. The empirical nature of this therapeutic stance requires the therapist and patient to work together as an investigative team to develop hypotheses about cognitive and behavioral patterns that can be tested by examining data. Such hypothesis testing can lead to explorations of alternative ways of thinking and behaving.

Implicit in this model is the conviction that learning is possible on the part of the patient. Because depression biases cognitive processes, therapists can help the patient to examine the evidence more realistically for his or her distorted attitudes and beliefs. The therapist proves this to the patient through behavioral experiments that can lead to demonstrable benefits for the patient.

Compared with other types of psychotherapy, in the initial sessions of cognitive therapy, the therapist spends more time teaching and explaining cognitive therapy. As the patient comes to understand the model and can apply his or her newly learned cognitive therapy techniques appropriately when needed, the therapist becomes less active to allow the patient to lead the collaborative team.

Beck and colleagues (Clark et al. 1999; Wright et al. 2004) have recommended several strategies to enhance collaborative empiricism:

- Adjusting the therapist's level of activity to match the patient's symptom severity or phase of treatment
- Encouraging the use of self-help procedures
- Attending to "nonspecific" psychotherapeutic variables—respect for the patient, empathy, equanimity, kindness, and good listening skills
- Using feedback from the patient and summarizing at key points in the session to ensure that the patient and therapist are on the same track
- Devising coping strategies for the patient to help him or her deal with real problems or implementing a plan of action to address maladaptive behaviors
- Recognizing and interpreting behaviors traditionally thought to reflect transference phenomena according to the cognitive therapy model
- Customizing the therapeutic intervention to the intellectual and emotional level of the patient or to the phase of depression the patient is currently experiencing
- Using humor judiciously to point out the dysfunctional aspects of cognitive distortions and maladaptive behaviors
- Recognizing the individual and cultural differences, social attitudes, and expectations that each person brings to therapy (Wright and Davis 1994)

Psychoeducation

Psychoeducation, although not unique to cognitive therapy, is another characteristic of this modality. The initial session includes a description of the therapy and its methods and almost always ends with provision of an informational pamphlet about cognitive therapy (A. T. Beck and Greenberg 1974). Further psychoeducation is implemented during the course of therapy by blending information about depression and its treatment within sessions in a manner that does not emphasize formal teaching. Beginning in the first session, the therapist explains and demonstrates the basic concepts of cognitive therapy with

examples based on the patient's symptomatology, history, or patterns of cognition and behavior. By using situations, feelings, and thoughts from the patient's experience to explain the basic principles, the therapist ensures that the learning process is relevant and increases the likelihood that new modes of thinking will be used. As the patient acculturates to the methods of cognitive therapy and shows competency with its techniques, the therapist can use less active methods, such as Socratic questioning techniques (discussed in the "Socratic Questioning" subsection later in this chapter). Furthermore, the patient's expectations for the therapy are fully explored, problems are defined, and goals for the therapy are established. This process, in itself, models a problem-solving methodology for the patient that is a critical cognitive therapy skill.

Homework

Homework is a defining characteristic of all models of CBT. The primary rationale for homework is to give the patient an opportunity to practice and reinforce the strategies learned within a session. Evidence shows that homework compliance increases the likelihood of a favorable treatment outcome (Burns and Spangler 2000; Whisman 1993). In addition to the initial reading assignment (A. T. Beck and Greenberg 1974), other books such as *Feeling Good* (Burns 1980), *The Feeling Good Handbook* (Burns 1990), *Mind Over Mood* (Greenberger and Padesky 1995), and *Getting Your Life Back* (Wright and Basco 2001) can be used to guide homework assignments. We advocate the use of a notebook to document in-session discussions and to organize homework and other assignments. In this way, the notebook becomes a personal "instruction manual" that summarizes the techniques and methods learned and applied in therapy. In the future, computer-assisted assignments are likely to be used in the early stages of a therapy's development to augment the therapeutic process (Locke and Rezza 1996; Wright and Wright 1997; Wright et al. 2001).

Modifying Automatic Negative Thoughts

A primary task of the early sessions of cognitive therapy is to help the patient recognize automatic negative thoughts and begin to challenge and modify them. A seasoned therapist will begin to note and record the patient's automatic negative thoughts as the psychiatric history is obtained. Often, a salient and prominent automatic negative thought can be used psychoeducationally to illustrate the cognitive therapy model in the first session.

The most important automatic negative thoughts, or

FIGURE 22–2. Sample Daily Record of Dysfunctional Thoughts.

Situation/ behavior	Feelings	Thoughts (automatic negative thoughts)	Cognitive distortion	Strength of belief
"My boss looked sternly at me." (He is anxious to get his new computer.)	Ashamed Anxious Sad and low	"He thinks I am stupid." Rule: "If others are angry with me, it must be because I am stupid."	1. Disregarded the positive (a history of good work evaluations) 2. "Jumped to conclusions" or used "mind-reading" (made an assumption not based on evidence) 3. Used personalization (external events are my fault)	Originally: 90% After automatic negative thought examined and modified: <30%

Realistic alternative:
"Just because my boss was impatient over his new computer arriving does not mean that I did something wrong."

"hot thoughts," are associated with strong affects; A. T. Beck (1991) thus referred to emotion as the "royal road to cognition." Often, "hot cognitions" are identified while reviewing the symptom review inventory or mood shifts noted in the Weekly Activity Schedule. Standard questions to elicit automatic negative thoughts are as follows: "What thoughts ran through your mind during that time you were feeling so depressed? Is it possible to speak those thoughts out loud?" Of course, witnessing a patient's sudden mood shift during the session will provide an invaluable opportunity to examine the patient's thoughts. The automatic negative thought associated with the shift in emotion is identified and can be examined for its accuracy or for examples of cognitive errors (see Table 22–1). To facilitate this process, a second form, the Daily Record of Dysfunctional Thoughts (also called a Five-Column Sheet; Figure 22–2), is used within sessions and for homework assignments.

For example, when reviewing her mood symptoms, Ms. A stated that she had felt most depressed this past week on Tuesday during work. In fact, she became tearful recalling the incident—her boss had "looked sternly at me" after he inquired about a purchase order and a piece of office equipment he was expecting. She became sullen and withdrawn, avoiding any further contact with him that day. "Luckily for me," she reported, "it came in the next morning."

One of Ms. A's automatic negative thoughts was identified: "He thinks I'm stupid." Next, the evidence for her belief was examined. First, the boss had never said anything to her about her intelligence being inadequate, and she has always had good work evaluations from him ("disregarding the positive"). Second, it appeared that Ms. A may have

"jumped to conclusions" or used "mind reading" to assume her boss's real thoughts (negative) about her. Third, Ms. A may have "personalized" this situation by interpreting his behavior as indicating a negative aspect of her abilities. A dysfunctional attitude could be identified: "If others are angry with me, then it must be because I'm stupid," which would be addressed later in the course of therapy. In summary, a realistic alternative to her automatic negative thought would be identified, such as: "Just because my boss was impatient over his new computer arriving doesn't mean that I did something wrong. And if I didn't do anything wrong, there's no reason to think I'm stupid."

The fourth and fifth columns of the Daily Record of Dysfunctional Thoughts concern developing rational alternatives to the automatic negative thoughts and evaluating the effect of the intervention on feelings of depression or anxiety. Specifically, the patient is asked to rate the strength of his or her belief in the thought—at the time it occurred (e.g., 90%) and after the automatic negative thought is examined and modified (e.g., 30%). Furthermore, patients are taught to question, "What does the automatic negative thought mean about you?" Such inquiries lead to identification of the patient's beliefs, which can then be discussed and examined for whether they aid or inhibit the patient in achieving his or her goals.

Socratic Questioning

Guided discovery or Socratic questioning is an important technique used to examine automatic negative thoughts and to uncover "silent" assumptions and dysfunctional attitudes (A. T. Beck et al. 1979; Overholser 1993a, 1993b, 1993c). Cognitive therapy uses the principles of rational inquiry and inductive reasoning, grounded in the collaborative empirical stance, to help the patient learn to challenge the validity of his or her thoughts and feelings. Gentle, nonconfrontational questions are used to engage the patient in inquiry into the evidence for his or her automatic negative thoughts, with the goal of modifying his or her biased or distorted cognitive style ("And if that were true, what would that really say about you, your place in the world, or your future?"). Few formal guidelines exist for Socratic questioning (Overholser 1993a), and effectiveness in using this technique comes with time and practice. Permissive phrases such as "Is it okay if we talk about…" or "Do you mind if I ask you a question about…?" can be used to respectfully address difficult problem areas. The responses to such questioning can be used to guide the patient to new ways of approaching problems and modifying automatic negative thoughts, rules, and beliefs. When long-standing, learned behaviors can be questioned by the patient, they are open to modification. Alternative interpretations and behaviors can be proposed as reasonable options available if the patient so chooses.

Imagery Techniques and Role-Playing

Some patients do not respond well to Socratic questioning, and imagery techniques and role-playing may be helpful in those circumstances. For some patients, visualization techniques are helpful in eliciting distressing situations. Imagining the scene of a situation that was associated with strong emotional reaction can aid in identifying the automatic negative thought. Some patients need prompts to visualize scenes. These can be framed as helpful questions, such as 1) "What can you tell me about the physical details of the setting?" 2) "What occurred immediately before the interaction?" and 3) "Can you describe the other people in the scene?" (Wright et al. 2004). Role-playing allows the patient and therapist to play out interpersonal vignettes and thereby to help elicit automatic negative thoughts. The therapist can play the antagonist in the patient's description of a distressing situation and monitor the patient's reactions and cognitions. Once identified, automatic negative thoughts can be analyzed. The therapist can also play the patient, adopting the patient's coping strategies (sometimes exaggerating them) to make them obvious to the patient.

Examining the Evidence and Generating Realistic Thoughts

The collaborative empirical relationship provides a safe haven where patients can learn to examine the evidence for, and against, their automatic negative thoughts. The use of Socratic questioning provides a technique for doing so.

Thus, the collaborative team can examine the validity of a patient's automatic negative thoughts in an emotionally "uncharged" environment. We use the scientific method to model a rational approach to questioning the validity of beliefs. The patient is instructed to treat cognitions as hypotheses to be tested rather than as established facts. Patients are taught to make pro and con lists of pieces of evidence that support or refute the hypothesis in question. Each of these lists is kept in the notebook and can be added to over time—modeling the longitudinal need to continue to attend to this process after therapy ends. The therapist can assign hypotheses to be examined as homework assignments, helping patients to acquire and exercise the skill set in between sessions and to apply their analytic skills to new problems. Thus, the patient moves from general, negatively biased, unchanging, and global interpretations to more specific, factually based statements.

After the patient identifies the conflicting evidence for the dysfunctional automatic negative thought, he or she is guided to make a "realistic alternative" revision of the automatic negative thought that is factually based. Socratic questioning, psychoeducation, use of the Daily Record of Dysfunctional Thoughts, and identification of maladaptive beliefs are techniques that help the patient to think in a more adaptive and functional manner. Gradually, these changes in cognition are reinforced through practice and rehearsal. Incrementally, the patient replaces dysfunctional automatic negative thoughts with corresponding and more adaptive and satisfying realistic alternatives.

Examining Rules, Core Beliefs, and Schemas

As patients begin to master use of the Daily Record of Dysfunctional Thoughts, the therapist can begin to encourage them to look for common themes that point to the rules and beliefs that may underpin negative thinking. The techniques used to examine automatic negative thoughts also can be applied to the rational examination of rules, beliefs, and schemas. Most patients are unaware of the rules that guide their behaviors. Patients can use the scientific method to test the validity of their rules and to examine their usefulness. This method often leads to an examination of their "core beliefs," those bedrock beliefs about their adequacy, ability to be loved or to love, and ability to trust. The beliefs are also tested through rational inquiry, and hypothetical alternative beliefs can be generated and then examined in vivo.

Schemas define the patient's reality by incorporating the patient's most strongly held beliefs. As a consequence, schemas are often highly resistant to change because, in essence, they describe the patient's most adaptive solutions to life problems confronted in the past. Nonetheless, schemas can be examined and analyzed for common themes. These themes can be related to the patient's early childhood experiences, helping him or her to identify the sources of his or her dysfunctional core beliefs. Then, consistent with the learning model, these themes can be examined for veracity and utility. The patient then can generate new, and more adaptive, strategies for problem solving and emotional regulation. Young (1999) described in depth the cognitive therapy approach to schema-focused therapy.

Behavioral Techniques

Even in cognitive therapy, behavioral techniques are used to counteract the behavioral inactivation component (anhedonia, lethargy, and amotivation symptoms) of depression. A useful guiding principle is that the greater the degree of a patient's behavioral inactivation, the greater the emphasis on behavioral techniques. Rehm (1977) described depression as a deficit state characterized by a lack of adaptive self-reinforcement. Some investigators (Weiss and Simson 1985; Willner 1991) believe that neurobiological changes accompanying prolonged stress underpin such dampened hedonic capacity. Thus, the fundamental problem may be decreased reward salience rather than decreased exposure to rewarding activities. This view complements those of Seligman (1975) pertaining to learned helplessness as a model for the etiology of depression. When cognitive and behavioral techniques are combined, we can treat deficits in these biological and behavioral domains (Friedman et al. 2003; Wright and Thase 1992).

Behavioral activation strategies include activity scheduling, graded task assignments, and mastery-pleasure exercises. Behavioral activation techniques are used to actively overcome the lethargy cycle of depression, in which amotivation and indecisiveness, fatigue, lethargy, and anhedonia reinforce automatic negative thoughts and beliefs of inadequacy and failure. This cycle becomes self-reinforcing, as worry and inactivity lead to sleep-cycle disintegration, which promotes further biological dysregulations that compromise subjective appraisals of well-being.

One way to reverse this cycle is to engage the patient in planned activities that substantially increase the patient's access to reinforcement. The basic tool for this process is called the Weekly Activity Schedule, a calendar-like template that is used to help the patient document how he or she spends time and to schedule new activities. A Weekly Activity Schedule is included in the first psychoeducationally oriented homework assignment, the *Coping With Depression* pamphlet (A. T. Beck and Green-

berg 1974). The patient is instructed to fill in the hourly grid with his or her activities. The therapist examines the activities the patient engaged in over the past week. The patient is taught to appraise realistically the mastery and pleasure he or she experienced while performing these activities. In so doing, the patient comes to see that an adequate degree of mastery can be achieved even when we derive little pleasure from an activity. Conversely, some activities may be very pleasurable even when we cannot completely master them.

To enhance his or her sense of competence, the patient is taught to examine situations realistically for their degree of mastery and pleasure. To accomplish tasks effectively, the patient must have realistic goals. He or she must learn to have realistic expectations of his or her abilities. Realistic expectations can be deduced from activities that were successfully completed in the past, and they can be modified for the depressed state. Patients learn that depression interferes with successful performance of usual activities and that standards must be revised to take into account the need for lower expectations. (When the patient is depressed, the coda needs to be that activities are "harder to do, take longer to do...but they can nonetheless be accomplished.") The therapist must design tasks and assignments that give the patient the opportunity to reestablish self-efficacy, particularly the morale to view oneself as an active problem solver. This is done in a graded manner, slowly increasing the complexity and difficulty of the tasks assigned to the patient in proportion to both his or her ability and the degree of improvement in the depression. Exploring with the patient those efficient coping strategies he or she once used but abandoned in the current depressed state provides a source of possible tasks to be reintroduced into daily activities. It is important to assign pleasurable activities to the patient as well.

A typical early homework assignment is to identify a pleasurable activity and have the patient schedule it in the Weekly Activity Schedule. As homework, the patient monitors the mastery and pleasure he or she actually attains while engaged in the activity. By self-monitoring his or her hedonic capacity with the Weekly Activity Schedule, the patient learns how expectations and predictions lead to specific mood states and behavioral outcomes.

Intensity and Duration of Cognitive Therapy

Outpatient cognitive therapy usually is conducted twice weekly for the first month and weekly thereafter for a course of 16 to 20 sessions. J.S. Beck (1995) reminds us that termination begins in the first session. As the patient's depression improves, successively longer intervals between sessions can be scheduled to provide the patient the opportunity to use cognitive therapy self-help skills successfully with progressively less therapeutic support. The therapist assesses the patient's success in managing stresses and situations that previously elicited depressive thoughts. During this final phase of treatment, it is important to identify the obstacles that would inhibit the patient from using cognitive therapy self-help skills, to determine the patient's unique vulnerabilities, and to develop a self-management plan to overcome these obstacles. The therapist fosters effective termination by reflecting on the gains the patient has made and the evidence that he or she can now effectively, and independently, manage his or her moods.

Continuation Cognitive Therapy

We have found that most patients who remit fully and rapidly during the acute phase of cognitive therapy do not require further treatment. The relapse risk following time-limited cognitive therapy can be predicted by the patient's pattern of symptoms during the final weeks of therapy. Specifically, patients who are able to achieve and maintain a symptomatic remission for 6 consecutive weeks prior to termination appear to have little risk of relapse (i.e., <10%), whereas patients who have less complete or more labile symptomatic courses are at substantially greater risk (i.e., >50% within 1 year) (Thase et al. 1992). This risk is moderated by lower levels of dysfunctional attitudes and increased by chronicity and an early age at onset. For such patients, an extended course of continuation-phase cognitive therapy has been shown to neutralize the heightened risk of relapse (Jarrett et al. 2001).

Jarrett formulated continuation cognitive therapy for the patients who remain at risk for relapse after acute-phase cognitive therapy. Considered from a learning perspective, acute-phase cognitive therapy teaches patients skills to restructure their attitudes about self, world, and future and to shift their attributional style to more flexible and specific explanations. Acute-phase cognitive therapy draws heavily from learning theory, emphasizing the acquisition, generalization, and maintenance of beneficial coping responses. Cognitive therapy uses behavioral rehearsal and guided practice to promote self-efficacy. From this perspective, incomplete remission reflects an idiosyncratic difference in the higher-risk patient's ability to learn these new strategies, which can be remedied by directed strategies to overcome the blocks to achieving therapeutic goals. In addition, the cognitive therapy model conceptualizes depressive vulnerability as the product of dysfunctional core beliefs and schemas in critical areas pertaining to attachment, approval, or loss, which are exacerbated in response to relevant or matching stressors. From this perspective, incomplete remission may reflect an underlying more serious and persistent cognitive vulnerability. Acute-phase cognitive therapy cannot fully examine or necessarily address the dysfunctional schemas associated with severe depression and anxiety and other severe Axis II disorders. For some patients, other specific CBT should be recommended; for example, dialectical behavior therapy for patients with borderline personality disorder or exposure therapy for obsessive-compulsive disorder. Otherwise, the schematic material can be addressed with continuation cognitive therapy.

Jarrett and Kraft (1997) have defined the theoretical principles to guide practice during continuation cognitive therapy. Whereas acute-phase cognitive therapy seeks to reduce symptoms, continuation cognitive therapy seeks to eliminate symptoms and prevent symptom relapse. Relapse prevention is accomplished through the learning of new skills to reduce or prevent depressive symptoms and to teach the patient to decrease the conditions that foster recurrence. Because the goal is complete recovery, the patient's cognitive and emotional vulnerabilities are identified. These can be explored and analyzed in terms of the patient's beliefs about himself or herself, the world, and the ability to change his or her future.

Continuation cognitive therapy recognizes that living with a recurrent and sometimes chronic illness has consequences and that this situation affects the patient's beliefs. The continuation cognitive therapist must identify the critical skills the patient needs to learn and match them with the characteristics of the patient and his or her environment that promote or impede the acquisition of new skills. These skills then must be generalized and implemented. New skill acquisition is evident when the patient can successfully negotiate situations that would have previously triggered depressive episodes. Over time, continued evidence that the acquired skills are being used constitutes relapse prevention. Dysfunctional schemas are restructured with logical analysis, experimentation, and empiricism to test alternative rules and beliefs. Finally, behavior changes are made that are associated with long-term positive outcomes. Patients show mastery of new skills through comprehension, role-playing, successful homework completion, and the use of these skills in new everyday situations.

Over the course of the therapy, the therapist encourages the generalization of critical cognitive therapy skills by the reduction in frequency of sessions and the gradual turning over of control of both the agenda and the session to the patient. The therapist uses fewer prompts, uses more Socratic questioning, and (consistent with the collaborative empiricism model) allows the patient to identify and analyze recent factors that might impede or promote the use of critical skills. Through the use of "stress inoculation," the therapist challenges the patient's reactions to premorbid stressors through the use of imaginal techniques, bibliotherapy, role-play, and homework assignments. Finally, termination is considered the final part of the generalization of skills process—when the patient is confident in his or her ability to use new skills, and the therapist accedes the locus of control to the patient.

Cognitive-Behavioral Analysis System of Psychotherapy

The Cognitive-Behavioral Analysis System of Psychotherapy (CBASP) (McCullough 2000) was developed specifically to address the problems encountered in the treatment of chronic depression and dysthymia that frequently lead to treatment failure in acute-phase CBT and other therapies. McCullough conceptualized chronic depression to be the product of dysfunctional cognitions of helplessness, hopelessness, and failure that are linked to a detached and maladaptive interpersonal style, which is reinforced by habitually poor social problem solving. In short, the chronically depressed patients' perceptual distortions produce behaviors that are incompatible with their desired outcomes. CBASP is a "person × environment" model of therapy, whereby helpless and hopeless perceptual biases prevent individuals from recognizing the connection between *what they do* and the *effects of what they do on others*. These patients repeatedly experience undesired outcomes as a result of their behaviors, reinforcing their beliefs in their inadequacy and ineffectuality. CBASP aims to establish explicitly, or reestablish, a connection between the person and his or her environment, which helps him or her learn new, adaptive coping styles to attain positive outcomes in his or her environment. CBASP assumes that 1) chronic depression is the result of a person's experience of long-term failure to cope adequately with life stressors; and 2) people can be taught to view their problems in terms of a "person × environment" perspective that results in behavior change, personal empowerment, and improved emotional self-regulation.

McCullough (2000) observed that many chronically depressed individuals function at a preoperational (i.e., prelogical and precausal) stage of thinking. Premises and conclusions are automatically and unconditionally accepted as true because the content is consistent with their affective state. Their thought patterns are generally unaffected by logical reasoning and the reality-based views of others. They do not appreciate cause-and-effect reasoning, and their conclusions are static, global, and unchanging. As is typical of patients with depression, they accept the veracity of their negative thoughts without question, assuming them to be true. As a consequence, any challenges to such thoughts are perceived as direct challenges to the person, leading to interpersonal difficulties and conflictual relationships.

These chronically depressed individuals lack empathy. They speak in monologues, which makes it difficult to engage with others, a particular problem in therapy. This often leads to frustration with others and a lack of emotional control when they are confronted with stressful situations, activating their ideas of helplessness and hopelessness and reinforcing their beliefs about failure.

CBASP teaches patients with preoperational thinking to think causally. It teaches them to engage in social problem solving at a higher developmental level, thereby instituting change. Patients begin to experience more positive outcomes and improvement in interpersonal relationships.

Strategies for Change

McCullough (2000) explained that the "person × environment" interaction maintains the chronicity of depression in these patients. Their preoperational thinking style leads to dysfunctional perceptions that repeatedly produce unpleasant and unwanted outcomes, which positively reinforce their globally negative beliefs. As a result of this understanding, McCullough realized the importance of motivation in overcoming helplessness and hopelessness and the negative reinforcement of their failure experiences. He realized that by teaching chronically depressed individuals to perceive the behavioral consequences of their interactions on others, he could help them obtain more desirable outcomes. They could then change their perceptions of the contingency relationships between their behavior and its consequences. The technique for doing this is to target the antecedent behaviors that produce relief or a decrease in misery and then reinforce these new and more adaptive behaviors. McCullough has devised several techniques for accomplishing these goals: the Situational Analysis, the Interpersonal Discrimination Exercise, the Interpersonal Transference Hypothesis, and the Significant Other List.

Situational Analysis

Situational Analysis is a central CBASP exercise in formal operations training that is used to modify behaviors. It is used both diagnostically and remedially. Diagnostically, the Situational Analysis helps identify the patient's contribution to maladaptive social encounters and various forms of interpersonal, cognitive, and behavioral pathology that result from the encounter. It serves as a remediation exercise once the pathological behaviors are identified because the behaviors can be targeted for change in a gradual manner until desired outcomes are achieved. As in Beckian cognitive therapy, the patients are taught to identify negative affects in the targeted Situational Analysis. Patients compare and contrast their typical problem-solving style with an alternative solution. The CBASP therapist then highlights the relief the patients have experienced and the specific cognitive and behavioral processes that precipitated that relief. In this manner, behavior change is modeled, and the individual is motivated to continue in a process of change through ongoing use of the Situational Analysis technique. See Table 22–5 for a description of the Situational Analysis technique.

Interpersonal Discrimination Exercise

The Interpersonal Discrimination Exercise is another core CBASP technique. This exercise teaches patients new cognitive and behavioral strategies for interacting with important people in their lives. The CBASP therapist uses the Interpersonal Discrimination Exercise to teach the patient formal operational thinking while increasing his or her motivation for change. The therapist uses data about the patient's intimate relationships to generate a cognitive-behavioral conceptualization of the patient. The therapist explores areas in which the patient believes his or her needs are not being met, situations that elicit thoughts of failure, and situations associated with the generation of negative affects.

An important part of the Interpersonal Discrimination Exercise strategy is based on management of the therapist–patient transference relationship as a model for appropriate interpersonal interaction. McCullough understands that long-standing helplessness and hopelessness are the cognitive correlates of chronic depression and that this problem permeates the treatment dyad. The chronically depressed patient enacts his or her helplessness in the session, "pulling" on the therapist to "fix" him or her. In reaction, therapists often have thoughts of failure and feelings of anger and frustration toward the patient. McCullough recognizes that this dynamic must be addressed for therapeutic change to occur. This position of hopelessness reinforces the lack of motivation and the behavioral inactivation characteristic of these patients. These patients come to therapy convinced of their inadequacy, armed with the evidence of many failure experiences, describing themselves in static, global, and unchanging negative terms. McCullough (2000) observed that these patients imposed past behavior

TABLE 22–5. Situational Analysis (SA)

Six therapist prompts are used to elicit an SA:

1. Describe what happened in the situation.
2. Describe your *interpretation(s)* of what happened.
3. Describe what *you* did in the situation.
4. Describe how the event came out for you; that is, what was the *actual outcome?*
5. Describe how you would have wanted the event to come out for you; that is, what is your *desired outcome?*
6. Explain whether you got what you wanted here (why/why not).

Examination of the situation in the SA:

1. How did each interpretation contribute to your obtaining the desired outcome? How did your behavior help you obtain the desired outcome?
2. What did you learn in going through this SA?
3. How does what you have learned in this situation apply to other similar situations?

patterns on the therapeutic relationship. As a result of early childhood experiences of neglect or abuse that are characteristic of the histories of these patients, they expect, in moments of severe distress, to be treated as they were in the past. They fear rejection by the therapist and, if they come to trust the therapist, that they will become dependent on and then ultimately be abandoned by the therapist. CBASP therapists use the Interpersonal Discrimination Exercise to explore these transference issues that inevitably arise in the treatment of such patients. The therapist compares in-session behavior with the patient's expectation about how the session would go. The therapist can identify, compare, and contrast actual versus expected outcomes of the patient's in-session behavior. Then the patient begins to perceive and enact new ways of behaving with other important people in his or her life according to what he or she has learned through the CBASP analysis of transference relationships. The CBASP therapist uses these data to construct Interpersonal Transference Hypotheses that explain maladaptive patterns of behavior. Issues relating to problems with intimacy, failure experiences, unmet emotional needs, ridicule and punishment, and fears of expressing negative affects can be explored in a methodical manner.

Significant Other List

Another important CBASP tool for determining the patient's range of interpersonal behaviors is the Significant Other List. This exercise helps the therapist learn about the major persons who have influenced the patient either positively or negatively. The patient creates a list of significant others, and each person on the list is examined to clarify the consequences of that relationship on the patient's belief system.

Evidence for the Efficacy of Cognitive-Behavioral Analysis System of Psychotherapy

A large multisite randomized trial compared CBASP with the antidepressant drug nefazodone, alone and in combination (Keller et al. 2000). The 681 patients with chronic nonpsychotic major depression were randomly assigned to CBASP, nefazodone, or both. At baseline, all patients had Hamilton Rating Scale for Depression (24-item) scores of at least 20, and remission was defined as a score of 8 or less at weeks 10 and 12. For patients who did not have a remission, a satisfactory response was defined as a reduction in score by at least 50% from baseline and a score of 15 or less. This analysis included all patients who attended at least one treatment session. The overall rate of response (both remission and satisfactory response) was 48% in both the nefazodone group and the CBASP group, compared with 73% in the combined therapy group ($P > 0.001$ for both comparisons). Among the 519 subjects who completed the study, the response rates were 55% in the nefazodone group and 52% in the CBASP group, compared with 85% in the combined therapy group ($P > 0.001$, effect size = 0.59; $P > 0.001$, effect size = 0.64, respectively).

These results are very impressive for several reasons. First, the response rate for the medication group was consistent with antidepressant response rates in other studies, lending credibility to this finding. Second, the degree of superiority of the combined CBASP and medication treatment group suggests a "clinically meaningful advantage" for such treatment in a group of patients who had active depression for many years. Pharmacotherapy produced more rapid effects (significant advantage at 4 weeks), but the psychotherapy had greater effect during the second part of the trial, and by week 12, the efficacy rates were similar. The nefazodone group had higher frequencies of adverse events, but the rate of withdrawal from the study was similar in all three groups. Keller and colleagues (2000) noted that the combined treatment was efficacious later in the study, suggesting that when medication and psychotherapy are administered together, they exert independent rather than synergistic mechanisms of action.

Limitations of this study included the lack of placebo control and the inability to mask patients and their therapists to their treatment group (a problem in all psychotherapy research). The rate of withdrawal was lower in the combined treatment group (21%) than in the nefazodone group (26%) and the CBASP group (24%), which may have biased the outcome comparisons. The restrictive inclusion criteria also may have limited the generalizability of the results.

In an attempt to replicate and advance the validity of this first major CBASP study, the National Institute of Mental Health has sponsored the Research Evaluating the Value of Augmenting Medications With Psychotherapy (REVAMP) program. This multisite randomized, parallel-group clinical trial is studying the efficacy of adjunctive psychotherapy for outpatients with chronic major depression whose symptoms fail to respond fully to a trial of antidepressant medication. The project has three specific aims: 1) to compare the efficacy of adding psychotherapy to a medication change (either switching or augmentation) with that of changing medication alone in patients with chronic depression who are either nonresponders or partial responders to an initial medication trial; 2) to test the specific efficacy of CBASP as an augmentation strategy by comparing it with supportive psychotherapy; and 3) to test a hypothesized mechanism of action of CBASP by examining whether patients receiving CBASP have significantly greater improvements in social problem solving than do patients receiving adjunctive supportive psychotherapy or continued medication alone and to explore whether changes in social problem solving mediate CBASP's efficacy in treating depression. The REVAMP study attempts to address some of the limitations of the CBASP-nefazodone study. The lack of a comparison psychotherapy in that study, or of a placebo comparator condition, is remedied with the comparison of CBASP with supportive psychotherapy.

Supportive psychotherapy (Markowitz et al. 1995) is a patient-centered psychotherapy that contains many of the "nonspecific" factors associated with most psychotherapies: reflective listening, helping patients feel understood, empathy, therapeutic optimism, and an acknowledgment of the patient's assets. However, unlike CBASP therapists, supportive psychotherapy therapists offer no explicit explanatory mechanism for treatment effect, and they do not focus on social problem solving. The supportive psychotherapy treatment manual proscribes interpersonal, cognitive, and psychodynamic interventions. Even though supportive psychotherapy is less structured than CBASP, the supportive psychotherapy group in the REVAMP study will parallel the CBASP group by completing 18 therapy sessions in 12 weeks.

The REVAMP study also uses a sequenced medication algorithm to optimize each patient's pharmacological response. Medications available in the treatment algorithm include sertraline, citalopram, bupropion, venlafaxine, mirtazapine, and lithium augmentation. The sequenced medication treatment model emphasizes monotherapies before combinations and those interventions that have already been studied in chronically depressed patients. It is hoped that these results will be generalizable and able to provide clinically important treatment recommendations for patients with chronic depression.

Conclusion

Recent years have seen significant advances in the treatment of chronic depression. The cognitive-behavioral therapies have broadened their treatment scope to address problems of recurrence and residual symptoms. CBASP offers additional techniques that address the specific cognitive, behavioral, and relational problems of patients with chronic depression. When CBT is combined with optimal pharmacotherapy, we may be able to effectively treat the chronic depressive disorders.

References

Abramson LY, Seligman MEP, Teasdale J: Learned helplessness in humans: critique and reformulation. J Abnorm Psychol 87:49–74, 1978

Beach SRH, O'Leary KD: Treating depression in the context of marital discord: outcome and predictors of response of marital therapy versus cognitive therapy. Behav Ther 23:507–528, 1992

Beck AT: Thinking and depression. Arch Gen Psychiatry 9:324–333, 1963

Beck AT: Thinking and depression, 2: theory and therapy. Arch Gen Psychiatry 10:561–571, 1964

Beck AT: Depression: Clinical, Experimental, and Theoretical Aspects. New York, Harper & Row, 1967

Beck AT: Cognitive Therapy and the Emotional Disorders. New York, International Universities Press, 1976

Beck AT: Cognitive therapy: a 30-year retrospective. Am Psychol 46:368–375, 1991

Beck AT, Emery G: Anxiety Disorders and Phobias: A Cognitive Perspective. New York, Basic Books, 1985

Beck AT, Freeman A: Therapy of Personality Disorders. New York, Guilford, 1990

Beck AT, Greenberg RL: Coping With Depression. New York, Institute for Rational Living, 1974

Beck AT, Rush AJ, Shaw BF, et al: Cognitive Therapy of Depression. New York, Guilford, 1979

Beck AT, Hollon SD, Young JF, et al: Treatment of depression with cognitive therapy and amitriptyline. Arch Gen Psychiatry 42:142–148, 1985

Beck JS: Cognitive Therapy: Basics and Beyond. New York, Guilford, 1995

Beutler LE, Scogin F, Kirkish P, et al: Group cognitive therapy and alprazolam in the treatment of depression in older adults. J Consult Clin Psychol 55:550–556, 1987

Blackburn IM, Moore RG: Controlled acute and follow-up trial of cognitive therapy and pharmacotherapy in out-patients with recurrent depression. Br J Psychiatry 171:328–334, 1997

Blackburn IM, Bishop S, Glen AIM, et al: The efficacy of cognitive therapy in depression: a treatment trial using cognitive therapy and pharmacotherapy, each alone and in combination. Br J Psychiatry 139:181–189, 1981

Blackburn IM, Eunson KM, Bishop S: A two-year naturalistic follow-up of depressed patients treated with cognitive therapy, pharmacotherapy and a combination of both. J Affect Disord 10:67–75, 1986a

Blackburn IM, Jones S, Lewin RJP: Cognitive style in depression. Br J Clin Psychol 25:241–251, 1986b

Bowlby J: The role of childhood experience in cognitive disturbance, in Cognition and Psychotherapy. Edited by Mahoney MJ, Freeman A. New York, Plenum, 1985, pp 181–200

Burns DD: Feeling Good. New York, William Morrow, 1980

Burns DD: The Feeling Good Handbook. New York, Penguin Books, 1990

Burns DD, Spangler DL: Does psychotherapy homework lead to improvements in depression in cognitive-behavioral therapy or does improvement lead to increased homework compliance? J Consult Clin Psychol 68:46–56, 2000

Clark DA, Beck AT, Alford BA: Scientific Foundations of Cognitive Theory and Therapy of Depression. New York, Wiley, 1999, pp 76–112

Comas-Diaz L: Effects of cognitive and behavioral group treatment on the depressive symptomatology of Puerto Rican women. J Consult Clin Psychol 49:627–632, 1981

Covi L, Lipman RS: Cognitive-behavioral group psychotherapy combined with imipramine in major depression. Psychopharmacol Bull 23:173–177, 1987

DeMonbreun BG, Craighead WE: Distortion of perception and recall of positive and neutral feedback in depression. Cognit Ther Res 1:311–329, 1977

Depression Guideline Panel: Clinical Practice Guideline, Number 5. Depression in Primary Care, Vol 2: Treatment of Major Depression (AHCPR Publ No 93-0551). Rockville, MD, Agency for Health Care Policy and Research, 1993

DeRubeis RJ, Evans MD, Hollon SD, et al: How does cognitive therapy work? Cognitive change and symptom change in cognitive therapy and pharmacotherapy for depression. J Consult Clin Psychol 58:862–869, 1990

Deutscher S, Cimbolic P: Cognitive processes and their relationship to endogenous and reactive components of depression. J Nerv Ment Dis 178:351–359, 1990

Dobson KS, Block L: Historical and philosophical bases of the cognitive-behavioral therapies, in Handbook of Cognitive-Behavioral Therapies. Edited by Dobson KS. New York, Guilford, 1988, pp 3–38

Dobson KS, Shaw BF: Cognitive assessment with major depressive disorders. Cognit Ther Res 10:13–29, 1986

Elkin I, Shea MT, Watkins JT, et al: National Institute of Mental Health Treatment of Depression Collaborative Research Program: general effectiveness and treatments. Arch Gen Psychiatry 46:971–982, 1989

Fava GA, Grandi S, Zielezny R, et al: Cognitive behavioral treatment of residual symptoms in primary major depressive disorder. Am J Psychiatry 151:1295–1299, 1994

Fava GA, Rafanelli S, Grandi S, et al: Prevention of recurrent depression with cognitive behavioral therapy: preliminary findings. Arch Gen Psychiatry 55:816–820, 1998

Fleming BM, Thornton DW: Coping skills training as a component in the short-term treatment of depression. J Consult Clin Psychol 5:652–654, 1980

Freeman A, Simon KM, Beutler LE, et al (eds): Comprehensive Handbook of Cognitive Therapy. New York, Plenum, 1989

Friedman ES, Thase ME, Wright JH: Cognitive and Behavioral Therapies in Psychiatry, 2nd Edition, Vol 2. Edited by Tasman A, Kay J, Lieberman JA. West Sussex, England, Wiley, 2003

Gallagher E, Thompson LW: Treatment of major depressive disorder in older adult outpatients with brief psychotherapies. Psychotherapy: Theory, Research and Practice 19:482–490, 1982

Gemar MC, Segal ZV, Sagrati S, et al: Mood-induced changes on the implicit association test in recovered depressed patients. J Abnorm Psychol 110:282–289, 2001

Gloaguen V, Cottraux J, Cucherat M, et al: A meta-analysis of the effects of cognitive therapy in depressed patients. J Affect Disord 49:59–72, 1998

Greenberger D, Padesky CA: Mind Over Mood: A Cognitive Therapy Treatment Manual for Clients. New York, Guilford, 1995

Hogg JA, Deffenbacher JL: A comparison of cognitive and interpersonal-process group therapies in the treatment of depression among college students. J Couns Psychol 35:304–310, 1988

Hollon SD, DeRubeis SJ, Evans MD, et al: Cognitive therapy and pharmacotherapy for depression singly and in combination. Arch Gen Psychiatry 49:774–781, 1992

Ingram RE, Kendall PC: The cognitive side of anxiety. Cognit Ther Res 11:523–536, 1987

Jacobson NS, Fruzzetti AE, Dobson K, et al: Marital therapy as a treatment for depression. J Consult Clin Psychol 59:547–557, 1991

Jarrett R, Kraft D: Prophylactic cognitive therapy for major depressive disorder. In Session: Psychotherapy in Practice 3:65–79, 1997

Jarrett RB, Schaffer M, McIntire D, et al: Treatment of atypical depression with cognitive therapy or phenelzine: a double-blind, placebo-controlled trial. Arch Gen Psychiatry 56:431–437, 1999

Jarrett RB, Kraft D, Doyle J, et al: Preventing recurrent depression using cognitive therapy with and without a continuation phase: a randomized clinical trial. Arch Gen Psychiatry 58:381–388, 2001

Keller MB, McCullough JP, Klein DN, et al: A comparison of nefazodone, the cognitive-behavioral-analysis system of psychotherapy, and their combination for the treatment of chronic depression. N Engl J Med 342:1462–1470, 2000

Kendall PC, Hollon SD: Anxious self-talk: development of the Anxious Self-Statement Questionnaire (ASSQ). Cognit Ther Res 13:81–93, 1989

LeDoux J: Fear and the brain: where have we been, and where are we going? Biol Psychiatry 44:1229–1238, 1988

LeFebvre MF: Cognitive distortion and cognitive errors in depressed psychiatric and low back pain patients. J Consult Clin Psychol 49:517–525, 1981

Locke SE, Rezza ME: Computer-based education in mental health. MD Comput 13:10–18, 20–45, 102, 1996

Markowitz JC, Klerman GL, Clougherty KF, et al: Individual psychotherapies for depressed HIV-positive patients. Am J Psychiatry 152:1504–1509, 1995

McCullough JP: Treatment for Chronic Depression: Cognitive Behavioral Analysis System of Psychotherapy. New York, Guilford, 2000

McKnight DL, Nelson-Gray RO, Barnhill J: Dexamethasone suppression test and response to cognitive therapy and antidepressant medication. Behav Ther 23:99–111, 1992

Metalasky GI, Halberstad LJ, Abramson LY: Vulnerability to depressive mood reactions: toward a more powerful test of diathesis-stress and causal mediation components of the reformulated theory of depression. J Pers Soc Psychol 52:386–393, 1987

Miranda J, Persons JB: Dysfunctional attitudes are mood-state dependent. J Abnorm Psychol 97:76–79, 1999

Miranda J, Persons JB, Byers CN: Endorsement of dysfunctional beliefs depends upon current mood state. J Abnorm Psychol 99:237–241, 1990

Murphy GE, Simons AD, Wetzel RD, et al: Cognitive therapy and pharmacotherapy: singly and together in the treatment of depression. Arch Gen Psychiatry 41:33–41, 1984

Murphy GE, Carney RM, Knesevich MA, et al: Cognitive behavior therapy, relaxation training, and tricyclic antidepressant medication in the treatment of depression. Psychol Rep 77:403–420, 1995

Overholser JC: Elements of the Socratic method, I: systematic questioning. Psychotherapy 30:67–74, 1993a

Overholser JC: Elements of the Socratic method, II: inductive reasoning. Psychotherapy 30:78–85, 1993b

Overholser JC: Elements of the Socratic method, III: universal definitions. Psychotherapy 31:286–293, 1993c

Paykel ES, Scott J, Teasdale JD, et al: Prevention of relapse in residual depression by cognitive therapy. Arch Gen Psychiatry 56:829–835, 1999

Persons JB: Cognitive Therapy in Practice: A Case Formulation Approach. New York, WW Norton, 1989

Persons JB, Davidson J, Tompkins MA: Essential Components of Cognitive-Behavior Therapy for Depression. Washington, DC, American Psychological Association, 2001

Peterson C, Villanova P, Raps CS: Depression and attributions: factors responsible for inconsistent results in the published literature. J Abnorm Psychol 94:165–168, 1985

Propst LR, Ostrom R, Watkins P, et al: Comparative efficacy of religious and nonreligious cognitive-behavioral therapy for the treatment of clinical depression in religious individuals. J Consult Clin Psychol 60:94–103, 1992

Rehm LP: A self-control model of depression. Behav Ther 8:787–804, 1977

Rizley R: Depression and distortion in the attribution of causality. J Abnorm Psychol 87:32–48, 1978

Ross M, Scott M: An evaluation of the effectiveness of individual and group cognitive therapy in the treatment of depressed patients in an inner city health centre. J R Coll Gen Pract 35:239–242, 1985

Rude SS: Relative benefits of assertion or cognitive self-control treatment for depression as a function of proficiency in each domain. J Consult Clin Psychol 54:390–394, 1986

Rush AJ, Watkins JT: Cognitive therapy with psychologically naive depressed outpatients, in New Directions in Cognitive Therapy. Edited by Emery G, Hollon SD, Bedrosian C. New York, Guilford, 1981, pp 5–28

Rush AJ, Beck AT, Kovacs M, et al: Comparative efficacy of cognitive therapy and pharmacotherapy in the treatment of depressed outpatients. Cognit Ther Res 1:17–37, 1977

Scott MJ, Stradling SG: Group cognitive therapy for depression produces clinically significant reliable change in community-based settings. Behavioural Psychotherapy 18:1–19, 1990

Segal ZV: Appraisal of the self-schema construct in cognitive models of depression. Psychol Bull 103:147–162, 1988

Segal ZV, Gemar MC, Williams S: Differential cognitive response to a mood challenge following successful cognitive therapy or pharmacotherapy for unipolar depression. J Abnorm Psychol 108:3–10, 1999

Seligman MEP: Helplessness: On Depression, Development, and Death. San Francisco, CA, WH Freeman, 1975

Selmi PM, Klein MH, Greist JH, et al: Computer-administered cognitive-behavioral therapy for depression. Am J Psychiatry 147:51–56, 1990

Shapiro DA, Barkham M, Rees A, et al: Effects of treatment duration and severity of depression on the effectiveness of cognitive-behavioral and psychodynamic-interpersonal psychotherapy. J Consult Clin Psychol 62:522–534, 1994

Shaw BF: Comparison of cognitive therapy and behavior therapy in the treatment of depression. J Consult Clin Psychol 45:543–551, 1977

Simons AD, Garfield SL, Murphy CE: The process of change in cognitive therapy and pharmacotherapy for depression. Arch Gen Psychiatry 41:45–51, 1984

Steuer JL, Mintz J, Hammen CL, et al: Cognitive-behavioral and psychodynamic group psychotherapy in treatment of geriatric depression. J Consult Clin Psychol 52:180–189, 1984

Sweeney PD, Anderson K, Bailey S: Attributional style in depression: a meta-analysis review. J Pers Soc Psychol 50:974–991, 1986

Teasdale JD: Negative thinking in depression: cause, effect, or reciprocal relationship? Advanced Behavior Research and Therapy 5:3–25, 1983

Teasdale JD, Fennell MJV, Hibbert GA, et al: Cognitive therapy for major depressive disorder in primary care. Br J Psychiatry 144:400–406, 1984

Thase ME: Depression-focused psychotherapies, in Treatments of Psychiatric Disorders, 3rd Edition, Vol 2. Gabbard GO, Editor-in-Chief. Washington, DC, American Psychiatric Press, 2001, pp 1181–1226

Thase ME, Beck AT: Cognitive therapy: an overview, in The Cognitive Milieu: Inpatient Applications to Cognitive Therapy. Edited by Wright JH, Thase ME, Ludgate J, et al. New York, Guilford, 1993, pp 3–34

Thase ME, Simons AD, McGeary J, et al: Relapse after cognitive-behavior therapy of depression: potential implications for longer courses of treatment? Am J Psychiatry 149:1046–1052, 1992

Thompson LW, Gallagher D, Steinmetz-Breckenridge J: Comparative effectiveness of psychotherapies for depressed elders. J Consult Clin Psychol 55:385–390, 1987

Watkins JT, Rush AJ: Cognitive response test. Cognit Ther Res 7:425–436, 1983

Weiss JM, Simson PG: Neurochemical mechanisms underlying stress-induced depression, in Stress and Coping. Edited by Field TM, McCabe PM, Schneiderman N. Hillsdale, NJ, Lawrence Erlbaum, 1985, pp 93–113

Wenzloff RM, Grozier SA: Depression and the magnification of failure. J Abnorm Psychol 97:90–93, 1988

Whisman MS: Mediators and moderators of change in cognitive therapy of depression. Psychol Bull 114:248–265, 1993

Willner P: Animal models as simulations of depression. Trends Pharmacol Sci 12:131–136, 1991

Wilson PH, Goldin JC, Charbonneau-Powis M: Comparative efficacy of behavioral and cognitive treatments of depression. Cognit Ther Res 7:111–124, 1983

Wright JH, Basco MR: Getting Your Life Back: The Complete Guide to Depression. New York, Free Press, 2001

Wright JH, Beck AT: Cognitive therapy of depression: theory and practice. Hosp Community Psychiatry 34:1119–1127, 1983

Wright JH, Davis D: The therapeutic relationship in cognitive-behavioral therapy: patient perceptions and therapist responses. Cognitive Behavior Practice 1:25–45, 1994

Wright JH, Thase ME: Cognitive and biological therapies: a synthesis. Psychiatr Ann 22:451–458, 1992

Wright JH, Wright AS: Computer-assisted psychotherapy. J Psychother Pract Res 6:315–329, 1997

Wright JH, Wright AS, Basco MR, et al: Controlled trial of computer-assisted cognitive therapy for depression. Poster presented at World Congress of Cognitive Therapy, Vancouver, Canada, July 2001

Wright JH, Beck AT, Thase ME: Cognitive therapy, in The American Psychiatric Publishing Textbook of Clinical Psychiatry, 4th Edition. Edited by Hales RE, Yudofsky SC. Washington, DC, American Psychiatric Publishing, 2004, pp 1245–1284

Young JE: Cognitive Therapy for Personality Disorders: A Schema-Focused Approach. Sarasota, FL, Professional Resource Exchange, 1999

Young JE, Lindermann MD: An integrative schema-focused model for personality disorders. Journal of Cognitive Psychotherapy 6:11–23, 1992

Zautra JH, Geunther RT, Chartier GM: Attributions for real and hypothetical events: their relation to self-esteem and depression. J Abnorm Psychol 94:530–540, 1985

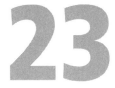

Interpersonal Psychotherapy for Depression and Dysthymic Disorder

JOHN C. MARKOWITZ, M.D.

MOOD DISORDERS ARE where interpersonal psychotherapy (IPT) began. In the 1970s, the late Gerald L. Klerman, M.D., Myrna M. Weissman, Ph.D., and colleagues were planning a randomized trial comparing pharmacotherapy and placebo for outpatients with major depressive disorder (MDD). Recognizing that many depressed patients received psychotherapy as part of their treatment, Klerman and Weissman decided to add psychotherapy to the study. They then realized that they had no gauge of what constituted typical psychotherapy in the community. These researchers decided to devise their own standardized treatment, which they hoped would not be too removed from community practice but also would rely on interpersonal theory and, more particularly, on empirical research on interpersonal aspects of depression.

Klerman, Weissman, and colleagues developed a manual for this treatment (Klerman et al. 1984) and trained therapists to use it. The resultant psychotherapy worked as well as tricyclic antidepressant medication and better than control conditions, and the combination of this psychotherapy with pharmacotherapy had advantages over either monotherapy alone (Klerman et al. 1974). Moreover, patients who received this interpersonally focused therapy developed new social skills over time; patients who received medication alone did not develop these skills. What became known as IPT has subsequently shown efficacy for major depression in repeated randomized, controlled trials and for other subtypes of mood, and increasingly for nonmood, disorders as well (Weissman et al. 2000). In this chapter, I review basic aspects of IPT and its application to acute and chronic unipolar mood disorders.

Portions of this chapter were adapted from Markowitz JC: "Interpersonal Psychotherapy," in *The American Psychiatric Publishing Textbook of Clinical Psychiatry*, 4th Edition. Edited by Hales RE, Yudofsky SC. Washington, DC, American Psychiatric Publishing, 2003, pp. 1207–1223. Used with permission.

History and Early Work

The history of IPT has consisted of a series of randomized clinical trials, beginning with trials in mood disorders. Until recently, IPT paradoxically had been very well researched but little practiced: it was almost purely a research intervention. Its research successes and recommendation by treatment guidelines (e.g., Depression Guideline Panel 1993; Karasu et al. 1993), however, have led to increasing interest and demand for training from clinicians. IPT has spread to different diagnoses, formats, and cultures. One of the few empirically validated antidepressant psychotherapies, IPT has been tested in key studies such as the National Institute of Mental Health (NIMH) Treatment of Depression Collaborative Research Program (Elkin et al. 1985, 1989). The IPT manual has been translated into several languages, and this treatment has proved transportable to European, South American, and African settings. Developed as an individual psychotherapy, IPT also shows promise in group, couples, and telephone formats.

Theoretical Model and Hypothesized Mechanisms

An eclectic treatment, IPT derives from several sources. One root is the interpersonal theory that arose in the United States after World War II. In contrast to the then-prevailing intrapsychically focused psychoanalytic thinking, psychiatrists such as Adolf Meyer, Harry Stack Sullivan (1953), Erich Fromm, and Frieda Fromm-Reichmann emphasized the status of humans as social beings and the effects of environment and current life events on psychopathology. Bowlby (1973, 1988) underscored the importance of attachment to primary caregivers as the basis for understanding affective responses to stress and to attachment in adult relationships. This theory provides a background for understanding IPT.

Research on psychosocial aspects of mood disorders confirmed the importance of life events as both precipitants and consequences of depression and indicated that social supports protect against depressive episodes (G.W. Brown and Harris 1978; see also Williams and Neighbors, Chapter 9, in this volume). Furthermore, research had connected the onset of mood disorders with life events such as the deaths of significant others (*complicated bereavement*), struggles with significant others (*role disputes*), and important life changes such as geographic moves, marriage or divorce, and beginning or ending jobs

(*role transitions*) (Klerman et al. 1984). Negative life events are even more likely to follow the onset of depression than to precede it. Depressed patients withdraw socially, talk less to other people, and function less well in social and work settings. Regardless of whether a life event triggers a depressive episode, negative life events tend to follow its onset, confirming the patient's sense that life is spiraling downward and out of control.

IPT was developed as a simple, practical treatment by researchers. Its structure followed the logic of extant research on interpersonal aspects of depression. Patients are given the diagnosis of MDD according to standard diagnostic criteria (American Psychiatric Association 2000). Treatment focuses on problem areas defined as stressful triggers or consequences of depressive episodes: complicated bereavement following the death of a loved one, a struggle with a significant other, a major life change, or social isolation. The treatment does not demand a causal relation between mood event and life situation—the etiology of all psychiatric syndromes remains unknown and is surely multifaceted—but simply notes the association of the two. This connection between life situation and mood is one that many depressed patients forget; they guiltily blame themselves for their illness, its symptoms, and what is going wrong in their lives. IPT therapists encourage patients to see that by handling a situation well, they can make life go right and thereby improve their mood.

The mechanisms that make IPT efficacious are unknown. Research on IPT has been almost exclusively outcome research, designed to test whether the treatment works, rather than dismantling or process research to explore why it works; hence, more is known about appropriate target diagnoses for IPT than about its active ingredients. Nonetheless, IPT provides several likely helpful factors:

- The IPT therapist names the illness (e.g., major depression) and explicitly reassures the patient that what he or she is experiencing is a treatable illness, not the patient's fault. This medical model gives the patient a temporary "sick role" (Parsons 1951) and shifts blame for symptoms from the overly guilty depressed patient to the syndrome.
- IPT helps the patient to understand connections between affects and actions in the interpersonal arena and to put them to effective use. This is a relatively simple and plausible central focus that even a depressed patient with concrete thinking and poor ability to concentrate can grasp.
- IPT focuses on building interpersonal skills such as self-assertion, effective expression of anger, and social risk-taking. Many depressed patients lack these important practical skills.

- The focus on understanding and confronting current interpersonal difficulties leads to "success experiences," victorious interpersonal encounters (J. Frank 1971). These successes give the patient a greater sense of competence, agency, and control over his or her environment.
- IPT therapists assign no homework. This means that patients cannot fail to complete assignments, a frequent occurrence in other therapies that makes noncompliant patients feel like failures.
- IPT focuses outside the office rather than on the therapeutic relationship. This has at least two positive consequences. First, therapists foster a positive therapeutic alliance; avoiding interpretations of the therapeutic relationship minimizes the risk of therapeutic ruptures (Safran and Muran 2000). Second, as termination approaches, patients can clearly see that they have done the hard work on, and hence deserve the credit for, their improved daily functioning and symptomatic gains.
- Therapeutic optimism, an important aspect of the IPT therapist's stance, is bolstered by research that IPT works.

Conducting Interpersonal Psychotherapy

Techniques

IPT therapists define depression as a treatable *medical illness* that is not the patient's fault. This definition displaces burdensome guilt from the patient to the illness. It also provides hope for improvement: an illness is far more treatable than a self-perceived intrinsic flaw. The IPT therapist uses DSM-IV-TR (American Psychiatric Association 2000) to diagnosis a mood disorder and a rating scale such as the Hamilton Rating Scale for Depression (Ham-D; Hamilton 1960) or Beck Depression Inventory (BDI; Beck 1978) to assess and explain depressive symptoms. These instruments provide psychoeducation to help the patient to recognize that he or she is struggling with a common disorder with a predictable set of symptoms. The Ham-D and BDI have been used for decades, reinforcing the problem is not a personal flaw but a long-recognized syndrome. The therapist gives the depressed patient the sick role (Parsons 1951), which excuses what the illness prevents him or her from doing, while entailing responsibility to work in treatment to recover the lost healthy role. By solving an interpersonal problem—addressing complicated bereavement, a role dispute or transition, or an interpersonal deficit—the IPT patient can both improve his or her life situation and relieve symptoms of the depressive episode. This coupled formula has been validated in randomized, controlled trials and can be offered with confidence and optimism.

IPT is an eclectic therapy that uses techniques seen in other treatment approaches yet can be clearly distinguished from other therapies by adherence ratings (Hill et al. 1992; Markowitz et al. 2000b). Its medical model of depressive illness mimics, and makes it highly compatible with, pharmacotherapy. Marital therapists find its approach to interpersonal issues familiar. IPT shares role-playing and a here-and-now focus with cognitive-behavioral therapy (CBT; Beck et al. 1979; Markowitz 2001). Akin to CBT as a time-limited, syndrome-targeted treatment, IPT is less structured, assigns no homework, and focuses on interpersonal problem areas and associated affect rather than automatic thoughts and core beliefs. IPT overlaps with psychodynamic psychotherapies, and many early IPT research therapists came from psychodynamic backgrounds. Yet IPT also meaningfully differs from psychodynamic therapies in its focus on the present, not the past; its focus on real-life change rather than self-understanding; its medical model; and its avoidance of interpreting dreams and the transference (Markowitz et al. 1998b). No one technique or tactic makes IPT a unique and coherent approach; its overall strategies do.

Each of the four IPT interpersonal problem areas has discrete, if overlapping, goals for the therapist and patient to pursue. The therapist repeatedly helps the patient relate life events to mood and other symptoms. In each session after the first one, an *opening question* elicits an interval history of mood and events and focuses treatment on them. Other techniques include

- *Communication analysis*—the reconstruction and evaluation of recent, affectively charged interpersonal encounters
- *Exploration of the patient's wishes and options*—to pursue these in interpersonal situations
- *Decision analysis*—to help the patient choose among options
- *Role-playing*—to help patients rehearse tactics for real life

IPT focuses on current interpersonal relationships in the patient's immediate social context. The IPT therapist attempts to intervene in symptom formation and social dysfunction associated with depression rather than aspects of personality. Personality is difficult to accurately assess during an episode of an Axis I disorder such as depression (Hirschfeld et al. 1983). IPT does build new social skills (Weissman et al. 1974, 1981), which may be as valuable as changing personality traits.

TABLE 23–1.   Phases of interpersonal psychotherapy (IPT)

I. Early phase

    A. Deal with the depression.

        1. Review depressive symptoms.

        2. Name the syndrome: formal diagnosis.

        3. Provide psychoeducation about depression and its treatment.

        4. Give patient the "sick role."

        5. Evaluate the need for medication.

    B. Relate depression to interpersonal context: interpersonal inventory.

        1. Determine nature of interaction with significant persons.

        2. Identify reciprocal expectations of patient and significant others and whether these were fulfilled.

        3. Discuss satisfying and unsatisfying aspects of relationships.

        4. Detect recent changes in key relationships.

        5. Determine changes patient desires in relationships.

    C. Identify the major problem area.

        1. Determine problem area related to current episode and set treatment goals.

        2. Identify which relationship is related to the episode and what might change in it.

    D. Explain IPT concepts and contract.

        1. Outline understanding of the problem: formulation.

        2. Agree on treatment goals (focal problem area):

            a. *brief* treatment (time limit)

            b. target is depression (not character)

        3. Describe IPT procedures: here-and-now focus, need to discuss important concerns, review of current interpersonal relationships, discussion of practical aspects of treatment.

II. Middle phase

    A. Use specific strategies for treating grief, role disputes, role transitions, or interpersonal deficits.

III. Termination phase

    A. Consolidate gains.

    B. Foster independence.

    C. Address guilt (and blame therapy) if the patient's symptoms did not respond.

    D. Review risk of relapse and recurrence.

    E. Recontract for continuation and maintenance treatment if appropriate.

Phases of Treatment

As an acute treatment, IPT has three phases (see Table 23–1) (Weissman et al. 2000). The *early phase*, usually lasting no more than three sessions, sets the stage for what follows. The therapist reviews symptoms, diagnoses depression by standard criteria (American Psychiatric Association 2000), and gives the patient the sick role. The psychiatric history includes an "interpersonal inventory," a careful cataloguing of the patient's past and current social functioning and close relationships, including their patterns and mutual expectations. Initial sessions elucidate changes in relationships proximal to the onset of symptoms: for example, death of a loved one, children leaving home, worsening marital strife, or isolation from a confidant. The therapist looks for meaningful life events such as a career change or onset of a medical illness. This review provides a framework for understanding the social and interpersonal context of the depressive symptoms, and this framework becomes the basis of a treatment focus.

In clinical practice, the therapist assesses the need for medication on the basis of symptom severity, illness history and response to treatment, and patient preference. The therapist then educates the patient about the constellation of symptoms that define MDD, their psychosocial concomitants, and what the patient may expect from treatment. A formulation links the depressive syndrome to the patient's interpersonal situation (Markowitz and Swartz 1997), centered on one of four interpersonal problem areas: 1) grief, 2) interpersonal role disputes, 3) role transitions, or 4) interpersonal deficits (Table 23–2). With the patient's explicit acceptance of this formulation as a treatment focus, therapy enters the middle phase.

Any formulation perforce simplifies a patient's complex life story. Although many patients present with multiple interpersonal problems, the formulation isolates one or at most two salient problems related to the patient's mood disorder, either as a precipitant or as a consequence, and weaves them into an organizing fiction. More than two foci in a brief psychotherapy means no focus at all. Choice of focal problem area depends on clinical acumen, although research has shown that IPT therapists agree in choosing such areas (Markowitz et al. 2000a). Patients seem to find the foci credible.

In the *middle phase*, the IPT therapist pursues strategies appropriate to the focal interpersonal problem area (Weissman et al. 2000). To address grief (complicated bereavement following the death of a loved one), the therapist facilitates the catharsis of mourning and helps the patient to find new activities and relationships to compensate for the loss. For role disputes (conflicts with a spouse, other family member, boss, co-worker, or friend), the therapist helps the patient to explore the relationship, the nature of the dispute, whether it has reached an impasse, and available options to resolve it. If these options fail, the therapist and patient may conclude that the relationship has reached an impasse and consider ways to change the impasse or to end the relationship.

A role transition is a change in life status: e.g., the beginning or ending of a relationship or career, moving, being promoted, retiring, graduating, or receiving a diagnosis of a medical illness. The patient learns to manage the change by mourning the loss of the old role while recog-

TABLE 23–2. Interpersonal psychotherapy problem areas

Problem area	Definition
Grief (complicated bereavement)	Death of a significant other
Role disputes	Struggle with a significant other
Role transitions	Life event that changes perceived social role
Interpersonal deficits	No life events; social isolation (used only if none of the above is appropriate)

nizing positive and negative aspects of the new role he or she is assuming and taking steps to master it. The residual fourth IPT problem area, interpersonal deficits, categorizes patients who lack one of the first three problem areas (i.e., without recent life events). This least-defined focus, an anomalous non–life-event-based category for a life-event-based therapy, defines the patient as lacking the social skills to initiate or sustain relationships. Its goal is to help the patient develop new relationships and skills. Some patients who appear to fit this category may have dysthymic disorder, for which other IPT strategies have been developed (Markowitz 1998).

IPT sessions address current, here-and-now problems. Sessions open with the question: "How have things been since we last met?" This orients the patient to recent interpersonal events and recent mood, which the therapist helps the patient to connect. Therapists sympathize with patients' suffering while taking an active, supportive, and hopeful stance to counter the depressed patient's pessimism. They elicit and emphasize the options for change in the patient's life, options that the depressive episode often has kept the patient from seeing or exploring fully. Understanding the situation does not suffice; therapists stress the need for patients to *test* these options to improve their lives and simultaneously treat their depressive episodes. Enacting a practical solution to the patient's focal interpersonal crisis within the envelope of the time-limited treatment is the implicit homework of IPT.

The *termination phase* of IPT, the last few sessions of acute treatment or last months of maintenance treatment, supports the patient's newly regained sense of competence by recognizing and consolidating therapeutic gains. The therapist enhances the patient's self-esteem and independence by underscoring that the patient's depressive episode has improved through the patient's actions in changing a life situation. Moreover, the patient achieved this at a time when he or she had felt weakest. The therapist also helps the patient to anticipate triggers for and responses to depressive symptoms that might arise in the future. Relative to psychodynamic therapy, IPT deemphasizes termination: it is a graduation from successful treatment, a role transition that, like most, is bittersweet. The sadness of separation is distinguished from depressive feelings. If the patient has not improved, the therapist emphasizes that the treatment has failed, not the patient, and that alternative effective treatment options exist. Patients with multiple prior depressive episodes or significant residual symptoms, who successfully complete acute treatment but remain at high risk for recurrence, may contract for maintenance therapy as acute treatment draws to a close.

Indications and Contraindications

Research on psychotherapy outcome has lacked the resources available to pharmaceutical companies, whose products are accordingly better studied. Nonetheless, a series of randomized, controlled trials comparing IPT with control conditions have defined the efficacy of IPT for patients with mood disorders. Indications for IPT thus have been determined not by random application but by randomized, controlled trials. For some patient subgroups, IPT has been adapted in separate treatment manuals (e.g., Markowitz 1998; Mufson et al. 1993).

Still more interesting are comparative trials of IPT with CBT and medication, which have provided some data on differential therapeutics. No absolute contraindications exist for using IPT with nondelusional depressed outpatients, yet no treatment is ideal for all patients. Given a choice between two treatments of already established efficacy, the clinician must determine which factors may predict better outcome for patients with a given diagnosis (Frances et al. 1984). In this section, I document the efficacy of IPT for patients with unipolar, nondelusional mood disorders, first addressing acute and then chronic forms of depression (see Table 23–3).

Acute Treatment of Major Depression

IPT was first studied as an acute antidepressant treatment in a four-cell, 16-week randomized trial comparing IPT, amitriptyline, their combination, and a nonscheduled control treatment for 81 outpatients with MDD (DiMascio et al. 1979; Weissman et al. 1979). Amitriptyline worked more quickly, but IPT and amitriptyline did not significantly differ in symptom reduction at the end of treatment. Each reduced symptoms more efficaciously than did the control treatment, and combined amitrip-

---

TABLE 23–3. Empirically based indications for interpersonal psychotherapy

Major depression

    Acute

    Recurrent (prophylaxis)

    Geriatric patients

    Adolescent patients

    Human immunodeficiency virus–positive patients

    Primary care patients

    Antepartum and postpartum depressed women

    Conjoint therapy for depressed married women

Dysthymic disorder[a]

Bipolar disorder (adjunctive treatment)[a,b]

Interpersonal counseling for subsyndromal depression

[a]Preliminary results encouraging.
[b]See Chapter 25, this volume.

---

tyline-IPT was more efficacious than either active monotherapy. Not surprisingly, patients with psychotic depression who received IPT alone fared poorly. On naturalistic follow-up at 1 year, many patients had sustained improvement from the brief IPT intervention, and IPT patients had developed significantly better psychosocial functioning, regardless of whether they had received medication. This effect on social function was not found for amitriptyline alone, nor had it been evident for IPT immediately after the 16-week trial (Weissman et al. 1981).

In the ambitious, multisite NIMH Treatment of Depression Collaborative Research Program (Elkin et al. 1989), investigators randomly assigned 250 outpatients with MDD to 16 weeks of IPT, CBT, or clinical management with either imipramine or pill placebo. Most subjects completed at least 15 weeks or 12 treatment sessions. More mildly depressed patients (defined by baseline 17-item Ham-D score <20) improved equally in all treatments. Among more depressed patients (Ham-D score ≥20), imipramine worked fastest and most consistently outperformed placebo. IPT was comparable to imipramine on several outcome measures, including Ham-D, and superior to placebo for the more depressed patients. CBT was not superior to placebo among the more depressed patients.

Klein and Ross (1993) reanalyzed the NIMH Treatment of Depression Collaborative Research Program data with the Johnson-Neyman technique and found that medication outperformed the psychotherapies, which were superior to placebo, especially among more impaired patients. The authors found CBT inferior to IPT for patients with BDI scores greater than 30, a score demarcating the boundary between moderate and severe depression.

In a naturalistic follow-up study of Treatment of Depression Collaborative Research Program subjects at 18 months posttreatment, Shea and colleagues (1992) found no significant difference across treatments in recovery among patients who had remitted (i.e., those who had minimal or no symptoms after treatment and sustained this improvement during follow-up). Thirty percent of CBT, 26% of IPT, 20% of placebo, and 19% of imipramine subjects who had acutely remitted remained in remission during that time span. Of the subjects who had acutely remitted, relapse rates over the 18 months were 36% for CBT, 33% for IPT, 50% for imipramine (albeit medication had been stopped at 16 weeks), and 33% for placebo. The authors concluded that, for many patients, 16 weeks of treatment were insufficient to achieve lasting recovery.

IPT seems to work outside of the United States as well. In a trial in the Hague, the Netherlands, Blom and colleagues (1996) first undertook a pilot trial and have since completed a randomized trial of IPT, nefazodone, and their combination for 191 subjects with MDD (Blom et al. 2004). Preliminary results suggest that all three treatments had similar benefit.

Geriatric Depression

IPT was first used with 30 geriatric depressed patients to enhance compliance in a 6-week pharmacotherapy trial and to enhance the pill placebo control group (Rothblum et al. 1982; Sholomskas et al. 1983). The investigators noted grief and role transitions as the modal treatment foci. They suggested modifications of IPT for older depressed patients, including flexible duration of sessions, more practical advice and concrete support (e.g., arranging transportation, calling physicians), and recognizing that major role changes may be impractical and detrimental (e.g., divorce at age 75). The 6-week trial comparing IPT with nortriptyline in depressed elderly patients showed some advantages for IPT, largely because of higher attrition in the medication group from nortriptyline's side effects (Sloane et al. 1985).

Depressed Adolescents

Mufson et al. (1993) modified IPT to incorporate adolescent developmental issues. The researchers conducted an open feasibility and follow-up trial and then a controlled

12-week clinical trial comparing IPT for depressed adolescents (IPT-A) and clinical monitoring in 48 clinic-referred adolescents, ages 12–18, who met DSM-III-R (American Psychiatric Association 1987) criteria for MDD. Patients were rated biweekly by a blinded independent evaluator to assess symptomatology, social functioning, and social problem-solving skills. Of the 48 patients, 32 (21 IPT-A, 11 control) completed the protocol.

Patients receiving IPT-A reported significantly greater improvement in depressive symptoms and social functioning, including functioning with friends and problem-solving skills. In the intent-to-treat sample, 75% of the IPT-A patients met the recovery criterion (Ham-D score ≤6), compared with 46% of the control subjects. The findings support the feasibility, patient acceptance, and efficacy of 12 weeks of IPT-A with acutely depressed adolescents in reducing depressive symptomatology and improving social functioning and interpersonal problem-solving skills (Mufson et al. 1999).

Mufson and colleagues (2004) subsequently tested IPT-A in a large-scale effectiveness study in New York City school-based clinics; 12 sessions of IPT-A delivered by school counselors were compared with treatment as usual over 16 weeks. Adolescents with mood disorders who received IPT-A (N=63) again showed greater improvements than did those receiving usual treatment on independent, clinician, and self-report ratings of symptoms and social functioning. Thus, IPT-A has shown benefits in both efficacy and effectiveness trials. Mufson and colleagues (2004) also have developed a group format for depressed adolescents, which might have economic benefits and take advantage of teenage peer support.

Rosselló and Bernal (1999) at the University of Puerto Rico compared IPT (n=22), CBT (n=25), and a waiting-list control condition (n=24) in a 12-week randomized, controlled trial for adolescents, ages 13–18, who met DSM-III-R criteria for MDD, dysthymia, or both. The investigators did not use Mufson's IPT-A adaptation. Both IPT and CBT were more efficacious than the waiting list in reducing adolescents' self-rated depressive symptoms. IPT was more efficacious than CBT in increasing self-esteem and social adaptation. Effect sizes for improvement were 0.73 for IPT and 0.43 for CBT.

Depressed HIV-Positive Patients

Markowitz et al. (1992) modified IPT for depressed patients with human immunodeficiency virus (IPT-HIV) in the early years of the epidemic, when acquired immunodeficiency syndrome (AIDS) appeared to be an acute and lethal illness rather than the chronic disease it has now become. The adaptation emphasized common concerns among this population about illness and death, grief, and role transitions. A 16-week randomized trial of 101 subjects compared IPT-HIV, CBT, supportive psychotherapy, and imipramine plus supportive psychotherapy (Markowitz et al. 1998a). As with the subset of more severely depressed subjects in the Treatment of Depression Collaborative Research Program study (Elkin et al. 1989), all treatments were associated with symptom reduction, but IPT and imipramine plus supportive psychotherapy produced significantly greater symptomatic and functional improvement than CBT or supportive psychotherapy. Many patients reported improvement in neurovegetative symptoms that they had mistakenly attributed to HIV infection.

Depressed Primary Care Patients

Schulberg and colleagues compared IPT with pharmacotherapy for depressed primary care medical patients (Schulberg et al. 1996). The investigators integrated IPT into the primary care center. Not only did nurses take vital signs before sessions, but primary care patients received treatment for major depression without having to go to a "shrink": the mental health care came to them. If patients were medically hospitalized, attempts were made to continue IPT in the hospital.

Patients with MDD (N=276) were randomly assigned to receive IPT, nortriptyline, or primary care physicians' usual care. IPT was given weekly for 16 weeks and then monthly for 4 months (Schulberg et al. 1996). Depressive symptoms declined more rapidly with either nortriptyline or IPT than with usual care. About 70% of those who completed the trial who had received nortriptyline or IPT, but only 20% of those who had received usual care, had recovered after 8 months. Subjects with a history of comorbid panic disorder had a poorer response across treatments than did those without a panic history (C. Brown et al. 1996), a finding subsequently corroborated by E. Frank and colleagues (2000).

Antepartum and Postpartum Depression

Pregnancy and nursing are key role transitions for women of childbearing age, who are prime candidates for depressive episodes (see Kornstein and Sloan, Chapter 41, in this volume). Even though most antidepressant medications may carry little risk of teratogenesis and not all are detectable in breast milk, physicians are reluctant to prescribe medication, and patients are reluctant to accept it during pregnancy and nursing. Thus, peripartum depression is an ideal target for IPT.

Spinelli (1997) at Columbia University tested IPT in women with antepartum depression. She added "complicated pregnancy" as a fifth interpersonal problem area. Timing and duration of sessions are adjusted in response to bed rest, delivery, obstetrical complications, and child care. As with depressed HIV-positive and primary care patients, telephone sessions and hospital visits are sometimes necessary (Spinelli 1997). In a 16-week trial of IPT compared with a relatively weak, "nontherapeutic control group" of parent education sessions, Spinelli and Endicott (2003) treated 50 depressed women of generally low socioeconomic status. They reported benefits for IPT in this pilot controlled trial for a high-risk, in-need population. Patients showed modest but meaningful gains on the Ham-D and other scales.

O'Hara and colleagues (2000) compared IPT with a waiting-list control in 120 women with postpartum depression in a 12-week trial with an 18-month follow-up. The research assessed both the symptom states of the postpartum mothers and their interactions with their infants (Stuart and O'Hara 1995). Of the IPT group, 38% met Ham-D and 44% met BDI remission criteria, compared with 14% on each measure for the control group. Sixty percent of IPT patients, in contrast to 16% of control subjects, reported more than a 50% reduction in BDI score. Mothers receiving IPT showed significantly improved social adjustment relative to the control group.

Klier and colleagues (2001) treated 17 women with postpartum depression in nine weekly 90-minute group sessions followed by an hour-long individual termination session. Scores on the 21-item Ham-D declined from 19.7 to 8.0, suggesting the efficacy of this approach. In an exciting study of IPT as prevention, Zlotnick and colleagues (2001) treated 37 women at risk for postpartum depression with either four 60-minute sessions of an IPT-based group or usual treatment. Six of the 18 women in usual care developed depression by 3 months postpartum, compared with none of the 17 IPT group patients.

Conjoint Interpersonal Psychotherapy for Depressed Patients With Marital Disputes

Stressful changes in relationships such as marital conflict, separation, and divorce can precipitate or complicate depressive episodes (Rounsaville et al. 1979). Treating marital role disputes in individual IPT often has the feel of unilateral couples therapy (Weissman et al. 2000), so extending IPT to a couples format was not difficult. Weissman and Klerman (1993) developed a manual for conjoint therapy for depressed patients with marital disputes (IPT-CM). IPT-CM includes the spouse in all sessions and focuses on the current marital dispute. Eighteen patients with MDD linked to onset or exacerbation of marital disputes were randomly assigned to 16 weeks of either individual IPT or IPT-CM. Patients showed similar reductions in depressive symptoms in both treatments, but patients receiving IPT-CM reported significantly better marital adjustment, marital affection, and sexual relationships (Foley et al. 1989). These pilot findings require replication with a larger sample and other control groups.

Interpersonal Counseling

Many primary care patients report psychiatric symptoms but do not meet full criteria for a psychiatric disorder. Their symptoms can be debilitating and, if ignored or misdiagnosed, may result in wasted use of medical procedures (Wells et al. 1989). Interpersonal counseling is a truncated form of IPT, designed for use by medical personnel without formal psychotherapy experience to treat distressed primary care patients who do not meet full criteria for psychiatric syndromes. Interpersonal counseling was initially a one- to six-session intervention for nurse practitioners. The first session lasts up to 30 minutes; subsequent sessions are briefer.

The interpersonal counseling therapist assesses the patient's current functioning, recent life events, occupational and familial stressors, and changes in interpersonal relationships. Such events provide the context in which emotional and bodily symptoms presumably occur. Klerman and colleagues (1987) randomized 128 patients in a primary care clinic who scored 6 or higher on the Goldberg General Health Questionnaire (GHQ) to interpersonal counseling or to usual care. Over an average of 3 months, interpersonal counseling subjects, often after receiving only one or two sessions, showed significantly greater symptom relief on the GHQ than did control subjects, especially mood improvement. Interpersonal counseling subjects subsequently used more mental health services, implying new awareness of their psychiatric symptomatology.

Mossey et al. (1996), noting that subsyndromal depressive symptoms delayed recovery of hospitalized elderly patients, conducted a 10-session trial of interpersonal counseling for elderly hospitalized medical patients with minor depression. Patients were seen for hour-long sessions flexibly adjusted to the patient's medical status. Seventy-six hospitalized patients older than 60, who had depressive symptoms on two consecutive assessments but did not meet full criteria for MDD, were randomly assigned to either interpersonal counseling or usual care. Researchers also monitored a euthymic, untreated, geriatric control group. Patients found interpersonal counseling feasible and tolerable. After 3 months, assessments showed nonsignificantly greater improvement on all out-

come variables for interpersonal counseling relative to usual care, whereas control subjects showed a slight symptomatic worsening. Rehospitalization rates were virtually identical (11%–15%) for the interpersonal counseling and euthymic control groups and significantly less than those for the cohort in usual care (50%). Differences between interpersonal counseling and usual care groups reached statistical significance at 6 months on depressive symptom reduction and self-rated health but not physical or social functioning. The investigators thought that 10 sessions were insufficient for some patients and that maintenance interpersonal counseling might have been useful.

In a fascinating study in an area of Uganda ravaged by poverty, HIV, and depression, Bolton and colleagues (2003) used a dilute version of group IPT to treat depressed women. For lack of mental health professionals, treatment was conducted by local college graduates trained in what might be considered a form of interpersonal counseling. Researchers randomized assignment to either the interpersonal intervention or usual care by village rather than by depressed individual. Despite potential cultural differences, the interpersonal counseling group had a huge benefit relative to usual care, which was apparently minimal treatment. That the treatment had benefits for the village as a whole, even for villagers who had not participated in groups, is impressive. IPT proved transportable to this very different culture presumably because of its practical, present-focused emphasis on interpersonal relationships and problems, without having to teach what would have been an alien theory of cognition or unconscious drives, for example.

Other Formats

Wilfley and colleagues (2000) have defined group IPT as a treatment format. Swartz and colleagues (2004) have tested IPT in a briefer, eight-session format for MDD with promising results. Weissman (1995) has developed a handbook of IPT for patients that includes psychoeducation and worksheets. Its utility has not been formally researched.

Differential Therapeutics

If two treatments have shown efficacy in treating depression, for which patients will one treatment likely yield a better outcome than the other? Outcome studies comparing such treatments are beginning to identify factors that moderate, or predict, treatment outcome (see Table 23–4). The NIMH Treatment of Depression Collaborative Research Program, which compared IPT, CBT, and imipramine, suggested such moderating factors. Sotsky and colleagues (1991) found that Treatment of Depression Collaborative Research Program depressed patients with low baseline levels of social dysfunction responded well to IPT, whereas those with severe social deficits (probably equivalent to the "interpersonal deficits" problem area) responded less well. In contrast, patients with greater symptom severity and difficulty in concentrating responded poorly to CBT. Initial severity of major depression and of impaired functioning predicted superior response to IPT and to imipramine. Imipramine worked most efficaciously for patients with difficulty functioning at work, likely reflecting its faster onset of action. Patients with atypical depression responded better to IPT or CBT than to imipramine or placebo (Shea et al. 1999).

In the trial of HIV-positive patients with depressive symptoms, IPT yielded a better outcome than CBT (Markowitz et al. 1998a). This was not explainable by therapist adherence or competence, which was excellent for all treatments. Rather, IPT appeared a good "fit" for depressed HIV-positive patients, who had many of the upsetting life events that IPT addresses. In contrast, CBT therapists were in the relatively difficult position of cautioning against "catastrophizing" patients who in fact faced catastrophic situations. Thus, the context of particular patients may favor one therapy over another: patients without life events might fare better in CBT than in IPT.

Barber and Muenz (1996) studied patients who completed the Treatment of Depression Collaborative Research Program and found that IPT was more efficacious than CBT for patients with obsessive personality traits, whereas CBT worked better for avoidant patients. These findings did not hold for all subjects entered in the study (i.e., the intention-to-treat sample). Biological factors also may affect outcome: abnormal electroencephalogram sleep profiles predicted significantly poorer response to IPT than for patients with normal sleep parameters (Thase et al. 1997). E. Frank and colleagues (1991) found that psychotherapist adherence to a focused IPT approach may enhance outcome. The replication and further elaboration of these predictive factors deserve ongoing study.

Chronic Depressions

A significant proportion of all depressions is chronic, and this chronicity may take two forms. First, most individuals who have a single episode of MDD have a greater than even chance of having a second lifetime episode; the more episodes one has, the greater the risk of subsequent episodes (Boland and Keller 2002; see Stewart et al., Chapter 33, in this volume). Patients with recurrent MDD require

not only acute remission of symptoms but also prevention of relapse and recurrence. IPT is the first psychotherapy to have been tested as a maintenance treatment to prevent recurrence of depressive episodes. Second, many depressive episodes are chronic—either chronic MDD, dysthymic disorder, or so-called double depression, which is major depression superimposed on dysthymic disorder. Chronically depressed patients are still more hopeless and resigned than are acutely depressed patients, and the chronicity of their illness alters treatment strategies for their acute treatment.

Maintenance Prophylaxis for Recurrent Major Depressive Disorder

IPT was first tested in an 8-month, six-cell trial (Klerman et al. 1974; Paykel et al. 1976). A study of this length today would be considered a continuation treatment because the concept of long-term maintenance antidepressant treatment has lengthened. Acutely depressed outpatient women (N=150) who had responded (with 50% or greater symptom reduction by interviewer rating) to a 4- to 6-week acute trial of amitriptyline were randomly assigned to 8 months of weekly IPT, amitriptyline, placebo alone, combined IPT-amitriptyline, IPT-placebo, or no pill. Randomization to IPT or a low-contact psychotherapy condition occurred at entry into the continuation phase, whereas randomization to medication, placebo, or no pill occurred at the end of the second month of continuation treatment. Maintenance pharmacotherapy was found to prevent relapse and symptom exacerbation, whereas IPT improved social functioning (Weissman et al. 1974). The effects of IPT on social functioning did not appear for 6–8 months. Combined psychotherapy and pharmacotherapy had the best outcome.

Researchers in Pittsburgh, Pennsylvania, conducted two longer antidepressant maintenance trials of IPT (IPT-M). E. Frank et al. (1990, 1991) studied 128 outpatients with multiply and rapidly recurrent depression. Patients were given combined high-dose (>200 mg/day) imipramine and weekly IPT until they responded; the high-dose medication was continued while IPT was tapered to a monthly frequency during a 4-month continuation phase. Patients who remained in remission were then randomly assigned to 3 years of 1) ongoing high-dose imipramine plus clinical management, 2) high-dose imipramine plus monthly IPT, 3) monthly IPT alone, 4) monthly IPT plus placebo, or 5) placebo plus clinical management. High-dose imipramine, with or without further IPT, proved most efficacious, protecting more than 80% of the patients over 3 years. Most placebo patients relapsed within the first few months. Once-

---

TABLE 23–4. Prescribing interpersonal psychotherapy (IPT) and cognitive-behavioral therapy (CBT)

I. **Similarities**

    A. Common factors of psychotherapy

        1. Sense of feeling understood (**R**elationship)

        2. Framework for understanding (**R**ationale)

        3. Hope and optimism (**R**emoralization)

        4. Psychoeducation (**R**ecognition)

        5. Technique for getting better (**R**itual)

        6. Success experiences (**R**ecovering control)

    B. Common features of brief antidepressant psychotherapies

        1. Manualized

        2. Active

        3. Time-limited (with comparable time courses)

        4. Structured (CBT>IPT)

        5. Here-and-now, current focus

        6. Goals of self-assertion, mastery

        7. Ultimate goal of new skills for prophylaxis

        8. Can be combined with antidepressant medication

    C. Technical similarities

        1. Mobilizing patient to greater activity

        2. Linking mood to activities and reactions to events, albeit with different emphases

        3. Problem solving: "exploring options" vs. "empirical hypothesis testing"

        4. Addressing "expectations" vs. "assumptions" about others

        5. Role-playing

II. **Differences**

    A. IPT: medical model

    B. CBT: homework

    C. Focus on affect (IPT) vs. thoughts→affect (CBT); hence, more external vs. more intrapsychic approach

III. **Differential therapeutics of major depression: which works better for whom?**

Predictor	IPT if predictor is...	CBT if predictor is...
Life events	Present	Absent
Social dysfunction (baseline)	Low	Very high (interpersonal deficits)
Symptom severity (baseline)	Higher	Lower
Personality traits	Obsessive	Avoidant

monthly IPT, although less efficacious than medication, was statistically and clinically superior to the control condition in this high-risk patient population.

Reynolds et al. (1999) conducted a second 3-year maintenance study for geriatric patients with recurrent depression; they used IPT and nortriptyline in a design similar to that used in the E. Frank et al. (1990) study. The IPT manual was modified to allow more flexible length of sessions, under the assumption that some elderly patients might have difficulty tolerating 50-minute sessions. The investigators found that geriatric patients needed to address early life relationships in psychotherapy, digressing from the here-and-now focus of IPT. Like Sholomskas et al. (1983), Reynolds and colleagues believed that therapists needed to help patients solve practical problems while acknowledging that some problems may not be resolvable, such as existential late-life issues or lifelong psychopathology (Rothblum et al. 1982). Elderly depressed patients whose sleep quality normalized by the early continuation phase had an 80% chance of remaining well during the first year of maintenance treatment. Response rates were similar for patients who subsequently received either nortriptyline or IPT.

The acute treatment sample comprised 187 patients, aged 60 years or older, with recurrent MDD. These patients received combined IPT and nortriptyline. One hundred seven who remitted and then achieved recovery after continuation therapy were randomly assigned to one of four 3-year maintenance conditions: 1) medication clinic with nortriptyline alone, with steady-state nortriptyline plasma levels maintained in a therapeutic window of 80–120 ng/mL; 2) medication clinic with placebo; 3) monthly maintenance IPT with placebo; or 4) monthly maintenance IPT plus nortriptyline. Recurrence rates were 90% for placebo, 64% for IPT with placebo, 43% for nortriptyline alone, and 20% for combined treatment. Each monotherapy was statistically superior to placebo, whereas combined therapy showed superiority to IPT alone and a trend for superiority over nortriptyline alone. Patients in their 70s were more likely to have a recurrence, and to do so more quickly, than patients in their 60s. This study corroborated the maintenance findings of E. Frank and colleagues, with the difference that combined treatment showed advantages over pharmacotherapy alone for the geriatric population.

In both maintenance studies, the comparison of high-dose tricyclic antidepressants with low-dose maintenance IPT is easy to misinterpret. No previous maintenance studies had ever used either such high doses of medication or so low a dose of psychotherapy. Had the medication been lowered comparably to the reduced psychotherapy dosage, recurrence in the medication groups might well have been greater; had psychotherapy been more intensive, recurrence rates might have declined. Because there were no precedents for this research, the choice of a monthly dosing interval for maintenance IPT was reasonable and indeed showed some benefit. Several studies have since begun to test the effects of differing maintenance doses of psychotherapy.

These difficult, protracted studies have yielded exciting results. They showed that psychotherapy not only works acutely but also can continue working to ward off the return of a typically recurrent illness. These research trials also have contributed to knowledge of differential therapeutics by assessing potential moderators of outcome.

Dysthymic Disorder

Dysthymic disorder is a syndrome, often of early onset, with high debility and comorbidity (see Stewart et al., Chapter 33, in this volume). Because dysthymic individuals often have been ill from an early age, they tend to accept their symptoms as part of themselves, an internal defect, and may not seek appropriate treatment. Early onset of symptoms retards the development of social skills. Moreover, because they often struggle through life without the evident collapse of a major depression, people around them also may accept that they have nervous or melancholy characters and not press them to find treatment. Thus, many dysthymic individuals become patients late in the course of chronic illness and are resigned to their condition.

From an IPT perspective, dysthymic patients present an additional problem. As the description of IPT earlier in this chapter indicates, the IPT model connects recent life events with recent mood changes. This model nicely fits acute depression but makes less sense for the often decades-long chronic depressions. Accordingly, Markowitz (1998) modified IPT for dysthymic disorder (IPT-D), taking advantage of the patient's sense that the illness was part of his or her character. IPT-D encourages patients to reconceptualize what they consider their lifelong character flaws as ego-dystonic, chronic mood-dependent symptoms: as a chronic but treatable "state" rather than an immutable "trait." Therapy itself is defined as an "iatrogenic role transition" from believing oneself flawed in personality to recognizing and treating the mood disorder. Markowitz (1994, 1998) openly treated 17 pilot subjects with 16 sessions of IPT-D: none worsened, and 11 subjects remitted.

On the basis of these pilot results, investigators at Weill Medical College of Cornell University conducted a randomized trial comparing 16 weeks of IPT-D alone, sertraline plus clinical management, supportive psychotherapy, and combined IPT and sertraline for 86 patients with "pure" dysthymic disorder (i.e., no major depression within the prior 6 months). Preliminary results in this underpowered trial found improvement across cells, with no statistically significant advantages for any condition, although post hoc analyses showed some advantages for the pharmacotherapy cells (Markowitz 2003). Other studies at Cornell University are comparing IPT with supportive psychotherapy for double depression and IPT plus Alcoholics Anonymous (AA) meetings with supportive psychotherapy plus AA meetings for chronically depressed patients with secondary alcohol abuse.

Browne and associates (2002) conducted one of the largest psychotherapy studies ever, treating 707 patients with DSM-IV (American Psychiatric Association 1994) dysthymic disorder. Most patients (68%) were women, with a mean age in the early 40s. Half had early-onset (before age 21) dysthymic disorder, a third had current double depression, and two-thirds had a history of double depression. Patients were randomized to sertraline (50–200 mg/day) alone, IPT alone, or combined IPT plus sertraline. Median dosages of sertraline were 100 mg/day in the sertraline-only group and 150 mg/day in the combined treatment cell. Treatment dosage in this community study was not fully balanced; IPT treatment (not adapted as described above) consisted of up to 12 (mean=10) 1-hour sessions over 6 months, whereas sertraline treatment usually endured for the 2 years of the study. Thus, the study compared acute psychotherapy with acute and maintenance pharmacotherapy.

Treatment outcome considered both symptoms and economics. Response was defined as 40% or greater decrease on the Montgomery-Åsberg Rating Scale for Depression (Montgomery and Åsberg 1979). (Many studies require a 50% decrement for response.) Of the 586 patients completing the 6-month acute phase, 60% of the sertraline-alone, 58% of the combined treatment, and 47% of the IPT-alone patients met response criteria. Sertraline, alone or combined with IPT, was significantly more efficacious than IPT alone. At 2-year follow-up ($n=525$), IPT continued to lag in outcome, but both IPT groups had lower health and social services costs than did the sertraline-alone group, making the combination of IPT and sertraline most cost-effective. Concomitant IPT also decreased the likelihood of patients discontinuing their sertraline (Browne et al. 2002).

The first of these studies was underpowered. The second was large but included no control condition and a dosage imbalance between IPT and pharmacotherapy. The two trials did not provide definitive evidence of the utility of IPT for chronic and persistent depression but suggested that its benefits may be modest (Markowitz 2003).

Integration of Psychotherapy and Pharmacotherapy

There has been an historic tension between psychotherapists and pharmacotherapists, whose theories of psychopathology often conflict. Such is not the case for IPT. Pharmacotherapy and IPT are easily combined and share a medical model of illness. From its inception, IPT has been used in contrast to and in combination with antidepressant medication. IPT therapists compare mood disorders to other medical diatheses, such as hypertension, asthma, or diabetes, syndromes for which both pharmacological and behavioral interventions are often combined. In similar fashion, patients with mood disorders may benefit from pharmacotherapy, which relieves symptoms faster and provides the best tested protection against depressive recurrence and relapse, and from IPT, which may help patients solve current life dilemmas, reduce external stressors, and strengthen interpersonal functioning.

The literature on combined treatment of depression with pharmacotherapy and psychotherapy does not always show advantages for combined treatment, but combined treatment never fares worse than monotherapy. Many studies have been underpowered—treating too few patients to show a difference between already efficacious monotherapies and their combination (Hollon et al. 2002). Because treatment with either medication or IPT frequently works well enough, combined treatment probably should be reserved for more chronic, severe, or treatment-resistant patients (Rush and Thase 1999). Some of the studies already described tested IPT in comparison to and in combination with pharmacotherapy. Two more studies of chronic depression treatment follow.

Feijò de Mello and colleagues (2001) in São Paolo, Brazil, randomly assigned 35 dysthymic outpatients to either moclobemide alone or moclobemide plus 16 weekly sessions of IPT. Both groups improved. There was a nonsignificant trend for greater improvement on the Ham-D and Montgomery-Åsberg Rating Scale for Depression in the combined treatment group. Given the small sample size, the lack of statistically significant differences is not surprising, but the study at least hints that combined treatment might benefit chronically depressed patients.

Hellerstein and colleagues (2001) developed a manual for cognitive-interpersonal group therapy for chronic depression (CIGP-CD), a group therapy for dysthymic patients. As the name suggests, CIGP-CD combines cognitive and interpersonal strategies, as well as psychoeducation, in a group format. The researchers tested CIGP-CD in a pilot randomized trial for fluoxetine responders. Twenty male and 20 female subjects with pure, early-onset DSM-III-R dysthymia were openly treated for 8 weeks with fluoxetine 20–80 mg/day (mean dose=38 mg/day). Subjects who had a 40% or greater decrease in Ham-D score and a Clinical Global Impression Scale score of 1 (very much improved) were randomly assigned to either continued medication alone or medication plus CIGP-CD for 16 weeks. CIGP-CD groups of about 10 patients met weekly for 90-minute sessions. No significant group differences were seen on depressive symptom measures at follow-up. However, there were trends (P=0.06) for further gains at 24 weeks in the augmented group therapy condition over medication alone in global functioning (measured by Global Assessment of Functioning Scale), personality functioning (on the Inventory of Interpersonal Problems and other measures), and overall domains. Thus, again, an interpersonally based psychotherapy may have had augmentation benefits when added to medication for chronic depression.

Conclusion

IPT began some 30 years ago as a treatment for outpatients with major depression. IPT has since repeatedly shown efficacy for such patients and has expanded its indications for particular subtypes of depression. Future research should continue to define indications for and limitations of IPT and its differential application in relation to and in combination with other antidepressant treatments. Its increasing spread among mental health clinicians reflects these achievements but also poses challenges. How will a treatment that has been delivered mainly by highly trained research therapists fare in clinical practice? The International Society for Interpersonal Psychotherapy (http://www.interpersonalpsychotherapy.org) is attempting to organize training standards for IPT as it spreads around the world.

References

American Psychiatric Association: Diagnostic and Statistical Manual of Mental Disorders, 3rd Edition, Revised. Washington, DC, American Psychiatric Association, 1987

American Psychiatric Association: Diagnostic and Statistical Manual of Mental Disorders, 4th Edition. Washington, DC, American Psychiatric Association, 1994

American Psychiatric Association: Diagnostic and Statistical Manual of Mental Disorders, 4th Edition, Text Revision. Washington, DC, American Psychiatric Association, 2000

Barber JP, Muenz LR: The role of avoidance and obsessiveness in matching patients to cognitive and interpersonal psychotherapy: empirical findings from the Treatment for Depression Collaborative Research Program. J Consult Clin Psychol 64:951–958, 1996

Beck AT: Depression Inventory. Philadelphia, PA, Center for Cognitive Therapy, 1978

Beck AT, Rush AJ, Shaw BF, et al: Cognitive Therapy of Depression. New York, Guilford, 1979

Blom MBJ, Hoencamp E, Zwaan T: Interpersoonlijke psychotherapie voor depressie: Een pilot-onderzoek [Interpersonal psychotherapy for depression: a pilot study]. Tijdschrift voor Psychiatr 38:398–402, 1996

Blom MBJ, Jonker K, Hoencamp E, et al: Combination of IPT and medication in depressed outpatients: is it the best we can do? Symposium presentation at the annual meeting of the American Psychiatric Association, New York, NY, May 2004

Boland RJ, Keller MB: Course and outcome of depression, in Handbook of Depression, 2nd Edition. Edited by Gotlib IH, Hammen CL. New York, Guilford, 2002, pp 43–60

Bolton P, Bass J, Neugebauer R, et al: Group interpersonal psychotherapy for depression in rural Uganda: a randomized controlled trial. JAMA 289:3117–3124, 2003

Bowlby J: Attachment and Loss, Vol 1: Separation: Anxiety and Anger. New York, Basic Books, 1973

Bowlby J: A Secure Base: Parent-Child Attachment and Healthy Human Development. New York, Basic Books, 1988

Brown C, Schulberg HC, Madonia MJ, et al: Treatment outcomes for primary care patients with major depression and lifetime anxiety disorders. Am J Psychiatry 153:1293–1300, 1996

Brown GW, Harris TO: Social Origins of Depression: A Study of Psychiatric Disorder in Women. London, Tavistock, 1978

Browne G, Steiner M, Roberts J, et al: Sertraline and/or interpersonal psychotherapy for patients with dysthymic disorder in primary care: 6-month comparison with longitudinal 2-year follow-up of effectiveness and costs. J Affect Disord 68:317–330, 2002

Depression Guideline Panel: Clinical Practice Guideline. Depression in Primary Care, Vols 1–4 (AHCPR Publ No 93-0550–93-0553). Rockville, MD, Agency for Health Care Policy and Research, 1993

DiMascio A, Weissman MM, Prusoff BA, et al: Differential symptom reduction by drugs and psychotherapy in acute depression. Arch Gen Psychiatry 36:1450–1456, 1979

Elkin I, Parloff MB, Hadley SW, et al: NIMH Treatment of Depression Collaborative Research Program. Arch Gen Psychiatry 42:305–316, 1985

Elkin I, Shea MT, Watkins JT, et al: National Institute of Mental Health Treatment of Depression Collaborative Research Program: general effectiveness of treatments. Arch Gen Psychiatry 46:971–982, 1989

Feijò de Mello M, Myczowisk LM, Menezes PR: A randomized controlled trial comparing moclobemide and moclobemide plus interpersonal psychotherapy in the treatment of dysthymic disorder. J Psychother Pract Res 10:117–123, 2001

Foley SH, Rounsaville BJ, Weissman MM, et al: Individual versus conjoint interpersonal psychotherapy for depressed patients with marital disputes. International Journal of Family Psychiatry 10:29–42, 1989

Frances A, Clarkin JF, Perry S: Differential Therapeutics in Psychiatry: The Art and Science of Treatment Selection. New York, Brunner/Mazel, 1984

Frank E: Interpersonal psychotherapy as a maintenance treatment for patients with recurrent depression. Psychotherapy 28:259–266, 1991

Frank E, Kupfer DJ, Perel JM, et al: Three-year outcomes for maintenance therapies in recurrent depression. Arch Gen Psychiatry 47:1093–1099, 1990

Frank E, Kupfer DJ, Wagner EF, et al: Efficacy of interpersonal psychotherapy as a maintenance treatment of recurrent depression. Arch Gen Psychiatry 48:1053–1059, 1991

Frank E, Shear MK, Rucci P, et al: Influence of panic-agoraphobic spectrum symptoms on treatment response in patients with recurrent major depression. Am J Psychiatry 157:1101–1107, 2000

Frank J: Therapeutic factors in psychotherapy. Am J Psychother 25:350–361, 1971

Hamilton M: A rating scale for depression. J Neurol Neurosurg Psychiatry 25:56–62, 1960

Hellerstein DJ, Little SA, Samstag LW, et al: Adding group psychotherapy to medication treatment in dysthymia: a randomized prospective pilot study. J Psychother Pract Res 10:93–103, 2001

Hill CE, O'Grady KE, Elkin I: Applying the Collaborative Study Psychotherapy Rating Scale to rate therapist adherence in cognitive-behavior therapy, interpersonal therapy, and clinical management. J Consult Clin Psychol 60:73–79, 1992

Hirschfeld RMA, Klerman GL, Clayton PJ, et al: Assessing personality: effects of the depressive state on trait measurement. Am J Psychiatry 140:695–699, 1983

Hollon SD, Thase ME, Markowitz JC: Treatment and prevention of depression. Psychological Science in the Public Interest 3(2):39–77, 2002

Karasu TB, Docherty JP, Gelenberg A, et al: Practice guideline for major depressive disorder in adults. Am J Psychiatry 150 (suppl):1–26, 1993

Klein DF, Ross DC: Reanalysis of the National Institute of Mental Health Treatment of Depression Collaborative Research Program general effectiveness report. Neuropsychopharmacology 8:241–251, 1993

Klerman GL, DiMascio A, Weissman MM, et al: Treatment of depression by drugs and psychotherapy. Am J Psychiatry 131:186–191, 1974

Klerman GL, Weissman MM, Rounsaville BJ, et al: Interpersonal Psychotherapy of Depression. New York, Basic Books, 1984

Klerman GL, Budman S, Berwick D, et al: Efficacy of a brief psychosocial intervention for symptoms of stress and distress among patients in primary care. Med Care 25:1078–1088, 1987

Klier CM, Muzik M, Rosenblum KL, et al: Interpersonal psychotherapy adapted for the group setting in the treatment of postpartum depression. J Psychother Pract Res 10:124–131, 2001

Markowitz JC: Psychotherapy of dysthymia. Am J Psychiatry 151:1114–1121, 1994

Markowitz JC: Interpersonal Psychotherapy for Dysthymic Disorder. Washington, DC, American Psychiatric Press, 1998

Markowitz JC: Learning the new psychotherapies, in Treatment of Depression: Bridging the 21st Century. Edited by Weissman MM. Washington, DC, American Psychiatric Publishing, 2001, pp 281–300

Markowitz JC: Interpersonal psychotherapy for chronic depression. J Clin Psychol 59:847–858, 2003

Markowitz JC, Swartz HA: Case formulation in interpersonal psychotherapy of depression, in Handbook of Psychotherapy Case Formulation. Edited by Eells TD. New York, Guilford, 1997, pp 192–222

Markowitz JC, Klerman GL, Perry SW, et al: Interpersonal psychotherapy of depressed HIV-positive outpatients. Hosp Community Psychiatry 43:885–890, 1992

Markowitz JC, Kocsis JH, Fishman B, et al: Treatment of HIV-positive patients with depressive symptoms. Arch Gen Psychiatry 55:452–457, 1998a

Markowitz JC, Svartberg M, Swartz HA: Is IPT time-limited psychodynamic psychotherapy? J Psychother Pract Res 7:185–195, 1998b

Markowitz JC, Leon AC, Miller NL, et al: Rater agreement on interpersonal psychotherapy problem areas. J Psychother Pract Res 9:131–135, 2000a

Markowitz JC, Spielman LA, Scarvalone PA, et al: Psychotherapy adherence of therapists treating HIV-positive patients with depressive symptoms. J Psychother Pract Res 9:75–80, 2000b

Montgomery SA, Åsberg M: A new depression scale designed to be sensitive to change. Br J Psychiatry 134:382–389, 1979

Mossey JM, Knott KA, Higgins M, et al: Effectiveness of a psychosocial intervention, interpersonal counseling, for sub-dysthymic depression in medically ill elderly. J Gerontol A Biol Sci Med Sci 51:M172–M178, 1996

Mufson L, Moreau D, Weissman MM: Interpersonal Therapy for Depressed Adolescents. New York, Guilford, 1993

Mufson L, Weissman MM, Moreau D, et al: Efficacy of interpersonal psychotherapy for depressed adolescents. Arch Gen Psychiatry 56:573–579, 1999

Mufson L, Dorta KP, Wickramaratne P, et al: A randomized effectiveness trial of interpersonal psychotherapy for depressed adolescents. Arch Gen Psychiatry 661:557–584, 2004

Mufson L, Gallagher T, Dorta KP, et al: A group adaptation of interpersonal psychotherapy for depressed adolescents. Am J Psychother 58:220–237, 2004

O'Hara MW, Stuart S, Gorman LL, et al: Efficacy of interpersonal psychotherapy for postpartum depression. Arch Gen Psychiatry 57:1039–1045, 2000

Parsons T: Illness and the role of the physician: a sociological perspective. Am J Orthopsychiatry 21:452–460, 1951

Paykel ES, DiMascio A, Klerman GL, et al: Maintenance therapy of depression. Pharmakopsychiatrie Neuropsychopharmakologie 9:127–136, 1976

Reynolds CF III, Frank E, Perel JM, et al: Nortriptyline and interpersonal psychotherapy as maintenance therapies for recurrent major depression: a randomized controlled trial in patients older than fifty-nine years. JAMA 281:39–45, 1999

Rosselló J, Bernal G: The efficacy of cognitive-behavioral and interpersonal treatments for depression in Puerto Rican adolescents. J Consult Clin Psychol 67:734–745, 1999

Rothblum ED, Sholomskas AJ, Berry C, et al: Issues in clinical trials with the depressed elderly. J Am Geriatr Soc 30:694–699, 1982

Rounsaville BJ, Weissman MM, Prusoff BA, et al: Marital disputes and treatment outcome in depressed women. Compr Psychiatry 20:483–490, 1979

Rush AJ, Thase ME: Psychotherapies for depressive disorders: a review, in Depressive Disorders. Edited by Maj M, Sartorius N. New York, Wiley, 1999, pp 161–206

Safran JD, Muran JC: Negotiating the Therapeutic Alliance. New York, Guilford, 2000

Schulberg HC, Block MR, Madonia MJ, et al: Treating major depression in primary care practice. Arch Gen Psychiatry 53:913–919, 1996

Shea MT, Elkin I, Imber SD, et al: Course of depressive symptoms over follow-up: findings from the National Institute of Mental Health Treatment for Depression Collaborative Research Program. Arch Gen Psychiatry 49:782–794, 1992

Shea MT, Elkin I, Sotsky SM: Patient characteristics associated with successful treatment: outcome findings from the NIMH Treatment of Depression Collaborative Research Program, in Psychotherapy Indications and Outcomes. Edited by Janowsky DS. Washington, DC, American Psychiatric Press, 1999, pp 71–90

Sholomskas AJ, Chevron ES, Prusoff BA, et al: Short-term interpersonal therapy (IPT) with the depressed elderly: case reports and discussion. Am J Psychother 36:552–566, 1983

Sloane RB, Stapes FR, Schneider LS: Interpersonal therapy versus nortriptyline for depression in the elderly, in Clinical and Pharmacological Studies in Psychiatric Disorders. Edited by Burrows GD, Norman TR, Dennerstein L. London, John Libbey, 1985, pp 344–346

Sotsky SM, Glass DR, Shea MT, et al: Patient predictors of response to psychotherapy and pharmacotherapy: findings in the NIMH Treatment of Depression Collaborative Research Program. Am J Psychiatry 148:997–1008, 1991

Spinelli M: Interpersonal psychotherapy for depressed antepartum women: a pilot study. Am J Psychiatry 154:1028–1030, 1997

Spinelli MG, Endicott J: Controlled clinical trial of interpersonal psychotherapy versus parenting education program for depressed pregnant women. Am J Psychiatry 160:555–562, 2003

Stuart S, O'Hara MW: IPT for postpartum depression. J Psychother Pract Res 4:18–29, 1995

Sullivan HS: The Interpersonal Theory of Psychiatry. New York, WW Norton, 1953

Swartz HA, Frank E, Shear MK, et al: A pilot study of brief interpersonal psychotherapy for depression among women. Psychiatr Serv 55:448–450, 2004

Thase ME, Buysse DJ, Frank E, et al: Which depressed patients will respond to interpersonal psychotherapy? The role of abnormal EEG profiles. Am J Psychiatry 154:502–509, 1997

Weissman MM: Mastering Depression: A Patient Guide to Interpersonal Psychotherapy. Albany, NY, Graywind Publications, 1995 (Currently available through The Psychological Corporation, Order Service Center, P.O. Box 839954, San Antonio, TX 78283-3954; tel. 1-800-228-0752, fax 1-800-232-1223)

Weissman MM, Klerman GL: Conjoint interpersonal psychotherapy for depressed patients with marital disputes, in New Applications of Interpersonal Psychotherapy. Edited by Klerman GL, Weissman MM. Washington, DC, American Psychiatric Press, 1993, pp 103–127

Weissman MM, Klerman GL, Paykel ES, et al: Treatment effects on the social adjustment of depressed patients. Arch Gen Psychiatry 30:771–778, 1974

Weissman MM, Prusoff BA, DiMascio A, et al: The efficacy of drugs and psychotherapy in the treatment of acute depressive episodes. Am J Psychiatry 136:555–558, 1979

Weissman MM, Klerman GL, Prusoff BA, et al: Depressed outpatients: results one year after treatment with drugs and/or interpersonal psychotherapy. Arch Gen Psychiatry 38:52–55, 1981

Weissman MM, Markowitz JC, Klerman GL: Comprehensive Guide to Interpersonal Psychotherapy. New York, Basic Books, 2000

Wells KB, Stewart A, Hays RD, et al: The functioning and well-being of depressed patients: results from the Medical Outcomes Study. JAMA 262:914–919, 1989

Wilfley DE, MacKenzie RK, Welch RR, et al: Interpersonal Psychotherapy for Group. New York, Basic Books, 2000

Zlotnick C, Johnson SL, Miller IW, et al: Postpartum depression in women receiving public assistance: pilot study of an interpersonal-therapy-oriented group intervention. Am J Psychiatry 158:638–640, 2001

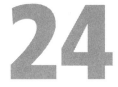

Psychoanalytic and Psychodynamic Psychotherapy for Depression and Dysthymia

GLEN O. GABBARD, M.D.

TANYA J. BENNETT, M.D.

History

The history of psychoanalytic and psychodynamic approaches to depression begins with Sigmund Freud's classic work "Mourning and Melancholia" (Freud 1917/1963). Central to Freud's view was that early losses in childhood led to later vulnerability to depression in adulthood. He also observed that the marked self-depreciation so common in depressed patients was the result of anger turned inward. More specifically, he conceptualized that rage is directed internally because the self of the patient has identified with the lost object. In Freud's words, "Thus the shadow of the object fell upon the ego, and the latter could henceforth be judged by a special agency, as though it were an object, the forsaken object" (Freud 1917/1963, p. 249). In 1923, Freud noted that taking a lost object inside and identifying with it may be the only way that some people can give up an important figure in their lives. That same year, in "The Ego and the Id," he

postulated that melancholic patients have a severe superego, which he related to their guilt over having shown aggression toward loved ones (Freud 1923/1961).

Karl Abraham (1924/1927) elaborated on Freud's ideas by linking present with past. He suggested that depressed adults experienced a severe blow to their self-esteem during childhood and that adult depression is triggered by a new loss or new disappointment that stirs intense negative feelings toward both past and present figures who have hurt the patient through either real or imagined withdrawal of love.

The next significant development in the psychoanalytic understanding of depression was the work of Melanie Klein (1940/1975). In her model, depression was linked to a developmental failure around the depressive position. Adults with depression were vulnerable because they had never adequately resolved their early concern that they had destroyed loving figures in their environment, such as their parents, through their own destructiveness and greed. They believed that as a consequence of that destruction, they were persecuted by hated bad objects that remained active internally. This feeling of being persecuted by bad internal objects while longing for the lost good objects that they had destroyed constitutes the essence of the depressive position, which Klein viewed as reactivated in adult depression. Patients may feel worthless because they sense that they have changed their good internal parents into persecuting, rageful parents as a result of their own destructive impulses and fantasies.

In the 1950s, the contributions of Bibring (1953) appeared and differed substantially from those of Freud and Klein regarding the role of aggression. Bibring believed that depression was better understood as a primary affective state unrelated to the aggression turned inward that Freud and Klein emphasized. He viewed melancholic states as arising from the tension between ideals and reality. Three highly invested narcissistic aspirations—to be worthy and loved, to be strong or superior, and to be good and loving—are held up as standards of conduct. However, the ego's awareness of its actual or imagined inability to measure up to these standards produces depression. As a result, the depressed person feels helpless and powerless. Bibring believed that any wound to one's self-esteem might precipitate a clinical depression. Hence, narcissistic vulnerability was a key to his understanding of what set a depressive process in motion. He did not view the superego as having a key role in the process.

After studying the records of depressed children at the Hampstead Clinic in the United Kingdom, Sandler and Joffe (1965) concluded that the children became depressed when they thought that they had lost something essential to self-esteem but felt helpless to do anything about the loss. They emphasized that the loss was more than just a real or an imagined love object but also a state of well-being conferred on them by the object. This state becomes a type of "Paradise Lost" that becomes idealized and intensely desired, even though it is unattainable.

Jacobson (1971) built on Freud's formulation by suggesting that depressed patients actually behave as if they were the worthless lost love object, even though they do not assume all the characteristics of that lost person. Eventually, this bad internal object—or the lost external love object—is transformed into a sadistic superego. A depressed patient then becomes "a victim of the superego, as helpless and powerless as a small child who is tortured by his cruel, powerful mother" (Jacobson 1971, p. 252).

Arieti (1977) postulated a preexisting ideology in persons who become severely depressed. He observed in treating severely depressed patients that they often had a pattern of living for someone else instead of for themselves. He termed the person for whom they lived the *dominant other*. The spouse is often the dominant other in this formulation, but sometimes an ideal or an organization can serve the same function. He used the term *dominant goal* or *dominant etiology* when a transcendent purpose or aim occupied this place in the individual's psychological world. These individuals feel that living for someone or something else is not working out for them, but they feel unable to change. They may believe that life is worthless if they cannot elicit the response they wish from the dominant other or if they cannot achieve their impossible goal.

Much can be learned about depression from attachment theory. John Bowlby (1969) viewed the child's attachment to his or her mother as necessary for survival. When attachment is disrupted through loss of a parent or through an unstable ongoing attachment to the parent, children view themselves as unlovable and their mothers or caregivers as undependable and abandoning. Hence, in adult life, such children may become depressed whenever they experience a loss because it reactivates the feelings of being an unlovable and abandoned failure.

Several themes run throughout the various psychodynamic formulations, which are summarized in Table 24–1.

Almost all psychoanalytic views emphasize a fundamental narcissistic vulnerability or fragile self-esteem in depressed patients (Busch et al. 2004). Anger and aggression are also implicated in most theories, particularly in connection with the guilt and self-denigration that they produce. In addition, the seeking of a highly perfectionistic caregiving figure with the certainty that one will not find such a person is a part of the depressive picture. A demanding and perfectionistic superego appears to play a central role and can become tormenting in its demands on the individual. In some cases, a vicious cycle is established (Busch et al. 2004). Someone who is depressed may try to compensate by idealizing either oneself or a significant other. This idealization, however, only increases the likelihood of eventual disappointment, which then triggers depression because these high standards have not been met. This failure also leads to devaluation of the self and self-directed anger.

An Integrated Theoretical Model and Hypothesized Mechanisms

Psychodynamic approaches to understanding depression today recognize that mood disorders are strongly influenced by genetic and biological factors (Gabbard 2000). In fact, depressive illness serves as an ideal model to study how genes and environment interact to produce clinical syndromes.

TABLE 24–1. Major contributions to psychodynamic models of depression and dysthymia

Freud (1917/1963)	Anger turned inward
Abraham (1924/1927)	Present loss reactivates childhood blow to self-esteem
Klein (1940/1975)	Developmental failure during depressive position
Bibring (1953)	Tension in the ego between ideals and reality
Sandler and Joffe (1965)	Helplessness in response to childhood loss of real or imagined love object
Bowlby (1969)	Loss reactivates feeling of being unlovable and abandoned secondary to insecure attachment
Jacobson (1971)	Lost love object transformed into sadistic superego
Arieti (1977)	Living for dominant other

Kendler and colleagues (1995) followed up female-female twin pairs of known zygosity to determine whether an etiological model could be developed to predict major depressive episodes. The most compelling model to emerge from their findings was the following: sensitivity to the depression-inducing effects of stressful life events appears to be under genetic control. For example, when the individuals at lowest genetic risk for major depression were examined, they had a probability of onset of major depression per month of only about 0.5% in the absence of a stressful life event. When these individuals were exposed to a stressor, however, the probability increased to 6.2%. In those individuals who were at the highest genetic risk, the probability of onset of depression per month was only 1.1% without exposure to a life stressor, but the risk rose dramatically—to 14.6%—when a stressful life event was present.

Further support for this model was provided by a prospective study of 1,037 children from New Zealand (Caspi et al. 2003). These investigators found that a functional polymorphism in the promoter region of the serotonin transporter (5-HTT) gene was found to moderate the influence of stressful life events on depression.

In a subsequent analysis (Kendler et al. 1999), the investigators found that about one-third of the association between stressful life events and onset of depression was *noncausal* because those individuals predisposed to major depression select themselves into high-risk environments. For example, persons with a temperament high in neurot-

icism may alienate others and thus cause a breakup of a significant relationship.

The most powerful stressors appeared to be death of a close relative, assault, serious marital problems, and divorce or breakup (see Williams, Chapter 9, in this volume). However, considerable evidence also suggests that early experiences of abuse, neglect, or separation may create a neurobiological sensitivity that predisposes individuals to respond to stressors in adulthood by developing a major depressive episode. For example, Kendler et al. (1992) documented an increased risk for major depression in those women who had experienced maternal or paternal separation in childhood or adolescence. In subsequent work, Kendler et al. (2001) found other gender differences regarding the depressogenic effect of stressful life events. Men were more sensitive to the depressogenic effects of divorce or separation and work problems, whereas women were more sensitive to the depressogenic effects of problems encountered with individuals in their proximal network.

As Nemeroff (1999) has pointed out, Freud's view that early loss created a vulnerability that predisposed one to depression in adulthood has been confirmed by recent research (see Williams, Chapter 9, in this volume). Agid et al. (1999) reported a case–control study in which rates of early parental loss as a result of parental death or permanent separation before age 17 years were evaluated in patients with various adult psychiatric disorders. Loss of a parent during childhood significantly increased the likelihood of developing major depression during adult life. The effect of loss due to permanent separation was more striking than loss due to death, as was loss before age 9 years compared with later childhood and adolescence. In addition, Gilman et al. (2003) found that parental divorce in early childhood was associated with a higher lifetime risk of depression. Not only early childhood losses appear to increase vulnerability to depression. Both physical and sexual abuse have been independently associated with adult depression in women (Bernet and Stein 1999; Bifulco et al. 1998, 2000; Brown 1993; Brown and Eales 1993). Women with a history of child abuse or neglect are twice as likely as those without such a history to have negative relationships and low self-esteem in adulthood (Bifulco et al. 1998). Those abused or neglected women who have these negative relationships and low self-esteem in adulthood are then 10 times more likely to experience depression.

The early trauma that appears to be relevant to a significant number of adults with depression can lead to permanent biological alterations. Vythilingam et al. (2002) found that depressed women with childhood abuse had an 18% smaller mean left hippocampal volume than did nonabused depressed subjects and a 15% smaller mean left hippocampal volume than did healthy subjects. In addition, a good deal of research has documented that corticotropin-releasing factor (CRF), which induces the pituitary to secrete corticotropin, is consistently elevated in the cerebrospinal fluid of depressed patients compared with nondepressed control subjects (Heim et al. 2000; Nemeroff 1998a). These observations suggest a diathesis-stress model for mood disorders. In other words, a genetic substrate might serve to diminish monoamine levels in synapses or to increase reactivity of the hypothalamic-pituitary-adrenal (HPA) axis to stress. If no serious stress affects the individual, the genetically determined threshold is not necessarily sufficient to induce depression. However, experiences of neglect or abuse in childhood may activate the stress response and induce elevated activity in CRF-containing neurons, which are responsive to stress and excessively active in depressed persons. These cells can become supersensitive in certain individuals, reacting dramatically to even mild stressors. Hammen et al. (2000) confirmed that in adult women, childhood adversity appears to sensitize women to stressor-induced depression in adult life.

In an elegantly designed study, Heim et al. (2000) studied 49 healthy women ages 18–45 years who were taking no hormonal or psychotropic medications. They divided them into four groups: 1) those with no history of child abuse or psychiatric disorder, 2) those with current major depression who were sexually or physically abused as children, 3) those without current major depression who were sexually or physically abused as children, and 4) those with current major depression but no history of childhood abuse. Those women in the study with a history of childhood abuse had increased pituitary, adrenal, and autonomic responses to stress compared with control subjects. This effect was particularly significant in women with current symptoms of depression and anxiety. Women with a history of childhood abuse and a current major depression diagnosis had a more than sixfold greater corticotropin response to stress than did age-matched control subjects. The investigators concluded that the HPA axis and autonomic nervous system hyperreactivity related to CRF hyposecretion is a persistent consequence of childhood abuse that may contribute to the diathesis for adult depression.

The early stressors in childhood are inherent in a psychodynamic model that views adult pathology as related to early traumas. However, the psychoanalytic perspective also takes into account the meaning of a particular stressor. Clinicians must keep in mind that what may seem like a relatively mild stressor to an outside observer may have powerful conscious or unconscious meanings to the patient that greatly amplify its effect. Hammen (1995) noted that "the field has reached considerable consensus that it is not the mere occurrence of a negative life event, but rather the person's interpretation of the meaning of the event and its significance in the context of its occurrence" (p. 98). In a longitudinal study of the link between depressive reactions and stressors, Hammen and colleagues (1985) found that those stressors whose content matched the patient's area of self-definition were particularly likely to precipitate depressive episodes. In other words, in someone whose sense of self is partly defined by social connectedness, loss of a significant interpersonal relationship may precipitate a major depression. If someone's self-worth is especially linked to mastery and achievement, such a person might be more likely to have a depressive episode in response to a perceived failure in work or in school.

A recent report from Kendler et al. (2003) also suggests that life events with particular meanings to the individual may be more closely linked to the onset of major depression in adult patients. In interviews with their twin sample from the population-based Virginia Twin Registry, Kendler and colleagues found that onset of major depression was predicted by higher ratings of loss and humiliation in the stressors. They also noted that events with a combination of humiliation (because of a separation initiated by a significant other) and loss were more depressogenic than were pure loss events such as death. Humiliating events that directly devalue the individual in a core role were strongly linked to a risk for depressive episodes. Hence, a psychodynamic clinician would want to explore the meaning of all stressors to determine the unique way that the stressor affected the patient.

A contemporary psychodynamic model of depression would understand that early traumatic experiences leave the child to develop problematic self and object representations. In the case of physical and sexual abuse, the child internalizes a bad self, deserving of abuse, who feels hypervigilant about victimization. The object representation is likely to be that of an abusive, punitive figure that attacks the self. The feeling of being tormented or persecuted by this abusive internal object fits well with observations of a punitive superego. Similarly, early loss of a parent leads a child to develop a sense of an abandoned self that cannot have its needs met in the usual way by a parent. The child also internalizes an abandoning object representation and grows up with a sense of loss and longing that becomes reactivated with any adult stressor involving loss. Hence, the effects of losses are magnified when they occur in adult life. Because a child's self-esteem is largely based on how the child is treated in early family interactions, a vulnerable self-esteem is also a legacy of childhood loss and trauma. The forging of the child's personality in the context of problematic relationships with parents and other significant figures will likely result in adult relational difficulties. Hence, adults with this background may have difficulties forming and maintaining relationships and thus be more vulnerable to loss and narcissistic injury from others.

The study of defense mechanisms is another component of psychoanalytic theory that is relevant to a psychodynamic model of depression. Defense mechanisms are established early in life to manage painful affect states. The work of Kwon (1999; Kwon and Lemmon 2000) suggests that certain defense mechanisms may contribute to the development of depression, whereas others may help protect against depression. Turning against the self, which involves exaggerated and persistent self-criticism, is an immature defense that has an additive effect on negative attributional style in the development of dysphoria. Other immature defense mechanisms also appear to increase the risk for depression and other psychiatric disorders (Vaillant and Vaillant 1992). In contrast, certain higher-level defense mechanisms, such as *principalization* (also called *intellectualization*), which involves the reinterpretation of reality through general and abstract principles, may positively moderate the influence of attributional styles on levels of dysphoria. Hence, adding a psychodynamic perspective on defenses may facilitate understanding and treatment of depression (Hayes et al. 1996; Jones and Pulos 1993).

Yet another principle of psychodynamic thinking is a focus on what is unique about each patient as opposed to seeing patients as part of one large group. In this regard, psychodynamic models of depression take into account unique qualities of defense mechanisms and object relations in each depressed person. For example, Blatt (1998, 2004) studied large populations of depressed patients and noted that two underlying psychodynamic types emerged from his work. The *anaclitic* type is characterized by feelings of helplessness, loneliness, and weakness related to chronic fears of being abandoned and unprotected. These individuals have longings to be nurtured, protected, and loved. They are characterized by vulnerability to disruptions of interpersonal relationships, and they typically use the defense mechanisms of denial, disavowal, displacement, and repression. By contrast, *introjective* patients who are depressed are primarily concerned with self-development. Intimate relationships are viewed as secondary, and they use different defense mechanisms: intellectualization, reaction formation, and rationalization. They are exceedingly perfectionistic and competitive and are excessively driven to achieve in work and school. The anaclitic types manifest their depression primarily in dys-

phoric feelings of abandonment, loss, and loneliness. The introjective types manifest their depression in feelings of guilt and worthlessness. They also have a sense of failure and a perception that their sense of autonomy and control has been lost.

The integrated psychodynamic model outlined here is relevant to understanding psychodynamic themes in suicide as well. For example, abuse in childhood appears to be a strong risk factor for the development of impulsivity and suicide attempts (Brodsky et al. 2001; Davidson et al. 1996; McHolm et al. 2003). The psychodynamic literature on suicide (Asch 1980; Meissner 1986) reports that a recurring theme in the object relations of suicidal patients is the drama between a sadistic tormentor and a tormented victim. The role of early abuse helps explain how the depressed suicidal patient may feel persecuted by what Asch (1980) referred to as "the hidden executioner." Some suicides may be motivated by relief from the persecution. Many suicidal patients also show strong dependency yearnings toward a lost object (Dorpat 1973), so that suicide may in some cases be motivated by strong reunion fantasies with a significant figure who has been lost. Finally, the way in which a patient manages aggression may be central to suicidal motivation. Depressed patients often feel that suicide is a way of taking revenge against their parents, a spouse, or others they think have significantly failed them (Gabbard 2000). In other words, the perception by the patient that he or she has experienced a severe narcissistic injury leads to narcissistic rage and revenge fantasies.

Principles of Technique

Although the term *psychodynamic* originally had a broader meaning than *psychoanalytic*, the two terms are commonly used interchangeably today. They refer to a psychotherapy that is based on a set of core principles:

1. *Much of mental life is unconscious.* This principle underscores the notion that the causes of suffering in emotional disturbances are often unclear to the patient. Meanings attached to particular stresses, for example, may not be available to the patient's conscious awareness.
2. *Past is prologue.* This phrase refers to the fact that all psychoanalytic theories have a basis in early developmental understanding. The traumas of childhood can be reactivated by stressful events as an adult. Similarly, the patterns of relationships between a child and significant others in the child's life will repeat themselves throughout each subsequent developmental phase. Thus, a child who is repeatedly criticized and humiliated by his father

will grow up anticipating that other male authority figures will behave toward him in a similar manner.

3. *Transference*. This concept follows directly from the first two. A person who comes to psychotherapy will relate to the therapist in a way that is shaped by past relationships with similar figures. Transference is initially unconscious until the patient starts to become aware of the patterns being repeated from long ago. Thus, qualities are attributed to the therapist that may belong to people from the patient's past. The analysis of the transference developments in psychotherapy constitutes one of the major technical strategies of a psychoanalytic psychotherapist.

4. *Countertransference*. Psychoanalytic or psychodynamic therapy is fundamentally treatment that takes into consideration a two-person model. In other words, just as patients have transferences to therapists, therapists have transferences to patients. This is called *countertransference*. This phenomenon is considered a joint creation in the sense that part of countertransference grows out of the therapist's past relationships, and another aspect of it is a direct response to what the patient evokes in the therapist. In this regard, countertransference also provides useful information about what is happening within the patient.

5. *Resistance*. Psychodynamic therapists recognize that patients are often ambivalent about getting better. Hence, they may unconsciously struggle against the therapy or the therapist. They may forget appointments, forget to fill a prescription, come late to sessions, talk about the weather or news events instead of their problems, and reject observations offered by the therapist. Resistance can have multiple meanings, and a psychoanalytic psychotherapist tries to help the patient understand resistance rather than simply remove it by exhortation.

In the practice of psychoanalytic and psychodynamic variations on psychotherapy, therapists formulate the patient's core conflicts by carefully observing what develops into therapeutic relationships. They also recognize that there are two persons in the room and both are contributing to the interaction. Therefore, psychodynamic therapists continually monitor how they may be affecting the process of therapy. They seek to understand resistance, transference, and the unconscious sources of the patient's symptoms. A succinct definition of psychoanalytic psychotherapy is "a therapy that involves careful attention to the therapist–patient interaction, with thoughtfully timed interpretation of transference and resistance embedded in a sophisticated appreciation of the therapist's contribution to the two-person field" (Gunderson and Gabbard 1999, p. 685).

Psychoanalytic and Psychodynamic Approaches to Depression and Dysthymia

The application of psychodynamic techniques to depression and dysthymia follows directly from the conceptual model outlined earlier. A psychodynamic therapist would carefully evaluate the nature of the stressor that appeared to trigger a depression. Did the stressor involve humiliation and loss? Did it reawaken early childhood losses or traumas? What was the particular meaning of the stressor to the patient? The dynamic therapist would want to know what the patient associates with the stressor. Is the event reminiscent of other feelings, thoughts, or fantasies that have been present in the patient's mind? A dynamic therapist also might encourage the patient to bring in dreams that may shed light on what is occurring unconsciously.

In the course of history-taking and evaluation of the stressor, psychodynamic therapists also listen closely to the themes that occur around relationship patterns and the patient's self-esteem. These therapists would consider the various psychodynamic themes enumerated earlier as they assess which themes may most accurately be involved in the pathogenesis of the patient's depression. Is the patient's anger turned inward? Is he or she concerned that his or her destructiveness or greed has harmed loved ones? Does he or she have a perfectionistic view of the self that seems impossible to attain? Is the patient tormented by a vicious and unrelenting superego that is constantly expecting more than the patient can deliver? Is he or she pining for lost love objects in the present or the past that makes the patient feel hopeless? Has the patient lived for a "dominant other" rather than fulfilling his or her own unique dreams and desires? Is the depression more the anaclitic type, with prominent feelings of helplessness, weakness, and loneliness, or is it more the introjective type, in which self-development seems to be of greater importance than finding a nurturing and protective love object? Similarly, what defense mechanisms does the patient use to manage painful affect states?

While exploring these themes in the patient's life narrative, the psychodynamic therapist also would be carefully observing transference, countertransference, and resistance phenomena. The way the patient relates to the therapist and the feelings evoked in the therapist by the patient will provide clues to familiar patterns of relationship problems that occur outside the therapy. The pattern of resistance may reflect the patient's defenses in other life situations as well. Eventually, the therapist develops a formulation of the patient's difficulties that involves both the early developmental issues and the current situation. The meaning of the stressor will probably figure prominently into the formulation. Often, core conflicts in relationships will become apparent and serve as a centerpiece of the patient's depression. Luborsky (1984) described this as the core conflictual relationship theme. This model generally takes the form of the patient's wishes, expectations, or fantasies about others; the perceived reaction of the other person; and the patient's response to that reaction. These themes generally emerge in the transference and countertransference embedded in the therapeutic process. A case example will illustrate:

> Mr. A became depressed after he had been passed over for a promotion in the workplace. He told Dr. B that it was just one more example of how he could never measure up to the expectations of others. In providing his history, Mr. A noted that his father was a high-ranking military officer, who was harsh in his criticisms of Mr. A and who was always expecting him to do better. If Mr. A ever came home with a report card that was less than perfect, his father would give him the "third degree" about why he had gotten B's instead of A's. He viewed his boss in the same way—namely, that he could never please his boss because the expectations placed on him were beyond his grasp or capabilities.
>
> This same pattern began emerging in the transference to Dr. B by the fourth session, when Mr. A said to his therapist, "I'm afraid I'm not doing this right. You want me to bring in my fantasies, dreams, and help figure out the causes of my depression, but I can't seem to remember my dreams, and I am worried that I am never talking about what I'm supposed to talk about here." Dr. B helped Mr. A formulate a core conflictual relationship theme. He had a desperate desire to please male authority figures by measuring up to their expectations. However, he anticipated that all such figures would be disappointed with his performance, so he responded with self-depreciation and a kind of hopelessness as a way of criticizing himself to fend off the criticism of the male authority figures. Dr. B interpreted this pattern by pointing out the similarity in what was transpiring with him, what had transpired in the past with his father, and what transpired recently with his boss when he was passed over for the promotion.

Interpretation of how unconscious conflicts and patterns of relationships repeat themselves again and again is a key practice principle in psychoanalytic psychotherapy. As in this case example, Dr. B made connections between the transference relationship, the patient's early life, and the current relationships in the patient's life outside of therapy. Mechanisms of change are not well understood, but we can speculate that the neural networks containing representations of self and other are modified such that newer representations gradually become more prominent

than the old, maladaptive ones (Gabbard and Westen 2003). Moreover, associations between affect states and those representations may be altered as well.

As therapy proceeds, the patient's defenses against distressing emotions also will be addressed. For example, in the case of Mr. A, Dr. B eventually pointed out how Mr. A defended against his own anger by turning the anger against himself in the form of self-depreciation. The psychotherapy helped Mr. A recognize that he had smoldering, long-standing rage at his father as well as at his boss.

Space considerations preclude a more detailed discussion of the principles of technique in the psychodynamic treatment of depression, but interested readers are referred to a well-written manual by Busch and colleagues (2004). The principles outlined here for depression are also useful in dysthymia. The major differences are that dysthymia is a chronic, long-standing condition in which discrete stressors may be more difficult to identify. However, the same psychodynamic themes will emerge in the therapy, and the same interpretative strategies are useful. Therapists may encounter more resistance with dysthymic patients because the chronic patterns have become more entrenched. Therefore, more of a working-through process may be necessary, in which the patient and therapist examine together the recurrent patterns of self-defeating and self-depreciating behavior and try to sort out what perpetuates the patterns. Is the patient guilty and, therefore, feeling that punishment and unhappiness are well deserved? Does he or she have a fantasy of defeating the therapist as a way of exacting revenge on parents or others who have disappointed the patient? These issues often take a much longer time to work through than the treatment of an uncomplicated major depressive episode. Childhood trauma and adversity, comorbid anxiety disorders, features of depressive personality, and Cluster C personality disorders all may contribute to a poorer prognosis in patients with dysthymic disorder (Hayden and Klein 2001).

Broadly speaking, two varieties of psychoanalytic or psychodynamic psychotherapy for depression exist. *Brief dynamic therapy* is generally time-limited from the beginning to fewer than 20 episodes. *Long-term* or *open-ended psychodynamic* or *psychoanalytic therapy* has no predetermined length. The therapist and patient agree to explore themes that are relevant to the patient's depression or dysthymia until the treatment goals have been accomplished and a mutual agreement for termination is reached.

Whether the therapy is brief or long term, most psychodynamic therapists readily use antidepressant medications as part of the overall treatment plan. Decades ago, there were concerns that medication might interfere with the patient's suffering in such a way that the patient would lose motivation for psychotherapy, but those fears are now widely held to be unfounded (Gabbard and Kay 2001). In fact, antidepressant medication is generally thought to facilitate the psychotherapy because it may address vegetative symptoms such as sleep disturbance, loss of appetite, and psychomotor retardation more rapidly and facilitate a more collaborative state of mind in the patients for purposes of the psychotherapy. Moreover, a substantial number of patients with dysthymia may have their conditions exacerbated by decompensating into a major depressive episode, the so-called double depression (Keller and Shapiro 1982; D.N. Klein et al. 2000). Hence, the dynamic therapist may need to address both chronic and acute elements of the depressive picture in the patient.

Research Findings

Psychoanalytic or psychodynamic psychotherapy for depression and dysthymia has a smaller research base than cognitive-behavioral therapy (CBT) and interpersonal psychotherapy. Psychoanalytic psychotherapy research presents many unique challenges and thus can be problematic. Defining therapeutic interventions unique to psychoanalytic psychotherapy, standardizing these techniques among well-trained therapists, allowing for the open-ended and often long-term nature of the work, selecting appropriate controls, and dealing with objections to random assignments all make research in this field intrinsically difficult.

Despite the complexities and difficulties intrinsic to the work, the number of studies in the literature that focus on psychoanalytic and psychodynamic psychotherapy for depression is growing. Early studies used brief dynamic therapy as a comparison group to assess and usually validate another therapeutic approach. More recent rigorous controlled studies have shown that psychodynamic psychotherapy is at least as effective when compared with other therapeutic modalities in short-term studies, and combination treatment (therapy plus medication) is superior to pharmacotherapy alone. "Dose-dependent" effects are generally not shown because long-term studies have not yet been performed.

In an investigation of 66 clinically depressed caregivers of elderly family members (Gallagher-Thompson and Steffen 1994), random assignment was made to one of two treatment cells: brief psychodynamic therapy or CBT. Initial diagnoses of major, minor, or intermittent depressive disorder were made according to the Schedule for Affective Disorders and Schizophrenia (SADS). Measures of change included the Beck Depression Inventory

(BDI), Hamilton Rating Scale for Depression (Ham-D), and (because the caregivers' mean age was 62 years) the Geriatric Depression Scale (GDS). Brief psychodynamic therapy focused on separation-individuation issues, and CBT focused on developing skills and coping strategies relevant to the demands of caregiving. At posttreatment (after 20 sessions), 71% of the caregivers were no longer clinically depressed, and 8% had diagnostic changes from major to minor depressive disorder ($n=52$, $P=0.19$). Overall, no differences were found between the two treatment groups ($n=54$, $P=0.19$).

Similar findings were reported in the second Sheffield Psychotherapy Project (Shapiro et al. 1994, 1995). In this randomized, controlled trial conducted in the United Kingdom, 117 clinically depressed patients were stratified according to pretreatment severity and randomly assigned within these groups to either 8 or 16 sessions of psychodynamic interpersonal therapy or CBT. Depression severity was determined via prescreening BDI scores as follows: low severity (16–20), moderate severity (21–26), and high severity (≥ 27). The authors defined psychodynamic interpersonal therapy as "exploratory" therapy on the basis of Hobson's (1985) conversational model and CBT as "prescriptive" therapy, in which a broad range of techniques and strategies is provided to the patient.

Improvement was assessed with several measures, including the BDI, Symptom Checklist–90—Revised Depression Subscale (SCL-90-R-D) and Global Severity Index (SCL-90-R-GSI), Inventory of Interpersonal Problems (IIP), Social Adjustment Scale Self-Report Social Subscale (SAS-SOC), Self-Esteem Measure (SE), and Present State Examination, Symptom Total Score (PSE). Both treatments were found to be equally effective on all measures, with the exception of the BDI (BDI score: CBT, adjusted mean [M_{adj}] $=7.99$; psychodynamic interpersonal therapy, $M_{adj}=11.51$; $P=0.05$). In general, both treatments appeared to exert their effects with equal rapidity. Patients who had only mild or moderate depression had the same outcome regardless of whether they received 8 or 16 weeks of therapy. However, in the severely depressed patients, significantly superior outcomes were noted when 16 weeks of therapy were provided, regardless of type of treatment. Adjusted means and tests of severity multiplied by duration interaction for the high-severity subgroup showed the following: 8 sessions, BDI $M_{adj}=19.83$; and 16 sessions, BDI $M_{adj}=9.29$ ($P<0.05$ for simple effect of duration, $P=0.03$ for interaction effect).

At 1-year follow-up by mail ($n=104$), no overall differences were found in either outcome or maintenance of gains between the two types of therapy. Despite no significant difference between 8- and 16-session CBT, longer periods of therapy did appear to be associated with better long-term outcomes in the case of psychodynamic interpersonal therapy. After 1 year, adjusted means and tests of treatment multiplied by duration interaction showed the following: BDI CBT, M_{adj}=6.72 and 7.55 for 8 and 16 sessions, respectively; and BDI psychodynamic interpersonal therapy, M_{adj}=11.39 and 5.21 for 8 and 16 sessions, respectively (for simple effect of duration, P=0.89 [CBT] and 0.03 [psychodynamic interpersonal therapy]; for simple effect of treatment, P=0.05 [8 sessions] and 0.33 [16 sessions]; and for interaction effect, P=0.04). No significant interaction was found between severity and duration, as had been noted in the analyses of short-term effects ($P \geq 0.15$ on all measures).

In another randomized, controlled trial comparing very brief cognitive-behavioral and psychodynamic interpersonal therapy for subsyndromal depression, Barkham et al. (1999) developed a "two-plus-one (2+1) model": two 1-hour sessions 1 week apart followed by a third 1-hour session 3 months later. The 116 patients were stratified according to severity on the basis of BDI scores as stressed (4–9), subclinical (10–15), or low-level clinical depression (16–25). Measures of change included the BDI, SCL-90-R, and IIP-32. All treatment groups improved, and no significant differences were seen between treatment modalities (post–session 3 effect size difference was 0.15). At 1-year follow-up, a significant advantage for CBT appeared on the BDI, and the effect size difference between treatments at this time was 0.57. This effect, however, did not approach significance on the SCL-90-R or IIP-30 (all F<1).

A randomized, controlled study of the effects of brief psychodynamic interpersonal therapy compared with usual care after deliberate self-poisoning (Guthrie et al. 2001) in the United Kingdom showed significantly less suicidal ideation and fewer attempts at self-harm at 6-month follow-up compared with control subjects. The 119 patients between ages 18 and 65 who had presented to an emergency department after intentionally poisoning themselves were divided into two groups. The psychotherapy intervention consisted of four 50-minute sessions of psychodynamic interpersonal therapy delivered by nurse therapists in the patient's home within 1 week of presentation. Therapy reportedly focused on identifying and promoting the resolution of interpersonal difficulties that worsen psychological stress. Control patients received "usual care," which most often consisted of referral back to their general practitioner. Suicidal ideation was assessed with the Beck Scale for Suicide Ideation (BSSI), and a difference of 5 points was considered by the authors to be clinically significant. Attempts at self-harm were evaluated by self-report and cross-referenced with the emergency department database. At 6-month follow-up

(n=95), the mean scores on the BSSI for the intervention and control groups were 7.9 and 12.8, respectively (P=0.005), and 9% (n=5) of the patients in the intervention group had harmed themselves versus 28% (n=17) in the control group (P=0.009).

A recent controlled trial of the short- and long-term effect of psychological treatment for postpartum depression (Cooper et al. 2003) compared the effects of nondirective counseling, CBT, or psychodynamic therapy in relation to a control condition of routine primary care. Women with postpartum depression (N=193) were randomly assigned to one of these four groups. Nondirective counseling offered women an opportunity to discuss any current concerns. CBT was aimed at the identification and management of parenting problems and improving the quality of the mother–infant interaction. Psychodynamic therapy focused on exploring the mother's early attachment history to promote her understanding of attachment issues related to her own infant. Therapy started at 8 weeks postpartum, the period during which depression is likely to be routinely detected, and continued on a weekly basis to 18 weeks postpartum. Posttreatment (4.5 months), all three treatment groups had significantly lower scores on the Edinburgh Postnatal Depression Scale compared with control subjects. Mean scores for the treatment groups were 8.9 (psychodynamic therapy [n=45], P=0.003), 9.4 (CBT [n=42], P=0.003), and 9.9 (counseling [n=47], P=0.02), compared with the control group score of 11.3 (n=50). Only psychodynamic therapy, however, was shown to be significantly superior to the control condition in reducing the rate of depression according to the Structured Clinical Interview for DSM-III-R (SCID). In the psychodynamic therapy group, 70% were no longer depressed compared with 40% in the control group (P=0.002).

The most recent meta-analytic review of the efficacy of short-term psychodynamic psychotherapy specifically in major depression (DSM-III; American Psychiatric Association 1980) compared with CBT or behavior therapy (Leichsenring 2001) included only studies in which 13 or more therapy sessions were performed, and more than 20 patients were treated. Eleven independent studies, including four follow-up studies, were reviewed, and six studies met the inclusion criteria. No significant differences were detected among therapy modalities with regard to improvements in depressive symptoms, general psychiatric symptoms, and social functioning or patients' reports of remitted symptoms or improvement after treatment. Only three of the selected studies provided the necessary data to determine effect sizes. When these were converted into percentages of nonoverlap of the distributions, the effects of short-term psychodynamic psychotherapy were interpreted as follows: the average depressed patient is better off after treatment than 82%–100% of depressed patients before treatment in terms of depressive symptoms, 82%–100% in terms of other psychiatric symptoms, and 75%–96% in terms of social functioning. The author concluded that, in general, short-term psychodynamic psychotherapy and CBT or behavior therapy appear to be equally effective in the treatment of depression. However, he cautioned that one should not assume that all forms of short-term psychodynamic psychotherapy and CBT or behavior therapy are equally effective in all groups of patients. In addition, he suggested that 16–20 sessions in any modality appear insufficient to maintain lasting remission, and future studies are needed to address not only specific versions of short-term psychodynamic psychotherapy but also the effects of longer treatments of depression.

A review of the treatment of depression in late life (Karel and Hinrichsen 2000) confirmed that psychodynamic psychotherapy is more effective than no treatment and appears to be just as effective when compared with other types of psychotherapy. The authors discussed various psychotherapy treatments, including cognitive-behavioral, interpersonal, psychodynamic, life review, group, and family interventions, in terms of overall efficacy, problems specific to older adults, background, and empirical support. The paucity of the current research and the need for more studies focusing on geriatric depression were emphasized in this review, as well as in a meta-analysis of pharmacological and psychological treatments for depressed older patients (Gerson et al. 1999). All data published between January 1974 and February 1998 regarding the treatment of depression in patients older than 55 were included. The authors noted that compared with the data on pharmacological treatments, those for psychological treatments (cognitive-behavioral, behavior, and psychodynamic therapies) are indeed very limited. All appear significantly better than placebo, and in the meta-analysis, response rates did not differ significantly when compared with pharmacological treatments. The authors noted, however, that direct comparison data were lacking and that no firm conclusions could be made.

One novel study on short-term psychodynamic psychotherapy for depression described its effectiveness in a naturalist setting with a hybrid effectiveness/efficacy treatment research model (Hilsenroth et al. 2003). Twenty-one patients with major depressive disorder, depressive disorder not otherwise specified, dysthymia, or adjustment disorder with depressed mood received once- or twice-weekly sessions. Unlike most previous studies, patients with comorbidities were not excluded. In addi-

tion, treatment duration was not fixed, as is the case in randomized, controlled trials, but was determined by clinician, patient, and progress in the work. All patients completed a minimum of 9 sessions, and the mean number of sessions was 30 during an average 7-month period.

DSM-IV (American Psychiatric Association 1994) depressive and global symptomatology and relational, social, and occupational functioning were assessed with clinician ratings and self-reports pre- and posttreatment. Specific measures included the DSM-IV major depressive episode symptoms, SCL-90-R-D, SCL-90-R-GSI, SCL-90-R Interpersonal Sensitivity Subscale (INT), Global Assessment of Functioning (GAF) Scale, Global Assessment of Relational Functioning (GARF), Social and Occupational Functioning Assessment Scale (SOFAS), and Global Adjustment Score of the Social Adjustment Scale (SASG). Statistically significant positive changes occurred in all areas of functioning. Depressive symptoms, as assessed by both clinicians and patients, significantly decreased pre- to posttreatment ($P<0.001$; major depressive episode effect size=2.15, $n=21$; SCL-90-R-D effect size=1.38, $n=20$). Most interestingly, a significant direct process–outcome link was observed between psychodynamic interpersonal therapeutic techniques and improvement in depressive symptoms. Specifically, results of one stepwise regression analysis showed that the mean for the Comparative Psychotherapy Process Scale: Psychodynamic-Interpersonal Process Subscale (CPPS-PI) item focusing on the therapist encouraging the patient to "experience and express emotion in the session" was significantly related to improvement in depressive symptomatology (major depressive episode symptoms) ($R=0.62$, $R^2=0.39$, $F=12.09$, $P=0.003$). A second stepwise regression analysis showed that the CPPS-PI item regarding the therapist addressing "the patient's avoidance of important topics and shifts in mood" also was significantly related to improvement on the SCL-90-R-D ($R=0.51$, $R^2=0.26$, $F=6.35$, $P=0.02$). Conversely, mean CPPS Cognitive-Behavioral Process Subscale interventions were not significant and negatively related to positive change in depressive symptoms reported on the major depressive episode symptoms and SCL-90-R-D (both $r=-0.33$, $P=0.15$). The authors acknowledged the limitations of the small sample size and mild to moderate levels of impairment. Nonetheless, the study is a first in terms of addressing effectiveness in a naturalistic setting.

More recent studies have started investigating combining psychotherapy with antidepressants in the treatment of depression. In one Dutch study, 167 outpatients with major depression were randomly assigned to receive 6-month clinical trials of antidepressants or combined therapy (de Jonghe et al. 2001). Initial antidepressant treatment was with fluoxetine, and a successive step protocol with amitriptyline and moclobemide was used for intolerance or inefficacy. Combination treatment added 16 sessions of short-term psychodynamic supportive psychotherapy. Efficacy was determined with the 17-item Ham-D in a semistructured interview by blinded independent observers; the Clinical Global Impression of Severity (CGI-S) and of Improvement (CGI-I) scales, as determined by the treating psychiatrists; and two self-rating scales, the SCL-90-R-D and the Quality of Life Depression Scale (QLDS). Statistically significant differences in success rates, consistently favoring combination therapy, were apparent at 8, 16, and 24 weeks of treatment. At 6 months, 40% of the patients taking antidepressants alone had stopped taking their medication, whereas 22% of those with combination therapy had stopped taking their medication. The mean success rate was 41% for the pharmacotherapy group and almost 60% for the combination therapy group at 24 weeks. Patients undergoing combined treatment were less likely to stop taking their medication or drop out of treatment and were therefore significantly more likely to recover.

Another study supporting the superiority of combination therapy over pharmacotherapy alone for major depression was performed by Burnand et al. (2002). In this Swiss study, 74 patients were randomly assigned to receive clomipramine-alone ($n=39$) or clomipramine and psychodynamic psychotherapy ($n=35$) treatment groups in an acute outpatient treatment setting for 10 weeks. Patients in the clomipramine-alone group received supportive care that was comparable to the amount of structured psychotherapy that the combination group received. Improvement was noted in both groups. However, patients in the combination treatment group had lower rates of treatment failure, which was defined as a major depressive episode at 10 weeks (9%, or 3 patients, compared with 28%, or 11 patients, in the clomipramine-alone group, $P=0.04$) and better work adjustment at 10 weeks (Hamilton Rating Scale for Depression Adjustment to Work subscale: 1.7 ± 0.8 compared with 2.1 ± 0.8, $P=0.04$). In addition, those in the combination treatment group appeared to have lower rates (6%, or 2 patients, vs. 23%, or 9 patients, $P=0.05$) and fewer days of hospitalization (mean$\pm$SD$=1.1\pm2.2$ vs. 3.2 ± 5.9, $P=0.04$). Short-term psychodynamic psychotherapy also proved cost-effective: cost savings of \$2,311/patient in the combined treatment group resulted from fewer lost workdays (mean savings of \$1,846/patient) and less hospitalization (mean savings of \$465/patient). For patients with prestudy stable employment, the indirect savings were even higher (\$3,394/patient). This amount exceeded the cost of providing the psychotherapy (mean total cost per patient = \$1,023: psychotherapy sessions \$570, psychoeducation \$114, psychotherapy supervision \$339).

Cost-effectiveness of short-term psychodynamic psychotherapy had been suggested in a study of 110 nonpsychotic patients who had been unresponsive to routine treatment with a mental health specialist over a 6-month period (Guthrie et al. 1999); 75.5% were found to have a depressive illness. All patients were randomly assigned to 8 weekly sessions of psychodynamic interpersonal psychotherapy or a control condition of usual care from their psychiatrist. Psychodynamic interpersonal psychotherapy was considered exploratory therapy, modeled after Hobson (1985), and was described by the authors as focusing more on the therapeutic relationship as a tool for addressing interpersonal issues rather than interpreting the transference. Usual care was defined as routine outpatient consultations of 15–30 minutes with referral options as needed (CBT, community alcohol resources, anxiety management, day hospitalization, or inpatient admission). At 6-month follow-up, those receiving therapy had significantly greater improvement than did control subjects in social functioning, as assessed by the 36-item Short-Form Health Survey Social Functioning Subscale (SF-36-SF). The mean score for the psychotherapy group was 48.9 ($n=42$) compared with 29.7 ($n=34$) for the control group ($P=0.002$). Significant improvement also occurred on measures of psychological stress (SCL-90-R-GSI and SCL-90-R-D). Mean SCL-90-R-GSI and SCL-90-R-D scores for the psychotherapy group were 1.76 and 2.16 ($n=42$, $P=0.03$), respectively, and 2.05 and 2.44 ($n=34$, $P=0.03$), respectively, for the control group. No significant differences were seen on any other SF-36 subscales (Physical Function, Physical Role Limitation, Mental Role Limitation, Mental Health, Energy and Vitality, Pain, and Health Perceptions). The psychotherapy group also showed significant reductions in health care use (inpatient days, family physician contacts, practice nurse contacts, number of prescription medications, and informal care required from relatives measured in hours per week) in the 6 months after treatment compared with control subjects. The direct treatment costs were compared with the use of geometric means. For the 3-month period prior to intervention (baseline) and the intervention phase, means were similar between groups (baseline: \$752 for the psychotherapy group, $n=55$; \$786 for the control group, $n=55$, $P=0.78$; intervention phase: \$664 for the psychotherapy group, $n=52$; \$537 for the control group, $n=51$, $P=0.29$). At 6-month follow-up, the total direct treatment and nontreatment costs were significantly lower for the psychotherapy group (\$1,006 for the psychotherapy group, $n=52$; \$1,567 for the control group, $n=49$, $P=0.04$). The total costs for the intervention phase and the 6-month follow-up period were not significantly different between the two groups ($1,959 for the psychotherapy group, $n=51$; $2,465 for the control group, $n=47$, $P=0.21$). The additional cost of the therapy was made up by the reductions in health care expenditures in 6 months.

Despite the growing number of research studies focusing on psychodynamic psychotherapy, the generalizability of results remains questionable given the variety of therapeutic subtypes termed *psychodynamic*. A recent investigation into the validity of controlled clinical trials of psychotherapy (Ablon and Jones 2002) highlighted several concerns. The authors questioned the premise that when a patient undergoing psychotherapy in a controlled clinical trial improves, the change is the result of the specific therapeutic intervention. They hypothesized that specific modalities such as brief psychodynamic therapy and CBT actually overlap in terms of applied strategies and intervention techniques. In an elegantly designed study, they enlisted expert therapists to create ideal "prototypes" of interpersonal psychotherapy and CBT regimens with the Psychotherapy Process Q-Set, an instrument designed to provide a standard language for treatment description. A separate panel of clinicians then scored actual transcripts of sessions that used both modalities, which had been conducted as part of the National Institute of Mental Health (NIMH) Treatment of Depression Collaborative Research Program, to determine to what extent the actual sessions correlated with the ideal prototypes.

The results showed that both forms of therapy sessions adhered more to the CBT prototype. Correlations between ideal psychotherapy regimens (Q-prototypes) and actual therapy administered (Q-sort ratings) were transformed into z scores, which represented the degree to which an hour of therapy correlated with the ideal regimen (CBT or interpersonal psychotherapy). In both the CBT and the interpersonal psychotherapy groups, the correlation was high between the Q-sort ratings of the session transcripts and the CBT prototype (CBT z score mean=0.64, SD=0.28, $n=29$; interpersonal psychotherapy z score mean=0.57, SD=0.24, $n=35$). The correlation with the interpersonal psychotherapy prototype was small for the CBT group (z score mean=0.18, SD=0.10) and moderate for the interpersonal psychotherapy group (z score mean=0.39, SD=0.11). The correlation with the interpersonal psychotherapy prototype was significantly higher in the interpersonal psychotherapy group compared with the CBT group ($P<0.001$), but the correlation with the CBT prototype was not significantly different between the two groups.

The authors concluded that one cannot rely on "brand names" of therapy, and they emphasized the importance of these findings to psychotherapy research. If it is not possible, even with prototypes, to control the process of psychotherapy, then legitimate conclusions cannot be made about cause and effect—a basic assumption of the controlled trial method. The authors suggested that controlled trials may be effective in comparison studies between therapy and medication or combination therapy but are dubious when studying psychotherapy alone.

Randomized, controlled studies investigating long-term psychodynamic therapy and psychoanalysis with depressed patients remain unavailable. Many clinicians recognize that a subgroup of depressed patients will require such treatment. Blatt et al. (1995) reanalyzed data from the NIMH Treatment of Depression Collaborative Research Program and found that highly perfectionistic and self-critical patients (i.e., the introjective subtype of depressed patients) did not respond well to any of the four treatment cells, which included 16 weeks of cognitive therapy, 16 weeks of interpersonal therapy, 16 weeks of imipramine plus clinical management, and 16 weeks of placebo plus clinical management. Factor analysis of the Dysfunctional Attitude Scale (DAS), which had been administered at intake, indicated that DAS Perfectionism, a self-critical factor, had significantly negative relations with all outcome measures (depression, general clinical functioning, and social adjustment) in all four treatment cells. For each of the five specific measures (BDI and Ham-D for depression, SCL-90 Total and GAF Scale for general clinical functioning, and SAS for social adjustment), higher pretreatment levels of DAS Perfectionism predicted higher levels of depression and greater impairment at termination regardless of treatment cell ($P=0.032$–0.004; BDI, Ham-D, SCL-90 Total $n=154$; GAF Scale $n=144$; SAS $n=143$).

Two naturalistic follow-up studies (Blatt 1992; Blatt et al. 1994) suggested that long-term psychodynamic therapy may be effective with the self-critical and perfectionistic patients who do not respond to brief modalities. Many of these patients probably have significant obsessive-compulsive or narcissistic characterological traits. These perfectionistic patients also may be at high risk for suicide (Blatt 1998; Hewitt et al. 1997), so the investment of time, energy, and resources may be well justified. Further research is needed to confirm this hypothesis. Although brief psychodynamic therapy is well supported by rigorous research, long-term psychoanalytic therapy awaits validation by controlled studies. Researchers face formidable challenges in designing and implementing such studies. These challenges are outlined in Table 24–2 (Gabbard et al. 2002).

TABLE 24–2. Challenges of long-term psychoanalytic psychotherapy research

Developing reliable and valid outcome measures

Convincing patients to accept random assignments

Identifying suitable control conditions

The longer the study period, the greater the risk that high dropout rate will compromise the statistical analysis

The longer the study period, the more likely that interfering life events (divorce, death of family members, serious illness) will influence outcome

May be prohibitively expensive

Therapist adherence to manualized technique

Indications and Contraindications

Thase et al. (1997) found a highly significant advantage for combining psychotherapy and medication in the more severe recurrent depressions. However, when the milder forms of depression were studied, combined therapy was not more effective than psychotherapy alone. Medication is often ineffective in minor depression, and these patients may need psychotherapy to be restored to normal functioning. In a mild depression without comorbid conditions, brief psychodynamic psychotherapy has been shown to be as effective as brief CBT (Gallagher-Thompson and Steffen 1994).

Some depressed patients will not comply with their prescribed medication for a variety of reasons, including that they feel that they do not deserve to get better or that taking medication stigmatizes them as having a mental illness. de Jonghe et al. (2001) concluded that combination treatment offered significant advantages compared with pharmacotherapy alone in patients with major depression. The patients in the combined group were significantly more compliant with medication and treatment in general and thus were more likely to recover. One major advantage to combined treatment, then, is the ability to directly address noncompliance issues in a more effective and timely manner as part of the psychotherapeutic process.

Some patients adamantly refuse to take medications, cannot take medications because of preexisting medical conditions, or cannot tolerate side effects. Psychodynamic approaches may be necessary to understand the meaning of medications and the reasons for refusal in such cases. Clinical experience has shown that some patients will accept medications after a pre-paratory phase of psychodynamic psychotherapy.

Other patients may be partially or completely refractory to any somatic treatment. Long-term psychodynamic psychotherapy may be indicated in cases of treatment failures with multiple medication trials and/or brief therapies. Clinicians assessing these patients should have a high index of suspicion for three discrete categories (Gabbard 2000): 1) Axis I major depression with Axis II comorbidity, 2) depressive personality, and 3) characterological depression in the context of personality disorders. In terms of the first category, several studies (Duggan et al. 1991; Reich and Green 1991; Shea et al. 1990) suggested that certain personality disorders may contribute to a tendency to maintain depression once it has already occurred, and characterological factors also may be responsible for poor medication compliance. Psychodynamic psychotherapy may be necessary in combination with medication to treat this population effectively.

With reference to the second category, much controversy has revolved around whether depressive personality disorder is truly distinct from dysthymia. Data suggest that the distinction between the two is valid and clinically useful (Phillips et al. 1998) and that the duration of psychotherapy is significantly longer for subjects who have depressive personality disorder than for those who do not. Dysthymic patients also may need combination treatment for optimal response. A trial of psychodynamic psychotherapy may be helpful in such cases to clarify diagnoses, define comorbidities, and promote recovery.

The third category refers primarily to patients with severe personality disorders, especially borderline, who complain of "depression" yet fail to meet DSM-IV-TR (American Psychiatric Association 2000) criteria for an Axis I disorder. These patients present unique treatment challenges for both the psychotherapist and the pharmacotherapist, and the American Psychiatric Association practice guideline (Oldham et al. 2001) recommends combined treatment.

The main indications and contraindications to psychodynamic psychotherapy for depression and dysthymia are the indications and contraindications for psychodynamic psychotherapy in general (Gabbard 2000). These are summarized in Table 24–3.

Conclusion

Psychoanalytic or psychodynamic therapy is widely used for depression and dysthymia. This modality has received less empirical support than other psychotherapies for mood disorders. However, in the last decade, more rigor-

TABLE 24–3. Indications and contraindications for psychodynamic psychotherapy

Indications	Contraindications
Strong motivation to understand	Poor motivation
Significant suffering	Tenuous ability to form therapeutic alliance
Tolerance for frustration	Low intelligence
Capacity for insight (psychological mindedness)	Lack of psychological mindedness
Intact reality testing	Poor reality testing
Ability to regress in the service of the ego	Organically based cognitive dysfunction
Meaningful object relations	
Good impulse control	
Ability to sustain a job	

ous research has begun to confirm its efficacy, especially for brief dynamic therapy. Long-term dynamic therapy is commonly used in the treatment of depression complicated by Axis II psychopathology and in cases refractory to brief treatments. Further research is needed to confirm the effectiveness of the modality for these situations.

References

Ablon JS, Jones EE: Validity of controlled clinical trials of psychotherapy: findings from the NIMH Treatment of Depression Collaborative Research Program. Am J Psychiatry 159:775–783, 2002

Abraham K: A short study of the development of the libido, viewed in light of mental disorders (1924), in Selected Papers on Psychoanalysis. London, Hogarth Press, 1927, pp 418–501

Agid O, Shapiro B, Zislan J, et al: Environment and vulnerability to major psychiatric illness: a case control study of early parental loss in major depression, bipolar disorder, and schizophrenia. Mol Psychiatry 4:163–172, 1999

American Psychiatric Association: Diagnostic and Statistical Manual of Mental Disorders, 3rd Edition. Washington, DC, American Psychiatric Association, 1980

American Psychiatric Association: Diagnostic and Statistical Manual of Mental Disorders, 4th Edition. Washington, DC, American Psychiatric Association, 1994

American Psychiatric Association: Diagnostic and Statistical Manual of Mental Disorders, 4th Edition, Text Revision. Washington, DC, American Psychiatric Association, 2000

Arieti S: Psychotherapy of severe depression. Am J Psychiatry 134:864–868, 1977

Asch SS: Suicide and the hidden executioner. Int Rev Psychoanal 7:51–60, 1980

Barkham M, Shapiro DA, Hardy GE, et al: Psychotherapy in two plus one sessions: outcomes of a randomized controlled trial of cognitive-behavioral and psychodynamic-interpersonal therapy for subsyndromal depression. J Consult Clin Psychol 67:201–211, 1999

Bernet CZ, Stein MB: Relationship in childhood maltreatment to the onsetting course of major depression in adulthood. Depress Anxiety 9:169–174, 1999

Bibring E: The mechanism of depression, in Affective Disorders: Psychoanalytic Contributions to Their Study. Edited by Greenacre P. New York, International Universities Press, 1953, pp 13–48

Bifulco A, Brown GW, Moran P, et al: Predicting depression in women: the role of past and present vulnerability. Psychol Med 28:39–50, 1998

Bifulco A, Bernazzani O, Moran P, et al: Lifetime stresses and recurrent depression: preliminary findings of the adult. Soc Psychiatry Psychiatr Epidemiol 35:264–275, 2000

Blatt SJ: The differential effect of psychotherapy and psychoanalysis with anaclitic and introjective patients: the Menninger Psychotherapy Research Project revisited. J Am Psychoanal Assoc 40:691–724, 1992

Blatt SJ: Contributions of psychoanalysis to the understanding and treatment of depression. J Am Psychoanal Assoc 46:723–752, 1998

Blatt SJ: Experiences of Depression: Theoretical, Clinical and Research Perspectives. Washington, DC, American Psychological Association, 2004

Blatt SJ, Ford R, Berman WH, et al: Therapeutic Change: An Object Relations Perspective. New York, Plenum, 1994

Blatt SJ, Quinlan DM, Pilkonis PA, et al: Impact of perfectionism and the need for approval in the brief treatment of depression: the National Institute of Mental Health Treatment of Depression Collaborative Research Program revisited. J Consult Clin Psychol 63:125–132, 1995

Bowlby J: Attachment and Loss, Vol 1: Attachment. New York, Basic Books, 1969

Brodsky BS, Oqendo M, Ellis SP, et al: The relationship of childhood abuse to impulsivity and suicidal behavior in adults with major depression. Am J Psychiatry 158:1871–1877, 2001

Brown G: Life events and affective disorder: replications and limitations. Psychosom Med 55:248–259, 1993

Brown G, Eales M: Etiology of anxiety and depressive disorders in an inner-city population. Psychol Med 23:155–165, 1993

Burnand Y, Andreoli A, Kolatte E, et al: Psychodynamic psychotherapy and clomipramine in the treatment of depression. Psychiatr Serv 53:585–590, 2002

Busch FN, Rudden M, Shapiro T: Psychodynamic Treatment of Depression. Arlington, VA, American Psychiatric Publishing, 2004

Caspi A, Sugden K, Moffitt TE, et al: Influence of life stress on depression: moderation by a polymorphism in the 5-HTT gene. Science 301:386–389, 2003

Cooper PJ, Murray L, Wilson A, et al: Controlled trial of the short- and long-term effect of psychological treatment of post-partum depression, I: impact on maternal mood. Br J Psychiatry 182:412–419, 2003

Davidson JRT, Hughes D, George LK, et al: The association of sexual assault and attempted suicide within the community. Arch Gen Psychiatry 53:550–555, 1996

de Jonghe F, Kool S, van Aalst G, et al: Combining psychotherapy and antidepressants in the treatment of depression. J Affect Disord 64:217–229, 2001

Dorpat TL: Suicide, loss, and mourning. Suicide Life Threat Behav 3:213–224, 1973

Duggan CF, Lee AS, Murray RM: Do different subtypes of hospitalized depressives have different long-term outcomes? Arch Gen Psychiatry 48:308–312, 1991

Freud S: Mourning and melancholia (1917), in The Standard Edition of the Complete Psychological Works of Sigmund Freud, Vol 14. Translated and edited by Strachey J. London, Hogarth Press, 1963, pp 237–260

Freud S: The ego and the id (1923), in The Standard Edition of the Complete Psychological Works of Sigmund Freud, Vol 19. Translated and edited by Strachey J. London, Hogarth Press, 1961, pp 1–66

Gabbard GO: Psychodynamic Psychotherapy in Clinical Practice, 3rd Edition. Washington, DC, American Psychiatric Press, 2000

Gabbard G, Kay J: The fate of integrated treatment: whatever happened to the biopsychosocial psychiatrist? Am J Psychiatry 158:1956–1963, 2001

Gabbard G, Westen D: Rethinking therapeutic action. Int J Psychoanal 84:823–841, 2003

Gabbard G, Gunderson J, Fonagy P: The place of psychoanalytic treatments within psychiatry. Arch Gen Psychiatry 59:505–510, 2002

Gallagher-Thompson D, Steffen AM: Comparative effects of cognitive-behavioral and brief psychodynamic psychotherapies for depressed family caregivers. J Consult Clin Psychol 62:543–549, 1994

Gerson S, Belin TR, Kaufman A, et al: Pharmacological and psychological treatments for depressed older patients: a meta-analysis and overview of recent findings. Harv Rev Psychiatry 7:1–28, 1999

Gilman SE, Kawachi I, Fitzmaurice GM, et al: Family disruption in childhood and risk of adult depression. Am J Psychiatry 160:939–946, 2003

Gunderson JG, Gabbard GO: Making the case for psychoanalytic therapies in the current psychiatric environment. J Am Psychoanal Assoc 47:679–704, 1999

Guthrie E, Moorey J, Margison F, et al: Cost-effectiveness of brief psychodynamic-interpersonal therapy in high utilizers of psychiatric services. Arch Gen Psychiatry 56:519–526, 1999

Guthrie E, Kapur N, Mackway-Jones K, et al: Randomised controlled trial of brief psychological intervention after deliberate self poisoning. BMJ 323:135–137, 2001

Hammen CL: Stress and the course of unipolar and bipolar disorders, in Does Stress Cause Psychiatric Illness? Edited by Mazure CM. Washington, DC, American Psychiatric Press, 1995, pp 87–110

Hammen C, Marks T, Mayol A, et al: Depressive self-schemas, life stress, and vulnerability to depression. J Abnorm Psychol 94:308–319, 1985

Hammen C, Henry R, Daley S: Depression and sensitization to stressors among young women as a function of childhood adversity. J Consult Clin Psychol 68:782–787, 2000

Hayden ED, Klein DM: Outcome of dysthymic disorder at five-year followup: the effect of familial psychopathology, early adversity, personality, comorbidity, and chronic stress. Am J Psychiatry 158:1864–1870, 2001

Hayes AM, Castonguay LG, Goldfried MR: Effectiveness of targeting vulnerability factors of depression in cognitive therapy. J Consult Clin Psychol 64:623–627, 1996

Heim C, Newport DJ, Heit S, et al: Pituitary-adrenal and autonomic responses to stress in women after sexual and physical abuse in childhood. JAMA 284:592–597, 2000

Hewitt PL, Newton J, Fett GL, et al: Perfectionism and suicide ideation in adolescent psychiatric patients. J Abnorm Child Psychol 25:95–101, 1997

Hilsenroth MJ, Ackerman SJ, Blagys MD, et al: Short-term psychodynamic psychotherapy for depression: an examination of statistical, clinically significant, and technique-specific change. J Nerv Ment Dis 191:349–357, 2003

Hobson RF: Forms of Feeling: The Heart of Psychotherapy. New York, Basic Books, 1985

Jacobson E: Transference problems in depressives, in Depression: Comparative Studies of Normal, Neurotic, and Psychotic Conditions. Edited by Jacobson E. New York, International Universities Press, 1971, pp 242–263

Jones EE, Pulos SM: Comparing the process of psychodynamic and cognitive behavioral therapies. J Consult Clin Psychol 61:306–316, 1993

Karel MJ, Hinrichsen G: Treatment of depression in late life: psychotherapeutic interventions. Clin Psychol Rev 20:707–729, 2000

Keller MB, Shapiro RW: Double depression: superimposition of acute depressive episodes on chronic depressive disorders. Am J Psychiatry 139:438–442, 1982

Kendler KS, Neale MC, Kessler RC, et al: Childhood parental loss and adult psychopathology in women: a twin study perspective. Arch Gen Psychiatry 49:109–116, 1992

Kendler KS, Kessler RC, Walters EE, et al: Stressful life events, genetic liability, and onset of an episode of major depression in women. Am J Psychiatry 152:833–842, 1995

Kendler KS, Karkowski LM, Prescott CA: Causal relationship between stressful life events and the onset of major depression. Am J Psychiatry 156:837–841, 1999

Kendler KS, Thornton LM, Prescott CA: Gender differences in the rates of exposure to stressful life events and sensitivity to their depressogenic effects. Am J Psychiatry 158:587–593, 2001

Kendler KS, Hettema JM, Butera F, et al: Life event dimensions of loss, humiliation, entrapment, and danger in the prediction of onsets of major depression and generalized anxiety. Arch Gen Psychiatry 60:789–796, 2003

Klein DN, Schwartz JE, Rose S, et al: Five-year course and outcome of dysthymic disorder: a prospective naturalistic follow-up study. Am J Psychiatry 157:931–939, 2000

Klein M: Mourning and its relation to manic-depressive states (1940), in Love, Guilt and Reparation and Other Works 1921–1945. New York, Free Press, 1975, pp 344–369

Kwon P: Attributional style and psychodynamic defense mechanisms: toward an integrative model of depression. J Pers 67:645–658, 1999

Kwon P, Lemmon KE: Attributional style and defense mechanisms: a synthesis of cognitive and psychodynamic factors in depression. J Clin Psychol 56:723–735, 2000

Leichsenring F: Comparative effects of short-term psychodynamic psychotherapy and cognitive-behavioral therapy in depression: a meta-analytic approach. Clin Psychol Rev 21:401–419, 2001

Luborsky L: Principles of Psychoanalytic Psychotherapy: A Manual for Supportive Expressive Treatment. New York, Basic Books, 1984

McHolm AE, MacMillan HL, Jamieson E: The relationship between childhood physical abuse and suicidality among depressed women: results from a community sample. Am J Psychiatry 160:933–938, 2003

Meissner WW: Psychotherapy and the Paranoid Process. Northvale, NJ, Jason Aronson, 1986

Nemeroff C: The neurobiology of depression. Sci Am 278:42–49, 1998a

Nemeroff C: The pre-eminent role of early untoward experience on vulnerability to major psychiatric disorders: the nature-nurture controversy revisited and soon to be resolved. Mol Psychiatry 4:106–108, 1999

Oldham JM, Phillips KA, Gabbard GO, et al: Practice Guideline for the Treatment of Patients With Borderline Personality Disorder. Washington, DC, American Psychiatric Association, 2001

Phillips KA, Gunderson JG, Triebwasser J, et al: Reliability and validity of depressive personality disorder. Am J Psychiatry 155:1044–1048, 1998

Reich JH, Green AI: Effect of personality disorders on outcome of treatment. J Nerv Ment Dis 179:74–82, 1991

Sandler J, Joffe WG: Notes on childhood depression. Int J Psychoanal 46:88–96, 1965

Shapiro DA, Barkham M, Rees A, et al: Effects of treatment duration and severity of depression on the effectiveness of cognitive-behavioral and psychodynamic-interpersonal psychotherapy. J Consult Clin Psychol 62:522–534, 1994

Shapiro DA, Barkham M, Rees A, et al: Effects of treatment duration and severity of depression on the maintenance of gains after cognitive-behavioral and psychodynamic interpersonal psychotherapy. J Consult Clin Psychol 63:378–387, 1995

Shea MT, Pilkonis PA, Beckham E, et al: Personality disorders and treatment outcome in the NIMH Treatment of Depression Collaborative Research Program. Am J Psychiatry 147:711–718, 1990

Thase ME, Greenhouse JB, Frank E, et al: Treatment of major depression with psychotherapy or psychotherapy-pharmacotherapy combinations. Arch Gen Psychiatry 54:1009–1015, 1997

Vaillant GE, Vaillant CA: A cross-validation of two methods of investigating defenses, in Ego Mechanisms of Defense: A Guide for Clinicians and Researchers. Edited by Vaillant GE. Washington, DC, American Psychiatric Press, 1992, pp 159–170

Vythilingam M, Heim C, Newport J, et al: Childhood trauma associated with smaller hippocampal volume in women with major depression. Am J Psychiatry 159:2072–2080, 2002

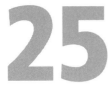

Psychotherapy for Bipolar Disorder

HOLLY A. SWARTZ, M.D.

ELLEN FRANK, PH.D.

DAVID J. KUPFER, M.D.

OF THE SERIOUS psychiatric conditions, bipolar disorder has long been considered among the most "biological." Driven by the apparent absence of an overt connection between manifestations of its psychopathology and antecedent psychological stressors, as well as the strong likelihood of a genetic etiology, clinical researchers have historically regarded bipolar disorder as a medical condition amenable only to somatic interventions. The introduction of lithium carbonate in 1949 (Cade 1949) to treat bipolar disorder and its early success in clinical trials reinforced the notion that this disorder could be managed with medication alone. Positive experiences with major and minor tranquilizers led further credence to this approach. The established efficacy of pharmacotherapy coupled with an absence of data on bipolar-specific psychosocial interventions further encouraged psychiatrists to rely primarily on medications to treat this illness. This cycle has been perpetuated because most of the progress

in the treatment of bipolar disorder during the latter half of the twentieth century rested on advances in psychopharmacological, rather than psychosocial, interventions.

If one considers the major symptom domains of bipolar I disorder, it is not surprising that psychosocial interventions were largely overlooked by researchers as tools for managing this disorder. As shown in Figure 25–1, the symptoms of bipolar disorder can be divided into four domains: 1) manic mood and associated behaviors, 2) psychotic symptoms, 3) dysphoric or negative mood and associated behaviors, and 4) cognitive symptoms (a set of symptoms that has only recently been recognized as a separate domain that may require specific treatment) (Sweeney et al. 2000; Tavares et al. 2003). It seems, at first glance, that psychotherapy is unlikely to have much of an effect on these symptoms. For instance, manic mood and its associated behaviors and psychotic symptoms appear to be driven "internally" and are therefore unlikely to

Supported in part by National Institute of Mental Health grants MH30915, MH29618, and MH64518. The authors also would like to thank John Scott, A.M., for his statistical assistance.

respond to a behavioral or psychological intervention. Similarly, the cognitive symptoms endemic to bipolar disorder, such as distractibility and rapid thoughts, specifically interfere with processing of information and are therefore very unlikely to resolve with a "talking" intervention. Although dysphoric mood and its associated behaviors overlap considerably with nonbipolar depressive states, and psychosocial interventions have been shown to play an important role in the management of these syndromes, antidepressant medications are clearly central to the treatment of depression. Thus, pharmacology is the mainstay of treatment for all four domains of bipolar symptomatology. If medications are so important to the management of this illness, what, then, is the role of psychotherapy in treating bipolar disorder?

Historical Perspective

Although rarely the focus of systematic inquiry, psychotherapy was routinely offered throughout the twentieth century to patients who had bipolar disorder. As pharmacotherapy ascended to the forefront of bipolar illness management, psychotherapy continued to be provided to individuals with bipolar spectrum disorder. Most of these treatments were based on the prevailing psychotherapeutic paradigm of the era (i.e., psychoanalysis). Not surprisingly, psychoanalysis had little to offer manic patients who, by definition, have marked impairments in insight. Although psychotherapy played a greater role in the management of bipolar depression and bipolar spectrum disorder, early practitioners of psychotherapy for bipolar disorder concluded that "[w]hereas it appeared to work with the schizophrenic, it was not generally successful with the manic-depressive" (Fromm-Reichmann 1949, p. 158). These treatment failures further reinforced the concept that bipolar disorder was best treated primarily—if not exclusively—with pharmacotherapy.

In the latter part of the twentieth century, clinicians began using psychodynamic techniques to explore not only the manic-depressive character but also the psychological consequences of the illness. These treatments are reviewed in the comprehensive monograph *Manic-Depressive Illness* by Goodwin and Jamison (1990). In their chapter on psychotherapy, they suggest that rather than serving as a tool for symptom management, psychotherapy is typically used to help individuals adjust to the long-term sequelae of bipolar (manic-depressive) illness. Although they argue that this approach is very helpful to patients, they acknowledge that few data are available to support their assertion. Before 1990, psychotherapy fo-

cused on the following issues: anger, denial and ambivalence surrounding both the illness and its treatment, disappointments associated with less than complete treatment success, frustrations associated with lithium treatment, fears of recurrence, the dilemma of distinguishing between abnormal and normal moods, developmental tasks that may have been delayed because of psychiatric morbidity, problems with family and relationships, and concerns about the heritability of the disease. Following their exhaustive review of the literature, Goodwin and Jamison concluded—based on many anecdotes and scant research data—that manic-depressive disease should be treated with a combination of lithium or other medications and adjunctive psychotherapy. They could not systematically review controlled trials of targeted, specific psychotherapies for bipolar disorder because at the time their landmark book was written, none of these studies had been conducted.

Unlike the psychodynamic therapies of the previous decades that focused on intrapsychic conflicts and acquisition of insight, contemporary bipolar-specific psychotherapies use more directive and symptom-focused strategies, such as encouragement of medication adherence, provision of psychoeducation, involvement of family members, development of strategies for relapse prevention, exploration of the reciprocal relation between mood and either cognitions or interpersonal relationships, and establishment of regular sleep-wake cycles. Virtually all of these approaches can be traced to earlier psychotherapies for patients with major psychiatric disorders, such as work conducted with patients who have schizophrenia and other psychotic disorders or treatments developed for unipolar depression. Many "new" psychosocial interventions for bipolar disorder borrow from therapies developed for patients with schizophrenia, appropriating techniques such as provision of psychoeducation and intervention with family members (Anderson et al. 1980; Hogarty 2002; Pitschel-Walz et al. 2001). The best developed family therapy for bipolar disorder, family-focused therapy (Miklowitz et al. 2000), was specifically modeled on family interventions for schizophrenia developed by Michael Goldstein and colleagues at University of California–Los Angeles (Goldstein and Miklowitz 1995). The work of Aaron Beck and colleagues (1979) in cognitive psychotherapy for unipolar depression and that of Klerman and colleagues (1984) in interpersonal psychotherapy (IPT) for unipolar depression were both adapted and modified to address the symptoms (especially depressive symptoms) of bipolar disorder.

Regulation of sleep-wake cycles and daily routines is perhaps the single therapeutic approach to bipolar disorder that did *not* evolve from an earlier psychotherapy.

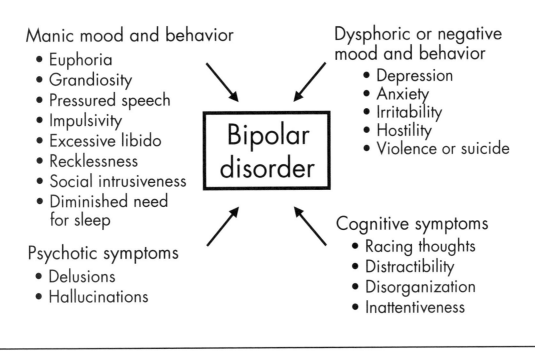

Manic mood and behavior
- Euphoria
- Grandiosity
- Pressured speech
- Impulsivity
- Excessive libido
- Recklessness
- Social intrusiveness
- Diminished need for sleep

Psychotic symptoms
- Delusions
- Hallucinations

Dysphoric or negative mood and behavior
- Depression
- Anxiety
- Irritability
- Hostility
- Violence or suicide

Cognitive symptoms
- Racing thoughts
- Distractibility
- Disorganization
- Inattentiveness

Bipolar disorder

FIGURE 25–1. **Symptom domains of bipolar disorder.**
Source. Reprinted from Perry A, Tarrier N, Morriss R, et al: "Randomised Controlled Trial of Efficacy of Teaching Patients With Bipolar Disorder to Identify Early Symptoms of Relapse and Obtain Treatment." *British Medical Journal* 318:149–153, 1999. Used with permission.

This approach was originally developed by Frank and colleagues (2000) at the University of Pittsburgh as a component of an interpersonally focused psychotherapy for bipolar disorder but has been integrated into several other bipolar-specific psychotherapies as well. Although some clinical trials testing these bipolar-specific psychotherapies have been completed or are under way, few of these evidence-based psychotherapies are available in nonresearch clinical settings.

Limitations in Establishing Efficacy of Psychosocial Treatments for Bipolar Disorder

Why, until recently, have there been so few formal psychotherapy trials for bipolar disorder? Several factors make it difficult to conduct psychotherapy studies in patients with bipolar disorder, in turn making it difficult to establish evidence-based guidelines for patient care. Some of these factors are logistical issues (such as previous long lengths of stay in an inpatient setting), and others represent methodological or conceptual challenges (such as the absence of well-defined end points for clinical trials in bipolar disorder). We discuss these issues below.

Duration of Hospitalization

Before 1990, psychiatric patients were usually hospitalized for long periods; in the current era, acute hospitalizations are too brief to permit initiation of a psychotherapy trial (for a notable exception, see Clarkin et al. 1990). The symptoms that lead to hospitalization are typically mania and psychosis—manifestations of the illness that are best managed with medications rather than psychotherapy. Hospitalization is not the optimal setting in which to study an intervention designed to help patients and their families cope with the multiple challenges of having a chronic illness, such as enduring impairments in functioning, ongoing cycling of mood states, and risk of recurrence. Furthermore, although treatment adherence typically emerges as a major treatment issue after discharge, it is less commonly encountered within the carefully monitored setting of an inpatient unit. Finally, while patients are still struggling to recover from an acute episode, it is difficult to implement psychotherapeutic techniques designed to help them identify specific early warning signs of the next depressive or manic episode.

Appropriate Outcomes

To establish treatment efficacy of either pharmacotherapy or psychotherapy, it is imperative that the investigator specify an appropriate outcome or end point. In bipolar disorder, is the appropriate outcome improvement in depression symptoms? Absence of manic symptoms? A symptom-free interval of 2 months? Two years? Return to previous level of functioning? Defining appropriate outcomes in bipolar disorder is complicated by the fact that this disease is a "moving target," with the absence of one set of symptoms being necessary but not sufficient to establish clinical improvement. Because the specification of outcome measures is much more complicated in bipolar disorder than in unipolar disorder, studies are more difficult to conduct and interpret. In addition, psychotherapy interventions are likely to affect domains of function beyond mood and neurovegetative symptoms. Changes in quality of relationships, self-confidence, and vocational performance are difficult to measure yet may be important outcomes for psychotherapy studies. These issues have significantly limited the number of research studies—especially psychotherapy studies—conducted with individuals who have bipolar disorder.

Role of Placebo

The optimal strategy for establishing efficacy of a new treatment is to show a statistically significant (and clinically meaningful) effect relative to placebo. In pharmacotherapy trials for bipolar disorder, few placebo-controlled studies have been done aside from those required by the U.S. Food and Drug Administration to register compounds for the acute mania indication. Given the very destructive nature of bipolar symptoms and low likelihood of placebo response, many have questioned the ethics of conducting these placebo-controlled studies in individuals with bipolar disorder. In the acute phase of bipolar disorder, it is possible to design both ethical and scientifically sound placebo-controlled clinical trials that use prespecified exit criteria that serve as both data end points (outcomes) and a safety valve for individuals who do not respond to or tolerate the compound (Frank et al. 2001). In the maintenance phase of the illness, however, it is much more difficult to envision a truly ethical, placebo-controlled clinical trial: the long study duration that is required to show efficacy of prophylaxis would require that the investigator expose an individual with documented bipolar disorder to an inactive compound for many months or even years, with the attendant high likelihood of subjecting previously euthymic patients to a new and debilitating episode of depression or mania. Yet in the absence of placebo-controlled trials, it is very difficult to establish the efficacy of new compounds or interventions that prevent episode recurrence.

With respect to psychotherapy, the issue of what constitutes a placebo is even more complicated than in pharmacotherapy trials. There is little consensus within the field on the definition of an appropriate control condition for psychotherapy studies. Among studies that have been conducted to establish the efficacy of a targeted psychotherapy (in bipolar disorder and other disorders), investigators have used a wide range of control conditions, varying from almost no treatment to very active treatments that include many nonspecific psychotherapeutic elements, such as support and empathy. Although one study may show an apparently large effect relative to a very inactive control (such as a waiting list), another study may seem to have little effect because the comparison condition is very active and includes many of the nonspecific elements of good bipolar disease management. This presents challenges to clinicians and policy-makers attempting to interpret these findings: an apparently weak treatment effect may be driven not by the treatment itself but by the relatively robust effects of the comparator condition.

The challenge in conducting long-term prevention studies in bipolar disorder is even greater than the challenges associated with acute treatment studies. In maintenance studies, if the control condition is not associated with at least a 50% recurrence rate within a year of treatment, then it is very difficult to generate enough power in the study (i.e., enroll enough subjects) to detect a significant signal from the active condition. Thus, a "weak" control condition will allow the investigator to more easily establish that a treatment works—but raises both ethical issues and the question of its working in comparison to a substandard comparison intervention.

Phase-Specific Treatment Effects

Some interventions for bipolar disorder—whether pharmacological or psychotherapeutic—may be efficacious for only one pole or one phase of the disorder. For instance, a compound that is extremely useful for acute mania may fail to prevent future episodes of mania or depression; a compound that is effective for acute depression may not only fail to treat mania but also induce mania under certain circumstances. In a similar way, the psychotherapeutic approaches may have acute effects, mania-specific effects, depression-specific effects, prophylactic effects, or a combination thereof. Investigators are faced with the difficult task of defining what their "target pole" will be and designing studies to appropriately measure these effects.

To complicate matters further, some psychotherapies are intended for acutely ill patients, some are for patients in remission, and still others accommodate patients who are *either* symptomatic or in remission. It is difficult to compare across trials on end points such as manic symptoms and time to recurrence when some studies enroll patients who are in an episode, whereas others require that patients be out of an episode for a specified time before entering the trial. To our knowledge, no study has yet been designed to evaluate the optimal time(s) in the course of illness to initiate psychotherapy, and existing data shed little light on this issue.

Combining Medication and Psychotherapy

Unlike the treatment of unipolar depression, for which successful trials have been conducted of psychotherapy alone, psychotherapy trials in bipolar I disorder will always involve pharmacotherapy as well as psychotherapy. Therefore, all clinical trials must be designed so that the investigator can analyze effectively the effects of combination treatments, augmentation strategies, or sequenced treatments. The complexity of these designs generally requires the investigator to enroll very large numbers of subjects in order to disentangle the effects of each modality. Although multisite studies may permit enrollment of adequate numbers of subjects to resolve these issues, it is especially difficult to ensure integrity of therapist training and reliability of psychotherapy quality when multiple sites are involved. Because a considerable amount of heterogeneity in treatment sites with respect to psychotherapy treatment in depression has been reported (Elkin et al. 1989), one would expect similar, if not greater, difficulties in conducting these trials in bipolar disorder.

The large, multisite National Institute of Mental Health project Systematic Treatment Enhancement Program (STEP) for Bipolar Disorder is currently evaluating three different psychotherapies (Sachs et al. 2003). To date, the three therapy modalities appear to have been delivered reliably at each of the sites—although it requires considerable persistence and effort to maintain these standards (G.S. Sachs, personal communication, December 2003).

Relevant Statistical Models to Capture the Variability in Bipolar Illness

Because of the inherent variability in the illness itself, outcomes in clinical trials of bipolar disorder are strongly influenced by underlying "normal" fluctuations in mood. In psychotherapy studies, trials are further confounded by the overlapping effects of concurrently administered medication and psychotherapy. Thus, to detect psychotherapy effects over time, investigators are likely to rely on the application of sophisticated statistical models to elucidate significant trends within complex data sets.

A recent review outlined the limitations of some of the statistical methods commonly used to evaluate data sets

from bipolar disorder trials (Hennen 2003). The author noted that studies of patients with bipolar disorder are associated with many nonrandom missing observations, time-varying outcomes, and a high degree of intraindividual variability and instability. To account for these sample characteristics, Hennen argued that investigators should 1) design longitudinal (rather than cross-sectional) studies to capture fluctuations in illness course over time, 2) use continuous (rather than binary) outcome measures to capture variability over time, 3) minimize missing data, and 4) enroll enough subjects in trials to compensate for low signal-to-noise ratios. He further suggested that relevant data analytical methods should tolerate a relatively high percentage of missing data, use all available data points (rather than end points only), and adjust for baseline severity levels. Methods favored by Hennen include time-to-event (survival analysis) modeling, random effects, generalized estimated equation regression modeling, and analysis of variance with repeated measures.

Post and Luckenbaugh (2003) argued that novel study designs—rather than conventional parallel-group randomized, controlled trials—may be better suited to elucidating treatment effects in bipolar disorder. They suggested that crossover trial designs may address some of the difficulties associated with the study of bipolar disorder because each subject acts as his or her own control. Although this approach may raise some special problematic issues in psychotherapy trials (see Frank et al. 1999), it also may help to reduce the number of subjects required per study. They suggested several novel analytical approaches to examining data generated by crossover design studies, including 1) ratio of number of episodes to observed trial length, 2) ratio of euthymic to noneuthymic days, 3) standard deviation of episode duration or of euthymic interval, and 4) sequential probability ratio test, which models confidence intervals for expected changes from the baseline mean value and stops the trial when the cumulative sum of observations exceeds the expected level of change. They also acknowledged that polypharmacy is the current norm in the management of bipolar disorder (Post et al. 2003) and that statistical methods used by oncologists to compare complex chemotherapy combination regimens may offer psychiatrists a model by which to evaluate the complex regimens currently prescribed for patients with bipolar disorder.

Moving to the Present Era: New Challenges

In the past two decades, there has been a radical shift in the way we conceptualize the major challenges associated with the management of bipolar disorder. Through the 1980s, researchers focused on improving pharmacological treatments for the acute phase of bipolar disorder, specifically manic symptoms. It has become apparent, however, that the biggest challenges in treating bipolar disorder are not acute illness and mania (which are very disruptive but can be brought under control relatively quickly) but rather chronic depressive symptoms (Post et al. 2003), failure to recover function despite symptomatic improvement (Goldberg et al. 1995), and prevention of subsequent episodes in this highly recurrent disorder (Sachs and Rush 2003). Multiple episodes—especially depressive episodes—predict poor long-term outcomes (Post et al. 2003); thus, a primary treatment goal must be episode prevention.

In addition to the challenge of preventing episodes over time, it is now clear that the predominant dysfunctional mood state in bipolar disorder is depression, not mania (Judd et al. 2002), and subsyndromal depressive symptoms that persist over time are proving to be an especially problematic feature of bipolar disease. These subacute depressive syndromes are clearly associated with decreased vocational and interpersonal functioning (Coryell et al. 1993) and may represent a risk for subsequent syndromal episodes (Bauwens et al. 1991; Gitlin et al. 1995). Finally, recovery from acute episodes is not necessarily associated with functional improvement (Tohen et al. 2000), suggesting that symptom control alone may not suffice for many patients.

Thus, contemporary treatments for bipolar disorders must address the problems of chronic depressive symptoms, failure to recover function despite symptom improvement, and the high risk of recurrence over time (Sachs and Rush 2003). As pharmacotherapeutic options have grown more plentiful, their limitations in these areas also have grown more apparent. It seems increasingly likely that bipolar-specific psychotherapy, in combination with medication, will play an important role in addressing these lacunae in our current treatment armamentarium, and the efficacy of bipolar-specific psychotherapies should be assessed in these domains.

Approach by Levels of Intensity (Review of Current Studies)

In a prior review of the existing literature on psychotherapy for bipolar disorder, we found a paucity of randomized, controlled clinical trials, most of which were conducted in the latter part of the 1990s (Swartz and Frank 2001). Most of the earlier reports consisted of case studies

or results from trials that used relatively weak study designs (i.e., matched case–control studies or retrospective reviews). Fortunately, in the past 10 years, there has been a large increase in the number of randomized, controlled clinical trials that have used manual-based psychotherapies for bipolar disorder (Zaretsky 2003). These trials have been conducted in the United Kingdom, Spain, and the United States and include interventions of varying intensity and duration. Psychotherapies that have been tested in randomized, controlled trials include psychoeducation, cognitive-behavioral psychotherapy, marital and family therapy, and IPT administered in conjunction with social rhythm therapy.

We have previously discussed the fact that several common strategies are used across these bipolar-specific psychotherapies, including education about the illness and medications, a careful review of medication side effects, the promotion (to varying degrees) of regular sleep-wake cycles, daily monitoring of mood states, relapse prevention (again, to varying degrees), and involvement of family members or significant others. Despite these common factors, outcomes among these trials appear variable; studies report differential effects on bipolar-specific end points such as acute mania, acute depression, depressive recurrences, and manic recurrences. As reviewed later in this chapter, psychotherapies that differ in level of intensity and nature of the intervention also may differ in their effect on the illness. Table 25–1 summarizes the calculated effect size of each intervention and the targeted outcome of each trial. Virtually all of these trials reported a small to medium effect size. It should be underscored, however, that these trials differed in clinical end points and control conditions; therefore, effect sizes are not necessarily comparable across trials.

Psychoeducation

Perry et al. (1999) tested a 7- to 12-session individual psychotherapy that focused on psychoeducation. They enrolled a group of remitted patients with the aim of teaching them to recognize early symptoms of relapse and the value of seeking treatment to prevent the episode. The treatment was administered by "a research psychologist with little previous clinical experience" (p. 150). The primary end point of this study was time to manic relapse. Time to manic relapse was significantly different in the experimental treatment compared with a control group that did not receive the individual treatment sessions (see Figure 25–2). Of the control group, 46% had a manic relapse within 12 months compared with 18% of the experimental group. Additional analyses found no significant difference in time to first depressive relapse or the

TABLE 25–1.   Effect sizes of psychosocial treatments

Psychotherapy	Outcome/end point	Effect size (Cohen's *d* or *w*)[a]	Number needed to treat[b]
Psychoeducation (Perry et al. 1999)	Manic relapse	0.30	4
Psychoeducation (Perry et al. 1999)	Depressive relapse	0.16	—
Psychoeducation (Colom et al. 2003)	Relapse during treatment phase	0.22	5
Psychoeducation (Colom et al. 2003)	Relapse during 2-year follow-up phase	0.32	4
Care management (Simon et al. 2005)	Number of weeks with manic symptoms	0.14	—
Cognitive therapy (Lam et al. 2003)	Relapse or recurrence (over 1 year)	0.32	4
Cognitive therapy (Scott et al. 2001)	Relapse or recurrence (over 18 months)	0.45	3
Family therapy (Miklowitz et al. 2003)	Relapse or recurrence (over 2 years)	0.17	6

[a]Effect size of less than 0.20 is considered small; 0.2–0.5 is considered moderate; greater than 0.5 is considered large (Cohen 1988).

[b]Number needed to treat refers to the number of patients who would need to be treated in order to prevent one adverse outcome (Gordis 2000).

number of depressive relapses. Of the control group, 31% experienced a new depressive episode within 12 months compared with 48% of the experimental group, although this difference was not statistically significant. Interestingly, the authors reported that teaching patients to recognize prodromes and seek early treatment also resulted in improvement in their social function and performance in employment.

Colom and colleagues (2003) in Barcelona, Spain, recently completed a randomized, controlled trial comparing 21 sessions of group psychoeducation with 21 sessions of unstructured group meetings (in addition to standard pharmacotherapy) to prevent recurrence in subjects with a 6-month history of remission from bipolar disorder (see Figure 25–3). The 120 euthymic bipolar I and II outpatients were randomly assigned to one of the two study conditions, treated for 20 weeks, and followed up for 2 years. The authors concluded that group psychoeducation represented an efficacious intervention and significantly reduced the number of recurrences. During the treatment phase, 60% of the control group had a recurrence compared with 38% of the psychoeducation group (*P*=0.05). At the end of the follow-up phase 2 years later, 92% of the control group had had a recurrence compared with 67% of the psychoeducation group (*P*<0.001). The individuals assigned to group psychoeducation had a significant reduction in the total number of recurrences, number of depressive recurrences, and number of hypomanic episodes but no overall difference in the number of manic episodes compared with the control group.

Two other major studies emphasize education and dis-

ease management without use of a specific psychotherapeutic approach. The multisite VA [U.S. Department of Veterans Affairs] Cooperative Study conducted by Bauer and colleagues (2001) will compare an easy-access treatment program with usual VA care. The study has not yet been completed, and results are not yet available. Simon and colleagues (2002) conducted a population-based care program for more than 400 patients with bipolar disorder (I and II) in four behavioral health clinics in a group-model managed care organization during a 3-year period. Individuals were randomly assigned to continue usual care or to receive usual care plus a systematic care management program. The systematic care management program included assessment and care planning; monthly telephone monitoring, which included a brief review of symptoms and medication monitoring; feedback and coordination with the mental health treatment team; and a structured group psychoeducational program, all of which were provided by a nurse care manager (Simon et al. 2002). This intervention was provided in addition to usual mental health treatment with psychopharmacologists and psychotherapists. In a report of the first 12 months of follow-up, primary outcomes included depression and mania symptom scores averaged over time. Over 12 months, participants in the intervention group had lower mean mania ratings. In addition, patients assigned to the intervention group spent approximately 1.7 weeks in a manic or hypomanic episode compared with 2.6 weeks for the control group. Interestingly, the depression ratings did not differ significantly between the two groups over 12 months, but depression scores showed

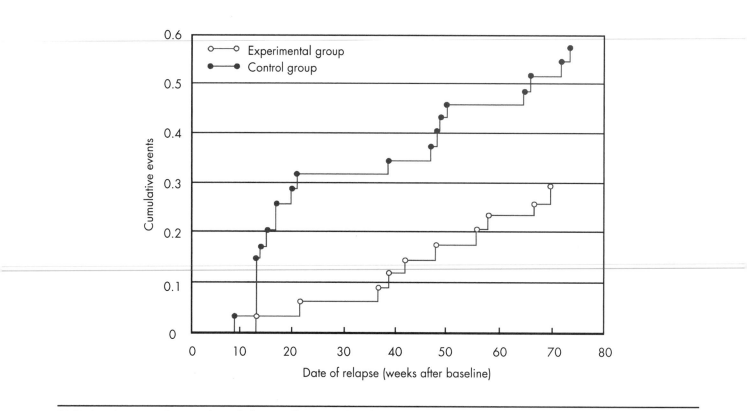

FIGURE 25–2. **Event plot of time to first manic relapse in experimental and control groups.**

Source. Reprinted from Perry A, Tarrier N, Morriss R, et al: "Randomised Controlled Trial of Efficacy of Teaching Patients With Bipolar Disorder to Identify Early Symptoms of Relapse and Obtain Treatment." *British Medical Journal* 318:149–153, 1999. Used with permission from the BMJ Publishing Group.

a larger decline over time in the intervention group compared with those assigned to usual care (Simon et al. 2005). In this study, patients were in a wide range of mood states at time of enrollment; therefore, it is difficult to evaluate rates of relapse in this group and also to compare this study with others that use recurrence as a primary end point.

Cognitive-Behavioral Therapy

The next group of studies tested various models of cognitive and behavior therapy for bipolar disorder. Most of these interventions, in addition to the common bipolar strategies discussed earlier, use daily mood diaries, focus on the automatic negative thoughts associated with the illness, and use cognitive strategies to address barriers to treatment adherence. Pilot studies conducted by Scott (2001) provided initial evidence suggesting that cognitive therapy may be useful for the management of bipolar disorder, and two subsequent randomized, controlled trials have been published confirming the utility of this approach.

Lam and colleagues (2003) randomly assigned 103 patients with bipolar I disorder to cognitive therapy or standard care, in addition to pharmacotherapy. At the time of entry to the study, patients were not in an episode of mania or depression, but 56% of the subjects had mild to moderate levels of depressive symptoms on the Beck Depression Inventory. Both groups received "minimal psychiatric care," defined as mood stabilizers at therapeutic levels and regular psychiatric follow-up. Those assigned to the cognitive therapy group also received an average of 14 sessions of cognitive therapy during the first 6 months and two booster sessions in the second 6 months. No attempt was made to control for the nonspecific aspects of additional professional attention received by the cognitive therapy group. Over a 12-month period, the cognitive therapy group had significantly fewer bipolar episodes (manic, depressed, or mixed) and hospital admissions for an episode of bipolar disorder (see Figure 25–4). Over 12 months, 75% of the patients in the control group had a recurrence compared with 44% in the cognitive therapy group. Patients in the cognitive therapy condition spent two-thirds fewer days in an episode (manic or

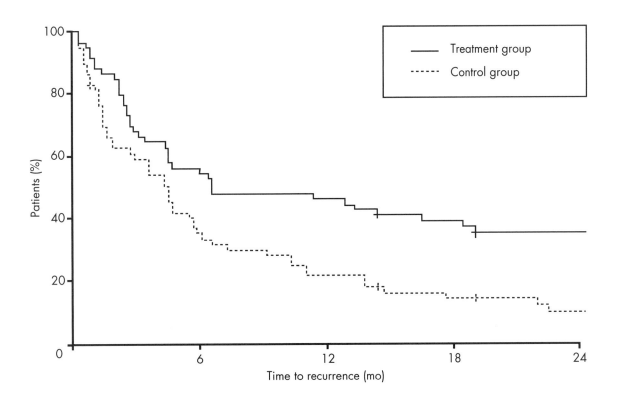

FIGURE 25–3. **Survival curves for recurrence with mania, depression, or mixed episode.**

Log rank$_1$=9.3; $P<0.003$.

Source. Reprinted, with the permission of the publisher and the authors, from Colom F, Vieta E, Martinez-Aran A, et al: "A Randomized Trial on the Efficacy of Group Psychoeducation in the Prophylaxis of Recurrences in Bipolar Patients Whose Disease Is in Remission." *Archives of General Psychiatry* 60:402–407, 2003. Copyright © 2003, American Medical Association. All rights reserved.

depressed) compared with control subjects, and the number of patients hospitalized for bipolar episodes was one-half in the cognitive therapy group compared with the control group. Patients completed the Coping With Prodromes Interview, a semistructured interview that asks patients to identify their early warning signs of an impending depression or mania episode. Patient responses were rated on a 7-point scale, ranging from 0 (poor) to 6 (extremely well). On this measure, patients in the cognitive therapy group scored significantly higher than did patients in the control group on coping with manic prodromes at both month 6 and month 12. The group difference favoring the cognitive therapy group in coping with depression prodromes at month 6 was lost by month 12.

Scott and colleagues (2001) randomly assigned 42 subjects meeting criteria for bipolar I or II disorder to 25 sessions of cognitive therapy or a 6-month wait-list control that was then followed by cognitive therapy. The baseline characteristics of the sample were very heterogeneous: 11 subjects met diagnostic criteria for a depressive

episode, 3 for rapid-cycling disorder, 2 for hypomania, and 1 for a mixed state. Twelve subjects met criteria for drug and/or alcohol problems or dependence. About 60% of the sample met criteria for a personality disorder. At 6 months, those assigned to cognitive therapy showed greater reduction in depressive symptoms—but not manic symptoms—relative to the wait-list control subjects. Those who received cognitive therapy (either assigned initially to cognitive therapy or assigned after the waiting list) had a 60% reduction in relapse rates compared with the 18 months prior to commencing cognitive therapy (66% vs. 21%). The cognitive therapy was administered by highly trained clinicians.

Family Therapy

Miklowitz and colleagues developed a 21-session family intervention—family-focused therapy (FFT)—that is administered to patients and their families over a 9-month period. FFT emphasizes psychoeducation, communica-

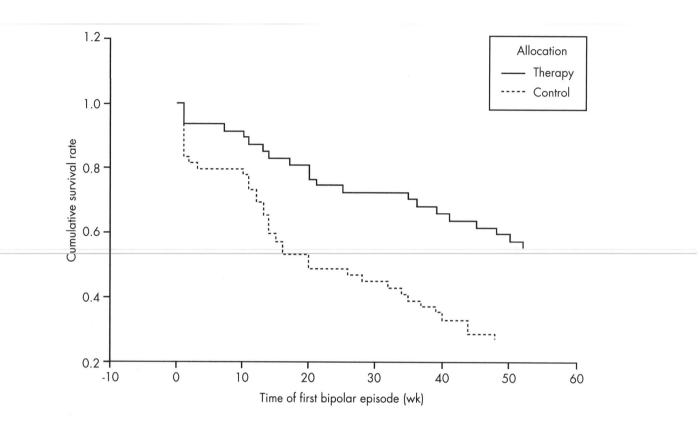

FIGURE 25–4.   **Survival curves from Cox regression intention-to-treat analysis.**

After controlling for medication compliance, the hazard ratio for relapse was 0.40 (95% confidence interval=0.21–0.74; P=0.004).

Source.   Reprinted with permission from Lam DH, Watkins ER, Hayward P, et al: "A Randomized Controlled Study of Cognitive Therapy for Relapse Prevention for Bipolar Affective Disorder." *Archives of General Psychiatry* 60:145–152, 2003. Copyright © 2003, American Medical Association. All rights reserved.

tion skills, and problem-solving skills, specifically around problematic family issues (Miklowitz and Hooley 1998). The 101 patients meeting criteria for bipolar I disorder who had had an episode of mania or depression within the preceding 3 months were randomly assigned to either FFT (*n*=31) or a less-intensive crisis management condition (*n*=70) (Miklowitz et al. 2003). The assignment to FFT was associated with significantly fewer relapses and a longer time to relapse than in those assigned to crisis management (see Figure 25–5). A hazard ratio of 0.38 reflects a threefold higher rate of survival in the FFT group over 2 years (52%) than in the crisis management group (17%). Compared with crisis management, assignment to FFT was associated with lower relapse rates (35% in FFT vs. 54% in crisis management) and a longer average duration of survival (73.5 weeks for FFT vs. 53.2 weeks for crisis management). Furthermore, FFT was associated with

lower levels of depressive and manic symptoms over 2-year follow-up. Notably, the benefits of the family intervention extended beyond the 9-month period of active treatment, with persistence of effects over the 2-year follow-up period.

Interpersonal and Social Rhythm Therapy

Interpersonal and social rhythm therapy (IPSRT) was developed by Frank and colleagues (2000) to help patients with bipolar disorder to address interpersonal problems and regulate their social rhythms. It combines the well-established principles of IPT for unipolar depression (Weissman et al. 2000) with a behavioral strategy designed to regularize daily routines (social rhythm therapy) and psychoeducation to enhance adherence to medication regimens. IPSRT focuses on 1) the identification

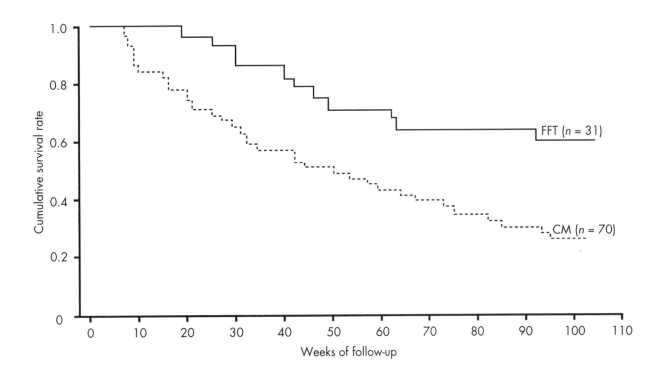

and management of affective symptoms; 2) the link between mood and life events; 3) the maintenance of regular daily rhythms as elucidated by the Social Rhythm Metric; 4) the identification and management of potential precipitants of rhythm dysregulation, with special attention to interpersonal triggers; and 5) the facilitation of mourning the lost healthy self (Frank et al. 2000).

A single large trial of IPSRT has recently concluded at the University of Pittsburgh in Pennsylvania. Acutely ill bipolar patients received medication and were randomly assigned to either IPSRT or intensive clinical management. Once stabilized (defined as 4 weeks of symptom scores averaging 7 or less on the Hamilton Rating Scale for Depression and 7 or less on the Bech-Rafaelsen Mania Scale [Bech et al. 1979] while receiving a stable medication regimen), patients were reassigned to either IPSRT or intensive clinical management (in conjunction with the medication regimen that led to stabilization) for 2 years of monthly maintenance treatment. Thus, this study in-

cluded both acute and maintenance phases. Several findings emerged from analyses conducted thus far, and additional results are forthcoming (Frank et al., in press). In this trial, half the patients received the same therapy intervention throughout the trial, and the other half received a sequence of psychotherapies (either IPSRT followed by intensive clinical management or intensive clinical management followed by IPSRT). This change in psychotherapy treatment at the time of entry into the maintenance phase was associated with a significantly greater likelihood of recurrence regardless of sequence order (Frank et al. 1999). We concluded that instability contributes to morbidity in bipolar disorder and that treatment approaches that increase stability improve outcome. The admittedly unexpected finding that altered treatment—rather than the content of the treatment per se—affects risk for recurrence underscores the insidious effects of instability in this population.

These findings have interesting ramifications for the

design of a comparative psychotherapy trial involving a sequence of interventions (Curtin 2003). Also, note that the overall recurrence rate in this investigation over a study period of 2 years, regardless of treatment assignment, was lower than in many of the studies already discussed in this chapter. This raises questions about the relatively high potency of the intensive clinical management condition, an active treatment that was administered by expert therapists and included education about bipolar disorder, education about medications used to treat bipolar disorder, education about basic sleep hygiene, careful review of side effects, medical and behavioral management of side effects, support, education about early warning signs of impending episodes and use of rescue medication, and a 24-hour on-call service. It is clear that this so-called control condition involved a substantial amount of nonspecific psychotherapy and psychoeducation.

Conclusion

Over the past few years, the number of randomized, controlled clinical trials of psychotherapy for bipolar disorder has burgeoned. Cumulatively, the data indicate that psychotherapy should play an important role in the management of bipolar disorder; however, many specific issues regarding psychotherapy and bipolar disorder remain unclear. Table 25–2 suggests that different treatments may have differential effects on specific phases of the disorder, depending on study design (i.e., whether patients were euthymic or in an episode at time of enrollment;

duration of follow-up) and specific features of the intervention. It appears that strategies that are less intensive or rely on less highly trained therapists have an effect on mania but not on depression. In contrast, the more intensive interventions that use highly trained therapists seem to have greater effects across the phases of the disorder. Relational strategies, such as interpersonally and family-focused treatments, as well as cognitive therapy or psychoeducation delivered by skilled therapists, may have greater effects on the depressive symptomatology, whereas the behavioral treatments administered by less-skilled therapists may have some effect on manic symptoms but little effect on depression. This may have important public health and public policy implications because most bipolar patients experience protracted depressions and only relatively brief manias, yet the number of skilled therapists trained to administer these empirically based psychotherapies is extremely limited.

Several common themes are critical to the success of any adjunctive psychotherapeutic intervention for bipolar disorder, including psychoeducation, medication side-effect monitoring, regulating the sleep-wake cycle, daily monitoring of mood states, attention to the patient's social support system, and a continuing focus on early warning symptoms. We cannot yet separate the specific ingredients from the common ones across treatments, but it appears that different therapies have different effects (Swartz 2002). This raises questions such as "What are the active ingredients of bipolar-specific psychotherapy?"; "Do bipolar-specific psychotherapies exert their effects directly, or is the effect mediated by treatment adherence?"; and "Which approaches work for whom?"

TABLE 25–2. Differential effects of psychotherapies

Therapy type (investigator)	Experienced therapists?	Effect on recurrence or relapse?		Effect on symptoms?	
		Mania	**Depression**	**Mania**	**Depression**
Individual psychoeducation (Perry)	No	Yes	No	—	—
Group psychoeducation (Colom)	Yes	No	Yes	—	—
Care management (Simon)	No	—	—	Yes	No
Cognitive therapy (Lam)	Yes	Yes	Yes	—	—
Cognitive therapy (Scott)	Yes	—	—	No	Yes
Family therapy (Miklowitz)	Yes	Yes	Yes	Yes	Yes
Interpersonal therapy (Frank)	Yes	Yes	Yes	Yes	Yes
Intensive clinical management (Frank)	Yes	Yes	Yes	Yes	Yes

Note. — indicates no data available or parameter not measured.

Our review illustrates that it is difficult to compare across studies because of variability in end points (recurrence vs. change in symptoms) and lack of comparability of the intensities of control conditions. To tease apart these effects, psychotherapy studies may need to focus initially on only a single aspect of the disorder at the time of study. We also may need to perform studies outside of tertiary settings specializing in bipolar disease management because the nonspecific factors of bipolar disorder psychoeducation and psychotherapy are becoming a part of routine practice in these settings, which may make it very difficult to show differences between specific psychotherapeutic approaches. Evaluation of studies must include an evaluation of the control condition and the active condition.

Investigators such as Bauer and Simon have initiated effectiveness trials that are currently ongoing. At the University of Pittsburgh, we recently established the Bipolar Disorder Center for Pennsylvanians, at which individuals will receive either algorithm-driven psychopharmacological intervention or algorithm-driven psychopharmacological intervention plus an enhanced clinical intervention. The enhanced clinical intervention, a modified version of the intensive clinical management intervention described earlier in this chapter, consists of 10 basic therapeutic strategies, each of which can be adapted to the specific needs of the subpopulations being studied in the randomized trial. These 10 central components of the enhanced intervention are listed in Table 25–3. In addition, there are specific intervention modules for youths, elderly patients, and African American patients in order to meet the unique needs of these populations. For instance, the approach used with youths includes a focus on differentiating bipolar symptoms from normal, developmentally appropriate behaviors such as tantrums and adolescent moodiness. The approach used with an older population includes a focus on physical comorbidities, current life transitions (i.e., bereavement or retirement), and complicated medication regimens. With African American patients, therapists anticipate and explore patient mistrust of nonblack therapists and medications while actively inviting African American patients to share their perspectives on symptoms, treatment, and clinical progress.

We have virtually no data on the role of psychotherapy in bipolar disorder across the life span. If we posit that early intervention for bipolar disorder in childhood and adolescence will become more common in the future as we develop better tools to identify the disorder in those at risk, we will need to consider introducing psychotherapy to engage these young people in their treatment and to help them meet developmental milestones despite the additional burden of having bipolar disorder (Goldberg-

TABLE 25–3. Ten key elements of enhanced clinical intervention

1. Education about the mood disorder
2. Education about medications used to treat the disorder
3. Education about basic sleep and social rhythm hygiene
4. Education about the use of rescue medications
5. Careful review of symptoms
6. Careful review of side effects
7. Medical and behavioral management of side effects
8. 24-Hour on-call service
9. Discussion of early warning signs of impending episodes
10. Nonspecific support

Arnold and Fristad 2003). At the other end of the life span, there is increasing recognition of bipolar disorder in geriatric populations; in these patients, the management of concurrent medical disease increases the likelihood of drug-drug interactions. It seems likely that psychotherapy will play an important role in the long-term treatment of bipolar disorder in this age group as well.

Further work on the role of psychotherapy in the treatment of bipolar disorder is particularly important because pharmacotherapy to date has not proven to be a "magic bullet" for symptom resolution and complete recovery associated with full functioning. It seems increasingly likely that psychotherapy will play an important role in helping patients to achieve a full recovery from their illness. Therefore, it is incumbent on all of us to better understand the effect of psychotherapeutic strategies on symptoms and functioning and to continue to develop better psychosocial tools that can be used in conjunction with pharmacotherapy to improve outcomes in bipolar disorder.

References

Anderson CM, Hogarty GE, Reiss DJ: Family treatment of adult schizophrenic patients: a psycho-educational approach. Schizophr Bull 6:490–505, 1980

Bauer MS, Williford WO, Dawson EE, et al: Principles of effectiveness trials and their implementation in VA Cooperative Study #430: 'Reducing the Efficacy-Effectiveness Gap in Bipolar Disorder.' J Affect Disord 67:61–78, 2001

Bauwens F, Tracy A, Pardoen D, et al: Social adjustment of remitted bipolar and unipolar out-patients: a comparison with age- and sex-matched controls. Br J Psychiatry 159:239–244, 1991

Bech P, Bolwig TG, Kramp P, et al: The Bech-Rafaelsen Mania Scale and the Hamilton Depression Scale: evaluation of homogeneity and inter-observer reliability. Acta Psychiatr Scand 59:420–430, 1979

Beck AT, Rush AJ, Shaw BF, et al: Cognitive Therapy of Depression. New York, Guilford, 1979

Cade JFL: Lithium salt in the treatment of psychotic excitement. Med J Aust 2:349–352, 1949

Clarkin JF, Glick ID, Haas GL, et al: A randomized clinical trial of inpatient family intervention, V: results for affective disorders. J Affect Disord 18:17–28, 1990

Cohen J: Statistical Power Analysis for Behavioral Sciences, 2nd Edition. Hillsdale, NJ, Lawrence Erlbaum Associates, 1988

Colom F, Vieta E, Martinez-Aran A, et al: A randomized trial on the efficacy of group psychoeducation in the prophylaxis of recurrences in bipolar patients whose disease is in remission. Arch Gen Psychiatry 60:402–407, 2003

Coryell W, Scheftner W, Keller M, et al: The enduring psychosocial consequences of mania and depression. Am J Psychiatry 150:720–727, 1993

Curtin F: Bipolar disorder and crossover design. J Clin Psychopharmacol 23:319–320, 2003

Elkin I, Shea MT, Watkins JT, et al: National Institute of Mental Health Treatment of Depression Collaborative Research Program: general effectiveness of treatments. Arch Gen Psychiatry 46:971–982, 1989

Frank E, Swartz HA, Mallinger AG, et al: Adjunctive psychotherapy for bipolar disorder: effects of changing treatment modality. J Abnorm Psychol 108:579–587, 1999

Frank E, Swartz HA, Kupfer DJ: Interpersonal and social rhythm therapy: managing the chaos of bipolar disorder. Biol Psychiatry 48:593–604, 2000

Frank E, Kupfer DJ, Gerebtzoff A, et al: The development of study exit criteria for evaluating antimanic compounds. J Clin Psychiatry 62:421–425, 2001

Frank E, Kupfer DJ, Thase ME, et al: Two year outcomes for interpersonal and social rhythm therapy in individuals with bipolar I disorder. Arch Gen Psychiatry (in press)

Fromm-Reichmann F: Intensive psychotherapy of manic-depressives. Confin Neurol 9:158–165, 1949

Gitlin MJ, Swendsen J, Heller TL, et al: Relapse and impairment in bipolar disorder. Am J Psychiatry 152:1635–1640, 1995

Goldberg JF, Harrow M, Grossman LS: Course and outcome in bipolar affective disorder: a longitudinal follow-up study. Am J Psychiatry 152:379–384, 1995

Goldberg-Arnold JS, Fristad MA: Psychotherapy for children with bipolar disorder, in Bipolar Disorder in Childhood and Early Adolescence. Edited by Geller B, DelBello MP. New York, Guilford, 2003, pp 272–294

Goldstein MJ, Miklowitz DJ: The effectiveness of psychoeducational family therapy in the treatment of schizophrenic disorders. J Marital Fam Ther 21:361–376, 1995

Goodwin F, Jamison K: Manic-Depressive Illness. New York, Oxford University Press, 1990

Gordis L: Epidemiology, 2nd Edition. Philadelphia, PA, WB Saunders, 2000

Hennen J: Statistical methods for longitudinal research on bipolar disorders. Bipolar Disord 5:156–168, 2003

Hogarty GE: Personal therapy: a practical psychotherapy for the stabilization of schizophrenia, in Treating Chronic and Severe Mental Disorders: A Handbook of Empirically Supported Interventions. Edited by Hofmann SG, Tompson MC. New York, Guilford, 2002, pp 53–68

Klerman GL, Weissman MM, Rounsaville BJ, et al: Interpersonal Psychotherapy of Depression. New York, Basic Books, 1984

Judd LL, Akiskal HS, Schettler PJ, et al: The long-term natural history of the weekly symptomatic status of bipolar I disorder. Arch Gen Psychiatry 59:530–537, 2002

Lam DH, Watkins ER, Hayward P, et al: A randomized controlled study of cognitive therapy for relapse prevention for bipolar affective disorder: outcome of the first year. Arch Gen Psychiatry 60:145–152, 2003

Miklowitz DJ, Hooley JM: Developing family psychoeducational treatments for patients with bipolar and other severe psychiatric disorders: a pathway from basic research to clinical trials. J Marriage Fam Couns 24:419–435, 1998

Miklowitz DJ, Simoneau TL, George EA, et al: Family focused treatment of bipolar disorder: one year effects of a psychoeducational program in conjunction with pharmacotherapy. Biol Psychiatry 48:582–592, 2000

Miklowitz DJ, George EL, Richards JA, et al: A randomized study of family focused psychoeducation and pharmacotherapy in the outpatient management of bipolar disorder. Arch Gen Psychiatry 60:904–912, 2003

Perry A, Tarrier N, Morriss R, et al: Randomised controlled trial of efficacy of teaching patients with bipolar disorder to identify early symptoms of relapse and obtain treatment. BMJ 318:149–153, 1999

Pitschel-Walz G, Leucht S, Bauml J, et al: The effect of family interventions on relapse and rehospitalization in schizophrenia—a meta-analysis. Schizophr Bull 27:73–92, 2001

Post RM, Luckenbaugh DA: Unique design issues in clinical trials of patients with bipolar affective disorder. J Psychiatr Res 37:61–73, 2003

Post RM, Denicoff KD, Leverich GS, et al: Morbidity in 258 bipolar outpatients followed for 1 year with daily prospective ratings on the NIMH life chart method. J Clin Psychiatry 64:680–690, 2003

Sachs GS, Rush AJ: Response, remission, and recovery in bipolar disorders: what are the realistic treatment goals? J Clin Psychiatry 64 (suppl 6):18–22, 2003

Sachs GS, Thase ME, Otto MW, et al: Rationale, design, and methods of the Systematic Treatment Enhancement Program for bipolar disorder. Biol Psychiatry 53:1028–1042, 2003

Scott J: Cognitive therapy as an adjunct to medication in bipolar disorder. Br J Psychiatry 178 (suppl 41):S164–S168, 2001

Scott J, Garland A, Moorhead S: A pilot study of cognitive therapy in bipolar disorders. Psychol Med 31:459–467, 2001

Simon GE, Ludman E, Unuetzer J, et al: Design and implementation of a randomized trial evaluating systematic care for bipolar disorder. Bipolar Disord 4:226–236, 2002

Simon GE, Ludman EJ, Unutzer J, et al: Randomized trial of a population-based care program for people with bipolar disorder. Psychol Med 35:13–14, 2005

Swartz HA: Convergent strategies or phase-specific interventions?, in Evidence and Experience in Psychiatry, Vol V: Bipolar Disorder. Edited by Maj M, Akiskal HS, Lopez-Ibor JJ, et al. Chichester, UK, Wiley, 2002, pp 322–324

Swartz HA, Frank E: Psychotherapy for bipolar depression: a phase-specific strategy? Bipolar Disord 3:11–22, 2001

Sweeney JA, Kmiec JA, Kupfer DJ: Neuropsychologic impairments in bipolar and unipolar mood disorders on the CANTAB neurocognitive battery. Biol Psychiatry 48:674–684, 2000

Tavares JVT, Drevets WC, Sahakian BJ: Cognition in mania and depression. Psychol Med 33:959–967, 2003

Tohen M, Hennen J, Zarate CM Jr, et al: Two-year syndromal and functional recovery in 219 cases of first-episode major affective disorder with psychotic features. Am J Psychiatry 157:220–228, 2000

Weissman MM, Markowitz JC, Klerman GL: Comprehensive Guide to Interpersonal Psychotherapy. New York, Basic Books, 2000

Zaretsky A: Targeted psychosocial interventions for bipolar disorder. Bipolar Disord 5 (suppl 2):80–87, 2003

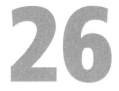

Psychotherapy for Depression in Children and Adolescents

V. ROBIN WEERSING, PH.D.

DAVID A. BRENT, M.D.

MOOD DISORDERS IN childhood and adolescence are disabling, distressing, and prevalent. By some estimates, more than one in five youths in the United States will have a significant episode of depression before they reach the end of puberty (Lewinsohn and Clarke 1999). The experience of depression in childhood and adolescence impairs youths' ability to form close and meaningful relationships, impedes school performance, and increases the risk of suicide attempts and completion (Brent et al. 1993; Gould et al. 1998; Rohde et al. 1994). In addition, the negative effects of early-onset mood problems may proliferate through development and substantially interfere with youths' ability to reach their full adult potential. Depression in youth predicts a variety of long-term adverse outcomes, including poor work history, substance abuse, and recurrent episodes of disorder in adulthood (Rohde et al. 1994; Weissman et al. 1999).

Over the last decade, data have begun to accumulate on the efficacy of treatments for depression in youths. Results of structured psychosocial interventions appear quite promising, without raising the safety concerns associated with psychotropic medication use (see Emslie, Chapter 35, in this volume). Cognitive-behavioral therapy (CBT) has garnered particularly solid support, reliably outperforming wait lists, attention-placebo controls, and (for depressed teenagers) other types of psychotherapy (Brent et al. 1997; Wood et al. 1996). Additional data from two open trials (Mufson et al. 1994; Santor and Kusumaker 2001) and three recent randomized studies have suggested that interpersonal psychotherapy (IPT) for depression, an efficacious intervention with adults, also may produce positive outcomes in samples of depressed teenagers (Mufson et al. 1999, 2004; Rosselló and Bernal 1999). Efficacy data on other psychotherapeutic approaches are sparse and results less clear, with positive outcomes reported by some investigators (family therapy;

Preparation of this manuscript was facilitated by support to V. Robin Weersing from the William T. Grant Foundation, the Klingenstein Third Generation Foundation, and the National Institute of Mental Health (R01 MH064503-01A1).

Diamond et al. 2002) but not others (Brent et al. 1997).

In this chapter, we provide an overview and critique of the psychosocial treatment literature for youth depression. We begin with a summary of the major models of intervention. We then 1) review efficacy data from the 21 published randomized controlled trials of psychotherapy for depressed youth, 2) describe available data on mechanisms of treatment action, and 3) discuss significant moderators and predictors of treatment response.

Psychosocial Models of Intervention

Modern research on the etiology and maintenance of depression focuses on understanding the interplay between 1) biological vulnerability to acute stress reactions; 2) the experience of negative life events; 3) "depressogenic" cognitive interpretations of these events; and 4) learned, maladaptive behavioral responses to stress. As described later in this chapter, the psychosocial treatments developed for depressed youths focus on reducing life stress (when possible) and on modifying these last two pathogenic responses to stress: depressogenic thinking and maladaptive behavioral and social response sets.

Cognitive-Behavioral Therapy

Theories of Intervention

CBT is based primarily on a *cognitive-vulnerability model* of depression. The classic version of this model, developed by Beck and colleagues (1979), posits that depression is the result of traitlike, depressogenic "schemas" or working models of the self, world, and future. These schemas are thought to be formed early in life as the result of negative experiences. Under stressful circumstances similar to those that produced the schema, the schemas become active, and vulnerable individuals engage in irrational, overly negative thinking about their *current* stressful situations. As a result, feelings of depression build and deepen. The Beck model and other cognitive theories (e.g., learned helplessness; Abramson et al. 1978, 1989) were developed to describe and explain adult depression. However, evidence indicates that children and adolescents engage in the patterns of depressogenic thinking specified in cognitive theories (see Gladstone and Kaslow 1995) and that these modes of thinking may at least "weakly" predict later episodes of depression in youths rather than simply co-occur with or be a symptom of negative mood (e.g., Lewinsohn et al. 1997).

In addition to cognitive-vulnerability models, several behavioral theories of depression have been influential in the creation of CBT programs. The most prominent of these—

social learning theory (Lewinsohn et al. 1998)—suggests that depression is caused and maintained, in part, by the disruption in adaptive behavior patterns caused by stressful events. This disruption is more severe for individuals already weak in behavioral mood regulation skills (e.g., those unsure how to use pleasant activities to raise mood). Social learning theory is compatible with cognitive models. Indeed, in social learning models, depression may emerge from several possible diatheses (stressful events, maladaptive cognitions, behavioral withdrawal) that interact with other risk factors to disrupt adaptive behaviors and spiral mood downward.

CBT Techniques

CBT for youths targets these cognitive distortions and behavioral deficits to improve current mood and to prevent future episodes of depression. In Table 26–1, we briefly describe common CBT techniques and the general sequence of treatment. Specific CBT protocols vary in the extent to which they emphasize the primacy of cognitive (e.g., Brent et al. 1997) or behavioral (e.g., Lewinsohn et al. 1990) strategies. However, all the intervention programs 1) teach depressed youths specific CBT mood regulation skills, 2) encourage practice of skills within and between sessions, and 3) treat skill acquisition as an "experiment" in which youths will be coached by their therapists to make changes in their lives and then will collaboratively assess the extent to which the changes led to positive affective outcomes.

Developmental Adaptation of CBT

Thus far, our description of the CBT intervention model for youth depression has been quite similar to the CBT model used with depressed adults. This is not an accident. Most research on depression has been conducted in adult samples, and the resulting theories of pathology and intervention were later adapted for child and adolescent populations. In CBT, these developmental adaptations have focused on two characteristics of young patients likely to impede progress in cognitive therapy. Compared with adults, youths may have 1) less developed abstract reasoning and perspective taking skills and 2) less control over their personal environment. To better map onto youths' cognitive developmental level, CBT protocols

- Emphasize the use of concrete examples to teach abstract concepts (e.g., having youths identify depressogenic thoughts in cartoon strips; Clarke et al. 2001)
- Include frequent summaries and reviews of key points
- Have youths "teach" treatment lessons to their therapists or parents to cement learning (Asarnow et al. 2002)
- Administer quizzes to assess youths' understanding of treatment concepts

---

TABLE 26–1. Cognitive-behavioral therapy (CBT) for children and adolescents with depression: common techniques and typical sequence

---

1. **Psychoeducation**
   Providing youths (and parents) information about the characteristics and course of depression and the CBT model of depression (linking thoughts, feelings, and behavior)

2. **Affective education and mood monitoring**
   Teaching youths to monitor their moods and observe what makes them feel both happy and depressed

3. **Behavioral activation**
   Promoting engagement in activities that provide youths opportunities for mastery or pleasure, both for short-term mood regulation and to promote a long-term focus on creating a rewarding, nonstressful, and mood-elevating environment

4. **Cognitive restructuring**
   Helping youths to examine their thoughts and assumptions and assess the accuracy and affective consequences of their views; teaching youths to engage in "rational" thinking about themselves, the world, and their possibilities for the future

5. **Supplemental CBT techniques used in many programs**
   Teaching youths relaxation techniques to cope with continuing environmental stressors, providing social skills and conflict resolution training to enhance youths' adaptive behavioral repertoire, and teaching general problem-solving skills

---

To address youths' dependence on their environment, many CBT protocols include family components—ranging in intensity from brief family psychoeducation at the beginning of treatment (Brent et al. 1997) to complete parent curricula that teach a set of CBT skills parallel to those learned by the depressed youth (e.g., Asarnow et al. 2002; Clarke et al. 1999).

Interpersonal Therapies

The cognitive-vulnerability and social learning models of depression have spurred a great deal of research and formed the basis of most of the protocols developed to treat depression in youth. However, a small (four studies), but growing, body of work exists on interpersonal models of youth depression treatment. Underneath our "interpersonal" umbrella, we group social skills training (without other CBT elements), family therapies, and IPT. All three treatments target social aspects of depression, although the specific domain differs, as do the techniques used to effect change.

In this background section, we provide additional detail on the theoretical model and treatment techniques used in IPT for depressed adolescents. IPT for depressed adolescents has been tested in only a few studies of adolescents (two randomized trials and two open trials); however, IPT has a strong record of support in the treatment of adult depression, and results with teenagers have been promising. It seems likely that there will be significant additional research with IPT for depressed adolescents in adolescent samples in the years ahead. We summarize the treatment programs of the two published family therapy clinical trials and the one social skill protocol in the context of our review of efficacy studies.

Interpersonal Psychotherapy for Depressed Adolescents

The IPT for depressed adolescents model targets the resolution of psychosocial stresses that coincide with the onset of teenage patients' index depressive episode. Depressed youths experience a high level of severe psychosocial stress, are exposed to family conflict and parental marital conflict, and are dependent for their basic physical and emotional needs on mothers (and fathers) with high rates of psychopathology (see Hammen et al. 1999). In addition, specific, aversive family communication styles have been identified as significant predictors of depression in youths (e.g., Asarnow et al. 1993). Furthermore, in adolescents, first onset and recurrence of depression are often preceded by negative interpersonal events separate from the family, such as breakup of romantic relationships and loss of friendships (Lewinsohn and Clarke 1999). Unlike CBT, IPT for depressed adolescents does not claim a causal role for these environmental stresses in creating depression (e.g., by specifically triggering depressogenic thinking). Instead, patients are taught that depression and life stress frequently co-occur and that, regardless of the cause of depression (adversity, biology), alleviation of interpersonal problems will likely result in an attenuation of depressive symptoms.

In the first phase of IPT for depressed adolescents, the difficult environmental context of teenage patients' lives is categorized into one of five common problem areas: grief, role disputes, role transitions, interpersonal deficits, or issues with single-parent families (an adaptation from adult IPT; see Moreau et al. 1991). In the remainder of treatment, specific strategies are used for working through each of the problem areas over the course of 12 sessions, with an overall emphasis on restoring (or creating) meaningful, low-conflict social relationships. For example, in working with a stressful role transition (such as changing to a more challenging school), an IPT for depressed adolescents therapist may help the teenager 1) mourn the loss of his or her old, comfortable role; 2) discuss the challenges involved in the transition; 3) attempt to discover the benefits of the new role or, at least, form reasonable expectations about the new role; and 4) help the teenager's interpersonal system adjust to the role transition. This final task—interacting directly with the adolescent's family—is a modification of the adult IPT model, similar to the increased involvement of parents in developmental adaptations of CBT.

Review of Clinical Trials

In this section, we review clinical trials of psychosocial interventions for youth depression. Our search procedures[1] identified 21 published randomized, controlled trials of CBT, IPT for depressed adolescents, family therapy, and social skills training. In our set of randomized, controlled trials, we included several studies that could be classified as prevention, such as the Clarke et al. (2001) intervention with high-symptom offspring of depressed parents. We chose to include targeted prevention studies because the youths receiving treatment in these "preventive" interventions showed depression symptoms as severe as or more severe than youths in some of the treatment trials (e.g., Ackerson et al. 1998).

Efficacy of Cognitive-Behavioral Therapy

CBT is currently the most widely researched psychotherapeutic intervention for youth depression, with 17 of 21 clinical trials testing the effects of CBT programs. In Table 26–2, we provide information on sample demographics, treatment characteristics, and clinical outcomes of CBT for adolescent depression. Table 26–3 contains similar information for CBT studies in child samples. As can be seen in the two tables, CBT has been tested across

the developmental spectrum, and several recent studies included a substantial proportion of ethnic minority youths (Ackerson et al. 1998; Asarnow et al. 2002; Rosselló and Bernal 1999; Weisz et al. 1997). CBT interventions have been delivered in a variety of formats, including individual therapy (e.g., Brent et al. 1997), group treatment (e.g., Lewinsohn et al. 1990), self-guided cognitive bibliotherapy (Ackerson et al. 1998), and youth CBT with combined family education sessions (Asarnow et al. 2002) or parent groups (Clarke et al. 1999; Lewinsohn et al. 1990). The mean number of CBT sessions also varied across the studies, ranging from a low of 6 to a high of 25.

Overall, results of this diverse set of investigations have supported the efficacy of CBT. Clinical response to CBT ranges from 43% to 86% at posttreatment and from 56% to 100% at follow-up (point prevalence, unless otherwise noted in the table). Among randomized, controlled trials that used stringent criteria for full remission of depression diagnoses, outcomes were similar, with 58% of youths, on average, achieving remission at posttreatment. Effect sizes on dimensional measures of depression were in the moderate range (see Tables 26–2 and 26–3), although effects were not uniform across studies and were larger for adolescents than for children. Indeed, the evidence base for CBT effects in childhood is leaner in several respects. There are fewer studies overall in childhood samples, and only two investigations have been conducted in samples of children with diagnoses of depression; notably, these investigations included both children and adolescents. Clinical trials of depression in childhood also tend to be older than the adolescent studies and less methodologically rigorous (e.g., lacking intent-to-treat analyses or analyses of clinically significant change).

We next review and critique the methods and results of a subset of the CBT literature: the set of seven randomized, controlled trials testing the effects of CBT in samples of youths meeting formal diagnostic criteria for major depression or dysthymia.

Review of Studies in Diagnostic Samples

Of the CBT investigations conducted in samples of youths with diagnosed depression, three of the seven have been by Peter Lewisohn, Greg Clarke, and colleagues. All

---

[1]To compile our list of studies, we searched the major electronic indexes (PsycINFO, PubMed), crossing search terms for developmental level with those for psychotherapy and depression, and limiting our search to peer-reviewed journal articles published in English. We also reviewed reference lists of reviews of youth depression treatment (Lewinsohn and Clarke 1999; Reinecke et al. 1998) and meta-analyses of psychotherapy in children and adolescents (e.g., Weisz et al. 1995) and identified youth depression clinical trials. In addition, we hand-searched the last 6 months of issues of major journals that publish psychotherapy clinical trials (*Archives of General Psychiatry, Journal of the American Academy of Child and Adolescent Psychiatry, Journal of Consulting and Clinical Psychology, Journal of Clinical Child and Adolescent Psychology*, and *Behavior Therapy*).

TABLE 26–2.   Cognitive-behavioral therapy (CBT) for adolescents with depression

Study	N	Source of sample	Mean age (years)	% Minority	Treatment and control conditions	Mean sessions	Primary symptom measure	CBT effect size[a] (symptoms)	Definition of clinical response	% Responding at post-treatment	% Responding at longest follow-up
Ackerson et al. (1998)	30	Community, screened for symptoms	15.9	35	CBT book Wait list	4 wk 4 wk	CDI	1.05	Normal CDI	59 (includes wait list)	
Brent et al. (1997)	107	Clinic, diagnosed depression	15.6	17	CBT Family Supportive	12.1 10.7 11.2	BDI	CBT: 0.40	No mood diagnosis and normal BDI	60 38 39	94 77 74 (24 mo)
Clarke et al. (1995)	150	Community, screened for symptoms	15.3	7	CBT TAU	15 Variable	CES-D	0.34	Categorical measure only available at follow-up		85 74 (12 mo)
Clarke et al. (1999)	123	Community, screened for diagnosis	16.2	Not reported	CBT CBTP Wait list	16 16+9 —	BDI	CBT: 0.58 CBTP: 0.24	No mood diagnosis	65 69 48	
Clarke et al. (2001)	94	Community, offspring of depressed parents, screened for symptoms	14.6	6	CBT+TAU TAU	15 Variable	CES-D	0.46	No episodes of depression over follow-up		90 71 (12 mo)
Clarke et al. (2002)	88	Community, offspring of depressed parents, screened for diagnosis	15.3	9	CBT+TAU TAU	16 CBT 8 wk	CES-D	0.20	No mood diagnosis	58 53	90 92 (24 mo)
Lewinsohn et al. (1990)	69	Community, screened for diagnosis	16.2	Not reported	CBT CBTP Wait list	14 14+7 —	BDI	CBT: 0.92 CBTP: 1.45	No mood diagnosis	43 47 5	15–20 (combined CBT/CBTP estimate) (24 mo)

TABLE 26–2. Cognitive-behavioral therapy (CBT) for adolescents with depression (continued)

Study	N	Source of sample	Mean age (years)	% Minority	Treatment and control conditions	Mean sessions	Primary symptom measure	CBT effect size[a] (symptoms)	Definition of clinical response	% Responding at post-treatment	% Responding at longest follow-up
Reynolds and Coats (1986)	30	Community, screened for symptoms	15.7	0	CBT Relaxation Wait list	10 10 —	BDI	1.53	Normal BDI	83 75 0	100 100 44 (1 mo)
Rosselló and Bernal (1999)	71	Community, screened for diagnosis	14.7	100	CBT IPT-A Wait list	12 12 —	CDI	0.34	Normal CDI	59 82 —	
Vostanis et al. (1996a)	63	Clinic, diagnosed depression	12.7[b]	12	CBT Supportive	6 6	MFQ-P	0.51	No mood diagnosis	86 75	74 85 (24 mo)
Wood et al. (1996)	53	Clinic, diagnosed depression	14.2[b]	Not reported	CBT Relaxation	6.4 6.2	MFQ-P	0.40	"Clinical remission"	54 21	56 36 (6 mo)

Note. BDI=Beck Depression Inventory; CBT book=CBT delivered via a self-help manual; CBTP=cognitive-behavioral sessions and psychoeducation/CBT coaching for parents of depressed youths; CDI=Children's Depression Inventory; CES-D=Center for Epidemiological Studies Depression Scale; IPT-A=interpersonal psychotherapy for depressed adolescents; MFQ-P=Mood and Feelings Questionnaire, parent version; TAU=treatment as usual in the community; may include psychotherapy and/or medication.
[a]Effect sizes compare the outcome of CBT with the outcome of the lowest-order control group on the primary symptom measure at posttreatment.
[b]Study sample included both children and adolescents.

TABLE 26–3. Cognitive-behavioral therapy (CBT) for children with depression

Study	N	Source of sample	Mean age (years)	% Minority	Treatment and control conditions	Mean sessions	Primary symptom measure	CBT effect size[a] (symptoms)	Definition of clinical response	% Responding at post-treatment	% Responding at longest follow-up
Asarnow et al. (2002)	23	Community, screened for symptoms	10	43	CBTP / Wait list	10 / —	CDI	0.30	No categorical measure		
Butler et al. (1980)	56	Community, screened for symptoms	11.5	Not reported	Cognitive / Role-play / Attention / Wait list	10 / 10 / 10 / —		Insufficient information in article	No categorical measure		
Kahn et al. (1990)	68	Community, screened for symptoms	12.1	Not reported	CBT / Relaxation / Self-modeling / Wait list	12 / 12 / 12 / —	CDI	CBT: 1.64	Normal CDI	88 / 76 / 59 / 29	76 / 65 / 41 (1 mo)
Liddle and Spence (1990)	31	Community, screened for symptoms	9.2	Not reported	CBT / Attention / No treatment	8 / 8 / —	CDI	0.35	No categorical measure		
Stark et al. (1987)	29	Community, screened for symptoms	11.2	Not reported	Self-control / Problem-solving / Wait list	12 / 12 / —	CDI	Self-control: 1.19 Problem-solving: 1.00	Normal CDI	78 / 60 / 11	88 / 67 (2 mo)
Vostanis et al. (1996a)	63	Clinic, diagnosed depression	12.7[b]	12	CBT / Supportive	6 / 6	MFQ-P	0.51	No mood diagnosis	86 / 75	74 / 85 (24 mo)
Weisz et al. (1997)	48	Community, screened for symptoms	9.6	37	CBT / No treatment	8 / —	CDI	0.52	Normal CDI	50 / 16	62 / 31 (9 mo)
Wood et al. (1996)	53	Clinic, diagnosed depression	14.2[b]	Not reported	CBT / Relaxation	6.4 / 6.2	MFQ-P	0.40	"Clinical remission"	54 / 21	56 / 36 (6 mo)

Note. CBTP=cognitive-behavioral sessions and psychoeducation/CBT coaching for parents of depressed youths; CDI=Children's Depression Inventory; MFQ-P=Mood and Feelings Questionnaire, parent version.

[a]Effect sizes compare the outcome of CBT with the outcome of the lowest-order control group on the primary symptom measure at posttreatment.

[b]Study sample included both children and adolescents.

of these randomized, controlled trials tested variants of the Coping with Depression (CWD) Course, a comprehensive CBT program that includes psychoeducation, pleasant activity scheduling, social skills training, problem-solving training, and cognitive restructuring. CWD is a group therapy developed for depressed adults and adapted to be developmentally appropriate for adolescents (e.g., by including cartoon examples for cognitive restructuring). To further adapt the CWD model to optimize outcomes with teenagers, a multisession CBT parent curriculum was developed. In the first trial of this program, Lewinsohn et al. (1990) randomly assigned adolescents to 14 sessions of the CWD Course for depressed adolescents (CWD-A), 14 sessions of CWD-A plus 7 sessions of the parent group, or a wait-list control. As can be seen in Table 26–2, response to the two CWD-A conditions was nearly identical at posttreatment and was maintained over follow-up assessments (at 1, 6, 12, and 24 months). Results on dimensional rating scales were similar; parent sessions did not boost the efficacy of CWD-A, but both versions of CBT were superior to the wait list.

In 1999, Clarke et al. replicated the Lewinsohn et al. (1990) findings. The design of the active treatment phase of this study was identical to that in the Lewinsohn et al. study (with slight modifications to the CWD manual), and results of the randomized, controlled trial were very similar. CWD-A and CWD-A with parent sessions reduced depression significantly more than did a wait list on dimensional symptom measures and on presence of diagnosable depression at posttreatment and follow-up. Again, addition of parent sessions did not seem to improve the effects of teenage-only group CBT. In this trial, booster sessions (one to two sessions) were provided after the termination of the acute treatment phase. These booster sessions did not reduce the rate of depression recurrence for those who had remitted by the end of treatment; however, booster sessions did appear to assist teenagers who had not yet recovered from depression at the end of the acute treatment phase.

In their most recent trial with diagnosed youths, Clarke and colleagues (2002) tested the CWD-A intervention in a sample of adolescents at high risk for recurrent episodes of mood disorder: teenagers who 1) personally met criteria for major depression and/or dysthymia and 2) had at least one parent with a recent episode of depressive disorder. This study was conducted in a large health maintenance organization (HMO), and depressed adults were found through the HMO medical records system. Adolescent children of depressed parents were then screened for depression themselves. Youths with elevated symptoms of depression were enrolled in a treat-

ment/prevention study that showed very good effects (see Table 26–2; Clarke et al. 2001). Adolescents meeting criteria for diagnosable depression were enrolled in this study and randomly assigned to receive 1) HMO usual care, which could include psychotherapy, medication, or no services; or 2) a 16-session version of CWD-A in addition to usual HMO services. Youths who received the CWD-A program did not have better outcomes than teenagers in usual care on any measures of treatment response at any of the posttreatment assessments (immediate, 12 months, or 24 months). These results are surprising, given the consistent support for the CWD program found in other adolescent depression randomized, controlled trials and in the adult literature. Clarke et al. raised two possible explanations for the null effects: 1) the HMO usual care condition may have been a very stringent control group, given some data that depressed youths in HMOs receive medication management in line with best practice recommendations (see DeBar et al. 2000), and/or 2) depressed children of depressed parents may have very severe, treatment-resistant symptoms.

We next review randomized, controlled trials of diagnosed depression testing the effects of CBT programs other than CWD-A. In 1996, Wood et al. completed the first randomized, controlled trial with a sample of teenagers presenting for care at an outpatient service. Adolescent outpatients with major or minor depression diagnoses were randomly assigned to a short course of CBT or relaxation training. Despite the brevity of the treatment (five to eight sessions), 54% of the CBT group and 21% of the relaxation group were judged to be in remission at posttreatment. Similar results were obtained on self-report measures of depressive symptoms. The superior outcomes of CBT at posttreatment were maintained at 3-month follow-up, but these group differences dissipated by 6-month follow-up. This may be due, in part, to continued improvement in the relaxation group and to a subgroup within the CBT cell with a high relapse rate. In a follow-up to this original clinical trial, Kroll et al. (1996) found that the addition of monthly CBT booster sessions after acute treatment resulted in a lower relapse rate (20% vs. 50%).

In another clinically referred sample, Vostanis et al. (1996a) randomly assigned depressed adolescents to either individual CBT (similar to the Wood et al. protocol) or a supportive therapy control. As can be seen in Table 26–2, CBT and supportive therapy were equivalent with regard to proportion of youths no longer meeting depressive criteria posttreatment and over follow-up (9 and 24 months; Vostanis et al. 1996b, 1998). The apparent high rate of success for both CBT (86%) and supportive therapy (75%) is surprising, in light of the relatively low dose of treatment. Teenagers in both treatments attended a mean of only six sessions occurring over an extended time (1–5 months).

The randomized, controlled trial conducted by Brent and colleagues (1997) is the only investigation other than Wood et al. (1996) and Vostanis et al. (1996a, 1996b) to use a primarily clinic-referred sample of depressed youths (two-thirds clinic vs. one-third from newspaper advertisements). Brent et al. (1997) randomly assigned adolescents with major depression to CBT, family therapy, or a supportive therapy control. The number of CBT sessions (12–16 weekly) in the Brent et al. trial was more similar to CWD-A than to the very short interventions used in the Wood et al. and Vostanis et al. studies. At posttreatment, results of the Brent et al. trial indicated that CBT produced outcomes superior to those of the alternative interventions. At posttreatment, significantly more teenagers receiving CBT (83%) than supportive therapy (58%) no longer met diagnostic criteria for major depression. Full remission of depression (no diagnosis and sustained low symptoms for 3 weeks) also was more common after CBT (60%) than with either family (38%) or supportive (39%) therapy, and symptom relief was faster in CBT than in the other two treatments. By 2-year follow-up, however, differences in depression remission and recovery rates among the three treatments were not significant (Birmaher et al. 2000), although the descriptive data again favored CBT (94% in remission) over family (77%) and supportive (74%) therapy.

In the final randomized, controlled trial delivered in diagnosed samples of youths, Rosselló and Bernal (1999) compared the efficacy of CBT with IPT for depressed adolescents and with a wait-list control condition. The study took place in Puerto Rico, and both CBT and IPT for depressed adolescents were adapted to be culturally appropriate for the sample (for description, see Rosselló and Bernal 1996). Overall, results of the investigation indicated that CBT and IPT for depressed adolescents were superior to the wait list in reducing symptoms of depression, but the outcomes of the two active treatments could not be reliably differentiated. Interpretation of this study's results is hampered by several methodological shortcomings of the study. Both CBT and IPT for depressed adolescents were designed to be 12-session interventions, but attendance problems occurred in both treatments. Only 68% of the IPT and 52% of the CBT patients completed more than 7 treatment sessions, and despite this high attrition rate, intent-to-treat analyses were not conducted on the full randomized sample. In addition, the investigators did not repeat diagnostic assessments at posttreatment and instead defined "clinical response" as a normative cutoff value on the Children's

Depression Inventory that was only three points lower than the mean for the sample at intake. On the basis of this criterion, 59% of the adolescents in the CBT condition and 82% of the IPT patients achieved clinically significant improvement in depression symptoms by posttreatment; data were not provided for the wait-list condition. Although this study has several methodological difficulties, these results provide some of the first information on the efficacy of CBT for depressed Latino adolescents and the only extant comparison of CBT and IPT for depressed adolescents.

Summary of Findings

Overall, results of these seven treatment studies indicated that CBT programs can have significant and clinically meaningful effects. CBT is reliably superior to wait-list control conditions, performs better than some active treatments (family and supportive therapy [Brent et al. 1997]; relaxation [Wood et al. 1996]), and appears equivalent to others (HMO usual care [Clarke et al. 2002]; IPT for depressed adolescents [Rosselló and Bernal 1999]; supportive therapy [Vostanis et al. 1996a, 1996b, 1998]). As can be seen in Tables 26–2 and 26–3, findings from the additional 10 randomized, controlled trials conducted in samples of youths with elevated symptoms of depression are concordant with the results of the seven studies in diagnostic samples. CBT produces significant benefits for youths, although CBT performs better against wait-list and no-treatment control conditions (Ackerson et al. 1998; Asarnow et al. 2002; Weisz et al. 1997) and less well when compared with active treatment conditions (Butler et al. 1980; Kahn et al. 1990; Liddle and Spence 1990; Reynolds and Coats 1986; Stark et al. 1987). Furthermore, CBT effects may be stronger for adolescents than for children, although child and adolescent studies differed in several methodological respects that made outcome differences difficult to interpret (e.g., use of diagnostic vs. high-symptom samples). Across studies, CBT results appear strongest at posttreatment, and differences between CBT and active interventions may dissipate over extended follow-up. In addition, although CBT has emerged as an efficacious intervention, a substantial portion of youths remains clinically depressed following a course of CBT (17%–57%).

Efficacy of Interpersonal Treatments

IPT for Depressed Adolescents

To date, there have been three published randomized trials of IPT for depressed adolescents, two conducted by the developers of the treatment (Mufson et al. 1999,

2004) and the Rosselló and Bernal (1999) study comparing IPT for depressed adolescents and CBT. As discussed earlier, Rosselló and Bernal randomly assigned teenagers with diagnosable depression to IPT for depressed adolescents, CBT, or a wait list. At posttreatment, 82% of the youths receiving IPT for depressed adolescents were below a normative cutoff score on the Children's Depression Inventory compared with 59% of the teenagers receiving CBT, but this difference was not statistically significant. In general, IPT for depressed adolescents and CBT performed similarly, and both were better than the wait list in reducing depression. Results of this trial indicated that IPT for depressed adolescents may be efficacious; however, the study had substantial attrition and did not conduct intent-to-treat analyses, limiting confidence in the generalizability of results. Results of the Mufson et al. (1999, 2004) studies provide additional verification of the positive findings on IPT for depressed adolescents reported by Rosselló and Bernal (1999).

In the Mufson et al. (1999) trial, adolescents seeking services at an outpatient clinic were screened for major depression and randomly assigned to 12 weeks of IPT for depressed adolescents or once-a-month clinical monitoring (over a similar period). As can be seen in Table 26–4, 75% of the teenagers in the IPT for depressed adolescents condition met recovery criteria on the Hamilton Rating Scale for Depression at posttreatment compared with only 46% of the monitoring group. On the basis of diagnostic criteria, 88% of the youths receiving IPT for depressed adolescents were no longer depressed compared with 58% of the teenagers in the control condition. No data were available for follow-up. There was a differential attrition between groups, with a higher loss in the clinical monitoring condition (54%) as a result of patient dissatisfaction, noncompliance, and worsening clinical status. To address this issue, Mufson et al. conducted intent-to-treat analyses for the dimensional symptom measures, carrying the last score forward. The pattern of results continued to support the superiority of IPT for depressed adolescents.

Recently, Mufson and colleagues transported IPT to five school-based health clinics and tested the interventions' effectiveness when delivered by school counseling staff who had been randomly assigned to receive IPT training (Mufson et al 2004). All teens referred for mental health services at the clinics were screened for study participation. Youths were required to evidence high levels of depression symptoms, report significant impairment, and meet criteria for a depression-related diagnosis (including adjustment disorder with depressed mood). Of the 160 youths eligible for the study at baseline, 64 consented to participate and were randomly assigned to receive 12 weeks of IPT or usual school counseling services,

typically supportive psychotherapy. At post-treatment, adolescents who had received IPT were less depressed according to self-report and interviewer-rated symptom scales, evidenced less impairment, and reported improved social functioning. At 16 weeks, adolescents were interviewed over the phone, and IPT treatment gains were maintained. As can be seen in Table 26–4, the recovery rate for youths who received IPT in the school clinics was somewhat lower than the rates reported in the two IPT efficacy studies (Mufson et al 1999, Roselló and Bernal 1999). However, the results are within the range of effects reported across the CBT and IPT literature and are some of the only data available on the real-world effectiveness of an intervention for depressed youth.

Taken together, data from these three trials strongly suggest that IPT for depressed adolescents is likely superior to no treatment, wait-list conditions, and school counseling. However, the status of IPT for depressed adolescents compared with other active interventions, such as CBT, remains unclear, and there are no data from randomized trials on the maintenance of effects of IPT for depressed adolescents over long-term follow-up. In one of the open trials of IPT for depressed adolescents, investigators attempted to contact their treated sample 1 year after the end of therapy (Mufson and Fairbanks 1996; Mufson et al. 1994). A substantial portion of the sample was lost to follow-up (36%), but among youths they were able to contact, rates of major depression were low (10% point prevalence).

Family Therapy Models

Two different family therapy programs are included in our review. As discussed in the CBT section, in the Brent et al. (1997) clinical trial, depressed teenagers were randomly assigned to 16 sessions of CBT, family therapy, or supportive therapy. The family therapy protocol was based on the work of Alexander and Parsons (1982) and Robin and Foster (1989). In the first phase of treatment, the family therapist attempted to clarify the concerns that brought the family to the clinic and to redefine the adolescent patient's problem as a problem both for and of the entire family system. Dysfunctional patterns of interaction and communication were identified, and the relation between these family problems and the adolescent patient's symptoms was delineated. In the second phase of therapy, family members were encouraged to try out new patterns of interaction and were given practice assignments for both within sessions and homework. In the Brent et al. randomized, controlled trial, this family therapy program was not as effective as CBT in reducing depression symptoms, and family therapy produced a posttreatment remission rate similar to that in

TABLE 26–4. Interpersonal, family, and social skills treatments for adolescents with depression

Study	N	Source of sample	Mean age (years)	% Minority	Treatment and control conditions	Mean sessions	Primary symptom measure	Target treatment effect size[a] (symptoms)	Definition of clinical response	% Responding at post-treatment	% Responding at longest follow-up
Brent et al. (1997)	107	Clinic, diagnosed depression	15.6	17	Family Supportive CBT	10.7 11.2 12.1	BDI	0.07	No mood diagnosis and normal BDI	38 39 60	77 74 94 (24 mo)
Diamond et al. (2002)	32	Unclear, screened for diagnosis	14.9	69	Family Wait list	12 6 wk	BDI	0.75	No mood diagnosis	81 47	87 (includes wait list) (6 mo)
Mufson et al. (1999)	48	Clinic, diagnosed depression	15.8	71	IPT-A Monitoring	9.8 2.8	BDI	0.57	Normal Ham-D	75 46	
Mufson et al. (2004)	63	Community, screened for diagnosis	15.1	71	IPT-A School TAU	10.5 7.9	BDI	0.40	Normal Ham-D	50 34	No categorical measure at follow-up
Rosselló and Bernal (1999)	71	Community, screened for diagnosis	14.7	100	IPT-A CBT Wait list	12 12 —	CDI	0.74	Normal CDI	82 59 —	
Reed (1994)	18	Unclear, screened for diagnosis	16	72	Social skills Art and imagery	6 6	CDI	Insufficient information in article	"Holistic judgment" at follow-up (not blind)		55 0 2 mo

Note. BDI = Beck Depression Inventory; CBT = cognitive-behavioral therapy; CDI = Children's Depression Inventory; Ham-D = Hamilton Rating Scale for Depression; IPT-A = interpersonal psychotherapy for depressed adolescents; School TAU = school counseling services.

[a]Effect sizes compare the outcome of the target treatment (interpersonal, family, or social skills) with the outcome of the lowest-order control group on the primary symptom measure at posttreatment.

the supportive therapy control group (see Table 26–4). Over long-term follow-up (24 months), significant differences between family therapy and CBT dissipated.

The family therapy program developed by Diamond and colleagues (2002) focused less on specific family communication patterns and homework tasks and instead attempted to improve parent–teenager attachment and relationship quality. The patients were teenagers with major depression drawn from low-income, inner-city neighborhoods, and most youths had been exposed to community or personal violence. In the attachment-based family therapy model, therapists helped families discuss past conflicts that had damaged family trust, such as abandonment and abuse. After these trust-building exercises, families were coached in how to support adolescents' social development outside the family sphere. Compared with teenagers on the wait list, youths in the intervention group were less likely to have a mood diagnosis (81% vs. 47%) and more likely to have Beck Depression Inventory scores in the normal range (62% vs. 19%) after treatment. The length of treatment and wait list did differ substantially (12 weeks vs. 6 weeks), and to address this, Diamond et al. compared mid-treatment data from the family therapy condition with post-wait-list scores. Dimensional measures of depression and family functioning did not show a significant difference at this 6-week comparison point, but the proportion of youths in the normal range on the Beck Depression Inventory was significantly higher in the treatment group (56%) than on the wait list (19%).

Social Skills Programs

In our literature search, we found only one randomized study of social skills training with depressed youths (Reed 1994). In this randomized, controlled trial, teenagers with major depression or dysthymia were randomly assigned to a social skills training or an art therapy group. Social skills training consisted of specific skill-building exercises, in vivo role-play, feedback from group members and therapists, and discussion and encouragement about how to apply these skills at home and with peers. Very few data were provided on the outcomes of this program, although standardized symptom measures, such as the Children's Depression Inventory, were administered. Nonblind, "holistic" clinical ratings of the measures were conducted, and analyses of these ratings supported the efficacy of the program (see Table 26–4). The author also reported that scores on rating scales significantly favored the social skills group for the males in the sample. However, descriptive statistics were not provided, and no overall statistical test of social skills training versus the art therapy was done. In addition, sample size was very small (N=18).

Mechanisms of Treatment Action

In our pool of 21 clinical trials, we found only 2 investigations that attempted to test the mechanisms of therapeutic action thought to underlie their treatment models. The Brent et al. (1997) randomized, controlled trial of CBT, family therapy, and supportive therapy included several measures of cognitive and family processes, and Kolko et al. (2000) sought to assess whether treatments produced significantly greater changes in the processes thought to be specific to their intervention model and whether change in these specific processes mediated the effect of treatment on depression outcomes. Data on these questions were mixed. As hypothesized, CBT did have a significantly greater effect on cognitive distortions than did family or supportive therapy, but CBT was not superior to these alternative interventions in changing the specific cognitions of hopelessness. In addition, CBT was as effective as family therapy in changing several indices of adaptive family functioning, undermining the specificity hypothesis for both CBT and family treatment. Furthermore, the changes in cognitive distortions that were found to be specific to CBT did not mediate the effect of CBT on depression symptoms.

Somewhat stronger support for the role of specific cognitive change in CBT outcome comes from the Ackerson et al. (1998) bibliotherapy program. Ackerson and colleagues found that the youths who were given a CBT self-help book showed a reduction in depression symptoms 4 weeks later, relative to wait list. At posttreatment, teenagers receiving CBT also had a reduction in depressogenic thinking, as assessed by the Dysfunctional Attitudes Scale, but they did not show significant change in negative automatic thoughts (a different cognitive measure). Change in dysfunctional attitudes did mediate the effects of the intervention on youth-reported depression symptoms, but the conditions for mediation were not met for other measures of depression (i.e., interviewer ratings). Furthermore, the mediational finding for dysfunctional attitudes is weakened by the simultaneous measurement of mechanism and outcome at posttreatment; logically, to identify mediation, the treatment mechanism should be shown to temporally change before change in depression outcome (for discussion, see Weersing and Weisz 2002b).

Moderators and Predictors of Treatment Response

Several of the CBT clinical trials investigated predictors of treatment outcome, and the Brent et al. (1997) randomized, controlled trial examined variables that predicted response to CBT, family therapy, and supportive therapy. We were unable to find any investigations of predictors of treatment response to social skills training, and data for IPT are thin (e.g., the effects of age in Mufson et al. 2004). As a result, our discussion is primarily based on studies comparing CBT protocols with wait-list and no-treatment conditions. The significant predictor variables uncovered in our review may, therefore, be predictors of response to CBT or could predict response to psychotherapy for youth depression in general. When data indicated differential response to one form of intervention (i.e., evidence of treatment moderation), we highlight these findings.

Various indices of depression severity were related to poor outcomes of psychotherapy. Greater severity of depression symptoms at intake (Birmaher et al. 2000; Brent et al. 1998; Clarke et al. 1992), less engagement in and enjoyment of pleasant activities (Clarke et al. 1992), and more cognitive distortions and feelings of hopelessness (Brent et al. 1998; Clarke et al. 1992) all predicted poor response across treatment types (i.e., in studies of CBT, family therapy, and supportive therapy). Of these factors, hopelessness seems particularly pernicious. In addition to its negative association with posttreatment response, hopelessness predicted early removal from the Brent et al. (1998) clinical trial. In addition, hopelessness may account for two other findings in the Brent et al. (1997) randomized clinical trial. In the 1997 clinical trial, youths who were referred to the study from clinical sources had worse outcomes than did those who were recruited via advertisement; this result was accounted for in part by the higher rates of hopelessness in the clinically referred sample. Interestingly, hopelessness also may mediate the moderating effects of suicidality. In a reanalysis of the Brent data, Barbe and colleagues (2004) found that CBT produced significantly better outcomes than supportive therapy for depressed adolescents with current or lifetime suicidality. In the CBT condition, 87% of the youths with lifetime suicidality no longer met criteria for major depression at posttreatment, a response rate virtually identical to that in youths without a suicide history (85%). Conversely, youths in supportive therapy with a history of significant suicidality fared much more poorly (36% without major depressive disorder) in comparison with their nonsuicidal peers (74% without major depressive disorder). This outcome appears to be the result of the CBT protocol's superior effect on reducing hopelessness, compared with supportive treatment.

Poor functioning at intake (Jayson et al. 1998) and presence of comorbid psychiatric conditions also have been identified as predictors of poor CBT response. The relation between comorbidity and depression treatment response appears to be complex, and contradictory findings have been reported in the literature. In the treatment of depressed teenagers, comorbid anxiety has been found to predict negative outcome (e.g., Clarke et al. 1992), positive outcome (e.g., Rohde et al. 2001), and superior outcome to CBT compared with alternative interventions (treatment moderation; Brent et al. 1998). Similarly, comorbid disruptive behavior problems have been unrelated to outcome in some samples (Clarke et al. 1992) and predictive of poor treatment response in other studies (Rohde et al. 2001). The effects of major depression comorbid with dysthymia also have been unclear (see Brent et al. 1998; Clarke et al. 1992).

Finally, aspects of the family environment appear to affect depression treatment outcome. Across treatment types, parent–child conflict was associated with depression recurrence over follow-up in the Brent et al. (1997) randomized, controlled trial sample (Birmaher et al. 2000). Maternal depression also predicted poor outcome in several CBT trials (Clarke et al. 1992; Jayson et al. 1998), and the presence of maternal depression eliminated the significant difference favoring CBT over family and supportive therapies in the Brent et al. (1998) study. In addition, maternal depression may account for the poor outcome of the Clarke et al. (2002) investigation, in which the generally successful CWD CBT program did not outperform a usual care control condition. The Clarke et al. sample in this study was composed entirely of depressed youths who also had one or more parents with a history of depression.

Conclusion and Future Directions

Overall, compelling data appear to support the efficacy of CBT and IPT for depressed adolescents, and family therapy may be worth investigating further. However, this good news is tempered by the fact that substantial percentages of youths remain clinically depressed following "successful" treatment and that the positive effects of psychosocial interventions may fade over time. In addition, it appears that therapy for depressed children and adolescents is perhaps least efficacious with those who need it the most—youths experiencing severe bouts of depression and those with a high family loading for depressive illness.

Two major clinical trials have been undertaken to examine the effects of combined psychosocial and pharmacological treatments in samples of more severely depressed youths: the Treatment for Adolescents With Depression

Study (TADS) and the Treatment of SSRI Resistant Depression in Adolescents study (TORDIA). Recently published data on acute treatment effects in TADS suggest that the combination of CBT and fluoxetine may produce the greatest benefit for teens in terms of both depression outcomes (71% response rate) and suicidality (TADS 2004). In this sample, fluoxetine alone produced the next best response (61%), with CBT and pill placebo producing statistically equivalent results (43% vs. 35%). The surprisingly low response rate for CBT in TADS has provoked debate (Bridge and Brent 2004), and the field awaits additional analyses of moderating variables and long-term outcomes to help clarify the results of the trial. In addition, the results of the in-progress TORDIA investigation may provide much-needed guidance for the treatment of teens who have not responded to an adequate trial of a selective serotonin reuptake inhibitor, including the relative benefits of switching to another antidepressant and/or adding CBT in addition to medication (Brent 2005).

Our understanding of the mechanisms of action of psychosocial treatments for depressed children and adolescents has significant gaps. Almost no empirical data exist on therapy mechanism, and the investigations that have attempted to test mediational models have had little success in showing that the specific cognitive, behavioral, or family processes that form the theoretical base of the intervention models are indeed responsible for the therapeutic effects (see Ackerson et al. 1998; Kolko et al. 2000). Data from moderator studies further cloud the mechanism picture. The various intervention models reviewed in this chapter are all based on a deficit framework; that is, treatments are designed to remediate cognitive vulnerabilities, improve social skills, or reduce interpersonal stress and thereby improve mood and reduce depression. However, youths with serious cognitive distortions do not fare better in CBT, which targets cognitive distortions, and family therapy does not perform better than CBT or supportive therapy with the children of depressed mothers (although the generally superior effects of CBT are attenuated for these youths; see Brent et al. 1998). Indeed, the available data seem to support the opposite model: teenagers with few cognitive distortions and many pleasant activities may do better in CBT than their peers with deficits in these areas. This would seem to be an area sorely in need of additional research. Without a solid understanding of why treatment works, it is difficult to systematically refine existing therapy protocols or to develop new, more efficacious interventions for subgroups of youths who show poor response to current therapies (for discussion, see Weersing and Weisz 2002b).

Additional treatment research in samples of depressed children also would be of substantial benefit to the field.

Only eight CBT studies investigated the effects of therapy for depressed children, and two of these randomized, controlled trials included adolescents in their samples. Notably, these two studies are the only investigations of CBT for "childhood" depression that were conducted in clinically referred samples of youths with mood disorder diagnoses (i.e., rather than youths screened for high symptoms of depression). The need for additional research is also highlighted by the apparently poorer CBT outcomes found for children compared with adolescents. Furthermore, we were unable to find a single randomized, controlled trial that tested interpersonal skills, social skills, or family therapy for children with depression (cf. parent psychoeducation plus CBT; Asarnow et al. 2002). The literature's exclusive focus on CBT techniques seemed an odd circumstance, and an opportunity for investigation, given children's less developed abstract reasoning skills compared with teenagers and greater dependence on parents (many of whom also have depression).

Finally, it also would be very helpful to have a better sense of the *effectiveness* of psychosocial interventions for youth depression under conditions more representative of active clinical service. Of the 21 clinical trials for youth depression, only 12 tested the effects of treatment in samples of youths with diagnosable depressive illness, and only 4 enrolled youths through clinical service system referral routes (see Tables 26–2, 26–3, and 26–4). The Clarke et al. (2002) investigation did embed its treatment within a real-world service setting (an HMO) and compared the effects of CBT with a usual care condition; CBT was not more effective than usual care in this particular study (although this finding may be a result of sample characteristics, as discussed earlier). The results of the IPT effectiveness study are more promising, with IPT outperforming typical school counseling services across a range of outcome measures (Mufson et al 2004). However, apart from these two examples, the use of real-world clinical samples and settings is rare in the depression treatment literature. The need for effectiveness data is made more pressing by recent investigations indicating that community mental health care for depressed youths may produce outcomes no faster or better than the natural remission rate (see Weersing and Weisz 2002a) and that practicing therapists do not find that the research literature is a helpful source of information on how to best care for patients (Addis and Krasnow 2000). By conducting studies to directly test the effectiveness of our "best" interventions under real-world conditions, we may be able to address both of these issues—providing data more immediately useful for and compelling to practicing therapists and improving the quality of everyday mental health care for depressed youths.

References

Abramson LY, Seligman MEP, Teasdale J: Learned helplessness in humans: critique and reformulation. J Abnorm Psychol 87:49–74, 1978

Abramson LY, Metalsky GI, Alloy LB: Hopelessness depression: a theory-based subtype of depression. Psychol Rev 96:358–372, 1989

Ackerson J, Scogin F, McKendree-Smith N, et al: Cognitive bibliotherapy for mild and moderate adolescent depressive symptomatology. J Consult Clin Psychol 66:685–690, 1998

Addis ME, Krasnow AD: A national survey of practicing psychologists' attitudes toward psychotherapy treatment manuals. J Consult Clin Psychol 68:331–339, 2000

Alexander J, Parsons BV: Functional Family Therapy. Pacific Grove, CA, Brooks-Cole Publishing, 1982

Asarnow JR, Goldstein MJ, Tompson M, et al: One-year outcomes of depressive disorders in child psychiatric inpatients: evaluation of the prognostic power of a brief measure of expressed emotion. J Child Psychol Psychiatry 34:129–137, 1993

Asarnow JR, Scott CV, Mintz J: A combined cognitive-behavioral family education intervention for depression in children: a treatment development study. Cognit Ther Res 26:221–229, 2002

Barbe R, Bridge J, Birmaher B, et al: Suicidality and its relationship to treatment outcome in depressed adolescents. Suicide Life Threat Behav 34:44–55, 2004

Beck AT, Rush AJ, Shaw BF, et al: Cognitive Therapy of Depression. New York, Guilford, 1979

Birmaher B, Brent DA, Kolko D, et al: Clinical outcome after short-term psychotherapy for adolescents with major depressive disorder. Arch Gen Psychiatry 57:29–36, 2000

Brent DA: Treatment of SSRI-resistant depression in adolescents (abstract). Available at: http://crisp.cit.nih.gov. Accessed May 15, 2005.

Brent DA, Perper JA, Moritz G, et al: Psychiatric risk factors of adolescent suicide: a case control study. J Am Acad Child Adolesc Psychiatry 32:521–529, 1993

Brent DA, Holder D, Kolko D, et al: A clinical psychotherapy trial for adolescent depression comparing cognitive, family, and supportive treatments. Arch Gen Psychiatry 54:877–885, 1997

Brent DA, Kolko D, Birmaher B, et al: Predictors of treatment efficacy in a clinical trial of three psychosocial treatments for adolescent depression. J Am Acad Child Adolesc Psychiatry 37:906–914, 1998

Bridge JA, Brent DA: Adolescents with depression (letter). JAMA 292:2578, 2004

Butler L, Miezitis S, Friedman R, et al: The effect of two school-based intervention programs on depressive symptoms in preadolescents. Am Educ Rec J 17:111–119, 1980

Clarke G, Hops H, Lewinsohn PM, et al: Cognitive-behavioral group treatment of adolescent depression: prediction of outcome. Behav Ther 23:341–354, 1992

Clarke GN, Hawkins W, Murphy M, et al: Targeted prevention of unipolar depressive disorder in an at-risk sample of high school adolescents: a randomized trial of group cognitive interventions. J Am Acad Child Adolesc Psychiatry 34:312–321, 1995

Clarke GN, Rohde P, Lewinsohn PM, et al: Cognitive-behavioral treatment of adolescent depression: efficacy of acute group treatment and booster sessions. J Am Acad Child Adolesc Psychiatry 38:272–279, 1999

Clarke GN, Hornbrook M, Lynch F, et al: A randomized trial of a group cognitive intervention for preventing depression in adolescent offspring of depressed parents. Arch Gen Psychiatry 85:1127–1134, 2001

Clarke GN, Hornbrook M, Lynch F, et al: Group cognitive-behavioral treatment for depressed adolescent offspring of depressed parents in a health maintenance organization. J Am Acad Child Adolesc Psychiatry 41:305–313, 2002

DeBar LL, Clarke GN, O'Connor EA, et al: Pharmacoepidemiology of child and adolescent mood disorders in an HMO (abstract). J Child Adolesc Psychopharmacol 10:236, 2000

Diamond GS, Reis B, Diamond GM, et al: Attachment-based family therapy for adolescents: a treatment development study. J Am Acad Child Adolesc Psychiatry 41:1190–1196, 2002

Gladstone TRG, Kaslow NJ: Depression and attributions in children and adolescents: a meta-analytic review. J Abnorm Child Psychol 23:597–606, 1995

Gould MS, King R, Greenwald S, et al: Psychopathology associated with suicidal ideation and attempts among children and adolescents. J Am Acad Child Adolesc Psychiatry 37:915–923, 1998

Hammen C, Rudolph K, Weisz J, et al: The context of depression in clinic-referred youth: neglected areas in treatment. J Am Acad Child Adolesc Psychiatry 38:64–71, 1999

Jayson D, Wood A, Kroll L, et al: Which depressed patients respond to cognitive-behavioral treatment? J Am Acad Child Adolesc Psychiatry 37:35–39, 1998

Kahn JS, Kehle TJ, Jenson WR, et al: Comparison of cognitive-behavioral, relaxation, and self-modeling interventions for depression among middle school students. School Psych Rev 19:196–211, 1990

Kolko D, Brent D, Baugher M, et al: Cognitive and family therapies for adolescent depression: treatment specificity, mediation and moderation. J Consult Clin Psychol 68:603–614, 2000

Kroll L, Harrington R, Jayson D, et al: Pilot study of continuation cognitive-behavioral therapy for major depression in adolescent psychiatric patients. J Am Acad Child Adolesc Psychiatry 35:1156–1161, 1996

Lewinsohn PM, Clarke GN: Psychosocial treatments for adolescent depression. Clin Psychol Rev 19:329–342, 1999

Lewinsohn PM, Clarke GN, Hops H, et al: Cognitive-behavioral treatment for depressed adolescents. Behav Ther 21:385–401, 1990

Lewinsohn PM, Seeley JR, Gotlib IH: Depression-related psychosocial variables: are they specific to depression in adolescents? J Abnorm Psychol 106:365–375, 1997

Lewinsohn PM, Gotlib IH, Hautzinger M: Behavioral treatment of unipolar depression, in International Handbook of Cognitive and Behavioural Treatments for Psychological Disorders. Edited by Caballo VE. Oxford, UK, Pergamon/Elsevier Science Ltd, 1998, pp 441–488

Liddle B, Spence SH: Cognitive-behavior therapy with depressed primary school children: a cautionary note. Behavioural Psychology 18:85–102, 1990

Moreau D, Mufson L, Weissman M, et al: Interpersonal psychotherapy for adolescent depression: description of modification and preliminary application. J Am Acad Child Adolesc Psychiatry 30:642–651, 1991

Mufson L, Fairbanks J: Interpersonal psychotherapy for depressed adolescents: a one-year naturalistic follow-up study. J Am Acad Child Adolesc Psychiatry 35:1145–1155, 1996

Mufson L, Moreau D, Weissman M, et al: Modification of interpersonal psychotherapy with depressed adolescents (IPT-A): Phase I and II studies. J Am Acad Child Adolesc Psychiatry 33:695–705, 1994

Mufson L, Weissman MW, Moreau D, et al: Efficacy of interpersonal psychotherapy for depressed adolescents. Arch Gen Psychiatry 56:573–579, 1999

Mufson L, Dorta KP, Wickramaratne P, et al: A randomized effectiveness trial of interpersonal psychotherapy for depressed adolescents. Arch Gen Psychiatry 61:577–584, 2004

Reed MK: Social skills training to reduce depression in adolescents. Adolescence 29:293–302, 1994

Reinecke MA, Ryan NE, Dubois DL: Cognitive-behavioral therapy of depression and depressive symptoms during adolescence: a review and meta-analysis. J Am Acad Child Adolesc Psychiatry 37:26–34, 1998

Reynolds WM, Coats KI: A comparison of cognitive-behavioral therapy and relaxation training for the treatment of depression in adolescents. J Consult Clin Psychol 54:653–660, 1986

Robin AL, Foster SL: Negotiating Parent-Adolescent Conflict: A Behavioral-Family Systems Approach. New York, Guilford, 1989

Rohde P, Lewinsohn PM, Seeley JR: Are adolescents changed by an episode of major depression? J Am Acad Child Adolesc Psychiatry 33:1289–1298, 1994

Rohde P, Clarke GN, Lewinsohn PM, et al: Impact of comorbidity on a cognitive-behavioral group treatment for adolescent depression. J Am Acad Child Adolesc Psychiatry 40:795–802, 2001

Rosselló J, Bernal G: Adapting cognitive-behavioral and interpersonal treatments for depressed Puerto Rican adolescents, in Psychosocial Treatments for Child and Adolescent Disorders: Empirically Based Strategies for Clinical Practice. Edited by Hibbs ED, Jensen PS. Washington, DC, American Psychological Association, 1996, pp 157–185

Rosselló J, Bernal G: The efficacy of cognitive-behavioral and interpersonal treatments for depression in Puerto Rican adolescents. J Consult Clin Psychol 67:734–745, 1999

Santor D, Kusumaker V: Open trial of interpersonal therapy in adolescents with moderate to severe major depression: effectiveness of novice IPT therapists. J Am Acad Child Adolesc Psychiatry 40:236–240, 2001

Stark KD, Reynolds WM, Kaslow NJ: A comparison of the relative efficacy of self-control therapy and a behavioral problem-solving therapy for depression in children. J Abnorm Child Psychol 15:91–113, 1987

Treatment for Adolescents With Depression Study Team: Fluoxetine, cognitive-behavioral therapy, and their combination for adolescents with depression: Treatment for Adolescents With Depression Study (TADS) randomized controlled trial. JAMA 292:807–820, 2004

Vostanis P, Feehan C, Grattan E, et al: A randomised controlled outpatient trial of cognitive-behavioural treatment for children and adolescents with depression: 9-month follow-up. J Affect Disord 40:105–116, 1996a

Vostanis P, Feehan C, Grattan E, et al: Treatment for children and adolescents with depression: lessons from a controlled trial. Clin Child Psychol Psychiatry 1:199–212, 1996b

Vostanis P, Feehan C, Grattan E: Two-year outcome of children treated for depression. Eur Child Adolesc Psychiatry 7:12–18, 1998

Weersing VR, Weisz JR: Community clinic treatment of depressed youth: benchmarking usual care against CBT clinical trials. J Consult Clin Psychol 70:299–310, 2002a

Weersing VR, Weisz JR: Mechanisms of action in youth psychotherapy. J Child Psychol Psychiatry 43:3–29, 2002b

Weissman MM, Wolk S, Wickramaratne P, et al: Children with prepubertal-onset major depressive disorder and anxiety grown up. Arch Gen Psychiatry 56:794–801, 1999

Weisz JR, Weiss B, Han SS, et al: Effects of psychotherapy with children and adolescents revisited: a meta-analysis of treatment outcome studies. Psychol Bull 117:450–468, 1995

Weisz JR, Thurber CA, Sweeney L, et al: Brief treatment of mild-to-moderate child depression using primary and secondary control enhancement training. J Consult Clin Psychol 65:703–707, 1997

Wood A, Harrington R, Moore A: Controlled trial of a brief cognitive-behavioural intervention in adolescent patients with depressive disorders. J Child Psychol Psychiatry 37:737–746, 1996

PART 6

Integrative Management of Mood Disorders

SECTION EDITOR: A. JOHN RUSH, M.D.

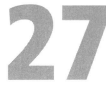

Guidelines for the Treatment of Major Depression

A. JOHN RUSH, M.D.

UNTIL THE 1980s, the medication management of major depressive disorder (MDD) was relatively straight-forward because only two classes of antidepressants were available: tricyclic antidepressants (TCAs) and mono-amine oxidase inhibitors (MAOIs). The clinician simply began with a tricyclic agent. If that agent was ineffective or poorly tolerated, a second TCA often was prescribed. Should that attempt fail, an MAOI was used, or for those with some but incomplete benefit, an augmenting agent (e.g., lithium, an anxiolytic, or a sedative-hypnotic) was added. Evidence to recommend one as opposed to another TCA was lacking. Side-effect profiles often were used to select among the options, with the notion that more-sedating agents might be preferred for the more anxious or more sleepless depressed patients on the basis of the unsubstantiated notions that greater efficacy, better tolerability, or better patient retention would ensue because of this choice. Conversely, more "activating" TCAs often were suggested for patients with more psychomotor retardation or anhedonia (Blackwell 1987).

Over the last two decades, a plethora of new antidepressant monotherapies, as well as a seemingly endless range of possible drug combinations, have led to a complex set of possible treatments. Furthermore, in the 1990s, wide

variations in physician practices were recognized in both general medicine (Andersen and Mooney 1990; Perrin et al. 1989; Wennberg 1984; Wennberg and Gittelshon 1973; Wennberg et al. 1987) and the care of depressed patients (Kramer et al. 2000; Ornstein et al. 2000). In response to wide variations in practice and with the aim of improving quality of care, practice guidelines for depressed patients were issued for primary care (Depression Guideline Panel 1993a, 1993b) and psychiatric practitioners (Altshuler et al. 2001; American Academy of Child and Adolescent Psychiatry 1998; American Psychiatric Association 1993, 2000b; Anderson et al. 2000; Ballenger 1999; Bauer et al. 2001, 2002a, 2002b; Canadian Psychiatric Association 2001; Crismon et al. 1999; Hirschfeld et al. 1997; Reesal and Lam 2001; Trivedi et al. 1998).

Guideline development also was supported by patients and families seeking predictable, higher-quality care. Furthermore, providers and organizations have sought to identify and implement more cost-efficient methods to achieve better outcomes (i.e., to maximize value for the health care dollar) (Woolf 1990). Many managed care organizations developed implicit incentives often based on explicit guidelines to constrain potentially cost-inefficient practice variations. These disease management protocols or "best practices" often were based largely on consensus rather than on direct evidence.

Only recently have researchers begun to evaluate prospectively the utility of implementing practice guidelines for depression in primary care (Katon et al. 1995, 1996, 1997, 1999; Unützer et al. 2002), psychiatric inpatients (Adli et al. 2002), and psychiatric outpatients (Rush et al. 1999a, 1999b; Trivedi et al. 2004a). In addition, a few controlled trials have been conducted to establish prospectively which of several treatment choices is preferred for patients not responding adequately to one or more previous treatments. These trials include smaller randomized trials for treatment-resistant depression (e.g., Shelton et al. 2001) and a large, ongoing multisite trial (Sequenced Treatment Alternatives to Relieve Depression; STAR*D) (M. Fava et al. 2003; Rush et al. 2004) (see http://www.star-d.org).

In this chapter, I review the concepts of treatment options, guidelines, and algorithms for MDD and highlight issues in developing and synthesizing the evidence and in implementing guidelines or algorithms. I provide a synopsis of medication guidelines and algorithms for adults with psychotic and nonpsychotic MDD and discuss the potential roles of psychotherapy in the treatment of MDD. The available evidence for the effectiveness of guidelines for clinical depression is reviewed, and clinical factors that likely affect the adaptation and potentially the effectiveness of these protocols are discussed. I conclude with comments on future directions in the evolution, implementation, and evaluation of guidelines for MDD.

Treatment Options, Guidelines, and Algorithms

The Institute of Medicine (1990) reviewed the concepts and terms used to specify various clinical treatment procedures for particular conditions. *Treatment options* refer to the different available treatments typically based on expert opinion, such as those enumerated in medical and psychiatric textbooks. The potential treatments are rarely compared or contrasted, little is said about the nature and certainty of the evidence supporting one or another treatment, and neither the sequencing of treatments nor the tactics used to implement optimally each treatment (e.g., starting dose, dose escalation, and adequate trial duration) is discussed.

With the growing emphasis on evidence-based medicine (Haynes et al. 1977; Rosenberg and Sackett 1996; Sackett 1997; Sackett and Rosenberg 1995), practice guidelines have been developed. *Practice guidelines* are "systematically developed statements to assist practi-

tioners and patient decisions about appropriate health care for specific clinical circumstances" (Institute of Medicine 1990, p. 8). Appropriate health care occurs "when the clinical benefit obtained outweighs the harm and cost involved" (Park et al. 1986). Woolf (1990) defined practice guidelines as "the official statements or policies of major organizations and agencies on the proper indications for performing a procedure or treatment or the proper management for specific clinical problems" (p. 1812). Thus, guidelines are patient care strategies developed to assist clinicians in clinical decision making.

The Institute of Medicine (1990) and the Agency for Health Care Policy and Research (AHCPR) (Clinton et al. 1994) recommended the following attributes for practice guidelines:

- *Validity:* Quality scientific and clinical evidence leads to the guidelines, which lead to projected outcomes.
- *Reliability/reproducibility:* Two groups of experts distill the same evidence to arrive at the same guidelines; recommendations are then interpreted and applied consistently in practice.
- *Clinical applicability:* The intended patient population is stated explicitly.
- *Clinical flexibility:* Guidance is given regarding variability among treatment options according to patient factors; guideline exceptions are specified.
- *Clarity:* Recommendations are stated clearly and are easy to follow.
- *Multidisciplinary process:* Key affected groups participate in guideline development.
- *Documentation:* The procedures used to develop the guidelines are specified.
- *Scheduled review:* A specific time frame for future review and possible revision is clearly stated.
- *Empirically tested:* Guidelines are empirically evaluated prospectively to assess their effect on patient outcomes.

Practice guidelines typically present specific treatment options along with the scientific evidence supporting the efficacy, safety, and tolerability of each treatment. Practice guidelines typically do not recommend specific sequences for the treatment options, although they may (if evidence is available) suggest patient groups for which a treatment is preferred or is to be avoided. Such practice guidelines are exemplified by those of the American Psychiatric Association (1993, 1994, 1997, 2000b), the AHCPR for depression in primary care (Depression Guideline Panel 1993a, 1993b), and the World Federation of Societies of Biological Psychiatry (Bauer et al. 2002a, 2002b).

Practice guidelines present a distillation of scientific information instead of expert opinions to make recommendations. However, research evidence typically lags behind or only partly addresses issues that clinicians confront on a daily basis. Most guidelines attempt to recommend preferred care—that is, care that is good for most individuals in most situations. But guidelines are based on group data, and they can only make group-based recommendations. To define *optimal* individual care, practitioners must appropriately adapt and tailor, or in some cases ignore, guideline recommendations—transforming preferred care (for a group) into optimal care (for an individual) (see Rush and Prien 1995). For example, most randomized, controlled trials are conducted for regulatory approval. Although they define the safety, tolerability, and efficacy of diverse treatments, they rarely provide definitive evidence in sufficient detail on when to choose or how to optimally implement a particular treatment for individual patients.

Algorithms, *clinical pathways*, or *disease management protocols* are more specific than guidelines because they often recommend specific treatments to be delivered in particular sequences. They specify not only the *strategies* (i.e., which treatments to use, in what order, and in what sequence) but also the *tactics* (i.e., how to implement each treatment strategy optimally). Algorithms are viewed as cognitive tools intended to assist, but not limit, clinical decision making (Jobson 1997; Kasper and Jobson 1997; Trivedi et al. 1998). A clinical algorithm often provides a flowchart to specify the clinical steps that might follow on the basis of a patient's clinical status and prior treatment response. Algorithm recommendations often rely on both scientific evidence and clinical judgment.

Rationale and Limitations of Guidelines or Algorithms

Table 27–1 highlights both the clinical and the administrative reasons for using guidelines or algorithms. They should improve clinical decision making (i.e., the quality of care), which should improve clinical outcomes, make more efficient use of resources, or both. Second, guidelines or algorithms should increase the consistency of care across both settings and clinicians so that a treatment trial (which may last 4–12 weeks) is conducted both well enough and long enough, so that a patient's response can be accurately gauged, and treatment plan revisions can be made when needed. Third, guidelines or algorithms provide a benchmark by which to define clinical outcomes achieved with a particular treatment plan. When a new treatment becomes available, it can be inserted into the algorithm at one step or another to determine empirically

where it best fits. For example, if a new antidepressant becomes available, it can be inserted after one or after two trials with available or generic agents to determine where it may fit.

Algorithms also may serve several key administrative goals, such as making optimal use of finite resources (i.e., improve the cost-efficiency of treatment) and making costs more predictable. Algorithms also can provide information by which to relate costs to specific treatments or to particular outcomes. With the insertion of a new treatment into an established stepwise sequence of care at various points, one also can gauge the cost benefit of the new treatment.

In essence, we hope that algorithms or guidelines will produce 1) a more rapid response, 2) a more complete response (i.e., symptom reduction, functional restoration), 3) lower patient attrition, and 4) lower side-effect burdens for more patients than usual care produces. Figure 27–1 provides a system perspective on the potential benefits of guidelines that improve the quality of care and clinical outcomes. Better care should reduce symptoms and improve function, resulting in less disability and less use of hospital, crisis, and emergency services (as well as courts, jails, prisons, and the welfare system), and it should reduce the risk of chronicity and secondary complications.

Algorithms also have inherent risks. The treatment recommendations may simply be wrong. Even if supported by randomized trials, the treatment may not produce better outcomes in representative patient groups, or the clinical consensus used to develop treatment recommendations (when scientific gaps exist) may be flawed. Alternatively, given the heterogeneity of depression, guideline recommendations may apply to only some but not other patient groups. Furthermore, treatment recommendations may increase cost with or without improving outcomes (Institute of Medicine 1990). At present, no randomized trials have compared one as opposed to another guideline or algorithm, but available evidence (see section "Efficacy and Effectiveness of Guidelines and Algorithms for Major Depressive Disorder" later in this chapter) indicates that depression guidelines are associated with better outcomes than is treatment as usual.

Issues in Developing Guidelines and Algorithms

Identifying and Synthesizing the Evidence

Various procedures have been used to develop guidelines or algorithms (Gilbert et al. 1998). These methods vary according to the following factors: 1) selection of topic,

TABLE 27–1. Rationale for developing and using guidelines

Clinical	Administrative
Facilitate clinical decision making	Improve cost-efficiency of treatment
Improve quality of care	Make costs more predictable
Improve clinical outcomes	Define costs related to specific treatments or outcomes
Make treatment plans consistent across sites and providers	Provide a basis for defining when new medications are cost-effective
Conveniently list options for appropriately tailoring treatment to individuals	Define where new treatments fit for optimal clinical outcomes
Provide adequate clinical documentation	Provide adequate clinical documentation

Source. Adapted from Rush et al 1998. This table is in the public domain and can be reproduced without permission, but appropriate citation is required.

2) who participates in algorithm development, 3) how the quality (certainty and relevance) of the available scientific literature is assessed, 4) how gaps in the scientific evidence are "filled in" in the absence of data, 5) how consensus is developed, 6) how and whether expert clinical judgment is used, and 7) how trade-offs between cost and clinical efficacy are considered.

Four major methods have been used to develop guidelines: informal consensus, formal consensus, evidence-based guideline development, and explicit guideline development (Woolf 1990, 1991). *Informal consensus* refers to an expert panel reaching consensus by open discussion—a global subjective judgment that may be of poor quality (Eddy 1992a).

Formal consensus, often used in the National Institutes of Health (NIH) Consensus Development Program, entails formal presentations of the evidence by experts, followed by an invited panel meeting to develop the guidelines in a closed session. These initial guideline recommendations are typically presented to an audience of the panelists' peers who may suggest further modest guideline revisions.

A variant of the formal process was pioneered by the RAND Corporation and subsequently (in a modified form) used by the Tri University Consortium (Kahn et al. 1997). This method entails the use of an expert panel, which is provided with background articles reviewing available scientific evidence relevant to the guideline topic, followed by a two-step process that uses the Delphi technique (Jones and Hunter 1995; Linstone 1978). Before the first meeting, each panelist assesses the appropriateness of several possible procedures for each of a series of indications and assigns a score from one to nine. The panel then meets and uses the scores to identify areas of disagreement. After thorough discussion, the panel res-

cores the evidence on the basis of this discussion. This method can produce a long list of appropriateness scores, which, according to Woolf (1990, 1991), can be a problem because it is difficult for clinicians to actually apply the results in practice.

Evidence-based guidelines grade the strength of recommendations according to the quality of the evidence, with grading rules established a priori. A systematic assessment of the certainty of the scientific evidence is typical of most guidelines. Level A (good research-based evidence) usually requires at least one or two randomized, controlled trials. Level B (fair research-based evidence) often entails open comparative trials or consecutive case series, for example. Level C (minimal research-based evidence) rests largely on case reports or clinical consensus (Depression Guideline Panel 1993b; Institute of Medicine 1990).

Practitioners are provided with weighted guidance as to the expected effectiveness of each treatment step. This approach has increased the scientific rigor of guidelines, but it often has led to an inability to produce recommendations because of frequent gaps in the scientific literature (Woolf 1990, 1991). Thus, neutral recommendations—neither for nor against a treatment—are often issued. The American Psychiatric Association (1993, 1994, 1997) used a modification of this approach, whereby levels of scientific credibility were provided for each recommendation, but a panel of experts reviewed the evidence and designed the guideline.

Work by Eddy (1990a, 1990b, 1990c, 1992b) has led to the use of more explicit methods for guideline development. These guideline developers specify the benefits, harms, and costs of potential interventions and derive explicit estimates of the probability of each outcome. Some critics argue that this method is too complex and requires too much time to develop the guidelines.

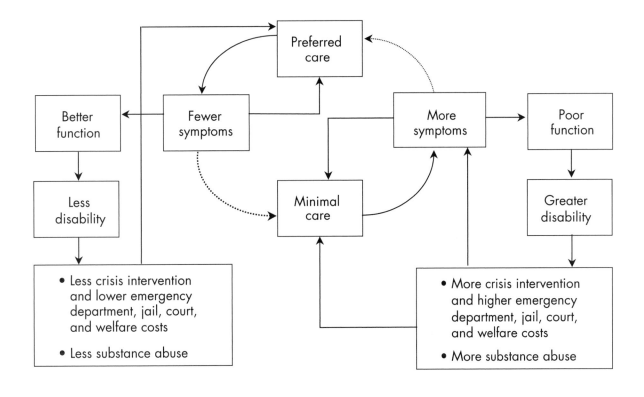

FIGURE 27–1.   Consequences of preferred versus minimal care.

Source.   Adapted from Rush et al 1998. This material is in the public domain and can be reproduced without permission, but appropriate citation is required.

Guideline Assumptions and Tensions

For both guidelines and algorithms, it is essential to specify explicitly the underlying assumptions and values that guide how to formulate, specify, and revise the recommendations (Cook and Giacomini 1999; Shaneyfelt et al. 1999). For example, one might suggest that staging treatments within an algorithm should begin with the simplest, least complicated treatments and move to more complicated treatment combinations only when patients have not responded to prior, less complicated interventions. An alternative principle could be to start with medications that are least costly on a per-pill basis (often disregarding longer-term overall costs of managing the illness).

Some of the assumptions used in developing the Texas Medication Algorithm Project (TMAP) algorithms (Chiles et al. 1999; Crismon et al. 1999; Dennehy and

Suppes 1999; Miller et al. 1999; Rush et al. 1998, 1999a, 1999b) serve to illustrate:

- Include only treatment options with proven efficacy.
- Use expert consensus only when gaps exist in the scientific literature.
- Include clinicians, patients and their families, advocates, administrators, and other decision makers in the development of the algorithms.
- Incorporate patient preference if treatments have similar efficacy and safety profiles (assumes patients' adherence increases if preference is exercised).
- Provide clinicians with choices among otherwise medically equivalent treatments.
- Use symptom ratings at key decision points to increase consistency in assessing outcomes at each algorithm stage.

The developers of guidelines also must deal with specific tensions that are an integral part of specifying guidelines

TABLE 27–2. Tensions in guideline development

Nomothetic (group) evidence versus ideographic (individual) decisions

Clinical consensus versus scientific evidence

General versus specific recommendations

Disorder-specific versus practice-specific recommendations

When and how to incorporate patient preference in the guideline recommendations

Preferred versus reimbursable practices

Cost-driven versus outcome-driven practices

Source. Adapted from Rush 2001b. Data from the Texas Medication Algorithm Project (Rush et al. 1999b). This material is in the public domain and can be reproduced without permission, but appropriate citation is required.

(Table 27–2). Guidelines may simply list treatment strategies or options with the relevant supporting evidence, providing some general evidence-based guidance as to when (for which patients, disorder types) the treatment is best or least well suited. Algorithms, on the other hand, typically provide more specific tactical information, such as recommendations on *how* to implement the treatment option once it is chosen. In either instance, the aim is to convert group-based (nomothetic) evidence, as reported in scientific studies, into recommendations applicable to individuals (ideographic decisions) (Rush and Prien 1995).

Other tensions in guidelines and algorithms include whether and to what degree to incorporate clinical consensus with or without scientific evidence, how specifically to define the target disorder (e.g., should we have separate guidelines for mild, moderate, severe, episodic, chronic, and single-episode MDD?), when and how to incorporate the role of patient preference, and whether and how to factor in issues of cost (e.g., to the treating agent or agency, to society, short- or long-term costs) (for a review, see Rush 2001b).

Perhaps the most vexing problem for guidelines and algorithms (for depression and other conditions) is whether to restrict guideline recommendations to only those treatments and treatment procedures that are currently reimbursed or that are common practice, or whether to recommend those treatments and treatment procedures with established efficacy and safety, independent of whether they are common practices or reimbursable. For example, most studies of cognitive therapy entail 12–20 sessions. Yet, reimbursement is often curtailed after 4–8 sessions, even though evidence for efficacy with so few sessions is lacking. Furthermore, evidence indicates that some who do not respond by session 6 or 8 will do so later (Rush and Thase 1999). Another example is illustrated by extended-release venlafaxine, which is often used clinically at doses in excess of those studied in randomized trials on the basis of clinical observations that higher doses produce greater efficacy. Should this common practice be recommended in the absence of controlled trial evidence?

Certainty and Applicability of Evidence

By definition, guideline and algorithm recommendations will be entirely suitable for some and wholly inappropriate for other patients (e.g., for those not included in any scientific reports). Thus, although the *certainty* of evidence is typically provided in guidelines (e.g., Institute of Medicine 2001), one also must judge the *applicability* of the evidence to the particular patient. The greater the specificity of the recommendation (e.g., specifying the starting dose and rate of dose adjustment), the greater the need for sophisticated basic and clinical knowledge and for substantial clinical experience to ensure the safe and proper adaptation of the recommendation to an individual patient.

The certainty of the available evidence may be high, yet the available evidence may have only minimal or modest applicability to the types of patients or types of depression being treated. For example, TCAs have clearly established efficacy in MDD but poorer efficacy than MAOIs in atypical depression (Quitkin et al. 1988, 1993; Thase et al. 1992a, 1995). Selective serotonin reuptake inhibitors (SSRIs) have established efficacy in MDD but may not be as effective if used as third-line treatments in patients whose symptoms have not responded to two prior treatments, one of which is another SSRI. Even though algorithms recommend options at multiple treatment steps for patients unresponsive to or not remitting with one or more prior treatments, only minimal evidence (even Level C) supports most treatment options after two prior treatments have resulted in unsatisfactory clinical outcomes.

To further elaborate on the issue of applicability, it is well known that efficacy trials for antidepressants typically engage symptomatic volunteers often recruited via media advertising. These subjects are often required to have no commonly occurring concomitant Axis I, II, or III conditions; to have no concurrent substance abuse; and to have no history of established treatment resistance. As a result, the applicability of efficacy and tolerability findings from these efficacy trial populations to more representative patient groups remains tenuous, even though the "level of evidence" is high (i.e., the scientific certainty of the findings is high, but the generalizability of the findings is questionable) (Rush and Prien 1995).

Population differences are only one important parameter that affects the applicability of guideline and algorithm recommendations. Another key difference between routine clinical care and efficacy studies are the clinical procedures (e.g., structured clinical interview to establish diagnosis, routine symptom severity assessment at each treatment visit to guide treatment implementation) that are typical for research studies but uncommon in daily practice. It is important to note that algorithms typically require a systematic assessment of symptom status at critical decision points to judge whether the treatment should be changed in dose, switched, or augmented.

Whether the procedural differences between efficacy trials and daily practice affect the clinical outcomes has yet to be fully studied. However, structured diagnostic interviewing may result in substantial disagreement with clinically rendered diagnoses (Basco et al. 2000), which would affect outcome. Furthermore, Kashner et al. (2003) found that structured interviewing changed the nature of subsequent visits and affected prescribing practices, with fewer medications being used, for example, for associated symptoms.

Procedural differences also include the timing and magnitude of dose adjustments. Efficacy trials often mandate dose increases at particular points during the acute trial. Practitioners, however, vary greatly as to when each chooses to raise the dose or even when to abandon the treatment. The timing of such decisions clearly will affect outcomes. Thus, procedural differences in prescribing affect the generalizability of efficacy trial results to daily practice.

Issues in Implementing Guidelines and Algorithms

Depression is typically a chronic or recurrent disorder. However, current practice procedures are often insufficient for the optimal implementation of a chronic disease management program. Such programs should include four essential elements: 1) practice design features, 2) patient education, 3) expert care (i.e., guideline-based care), and 4) information systems (Gilbert et al. 1998; Katon et al. 1997; Rush et al. 1999a, 1999b; Von Korff et al. 1998). *Practice design features* include appropriate appointment setting, patient reminders to keep appointments, follow-up procedures for missed appointments, and the specification of the roles for diverse providers in a multidisciplinary team. *Patient education* involves providing information about the disorder and the treatment options, setting realistic expectations about the possible treatment outcomes, developing skills in self-management, changing behavior, using social supports, and, most important, developing a clinician–patient partnership to manage the condition. *Expert care* requires education and decision support for clinicians and easy access to consultation should problems or obstacles arise. *Information systems* are needed to provide reminders and feedback to both clinicians and patients (e.g., a simplified outcome measure for providers and patients that facilitates revisions in the treatment plan, rapid access to new research that affects treatment decisions, and systems to reduce paperwork burden). Deficits in one or more of these critical parameters will likely affect clinical outcomes.

Broadly speaking, there are three major groups of obstacles to implementing depression treatment guidelines or algorithms: external obstacles, practitioner variables, and patient variables (Cabana et al. 2002). External obstacles include physical, fiscal, or procedural barriers to appropriate clinic visit frequency; appropriate clinic visit length; medication choices; access to specific medications, psychotherapies, or somatic treatments; or access to relevant consultation.

To ensure success with depression guidelines, these external barriers must be removed and incentives put in place to ensure that clinicians and the relevant treatment staff have sufficient time, skill, and support to implement the guideline recommendations.

Practitioner obstacles may include ignorance about the guidelines, beliefs that the guidelines are inappropriate or unsafe, or beliefs that they lack the skill or capacity to implement these guideline recommendations. Clearly, education, a chance to discuss and debate the guidelines, and an opportunity to test the guidelines with supervision or consultation being immediately available all help to address some of these potential obstacles.

Practitioner obstacles also can be reduced by providing credible, practical guidelines that allow a range of medically equivalent treatments and enough flexibility so that they can be tailored to each individual patient, taking into account the patient's treatment history, age, concomitant psychiatric or general medical conditions, and concomitant medications. By having several treatment options at various stages or steps in the algorithm, an algorithm or a guideline is applicable to a wide range of patients.

Even with evidence-based, credible, and straightforward depression guidelines, both *intelligent adherence* and *appropriate deviation* by clinicians are needed to optimally implement any guideline or algorithm. That is, guidelines or algorithms must be adapted to specific clinical situations, which requires both guideline and practitioner flexibility. For example, the algorithm may recommend that if a meaningful symptom reduction has not occurred by 6 weeks, the treatment type should be changed (e.g., Crismon et al. 1999). However, for some patients, perhaps those with more chronic, severe, or treatment-resistant depressions, a longer period may be needed before deciding that the initial treatment will not be successful. Thus, the timing of the critical decision point should be changed for selected patients.

A substantial degree of knowledge is required to implement, adapt, or even disregard, when appropriate, a guideline recommendation. For example, familiarity with drug-drug interactions, the effects of selected antidepressants on the cardiovascular system, and a compound of other pharmacological issues is essential for the safe and efficient adaptation of guidelines to individual patients.

Patients themselves also may present an obstacle to implementing guidelines. Direct, frequently repeated, stepwise educational opportunities (e.g., Toprac et al. 2000) to learn about the disorder, the treatment options, and the likely outcomes (both benefits and side effects) of each treatment can help patients participate in their care in an informal manner. Patient education of depressed patients has been shown both to reduce attrition and to improve symptomatic outcomes (Basco and Rush 1995). It is especially important that patients and clinicians be prepared for the likely probability that some patients may require two, three, or even more different treatments before one that is both highly effective and well tolerated is found.

Finally, guidelines or algorithms are living documents that require regular updating. For example, the American Psychiatric Association guidelines for MDD have been revised twice (American Psychiatric Association 1993, 2000b). Guidelines and algorithms should be revised often enough to ensure that they reflect key scientific evidence (thereby retaining credibility that fosters implementation) but not so often as to unnecessarily confuse clinicians without providing important and substantive, evidence-based changes.

Revisions should be based on the same process and as-

sumptions that engendered the initial guidelines, unless changes in the process and assumptions are stated in the revised versions. Typically, the availability of new treatments or of new scientifically sound information forms the rationale for guideline revisions. The greater the reliance of guidelines on clinical consensus, the shorter their shelf life, and the greater the threat to guideline credibility.

Treatment Algorithms for Major Depressive Disorder

There is no one preferred algorithm over another for MDD because no randomized comparisons of two or more algorithms are available. In this section, I present and discuss one algorithm (with some suggested minor modifications) that has been shown to be more effective in reducing depressive symptoms compared with treatment as usual as part of the TMAP (Crismon et al. 1999; Rush et al. 2003a; Trivedi et al., in press). The modifications are based on more recent Level B or C evidence and have not been evaluated by a consensus process. The algorithm is presented as an example to illustrate principles in developing such treatment plans.

The underlying principles (see subsection "Guideline Assumptions and Tensions" earlier in this chapter) rest on the notion of beginning with the simplest, medically safest, and most evidence-based treatments and then moving to the less-well-tested and/or more complex treatments (e.g., combinations of medications). The aim of treatment is to achieve sustained symptomatic remission (i.e., the virtual absence of depressive symptoms). The rationale for such an aim is well established given the evidence that depressive symptom remission, as opposed to response with residual symptoms, is associated with better day-to-day function (Agosti 1999; I.W. Miller et al. 1998; Riso et al. 1997; Simons et al. 1986) and a better prognosis (Faravelli et al. 1986; G.A. Fava 1999; Judd et al. 1998a, 1998b; Paykel et al. 1995, 1999; Thase et al. 1992b).

Treatment Algorithm for Nonpsychotic Major Depressive Disorder

Figure 27–2 provides an overview of the algorithm. Most stages or steps in the algorithm include a range of choices of antidepressant treatments. Clinicians and patients are free to select from among the choices presented on the basis of patient preference and clinician judgment (e.g., preference for one vs. another side-effect profile, desire for minimal drug-drug interactions). The treatments at each stage represent, in general, equivalent degrees of efficacy, tolerability, and safety in overdose. The treatments do differ in regard to side-effect profiles, ease of use (e.g., once- vs. twice-daily dosing), the probability of discontinuation symptoms (short half-life agents that block serotonin reuptake have a higher likelihood of discontinuation symptoms), and drug-drug interactions.

The clinician can begin with any of the seven stages proposed in the algorithm on the basis of the patient's history of treatment, clinical need for rapid response (e.g., by selecting electroconvulsive therapy [ECT] first), or evidence of preferential response of certain depressive subtypes to a class of medication (e.g., use of MAOIs as opposed to TCAs in atypical depression) (Depression Guideline Panel 1993b). The algorithm recommends that regardless of the stage chosen to begin with, for most patients, it is wise to proceed forward (e.g., stage 3 to stage 4) rather than backward (e.g., stage 3 to stage 2) once starting a stage. It is also important to obtain a definitive history of treatment (dose, duration, and response) by which to inform the choice of both stage and particular drug when initiating the algorithm. Importantly, however, patients with so-called treatment-resistant depression often have not had adequate doses or trial durations with prior medications (Bridges 1983; Brugha et al. 1992; Johnson 1974; Keller et al. 1982; Ketai 1976).

Stage 1

Stage 1 includes any of the available antidepressants except for TCAs and MAOIs. Substantial evidence indicates equivalent efficacy and medical safety in overdose among these stage 1 agents. Some post hoc analyses suggest that dual-action agents may produce higher remission rates (5%–7%) in depressed outpatients than do more selective agents (e.g., Entsuah et al. 2001; Thase et al. 2001), at least in 8-week trials. Other data (e.g., from a prospective comparison of imipramine and sertraline in a 12-week trial of chronic depression; Keller et al. 1998) indicate no difference in response or remission rates between a dual-action agent, imipramine, and the SSRI sertraline. Furthermore, in this study, for patients taking but not responding to imipramine who were crossed over to sertraline, response and remission rates were as high as for patients who did not respond initially to sertraline who were then crossed over to imipramine. However, two inpatient trials in Europe (DUAG 1 and 2; Danish University Antidepressant Group 1990, 1993) each reported greater response rates for the dual-action agent (clomipramine) than for the SSRI comparator, supporting the notion of greater efficacy for the dual-action agent. It is fair, I believe, to say that the issue is not yet resolved and will not be resolved until more prospective randomized

comparisons are available that take into account the treatment history of participants. Perhaps for some but not for other populations, a dual-action agent is more effective than the more selective agent. At any rate, the monotherapies recommended at stage 1 are supported by substantial randomized, controlled trial evidence, and selecting among them depends substantially on side effects, drug-drug interactions, likelihood of discontinuation of symptoms, and expected efficacy.

Selecting among antidepressant medication monotherapies for nonpsychotic depression remains more of an art than a science. Clues used by some practitioners are as follows:

- Select an agent that was previously shown to be effective and well tolerated for that individual.
- Select the same agent that was effective in a first-degree relative. This suggestion rests on the principle established in several trials for MAOIs versus TCAs (Mendels et al. 1983). It has not been evaluated for the newer agents.
- Select an agent with evidence of efficacy for both the depression and any co-occurring Axis I condition (Depression Guideline Panel 1993b) (e.g., select an SSRI over bupropion for depression co-occurring with obsessive-compulsive disorder). This recommendation rests on logic alone without data to support or deny its validity.
- Select an agent for which patients have a preference (usually based on the likelihood of different side effects, such as sexual dysfunction, somnolence, insomnia, or weight gain).

Other commonly used methods of selecting among antidepressants include attempting to match the side-effect profile with presenting symptoms (e.g., avoid activating antidepressants in persons with anxiety symptoms and MDD; avoid antidepressants that may cause some insomnia in depressed patients presenting with insomnia [Blackwell 1987]). However, these recommendations have not been supported. In fact, they have been found to be invalid in several retrospective data analyses (Rush et al. 2001a, 2001b; Simon et al. 1998; Stokes and Holtz 1997; Tollefson et al. 1994; Tyrer et al. 1980).

Stage 1A

If a clinical benefit that is short of remission occurs at stage 1 (or at subsequent stages), the option to augment or combine medications is provided. The best evidence for efficacy is with lithium augmentation, but that largely rests on randomized, placebo-controlled controlled trials

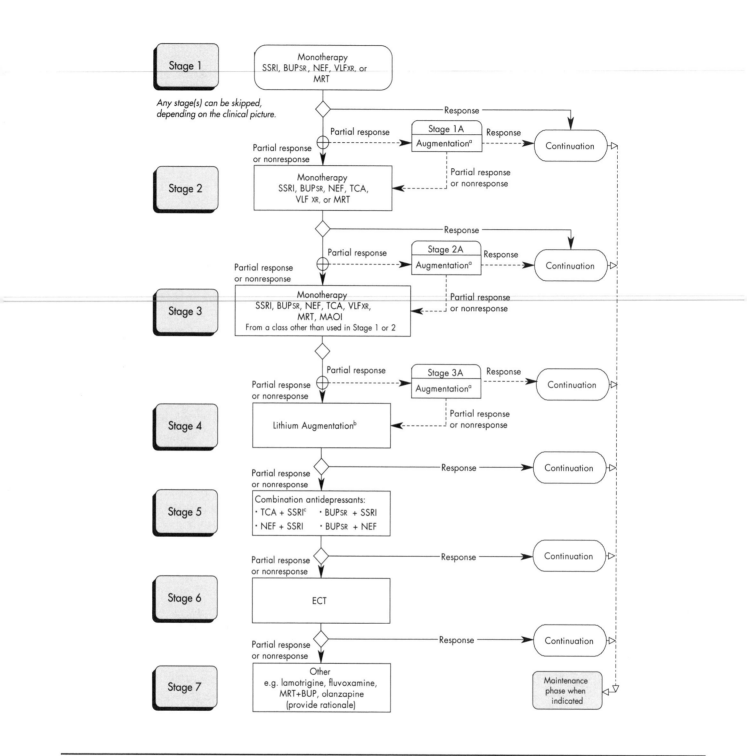

FIGURE 27–2.   Strategies for the treatment of major depression (nonpsychotic).

BUP_{SR}=bupropion sustained-release; ECT=electroconvulsive therapy; MAOI=monoamine oxidase inhibitor (consider TCA or VLF if not tried); MRT=mirtazapine; NEF=nefazodone; SSRI=selective serotonin reuptake inhibitor (fluoxetine, sertraline, paroxetine, citalopram); TCA=tricyclic antidepressant; VLF_{XR}=venlafaxine extended-release.

[a]Lithium, thyroid hormone, buspirone.

[b]Skip if lithium augmentation has already failed.

[c]Most studied combination.

Source.   Trivedi et al 2004a. This figure is in the public domain and may be reproduced without permission, but appropriate citation is required.

with lithium used to augment either a TCA or an MAOI. Other potential augmenting agents include buspirone (30–60 mg/day), which is supported by several uncontrolled case series (Bouwer and Stein 1997; Dimitriou and Dimitriou 1998; Jacobsen 1991; Joffe and Schuller 1993) but not by one randomized, placebo-controlled trial (Landen et al. 1998). A third augmentation option is with bupropion sustained-release (or extended-release), which is supported by post hoc chart reviews or by open trials (Bodkin et al. 1997; Marshall and Liebowitz 1996; Marshall et al. 1995; Spier 1998). Again, not all possible drug or augmentation combinations with either buspirone or bupropion have been evaluated.

When the algorithm was developed, some augmentation strategies were not recommended because of lack of data. Potential additional augmenting agents include the following. Triiodothyronine (T_3) (25–50 mg/day) has been shown to be as useful an augmenter as lithium in SSRI nonremitters (Joffe et al. 1993). Augmentation with mirtazapine (for SSRI nonremitters) is supported by a randomized, placebo-controlled trial (Carpenter et al. 2002). Other potential but less well-studied augmenters include stimulants (Nierenberg et al. 1998), folic acid (Coppen and Bailey 2000), and pramipexole (DeBattista et al. 2000).

Recent interest in the use of atypical antipsychotic agents as augmenting agents in nonpsychotic MDD was increased by a recent report (Shelton et al. 2001) that provided randomized, controlled trial evidence of the efficacy of the combination of fluoxetine and olanzapine in outpatients with nonpsychotic MDD whose symptoms had not remitted with fluoxetine alone (as well as two additional antidepressant monotherapies). An open case series suggested that risperidone also might be a useful SSRI augmenter (Ostroff and Nelson 1999). Nearly all of the atypical antipsychotic agents are under study as potential augmenting agents to SSRIs.

Tactical issues.   When to begin the augmentation, how long to continue the augmentation trial to determine whether it will be successful, and whether and when to stop the augmentation if it is successful are questions without definitive answers. Most studies suggest that response with a monotherapy should appear by 10–12 weeks, even for more chronically depressed patients. Remission typically follows response by 1–8 weeks, although in chronic depression, remission may occur even after 2–3 months for responders (Koran et al. 2001). Thus, if one reserves augmentation for those who have at least a response, then initiation of augmentation should not occur until 10–12 weeks after monotherapy is begun. Most augmentation trials suggest that effects should be

seen between 1 and 4 weeks after beginning the augmentation. Whether longer augmentation trials would result in even better outcomes is not clear. If augmentation is successful, most clinicians recommend continuing it for 4–9 months—the duration of continuation phase medication treatment—although no prospective data support or reject this suggestion.

Finally, if the initial augmentation trial is not successful, the probability of success with the second or third augmentation trial is not known. Some researchers believe that, as with monotherapy, the various augmentation strategies differ in regard to the target population for which each is successful. Again, we have no randomized sequenced augmentation comparisons to address this important issue.

Stages 2–7

Stage 2 basically provides the same options as stage 1, but TCAs are added. They are at stage 2, as opposed to stage 1, because of greater difficulties in tolerability and greater risk of death in the case of overdose. Stage 3 follows stage 2; MAOIs are added to the options available.

No prospective, controlled trials have been done for the third stage or beyond. Several caveats pertain to stages 2 and 3. The safety, tolerability, and efficacy of most augmentation strategies have not been prospectively evaluated under controlled conditions. The algorithm does *not* recommend mixing two or more augmentations together at the same time because both safety and efficacy for such polypharmacy are unknown. That is, if one augmentation fails, the augmentation should be stopped before the second augmentation is tried or before a switch to a new monotherapy may be chosen. Only lithium augmentation of MAOIs is recommended because of concern over safety issues.

Stage 4 mandates lithium augmentation (preferably with a TCA) because most of the controlled studies of lithium augmentation involve a TCA, but stage 4 allows for lithium augmentation with any monotherapy. Measuring lithium levels is strongly recommended for safety purposes.

Stage 5 entails a range of potential combinations of two antidepressants, most supported by Level B or C evidence. Whether combining atypical antipsychotic agents with SSRIs for nonpsychotic MDD should be relegated to stage 5 or should occur earlier is a clinical judgment, which should be based on the knowledge that all atypical antipsychotics have yet to undergo definitive, prospective, controlled trials.

Stage 6 requires ECT because of the consistent data for efficacy in highly treatment-resistant depressions

(Daly et al. 2001). Even so, the greater the level of treatment resistance, the lower the likelihood of success with ECT (or with any other treatment for that matter) (Prudic et al. 1990, 1996; Sackeim et al. 1990, 2000).

Stage 7 is based on case reports or small case series. These "treatments" have not been subjected to controlled comparisons. The "treatments" at this stage are basically educated guesses.

Treatment Algorithm for Psychotic Major Depressive Disorder

Figure 27–3 provides an algorithm for the treatment of psychotic depression. The premises for the algorithm are that

- Psychotherapy alone is not indicated.
- An antidepressant combined with an antipsychotic agent is the mainstay of treatment.
- Atypical antipsychotic agents may be used in lieu of typical antipsychotic agents, even though the Level A evidence rests largely on the use of typical antipsychotics. The exception is a recently published randomized, controlled trial of fluoxetine combined with olanzapine for psychotic depression, in which the combination exceeded the effects of either treatment alone (Corya et al. 2003).
- Before beginning ECT, a classic antipsychotic plus a tricyclic should be used given the relative abundance of randomized, controlled trials with this combination.
- ECT is clearly effective (and preferentially so) in psychotic depression, so it should come sooner rather than later in the algorithm (Petrides et al. 2001).

Strategic Issues

Whether one antipsychotic (typical or atypical) is better than another in psychotic depression has not been established in randomized, controlled trials. Whether one as opposed to another antidepressant is preferred is also unknown. Finally, whether augmenting strategies (and which ones) should be recommended is not known, although Belanoff et al. (2002) recently suggested that mifepristone might be useful in psychotic depression, and DeBattista et al. (2003, 2004) found that modafinil may be a useful and well-tolerated adjunct to standard antidepressants.

Tactical Issues

If an antipsychotic combined with an antidepressant is effective in the acute treatment phase, whether the antipsychotic dose can be lowered or even discontinued is not known. The Texas Consensus Conference Panel on

Medication Treatment of Major Depressive Disorder (Crismon et al. 1999) suggested an empirical trial of lowering the antipsychotic dose after 3–4 consecutive months of full remission with the combination. The expectation is that some patients will still require the full dose, but a minority may be able to continue in remission with a lower antipsychotic dose or even (in a few subjects) with the elimination of the antipsychotic. These recommendations rest entirely on clinical consensus, however.

Tactical Issues in Implementing Algorithms or Guidelines

Most or all of the algorithms suggested for MDD recommend diligent, specific, and timely assessments of symptomatic outcomes at critical decision points as each treatment step is implemented. This symptom assessment should entail a symptom-specific rather than a global judgment estimate of symptom status, at 4–6 weeks and at 9–12 weeks. Whether one scale is preferred over another has not been investigated, although an itemized symptom self-report more likely reflects an itemized clinician rating (the gold standard) than do either clinician or patient global ratings (Biggs et al. 2000; Shores-Wilson et al. 2002).

These critical decision points are based nearly entirely on clinical consensus, although some studies do indicate that about one-third of patients will respond after 4 weeks. For those with at least a 20% reduction by 4 (or 6) weeks, about 50% will respond, and 33% will remit, by 8–12 weeks (Nierenberg et al. 2000; Quitkin et al. 2003).

Symptom scales most easily used in practice are brief and preferably include all of the nine criteria symptom domains used to diagnose a major depressive episode by DSM-IV-TR (American Psychiatric Association 2000a). Such scales include the Patient Health Questionnaire (PHQ; Kroenke et al. 2001), the 16-item Quick Inventory of Depressive Symptomatology—Clinician Rating (QIDS-C$_{16}$) or Self-Report (QIDS-SR$_{16}$) (Rush et al. 2003b; Trivedi et al. 2004), the 30-item Inventory of Depressive Symptomatology—Clinician Rating (IDS-C$_{30}$) or Self-Report (IDS-SR$_{30}$) (Rush et al. 1986, 1996, 2000a; Trivedi et al. 2004), or the Beck Depression Inventory, 2nd Edition (BDI-II; Beck et al. 1961, 1996), among others (see American Psychiatric Association's *Handbook of Psychiatric Measures;* Rush et al. 2000b; Yonkers and Samson 2000 for a more extensive listing of possible rating scales) (see also Burt and IsHak 2002).

The Berlin Algorithm Project (Adli et al. 2003) recommends somewhat different medication steps for depressed inpatients, beginning with monotherapy, then lithium augmentation, then an irreversible MAOI, and

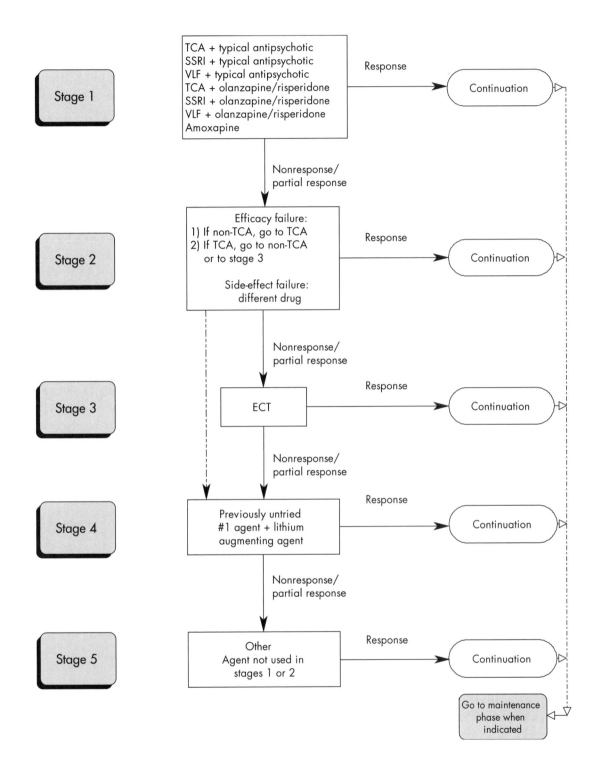

FIGURE 27–3. **Strategies for the treatment of major depression (psychotic).**

ECT=electroconvulsive therapy; SSRI=selective serotonin reuptake inhibitor; TCA=tricyclic antidepressant; VLF=venlafaxine.
Source. Trivedi et al 2004a. This figure is in the public domain and may be reproduced without permission, but appropriate citation is required.

then ECT. Of note, however, is the recommendation to measure symptomatic outcomes routinely at each treatment step to assess response. They recommend the Bech-Rafaelsen Melancholia Scale (Bech and Rafaelsen 1986).

Role of Psychotherapy

A major limitation of the Crismon et al. (1999) algorithm and its derivative (Figures 27–2 and 27–3) is the absence of a place for psychotherapy. The Crismon et al. algorithm was devised to focus on only medication because it was used to guide treatment in the TMAP (Rush et al. 2003a), wherein psychotherapy could not be made available in a consistent manner across sites. Since then, a consensus conference was held to define the role of psychotherapy in medication algorithms for depression. An extensive literature review was completed (Hollon et al. 2005), and the following recommendations were made:

1. Those psychotherapies with empirical evidence of efficacy in depression are cognitive (Beck et al. 1979), behavioral (Bellack et al. 1983; Lewinsohn and Clarke 1984; Lewinsohn et al. 1984; Nezu 1986; Rehm 1979), interpersonal (Weissman and Markowitz 2000; Weissman et al. 2002), and cognitive-behavioral analysis systems of psychotherapy (McCullough 1984, 2000, 2001, 2003).
2. These time-limited therapies should be delivered by appropriately trained and qualified therapists.
3. Combination antidepressant medication and depression-targeted, time-limited therapy is indicated in chronic depression (Keller et al. 2000). The therapy preferred for chronic depression is the cognitive-behavioral analysis system of psychotherapy (McCullough 1984, 2000, 2001, 2003), given the randomized, controlled trial evidence of efficacy (Keller et al. 2000).
4. For chronic depression, evidence (Schatzberg et al. 2005) indicates that the cognitive-behavioral analysis system of psychotherapy is effective even if medication (nefazodone) has not been successful. Thus, depression-targeted psychotherapies may be used as monotherapy at stages 1, 2, or 3. Furthermore, those doing better with therapy than with medication are those with chronic depression *and* a history of parental loss or abuse in childhood (Nemeroff et al. 2003). It could be readily argued that such therapy should be mandated at stage 1 for chronically depressed patients with such a childhood history.
5. Psychotherapy should be considered as an augmenting agent in those who achieve a response without remission to antidepressant monotherapy (GA. Fava et al. 1998; Paykel et al. 1999).

Role of Remission in Implementing Guidelines and Algorithms

It is widely accepted that full and sustained symptomatic remission is the goal of acute treatment for depression (Altshuler et al. 2001; American Academy of Child and Adolescent Psychiatry 1998; American Psychiatric Association 1993, 2000b; Anderson et al. 2000; Ballenger 1999; Bauer et al. 2001, 2002a, 2002b; Canadian Psychiatric Association 2001; Crismon et al. 1999; Hirschfeld et al. 1997; Reesal and Lam 2001; Trivedi et al. 1998). Even though remission is the aim of treatment, it is also widely recognized that sustained symptomatic remission is often difficult to achieve (Rush 2001a, 2001c).

In the course of implementing guideline recommendations, the clinician must decide at each new treatment step (whether an augmentation, a combination, or a switch) whether the individual patient has a reasonably good chance to do even better with the next treatment or whether the current treatment, even if it is associated with a benefit that is short of remission, is "as good as it gets" for this patient. Obviously, the next treatment step can be tried, and if it is unsuccessful, the clinician can return to the prior treatment if it produced better outcomes. However, given the number of medications and combinations, one could literally take a lifetime trying each alone and in combinations. The judgment as to when to conclude that maximal therapeutic benefit has been achieved for that patient is entirely uninformed by data.

Various factors likely affect the time to achieve remission, the likelihood of achieving remission, and even potentially the duration of remission, once achieved. These factors clearly include the type, dose, and duration of treatment, as well as pretreatment symptom severity and the degree of treatment resistance. Other factors likely include the presence or absence of concurrent Axis I, II, or III conditions; the level of psychosocial support and stressors; and the prior course of illness (e.g., chronic vs. acute illness).

It is well known that treatments differ in the timing of the onset of remission. For example, ECT often achieves remission in 1–3 weeks (Daly et al. 2001; Husain et al. 2004), whereas interpersonal psychotherapy (Klerman et al. 1984) or cognitive-behavioral therapy (Beck et al. 1979) may take 6–10 weeks. For medications, remission may begin within 4–12 weeks (or longer) after starting treatment (Trivedi et al. 2001). As would be expected, greater depressive symptom severity at pretreatment is typically associated with longer times to the onset of remission (Tedlow et al. 1998) and, therefore, to a lower probability of remission at earlier time points (e.g., at 6, 8, or 12 weeks).

The degree of treatment resistance affects the likelihood of and time to achieving remission independent of baseline depressive symptom severity (Sackeim 2001). The level of treatment resistance also may affect the stability of the remitted state (e.g., see Nierenberg et al. 1994).

Depressions that co-occur with certain Axis I (M. Fava et al. 1997), Axis II (Ezquiaga et al. 1999; Viinamaki et al. 2002), or Axis III conditions (Iosifescu et al. 2003; Keitner et al. 1991, 1992) are less likely to remit or may take longer to achieve remission compared with less complex depressions. Whether patients with more longstanding (i.e., chronic) depressions take longer to achieve remission or are less likely to remit with various treatments is suggested (M. Fava et al. 1997; Keller et al. 1998, 2000) but not yet unequivocally established.

The clinician implementing guideline-based care must take these clinical factors into account because they will affect the timing of critical decision points and the overall likelihood of achieving remission. For example, when confronted with a depressed patient with a chronic course, substantial baseline severity, and Axis I and II comorbidity, the clinician will need to change the timing of recommended critical decision points to later (e.g., look for a possible sign of response at 8–10 weeks, not 4–6 weeks; expect remission to be less likely, and if it is to occur, expect remission after 12–20 weeks of treatment).

Efficacy and Effectiveness of Guidelines and Algorithms for Major Depressive Disorder

The first studies to compare guideline-based care for depression with treatment as usual occurred in primary care settings (Katon et al. 1995). These studies implemented the AHCPR guidelines for the treatment of nonpsychotic MDD in primary care settings and provided the resources typically not available in primary care settings to implement the guidelines. This collaborative care model (Katon et al. 1999, 2002) entailed provision of staff to assess patient symptomatic outcome, ready access to psychiatric consultation, and sufficient staff to guide or assist the primary care providers in implementing the guidelines. Several studies of this approach by Katon have been conducted. In a recent report, enhanced care also entailed more patient education and greater visit frequency with a psychiatrist. Results showed that more patients receiving collaborative, guideline-based care stayed in treatment as compared with those receiving treatment as usual, and these patients had greater reduc-

tion in depressive symptoms and were more likely to have recovered at 3 and 6 months than were those receiving treatment as usual (Katon et al. 2002). Continued improvement in depression was noted at 28 months (Katon et al. 2002) for the moderate-severity group. For the high-severity group, benefits were noted at 6 months and at 12 months. No increase in the cost of care was reported for the collaborative group.

These findings have been corroborated by a recently published large multisite study (the Improving Mood-Promoting Access to Collaborative Treatment [IMPACT] study) (Unützer et al. 2002), which compared a collaborative care management program ($n=906$) in primary care settings for elderly outpatients with MDD with treatment as usual ($n=895$). This study provided a depression care specialist, whose duties included screening for patients, assisting in the clinical diagnosis, routinely measuring symptomatic patients' outcome with the PHQ (Kroenke et al. 2001) at each visit, following up to ensure adherence, educating patients, and providing problem-solving therapy (Nezu et al. 1989) for selected patients. Medications were delivered according to a prespecified three-step medication algorithm, consistent with American Psychiatric Association (2000b) guidelines and other algorithms (e.g., Crismon et al. 1999; Figure 27–2).

Results collected over a 12-month period following entry into treatment indicated that 45% of the intervention patients had a response as compared with 19% in the treatment as usual group. The intervention group had greater rates of treatment for depression, greater satisfaction with care, lower depression severity, less functional impairment, and greater quality of life. The intervention resulted in a net cost increase of $550 per patient per year. Both the Katon studies and the IMPACT study confirmed the efficacy of guideline-based care and illustrated the need for practice procedure changes to ensure the delivery of guideline-based care in primary care settings.

Further evidence of the clinical benefit of algorithms and guidelines over treatment as usual comes from the TMAP (Rush et al. 2003a; Suppes et al. 2003; Trivedi et al. 2004a). The TMAP was the first study to evaluate guidelines and algorithms in psychiatric outpatients with schizophrenia, bipolar disorder, or MDD treated in the public mental health sector. The intervention included specific medication treatment algorithms (Crismon et al. 1999; A.L. Miller et al. 1999; Suppes et al. 2001), the regular systematic assessment of symptoms and side effects at each medication visit (with the IDS-C$_{30}$ and IDS-SR$_{30}$) (Rush et al. 1986, 1996, 2000a; Trivedi et al. 2004b), the provision of a patient and family educational program (Toprac et al. 2000), and the provision of additional staff (the clinical research coordinator) to provide more frequent visits, closer follow-up of patients, and patient and family education and to guide physicians in the implementation of the algorithms.

Results (Trivedi et al. 2004a) showed a substantial clinically and statistically greater benefit in terms of depressive symptoms, function, and side-effect burden for the algorithm group (n=175) as compared with the treatment as usual group (n=175). Most dramatic differences were seen after 3 months of treatment. Both groups continued to improve over the year, and the algorithm group continued to sustain its advantage over treatment as usual.

The Berlin Algorithm Project is a three-phase project that evaluates algorithm-guided treatments for inpatients with depressive disorders treated by psychiatrists. Phase I is a 2-year pilot study to evaluate the effectiveness, feasibility, and acceptability of a standardized stepwise drug treatment regimen among algorithm users (Adli et al. 2002; Linden et al. 1994). The treatment steps in the algorithm, provided in sequence, are as follows:

1. Taper the previous unsuccessful medication.
2. Begin antidepressant monotherapy, including high doses if tolerated.
3. Augment with lithium.
4. Use an irreversible MAOI.
5. Initiate ECT.

Symptom assessment at each step is required (with the Bech-Rafaelsen Melancholia Scale; Bech and Rafaelsen 1986). Of 248 patients with depression, 119 (48%) were enrolled in the standardized stepwise drug treatment regimen protocol (129 [52%] were not included, mostly because of individualized treatment procedures). An intent-to-treat analysis showed that 38% of those enrolled achieved remission, whereas another 34% achieved response without remission in Phase I.

Phase II, a randomized, controlled, single-center study, compared the standardized stepwise drug treatment regimen with treatment as usual (Adli et al. 2002; Bauer et al. 2001). The standardized stepwise drug treatment regimen in this study included 10 steps. Standardized stepwise drug treatment was twice as likely to produce remission as was treatment as usual (P=0.004) (Adli et al. 2003). The remitted patients in standardized stepwise drug treatment had fewer switches than did those who remitted with treatment as usual, and polypharmacy was less frequent in standardized stepwise drug treatment regimen remitters than in treatment as usual remitters. Phase III, a nationwide randomized, controlled trial to compare two different algorithms with treatment as usual, is ongoing.

In summary, several comparative randomized, controlled trials recommend algorithm- or guideline-based

care over treatment as usual for MDD. The preferred algorithm, if there is one, is yet to be defined. Whether particular subgroups of patients with MDD would fare better with one as opposed to another algorithm deserves study.

To conduct trials comparing the effectiveness of algorithm- or guideline-based care, whether in the United States or Germany and whether in primary or psychiatric care settings, *changes in practice procedures* (and, in fact, often provision of additional resources to make these changes) were needed for the intervention group. The rationale for the changes was to ensure that guideline-based care was in fact being delivered. These changes largely reflect a shift to a chronic disease model of care for depression (Katon et al. 1995; Unützer et al. 2002). Thus, the differential advantage of algorithm- or guideline-based care over treatment as usual may be a result of one or more of the inherent differences in the practice procedures in these two groups. For the guideline-based care groups, these differences typically include greater visit frequency, the regular use of itemized symptom severity assessments at treatment visits to inform providers of the results of the current treatment step, specification of the recommended duration and doses of treatment, specification of critical decision points for each treatment step (i.e., time and symptom change-based cues for when to take the next treatment step), and greater use of patient education. Given the uniformly positive findings to date, these practice procedure changes can be recommended now. However, note that more intensive programs to manage depression, although more effective, also may be more costly (Badamgarav et al. 2003).

Conclusion and Future Directions

The development and evaluation of guidelines and algorithms for the treatment of depression has begun only within the last decade. Such efforts hold much promise in improving the quality, cost-efficiency, and clinical outcomes of care for depressed patients. Furthermore, several large studies provided evidence that such algorithm- or guideline-based care is associated with better outcomes than usual care in both primary care (Katon et al. 1995; Unützer et al. 2002) and psychiatric practice settings (Adli et al. 2003; Rush et al. 2003a; Trivedi et al. 2004a).

Every study of algorithms or guidelines, however, has had to incorporate practice changes to ensure the optimal delivery of care. These practice changes likely contribute substantially to better outcomes with the algorithm or guideline. These changes include the provision of 1) extra staff time to obtain repeated measurement of symptom response at each step in the algorithm and to pursue patients who miss appointments, 2) often a higher frequency of treatment visits and/or longer visits to ensure timely change in doses or types of treatment, 3) patient and family education, and 4) readily available medications recommended in the algorithm. Even with these changes, algorithm nonadherence by providers is not rare (Adli et al. 2003). Whether these occasions of algorithm nonadherence affect the clinical outcomes for the better or worse deserves study. It also would be essential to conduct studies to determine the independent contribution of practice procedure changes alone and of the treatment algorithms themselves on outcome.

Many other questions also remain unanswered, including 1) whether computer-assisted clinical decision support systems improve algorithm adherence and clinical outcomes; 2) whether one or another treatment sequence is recommended for a particular type of depression (e.g., early-onset versus later-onset MDD) (i.e., Is there a "best" algorithm for particular types of depression?); 3) when and how to decide that symptom remission for an individual patient is not attainable with current therapies; and 4) whether and which algorithm deviations negatively affect outcomes.

Perhaps the most important issue is to define the next best or preferred treatment choices in patients who have not responded adequately to one or more prior treatments in prospective controlled trials. For example, when is psychotherapy alone (or combined with medication) essential? Or, is a shift out of class following a failed SSRI trial more effective than a switch within class (i.e., from one SSRI to another)? The ongoing STAR*D trial (see http://www.star-d.org) should provide some answers to these questions (M. Fava et al. 2003; Lavori et al. 2001; Rush et al. 2004). This trial is comparing three augmentation treatments (bupropion sustained-release, buspirone, cognitive therapy) and four switch treatments (bupropion sustained-release, cognitive therapy, sertraline, and venlafaxine extended-release) following inadequate response to citalopram. This trial also is evaluating different switch and augmentation options at the third treatment step and two switch options at the fourth step.

Answers to these questions and the pursuit of more specific and effective algorithms and guidelines will require substantial multiyear research efforts. However, given the public health significance and the remarkable degree of disability and cost associated with depression, such investments are dearly needed and likely to further improve the care of these patients.

While work on algorithms and guidelines has begun in adults, analogous approaches have begun in children and adolescents (Hughes et al. 1999; Pliszka et al. 2003) and may be needed as well for the elderly or the medically frag-

ile depressed patient. Perhaps, in the near future, we may anticipate that the approach to the treatment of depression will evolve from an empirically informed, yet still trial-and-error, approach to a more selective, targeted approach that uses biological or genetic markers either to avoid potentially ineffective or poorly tolerated treatments or to select the preferred, most likely successful treatments. These advances should further increase the effectiveness and the cost-efficiency of the treatment of depression.

References

Adli M, Berghofer A, Linden M, et al: Effectiveness and feasibility of a standardized stepwise drug treatment regimen algorithm for inpatients with depressive disorders: results of a 2-year observational algorithm study. J Clin Psychiatry 63:782–790, 2002

Adli M, Rush AJ, Moller HJ, et al: Algorithms for optimizing the treatment of depression: making the right decision at the right time. Pharmacopsychiatry 36 (suppl 3):222–229, 2003

Agosti V: Predictors of persistent social impairment among recovered depressed outpatients. J Affect Disord 55:215–219, 1999

Altshuler LL, Cohen LS, Moline ML, et al: Expert Consensus Panel for Depression in Women: The Expert Consensus Guideline Series: Treatment of depression in women. Postgrad Med 111 (special issue):1–107, 2001

American Academy of Child and Adolescent Psychiatry: Practice parameters for the assessment and treatment of children and adolescents with depressive disorders. J Am Acad Child Adolesc Psychiatry 37 (suppl 10):63S–83S, 1998

American Psychiatric Association: Practice guideline for major depressive disorder in adults. Am J Psychiatry 150 (suppl 4):1–26, 1993

American Psychiatric Association: Practice guideline for the treatment of patients with bipolar disorder. Am J Psychiatry 151 (suppl 12):1–36, 1994

American Psychiatric Association: Practice guideline for the treatment of patients with schizophrenia. Am J Psychiatry 154 (suppl 4):1–63, 1997

American Psychiatric Association: Diagnostic and Statistical Manual of Mental Disorders, 4th Edition, Text Revision. Washington, DC, American Psychiatric Association, 2000a

American Psychiatric Association: Practice guideline for the treatment of patients with major depressive disorder (revision). Am J Psychiatry 157 (suppl 4):1–45, 2000b

Andersen TF, Mooney G (eds): The Challenge of Medical Practice Variations. London, England, Macmillan, 1990

Anderson IM, Nutt DJ, Deakin JFW: Evidence-based guidelines for treating depressive disorders with antidepressants: a revision of the 1993 British Association for Psychopharmacology guidelines. J Psychopharmacol 14:3–20, 2000

Badamgarav E, Weingarten SR, Henning JM, et al: Effectiveness of disease management programs in depression: a systematic review. Am J Psychiatry 160:2080–2090, 2003

Ballenger JC: Clinical guidelines for establishing remission in patients with depression and anxiety. J Clin Psychiatry 60 (suppl 22):29–34, 1999

Basco MR, Rush AJ: Compliance with pharmacotherapy in mood disorders. Psychiatr Ann 25:269–270, 278–279, 1995

Basco MR, Bostic JQ, Davies D, et al: Methods to improve diagnostic accuracy in a community mental health setting. Am J Psychiatry 157:1599–1605, 2000

Bauer M, Adli M, Kiesslinger U, et al: Algorithm-guided treatment vs. treatment as usual: randomized trial in inpatients with depression. Abstract presented at the 154th annual meeting of the American Psychiatric Association, New Orleans, LA, May 5–10, 2001

Bauer M, Whybrow PC, Angst J, et al: World Federation of Societies of Biological Psychiatry (WFSBP) guidelines for biological treatment of unipolar depressive disorders, part 1: acute and continuation treatment of major depressive disorder. World J Biol Psychiatry 3:5–43, 2002a

Bauer M, Whybrow PC, Angst J, et al: World Federation of Societies of Biological Psychiatry (WFSBP) guidelines for biological treatment of unipolar depressive disorders, part 2: maintenance treatment of major depressive disorder and treatment of chronic depressive disorders and subthreshold depressions. World J Biol Psychiatry 3:69–86, 2002b

Bech P, Rafaelsen OJ: The Melancholia Scale: development, consistency, validity and utility, in Assessment of Depression. Edited by Sartorius N, Ban TA. Berlin, Germany, Springer, 1986, pp 259–269

Beck AT, Ward CH, Mendelson M, et al: An inventory for measuring depression. Arch Gen Psychiatry 4:561–571, 1961

Beck AT, Rush AJ, Shaw BF, et al: Cognitive Therapy of Depression. New York, Guilford, 1979

Beck AT, Steer RA, Brown GK: Beck Depression Inventory, 2nd Edition. San Antonio, TX, Psychological Corporation, 1996

Belanoff JK, Rothschild AJ, Cassidy F, et al: An open label trial of C-1073 (mifepristone) for psychotic major depression. Biol Psychiatry 52:386–392, 2002

Bellack AS, Hersen M, Himmelhoch JM: A comparison of social-skills training, pharmacotherapy and psychotherapy for depression. Behav Res Ther 21:101–107, 1983

Biggs MM, Shores-Wilson K, Rush AJ, et al: A comparison of alternative assessments of depressive symptom severity: a pilot study. Psychiatry Res 96:269–279, 2000

Blackwell B: Side effects of antidepressant drugs, in Psychiatry Update: The American Psychiatric Association Annual Review, Vol 6. Edited by Hales RE, Frances AJ. Washington, DC, American Psychiatric Press, 1987, pp 724–745

Bodkin JA, Lasser RA, Wines JD Jr, et al: Combining serotonin reuptake inhibitors and bupropion in partial responders to antidepressant monotherapy. J Clin Psychiatry 58:137–145, 1997

Bouwer C, Stein DJ: Buspirone is an effective augmenting agent of serotonin selective re-uptake inhibitors in severe treatment-refractory depression. S Afr Med J 87 (4 suppl):534–537, 540, 1997

Bridges PK: "…and a small dose of an antidepressant might help." Br J Psychiatry 142:626–628, 1983

Brugha TS, Bebbington PE, MacCarthy B, et al: Antidepressants may not assist recovery in practice: a naturalistic prospective study. Acta Psychiatr Scand 86:5–11, 1992

Burt T, IsHak WW: Outcome measurement in mood disorders, in Outcome Measurement in Psychiatry: A Critical Review. Edited by IsHak WW, Burt T. Washington, DC, American Psychiatric Publishing, 2002, pp 155–190

Cabana MD, Rushton JL, Rush AJ: Implementing practice guidelines for depression: applying a new framework to an old problem. Gen Hosp Psychiatry 24:35–42, 2002

Canadian Psychiatric Association: Clinical guidelines for the treatment of depressive disorders. Can J Psychiatry 46 (suppl 1):13–90, 2001

Carpenter LL, Yasmin S, Price LH: A double-blind, placebo-controlled study of mirtazapine augmentation for refractory depression. Biol Psychiatry 51:183–188, 2002

Chiles JA, Miller AL, Crismon ML, et al: The Texas Medication Algorithm Project: development and implementation of the schizophrenia algorithm. Psychiatr Serv 50:69–74, 1999

Clinton JJ, McCormick K, Besteman J: Enhancing clinical practice: the role of practice guidelines. Am Psychol 49:30–33, 1994

Cook D, Giacomini M: The trials and tribulations of clinical practice guidelines. JAMA 281:1950–1951, 1999

Coppen A, Bailey J: Enhancement of the antidepressant action of fluoxetine by folic acid: a randomised, placebo controlled trial. J Affect Disord 60:121–130, 2000

Corya SA, Andersen SW, Detke HC, et al: Long-term antidepressant efficacy and safety of olanzapine/fluoxetine combination: a 76-week open-label study. J Clin Psychiatry 64:1349–1356, 2003

Crismon ML, Trivedi M, Pigott TA, et al: The Texas Medication Algorithm Project: report of the Texas Consensus Conference Panel on Medication Treatment of Major Depressive Disorder. J Clin Psychiatry 60:142–156, 1999

Daly JJ, Prudic J, Devanand DP, et al: ECT in bipolar and unipolar depression: differences in speed of response. Bipolar Disord 3:95–104, 2001

Danish University Antidepressant Group: Paroxetine: a selective serotonin reuptake inhibitor showing better tolerance, but weaker antidepressant effect than clomipramine in a controlled multicenter study. J Affect Disord 18:289–299, 1990

Danish University Antidepressant Group: Moclobemide: a reversible MAO-A-inhibitor showing weaker antidepressant effect than clomipramine in a controlled multicenter study. J Affect Disord 28:105–116, 1993

DeBattista C, Solvason HB, Breen JA, et al: Pramipexole augmentation of a selective serotonin reuptake inhibitor in the treatment of depression. J Clin Psychopharmacol 20:274–275, 2000

DeBattista C, Doghramji K, Menza MA, et al: Adjunct modafinil for the short-term treatment of fatigue and sleepiness in patients with major depressive disorder: a preliminary double-blind, placebo-controlled study. J Clin Psychiatry 64:1057–1064, 2003

DeBattista C, Lembke A, Solvason HB, et al: A prospective trial of modafinil as an adjunctive treatment of major depression. J Clin Psychopharmacol 24:87–90, 2004

Dennehy EB, Suppes T: Medication algorithms for bipolar disorder. Journal of Practical Psychiatry and Behavioral Health 5:142–152, 1999

Depression Guideline Panel: Clinical Practice Guideline, Number 5: Depression in Primary Care, Vol 1: Detection and Diagnosis (AHCPR Publ No 93-0550). Rockville, MD, Agency for Health Care Policy and Research, 1993a

Depression Guideline Panel: Clinical Practice Guideline, Number 5. Depression in Primary Care, Vol 2: Treatment of Major Depression (AHCPR Publ No 93-0551). Rockville, MD, Agency for Health Care Policy and Research, 1993b

Dimitriou EC, Dimitriou CE: Buspirone augmentation of antidepressant therapy. J Clin Psychopharmacol 18:465–469, 1998

Eddy DM: Guidelines for policy statements: the explicit approach. JAMA 263:2239–2240, 1990a

Eddy DM: Practice policies—what are they? JAMA 263:877–880, 1990b

Eddy DM: Practice policies—where do they come from? JAMA 263:1265–1275, 1990c

Eddy DM: Clinical decision making: from theory to practice: applying cost-effectiveness analysis: the inside story. JAMA 268:2575–2582, 1992a

Eddy DM: A Manual for Assessing Health Practices and Designing Practice Policies. Philadelphia, PA, American College of Physicians, 1992b

Entsuah AR, Huang H, Thase ME: Response and remission rates in different subpopulations with major depressive disorder administered venlafaxine, selective serotonin reuptake inhibitors, or placebo. J Clin Psychiatry 62:869–877, 2001

Ezquiaga E, Garcia A, Pallares T, et al: Psychosocial predictors of outcome in major depression: a prospective 12-month study. J Affect Disord 52:209–216, 1999

Faravelli C, Ambonetti A, Pallanti S, et al: Depressive relapses and incomplete recovery from index episode. Am J Psychiatry 143:888–891, 1986

Fava GA: Subclinical symptoms in mood disorders: pathophysiological and therapeutic implications. Psychol Med 29:47–61, 1999

Fava GA, Rafanelli C, Grandi S, et al: Prevention of recurrent depression with cognitive behavioral therapy: preliminary findings. Arch Gen Psychiatry 55:816–820, 1998

Fava M, Uebelacker LA, Alpert JE, et al: Major depressive subtypes and treatment response. Biol Psychiatry 42:568–576, 1997

Fava M, Rush AJ, Trivedi MH, et al: Background and rationale for the sequenced treatment alternatives to relieve depression (STAR*D) study. Psychiatr Clin North Am 26:457–494, 2003

Gilbert DA, Altshuler KZ, Rago WV, et al: Texas Medication Algorithm Project: definitions, rationale and methods to develop medication algorithms. J Clin Psychiatry 59:345–351, 1998

Haynes RB, Taylor DW, Sackett DL: Compliance in Health Care. Baltimore, MD, Johns Hopkins University Press, 1977

Hirschfeld RM, Keller MB, Panico S, et al: The National Depressive and Manic-Depressive Association consensus statement on the undertreatment of depression. JAMA 277:333–340, 1997

Hollon SD, Jarrett RB, Nierenberg AA, et al: Psychotherapy and medication in the treatment of adult and geriatric depression: which monotherapy or combined treatment? J Clin Psychiatry 66:455–468, 2005

Hughes CW, Emslie GJ, Crismon ML, et al: The Texas Children's Medication Algorithm Project: report of the Texas Consensus Conference Panel on medication treatment of childhood major depressive disorder. J Am Acad Child Adolesc Psychiatry 38:1442–1454, 1999

Husain MM, Rush AJ, Fink M, et al: Speed of response and remission in major depressive disorder with acute electroconvulsive therapy (ECT): a Consortium for Research in ECT (CORE) report. J Clin Psychiatry 65:485–491, 2004

Institute of Medicine Committee on Quality of Health Care in America: Crossing the Quality Chasm: A New Health System for the 21st Century. Washington, DC, National Academies Press, 2001

Institute of Medicine Committee to Advise the Public Health Service on Clinical Practice Guidelines, in Clinical Practice Guidelines: Directions for a New Program. Edited by Field MJ, Lohr KN. Washington, DC, National Academy Press, 1990

Iosifescu DV, Nierenberg AA, Alpert JE, et al: The impact of medical comorbidity on acute treatment in major depressive disorder. Am J Psychiatry 160:2122–2127, 2003

Jacobsen FM: Possible augmentation of antidepressant response by buspirone. J Clin Psychiatry 52:217–220, 1991

Jobson K: International Psychopharmacology Algorithm Project: algorithms in psychopharmacology. International Journal of Psychiatry in Clinical Practice 1 (suppl 1):S3–S4, 1997

Joffe RT, Schuller DR: An open study of buspirone augmentation of serotonin reuptake inhibitors in refractory depression. J Clin Psychiatry 54:269–271, 1993

Joffe RT, Singer W, Levitt AJ, et al: A placebo-controlled comparison of lithium and triiodothyronine augmentation of tricyclic antidepressants in unipolar refractory depression. Arch Gen Psychiatry 50:387–393, 1993

Johnson DAW: A study of the use of antidepressant medication in general practice. Br J Psychiatry 125:186–192, 1974

Jones J, Hunter D: Consensus methods for medical and health services research. BMJ 311:376–380, 1995

Judd LL, Akiskal HS, Maser JD, et al: Major depressive disorder: a prospective study of residual subthreshold depressive symptoms as predictor of rapid relapse. J Affect Disord 50:97–108, 1998a

Judd LL, Akiskal HS, Maser JD, et al: A prospective 12-year study of subsyndromal and syndromal depressive symptoms in unipolar major depressive disorders. Arch Gen Psychiatry 55:694–700, 1998b

Kahn D, Docherty J, Carpenter D, et al: Consensus methods in practice guideline development: a review and description of a new method. Psychopharmacol Bull 33:631–639, 1997

Kashner TM, Rush AJ, Suris A, et al: Impact of structured clinical interviews on physicians' practices in community mental health settings. Psychiatr Serv 54:712–718, 2003

Kasper S, Jobson K: First European Meeting for Algorithms on the Psychopharmacology of Psychiatric Disorders. International Journal of Psychiatry in Clinical Practice 1 (suppl 1):S1, 1997

Katon W, Von Korff M, Lin E, et al: Collaborative management to achieve treatment guidelines: impact on depression in primary care. JAMA 273:1026–1031, 1995

Katon W, Robinson P, Von Korff M, et al: A multifaceted intervention to improve treatment of depression in primary care. Arch Gen Psychiatry 53:924–932, 1996

Katon W, Von Korff M, Lin E, et al: Population-based care of depression: effective disease management strategies to decrease prevalence. Gen Hosp Psychiatry 19:169–178, 1997

Katon W, Von Korff M, Lin E, et al: Stepped collaborative care for primary care patients with persistent symptoms of depression: a randomized trial. Arch Gen Psychiatry 56:1109–1115, 1999

Katon W, Russo J, Frank E, et al: Predictors of nonresponse to treatment in primary care patients with dysthymia. Gen Hosp Psychiatry 24:20–27, 2002

Keitner GI, Ryan CE, Miller IW, et al: 12-Month outcome of patients with major depression and comorbid psychiatric or medical illness (compound depression). Am J Psychiatry 148:345–350, 1991

Keitner GI, Ryan CE, Miller IW, et al: Recovery and major depression: factors associated with twelve-month outcome. Am J Psychiatry 149:93–99, 1992

Keller MB, Klerman GL, Lavori PW, et al: Treatment received by depressed patients. JAMA 248:1848–1855, 1982

Keller MB, Gelenberg AJ, Hirschfeld RM, et al: The treatment of chronic depression, part 2: a double-blind, randomized trial of sertraline and imipramine. J Clin Psychiatry 59:598–607, 1998

Keller MB, McCullough JP, Klein DN, et al: A comparison of nefazodone, the cognitive behavioral-analysis system of psychotherapy, and their combination for the treatment of chronic depression. N Engl J Med 342:1462–1470, 2000

Ketai R: Family practitioners' knowledge about treatment of depressive illness. JAMA 235:2600–2603, 1976

Klerman GL, Weissman MM, Rounsaville BJ, et al: Interpersonal Psychotherapy of Depression. New York, Basic Books, 1984

Koran LM, Gelenberg AJ, Kornstein SG, et al: Sertraline versus imipramine to prevent relapse in chronic depression. J Affect Disord 65:27–36, 2001

Kramer TL, Daniels AS, Zieman GL, et al: Psychiatric practice variations in the diagnosis and treatment of major depression. Psychiatr Serv 51:336–340, 2000

Kroenke K, Spitzer RL, Williams JBW: The PHQ-9: validity of a brief depression severity measure. J Gen Intern Med 16:606–613, 2001

Landen M, Bjorling G, Agren H, et al: A randomized, double-blind, placebo-controlled trial of buspirone in combination with an SSRI in patients with treatment-refractory depression. J Clin Psychiatry 59:664–668, 1998

Lavori PW, Rush AJ, Wisniewski SR, et al: Strengthening clinical effectiveness trials: equipoise-stratified randomization. Biol Psychiatry 50:792–801, 2001

Lewinsohn PM, Clarke GN: Group treatment of depressed individuals: the "Coping with Depression" course. Adv Behav Res Ther 6:99–114, 1984

Lewinsohn PM, Antonuccio DA, Steinmetz J, et al: The Coping with Depression Course: A Psychoeducational Intervention for Unipolar Depression. Eugene, OR, Castalia Press, 1984

Linden M, Helmchen H, Mackert A, et al: Structure and feasibility of a standardized stepwise drug treatment regimen (SSTR) for depressed inpatients. Pharmacopsychiatry 27 (suppl 1):51–53, 1994

Linstone HA: The Delphi technique, in Handbook of Futures Research. Edited by Fowles RB. Westport, CT, Greenwood, 1978, pp 273–300

Marshall RD, Liebowitz MR: Paroxetine/bupropion combination treatment for refractory depression. J Clin Psychopharmacol 16:80–81, 1996

Marshall RD, Randall D, Johannet CM, et al: Bupropion and sertraline combination treatment in refractory depression. J Psychopharmacol 9:284–286, 1995

McCullough JP Jr: Cognitive-behavioral analysis system of psychotherapy: an interactional treatment approach for dysthymic disorder. Psychiatry 47:234–250, 1984

McCullough JP Jr: Treatment for Chronic Depression: Cognitive-Behavioral Analysis System of Psychotherapy. New York, Guilford, 2000

McCullough JP Jr: Skills Training Manual for Diagnosing and Treating Chronic Depression: Cognitive Behavioral Analysis System of Psychotherapy. New York, Guilford, 2001

McCullough JP Jr: Treatment for chronic depression using Cognitive Behavioral Analysis System of Psychotherapy (CBASP). J Clin Psychol 59:833–846, 2003

Mendels J, Amin MM, Chouinard G, et al: A comparative study of bupropion and amitriptyline in depressed outpatients. J Clin Psychiatry 44 (5 pt 2):118–120, 1983

Miller AL, Chiles JA, Chiles JK, et al: The Texas Medication Algorithm Project (TMAP) schizophrenia algorithms. J Clin Psychiatry 60:649–657, 1999

Miller IW, Keitner GI, Schatzberg AJ, et al: The treatment of chronic depression, part 3: psychosocial functioning before and after treatment with sertraline or imipramine. J Clin Psychiatry 59:608–619, 1998

Nemeroff CB, Heim CM, Thase ME, et al: Differential responses to psychotherapy versus pharmacotherapy in patients with chronic forms of major depression and childhood trauma. Proc Natl Acad Sci U S A 100:14293–14296, 2003

Nezu AM: Efficacy of a social problem-solving therapy approach for unipolar depression. J Consult Clin Psychol 54:196–202, 1986

Nezu AM, Nezu CM, Perri MG: Problem-Solving Therapy for Depression: Theory, Research, and Clinical Guidelines. New York, Wiley, 1989

Nierenberg AA, Dougherty D, Rosenbaum JF: Dopaminergic agents and stimulants as antidepressant augmentation strategies. J Clin Psychiatry 59 (suppl 5):60–63; discussion 64, 1998

Nierenberg AA, Feighner JP, Rudolph R, et al: Venlafaxine for treatment-resistant unipolar depression. J Clin Psychopharmacol 14:419–423, 1994

Nierenberg AA, Farabaugh AH, Alpert JE, et al: Timing of onset of antidepressant response with fluoxetine treatment. Am J Psychiatry 157:1423–1428, 2000

Ornstein S, Stuart G, Jenkins R: Depression diagnoses and antidepressant use in primary care practices: a study from the Practice Partner Research Network (PPRNet). J Fam Pract 49:68–72, 2000

Ostroff RB, Nelson JC: Risperidone augmentation of selective serotonin reuptake inhibitors in major depression. J Clin Psychiatry 60:256–259, 1999

Park RE, Fink A, Brook RH, et al: Physician ratings or appropriate indications for six medical and surgical procedures. Am J Public Health 76:766–772, 1986

Paykel ES, Ramana R, Cooper Z, et al: Residual symptoms after partial remission: an important outcome in depression. Psychol Med 25:1171–1180, 1995

Paykel ES, Scott J, Teasdale JD, et al: Prevention of relapse in residual depression by cognitive therapy: a controlled trial. Arch Gen Psychiatry 56:829–835, 1999

Perrin JM, Homer CJ, Berwick DM, et al: Variations in rates of hospitalization of children in three urban communities. N Engl J Med 320:1183–1187, 1989

Petrides G, Fink M, Husain MM, et al: ECT remission rates in psychotic versus nonpsychotic depressed patients: a report from CORE. J ECT 17:244–253, 2001

Pliszka SR, Lopez M, Crismon ML, et al: A feasibility study of the Children's Medication Algorithm Project (CMAP) algorithm for the treatment of ADHD. J Am Acad Child Adolesc Psychiatry 42:279–287, 2003

Prudic J, Sackeim HA, Devanand DP: Medication resistance and clinical response to electroconvulsive therapy. Psychiatry Res 31:287–296, 1990

Prudic J, Haskett RF, Mulsant B, et al: Resistance to antidepressant medications and short-term clinical response to ECT. Am J Psychiatry 153:985–992, 1996

Quitkin FM, Stewart JW, McGrath PJ, et al: Phenelzine versus imipramine in the treatment of probable atypical depression: defining syndrome boundaries of selective MAOI responders. Am J Psychiatry 145:306–311, 1988

Quitkin FM, Stewart JW, McGrath PJ, et al: Columbia atypical depression: a subgroup of depressives with better response to MAOI than to tricyclic antidepressants or placebo. Br J Psychiatry Suppl 21:30–34, 1993

Quitkin FM, Petkova E, McGrath PJ, et al: When should a trial of fluoxetine for major depression be declared failed? Am J Psychiatry 160:734–740, 2003

Reesal RT, Lam RW: CANMAT Depression Work Group: clinical guidelines for the treatment of depressive disorders, II: principles of management. Can J Psychiatry 46 (suppl 1)21S–28S, 2001

Rehm LP: Behavior Therapy for Depression. New York, Academic Press, 1979

Riso LP, Thase ME, Howland RH, et al: A prospective test of criteria for response, remission, relapse, recovery, and recurrence in patients treated with cognitive behavior therapy. J Affect Disord 43:131–142, 1997

Rosenberg WM, Sackett DL: On the need for evidence-based medicine. Therapie 51:212–217, 1996

Rush AJ: Management of treatment-resistant depression (Introduction). J Clin Psychiatry 62 (suppl 18):3, 2001a

Rush AJ: Practice guidelines and algorithms, in Treatment of Depression: Bridging The 21st Century. Edited by Weissman MM. Washington, DC, American Psychiatric Publishing, 2001b, pp 213–240

Rush AJ: Recognizing treatment-resistant depression (Introduction). J Clin Psychiatry 62 (suppl 16):3–4, 2001c

Rush AJ, Prien R: From scientific knowledge to the clinical practice of psychopharmacology: can the gap be bridged? Psychopharmacol Bull 31:7–20, 1995

Rush AJ, Thase ME: Psychotherapies for depressive disorders: a review, in WPA Series: Evidence and Experience in Psychiatry, Vol 1: Depressive Disorders. Edited by Maj M, Sartorius N. Chichester, UK, Wiley, 1999, pp 161–206

Rush AJ, Giles DE, Schlesser MA, et al: The Inventory for Depressive Symptomatology (IDS): preliminary findings. Psychiatry Res 18:65–87, 1986

Rush AJ, Gullion CM, Basco MR, et al: The Inventory of Depressive Symptomatology (IDS): psychometric properties. Psychol Med 26:477–486, 1996

Rush AJ, Crismon ML, Toprac MG, et al: Consensus guidelines in the treatment of major depressive disorder. J Clin Psychiatry 59 (suppl 20):73–84, 1998

Rush AJ, Crismon ML, Toprac MG, et al: Implementing guidelines and systems of care: experiences with the Texas Medication Algorithm Project (TMAP). Journal of Practical Psychiatry and Behavioral Health 5:75–86, 1999a

Rush AJ, Rago WV, Crismon ML, et al: Medication treatment for the severely and persistently mentally ill: the Texas Medication Algorithm Project. J Clin Psychiatry 60:284–291, 1999b

Rush AJ, Carmody T, Reimitz P-E: The Inventory of Depressive Symptomatology (IDS): clinician (IDS-C) and self-report (IDS-SR) ratings of depressive symptoms. Int J Methods Psychiatr Res 9:45–59, 2000a

Rush AJ, Pincus HA, First MB, et al (Task Force for the Handbook of Psychiatric Measures): Handbook of Psychiatric Measures. Washington, DC, American Psychiatric Association, 2000b

Rush AJ, Batey SR, Donahue RM, et al: Does pretreatment anxiety predict response to either bupropion SR or sertraline? J Affect Disord 64:81–87, 2001a

Rush AJ, Trivedi MH, Carmody TJ, et al: Response in relation to baseline anxiety levels in major depressive disorder treated with bupropion sustained release or sertraline. Neuropsychopharmacology 25:131–138, 2001b

Rush AJ, Crismon ML, Kashner TM, et al: Texas Medication Algorithm Project, Phase 3 (TMAP-3): rationale and study design. J Clin Psychiatry 64:357–369, 2003a

Rush AJ, Trivedi MH, Ibrahim HM, et al: The 16-Item Quick Inventory of Depressive Symptomatology (QIDS), clinician rating (QIDS-C), and self-report (QIDS-SR): a psychometric evaluation in patients with chronic major depression. Biol Psychiatry 54:573–583, 2003b

Rush AJ, Fava M, Wisniewski SR, et al for the STAR*D Investigators Group: Sequenced Treatment Alternatives to Relieve Depression (STAR*D): rationale and design. Control Clin Trials 25:119–142, 2004

Sackeim HA: The definition and meaning of treatment-resistant depression. J Clin Psychiatry 62 (suppl 16):10–17, 2001

Sackeim HA, Prudic J, Devanand DP, et al: The impact of medication resistance and continuation pharmacotherapy on relapse following response to electroconvulsive therapy in major depression. J Clin Psychopharmacol 10:96–104, 1990

Sackeim HA, Prudic J, Devanand DP, et al: A prospective, randomized, double-blind comparison of bilateral and right unilateral electroconvulsive therapy at different stimulus intensities. Arch Gen Psychiatry 57:425–434, 2000

Sackett DL: Evidence-Based Medicine: How to Practice and Teach EBM. New York, Churchill Livingstone, 1997

Sackett DL, Rosenberg WM: The need for evidence-based medicine. J R Soc Med 88:620–624, 1995

Schatzberg AF, Rush AJ, Arnow BA, et al: Chronic depression: medication (nefazodone) or psychotherapy (CBASP) is effective when the other is not. Arch Gen Psychiatry 62:513–520, 2005

Shaneyfelt TM, Mayo-Smith MF, Rothwangle J: Are guidelines following guidelines? The methodological quality of clinical practice guidelines in the peer-reviewed medical literature. JAMA 281:1900–1905, 1999

Shelton RC, Tollefson GD, Tohen M, et al: A novel augmentation strategy for treating resistant major depression. Am J Psychiatry 158:131–134, 2001

Shores-Wilson K, Biggs MM, Miller AL, et al: Itemized clinician ratings versus global ratings of symptom severity in patients with schizophrenia. Int J Methods Psychiatr Res 11:45–53, 2002

Simon GE, Heiligenstein JH, Grothaus L, et al: Should anxiety and insomnia influence antidepressant selection: a randomized comparison of fluoxetine and imipramine. J Clin Psychiatry 59:49–55, 1998

Simons AD, Murphy GE, Levine JL, et al: Cognitive therapy and pharmacotherapy for depression: sustained improvement over one year. Arch Gen Psychiatry 43:43–48, 1986

Spier SA: Use of bupropion with SRIs and venlafaxine. Depress Anxiety 7:73–75, 1998

Stokes PE, Holtz A: Fluoxetine tenth anniversary update: the progress continues. Clin Ther 19:1135–1250, 1997

Suppes TA, Swann C, Dennehy EB, et al: Texas Medication Algorithm Project: development and feasibility testing of a treatment algorithm for patients with bipolar disorder. J Clin Psychiatry 62:439–447, 2001

Suppes T, Rush AJ, Dennehy EB, et al: Texas Medication Algorithm Project, Phase 3 (TMAP-3): clinical results for patients with a history of mania. J Clin Psychiatry 64:370–382, 2003

Tedlow J, Fava M, Uebelacker L, et al: Outcome definitions and predictors in depression. Psychother Psychosom 67:266–270, 1998

Thase ME, Frank E, Mallinger AG, et al: Treatment of imipramine-resistant recurrent depression, III: efficacy of monoamine oxidase inhibitors. J Clin Psychiatry 53:5–11, 1992a

Thase ME, Simons AD, McGeary J, et al: Relapse after cognitive behavior therapy of depression: potential implications for longer courses of treatment. Am J Psychiatry 149:1046–1052, 1992b

Thase ME, Trivedi MH, Rush AJ: MAOIs in the contemporary treatment of depression. Neuropsychopharmacology 12:185–219, 1995

Thase ME, Entsuah AR, Rudolph RL: Remission rates during treatment with venlafaxine or selective serotonin reuptake inhibitors. Br J Psychiatry 178:234–241, 2001

Tollefson GD, Greist JH, Jefferson JW, et al: Is baseline agitation a relative contraindication for a selective serotonin reuptake inhibitor: a comparative trial of fluoxetine versus imipramine. J Clin Psychopharmacol 14:385–391, 1994

Toprac MG, Rush AJ, Conner TM, et al: The Texas Medication Algorithm Project Patient and Family Education Program: a consumer-guided initiative. J Clin Psychiatry 61:477–486, 2000

Trivedi MH, DeBattista C, Fawcett J, et al: Developing treatment algorithms for unipolar depression in cyberspace: International Psychopharmacology Algorithm Project (IPAP). Psychopharmacol Bull 34:355–359, 1998

Trivedi MH, Rush AJ, Pan JY, et al: Which depressed patients respond to nefazodone and when? J Clin Psychiatry 62:158–163, 2001

Trivedi MH, Rush AJ, Crismon ML, et al: Clinical results for patients with major depressive disorder in the Texas Medication Algorithm Project. Arch Gen Psychiatry 61:669–680, 2004a

Trivedi MH, Rush AJ, Ibrahim HM, et al: The Inventory of Depressive Symptomatology, Clinician Rating (IDS-C) and Self-Report (IDS-SR), and the Quick Inventory of Depressive Symptomatology, Clinician Rating (QIDS-C) and Self-Report (QIDS-SR) in public sector patients with mood disorders: a psychometric evaluation. Psychol Med 34:73–82, 2004b

Tyrer PJ, Lee I, Edwards JG, et al: Prognostic factors determining response to antidepressant drugs in psychiatric out-patients and general practice. J Affect Disord 2:149–156, 1980

Unützer J, Katon W, Callahan CM, et al: Collaborative care management of late-life depression in the primary care setting: a randomized controlled trial. JAMA 22:2836–2845, 2002

Viinamaki H, Hintikka J, Tanskanen A, et al: Partial remission in major depression: a two-phase; 12-month prospective study. Nord J Psychiatry 56:33–37, 2002

Von Korff M, Katon W, Bush T, et al: Treatment costs, cost offset, and cost-effectiveness of collaborative management of depression. Psychosom Med 60:143–149, 1998

Weissman MM, Markowitz JC: Interpersonal psychotherapy for depression, in Handbook of Depression. Edited by Gotlib IH, Hammen CL. New York, Guilford, 2002, pp 404–421

Weissman MM, Markowitz JC, Klerman GL: Comprehensive Guide to Interpersonal Psychotherapy. New York, Basic Books, 2000

Wennberg JE: Dealing with medical practice variations: a proposal for action. Health Aff (Millwood) 3:6–32, 1984

Wennberg JE, Gittelshon A: Small-area variation in health care delivery. Science 182:1102–1108, 1973

Wennberg JE, Freeman JL, Culp WJ: Are hospital services rationed in New Haven or over-utilised in Boston? Lancet 1:1185–1189, 1987

Woolf SH: Practice guidelines: a new reality in medicine, I: recent developments. Arch Intern Med 150:1811–1818, 1990

Woolf SH: Manual for Clinical Practice Guideline Development (AHCPR Publ 91-0007). Rockville, MD, Agency for Health Care Policy and Research, 1991

Yonkers KA, Samson J: Mood disorders measures, in Handbook of Psychiatric Measures. Edited by Rush AJ, Pincus HA, First MB, et al. Washington, DC, American Psychiatric Association, 2000, pp 515–548

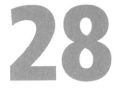

Guidelines for the Treatment of Bipolar Disorder

DAVID J. MUZINA, M.D.

JOSEPH R. CALABRESE, M.D.

BIPOLAR DISORDER IS a chronic, severe, and sometimes life-threatening mental illness that presents numerous treatment challenges. The manner in which psychiatry has classified bipolar disorder has had direct and significant effects on suggested pharmacological treatment strategies. The 1899 publication of Kraepelin's view of manic-depressive insanity, bringing together depressive and bipolar disorders, dominated epidemiological and clinical research on affective disorders, as well as the bipolar treatment paradigms, until the early 1970s (Kraepelin 1899). Identification and diagnosis of specific phases of illness, either manic or depressive, led to treatments prescribed specifically for that affective pole of illness.

Research has progressively reshaped our understanding of bipolar disorder as a diagnostic entity separate from other mood disorders, with its own complex intradiagnostic subtypes. The separation of bipolar disorder into type I and type II in 1976 (Dunner et al. 1976) was quickly followed by the description of a bipolar spectrum of disorders with six subgroups: mania and depression, hypo-

mania and depression, cyclothymic personality, hypomania or mania precipitated by drugs, depression with a family history of bipolar disorder, and mania without depression (Klerman 1981). Ongoing, recent work by leaders in the discipline of bipolar disorder, such as Angst and Akiskal, has further contributed to our understanding of bipolar disorder as an illness with a complex interrelation and commingling of various affective states, not just a mood disorder marked purely by classic manic and/or depressive presentations (Akiskal and Pinto 1999; Akiskal et al. 2000; Angst and Ernst 1993; Angst et al. 2003).

The treatment of bipolar disorder has since taken on added complexity, going beyond the resolution of acute episodes to designing strategies that prevent future episodes or that result in the reduction of episode frequency and severity. Treatments that do not potentially aggravate the short- or long-term course of illness must be considered, making the use of traditional antidepressants an ongoing controversial issue.

Any attempt to provide guidelines for the treatment of

bipolar disorder in 2004 and beyond should focus on overall symptom presentation, individual patterns of illness, and prevention of future relapses rather than just management of acute phases of mania and/or depression. Evidence-based guidelines recommended by the British Association for Psychopharmacology call for addressing the long-term treatment needs early in the course of treatment because of the high risk of relapse and progression of illness to more frequent episodes (Goodwin 2003).

Review of recently published guidelines for the treatment of bipolar disorder significantly contributed to the formulation of the guidelines suggested in this chapter (American Psychiatric Association 2002; Goodwin 2003; Grunze et al. 2002; Suppes et al. 2002). Table 28–1 summarizes the fundamentals of management of bipolar disorder, as proposed by Goodwin (2003).

We attempt to provide practical guidelines for the pharmacological treatment of bipolar disorder. In some ways, our attempts will be constrained by the traditional approach of selecting treatment according to phase of illness. However, we hope to focus on overall symptom presentation and discuss medications used in the treatment of bipolar disorder according to their abilities to stabilize mood from below and above baseline to provide the most practical yet evidence-based approach to managing the spectrum of bipolar disorder.

A New Nomenclature: Stabilization of Mood From Below and Above Baseline

The traditional emphasis on the acute management of bipolar mania in bipolar disorder does not adequately direct attention to the critical unmet needs in the therapeutics of the illness or the differential spectra of efficacy of the available treatments. A new nomenclature has been proposed that conceptualizes bipolar disorder as an aberration of mood, behavior, and cognition from baseline (euthymia), with *below baseline* referring to depressive states and *above baseline* referring to hypomanic and manic states (Ketter and Calabrese 2002). Subsyndromal mood depressions and elevations are easily described with this new nomenclature, as are treatments; mood stabilizers can correct mood aberrations in one or both directions to varying extents. This nomenclature thus emphasizes the importance of medication management plans that often use combination strategies to achieve a broad spectrum of coverage through their complementary differential spectra of therapeutic efficacy.

For treatment of those aberrant states of mood, be-

havior, and cognition that deviate above the euthymic baseline, the term *Class A* mood stabilizers has been suggested to define agents that 1) stabilize mood from *above* baseline and 2) possess short- and long-term antimanic properties without worsening of depression or destabilizing the overall course of illness. For those aberrant states that deviate below the euthymic baseline, the term *Class B* mood stabilizers has been suggested to define agents that 1) stabilize mood from *below* baseline and 2) possess short- and long-term antidepressant properties without inducing switches into mania or destabilizing the overall course of illness (Ketter and Calabrese 2002).

Stabilization of Mood From Above Baseline

The clinical approach to managing mood states that are pathologically above the healthy euthymic baseline encompasses treatment for clearly defined mania, hypomania, psychotic mania, mixed states, and subsyndromal mood elevations. With consideration to expanding definitions of bipolar disorder or spectrum bipolar disorders, stabilizing mood from above baseline also would refer to states described as hypomania or mania precipitated by drugs, schizo-bipolar disorder, chronic refractory hypomania, hypomania associated with minor depression, and hyperthymic and cyclothymic personalities (Akiskal 2002; Angst 1997; Angst et al. 2003).

We propose guidelines for the management of above-baseline mood states and symptoms with Class A mood stabilizers, focusing first on the acute stabilization phase and then on long-term maintenance treatment. A critical review of the evidence base for these suggested guidelines follows in later sections on medications in this chapter.

Acute Stabilization of Above-Baseline Mood States and Symptoms

Classic manic, hypomanic, and mixed bipolar episodes, as defined by DSM-IV-TR (American Psychiatric Association 2000), share characteristic traits of hyperactive behavior and/or thoughts, tendencies for impulsivity and lability, various mood elevations and irritabilities, and degrees of functional impairment or distress. Spectra bipolar states, atypical bipolar disorders, and rapid-cycling conditions (as described by Angst, Akiskal, and others) often are associated with above-baseline disturbances that cause significant functional impairment or distress despite lacking clear DSM-IV-TR–proposed criteria for duration, severity, or frequency of symptoms.

TABLE 28–1. Fundamentals of bipolar patient management (British Association for Psychopharmacology guidelines)

Diagnosis	Accurate diagnosis of illness and phase of illness is fundamental to sound management of bipolar disorder.
Access to services and the safety of the patient and others	The diagnosis of mania should prompt consideration of hospitalization or intensive outpatient management because of the frequent impairment in judgment associated with manic phases. Suicidal ideation and risk assessment must be performed at every visit. Collateral information from family or other third parties should be sought if any doubt exists about safety issues.
Enhanced care	The clinician should establish and maintain a therapeutic alliance.
	The clinician must educate himself or herself and then the patient and his or her family about the disorder.
	The clinician should enhance treatment adherence while respecting patient preferences, use of known tolerabilities of medicines, and education about the need for long-term maintenance.
	The clinician should promote awareness of stressors, sleep disturbance and early signs of relapse, and regular patterns of activity.
	The clinician must evaluate and manage functional impairments.

Source. Adapted from Goodwin (2003).

Regardless of distinct diagnostic classification, use of an overall symptom management strategy can unify the pharmacotherapeutic approach to all of these states. Table 28–2 lists options for acute treatment of above-baseline mood states or symptoms, including Class A mood stabilizers that are approved by the U.S. Food and Drug Administration (FDA) and others that are likely effective.

The initial step in determining first choice of mood stabilizer for above-baseline mood disturbances should involve assessment of the severity of symptoms, which may guide need for monotherapy or combination therapy. Patients with hypomanic to mild manic presentations may be candidates for monotherapy, whereas patients with more severe manic or mixed episodes usually should receive urgent treatment with combined Class A mood stabilizers. Other considerations, such as first episode or breakthrough episode, rapid cycling or refractory illness, and patient preference and tolerability issues affect decisions for initial management choices, as described in Table 28–3 (mania) and Table 28–4 (hypomania).

Lithium or divalproex is recommended in combination with an atypical antipsychotic such as olanzapine for the initial acute management of any first-episode, above-baseline mood disturbance beyond hypomania or limited mania. These treatments have the most data to support their use, although alternative Class A mood stabilizers may be used instead if patient preference or tolerability issues prevail. In breakthrough episodes, assurance of medication adherence and optimum dosing should be pursued before moving on to combination therapies. Rapid-cycling patients frequently require combination therapies

with two or more Class A agents. Antidepressants generally should be avoided in these patients and in those with treatment-refractory above-baseline mood symptoms because of their potential to aggravate hypomanic-manic symptoms or to produce rapid cycling.

TABLE 28–2. Class A mood stabilizers for management of above-baseline mood states and symptoms

Approved for use in acute episodes	Likely effective alternatives
Lithium	Clozapine
Divalproex sodium/ valproate	Conventional antipsychotics
Olanzapine	Lamotrigine (hypomania >mania)
Chlorpromazine	
Quetiapine	Oxcarbazepine
Risperidone	
Aripiprazole	
Carbamazepine extended release	
Ziprasidone	

Approved for prophylactic treatment	Likely effective alternatives
Lithium	Carbamazepine
Lamotrigine (depression >mania)	Divalproex sodium/ valproate
Olanzapine	Oxcarbazepine
	Other atypical antipsychotics

Prevention of Above-Baseline Mood States and Symptoms—Maintenance Treatments

The long-term objective of maintenance therapy for bipolar disorder is to prevent recurrence of disruptive mood episodes. Prevention of acute bipolar manic and hypomanic episodes through maintenance treatment is critical to improving the poor long-term outcomes in bipolar patients. In this area, there is significant debate as to the most appropriate treatments for prevention of future above-baseline (e.g., manic) mood disturbances. The most common practice in the United States is the continuation of the medication(s) that resolved an acute manic or hypomanic episode, although limited evidence supports this practice, except for lithium. More commonly in Europe, psychiatrists will treat acute manic episodes largely with typical antipsychotics and then discontinue the antipsychotic after resolution of the acute above-baseline phase of the illness followed by consideration of other medications for prophylactic treatment. Despite these differences, the consensus opinion and available data suggest that some form of maintenance pharmacotherapy should be prescribed following acute manic episodes or other frequently recurrent and disruptive states such as hypomania (Bowden et al. 2000b; Sachs et al. 2000).

Although lithium remains the gold standard for the prevention of future manic exacerbations of bipolar illness, emerging data suggest that other agents effective for acute mania may offer other prophylactic treatment options (Muzina and Calabrese, in press). The need for alternatives to lithium is clear because an estimated 20%–40% of patients do not respond sufficiently to it (Denicoff et al. 1997; O'Connell et al. 1991). In addition, undesirable side effects, adverse reactions, a narrow therapeutic index, and the increased risk of toxicity with overdose can make lithium therapy less than ideal for many patients. More important is our growing understanding of various types of bipolar disorder and unpredictable states, such as rapid cycling, dysphoric mania, and iatrogenic cycle acceleration, that pose significant additional challenges when attempting to prevent future exacerbations of bipolar illness.

Prophylactic therapy should be continued indefinitely, particularly for bipolar I disorder, because the risk for manic recurrence is high. Among Class A mood stabilizers, lithium is probably the most effective option, although the other antimanic agents (i.e., divalproex, olanzapine) should be considered if lithium is not tolerated or is ineffective. Combinations of Class A agents may be required in patients with breakthrough above-baseline mood disturbances. Breakthrough depressions suggest the need to combine Class A and Class B mood stabilizers for long-term prevention of relapse.

Stabilization of Mood From Below Baseline

The clinical approach to managing mood states that are pathologically below the healthy euthymic baseline encompasses treatment for clearly defined major depressive episodes with and without psychosis and mixed states. Recognition of a spectrum of bipolar disorders necessitates consideration of stabilizing mood from below baseline for states that have been termed *soft* bipolar disorders, such as depression with antidepressant-associated hypomania ("bipolar III"), atypical depressions with reversed vegetative signs, subsyndromal mood depressions, or recurrent brief depressions (Akiskal et al. 2000; Angst et al. 2003).

For treatment of those aberrant states of mood, behavior, and cognition that deviate below the euthymic baseline, *Class B* mood stabilizers are generally employed. We now discuss guidelines for treating below-baseline mood disturbances, focusing on first the acute stabilization phase and then on long-term maintenance treatment.

As Table 28–5 highlights, there are significantly fewer approved treatment options for bipolar depressive states compared with above-baseline mood disturbances. In addition, although some alternative, unapproved options exist, even fewer data are available to support their use with much confidence. Again, later sections of this chapter include an evidence base for these medication treatment guidelines.

Acute Stabilization of Below-Baseline Mood States and Symptoms (Bipolar Depression)

The recent FDA approval of the olanzapine-fluoxetine combination represents the first indicated therapy for the treatment of acute bipolar depression. The use of agents deemed "antidepressants" on the basis of efficacy in treatment trials for unipolar major depression has not been well studied for bipolar depression, much less for other below-baseline mood disturbances (Muzina and Calabrese 2003). Only 12 randomized, placebo-controlled trials of traditional antidepressants in the treatment of bipolar depression have been done between 1968 and 2001 (Ghaemi and Thase 2002). Only 5 of these studies reported the antidepressant studied to be more effective than placebo, although questions about study design and power among these studies can be raised.

In addition, tremendous uncertainty and debate exist about the potential danger of cycle acceleration or "switching" associated with the use of antidepressants by bipolar pa-

TABLE 28–3. Acute treatment of above-baseline mood states and symptoms (mania)

Illness characteristics	Management	
First episode (Patients with only mild mania may require only one antimanic agent)	*Choose one:* 1. Divalproex or 2. Lithium *Plus* 1. Olanzapine or 2. Quetiapine or 3. Risperidone	*Alternatives:* 1. Carbamazepine 2. Oxcarbazepine 3. Other atypical antipsychotics
Breakthrough episode during long-term maintenance medication treatment	Ensure compliance Optimize doses of both mood stabilizers Use adjunctive benzodiazepine If symptoms persist or worsen, add a third Class A mood stabilizer	
Part of rapid-cycling course	Ensure compliance Eliminate antidepressants Rule out thyroid disturbance or alcohol and drug abuse Two or more Class A mood stabilizers usually are needed Consider clozapine or electroconvulsive therapy	

tients. Although the phenomenon has not been rigorously studied, consensus is growing among United States psychiatrists that traditional antidepressants should be avoided in the treatment of acute bipolar depression, particularly if their action is not counteracted or "protected" by coadministration of known antimanic agents. The revised American Psychiatric Association "Practice Guideline for the Treatment of Patients With Bipolar Disorder" recommends with substantial clinical confidence the avoidance of antidepressant monotherapy for acute bipolar depression, instead recommending lithium or lamotrigine as first- and second-line treatment options (American Psychiatric Association 2002). Because of these guidelines, we focus the following discussion on potential Class B agents that can safely treat bipolar depressive disorders and do not include traditional antidepressant monotherapies. Traditional antidepressants should be considered only in combination with known antimanic (Class A) agents or as add-on therapy when Class B mood stabilizers have failed.

Tables 28–6 and 28–7 outline treatment guidelines for managing acute symptoms of below-baseline mood disturbance or "bipolar depression" in bipolar I and bipolar II disorder, respectively. Initiation of therapy in a patient with newly diagnosed bipolar depression may be directed by a history of mania versus hypomania, as well as by the presence of rapid cycling. In general, acute bipolar II depression initially can be treated with lamotrigine, whereas acute bipolar I depression should not be treated with lamotrigine monotherapy because of lamotrigine's relatively weaker prophylaxis against manic relapse compared with lithium (Calabrese et al. 2003). Severe acute bipolar I depression should

be treated with either the olanzapine-fluoxetine combination or a combination of lithium and lamotrigine. Less severe depression may respond to initial monotherapy with any of these agents, but careful monitoring is required. Patients with catatonic or psychotic features should receive aggressive treatment, with appropriate consideration of electroconvulsive therapy (ECT). Traditional antidepressants may be considered earlier on in the acute treatment course of bipolar II depression than in type I because of the probable lower risk of abnormal mood elevation or cycling in type II patients taking antidepressants. However, a history of rapid cycling or activation with antidepressants may preclude their safe use in many bipolar patients.

Prevention of Below-Baseline Mood States and Symptoms—Maintenance Treatments

Only two drug development efforts have conducted companion maintenance studies in both those patients presenting with mania and those patients presenting with depression. These studies examined the efficacy of lithium (Prien et al. 1973, 1974) and lamotrigine (Bowden et al. 2003; Calabrese et al. 2003) for prevention of mood episodes in manic versus depressed bipolar patients. The Phase III National Institute of Mental Health/Veterans Administration collaborative maintenance study also compared lithium with placebo and with imipramine monotherapy in recently depressed bipolar patients, observing that lithium prevented both mania and depression in patients with initial severe depression requiring hospitalization. Although imipramine also prevented

TABLE 28–4. Acute treatment of above-baseline mood states and symptoms (hypomania or limited mania)

Illness characteristics	Management	
First episode, mild symptoms	*Choose one:* 1. Divalproex 2. Lamotrigine 3. Lithium 4. Olanzapine 5. Quetiapine 6. Risperidone	*Alternatives:* 1. Carbamazepine 2. Oxcarbazepine 3. Other atypical antipsychotics
Breakthrough episode during long-term maintenance medication treatment	Ensure compliance (i.e., check medication levels) Optimize dose of monotherapy Use adjunctive benzodiazepine If symptoms persist or worsen, add a second Class A mood stabilizer	
Part of rapid-cycling course	Ensure compliance Eliminate antidepressants Rule out thyroid disturbance or alcohol and drug abuse Combined Class A mood stabilizers usually are needed	

TABLE 28–5. Class B mood stabilizers for management of below-baseline mood states and symptoms

Approved for use in acute episodes	Likely effective alternatives
Olanzapine-fluoxetine combination (OFC)	Lamotrigine Lithium Quetiapine Other atypical antipsychotics

Approved for prophylactic treatment	Possibly effective alternatives
Bipolar type I Lithium Lamotrigine Bipolar type II None	Carbamazepine Divalproex sodium/ valproate Olanzapine or OFC Oxcarbazepine Other atypical antipsychotics

depression, it did so by causing mania (Prien et al. 1973).

Given the highly recurrent nature of all bipolar disorder variants and the propensity for illness relapses to be depressive ones (Judd et al. 2002), the ability to prevent below-baseline mood disturbances could have a profound effect on ameliorating disease burden. The 2003 FDA approval of lamotrigine for the prevention of mood episodes associated with bipolar I disorder, with particular mention of preferen-

tial prophylaxis of depressive episodes, was a landmark event in the therapeutics of bipolar disorder. The availability of an approved treatment option other than lithium for this phase of preventive therapy is critical given the large unmet need in the treatment of bipolar depression and the relatively high rate of depressive relapse despite lithium maintenance.

Nevertheless, much uncertainty and unmet needs remain regarding maintenance treatment for bipolar depression that can prevent or delay depressive relapse without destabilizing the course of the bipolar illness. Significant debate still exists over the long-term use of antidepressants in bipolar disorder, for which controlled data are lacking to support efficacy. Data suggest an unacceptably high rate of manic relapse during long-term follow-up of patients taking antidepressants for maintenance, although co-therapy with a mood stabilizer such as lithium may reduce this risk (Prien et al. 1984).

At this time, it would appear that lamotrigine has the most potent efficacy for preventing depressive relapses and should be considered for all bipolar patients, with the exception of those with primarily recurrent manias. Lithium is also likely to be more effective than antiepileptics or atypical antipsychotics in preventing depression, although its potency for manic prophylaxis is much stronger. Traditional antidepressants should be used only in combination with known antimanic agents to minimize the risk of manic switches or cycle acceleration, and the duration of treatment with the antidepressant should be briefer than maintenance therapies for recurrent unipolar depression. Effective prophylaxis for most patients likely requires administering com-

TABLE 28–6. Acute treatment of below-baseline mood states and symptoms (bipolar I depression)

Illness characteristics	Management[a]
First episode, mild symptoms	*Choose one:*
	1. Olanzapine-fluoxetine combination (OFC) *Alternatives:* 1. Olanzapine or other atypical antipsychotic augmentation
	2. Lithium 2. Antiepileptic drug
	3. Lamotrigine 3. Combination with antidepressant
	4. Lithium plus lamotrigine
First episode, moderate or severe	OFC
	Use lithium plus lamotrigine
	Add-on olanzapine or atypical antipsychotic
	Add-on antiepileptic drug
	Add-on antidepressant (bupropion or SSRI)
	Thyroid augmentation
	ECT
Breakthrough episode during long-term maintenance medication treatment	Ensure compliance (i.e., check medication levels)
	Optimize dose of monotherapy
	Add-on lithium
	Add-on lamotrigine
	Add-on antiepileptic drug or atypical antipsychotic
	Add-on antidepressant (bupropion or SSRI)
	Thyroid augmentation
	ECT
Part of rapid-cycling course	Ensure compliance
	Eliminate antidepressants
	Rule out thyroid disturbance or alcohol and drug abuse
	Use lamotrigine plus lithium
	Add-on divalproex or atypical antipsychotic
	Thyroid augmentation
	ECT

Note. ECT=electroconvulsive therapy; SSRI=selective serotonin reuptake inhibitor.
[a]Recommendations based on combination of best evidence and clinical experience.

binations of currently available medications at the first illness episode and thereafter, with careful, regular monitoring for any warning signs of relapse while practicing the fundamental principles of managing patients with bipolar disorder (see Table 28–1).

Treatment of Bipolar Disorder in Women During Pregnancy and Lactation

Typically, pregnancy neither uniformly aggravates nor alleviates the risk of bipolar relapse. Treatment of acute episodes of depression or mania requires careful balancing of the potential teratogenic effects of medications with the harmful effects of an ill mother on the unborn child. Many women require maintenance treatment during pregnancy and during the vulnerable postpartum period, which is a time of increased risk for bipolar relapse and illness onset as well (American Psychiatric Association 2002). The revised 2002 American Psychiatric Association practice guideline contains a detailed review of recommendations that should be considered when making treatment decisions with bipolar women and their families during planned conception, pregnancy, postpartum, and breast-feeding phases of life (American Psychiatric Association 2002).

In general, the concept of "healthy moms make healthy babies" should be kept in mind when making treatment recommendations. Maternal stress, anxiety, and depression have been associated with an array of abnormalities in newborns, including lower birth weight (Hoffman and Hatch

TABLE 28–7.   Acute treatment of below-baseline mood states and symptoms (bipolar II depression)

Illness characteristics	Management[a]	
First episode, mild symptoms	*Choose one:* 1. Lamotrigine 2. Lithium 3. Olanzapine-fluoxetine combination (OFC)	*Alternatives:* 1. Olanzapine or other atypical antipsychotic augmentation 2. Combination with antidepressant
First episode, moderate or severe	Use lamotrigine plus lithium OFC Add-on olanzapine or atypical antipsychotic Add-on antidepressant (bupropion or SSRI) Thyroid augmentation ECT	
Breakthrough episode during long-term maintenance medication treatment	Ensure compliance (i.e., check medication levels) Optimize dose of monotherapy Add-on lamotrigine Add-on lithium Add-on antidepressant or atypical antipsychotic Thyroid augmentation ECT	
Part of rapid-cycling course	Ensure compliance Eliminate antidepressants Rule out thyroid disturbance or alcohol and drug abuse Use lamotrigine plus lithium Add-on divalproex or atypical antipsychotic Thyroid augmentation ECT	

Note.   ECT=electroconvulsive therapy; SSRI=selective serotonin reuptake inhibitor.
[a]Recommendations based on combination of best evidence and clinical experience.

2000; Paarlberg et al. 1999). Providing careful treatment to mothers may improve the health of the mother, child, and the mother–child dyad. Several strategies have been proposed to potentially reduce the harmful risks from medications in bipolar women, including 1) monotherapy with the lowest effective dose of a drug for the shortest period necessary, 2) periconceptional concomitant use of multivitamins with folate, 3) prescription of drugs with established safety records, and 4) avoidance of exposure to antimanic agents during the first trimester of pregnancy (Iqbal et al. 2001).

Medications

Lithium

Evidence

Since the introduction of lithium salts for the treatment of "psychotic excitement" in 1949 (Cade 1949) and subsequent approval by the FDA in 1970, lithium has been considered the cornerstone of bipolar disorder therapy, with particular utility for manic episodes. The short-term efficacy of lithium in the treatment of acute mania is supported by at least five placebo-controlled trials; studies indicate that about half of acutely manic patients respond well to lithium (Kukopulos et al. 1980; Small et al. 1988, 1991). The evidence supporting lithium's preventive efficacy against manic recurrences is substantial and dates back to 1970 (Angst et al. 1970; Baastrup et al. 1970). The Prien maintenance studies observed lithium's effectiveness for prophylaxis of mood episodes in the general population, although later analysis noted that lithium prevented mania but not depression in recently depressed patients (Prien et al. 1984; Shapiro et al. 1989). In a 2001 Cochrane meta-analysis of nine placebo-controlled studies (N=825), Burgess and colleagues (2001) concluded that lithium is effective in the prophylaxis of bipolar disorder relapse. Two large-scale, randomized, double-blind, placebo-controlled studies that used modern methods have further substantiated the role of lithium for preventing mood relapses in bipolar disorder, particularly for prophylaxis against manic recurrences (Bowden et al. 2003; Calabrese et al. 2003). Lithium extended the time until recurrence by 55%, as well as the time until intervention for a recurrent manic episode relative to placebo in these studies, solidifying the case for lithium as the most proven effective prophylactic treatment against above-baseline mood disturbances, such as mania.

Although lithium was noted to be the first-line recommendation for acute bipolar depression in the American Psychiatric Association (2002) practice guideline, only eight small placebo-controlled trials, with a total of 116 bipolar patients, have been done, and none have been completed since 1978. All used crossover designs, and seven of the eight trials reported that lithium was superior to placebo, with moderate to marked antidepressant response in 79% of the bipolar patients. Early studies consistently reported efficacy for lithium in the maintenance treatment of bipolar disorder (for review, see Muzina and Calabrese 2003). However, not until the recent large-scale lamotrigine trials have we understood the potential limitations within the range of lithium's prophylactic efficacy. The available data suggest that lithium has a much more robust potency against the development of any above-baseline mood disturbances, such as mania or hypomania, than it does against depressive relapses. Table 28–8 summarizes key issues in the use of lithium therapy in bipolar disorder.

Pretreatment Evaluation

Before beginning therapy with lithium, the following are recommended: general medical history, physical examination and weight measurement, serum urea nitrogen and creatinine determination, thyroid function studies, and pregnancy testing for women of childbearing potential. Lithium carries a teratogenicity Category D warning. Electrocardiogram for patients older than 40 and complete blood count measurement are also suggested (American Psychiatric Association 2002).

Dosing

For treatment of acute mania, lithium should be dosed to achieve therapeutic plasma concentrations between 0.8 and 1.2 mEq/L, avoiding toxic effects more commonly seen with levels exceeding 1.5 mEq/L. A routine initial dosing regimen is the administration of lithium carbonate 300 mg four times daily with trough plasma level determination on day 4 or 5 of treatment, targeting the therapeutic range and guarding against toxicity. When used to treat hypomania or to manage other acute above-baseline mood states, lower starting doses (300 mg

twice a day) and lower blood levels (0.6–0.8 mEq/L) may sufficiently stabilize mood over a period of several weeks to months. Similarly, lower doses and levels of lithium may be sufficient when combination pharmacotherapy strategies, such as lithium plus an anticonvulsant or antipsychotic, are used.

For maintenance treatment with lithium, serum levels between 0.8 and 1.2 mmol/L are recommended. Data from a randomized, double-blind, prospective trial indicated a 2.6 greater risk of manic relapse with the "low" dose strategy for prophylaxis (0.4–0.6 mmol/L) compared with standard dosing to serum lithium levels of 0.8–1.0 mmol/L (Gelenberg et al. 1989). Other reports also suggested that the lower dose range is less effective for preventing lesser manic or hypomanic episodes (Keller et al. 1992).

Although not well studied, most recommendations for the use of lithium to acutely manage below-baseline mood disturbances associated with bipolar disorder are to dose to a minimum serum lithium level of 0.8 mEq/L. In a double-blind, placebo-controlled study of bipolar depressed patients taking lithium, the addition of either paroxetine or imipramine was not effective in alleviating depressive symptoms in patients whose serum lithium levels were greater than 0.8 mEq/L (Nemeroff et al. 2001).

Although lithium is effective, clinical improvement is relatively slow, with an initial onset of therapeutic response generally occurring no sooner than 7–14 days after starting therapy with lithium. Additionally, lithium has a significant side-effect burden that complicates long-term management: 75% of lithium-treated patients experience adverse effects, predominantly affecting the thyroid, gastrointestinal, renal, and/or neurological systems (Janicak et al. 1997). These side effects may be less apparent during acute treatment with lithium than during maintenance treatment.

Side Effects and Drug Interactions

The most common side effects of lithium are nausea, vomiting, diarrhea, tremor, polydipsia, and polyuria. During acute treatment, gastrointestinal disturbances and tremor can be mitigated by slower dosing strategies. Worsening of any of these adverse effects or the development of bradycardia, syncope, confusion, or ataxic gait should alert the clinician to urgently assess lithium blood levels and consider necessary changes in dosing or treatment alternatives. The possibility of drug interactions with lithium always must be considered, particularly those that can increase adverse effects, such as thiazide diuretics, some antihypertensives, nonsteroidal anti-inflammatory drugs, and other psychotropics.

Long-term treatment with lithium may be compli-

TABLE 28–8.   Issues in the use of lithium for management of bipolar disorder

Pretreatment workup recommended	General medical history, physical examination and weight measurement, complete blood count, serum urea nitrogen and creatinine determination, thyroid function studies, pregnancy testing, electrocardiogram (patients older than 40)
Dosing	*Above-baseline mood disturbances:* Initiate 300 mg four times a day, adjust according to clinical response and serum lithium levels. May eventually be consolidated into single bedtime dose. Lower doses may be used for hypomania.
	Below-baseline mood disturbances: Similar dosing regimen recommended, particularly for bipolar I disorder. Lower doses may be attempted for bipolar II disorder or when used in combination with other Class B mood stabilizers.
Lithium level target	Trough serum level of 0.8–1.2 mEq/L; levels higher than 1.5 mEq/L may be toxic. Lower levels may be needed for hypomania. For depression, target level is 0.8–1.0 mEq/L.
Side effects	Most side effects can be reduced by lowering the lithium dose or adjusting the dosage schedule.
Postural tremor	Slower dosage titration, lower lithium level, β-blockers (i.e., propranolol 20–120 mg/day)
Gastrointestinal irritations	Slower dosage titration, lower lithium level, take lithium with food, use different lithium preparation
Polydipsia and polyuria	Consolidate to bedtime dose, lower lithium level, decrease dietary protein; thiazide or loop diuretics may help (more careful serum lithium monitoring required if used)
Weight gain	Nutritional measures to lower caloric intake, increase exercise
More serious adverse reactions: confusion, ataxia, bradycardia, syncope, skin reactions	If lowering dosage does not resolve these effects or lowering dose is not feasible because of ongoing mood symptoms, lithium discontinuation should be considered
Drugs that can increase levels of lithium	Angiotensin-converting enzyme inhibitors, Alprazolam, Amiloride, Ethacrynic acid, Fluoxetine, Ibuprofen, Indapamide, Indomethacin, Mefenamic acid, Naproxen, Phenylbutazone, Spironolactone, Sulindac, Thiazide diuretics, Triamterene, Zomepirac

cated by persistent side effects (described earlier), although the most serious potential adverse effects of impaired renal concentrating capacity or renal insufficiency, hypothyroidism, and cardiac conduction abnormalities necessitate precaution and routine monitoring.

Lithium levels may be decreased through drug interactions with caffeine, carbonic anhydrase inhibitors, osmotic diuretics, theophylline, and laxatives. Table 28–8 lists drug interactions that can increase serum lithium levels.

Antiepileptic Drugs

Divalproex Sodium

Evidence. Divalproex sodium (valproate, valproic acid) became the first anticonvulsant approved as a mood stabilizer by the FDA in 1995, after decades of case reports, open studies, and controlled trials culminated with a large-scale, randomized, double-blind, parallel-group study that found that divalproex was equivalent to lithium in superiority over placebo for the management of acute mania (Bowden et al. 1994). Divalproex was recommended as a first-line acute treatment option for euphoric mania and hypomania, mixed or dysphoric mania and hypomania, and psychotic mania in the Texas Medication Algorithm Project (Suppes et al. 2002). The revised American Psychiatric Association practice guideline lists divalproex as first-line pharmacological treatment of severe acute manic or mixed episodes when combined with an antipsychotic or as monotherapy for less ill patients (American Psychiatric Association 2002).

A general paucity of data remains to support the use of divalproex for bipolar maintenance treatment, particularly in comparison to lithium. A Cochrane meta-analysis of 19 studies determined that only one trial (Bowden et al. 2000a) met the inclusion criteria for a randomized controlled trial comparing divalproex with placebo or other mood stabilizers for specific use in maintenance therapy (Macritchie et al. 2001). The results of this meta-analysis were equivocal and led to the authors' recommendation to use lithium before divalproex for maintenance treatment. Since this report, reports from a 47-week, randomized, double-blind study comparing flexibly dosed olanzapine (5–20 mg/day) with divalproex (500–2,500 mg/day) for manic or mixed episodes of bipolar disorder have been published (Tohen et al. 2003). No placebo or comparator group was included. Rates of bipolar relapse did not differ, with approximately 40% of all patients experiencing a manic relapse during the study.

Divalproex does not contribute to any mood cycling or depression, and reports indicate its potential efficacy as an antidepressant (L.L. Davis et al. 1996; Ghaemi and Goodwin 2001; Kemp 1992). No placebo-controlled studies of the treatment of acute bipolar depression with divalproex have been published. Unpublished data from an 8-week trial indicated that divalproex was not more effective than placebo in treating bipolar depression (Sachs et al. 2001). However, multiple open divalproex trials in depression have detected some signal that there may be potential antidepressant activity for some patients during acute treatment of their below-baseline mood disturbances. Winsberg and colleagues (2001) conducted an open-label trial and observed that divalproex monotherapy appeared to be well tolerated and substantially benefited 63% of the patients with bipolar II depression. A more striking rate of antidepressant response to divalproex was seen in medication-naïve patients (82%) compared with mood stabilizer–naïve patients (38%) in this study.

As is the case with lithium, fewer data are available regarding the ability of divalproex to prevent depressive relapses than for above-baseline mood relapses. Clinical experience and data from open trials and add-on or combination mood stabilizer studies suggest that divalproex has a moderate degree of efficacy in decreasing depressive relapses, including patients with rapid cycling (Calabrese et al. 1990; Hirschfeld et al. 1999). A double-blind, parallel-group, multicenter study conducted over 52 weeks in 372 randomized bipolar I patients who met recovery criteria within 3 months of onset of an index manic episode were given divalproex, lithium, or placebo. The divalproex-treated group fared better on several dimensions of depressive morbidity, particularly in the prevention of depressive relapse among patients who responded to divalproex when initially manic and in patients with more severe bipolar illness (Gyulai et al. 2003).

Taken collectively along with the vast clinical experience of clinicians who have prescribed divalproex, these reports support classification of this agent as primarily a Class A mood stabilizer that can effectively treat not only manic, hypomanic, mixed, and rapid-cycling states but also other, less typical presentations of above-baseline mood disturbances and symptom complexes. As well, some data support Class B mood-stabilizing action for divalproex, particularly as preventive treatment of below-baseline mood disturbances, although further studies are needed.

Pretreatment evaluation. Before beginning therapy with divalproex, general medical history with special attention to any past problems of hepatic or hematological nature, baseline liver profile, and complete blood cell count are recommended. Pregnancy screening should be conducted before starting divalproex, particularly given its FDA black-box warning of teratogenicity Category D. The primary concern is the increased risk for neural tube defects, although growth retardation and hypoplasia of the midface and fingers are also thought to occur in some infants exposed to anticonvulsants in utero (Holmes et al. 2001).

Dosing. Divalproex can be dosed with either an oral-loading or a standard-titration strategy. For acute management of severely ill manic patients, divalproex oral loading with a therapeutic starting dose of 20–30 mg/kg/day is more rapidly effective than standard, gradual titration schedules (Hirschfeld et al. 1999, 2003; Keck et al. 1993). Oral loading typically achieves serum concentrations of valproic acid greater than 50 µg/mL by day 2, which represents the low end of the therapeutic range of serum concentrations for this agent of 50–125 µg/mL. This oral-loading strategy for divalproex has been shown to lead to a more rapid antimanic effect when compared with standard-titration divalproex, lithium, or placebo; it is also better tolerated than olanzapine and as well tolerated as lithium or standard-titration divalproex (Hirschfeld et al. 2003). Lower, divided doses are initially recommended (250 mg three times a day) for patients with less severe forms of above-baseline mood disturbances or in elderly patients.

Dosing strategies for preventing depression are not supported by investigative findings, but clinical experience and expert guidelines suggest minimum serum valproic acid levels of 50–60 μg/mL.

Side effects and drug interactions.   Adverse effects seen during initial therapy with divalproex are usually mild, transient, and easily managed. Gastrointestinal distress and sedation are the most commonly seen side effects during acute treatment, although other dose-related effects, including tremor and benign hepatic transaminase elevations, are occasionally encountered. Reduced dosage or slower upward titration can be helpful, in addition to use of divalproex sodium formulation or extended-release divalproex instead of valproic acid, which may lessen these side effects. Severe gastrointestinal distress can be alleviated by administration of a histamine-2 antagonist (Stoll et al. 1991), such as ranitidine or famotidine. Tremor may be minimized through dose reduction or concomitant β-blocker medication. The development of any significant or progressive abdominal distress, or of confusion or delirious states, during acute treatment with divalproex should alert the clinician to the possibility of rare but potentially serious adverse effects, such as irreversible hepatic failure, hemorrhagic pancreatitis, or hyperammonemic encephalopathy.

Problematic side effects during extended treatment with divalproex can include increased appetite with weight gain, essential-type tremor, and hair thinning or alopecia. Although rare, thrombocytopenia, potentially fatal hepatotoxicity, and pancreatitis have been reported, which necessitate routine blood monitoring. Complete blood count and liver and pancreatic enzymes should be checked every 6 months during divalproex therapy. Patients experiencing unexplained lethargy, vomiting, and mental status changes should have ammonia level determination performed promptly to exclude the possibility of hyperammonemic encephalopathy.

With the high propensity of divalproex to displace otherwise highly protein-bound drugs from their protein binding sites, clinicians must be aware of the possibility of clinically significant drug interactions. Divalproex also can inhibit the metabolism of other drugs cleared by the liver. Most notably, divalproex inhibits lamotrigine metabolism by 50%, resulting in the critical need to initiate lamotrigine at 50% lower doses when coadministered with divalproex.

Lamotrigine

Evidence.   Investigation into the efficacy of lamotrigine for the acute management of bipolar disorder episodes is ongoing, although the evidence for its preventive benefits—particularly for preventing depression—has led to its approval as a maintenance treatment for bipolar disorder. In three acute mania randomized trials, only one study suggested that lamotrigine was beneficial for acute mania. This study, however, lacked a placebo group and included a small sample size. Although the potential antimanic efficacy of lamotrigine has not yet been clearly established, it is thought likely to have only mild to moderate efficacy for manic symptoms, yet it may offer significant mood stabilization for rapid-cycling bipolar II disorder (Calabrese et al. 2001).

Open-label studies and case reports of the potential efficacy of lamotrigine before 1999 led to the first double-blind, placebo-controlled study of lamotrigine monotherapy in bipolar I depression (Calabrese et al. 1999). This study reported that lamotrigine was safe and effective for the treatment of bipolar depression, and it stimulated extensive further investigations into the spectrum of efficacy for this compound. Although not yet approved for the acute treatment of bipolar depression, the American Psychiatric Association practice guideline recommends lamotrigine for this use along with lithium.

Two large 18-month maintenance studies (Bowden et al. 2003; Calabrese et al. 2003) comparing lamotrigine, lithium, and placebo in recently manic and recently depressed bipolar I patients, respectively, provided clear and convincing evidence for the use of lamotrigine as a mood stabilizer. Both lithium and lamotrigine were superior to placebo in delaying the time until additional pharmacotherapy was required for treatment of a mood episode in recently manic or hypomanic patients with bipolar I disorder (Bowden et al. 2003). In recently depressed bipolar I patients, both lamotrigine and lithium were significantly superior to placebo in delaying time to intervention for any mood episode (Calabrese et al. 2003). Lamotrigine was superior to placebo in terms of delaying time to intervention for depressive episodes; lithium was not (Bowden et al. 2003; Calabrese et al. 2003). Compared with both lithium and placebo, lamotrigine had significantly greater efficacy for prolonging time to a depressive episode (Bowden et al. 2003; Calabrese et al. 2003). The results of these controlled maintenance studies support the use of lamotrigine to prevent mood episodes below baseline for bipolar I patients. In rapid-cycling bipolar patients, lamotrigine appears to be much more effective for prevention of bipolar II depression than for bipolar I depression (Calabrese et al. 2000). This finding is particularly relevant to the practical clinical management of bipolar rapid cycling, the hallmark of which appears to be depression (Calabrese et al. 2001).

These two lamotrigine maintenance studies were not powered to test lamotrigine's efficacy for above-baseline states. In the planned meta-analysis of these two studies, lamotrigine was significantly better than placebo in delaying time to intervention for mania, but the effect was modest, and lithium was significantly better than lamotrigine (Goodwin et al. 2003). Although lamotrigine may have mild to moderate prophylaxis against hypomania or mild mania, lamotrigine should not currently be considered as a maintenance monotherapy in patients with a history of recurrent manias. Patients with bipolar II disorder with prominent depression or rapid cycling may benefit greatly from lamotrigine therapy (Calabrese et al. 2001).

Pretreatment evaluation. No pretreatment laboratory tests are required before initiating lamotrigine, although routine physical examination, basic baseline chemistries, and pregnancy testing are advisable.

Dosing. Available evidence and expert opinion indicate that the target dose for lamotrigine in the treatment of acute bipolar depressive symptomatology should be 200 mg/day, although some patients may respond to a dose as low as 50 mg/day (Calabrese et al. 1999). Table 28–9 reviews dosing guidelines for lamotrigine in bipolar disorder. The presence of enzyme-inducing drugs, such as carbamazepine, requires doubling of the lamotrigine dose, whereas concomitant administration with divalproex requires a 50% reduction in lamotrigine dosing.

Side effects. The most common side effects observed with lamotrigine are dizziness, ataxia, somnolence, headache, diplopia, blurred vision, nausea, and vomiting (see package insert). These side effects are typically mild and rarely lead to treatment discontinuation. Decreasing the dose or slowing the rate of dose escalation may alleviate these bothersome side effects.

Following a careful and gradual dosage titration schedule reduces the risk of rash. A history of hypersensitivity to lamotrigine is the only contraindication to use. The risk of rash must be discussed before initiating therapy with lamotrigine. Lamotrigine-treated patients in mood disorder clinical trials have a reported rash rate of 8.3%, compared with 6.4% in the placebo-treated patients (Calabrese et al. 2002). Rates of serious rash were 0% with lamotrigine and 0.1% with placebo. In the open-label setting, the overall rate of rash for lamotrigine was 13.1% and of serious rash, 0.1%. One mild case of Stevens-Johnson syndrome was reported in a patient tak-

ing lamotrigine, and no cases of toxic epidermal necrolysis were seen. Any lamotrigine-treated patient developing any rash that cannot easily and rapidly be explained by a known other cause (i.e., contact dermatitis) should immediately discontinue lamotrigine and notify the treating physician before resuming therapy. In unclear or difficult cases, dermatological consultation should be obtained before restarting lamotrigine.

Carbamazepine

Evidence. Approximately 20 double-blind studies have examined the efficacy of carbamazepine or its 10-keto analog oxcarbazepine to date in mania (Muzina et al. 2002). The pooled data from five double-blind, randomized, controlled trials in mania indicated efficacy comparable to that of lithium with onset of response between 1 and 2 weeks for carbamazepine (Keck et al. 1998). Initial reports by Okuma (1993) and colleagues suggested that carbamazepine was effective in preventing bipolar relapse. A meta-analysis by J.M. Davis and colleagues (1999) on mood stabilizers in the prevention of recurrent affective disorders included 572 patients from 10 double-blind, randomized studies comparing carbamazepine with lithium. Over the 3-year study period, 55% of the carbamazepine-treated patients and 60% of the lithium-treated patients experienced a major affective relapse. This difference was not statistically significant, suggesting efficacy equal to that of lithium for overall maintenance therapy; however, the proportion of truly bipolar compared with recurrent unipolar patients cannot be determined from this meta-analysis.

Pretreatment evaluation. Before treatment with carbamazepine, a general history and physical examination should be performed, including screening for any history of liver disease or blood dyscrasias. Routine laboratory tests, including complete blood count, liver profile, and electrolytes with creatinine, should be obtained (American Psychiatric Association 2002).

Dosing and interactions. Serum levels of carbamazepine ranging from 3 to 14 µg/mL have been reported effective for acute mania (Okuma 1983; Petit et al. 1991; Post et al. 1980; Vasudev et al. 2000). The American Psychiatric Association practice guideline recommends beginning carbamazepine therapy at a total daily dose of 200–600 mg in divided doses, with incremental increases of 200 mg/day up to 1,000 mg/day, followed by careful monitoring of blood levels, side effects, and clinical efficacy (American Psychiatric Association 2002). Several factors affect carbamazepine blood levels beyond direct dosing, including

TABLE 28–9.   Lamotrigine dosing (mg/day) for bipolar disorder

Concomitant medication?	Weeks 1 and 2	Weeks 3 and 4	Week 5	Week 6	Week 7
Not taking divalproex or carbamazepine	25	50	100	200	200
Taking divalproex	25	25	50	100	100
Taking carbamazepine or phenytoin	50	100	200	300	300

autoinduction of metabolism and significant drug inter-actions, including increased clearance of oral contraceptives (see Table 28–10).

Side effects.   During acute treatment with carbamazepine, the most commonly observed side effects are nausea, fatigue, blurred vision, and ataxia. Less frequently, liver transaminase elevations, rash, hyponatremia, and blood dyscrasias may complicate treatment.

Oxcarbazepine

Evidence.   Controlled trials of oxcarbazepine have reported rates of clinical improvement in mania comparable to those of haloperidol and lithium (Emrich 1990; Emrich et al. 1985). Oxcarbazepine is very well tolerated and appears to allow reduction of the neuroleptic medication required for the treatment of mood and schizoaffective disorders, yet few clinical studies have been published (Dietrich et al. 2003). A recent naturalistic review reported that oxcarbazepine appeared effective in about one-half of patients and was well tolerated (Ghaemi et al. 2003). The Texas Medication Algorithm Project lists oxcarbazepine as a stage 2 medication alternative for treatment of mania or hypomania, preferring it to carbamazepine because of its better safety and tolerability profile. No controlled data on the efficacy of oxcarbazepine in the maintenance treatment of bipolar disorder have been published. Following the recommendations of the Texas Medication Algorithm Project to consider substituting oxcarbazepine for carbamazepine in the treatment of acute mania or other above-baseline mood disturbances because of improved safety and tolerability, similar comments could be made about maintenance treatment efforts.

Pretreatment evaluation, dosing, and interactions.   Oxcarbazepine is chemically related to carbamazepine but has a reduced risk for leukopenia, rash, cytochrome P450 drug interactions, and autoinduction of metabolism. Pretreatment workup may include routine laboratory tests, including sodium determination, because oxcarbazepine may contribute to hyponatremia (~2.5% incidence), but this is rarely a significant problem (Smith

TABLE 28–10.   Carbamazepine drug interactions

Carbamazepine decreases levels of

Antipsychotics

Benzodiazepines

Contraceptives

Corticosteroids

Lamotrigine

Thyroid hormone

Tricyclics

Increased levels of carbamazepine are caused by

Cimetidine

Diltiazem

Divalproex

Erythromycin

Fluoxetine

Fluvoxamine

Isoniazid

Propoxyphene

Verapamil

Decreased levels of carbamazepine are caused by

Phenobarbital

Phenytoin

Primidone

2001). Precautions are necessary for women taking oral contraceptives because the enzyme-inducing interaction of oxcarbazepine with ethinyloestradiol and levonorgestrel may interfere with contraceptive activity (Smith 2001). In general, therapy for manic or above-baseline mood disturbances can begin with oxcarbazepine, 150 mg twice a day, with increases of 300 mg/week as needed to a target range of 800–1,800 mg/day.

Atypical Antipsychotics

Emerging data on all of the atypical antipsychotics suggest that there may be a class effect for these agents in the management of mania, hypomania, mixed states, rapid cycling, and other atypical variants of above-baseline mood disturbances. Reports of efficacy in monotherapy, combination therapy, and add-on therapy study designs are in line with the American Psychiatric Association practice guideline that recommends first-line treatment of severe manic or mixed episodes with lithium or divalproex *plus* an antipsychotic. The guideline states that "atypical antipsychotics are preferred over typical antipsychotics because of their more benign side effect profile" (American Psychiatric Association 2002, p. 4).

Olanzapine

Evidence. With FDA approval in 2000, olanzapine became the first atypical antipsychotic, and the first antipsychotic since chlorpromazine, indicated for the treatment of mania associated with bipolar disorder. Preliminary data from several open-label studies of olanzapine in acutely manic patients led to two large placebo-controlled studies that supported olanzapine's use (McElroy et al. 1998; Ravindran et al. 1997; Tohen et al. 1999, 2000a; Zarate et al. 1998). Available data suggest that olanzapine brings about symptomatic remission from mania significantly earlier than divalproex (Tohen et al. 2003). A recent Cochrane Database System Review substantiated some superior efficacy for olanzapine over divalproex for acute mania but noted the increased risk of weight gain for olanzapine compared with divalproex (Rendell et al. 2003).

For the treatment of other above-baseline mood-disordered states, olanzapine also may possess a very broad range of therapeutic efficacy. In a recent open-label, uncontrolled 8-week trial of olanzapine monotherapy in 15 patients with hypomania without psychotic features, most patients experienced significant decreases in mania and more limited improvement of their depressive symptoms (Dennehy et al. 2003).

Adjunctive use of olanzapine for mania only partially responsive to either lithium or divalproex results in greater symptom reduction and acute treatment response rates than does placebo augmentation (68% vs. 45%) and also improves coexisting depressive (mixed) symptoms (Tohen et al. 2002a). In addition, olanzapine has been reported to be safe and effective for treatment of the acute manic and depressive symptoms associated with dysphoric mania and a rapid-cycling course (Gonzalez-Pinto et al. 2002; Sanger et al. 2003).

To date, one published open-label study (Sanger et al. 2001) and one randomized, double-blind study (Tohen et al. 2003) suggest that olanzapine may offer preventive efficacy in bipolar disorder, particularly for manic or hypomanic relapse.

Three randomized, controlled trials of olanzapine in maintenance treatment of bipolar disorder have been completed, and the following conclusions were made about the prevention of symptomatic depressive relapses:

- Depressive symptoms improved similarly between divalproex- and olanzapine-treated patients in a 47-week study of patients recovering from a manic episode (Tohen et al. 2003).
- Combination therapy—olanzapine plus either lithium or divalproex—was not significantly better at preventing depressive relapse than was either mood stabilizer alone (Tohen et al. 2002a).
- Depression relapse rates did not differ between olanzapine- and lithium-treated groups during 1-year follow-up from a manic episode (Tohen et al. 2000b).

Olanzapine is now approved by the FDA as maintenance therapy for bipolar disorder.

The results from a recent double-blind study in acute bipolar depression indicated that olanzapine alone and olanzapine in combination with fluoxetine improved depressive symptoms more than placebo did, whereas the olanzapine-fluoxetine combination was more effective than the olanzapine monotherapy (Tohen et al. 2002b). The dosages used in the olanzapine-fluoxetine combination group were olanzapine 6 or 12 mg/day plus fluoxetine 25 or 50 mg/day. The olanzapine-fluoxetine combination received approval by the FDA in December 2003 for the acute treatment of bipolar I depression.

The use of olanzapine to prevent depressive relapses requires further investigation, but these early data are encouraging. However, clinical experience continues to suggest that olanzapine's antimanic prophylactic efficacy in bipolar disorder is stronger than its ability to prevent depression. No data are available regarding newer atypical antipsychotics and their efficacy in preventing mood disturbances below the baseline in bipolar disorder.

Pretreatment evaluation, weight gain, and dosing. Before initiating olanzapine, basic medical history and examination, as well as baseline determination of fasting glucose level, weight, and lipid profile, are recommended. Acute therapy with olanzapine may be associated most commonly with sedation and increased appetite. Consolidating total daily dosage at bedtime or lowering the dose may reduce problematic daytime sedation. Initiation of education and dietary consultation may help longer-term weight management issues with some patients. Additional concern should arise for patients who are early rapid weight gainers, defined as 7% or greater weight gain at 2 weeks after initiation of olanzapine therapy, because this subgroup of olanzapine-treated patients may be at increased risk for ongoing weight gain. Maintenance therapy with olanzapine and any antipsychotic medication in bipolar patients must include careful and routine follow-up evaluation to guard against the development of tardive dyskinesia, despite the reduced incidence with atypical agents. Weight, serum lipid, and glucose levels should be monitored regularly in all patients to screen for development of obesity, hyperlipidemia, glucose intolerance, or diabetes. Patients should be weighed at every visit, and serum determinations of fasting lipids and glucose should be obtained every 3–6 months.

The antimanic dosage of olanzapine is thought to be 15 mg/day, although lower doses may be effective when used in combination with other mood stabilizers. During the initial treatment of a severe manic episode, doses of 30–40 mg/day may be required, which can be safely reduced once the acute episode has resolved.

Other Atypical Antipsychotics

Clozapine.   Although studies of clozapine are few, small, and open label, evidence is sufficient to clearly suggest its efficacy for acute mania as either monotherapy (Barbini et al. 1997; Calabrese et al. 1996) or add-on therapy (Suppes et al. 1999). These trials and clinical experience recommend clozapine in dose ranges of 300–600 mg/day, although lower doses of 100–200 mg/day may be appropriate when used as add-on therapy or in combination with other mood stabilizers. Usual precautions for blood monitoring and clozapine side effects must be observed.

Open-label studies of clozapine in treatment-refractory mood disorders such as bipolar disorder have consistently shown efficacy, including a report by Zarate and colleagues (1995) that 65% of the patients with refractory bipolar disorder were able to continue clozapine monotherapy and experienced fewer mood episodes and fewer hospitalizations. A recent study reported that 83.8% of treatment-refractory bipolar patients responded to clozapine during a naturalistic 48-month follow-up study; the bipolar patients had a more rapid rate of response and better functional outcome than did patients with schizoaffective disorder or schizophrenia who received clozapine (Ciapparelli et al. 2003).

Risperidone.   Multiple randomized, controlled trials of risperidone for treating acute mania have been carried out, beginning with the Segal et al. (1998) study that compared risperidone with haloperidol and lithium and found that all three agents significantly reduced manic symptoms by study end point of 4 weeks. Risperidone monotherapy or combined with another mood stabilizer has been shown to be an effective treatment for the hypomanic phase of bipolar II disorder (Vieta et al. 2001). In acute manic or mixed episodes, augmentation of the mood stabilizer (lithium or divalproex) with risperidone (mean modal dose=3.8 mg/day) was more efficacious than the mood stabilizer alone in reducing above-baseline mood symptoms, as measured by the Young Mania Rating Scale (Sachs et al. 2002a). In this study, risperidone was as efficacious as haloperidol as an augmentation to mood stabilizer therapy but produced significantly fewer extrapyramidal side effects. These findings were confirmed more recently by a double-blind comparison of risperidone and placebo added to a mood stabilizer in acutely manic patients, which reported considerable efficacy in the risperidone-treated group (Yatham et al. 2003). Relatively low doses (2–4 mg/day) of risperidone are needed for add-on or combination treatment strategies, whereas 4–8 mg/day or higher may be necessary if risperidone monotherapy is attempted in acute manic conditions. Risperidone has an FDA indication as monotherapy or adjunctive therapy with lithium or divalproex for the short-term treatment of acute manic or mixed episodes associated with bipolar I disorder.

A much smaller study has been reported that compared risperidone alone (1–6 mg/day), paroxetine alone (10–40 mg/day), and a risperidone-paroxetine combination for the treatment of bipolar depression that emerged in patients already taking a mood stabilizer (Stahl and Shelton 2001). In this unpublished study, the risperidone-paroxetine combination was more effective than paroxetine alone for depressive symptoms in the bipolar patients studied.

Quetiapine.   Quetiapine now has an FDA indication as monotherapy or adjunctive therapy with lithium or divalproex for the short-term treatment of acute manic episodes associated with bipolar I disorder, which is likely to translate to efficacy in other above-baseline disturbances in mood, such as hypomania and hyperthymic states. Case reports and open-label studies have suggested efficacy for treatment-resistant bipolar mania (Dunayevich and Strakowski 2000) and rapid-cycling bipolar disorder (Vieta et al. 2002a). Two recent double-blind, placebo-controlled studies of quetiapine monotherapy in acute mania both reported safety and efficacy (Brecher and Huizar 2003; Paulsson and Huizar 2003). These results support a previous study's findings that showed quetiapine in combination with lithium or divalproex to be significantly more effective than lithium or divalproex alone in treating bipolar mania (Sachs et al. 2002b). Quetiapine appears effective between 400 and 800 mg/day in the treatment of acute mania and associated above-baseline mood disturbances.

Ghaemi and colleagues (2002) reported the effect of quetiapine in an open trial on rapid cycling in 41 patients during all stages of bipolar disorder and observed that although depression rating scale scores improved somewhat, mania scores improved more consistently. However, the mean dose of quetiapine was only 170 mg/day.

Ziprasidone. Ziprasidone appears to have efficacy for the treatment of acute manic states according to a randomized, placebo-controlled 3-week trial of 210 patients with acute bipolar mania (Keck et al. 2003b). Ziprasidone at a mean dose of approximately 140 mg/day led to significant improvements in mania scores, associated psychotic features, and global ratings of improvement starting on day 2 and continuing throughout the study period. Ziprasidone received FDA approval in 2004 to treat acute bipolar I manic or mixed episodes.

Aripiprazole. The newest atypical antipsychotic already has been investigated for antimanic efficacy in a 3-week placebo-controlled, double-blind study of 262 hospitalized bipolar manic patients (Keck et al. 2003a). Aripiprazole monotherapy (15–30 mg/day) produced significant reduction in manic symptoms compared with placebo by day 4 of the study, and this statistically significant difference was maintained throughout the trial. Aripiprazole received FDA indication in 2004 for acute manic and mixed episodes associated with bipolar I disorder.

Studies with ziprasidone and aripiprazole in bipolar depressed states are in development or ongoing, with no published reports to date. Theoretically, the receptor activity profiles of these two atypical antipsychotics suggest that they may possess strong antidepressant properties, which may make them more likely to precipitate hypomanic or manic switching.

Benzodiazepines

Limited data support specific antimanic activity of benzodiazepines, despite their common use in the treatment of mania. Their clinical utility appears to be in the rapid relief of excitement, insomnia, anxiety, and agitation associated with manic or hypomanic states. A small double-blind, crossover trial with 12 acutely manic patients found clonazepam (mean dose=10.4 mg/day) to be as effective as lithium (mean dose=1,691 mg/day) in the management of acute mania (Chouinard 1987). A similar double-blind trial of clonazepam versus placebo found that clonazepam reduced manic, but not psychotic, symptoms and reduced the need for phenothiazine medication (Edwards et al. 1991). Intramuscular use of lorazepam has been reported safe and effective for manic agitation (Lenox et al. 1992). However, the

development of intramuscular atypical antipsychotics such as ziprasidone and olanzapine may offer more direct, clear treatments for agitation and manic psychosis.

Investigational and Novel Treatments

Very limited support exists for the use of gabapentin (Pande et al. 2000), topiramate (Keck and DelBello 2002), or levetiracetam for manic or hypomanic symptoms of bipolar disorder despite early enthusiasm for these newer anticonvulsants. Although gabapentin does not appear to be effective in the treatment of bipolar disorder, it may alleviate associated symptoms of anxiety and insomnia without aggravating the course of illness (Carta et al. 2003). Topiramate may offer some add-on efficacy for atypical or rapid-cycling bipolar disorders, and it helps limit or reduce weight gain associated with other mood stabilizers (Vieta et al. 2002b, 2003). Some more recent reports also suggested that levetiracetam may help with acute mania and rapid cycling when added to other partially effective treatments (Braunig and Kruger 2003; Grunze et al. 2003).

Several other agents have undergone preliminary investigations or suggested promise in the potential treatment of bipolar disorder with manic or above-baseline mood disturbances, including: zonisamide (Kanba et al. 1994), tiagabine (Schaffer et al. 2002), nimodipine (Pazzaglia et al. 1998), clonidine (Tudarache and Diacicov 1991), and L-tryptophan (Chouniard et al. 1985). None has been sufficiently tested to date to support their routine use in bipolar patients.

References

Akiskal H: Classification, diagnosis and boundaries of bipolar disorders: a review, in Bipolar Disorder. Edited by Maj M, Lopez-Ibor JJ, Sartorius N. Chichester, UK, Wiley, 2002, pp 1–52

Akiskal HS, Pinto O: The evolving bipolar spectrum: prototypes I, II, III, and IV. Psychiatr Clin North Am 22:517–534, vii, 1999

Akiskal HS, Bourgeois ML, Angst J, et al: Re-evaluating the prevalence of and diagnostic composition within the broad clinical spectrum of bipolar disorders. J Affect Disord 59 (suppl 1):S5–S30, 2000

American Psychiatric Association: Diagnostic and Statistical Manual of Mental Disorders, 4th Edition, Text Revision. Washington, DC, American Psychiatric Association, 2000

American Psychiatric Association: Practice guideline for the treatment of patients with bipolar disorder (revision). Am J Psychiatry 159 (4 suppl):1–50, 2002

Angst J: Recurrent brief psychiatric syndromes: hypomania, depression, anxiety and neurasthenia, in Basic and Clinical Science of Mental and Addictive Disorders. Edited by Judd LL, Saletu B, Filip V. Basel, Switzerland, Karger, 1997, pp 33–38

Angst J, Ernst C: Current concepts of the classification of affective disorders. Int Clin Psychopharmacol 8:211–215, 1993

Angst J, Weis P, Grof P, et al: Lithium prophylaxis in recurrent affective disorders. Br J Psychiatry 116:604–614, 1970

Angst J, Gamma A, Benazzi F, et al: Toward a re-definition of subthreshold bipolarity: epidemiology and proposed criteria for bipolar-II, minor bipolar disorders and hypomania. J Affect Disord 73:133–146, 2003

Baastrup PC, Poulsen JC, Schou M, et al: Prophylactic lithium: double blind discontinuation in manic-depressive and recurrent-depressive disorders. Lancet 2:326–330, 1970

Barbini B, Scherillo P, Benedetti F, et al: Response to clozapine in acute mania is more rapid than that of chlorpromazine. Int Clin Psychopharmacol 12:109–112, 1997

Bowden CL, Brugger AM, Swann AC, et al: Efficacy of divalproex vs lithium and placebo in the treatment of mania. The Depakote Mania Study Group. JAMA 271:918–924, 1994

Bowden CL, Calabrese JR, McElroy SL, et al: A randomized, placebo-controlled 12-month trial of divalproex and lithium in treatment of outpatients with bipolar I disorder. Divalproex Maintenance Study Group. Arch Gen Psychiatry 57:481–489, 2000a

Bowden CL, Lecrubier Y, Bauer M, et al: Maintenance therapies for classic and other forms of bipolar disorder. J Affect Disord 59 (suppl 1):S57–S67, 2000b

Bowden CL, Calabrese JR, Sachs G, et al: A placebo-controlled 18-month trial of lamotrigine and lithium maintenance treatment in recently manic or hypomanic patients with bipolar I disorder. Arch Gen Psychiatry 60:392–400, 2003

Braunig P, Kruger S: Levetiracetam in the treatment of rapid cycling bipolar disorder. J Psychopharmacol 17:239–241, 2003

Brecher M, Huizar K: Quetiapine monotherapy for acute mania associated with bipolar disorder. Poster presented at the 5th International Congress on Bipolar Disorder, Pittsburgh, PA, June 2003

Burgess S, Geddes J, Hawton K, et al: Lithium for maintenance treatment of mood disorders. Cochrane Database Syst Rev (3):CD003013, 2001

Cade J: Lithium salts in the treatment of psychotic excitement. Med J Aust 2:349–352, 1949

Calabrese JR, Delucchi GA: Spectrum of efficacy of valproate in 55 patients with rapid-cycling bipolar disorder. Am J Psychiatry 147:431–434, 1990

Calabrese JR, Kimmel SE, Woyshville MJ, et al: Clozapine for treatment-refractory mania. Am J Psychiatry 153:759–764, 1996

Calabrese JR, Bowden CL, Sachs GS, et al: A double-blind placebo-controlled study of lamotrigine monotherapy in outpatients with bipolar I depression. Lamictal 602 Study Group. J Clin Psychiatry 60:79–88, 1999

Calabrese JR, Suppes T, Bowden CL, et al: A double-blind, placebo-controlled, prophylaxis study of lamotrigine in rapid-cycling bipolar disorder. Lamictal 614 Study Group. J Clin Psychiatry 61:841–850, 2000

Calabrese JR, Shelton MD, Bowden CL, et al: Bipolar rapid cycling: focus on depression as its hallmark. J Clin Psychiatry 62 (suppl 14):34–41, 2001

Calabrese JR, Sullivan JR, Bowden CL, et al: Rash in multicenter trials of lamotrigine in mood disorders: clinical relevance and management. J Clin Psychiatry 63:1012–1019, 2002

Calabrese JR, Bowden CL, Sachs GS, et al: A placebo-controlled 18-month trial of lamotrigine and lithium maintenance treatment in recently depressed patients with bipolar I disorder. Lamictal 605 Study Group. J Clin Psychiatry 64:1013–1024, 2003

Carta MG, Hardoy MC, Hardoy MJ, et al: The clinical use of gabapentin in bipolar spectrum disorders. J Affect Disord 75:83–91, 2003

Chouinard G: Clonazepam in acute and maintenance treatment of bipolar affective disorder. J Clin Psychiatry 48 (suppl): 29–37, 1987

Chouinard G, Young SN, Annable L: A controlled clinical trial of L-tryptophan in acute mania. Biol Psychiatry 20:546–557, 1985

Ciapparelli A, Dell'Osso L, Bandettini di Poggio A, et al: Clozapine in treatment-resistant patients with schizophrenia, schizoaffective disorder, or psychotic bipolar disorder: a naturalistic 48-month follow-up study. J Clin Psychiatry 64:451–458, 2003

Davis JM, Janicak PG, Hogan DM: Mood stabilizers in the prevention of recurrent affective disorders: a meta-analysis. Acta Psychiatr Scand 100:406–417, 1999

Davis LL, Kabel D, Patel D, et al: Valproate as an antidepressant in major depressive disorder. Psychopharmacol Bull 32:647–652, 1996

Denicoff KD, Smith-Jackson EE, Disney ER, et al: Comparative prophylactic efficacy of lithium, carbamazepine, and the combination in bipolar disorder. J Clin Psychiatry 58:470–478, 1997

Dennehy EB, Doyle K, Suppes T: The efficacy of olanzapine monotherapy for acute hypomania or mania in an outpatient setting. Int Clin Psychopharmacol 18:143–145, 2003

Dietrich DE, Kropp S, Emrich HM: [Oxcarbazepine in the treatment of affective and schizoaffective disorders] (German). Fortschr Neurol Psychiatr 71:255–264, 2003

Dunayevich E, Strakowski SM: Quetiapine for treatment-resistant mania. Am J Psychiatry 157:1341, 2000

Dunner DL, Fleiss JL, Fieve RR: The course of development of mania in patients with recurrent depression. Am J Psychiatry 133:905–908, 1976

Edwards R, Stephenson U, Flewett T: Clonazepam in acute mania: a double blind trial. Aust N Z J Psychiatry 25:238–242, 1991

Emrich H: Studies with oxcarbazepine in acute mania. Int Clin Psychopharmacol 5:83–88, 1990

Emrich HM, Dose M, von Zerssen D: The use of sodium valproate, carbamazepine and oxcarbazepine in patients with affective disorders. J Affect Disord 8:243–250, 1985

Gelenberg AJ, Kane JM, Keller MB, et al: Comparison of standard and low serum levels of lithium for maintenance treatment of bipolar disorder. N Engl J Med 321:1489–1493, 1989

Ghaemi SN, Goodwin FK: Long-term naturalistic treatment of depressive symptoms in bipolar illness with divalproex vs. lithium in the setting of minimal antidepressant use. J Affect Disord 65:281–287, 2001

Ghaemi SN, Thase ME: Role of antiepileptics and atypical antipsychoticsóbipolar depression. Current Psychiatry 1:13–20, 2002

Ghaemi SN, Goldberg JF, Ko J, et al: Quetiapine treatment of rapid cycling bipolar disorder: an open prospective study. Paper presented at the 15th Congress of the European College of Neuropsychopharmacology, Barcelona, Spain, October 2002

Ghaemi SN, Berv DA, Klugman J, et al: Oxcarbazepine treatment of bipolar disorder. J Clin Psychiatry 64:943–945, 2003

Gonzalez-Pinto A, Tohen M, Lalaguna B, et al: Treatment of bipolar I rapid cycling patients during dysphoric mania with olanzapine. J Clin Psychopharmacol 22:450–454, 2002

Goodwin GM: Evidence-based guidelines for treating bipolar disorder: recommendations from the British Association for Psychopharmacology. J Psychopharmacol 17:149–173, 2003

Grunze H, Kasper S, Goodwin G, et al: World Federation of Societies of Biological Psychiatry (WFSBP) guidelines for biological treatment of bipolar disorders, part I: treatment of bipolar depression. World J Biol Psychiatry 3:115–124, 2002

Grunze H, Langosch J, Born C, et al: Levetiracetam in the treatment of acute mania: an open add-on study with an on-off-on design. J Clin Psychiatry 64:781–784, 2003

Gyulai L, Bowden CL, McElroy SL, et al: Maintenance efficacy of divalproex in the prevention of bipolar depression. Neuropsychopharmacology 28:1374–1382, 2003

Hirschfeld RM, Allen MH, McEvoy JP, et al: Safety and tolerability of oral loading divalproex sodium in acutely manic bipolar patients. J Clin Psychiatry 60:815–818, 1999

Hirschfeld RM, Baker JD, Wozniak P, et al: The safety and early efficacy of oral-loaded divalproex versus standard-titration divalproex, lithium, olanzapine, and placebo in the treatment of acute mania associated with bipolar disorder. J Clin Psychiatry 64:841–846, 2003

Hoffman S, Hatch MC: Depressive symptomatology during pregnancy: evidence for an association with decreased fetal growth in pregnancies of lower social class women. Health Psychol 19:535–543, 2000

Holmes LB, Harvey EA, Coull BA, et al: The teratogenicity of anticonvulsant drugs. N Engl J Med 344:1132–1138, 2001

Iqbal MM, Gunlapalli SP, Ryan WG, et al: Effects of antimanic mood-stabilizing drugs on fetuses, neonates, and nursing infants. South Med J 94:304–322, 2001

Janicak PG, Davis JM, Preskorn SH, et al: Principles and Practice of Psychopharmacotherapy, 2nd Edition. Baltimore, MD, Williams & Wilkins, 1997

Judd LL, Akiskal HS, Schettler PJ, et al: The long-term natural history of the weekly symptomatic status of bipolar I disorder. Arch Gen Psychiatry 59:530–537, 2002

Kanba S, Yagi G, Kamijima K, et al: The first open study of zonisamide, a novel anticonvulsant, shows efficacy in mania. Prog Neuropsychopharmacol Biol Psychiatry 18:707–715, 1994

Keck P, DelBello M: Advances in pharmacologic treatment: bipolar mania. Current Psychiatry Supplement, December 2002, pp 6–12

Keck PE Jr, McElroy SL, Tugrul KC, et al: Valproate oral loading in the treatment of acute mania. J Clin Psychiatry 54:305–308, 1993

Keck PE Jr, McElroy SL, Strakowski SM: Anticonvulsants and antipsychotics in the treatment of bipolar disorder. J Clin Psychiatry 59 (suppl 6):74–81; discussion 82, 1998

Keck PE Jr, Marcus R, Tourkodimitris S, et al: A placebo-controlled, double-blind study of the efficacy and safety of aripiprazole in patients with acute bipolar mania. Am J Psychiatry 160:1651–1658, 2003a

Keck PE Jr, Versiani M, Potkin S, et al: Ziprasidone in the treatment of acute bipolar mania: a three-week, placebo-controlled, double-blind, randomized trial. Am J Psychiatry 160:741–748, 2003b

Keller MB, Lavori PW, Kane JM, et al: Subsyndromal symptoms in bipolar disorder: a comparison of standard and low serum levels of lithium. Arch Gen Psychiatry 49:371–376, 1992

Kemp LI: Sodium valproate as an antidepressant. Br J Psychiatry 160:121–123, 1992

Ketter TA, Calabrese JR: Stabilization of mood from below versus above baseline in bipolar disorder: a new nomenclature. J Clin Psychiatry 63:146–151, 2002

Klerman GL: The spectrum of mania. Compr Psychiatry 22:11–20, 1981

Kraepelin E: Psychiatrie: Ein Lehrbuch für Studierende und Aerzte. 6. vollständig umgearbeitete Ausgabe [Psychiatry: A Textbook for Students and Physicians. 6th Revised Edition]. Leipzig, Germany, Verlag Johann Ambrosius Barth, 1899

Kukopulos A, Reginaldi D, Laddomada P, et al: Course of the manic-depressive cycle and changes caused by treatment. Pharmakopsychiatr Neuropsychopharmakol 13:156–167, 1980

Lenox RH, Newhouse PA, Creelman WL, et al: Adjunctive treatment of manic agitation with lorazepam versus haloperidol: a double-blind study. J Clin Psychiatry 53:47–52, 1992

Macritchie KA, Geddes JR, Scott J, et al: Valproic acid, valproate and divalproex in the maintenance treatment of bipolar disorder. Cochrane Database Syst Rev (3):CD003196, 2001

McElroy SL, Frye M, Denicoff K, et al: Olanzapine in treatment-resistant bipolar disorder. J Affect Disord 49:119–122, 1998

Muzina DJ, Calabrese JR: Recent placebo-controlled acute trials in bipolar depression: focus on methodology. Int J Neuropsychopharmacol 6:285–291, 2003

Muzina DJ, Calabrese JR: Maintenance therapies in bipolar disorder: focus on evidence from controlled data studies. Aust N Z J Psychiatry (in press)

Muzina DJ, El-Sayegh S, Calabrese JR: Antiepileptic drugs in psychiatry: focus on randomized controlled trial. Epilepsy Res 50:195–202, 2002

Nemeroff CB, Evans DL, Gyulai L, et al: Double-blind, placebo-controlled comparison of imipramine and paroxetine in the treatment of bipolar depression. Am J Psychiatry 158:906–912, 2001

O'Connell RA, Mayo JA, Flatow L, et al: Outcome of bipolar disorder on long-term treatment with lithium. Br J Psychiatry 159:123–129, 1991

Okuma T: Therapeutic and prophylactic effects of carbamazepine in bipolar disorders. Psychiatr Clin North Am 6:157–174, 1983

Okuma T: Effects of carbamazepine and lithium on affective disorders. Neuropsychobiology 27:138–145, 1993

Paarlberg KM, Vingerhoets AJ, Passchier J, et al: Psychosocial predictors of low birthweight: a prospective study. Br J Obstet Gynaecol 106:834–841, 1999

Pande AC, Crockatt JG, Janney CA, et al: Gabapentin in bipolar disorder: a placebo-controlled trial of adjunctive therapy. Gabapentin Bipolar Disorder Study Group. Bipolar Disord 2:249–255, 2000

Paulsson B, Huizar K: Quetiapine monotherapy for the treatment of bipolar mania. Poster presented at the 5th International Congress on Bipolar Disorder, Pittsburgh, PA, June 2003

Pazzaglia PJ, Post RM, Ketter TA, et al: Nimodipine monotherapy and carbamazepine augmentation in patients with refractory recurrent affective illness. J Clin Psychopharmacol 18:404–413, 1998

Petit P, Lonjon R, Cociglio M, et al: Carbamazepine and its 10,11-epoxide metabolite in acute mania: clinical and pharmacokinetic correlates. Eur J Clin Pharmacol 41:541–546, 1991

Post RM, Ballenger JC, Hare TA, et al: Lack of effect of carbamazepine on gamma-aminobutyric acid in cerebrospinal fluid. Neurology 30:1008–1011, 1980

Prien RF, Caffey EM Jr, Klett CJ: Lithium carbonate and imipramine in prevention of affective episodes: a comparison in recurrent affective illness. Arch Gen Psychiatry 29:420–425, 1973

Prien RF, Caffey EM Jr, Klett CJ: Factors associated with treatment success in lithium carbonate prophylaxis: report of the Veterans Administration and National Institute of Mental Health Collaborative Study Group. Arch Gen Psychiatry 31:189–192, 1974

Prien RF, Kupfer DJ, Mansky PA, et al: Drug therapy in the prevention of recurrences in unipolar and bipolar affective disorders: report of the NIMH Collaborative Study Group comparing lithium carbonate, imipramine, and a lithium carbonate-imipramine combination. Arch Gen Psychiatry 41:1096–1104, 1984

Ravindran AV, Jones BW, al-Zaid K, et al: Effective treatment of mania with olanzapine: 2 case reports. J Psychiatry Neurosci 22:345–346, 1997

Rendell JM, Gijsman HJ, Keck P, et al: Olanzapine alone or in combination for acute mania. Cochrane Database Syst Rev (3):CD004040, 2003

Sachs GS, Printz DJ, Kahn DA, et al: The Expert Consensus Guideline Series: Medication treatment of bipolar disorder 2000. Postgrad Med (spec No):1–104, 2000

Sachs G, Altshuler L, Ketter TA, et al: Divalproex versus placebo for the treatment of bipolar depression. Paper presented at the annual meeting of the American College of Neuropsychopharmacology, Honolulu, HI, December 2001

Sachs GS, Grossman F, Ghaemi SN, et al: Combination of a mood stabilizer with risperidone or haloperidol for treatment of acute mania: a double-blind, placebo-controlled comparison of efficacy and safety. Am J Psychiatry 159:1146–1154, 2002a

Sachs G, Mullen J, Devine N: Quetiapine vs placebo as adjunct to mood stabilizer for the treatment of acute mania. Bipolar Disord 4:61–133, 2002b

Sanger TM, Grundy SL, Gibson PJ, et al: Long-term olanzapine therapy in the treatment of bipolar I disorder: an open-label continuation phase study. J Clin Psychiatry 62:273–281, 2001

Sanger TM, Tohen M, Vieta E, et al: Olanzapine in the acute treatment of bipolar I disorder with a history of rapid cycling. J Affect Disord 73:155–161, 2003

Schaffer LC, Schaffer CB, Howe J: An open case series on the utility of tiagabine as an augmentation in refractory bipolar outpatients. J Affect Disord 71:259–263, 2002

Segal J, Berk M, Brook S: Risperidone compared with both lithium and haloperidol in mania: a double-blind randomized controlled trial. Clin Neuropharmacol 21:176–180, 1998

Shapiro DR, Quitkin FM, Fleiss JL: Response to maintenance therapy in bipolar illness: effect of index episode. Arch Gen Psychiatry 46:401–405, 1989

Small JG, Klapper MH, Kellams JJ, et al: Electroconvulsive treatment compared with lithium in the management of manic states. Arch Gen Psychiatry 45:727–732, 1988

Small JG, Klapper MH, Milstein V, et al: Carbamazepine compared with lithium in the treatment of mania. Arch Gen Psychiatry 48:915–921, 1991

Smith PE: Clinical recommendations for oxcarbazepine. Seizure 10:87–91, 2001

Stahl S, Shelton RC: Risperidone with and without paroxetine alone for bipolar depression. Paper presented at the annual meeting of the American College of Neuropsychopharmacology, Honolulu, HI, December 2001

Stoll A, Walton S, McElroy S: Histamine-2-receptor antagonists for the treatment of valproate-induced gastrointestinal distress. Ann Clin Psychiatry 3:301–304, 1991

Suppes T, Webb A, Paul B, et al: Clinical outcome in a randomized 1-year trial of clozapine versus treatment as usual for patients with treatment-resistant illness and a history of mania. Am J Psychiatry 156:1164–1169, 1999

Suppes T, Dennehy EB, Swann AC, et al: Report of the Texas Consensus Conference Panel on Medication Treatment of Bipolar Disorder 2000. J Clin Psychiatry 63:288–299, 2002

Tohen M, Sanger TM, McElroy SL, et al: Olanzapine versus placebo in the treatment of acute mania. Olanzapine HGEH Study Group. Am J Psychiatry 156:702–709, 1999

Tohen M, Jacobs TG, Grundy SL, et al: Efficacy of olanzapine in acute bipolar mania: a double-blind, placebo-controlled study. The Olanzapine HGGW Study Group. Arch Gen Psychiatry 57:841–849, 2000a

Tohen M, Marneros A, Bowden CL, et al: Olanzapine versus lithium in relapse prevention in bipolar disorder: a randomized double-blind controlled 12-month clinical trial. Paper presented at the European Stanley Foundation Bipolar Conference, Freiberg, Germany, September 2000b

Tohen M, Chengappa KN, Suppes T, et al: Efficacy of olanzapine in combination with valproate or lithium in the treatment of mania in patients partially nonresponsive to valproate or lithium monotherapy. Arch Gen Psychiatry 59:62–69, 2002a

Tohen M, Vieta E, Ketter TA, et al: Olanzapine and olanzapine-fluoxetine combination (OFC) in the treatment of bipolar depression. Paper presented at the 155th annual meeting of the American Psychiatric Association, Philadelphia, PA, May 18–23, 2002b

Tohen M, Ketter TA, Zarate CA, et al: Olanzapine versus divalproex sodium for the treatment of acute mania and maintenance of remission: a 47-week study. Am J Psychiatry 160:1263–1271, 2003

Tudorache B, Diacicov S: The effect of clonidine in the treatment of acute mania. Rom J Neurol Psychiatry 29:209–213, 1991

Vasudev K, Goswami U, Kohli K: Carbamazepine and valproate monotherapy: feasibility, relative safety and efficacy, and therapeutic drug monitoring in manic disorder. Psychopharmacology (Berl) 150:15–23, 2000

Vieta E, Gasto C, Colom F, et al: Role of risperidone in bipolar II: an open 6-month study. J Affect Disord 67:213–219, 2001

Vieta E, Parramon G, Padrell E, et al: Quetiapine in the treatment of rapid cycling bipolar disorder. Bipolar Disord 4:335–340, 2002a

Vieta E, Torrent C, Garcia-Ribas G, et al: Use of topiramate in treatment-resistant bipolar spectrum disorders. J Clin Psychopharmacol 22:431–435, 2002b

Vieta E, Goikolea JM, Olivares JM, et al: 1-Year follow-up of patients treated with risperidone and topiramate for a manic episode. J Clin Psychiatry 64:834–839, 2003

Winsberg ME, DeGolia SG, Strong CM, et al: Divalproex therapy in medication-naive and mood-stabilizer-naive bipolar II depression. J Affect Disord 67:207–212, 2001

Yatham LN, Grossman F, Augustyns I, et al: Mood stabilisers plus risperidone or placebo in the treatment of acute mania: international, double-blind, randomised controlled trial. Br J Psychiatry 182:141–147, 2003

Zarate CA Jr, Tohen M, Banov MD, et al: Is clozapine a mood stabilizer? J Clin Psychiatry 56:108–112, 1995

Zarate CA Jr, Narendran R, Tohen M, et al: Clinical predictors of acute response with olanzapine in psychotic mood disorders. J Clin Psychiatry 59:24–28, 1998

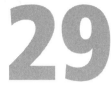

CHAPTER

Understanding and Preventing Suicide

J. JOHN MANN, M.D.

DIANNE CURRIER, PH.D.

SUICIDE IS CURRENTLY the eleventh leading cause of death in the United States and accounted for 29,350 deaths in 2000 (Arias and Smith 2003). It is the third leading cause of death in the 15- to 24-year age group despite a 21% decline from 1990 to 2000 (from 13.2 to 10.41 per 100,000) (National Center for Injury Prevention and Control 2003). Disproportionately high suicide rates are also found among the elderly, who constituted 12.6% of the population in 2000 but represented 18.1% of suicides (Arias and Smith 2003). In the United States, men commit suicide more than four times more frequently than do women (17.5 per 100,000/year and 4.1 per 100,000/year, respectively, in 2000) (National Center for Health Statistics 2004). No official national statistics are compiled on suicide attempts; however, it is estimated that 25 attempts occur for every death by suicide across all age groups, with rates varying from 100:1 to 200:1 in youths and 4:1 in the elderly (Arias and Smith 2003). Women have a higher rate of attempted suicide, with an estimated three female attempts for every male attempt in the United States in 2000 (Arias and Smith 2003).

On a global level, the World Health Organization (2001) estimated that approximately 814,000 individuals worldwide died by suicide in 2000. Suicide rates vary con-

siderably across countries, ranging from less than 1 per 100,000/year in Syria, Egypt, and Lebanon to more than 40 per 100,000/year in many countries that were part of the former Soviet Union (World Health Organization 2003). Worldwide, suicide rates rose dramatically between 1950 and 1995, with a 35% increase in males and a 10% increase in females (World Health Organization 2003). Recent data show some trend toward declining suicide rates in the 1995–1998 period in regions including the European Union, Japan, the United States, and Eastern Europe, although the rate remains substantially higher in eastern Europe than in the European Union (Levi et al. 2003). In the United States from 1990 to 2000, the overall suicide rate declined from 12.4 per 100,000 to 10.7 per 100,000. In contrast, the Russian Federation has seen a substantial increase in mortality from suicide over that period from 37.7 per 100,000 males in 1985–1995 to 58.3 in 1995–1998 and from 8.5 to 9.5 per 100,000 females. Many other countries formerly in the Soviet Union show similar trends (Levi et al. 2003).

The sex distribution of suicide also varies across countries. In 1990, the ratio of male to female suicides varied: 4:1 in the United States, 5:1 in sub-Saharan Africa, and 1.2:1 in India; China was the only country with lower rates in males than in females—0.9:1 (Reza et al. 2001). The reasons for differences in sex ratios for suicide are uncertain, but method of suicide is one factor. Widespread use of pesticides in rural China and Sri Lanka, a highly lethal method, means that most suicide attempts are fatal, and because women make more suicide attempts than men, the rate of completed suicide in women can exceed that in men. First-generation immigrants to Australia have reported suicide rates closer to those of their native countries (Cantor and Neulinger 2000), indicating cultural and ethnic influences on suicide rates, although this tends to fade in the second generation (Burvill and Woodings 1982).

Suicide and Mood Disorders

Those with mood disorders are at significantly higher risk for suicidal behavior. Studies have found that more than 90% of suicide victims had a psychiatric disorder at the time of suicide (Barraclough et al. 1974; Dorpat and Ripley 1960; Rich et al. 1988; Robins et al. 1959; Shaffer et al. 1996). That figure may well be higher given that such studies generally determine psychiatric diagnosis with the psychological autopsy method. That method involves a review of all available medical records and interviews with family members and friends of the deceased person to ascertain the victim's state of mind before death. This method has been shown to generate a valid psychiatric diagnosis (Kelly and Mann 1996). However, because informants are not always available, it is probable that even more than 90% of suicide victims had psychiatric disorders.

Risk for suicidal behavior varies according to type of psychiatric disorder. Approximately 60% of all suicides occur in relation to mood disorders (Barraclough et al. 1974; Dorpat and Ripley 1960; Isometsä et al. 1995a; Robins et al. 1959). Other psychiatric conditions associated with increased risk for suicidal behavior include schizophrenia (Drake et al. 1989), alcoholism (Murphy et al. 1992), substance abuse (Murphy 1988; Rich and Runeson 1995; Rich et al. 1988), and personality disorders (Henriksson et al. 1993), such as borderline personality disorder or antisocial personality disorder (Frances et al. 1986; Marttunen et al. 1991; Runeson 1989; Shaffer et al. 1996).

The lifetime mortality from suicide in discharged hospital populations varies across diagnoses from approximately 20% in manic depression or bipolar disorder to 15% in unipolar depression or major depressive disorder, 10% in schizophrenia, 18% in alcoholism, and 5%–10% in borderline and antisocial personality disorders (Frances et al. 1986; Jamison 1986; Johns et al. 1986;

Marttunen et al. 1991; Roy and Linnoila 1986; Roy et al. 1986). General psychiatric populations, as opposed to hospitalized patients, have lower lifetime mortality rates due to suicide (Bostwick and Pankratz 2000; Murphy and Wetzel 1990). Unsurprisingly, a diagnosis of mood disorder also carries an elevated risk for nonfatal suicide attempts. Epidemiological studies document lifetime rates of suicide attempt of 29.2% in bipolar disorder, 15.9% in unipolar disorder, and 4.2% in all other DSM-III (American Psychiatric Association 1980) Axis I disorders (Chen and Dilsaver 1996).

Although patients with mood disorders are clearly at higher risk for both suicide attempts and completions, most individuals with a psychiatric disorder, including mood disorders, never attempt suicide. Even high-risk groups, such as those with unipolar or bipolar mood disorders, have a lifetime suicide attempt rate substantially lower than 50%. The one exception may be major depression with comorbid alcoholism (Cornelius et al. 1996). Psychiatric disorder alone, then, is not sufficient explanation for suicidal behavior. Research has focused on discerning the clinical, biological, psychosocial, and other differences that distinguish individuals with psychiatric disorders who die by suicide from those who do not. Such differences may pertain to a predisposition, or diathesis, for suicidal behavior under conditions of a psychiatric illness.

Defining Suicidal Behavior

Suicidal behavior covers a spectrum of behaviors, including suicidal ideation, suicide attempts of varying degrees of intent and lethality, and completed suicide. *Suicidal ideation* refers to thoughts of harming or killing oneself, and the frequency, intensity, and duration of such thoughts can vary considerably. Although suicidal ideation without action is more prevalent than attempted or completed suicide (Stengel 1973), severe ideation can be an important indicator of risk for future suicide attempts. In particular, suicidal ideation that includes a specific plan or method for committing suicide is of greatest clinical concern. Our studies have suggested that the clinical profile of such patients resembles that of suicide attempters more so than those with suicidal ideation and no plan (Oquendo et al. 2004).

Suicide attempts vary in both *lethality* (i.e., the degree of medical lethality or damage resulting from a suicide attempt) and suicidal intent (i.e., the degree of preparation and the chances of discovery or rescue, reflecting the balance between the desire to die and the desire to live) (Beck et al. 1976). More highly lethal attempts usually involve more careful planning (including taking measures to avoid detection) and the use of more lethal methods such as firearms. In such attempts, survival may be the result of good fortune. Less lethal attempts more often occur in the context of a social crisis and usually contain a strong element of appeal for help (Stengel 1973). More highly lethal attempts have been recorded more often among men, whereas women tend to use less lethal suicide methods with a higher chance of survival. These less lethal attempts more commonly express an appeal for help insofar as they are conducted in a manner that favors discovery and rescue (Beck et al. 1976; Shearer et al. 1988). Those who make less lethal attempts are more impulsive, and prevention efforts need to address not only major depression and psychiatric syndromes but also problem solving and interpersonal relationships as potential therapeutic targets.

If differences in degree of intent and lethality distinguish different types of suicide attempts, suicide attempters and completers are also understood as two distinct populations. A degree of overlap is seen in the clinical profile of suicide attempts and completions, which contains that group of suicide attempters who survive very lethal attempts and who have the same clinical and psychosocial profile as suicide completers (Linehan 1986). This group is sometimes termed *failed suicides* and is a subgroup of suicide attempters. Investigation of this group is particularly relevant for insight into the etiology of completed suicide.

Studies have found that intent and lethality are correlated, whereby the higher the level of intent, the more lethal, or more medically damaging, the attempt is likely to be. In most studies, the degree of correlation is modest, indicating that important, unidentified factors determine the lethality of suicide attempts. More research into such factors may identify targets for therapeutic intervention and prevention.

One such approach has been the study of biological correlates of suicidal behavior. Correlations have been found among intent, lethality, and certain biological abnormalities associated with a higher risk for suicide (Beck et al. 1976; Mann et al. 1992, 1996b), as discussed in more detail below in the section "Neurobiology of Suicidal Behavior." Briefly, completed suicide correlates with a variety of indices of abnormal serotonin function in the brain, and higher intent and more lethal suicide attempts show the clearest correlation with lower serotonin function.

Intent and lethality are also related to the risk for future completed suicide among those who survive a suicide attempt (Beck et al. 1976). A previous suicide attempt is an important predictor of future suicide (Beck and Steer 1989) or suicide attempt (Leon et al. 1990), and subsequent suicide attempts may involve a greater degree of intent and lethality (Malone et al. 1995). The more serious the suicidal intent and the more lethal the suicide at-

tempt, the greater the risk of a future suicide. Although the presence of a previous suicide attempt is an important predictor of future suicidal behavior, it cannot be relied on as the sole indicator of future risk because more than two-thirds of suicides occur on the first attempt.

Prevention of suicide requires detection of high-risk individuals. One such group comprises those who have attempted suicide and survived. Another is nonattempters with other stigmata of risk, such as impulsive-aggressive traits, more pronounced subjective depression, suicidal ideation, hopelessness, a perception of fewer reasons for living, and low serotonin function.

Modeling Suicidal Behavior

Suicidal behavior is not the outcome of a single causative factor; rather, it is multidetermined, which makes prediction a complex and difficult task. To better understand, and thus to better predict, suicidal behavior, investigators have proposed various models to explain the interaction of identified risk factors. One such model is the diathesis-stress model (Mann et al. 1999). This model understands the diathesis as a predisposition to suicidal behavior in an individual. That is, a set of enduring conditions or traits constitutes a diathesis, the presence of which makes an individual more likely to engage in suicidal behavior when encountering a stressor than someone without the diathesis (Mann et al. 1999). Thus far, aggressive-impulsive traits and a tendency to pessimism (more suicidal ideation, hopelessness, subjective depression, a perception of fewer reasons for living) are two elements of the diathesis that have been identified.

Among the many types of stressors, the onset or acute worsening of a psychiatric disorder is nearly always present in attempters. Other stressors might include psychosocial crises, such as job loss or relationship breakdown. One method of discerning the factors that constitute the diathesis and that, therefore, may explain why some but not other individuals are prone to suicidal behavior is to compare suicide attempters and nonattempters with the same psychiatric diagnoses and with comparable severities of illness and to document the differences. This methodology has yielded considerable insight into clinical, psychosocial, and biological influences (e.g., see Mann et al. 1999).

Clinical Aspects of Suicidal Behavior

Clinical studies have identified two key differences between those with mood disorders who attempt suicide and those who do not. These two traits constitute part of the clinical characteristics of a diathesis for suicidal behavior. The first characteristic is that despite the same objective severity of psychiatric illness and a comparable number of adverse life events to those who do not attempt suicide, suicide attempters experience more subjective depression, hopelessness, and, importantly, more severe suicidal ideation. They also report fewer reasons for living relative to suicide nonattempters, such as significantly more adverse life events, despite a lack of objective evidence for such a view of their lives. Early studies identified a strong association between hopelessness and suicidal behavior (Beck et al. 1975; Wetzel 1976). This tendency toward greater hopelessness and suicidal ideation may have its own diathesis; that is, it may itself be the result of a predisposition for such a response to stressors. For example, Caspi et al. (2003) found that recent life events triggered major depression more frequently in individuals with a low-expressing form of the serotonin transporter gene compared with those who have the high-expressing variant of the gene.

The second clinical element of the diathesis for suicidal behavior is the presence of greater lifetime aggressivity and impulsivity (Mann et al. 1999). Suicidal individuals have been found not only to show more aggression toward others and their environment but also to be more impulsive in other ways involving relationships and personal decisions. This propensity for more acute distress in relation to stressors and a concomitant tendency for more severe suicidal ideation, combined with a greater likelihood of acting on powerful feelings, increase the likelihood of suicidal behavior. The diathesis for suicidal behavior is not confined to mood disorders; rather, it has been observed in suicide attempters and completers across diagnostic categories and is thus independent of specific psychiatric disorder (Mann et al. 1999).

Several other clinical factors and conditions have been strongly associated with higher risk for suicidal behavior. Lifetime or current comorbidity for substance abuse and alcoholism (Dulit et al. 1990; Marzuk and Mann 1988; Murphy 1988; Murphy and Wetzel 1990; Murphy et al. 1992; Rich et al. 1988; Roy and Linnoila 1986; Roy et al. 1990a, 1990b), a reported history of physical or sexual abuse during childhood (Brodsky et al. 1997), a history of a head injury or neurological disorder (Brent 1986; Breslau 1992; Breslau et al. 1991a; Farrer 1986; Schoenfeld et al. 1984), and cigarette smoking (Breslau et al. 1991b, 1993; Glassman 1993; Glassman et al. 1990; Mann et al. 1999) are all associated with a greater likelihood of suicidal behavior.

These factors converge with the diathesis on multiple levels; in some instances, these factors contribute to the development of the two principal clinical traits that characterize the diathesis, and in others, they manifest and perhaps intensify those traits. Evidence indicates that some of these factors are implicated in the development and functioning of the aggressive-impulsive aspect of the diathesis. For example, alcoholism and substance abuse, earlier-onset major depression, head injury, and cigarette smoking appear to be associated with greater aggression and impulsivity (Brent et al. 1994). These are not necessarily direct causal associations; contributory factors are often interrelated, and their contribution to the diathesis is mediated through those relations. Thus, head injuries occur more frequently in aggressive-impulsive individuals and in individuals with alcoholism and substance abuse. This is a bidirectional relation because alcoholism, substance abuse, and aggressive behaviors sometimes follow head injuries (Clifton et al. 1993; Elliott 1992; Frost 1994; Gorenstein and Newman 1980; McAllister 1992). Aggression or impulsivity as a trait, then, is exacerbated by certain conditions at the same time as its presence increases the likelihood of such conditions occurring. Thus, the diathesis for suicidal behavior can be detected as underlying diverse factors that clinical or biological studies have observed and can indicate elevated long-term risk for suicidal behavior in those with mood disorders or other psychiatric conditions.

The combination of these factors and traits can vary and perhaps explain other differences that have been documented in suicidal behavior. For example, more severe aggressive behaviors and alcoholism are both more commonly found in men (Mann et al. 1999; Murphy et al. 1992; Raine et al. 1997; Rich and Runeson 1995). Men are also more prone to head injuries. Thus, males are likely to make suicide attempts that are more lethal, perhaps because of the presence of a diathesis for more lethal suicidal behavior. This could account, in part, for the generally higher completed suicide rates reported in males compared with females. How and why the diathesis for suicidal behavior differs in males compared with females is an area for further study.

Genetic and Familial Aspects of Suicidal Behavior

Familial factors may contribute to the development of the diathesis for suicidal behavior through both genetic and environmental, or developmental, pathways and may act as more current stressors. Suicide has been found to cluster in families, and individuals who commit suicide or make suicide attempts have higher rates of suicidal acts in their families (Roy 1983). This is the case in comparison to both general population control subjects and psychiatric control subjects who have never attempted suicide.

Twin studies have shown a higher concordance rate for both suicide (Roy et al. 1991) and suicide attempts (Roy et al. 1995) in monozygotic compared with dizygotic twins, indicating a genetic contribution to the transmission of suicidal behavior. A role for genetics is further supported by adoption studies that have documented higher rates of suicide in the biological parents of adoptees who commit suicide, compared with the biological relatives of nonsuicidal adoptees (Schulsinger et al. 1979).

Although familial transmission of suicidal behavior might be partly the result of the heritability of mood disorders or other major psychiatric disorders associated with higher suicide risk, numerous family studies have found that suicidal behavior is, to a significant degree, transmitted independently of the transmission of mood disorders and other psychiatric disorders (Brent et al. 1996; Egeland and Sussex 1985; Johnson et al. 1998; Malone et al. 1995; Roy 1983, 1985; Runeson and Åsberg 2003; Tsuang 1983). We have hypothesized that those genetic factors may relate to the diathesis for suicidal behavior. Aggressive and impulsive traits are heritable, and it remains to be determined whether pessimism is heritable. In general, the heritability of suicide is comparable to the heritability of other major psychiatric disorders such as bipolar disorder and schizophrenia (Statham et al. 1998).

The specific genes that contribute to suicidal behavior independently of genes involved in psychiatric disorders themselves remain unknown. Candidate genes for suicidal behavior have been selected largely on the basis of biological correlates and examined in association and linkage studies. They include the gene for tryptophan hydroxylase (TPH; the rate-limiting biosynthetic enzyme for serotonin), the serotonin transporter, and the serotonin 1B (5-HT_{1B}) receptor and 5-HT_{2A} receptor genes. Although the results of such studies are often unreliable, promising associations between a polymorphism in the *TPH1* gene, suicide attempt behavior, and lower serotonergic function have been reported (for a review, see Mann et al. 2001). The *TPH1* gene expresses a form of TPH found in the pineal gland and outside the brain. *TPH2* is a newly discovered gene that is expressed in the brain, and preliminary studies link an intronic polymorphism to completed suicide and depression (Zill et al. 2004).

Several nongenetic familial factors potentially contribute to the development of the diathesis for suicidal behavior, including the effect of parenting and physical or sexual abuse (Brodsky et al. 1997). These may occur in the context of greater parental impulsivity and/or parental depression, alcoholism, and substance abuse, all of which can contribute to adverse parenting. Some evidence also shows that sexual abuse may be transmitted intergenerationally (Brent et al. 2002).

Recent genetic studies suggest that the diathesis for suicidal behavior might appear in the context of the interaction between environmental and genetic factors. For example, the short form of the serotonin transporter gene has a lower level of expression and is associated with increased risk for depression and suicidality in the face of stressful recent life events (Caspi et al. 2003). Family environment (in this case, adverse child rearing) in combination with a lower-expressing variant of the monoamine oxidase A gene can contribute to the development of antisocial behavior and more impulsivity in males but not females (Caspi et al. 2002; Huang et al. 2004). Finally, the effect of modeling of suicidal behavior in important family members has been suggested as a potential influence on risk for future suicidal behavior in children. However, recent family studies (Brent et al. 2002), as well as twin (Statham et al. 1998) and adoption (Schulsinger et al. 1979) studies, found little evidence that imitation or modeling plays a significant role in the familial transmission of suicidal behavior.

Neurobiology of Suicidal Behavior

Research has sought to identify biological differences between individuals with mood disorders who engage in suicidal behavior and those who do not. Investigations of several neurobiological systems have yielded promise, although no clear-cut biological predictor of suicide or suicide attempts has yet emerged. Given the complex causation of suicidal behavior, biological studies have sought connections between biological anomalies, the diathesis, and particular stressors.

The most extensively researched area of neurobiology in suicide is the serotonergic system, and altered serotonergic function has been associated with the diathesis for suicidal behavior (for a review, see Mann 1998). Suicide completers have been consistently documented as having impaired serotonergic function. Postmortem studies of the brains of suicide victims have localized abnormal serotonergic dysfunction to the ventromedial prefrontal cortex (Arango et al. 1995; Mann et al. 2000; Ono et al. 2002). The ventromedial prefrontal cortex is involved in the executive function of behavioral and cognitive inhibition (Burgess and Shallice 1996), and injuries to this brain area can result in disinhibition (Damasio et al. 1994). Low serotonergic input into this part of the brain may contribute to impaired inhibition and thus create a greater propensity to act on suicidal or aggressive feelings. In vivo brain imaging studies have linked prefrontal cortical activity and serotonin release to suicidal acts (Mann et al. 1996a) and impulsivity (Oquendo et al. 2003). Impaired cortical response is associated with suicidal and aggressive behaviors (Siever et al. 1999; Soloff et al. 2000). Thus, either less serotonin input or damage to the cortical neurons that are the target of that serotonin input can result in a predisposition to more aggression or suicidal behavior.

Externally directed aggression is associated with suicidal behavior, and both are independently associated with low serotonergic function (for reviews, see Mann 1995 and Stanley et al. 2000). Studies of cerebrospinal fluid (CSF) levels of the serotonin metabolite 5-hydroxyindoleacetic acid (5-HIAA) and behavioral traits in depressed suicide attempters also found that lower levels of serotonin were associated with greater aggression and hostility. Interestingly, among suicide attempters, only those who make more highly lethal attempts have a lower CSF level of 5-HIAA, indicating a serotonin deficit comparable to that in persons who completed suicides, whereas low-lethality attempters have CSF levels of 5-HIAA closer to those of nonattempters (Malone et al. 1996; Mann et al. 1992).

Serotonergic function is under substantial genetic control (Higley et al. 1993). However, interaction between genetics and environment is also crucial, as shown in animal studies. Peer-reared monkeys, compared with maternally raised monkeys, develop lower serotonergic activity that persists into adulthood and is reflected in greater impulsivity and aggression. This effect may be more striking in monkeys that have a lower-expressing variant of the serotonin transporter gene, indicating a gene–environment interaction.

A history of child abuse is associated with a greater risk for both mood disorders and suicidal behavior in adult life, the latter partly resulting from greater impulsiveness. Extrapolating from animal studies, one can hypothesize that adverse rearing such as child abuse resets serotonergic function at a lower level, an effect that persists into adulthood and increases the risk for suicidal behavior by favoring impulsiveness and development of mood disorders.

Given the degree of genetic regulation of serotonergic function, it has been suggested that genetic factors also might come into play in terms of the heritability of suicide through their effect on serotonergic function (Mann et al. 2001). The high-expressing variant of the monoamine oxidase A gene appears to protect against the development of aggressive and antisocial behaviors in adulthood in those exposed to adverse childhood experiences. Other candidate gene studies are necessary to complete this partial picture because any individual gene explains only a small part of the variance.

Serotonergic changes related to the aggressive aspect of

the diathesis for suicidal behavior are biological traits that remain relatively constant between depressive episodes. Moreover, abnormal serotonergic functioning has been observed in suicide completers and attempters with mood disorders, schizophrenia, and personality disorders (Cooper et al. 1992; Mann and Arango 1999; Mann et al. 2000), indicating a degree of independence from psychiatric diagnosis. Thus, abnormal serotonergic function may constitute a biological characteristic of the diathesis for suicidal behavior found in multiple psychiatric disorders.

With respect to other neurobiological systems, abnormal functioning in the noradrenergic system and the hypothalamic-pituitary-adrenal (HPA) axis has been associated with both major depression and suicidal behavior. Dysfunction in these systems appears to be state dependent rather than indicative of enduring traits and, as such, may be a potential predictor of periods when risk for suicidal behavior is more acute. Studies of the noradrenergic system have observed fewer noradrenergic neurons in the locus coeruleus in the brain stem of depressed suicide victims (Arango et al. 1996), along with indications of cortical noradrenergic overactivity such as lower α-adrenergic and high-affinity β_1-adrenergic receptor binding (Arango et al. 1993). Although data are limited about the role of the noradrenergic system in suicidal behavior (Ågren 1980), severe anxiety or agitation increases suicide risk and is associated with noradrenergic and HPA overactivity (Brown et al. 1987; Fawcett et al. 1997).

Noradrenergic dysfunction may be a developmental consequence, although nonspecific illness or stress effects cannot be ruled out. In rodent studies, restraint stress depletes norepinephrine, and exaggerated noradrenergic and cortisol stress responses are reported in adult depression (G.K. Weiss et al. 1994). Moreover, greater sympathetic responses to stress in adulthood have been observed in both rodents and humans exposed to adverse rearing or childhood abuse (Heim and Nemeroff 2001; Heim et al. 2001). Such a response would further decrease norepinephrine function if there were fewer noradrenergic neurons to begin with (J.M. Weiss et al. 1994). Thus, these biochemical findings potentially reflect a response of the brain noradrenergic system to the stress associated with an impending suicidal act in the context of a serious psychiatric illness. Although the noradrenergic system is partly under genetic control (Higley et al. 1993), its activity is state dependent insofar as it mediates acute stress responses to circumstances such as a psychiatric illness or severe suicidal ideation.

Major depression is often associated with hyperactivity of the HPA axis (Carroll et al. 1981), and suicidal patients in diagnostically heterogeneous populations have HPA axis abnormalities, most commonly dexamethasone resistance (Brunner et al. 2001; Bunney et al. 1969; Coryell and Schlesser 2001; Inder et al. 1997; Meltzer et al. 1984; Nemeroff et al. 1988; Roy 1992; Träskman-Bendz et al. 1992; van Heeringen et al. 2000). Longitudinal studies have found higher cortisol levels after dexamethasone suppression and HPA axis hyperactivity at baseline associated with as much as a 14-fold higher risk for eventual suicide (Brown et al. 1987; Coryell and Schlesser 2001). Studies of both the HPA axis and brain noradrenergic indices indicate deranged biological stress responses that may reflect the risk for suicide.

Evidence has linked very low cholesterol levels and suicide risk (Muldoon et al. 1990, 1993). Very small increases in the rate of suicidal behavior have been reported in individuals with very low cholesterol levels and in diet-based lowering of cholesterol levels (for a complete review, see Golomb 1998). Serotonergic function may play a mediating role in the relation between cholesterol and suicide. Studies of nonhuman primates on a low-cholesterol diet found lower serotonergic activity and increased aggressive behaviors (Kaplan et al. 1994; Muldoon et al. 1993). These associations have not yet been confirmed in human subjects, but they offer some explanation of how cholesterol levels might influence not only suicide risk but also accidental deaths, which also increase with cholesterol lowering (for reviews, see Muldoon et al. 1993 and Golomb 1998). Cholesterol level, in itself, however, has little utility as a predictor of suicidal behavior given the extremely small observed effect of low cholesterol on risk for suicide.

In interpreting the results of biological studies, it is important to distinguish in what context biological abnormalities affect suicidal behavior. Neurobiological changes may be associated with a primary psychiatric disorder, such as major depression or psychosis; may relate to the diathesis for suicidal behavior; or may be indicators of excessive stress experienced in the period leading up to a suicidal act.

Management of Suicidal Patients

Suicidal patients have a high level of contact with medical professionals; it is estimated that 50% of persons who have committed suicide sought professional help within 1 month of the act (Lester 1993). This high level of medical contact increases the opportunity for effective treatment intervention (Isacsson et al. 1995). In formulating a treatment and management strategy for suicidal patients, three principal aspects require attention: 1) diagnosis and treatment of existing psychiatric disorders, 2) assessment of suicide risk and removal of the means for suicide, and 3) specific treatment

to reduce the diathesis or propensity to attempt suicide (for a review, see Hirschfeld and Russell 1997).

Diagnosis and Treatment of Existing Psychiatric Disorders

Generally, there are two avenues through which suicidal patients come into contact with medical professionals. First, they might present seeking treatment for a psychiatric disorder (particularly mood or anxiety disorders), or second, they may present with a medical problem that brings them to either a general practitioner or an internist. The presence of major depression can be discerned through careful assessment of presenting symptoms, such as depressed mood, suicidal ideation, hopelessness, guilt, insomnia, tiredness, anorexia, weight loss, constipation, and poor concentration. Given the increased risk of suicidal behavior associated with major depression, prompt diagnosis and effective treatment are crucial. Studies have found that fewer than one in six patients who committed suicide in the course of a major depressive episode were receiving adequate antidepressant treatment (Isometsä et al. 1994). Thus, more effective recognition and treatment of depressive illnesses can potentially reduce suicide rates significantly (Rutz et al. 1989). This strategy has particular relevance in the United States, where most individuals who have a depressive illness, including those with a history of a suicide attempt, are not receiving antidepressant treatment (for a review, see Oquendo et al. 1999).

In the second scenario, patients present, often to the emergency department, seeking aid for low-lethality suicide attempts. It should not be assumed that the potential for further and more serious suicide attempts, or completion, is low because of the low lethality of the presenting attempt. Psychiatric evaluation, including questioning about past suicidal behavior, may identify more lethal suicide attempts. Moreover, less lethal attempts can be precursors to future, more serious attempts, and the presence of any attempt may indicate the presence of a diathesis, or predisposition, for suicidal behavior. Comorbid alcoholism or substance abuse also significantly increases the risk of suicide in mood disorders (Cornelius et al. 1995) and schizophrenia (Harkavy-Friedman et al. 1999). Detecting the presence of these disorders and instituting appropriate management and treatment can also diminish suicide risk.

Assessment of Suicide Risk and Removal of Means for Suicide

Predicting suicidal behavior is a complex and difficult task. Predictive models generally have not proven accurate or sensitive enough to have practical clinical value (for a review, see Amsel and Mann 2001). However, several factors have been identified that appear to have some degree of predictive power. Such factors may indicate the presence of a diathesis for suicidal behavior and a reaction to current stressors. A vulnerability, or diathesis, is indicated by a history of attempting suicide and the presence of suicidal behavior in family members. A history of attempting suicide indicates that, at some juncture, in the face of a stressor, the individual has shown a propensity to act on suicidal ideation. As discussed earlier, suicide has been shown to cluster in families and may be transmitted from one generation to the next (Egeland and Sussex 1985). Thus, the presence of a family history of suicidal behavior signals the potential transmission of both a psychiatric illness that could act as a stressor and the diathesis for suicidal behavior. A study of families in the Old Order Amish indicated that mood disorders and the propensity for suicide can run in families independently (Egeland and Sussex 1985).

A history of suicidal behavior together with current suicidal ideation is the best predictor of imminent risk. Suicidal ideation is a stronger predictor of short-term than of long-term risk (Goldstein et al. 1991; Pokorny 1983). Moreover, suicidal ideation that includes a plan for suicide or evidence of active preparation for a suicide attempt is a more serious portent of short-term risk. Detecting suicidal ideation may necessitate active inquiry on the part of clinicians, particularly among male patients, who are half as likely as females to report suicidal ideation to their doctor before suicide (Isometsä et al. 1995b). Additional information might be sought from available relatives regarding behaviors indicating planning for a suicide attempt or statements they may have heard from the patient suggesting that he or she has formulated a specific plan.

Systematic inquiry into current depression, hopelessness, and suicidal ideation will assist clinicians in assessment of the risk for impending suicidal behavior. The severity of all three is more pronounced in those with a diathesis for suicidal behavior. The presence of severe suicidal ideation, such as a plan for attempting suicide, may indicate a need for increased observation, up to and including hospitalization. Additionally, for patients who are identified as being at risk, steps should be taken to reduce the availability of a means for suicide, particularly the removal of guns from the house.

Specific Treatment to Reduce Diathesis

Given the evidence of a distinct etiology for suicidal behavior, treatment needs to be developed that focuses on the diathesis for suicidality rather than just the accompa-

nying psychiatric disorder. To date, a paucity of scientific evidence exists regarding treatments that may be beneficial specifically for suicidal behavior. However, recent evidence has emerged that for patients with bipolar or recurrent unipolar depressive disorders, lithium may have specific antisuicidal properties over and above its mood-stabilizing effects (Baldessarini et al. 1999; Nilsson 1999). Lithium is used to prevent the recurrence of either manic or depressive episodes, but it also appears to significantly reduce the risk for suicide and suicide attempts. This antisuicidal effect is particularly striking given the potential toxicity of lithium in overdose, suggesting that it also must reduce the number of suicide attempts (Baldessarini et al. 1999). Suicidal behavior has been shown to increase on discontinuation of lithium to the same rates as those seen prior to starting lithium. As such, it is recommended that lithium withdrawal be undertaken gradually over a period of weeks to reduce the chances of a recrudescence of suicidal behavior.

The antisuicidal properties of anticonvulsant mood stabilizers remain to be tested. In schizophrenia, however, evidence indicates that clozapine, an atypical antipsychotic, may reduce suicidal behavior independently of its antipsychotic therapeutic effects (Meltzer and Okayli 1995; Meltzer et al. 2003; Reid et al. 1998; Walker et al. 1997). Given the favorable side-effect and toxicity profile of atypical antipsychotics, data on their antisuicidal effects would be of great interest. Although the specific mechanisms whereby lithium and clozapine have potentially antisuicidal therapeutic effects are unknown, they may alter the diathesis for suicidal behavior via the serotonergic system on which both agents have pronounced effects. This hypothesis remains to be formally tested.

Conclusion

Identifying patients at risk for suicidal behavior and implementing treatment and intervention strategies is an urgent yet difficult task. It involves cognizance of both the long-term traits that predispose individuals to suicidal behavior and the more transient states that might precipitate that behavior. In terms of stressors, the onset of or failure to recover from a mood disorder is a powerful stressor, and psychosocial events also require consideration. Interventions available at this level include treatment of depression, substance use disorder, or psychosis; psychotherapy to strengthen coping skills; and improvement of the psychosocial support systems for the patient, including psychoeducation for the family. Indicators of heightened risk of suicide in the face of such stressors include a history of suicidal activity, a family history of suicidal behavior, and comorbid alcohol or substance abuse. Current suicidal ideation and active planning indicate potentially imminent risk. Long-term interventions might include effective antidepressant treatment, possibly with medication that has shown indications of antisuicidal effects; psychotherapies such as dialectical behavior therapy for borderline personality disorder; and the treatment of alcohol and substance abuse. Hospitalization and removal of the means of suicide may reduce imminent risk. Public health efforts to educate medical professionals, community workers, and the general population about both mental illness and suicide also may contribute to more effective identification of those at risk and more timely and effective intervention.

References

Ågren H: Symptom patterns in unipolar and bipolar depression correlating with monoamine metabolites in the cerebrospinal fluid, II: suicide. Psychiatry Res 3:225–236, 1980

American Psychiatric Association: Diagnostic and Statistical Manual of Mental Disorders, 3rd Edition. Washington, DC, American Psychiatric Association, 1980

Amsel L, Mann JJ: Suicide risk assessment and the suicidal process approach, in Understanding Suicidal Behaviour: The Suicidal Process Approach to Research and Treatment. Edited by van Heeringen K. Sussex, UK, Wiley, 2001, pp 163–181

Arango V, Ernsberger P, Sved AF, et al: Quantitative autoradiography of alpha 1- and alpha 2-adrenergic receptors in the cerebral cortex of controls and suicide victims. Brain Res 630:271–282, 1993

Arango V, Underwood MD, Gubbi AV, et al: Localized alterations in pre- and postsynaptic serotonin binding sites in the ventrolateral prefrontal cortex of suicide victims. Brain Res 688:121–133, 1995

Arango V, Underwood MD, Mann JJ: Fewer pigmented locus coeruleus neurons in suicide victims: preliminary results. Biol Psychiatry 39:112–120, 1996

Arias E, Smith BL: Deaths: preliminary data for 2001. Natl Vital Stat Rep 51:1–44, 2003

Baldessarini RJ, Tondo L, Hennen J: Effects of lithium treatment and its discontinuation on suicidal behavior in bipolar manic-depressive disorders. J Clin Psychiatry 60 (suppl 2):77–84, 1999

Barraclough B, Bunch J, Nelson B, et al: One hundred cases of suicide: clinical aspects. Br J Psychiatry 125:355–373, 1974

Beck AT, Steer RA: Clinical predictors of eventual suicide: a 5- to 10-year prospective study of suicide attempters. J Affect Disord 17:203–209, 1989

Beck AT, Kovacs M, Weissman A: Hopelessness and suicidal behavior: an overview. JAMA 234:1146–1149, 1975

Beck AT, Weissman A, Lester D, et al: Classification of suicidal behaviors, II: dimensions of suicidal intent. Arch Gen Psychiatry 33:835–837, 1976

Bostwick JM, Pankratz VS: Affective disorders and suicide risk: a reexamination. Am J Psychiatry 157:1925–1932, 2000

Brent DA: Overrepresentation of epileptics in a consecutive series of suicide attempters seen at a children's hospital, 1978–1983. J Am Acad Child Psychiatry 25:242–246, 1986

Brent DA, Johnson BA, Perper J, et al: Personality disorder, personality traits, impulsive violence, and completed suicide in adolescents. J Am Acad Child Adolesc Psychiatry 33:1080–1086, 1994

Brent DA, Bridge J, Johnson BA, et al: Suicidal behavior runs in families: a controlled family study of adolescent suicide victims. Arch Gen Psychiatry 53:1145–1152, 1996

Brent DA, Oquendo M, Birmaher B, et al: Familial pathways to early onset suicide attempt: risk for suicidal behavior in offspring of mood-disordered suicide attempters. Arch Gen Psychiatry 59:801–807, 2002

Breslau N: Migraine, suicidal ideation, and suicide attempts. Neurology 42:392–395, 1992

Breslau N, Davis GC, Andreski P: Migraine, psychiatric disorders, and suicide attempts: an epidemiologic study of young adults. Psychiatry Res 37:11–23, 1991a

Breslau N, Kilbey MM, Andreski P: Nicotine dependence, major depression, and anxiety in young adults. Arch Gen Psychiatry 48:1069–1074, 1991b

Breslau N, Kilbey MM, Andreski P: Nicotine dependence and major depression: new evidence from a prospective investigation. Arch Gen Psychiatry 50:31–35, 1993

Brodsky BS, Malone KM, Ellis SP, et al: Characteristics of borderline personality disorder associated with suicidal behavior. Am J Psychiatry 154:1715–1719, 1997

Brown RP, Stoll PM, Stokes PE, et al: Adrenocortical hyperactivity in depression: effects of agitation, delusions, melancholia, and other illness variables. Psychiatry Res 23:167–178, 1987

Brunner J, Stalla GK, Stalla J, et al: Decreased corticotropin-releasing hormone (CRH) concentrations in the cerebrospinal fluid of eucortisolemic suicide attempters. J Psychiatr Res 35:1–9, 2001

Bunney WE Jr, Fawcett JA, Davis JM, et al: Further evaluation of urinary 17-hydrocorticosteroids in suicidal patients. Arch Gen Psychiatry 21:138–150, 1969

Burgess PW, Shallice T: Response suppression, initiation and strategy use following frontal lobe lesions. Neuropsychologia 34:263–273, 1996

Burvill PW, Woodings TL: Suicide during 1961–70 migrants in Australia. Psychol Med 12:295–308, 1982

Cantor C, Neulinger K: The epidemiology of suicide and attempted suicide among young Australians. Aust N Z J Psychiatry 34:370–387, 2000

Carroll BJ, Feinberg M, Greden JF, et al: A specific laboratory test for the diagnosis of melancholia: standardization, validation, and clinical utility. Archives of General Psychiatry 38:15–22, 1981

Caspi A, McClay J, Moffitt TE, et al: Role of genotype in the cycle of violence in maltreated children. Science 297:851–854, 2002

Caspi A, Sugden K, Moffitt TE, et al: Influence of life stress on depression: moderation by a polymorphism in the 5-HTT gene. Science 301:386–389, 2003

Chen YW, Dilsaver SC: Lifetime rates of suicide attempts among subjects with bipolar and unipolar disorders relative to subjects with other Axis I disorders. Biol Psychiatry 39:896–899, 1996

Clifton GL, Kreutzer JS, Choi SC, et al: Relationship between Glasgow Outcome Scale and neuropsychological measures after brain injury. Neurosurgery 33:34–38, 1993

Cooper SJ, Kelly CB, King DJ: 5-Hydroxyindoleacetic acid in cerebrospinal fluid and prediction of suicidal behaviour in schizophrenia. Lancet 340:940–941, 1992

Cornelius JR, Salloum IM, Mezzich J, et al: Disproportionate suicidality in patients with comorbid major depression and alcoholism. Am J Psychiatry 152:358–364, 1995

Cornelius JR, Salloum IM, Day NL, et al: Patterns of suicidality and alcohol in alcoholics with major depression. Alcohol Clin Exp Res 20:1451–1455, 1996

Coryell W, Schlesser M: The dexamethasone suppression test and suicide prediction. Am J Psychiatry 158:748–753, 2001

Damasio H, Grabowski T, Frank R, et al: The return of Phineas Gage: clues about the brain from the skull of a famous patient. Science 264:1102–1105, 1994

Dorpat TL, Ripley HS: A study of suicide in the Seattle area. Compr Psychiatry 1:349–359, 1960

Drake RE, Bartels SJ, Torrey WC: Suicide in schizophrenia: clinical approaches, in Depression in Schizophrenics. Edited by Williams R, Dalby JT. New York, Plenum, 1989, pp 171–186

Dulit RA, Fyer MR, Haas GL, et al: Substance use in borderline personality disorder. Am J Psychiatry 147:1002–1007, 1990

Egeland JA, Sussex JN: Suicide and family loading for affective disorders. JAMA 254:915–918, 1985

Elliott FA: Violence: the neurologic contribution: an overview. Arch Neurol 49:595–603, 1992

Farrer LA: Suicide and attempted suicide in Huntington disease: implications for preclinical testing of persons at risk. Am J Med Genet 24:305–311, 1986

Fawcett J, Busch KA, Jacobs D, et al: Suicide: a four-pathway clinical-biochemical model. Ann N Y Acad Sci 836:288–301, 1997

Frances A, Fyer M, Clarkin J: Personality and suicide. Ann N Y Acad Sci 487:281–293, 1986

Frost EA: Perioperative management of the head trauma patient. Ann Acad Med Singapore 23:497–502, 1994

Glassman AH: Cigarette smoking: implications for psychiatric illness. Am J Psychiatry 150:546–553, 1993

Glassman AH, Helzer JE, Covey LS, et al: Smoking, smoking cessation, and major depression. JAMA 254:1546–1549, 1990

Goldstein RB, Black DW, Nasrallah A, et al: The prediction of suicide: sensitivity, specificity, and predictive value of a multivariate model applied to suicide among 1906 patients with affective disorders. Arch Gen Psychiatry 48:418–422, 1991

Golomb BA: Cholesterol and violence: is there a connection? Ann Intern Med 128:478–487, 1998

Gorenstein EE, Newman JP: Disinhibitory psychopathology: a new perspective and a model for research. Psychol Rev 87:301–315, 1980

Harkavy-Friedman JM, Restifo K, Malaspina D, et al: Suicidal behavior in schizophrenia: characteristics of individuals who had and had not attempted suicide. Am J Psychiatry 156:1276–1278, 1999

Heim C, Nemeroff CB: The role of childhood trauma in the neurobiology of mood and anxiety disorders: preclinical and clinical studies. Biol Psychiatry 49:1023–1039, 2001

Heim C, Newport DJ, Bonsall R, et al: Altered pituitary-adrenal axis responses to provocative challenge tests in adult survivors of childhood abuse. Am J Psychiatry 158:575–581, 2001

Henriksson MM, Aro HM, Marttunen MJ, et al: Mental disorders and comorbidity in suicide. Am J Psychiatry 150:935–940, 1993

Higley JD, Thompson WW, Champoux M, et al: Paternal and maternal genetic and environmental contributions to cerebrospinal fluid monoamine metabolites in rhesus monkeys (Macaca mulatta). Arch Gen Psychiatry 50:615–623, 1993

Hirschfeld RM, Russell JM: Assessment and treatment of suicidal patients. N Engl J Med 337:910–915, 1997

Huang YY, Cate SP, Battistuzzi C, et al: An association between a functional polymorphism in the monoamine oxidase A gene promoter, impulsive traits and early abuse experiences. Neuropsychopharmacology 29:1498–1505, 2004

Inder WJ, Donald RA, Prickett TC, et al: Arginine vasopressin is associated with hypercortisolemia and suicide attempts in depression. Biol Psychiatry 42:744–747, 1997

Isacsson G, Holmgren P, Wasserman D, et al: Antidepressants and suicide. BMJ 310:127, 1995

Isometsä E, Henriksson M, Heikkinen M, et al: Suicide and the use of antidepressants: drug treatment of depression is inadequate. BMJ 308:915, 1994

Isometsä E, Henriksson M, Marttunen M, et al: Mental disorders in young and middle aged men who commit suicide. BMJ 310:1366–1367, 1995a

Isometsä ET, Heikkinen ME, Marttunen MJ, et al: The last appointment before suicide: is suicide intent communicated? Am J Psychiatry 152:919–922, 1995b

Jamison KR: Suicide and bipolar disorders. Ann N Y Acad Sci 487:301–315, 1986

Johns CA, Stanley M, Stanley B: Suicide in schizophrenia. Ann N Y Acad Sci 487:294–300, 1986

Johnson BA, Brent DA, Bridge J, et al: The familial aggregation of adolescent suicide attempts. Acta Psychiatr Scand 97:18–24, 1998

Kaplan JR, Shively CA, Fontenot MB, et al: Demonstration of an association among dietary cholesterol, central serotonergic activity, and social behavior in monkeys. Psychosom Med 56:479–484, 1994

Kelly TM, Mann JJ: Validity of DSM-III-R diagnosis by psychological autopsy: a comparison with antemortem diagnosis. Acta Psychiatr Scand 94:337–343, 1996

Leon AC, Friedman RA, Sweeney JA, et al: Statistical issues in the identification of risk factors for suicidal behavior: the application of survival analysis. Psychiatry Res 31:99–108, 1990

Lester D: Restricting the availability of alcohol and rates of personal violence (suicide and homicide). Drug Alcohol Depend 31:215–217, 1993

Levi F, La Vecchia C, Saraceno B: Global suicide rates. Eur J Public Health 13:97–98, 2003

Linehan MM: Suicidal people: one population or two? Ann N Y Acad Sci 487:16–33, 1986

Malone KM, Haas GL, Sweeney JA, et al: Major depression and the risk of attempted suicide. J Affect Disord 34:173–185, 1995

Malone KM, Corbitt EM, Li S, et al: Prolactin response to fenfluramine and suicide attempt lethality in major depression. Br J Psychiatry 168:324–329, 1996

Mann JJ: Violence and aggression, in Psychopharmacology: The Fourth Generation of Progress. Edited by Bloom FE, Kupfer DJ. New York, Raven, 1995, pp 1919–1928

Mann JJ: The neurobiology of suicide. Nat Med 4:25–30, 1998

Mann JJ, Arango V: Neurobiology of suicidal behavior, in The Harvard Medical School Guide to Suicide Assessment and Intervention. Edited by Jacobs DG. San Francisco, CA, Jossey-Bass, 1999, pp 98–114

Mann JJ, McBride PA, Brown RP, et al: Relationship between central and peripheral serotonin indexes in depressed and suicidal psychiatric inpatients. Arch Gen Psychiatry 49:442–446, 1992

Mann JJ, Malone KM, Diehl DJ, et al: Demonstration in vivo of reduced serotonin responsivity in the brain of untreated depressed patients. Am J Psychiatry 153:174–182, 1996a

Mann JJ, Malone KM, Sweeney JA, et al: Attempted suicide characteristics and cerebrospinal fluid amine metabolites in depressed inpatients. Neuropsychopharmacology 15:576–586, 1996b

Mann JJ, Waternaux C, Haas GL, et al: Towards a clinical model of suicidal behavior in psychiatric patients. Am J Psychiatry 156:181–189, 1999

Mann JJ, Huang Y, Underwood MD, et al: A serotonin transporter gene promoter polymorphism (5-HTTLPR) and prefrontal cortical binding in major depression and suicide. Arch Gen Psychiatry 57:729–738, 2000

Mann JJ, Brent DA, Arango V: The neurobiology and genetics of suicide and attempted suicide: a focus on the serotonergic system. Neuropsychopharmacology 24:467–477, 2001

Marttunen MJ, Aro HM, Henriksson MM, et al: Mental disorders in adolescent suicide: DSM-III-R Axes I and II diagnoses in suicides among 13- to 19-year-olds in Finland. Arch Gen Psychiatry 48:834–839, 1991

Marzuk PM, Mann JJ: Suicide and substance abuse. Psychiatr Ann 18:639–645, 1988

McAllister TW: Neuropsychiatric sequelae of head injuries. Psychiatr Clin North Am 15:395–413, 1992

Meltzer HY, Okayli G: Reduction of suicidality during clozapine treatment of neuroleptic-resistant schizophrenia: impact on risk-benefit assessment. Am J Psychiatry 152:183–190, 1995

Meltzer HY, Perline R, Tricou BJ, et al: Effect of 5-hydroxytryptophan on serum cortisol levels in major affective disorders, II: relation to suicide, psychosis and depressive symptoms. Arch Gen Psychiatry 41:379–387, 1984

Meltzer HY, Alphs L, Green AI, et al: Clozapine treatment for suicidality in schizophrenia: International Suicide Prevention Trial (InterSePT). Arch Gen Psychiatry 60:82–91, 2003

Muldoon MF, Manuck SB, Matthews KA: Lowering cholesterol concentrations and mortality: a quantitative review of primary prevention trials. BMJ 301:309–314, 1990

Muldoon MF, Rossouw JE, Manuck SB, et al: Low or lowered cholesterol and risk of death from suicide and trauma. Metabolism 42 (suppl 1):45–56, 1993

Murphy GE: Suicide and substance abuse. Arch Gen Psychiatry 45:593–594, 1988

Murphy GE, Wetzel RD: The lifetime risk of suicide in alcoholism. Arch Gen Psychiatry 47:383–392, 1990

Murphy GE, Wetzel RD, Robins E, et al: Multiple risk factors predict suicide in alcoholism. Arch Gen Psychiatry 49:459–463, 1992

National Center for Health Statistics: Mortality data from the National Vital Statistics System. Available at: http://www.cdc.gov/nchs/about/major/dvs/mortdata.htm. Accessed October 2003.

National Center for Injury Prevention and Control: Welcome to WISQARS (Web-Based Injury Statistics Query and Reporting System). Centers for Disease Control and Prevention Web site. Available at: http://www.cdc.gov/ncipc/wisqars/. Accessed October 2003.

Nemeroff CB, Owens MJ, Bissette G, et al: Reduced corticotropin releasing factor binding sites in the frontal cortex of suicide victims. Arch Gen Psychiatry 45:577–579, 1988

Nilsson A: Lithium therapy and suicide risk. J Clin Psychiatry 60 (suppl 2):85–88, 1999

Ono H, Shirakawa O, Kitamura N, et al: Tryptophan hydroxylase immunoreactivity is altered by the genetic variation in postmortem brain samples of both suicide victims and controls. Mol Psychiatry 7:1127–1132, 2002

Oquendo MA, Malone KM, Ellis SP, et al: Inadequacy of antidepressant treatment of patients with major depression who are at risk for suicidal behavior. Am J Psychiatry 156:190–194, 1999

Oquendo MA, Placidi GP, Malone KM, et al: Positron emission tomography of regional brain metabolic responses to a serotonergic challenge and lethality of suicide attempts in major depression. Arch Gen Psychiatry 60:14–22, 2003

Oquendo MA, Galfalvy H, Russo S, et al: Prospective study of clinical predictors of suicidal acts after a major depressive episode in patients with major depressive disorder or bipolar disorder. Am J Psychiatry 161:1433–1441, 2004

Pokorny AD: Prediction of suicide in psychiatric patients: report of a prospective study. Arch Gen Psychiatry 40:249–257, 1983

Raine A, Buchsbaum M, LaCasse L: Brain abnormalities in murderers indicated by positron emission tomography. Biol Psychiatry 42:495–508, 1997

Reid WH, Mason M, Hogan T: Suicide prevention effects associated with clozapine therapy in schizophrenia and schizoaffective disorder. Psychiatr Serv 49:1029–1033, 1998

Reza A, Mercy JA, Krug E: Epidemiology of violent deaths in the world. Inj Prev 7:104–111, 2001

Rich CL, Runeson BS: Mental illness and youth suicide. Am J Psychiatry 152:1239–1240, 1995

Rich CL, Fowler RC, Fogarty LA, et al: San Diego Suicide Study, III: relationships between diagnoses and stressors. Arch Gen Psychiatry 45:589–592, 1988

Robins E, Murphy GE, Wilkinson RH Jr, et al: Some clinical considerations in the prevention of suicide based on a study of 134 successful suicides. Am J Public Health 49:888–899, 1959

Roy A: Family history of suicide. Arch Gen Psychiatry 40:971–974, 1983

Roy A: Family history of suicide in manic-depressive patients. J Affect Disord 8:187–189, 1985

Roy A: Hypothalamic-pituitary-adrenal axis function and suicidal behavior in depression. Biol Psychiatry 32:812–816, 1992

Roy A, Linnoila M: Alcoholism and suicide. Suicide Life Threat Behav 16:244–273, 1986

Roy A, Virkkunen M, Guthrie S, et al: Indices of serotonin and glucose metabolism in violent offenders, arsonists, and alcoholics. Ann N Y Acad Sci 487:202–220, 1986

Roy A, Lamparski D, De Jong J, et al: Cerebrospinal fluid monoamine metabolites in alcoholic patients who attempt suicide. Acta Psychiatr Scand 81:58–61, 1990a

Roy A, Lamparski D, DeJong J, et al: Characteristics of alcoholics who attempt suicide. Am J Psychiatry 147:761–765, 1990b

Roy A, Segal NL, Centerwall BS, et al: Suicide in twins. Arch Gen Psychiatry 48:29–32, 1991

Roy A, Segal NL, Sarchiapone M: Attempted suicide among living co-twins of twin suicide victims. Am J Psychiatry 152:1075–1076, 1995

Runeson B: Mental disorder in youth suicide: DSM-III-R Axes I and II. Acta Psychiatr Scand 79:490–497, 1989

Runeson B, Åsberg M: Family history of suicide among suicide victims. Am J Psychiatry 160:1525–1526, 2003

Rutz W, Von Knorring L, Wålinder J: Frequency of suicide on Gotland after systematic postgraduate education of general practitioners. Acta Psychiatr Scand 80:151–154, 1989

Schoenfeld M, Myers RH, Cupples LA, et al: Increased rate of suicide among patients with Huntington's disease. J Neurol Neurosurg Psychiatry 47:1283–1287, 1984

Schulsinger F, Kety SS, Rosenthal D, et al: A family study of suicide, in Origin, Prevention and Treatment of Affective Disorders. Edited by Schou M, Stromgren E. New York, Academic Press, 1979, pp 277–287

Shaffer D, Gould MS, Fisher P, et al: Psychiatric diagnosis in child and adolescent suicide. Arch Gen Psychiatry 53:339–348, 1996

Shearer SL, Peters CP, Quaytman MS, et al: Intent and lethality of suicide attempts among female borderline inpatients. Am J Psychiatry 145:1424–1427, 1988

Siever LJ, Buchsbaum MS, New AS, et al: d,l-Fenfluramine response in impulsive personality disorder assessed with [^{18}F]fluorodeoxyglucose positron emission tomography. Neuropsychopharmacology 20:413–423, 1999

Soloff PH, Meltzer CC, Greer PJ, et al: A fenfluramine-activated FDG-PET study of borderline personality disorder. Biol Psychiatry 47:540–547, 2000

Stanley B, Molcho A, Stanley M, et al: Association of aggressive behavior with altered serotonergic function in patients who are not suicidal. Am J Psychiatry 157:609–614, 2000

Statham DJ, Heath AC, Madden PA, et al: Suicidal behaviour: an epidemiological and genetic study. Psychol Med 28:839–855, 1998

Stengel E: Suicide and Attempted Suicide. Harmondsworth, Middlesex, UK, C Nicholls, 1973

Träskman-Bendz L, Ekman R, Regnell G, et al: HPA-related CSF neuropeptides in suicide attempters. Eur Neuropsychopharmacol 2:99–106, 1992

Tsuang MT: Risk of suicide in the relatives of schizophrenics, manics, depressives, and controls. J Clin Psychiatry 44:396–400, 1983

van Heeringen K, Audenaert K, Van de WL, et al: Cortisol in violent suicidal behaviour: association with personality and monoaminergic activity. J Affect Disord 60:181–189, 2000

Walker AM, Lanza LL, Arellano F, et al: Mortality in current and former users of clozapine. Epidemiology 8:671–677, 1997

Weiss GK, Ratner A, Voltura A, et al: The effect of two different types of stress on locus coeruleus alpha-2 receptor binding. Brain Res Bull 33:219–221, 1994

Weiss JM, Stout JC, Aaron MF, et al: Depression and anxiety: role of the locus coeruleus and corticotropin-releasing factor. Brain Res Bull 35:561–572, 1994

Wetzel RD: Hopelessness, depression, and suicide intent. Arch Gen Psychiatry 33:1069–1073, 1976

World Health Organization: Suicide, in The World Health Report 2001: Mental Health: New Understanding, New Hope. 2001. Available at: http://www.who.int/whr2001/2001/main/en/chapter2/002g.htm. Accessed October 2003.

World Health Organization: Suicide prevention: country reports. Available at: http://www.who.int/mental_health/prevention/suicide/country_reports/en. Accessed October 2003.

Zill P, Buttner A, Eisenmenger W, et al: Single nucleotide polymorphism and haplotype analysis of a novel tryptophan hydroxylase isoform (TPH2) gene in suicide victims. Biol Psychiatry 56:581–586, 2004

30

Suicide in Children and Adolescents

CYNTHIA R. PFEFFER, M.D.

THE NATIONAL HEALTH IMPLICATIONS of suicide among children and adolescents were not appreciated until the 1980s. Few among the general public realized that since 1969, the rates of suicide among adolescents and young adults, ages 15–24 years, had been increasing. Then, when national attention was drawn to clusters of suicide among teenagers in the 1980s, the public became more aware that suicide was the third leading cause of death among adolescents and young adults ages 15–24 years. Accidents resulted in the greatest incidence of death within that age group, and the second greatest incidence of death was from homicide (Arias et al. 2003).

A surge of research arose as a result of intense community concerns about the tragedy of youth suicide. This research focused on understanding the risk factors for youth suicide. Many suicide prevention programs were developed and implemented, primarily in schools nationwide. As a result of these initial and continuing research investigations, progress is being made in preventing youth suicide.

In this chapter, I highlight gains in delineating risk for suicide among children and adolescents and the types of efforts that have been proposed and applied to prevent children and adolescents from taking their own lives. I describe the epidemiological information about youth suicide and nonfatal suicidal acts. I highlight treatments that have been used in decreasing risk for childhood and adolescent suicide and outline youth suicide prevention strategies. Throughout this chapter, implications for research and clinical care are indicated.

Epidemiology of Suicide Among Children, Adolescents, and Young Adults

The high incidence of suicide among children, adolescents, and young adults continues to be worrisome. In 2001, which is the latest year that national suicide data were completely compiled for the United States, 3,971 adolescents and young adults ages 15–24 years in the United States committed suicide (Arias et al. 2003). The age-adjusted rate of suicide for this age group (9.9 per 100,000 individuals) was lower than the age-adjusted rate for all individuals (10.8 per 100,000 individuals) in that year in the United States. However, age-adjusted rates of suicide among adolescents and young adults ages 15–24 years are exceeded by those in older age groups. For

The author wishes to acknowledge support from Nanette L. Laitman and the William and Mildred Lasdon Foundation.

example, elderly persons have the highest age-adjusted rates of suicide in the United States (Arias et al. 2003). As is the case for all individuals who committed suicide in the United States, youths who were 15–24 years old committed suicide most frequently by using firearms. The age-adjusted rate for firearm suicide for this age group was 5.3 per 100,000 in 2001. This method of committing suicide is not characteristic of many other countries. It is a particular sociocultural phenomenon in the United States.

Although many are surprised that young children commit suicide, the incidence of suicide in children ages 5–14 years in the United States is currently disconcerting. In 2001, the age-adjusted suicide rate for children ages 5–14 years was 0.7 per 100,000 individuals. This represented 279 suicide deaths for this age group in that year. All of these suicides were among children between ages 10 and 14 years. This age-adjusted suicide rate was almost double the age-adjusted suicide rate of 0.4 per 100,000 individuals for this age group in 1979 (Gardner and Hudson 1996). It is not known why the suicide rates for children in this age group have been rising. The age-adjusted suicide rate by firearms for children ages 5–14 years in 2001 was 0.2 per 100,000 individuals. The fact that young children used this highly lethal method to commit suicide indicates the ready availability of firearms to such children.

Table 30–1 highlights trends in age-adjusted suicide rates from 1979 to 2001 for children ages 5–14 years, adolescents and young adults ages 15–24 years, and all ages combined. Important issues are evident. First, the trends in age-adjusted suicide rates for children ages 5–14 years differed from those for adolescents and young adults ages 15–24 years. Second, age-adjusted rates of suicide for children from 1979 to 2001 have been increasing. Third, age-adjusted suicide rates for adolescents and young adults ages 15–24 years have been decreasing in the last few years (1999–2001). Notably, the age-adjusted suicide rates for adolescents and young adults ages 15–24 years were higher in 1979–1993 and began to decrease in 1999. In general, age-adjusted suicide rates for all ages combined have been decreasing since 1979.

Reasons for the decrease in suicide rates for adolescents and young adults ages 15–24 years have not been conclusively discerned. Recent research suggests that the decrease in adolescent and young adult suicide rates may be related to the increased use of antidepressant medications to treat adolescent psychiatric disorders associated with risk for suicide (Olfson et al. 2003). Because this study used a cross-sectional research design, causality could not be ascribed to the effect of antidepressant medication treatment on adolescent and young adult suicide rates. Increased public awareness of youth suicide also may be associated with decreased suicide

TABLE 30–1. Age-adjusted suicide rates per 100,000 for children ages 5–14 years, youths ages 15–24 years, and all ages in 1979, 1992, 1993, 1999, 2000, and 2001

Year	Children	Youths	All ages
1979[a]	0.4	12.4	12.1
1992[a]	0.9	13.0	12.0
1993[a]	0.9	13.5	12.1
1999[b]	0.6	10.1	10.5
2000[b]	0.7	10.2	10.4
2001[b]	0.7	9.9	10.8

[a]Gardner and Hudson 1996.
[b]Arias et al. 2003.

rates among adolescents and young adults. The awareness of the high incidence of adolescent and young adult suicide may have enhanced the identification of youths at risk. Early identification of risk for youth suicide may have improved referrals of youths to treatment services. However, empirical evidence for this trend is not available because this has not been studied systematically.

Racial/ethnic differences exist for suicide rates among youths in the United States. For example, the suicide rates per 100,000 for adolescents and young adult males ages 15–24 years in 2001 were highest for American Indians or Alaskan natives (24.7), compared with white non-Hispanic individuals (19.6), African Americans (13.0), Hispanic individuals (9.5), or Asians or Pacific Islanders (9.1) (Arias et al. 2003). With regard to adolescent and young adult females ages 15–24 years in 2001, suicide rates per 100,000 were highest for Asians or Pacific Islanders (3.6), compared with white non-Hispanic individuals (3.3), Hispanic individuals (2.3), or African Americans (1.3). Data were not available for American Indian or Alaskan native females of this age group or for children ages 5–14 years (Arias et al. 2003).

In recent years, the national suicide rates for African American youths ages 15–24 years have been increasing in contrast to the decreasing suicide rates for white youths in the same age group. It has been suggested that African American youth suicide was increasing because of loss of protective traditional religious practices among African Americans, which was associated with changes in geographic locations of residence among African Americans (Shaffer 1994). As African American youths experience stresses similar to those of whites living in urban settings, African American youths appear to be more vulnerable to suicide than are those living in family-centered rural environments. Trends for racial/ethnic differences in suicide rates need to be explored. Therefore, an extensive amount of additional research regarding sociocultural changes among racial/ethnic groups of youths is necessary to address this epidemiological trend for African American youths in the United States.

Gender differences also exist for suicide rates in the United States. The trends in gender-specific suicide rates have been consistent since 1979 for children ages 5–14 years and for adolescents and young adults ages 15–24 years. In all ages, males (17.6 per 100,000) had higher suicide rates than females (4.1 per 100,000) in 2001 (Arias et al. 2003). As is the case for suicide rates for all ages, the suicide rates for males exceeded those for females in both children ages 5–14 years and youths ages 15–24 years.

Explanations for the higher suicide rates of males have not been clearly discerned. Some factors that may be related to the higher male suicide rates may be increased aggression among males. Different social roles for males, in which they are expected to cope with stress and not to discuss their personal concerns about their perceived stresses, may intensify their stress and isolation. This may lead to suicidal acts. Males have different rates of psychiatric disorders from those of females. For example, males have higher rates of substance abuse and impulsive-aggressive tendencies, which may lead to use of more lethal suicide methods, such as using firearms.

Although national data are not maintained for youth suicide attempts, epidemiological studies suggest trends in rates of nonfatal suicidal acts among high school students. For example, the Youth Risk Behavior Surveillance in the United States in 1999 surveyed adolescents in grades 9–12 to include a nationally representative sample (Kann et al. 2000). The sample included 15,349 adolescents. Approximately 19.3% of the high school students seriously thought of committing suicide within the year prior to the survey. Females (24.9%) had higher rates of suicidal ideation than did males (13.7%). Hispanic adolescents (17.7%) compared with white (12.4%) and African American (11.7%) adolescents had a higher frequency of suicidal planning.

Approximately 8.3% of the adolescents attempted suicide within the year prior to the survey. Females (10.9%) attempted suicide more frequently than males (5.7%). The higher rates of suicidal ideation and suicide attempts among females are a different trend from that of higher rates of completed suicide among males. Hispanic adolescents (12.8%) attempted suicide more frequently than did African American (7.3%) and white (6.7%) adolescents. The higher rates of nonfatal suicidal behavior in Hispanic adolescents than in white adolescents are distinctly different from the trend of white adolescents having higher rates of suicide than Hispanic adolescents. These data indicate the significant prevalence of nonfatal suicidal acts among adolescents. Nonfatal suicidal behavior is a risk factor for adolescent and young adult suicide.

Suicide Risk Factors for Children, Adolescents, and Young Adults

Several methods of research provide evidence for risk factors associated with childhood and youth suicide. A main research design is to collect retrospective data on the psychiatric state of children and adolescents who committed suicide by interviewing parents and others who knew the deceased child or adolescent. This psychological autopsy method is considered reliable in gathering data. Cross-sectional studies of child and adolescent suicide attempters offer data about nonfatal suicidal behavior. This design is highly reliable because the suicidal individual is evaluated directly. Cross-sectional studies usually are the first phase of prospective studies of suicidal children and youths. Prospective studies that follow up on the psychological status of suicidal children and adolescents offer the important advantage of identifying true risk factors. Factors that are evaluated before suicidal behavior occurs can be assessed for the degree of risk they impart for suicidal behavior. This approach enables inferences to be made about causality of suicidal behavior. Family studies provide evidence for risk factors associated with youth suicide. It may be inferred that risk factors identified through family studies may suggest heritable trends for suicide.

In the following subsections, I describe empirically identified psychopathological, environmental, and biological risk factors for suicide among children and adolescents.

Psychopathological Risk Factors for Suicide Among Children and Adolescents

The severity of psychopathology has been determined as a prominent risk factor for suicide among children and adolescents (Beautrais 2000). Table 30–2 summarizes psychopathological risk factors for suicide among children and adolescents.

Many psychological autopsy studies have suggested that approximately 90% of the children, adolescents, and young adults who committed suicide had psychiatric disorders (Brent et al. 1988, 1993a; Shaffer et al. 1996). The greatest risk for childhood and adolescent suicide was imparted by the presence of mood disorders, especially major depressive and bipolar disorders or their comorbidity with substance abuse disorders. Adolescents with a mood disorder diagnosis were at least 12 times more likely to

TABLE 30–2. Psychopathological risk factors for suicide among children and adolescents

Category	Specific risk factor
Psychiatric disorders	Major depressive disorder
	Bipolar disorder
	Comorbid substance abuse disorders
	Schizophrenia
	Personality disorders
Suicidal behavior	Prior suicide attempts
Behaviorial dyscontrol	Impulsivity
Cognitive dysfunction	Hopelessness
Family psychopathology	Suicidal behavior
	Substance abuse
	Violence
	Mood disorders

commit suicide than were adolescents without a history of a mood disorder (Shaffer et al. 1996). Psychological autopsy studies suggested that adolescents who committed suicide compared with nonsuicidal adolescents living in the community were between 20 and 27 times more likely to have a diagnosis of major depressive disorder (Brent et al. 1993a, 1999).

Adolescents who committed suicide were found in one study to be 9 times more likely to have a bipolar disorder compared with adolescents without suicidal behaviors (Brent et al. 1993a, 1999). These rates appeared similar to the rates reported in studies of adults, which indicated that approximately 10%–15% of the individuals with bipolar disorder committed suicide. However, another study reported a negligible risk for suicide imparted by presence of bipolar disorder (Shaffer et al. 1996). The results of this study may have been affected by the relatively low incidence of bipolar disorder among children and adolescents. Because bipolar disorder and schizophrenia usually have their onsets in late adolescence and young adulthood, the data from most psychological autopsy studies may have underestimated or lacked systematic information about risk for suicide imparted by bipolar disorder or schizophrenia. The risk for suicide imparted by bipolar disorder in these psychological autopsy studies may have been more difficult to approximate also because of difficulties in diagnosing this disorder in children and adolescents. For example, although some adolescent suicide victims were given diagnoses of bipolar disorder in psychological autopsy studies, even more of those adolescent suicide victims who were identified as having major depressive disorder may actually have been experiencing

the depressive state of bipolar disorder (Strober et al. 1993). These issues require additional clarification from studies that focus on the prospective course of mood disorders in children and adolescents.

Studies indicate that rates of suicide among adults who have schizophrenia are high. However, the low rate of schizophrenia in studies of adolescents who committed suicide precluded estimates of risk for suicide imparted by this psychiatric disorder.

Psychological autopsy studies also indicated that adolescent suicide victims were significantly more likely to have alcohol abuse (approximately fivefold greater prevalence) and substance abuse disorders (at least ninefold greater prevalence) than were adolescents without suicidal behavior (Brent et al. 1993a, 1999; Shaffer et al. 1996). Risk for suicide was especially high when substance abuse disorders were comorbid with mood disorders in adolescents. These results suggested that evaluation of suicidal intent among adolescents with a history of alcohol and/or drug abuse should be an essential feature of suicide prevention strategies.

Cross-sectional studies of children and adolescents indicated strong associations of major depressive disorder with nonfatal suicidal behavior. Prospective studies of children and adolescents also suggested that presence of major depressive disorder was a strong risk factor for childhood and adolescent suicidal behavior. For example, prospective evaluations of prepubertal children with diagnoses of major depressive disorder found that such children had an almost six times higher likelihood of attempting suicide when they were adolescents compared with prepubertal children without a history of major depressive disorder (Pfeffer et al. 1993). Other prospective research highlighted that prepubertal children with a diagnosis of major depression and those with a diagnosis of anxiety disorder, compared with prepubertal children without any psychiatric disorder, were threefold and twofold, respectively, more likely to attempt suicide in young adulthood (Weissman et al. 1999). Prospective study of representative community samples of adolescents suggested that adolescent males and females who had major depressive disorder were 12 and 15 times, respectively, more likely to have reported a suicide attempt than were adolescents without this disorder (Andrews and Lewinsohn 1992).

Prospective research indicated that adolescent males and females with alcohol abuse had approximately a 10-fold greater risk for a suicide attempt than did adolescents without alcohol abuse (Andrews and Lewinsohn 1992). The association of posttraumatic stress disorder and youth suicide has not been reported. However, it may be expected that such psychopathology, which involves intense states of anxiety, increases risk for suicidal behavior.

A prior suicide attempt is a risk factor for youth suicide. Approximately 33% of the adolescents who committed suicide had a history of suicide attempts (Brent et al. 1999; Shaffer et al. 1996). Specifically, adolescents who committed suicide were 17 times more likely to have a history of a suicide attempt than were adolescents who did not commit suicide (Brent et al. 1993a). Prospective studies of prepubertal children suggested that those who reported suicidal ideation and those who had attempted suicide were approximately at fourfold and sixfold increased risk, respectively, for a suicide attempt in adolescence than were prepubertal children without a history of suicidal behavior (Pfeffer et al. 1993).

Psychiatric symptoms of behavioral dyscontrol, with its hallmark indicator of impulsivity, increased risk for suicide among children and adolescents (Brent et al. 1993a; Shaffer et al. 1996). Psychological autopsy studies indicated that those suicide victims with major depressive disorder comorbid with disruptive behavior disorders, such as conduct disorder or attention-deficit/hyperactivity disorder, were at increased risk for suicide. It has not been determined what aspects of these disorders increased risk for suicide. However, it may be inferred that children and adolescents with such disruptive behavior disorders have increased levels of impulsivity and poor tolerance for frustration. These traits may be important for elevating risk for suicide.

Personality traits or personality disorders in adolescence that involve impulsivity, aggression, and mood instability (borderline, histrionic, and narcissistic personality disorders) or avoidance, dependence, and obsessive-compulsive symptoms (avoidant, dependent, and obsessive-compulsive personality disorders) have been identified as associated with adolescent suicide (Brent et al. 1994). Validation for the associations between these personality traits and personality disorders and suicidal behavior was provided in studies of young adults with suicidal ideation and suicide attempts (Johnson et al. 1999). For example, adolescents with borderline, histrionic, or narcissistic personality disorders were approximately at fourfold greater risk for suicidal ideation or a suicide attempt in early adulthood than were adolescents without these personality disorders (Johnson et al. 1999).

Cognitive dysfunction may increase risk for childhood and adolescent suicide. This has been prominently evident among adults who reported hopelessness (Beck et al. 1985). Specifically, a 10-year prospective study of adults who were psychiatrically hospitalized because of suicidal ideation suggested that hopelessness was significantly associated with suicide within 10 years of follow-up. Similar prospective studies of the role of hopelessness as a risk factor for suicide have not been conducted with children and adolescents. Individuals who reported hopelessness tended to feel despairing, worthless, incompetent, and guilty. These cognitive dysfunctions were among the risk elements for suicide.

Although not considered a psychiatric disorder, being gay, lesbian, or bisexual has implications for risk for adolescent and young adult suicidal behavior (Fergusson et al. 1999). Studies suggested that youths with such sexual orientations were at sixfold greater risk for adolescent suicide attempts than were youths without such sexual orientations (Remafedi et al. 1998). Investigators have suggested that youths who are gay, lesbian, or bisexual are at increased risk for suicidal behavior because they had the same psychiatric disorders as did heterosexual youths who committed suicide. Thus, as with heterosexual youths, being gay, lesbian, or bisexual carries risk for suicide when psychopathology is present.

Psychological autopsy studies have suggested that family psychopathology, including suicidal behavior, substance abuse, violence, and mood disorders, was associated with youth suicide (Brent et al. 1996). Similar psychiatric disorders among parents and siblings have been found to be associated with childhood and adolescent nonfatal suicidal behavior (Pfeffer et al. 1994, 1998b). These psychological autopsy and prospective studies suggested that suicide runs in families. Specifically, children and adolescents who committed suicide or nonfatal suicidal acts had higher rates of parents and siblings with suicidal behavior, including suicide completion. Risk imparted by family history of suicidal behavior appeared to be independent of the presence of psychiatric disorders (Brent et al. 1996; Pfeffer et al. 1994, 1998b). These studies suggested that separate mechanisms exist for suicide risk and for risk for psychiatric disorders. Specifically, parental and sibling history of suicidal behavior increased risk for adolescent suicide fivefold (Brent et al. 1996; Gould et al. 1996). The results of these studies suggest that heritable features of suicidal behavior among children and adolescents should be studied further.

Environmental Risk Factors for Suicide Among Children and Adolescents

The significance of cumulative psychosocial stress for risk for child and adolescent suicidal behavior has been validated in several studies. For example, children with major multiple negative life event experiences before adolescence were reported to have higher risk for a suicide attempt in adolescence than were children of similar age who did not experience multiple negative life event experiences (Pfeffer et al. 1993). Children with psychosocial adversities, such as maladaptive parenting and childhood maltreatment, had elevated risk for suicide attempts in late adolescence and young adulthood (Johnson et al. 2002).

Psychological autopsy studies have identified specific family problems and other negative life event experiences that were associated with adolescent suicide. Specifically, separation of family members increased risk for adolescent suicide approximately twofold (Gould et al. 1996). Risk for adolescent suicide was increased fourfold when the child had a history of communication problems with his or her mother and father (Gould et al. 1996). A history of paternal problems with law enforcement increased risk for adolescent suicide at least fourfold (Gould et al. 1996). Recent crises related to an adolescent being disciplined by the family increased risk fivefold (Gould et al. 1996). Adolescent school problems resulting in school suspension increased risk sevenfold (Gould et al. 1996).

Experiences of family loss increased risk approximately twofold (Gould et al. 1996). Although family loss may be a risk factor, divorce has not been identified as a significant risk factor for youth suicide (Gould et al. 1996). Furthermore, adolescents who lost a peer as a result of a peer's suicide had a sevenfold risk for suicidal ideation (Brent et al. 1993b). In general, prepubertal children who had problems with family, at school, and with friends had a four times greater risk for adolescent suicide attempts than did children without such problems (Pfeffer et al. 1993).

Physical and sexual abuse in childhood and adolescence imparted significant risk for suicide among adolescents and young adults. Research indicated that children experiencing sexual abuse had approximately six times greater risk for suicide than children who had not been sexually abused (Brown et al. 1999). Physical abuse and sexual abuse in childhood imparted a fivefold and sevenfold greater risk, respectively, for a suicide attempt in young adulthood (Johnson et al. 2002).

Biological Risk Factors for Suicide Among Children and Adolescents

Genetic and neurobiological features of suicide have been an important focus for research investigation. Most studies have described the primacy of the serotonergic neurotransmitter system as strongly associated with suicidal behavior (Kamali et al. 2001). These genetic and neurobiological studies have involved samples of adults, with a limited number of studies of children and adolescents. In general, methodological problems for including children in such studies have precluded their participation. This has limited the determination of whether genetic and neurobiological characteristics of suicidal behavior vary with regard to stages of human development.

Serotonergic candidate genes have been associated with suicidal behavior in studies of adults. These candidate genes included polymorphisms of the tryptophan hydroxylase (TPH) gene (Mann 1999) and the 102*C allele in the serotonin type 2A (5-HT$_{2A}$) receptor gene (Du et al. 2000). In contrast, studies of suicidal adolescents have not been clear in identifying genetic associations with adolescent suicidal behavior. For example, the serotonin transporter–linked promoter region (5-HTTLPR) polymorphism and the polymorphism A218C in intron 7 of the TPH gene were not found to be more prevalent among adolescents with suicidal behavior than among adolescents in the general population (Zalsman et al. 2001a, 2001b). The reason that no significant associations were identified among suicidal adolescents is not clear. These findings raise questions about whether there are etiological differences in the risk for suicidal behavior during different stages of human development.

A notable prospective study of a representative birth cohort that was followed up from childhood to young adulthood linked the effects of psychosocial stress and genetics with risk for suicidal behavior (Caspi et al. 2003). This study suggested that individuals with a specific 5-HTTLPR polymorphism and who experienced significant psychosocial stress in childhood were at significantly greater risk in young adulthood for suicidal acts than were individuals without this polymorphism. This study supported concepts that early severe adverse events may sensitize the central nervous system, which may increase vulnerability to subsequent psychopathology (Heim and Nemeroff 2001). The mechanisms for this sensitization of the central nervous system may be regulated by genetic variations.

Several studies indicated that biological factors among suicidal children and adolescents were indicators of serotonin neurotransmitter dysregulation. For example, higher levels of 5-HT$_{2A}$ receptors in the prefrontal cortex and hippocampus were identified in postmortem brains of adolescent suicide victims compared with the same brain regions of adolescents who were not suicide victims (Pandey et al. 2002). The prefrontal cortex and hippocampus are brain regions that are important in the regulation of human emotions, responses to stress, and cognitive functioning. Variations in functioning of these brain regions may account for emotional and cognitive features of risk for suicide.

Peripheral serotonergic dysfunctions among prepubertal psychiatric inpatients were associated with suicidal behavior (Pfeffer et al. 1998a). Specifically, prepubertal psychiatric inpatients who attempted suicide were found to have lower whole blood tryptophan levels compared with nonsuicidal prepubertal psychiatric inpatients (Pfeffer et al. 1998a). A heightened prolactin response to fenfluramine challenge was identified among adolescent suicide attempters compared with nonsuicidal adolescents (Greenhill et al. 1995).

Postmortem brain studies of adults suggested that dysregulation of the hypothalamic-pituitary-adrenal (HPA) axis and noradrenergic neurotransmitter functions may be state-dependent indicators of suicidal risk (Mann and Arango 1999). Evaluation of these issues in children and adolescents has been attempted on a limited basis.

Plasma cortisol levels prior to sleep onset were elevated among depressed adolescents with a history of a recent suicide attempt compared with levels among nonsuicidal depressed adolescents (Dahl et al. 1990). Higher levels of plasma cortisol in response to the dexamethasone suppression test were identified among prepubertal psychiatric inpatients who reported recent suicidal ideation or suicide attempts compared with levels among nonsuicidal psychiatric inpatients (Pfeffer et al. 1991). Because the HPA axis is involved in stress responses, these results may indicate that the suicidal children and adolescents who participated in these studies were experiencing greater stresses than were nonsuicidal children and adolescents. Lower platelet imipramine binding was seen among depressed suicidal children and adolescents compared with nonsuicidal depressed children of similar demographic background (Ambrosini et al. 1992). This study provided information that noradrenergic neurotransmitter regulation is disturbed among suicidal children and adolescents.

Identification and Assessment of Suicide Risk in Children and Adolescents

In a pioneering effort to advance suicide prevention strategies, the surgeon general of the United States (U.S. Public Health Service 1999) wrote a report suggesting that one of the most important suicide prevention methods is identification of those children and adolescents who are at risk for suicidal behavior. The report also noted that once such children and adolescents are identified as being at risk for suicide, immediate referral for intervention to reduce suicide risk is necessary. This report implied that effective methods to screen children and adolescents for suicide risk require development.

A public health orientation to suicide risk identification may provide the most effective strategy to reduce suicide in the United States. Therefore, population screening methods would need to be developed and evaluated for their efficacy in identifying children and adolescents who are truly at risk for suicide. Population screening methods need to involve the appraisal of specific suicide risk factors, such as psychiatric disorders, psychiatric

symptoms, and life event history. Because there have been few studies of biological indicators of suicide risk, no biological screening test is currently available for suicide risk.

A screening approach that has had consensus agreement is to use a cost-effective and time-effective method such as the use of self-report questionnaires to identify children and adolescents at risk for suicide. Specific risk factors, such as psychiatric disorders, psychiatric symptoms, and life event history, may be elicited with such approaches. Screening questionnaires could be administered to children and adolescents in schools or other places where large numbers of youths are present.

Screening questionnaires alone are not sufficient to identify children and adolescents at risk for suicide. Once screening questionnaires are administered and scored and specific children and adolescents are determined to be at risk for suicide, it is important to conduct direct assessments of these children and adolescents. This two-tiered screening approach may be used in places where children and adolescents are usually seen, such as at school or at pediatricians' offices.

Problems exist if only screening questionnaires are used to identify children and adolescents who are at risk for suicide. Specifically, questionnaires may overidentify those at risk and may cause distress in children and adolescents and their parents if they are told that they may be at increased risk for suicide (Pfeffer et al. 2000). Screening procedures have a high rate of false-positive identification of suicide risk. This rate may be reduced by conducting in-depth interviews of those identified on screening questionnaires as at risk for suicide. Another problem with all screening techniques is that their predictive ability has not been conclusively determined. Therefore, it is not possible to specify which children or adolescents identified as at risk for suicide will actually commit suicide. Additional research is necessary to evaluate the sensitivity, specificity, and predictive validity of suicide risk screening methods (Pfeffer et al. 2000).

Clinical assessment of suicide risk in children and adolescents should focus on identifying, during clinical interviews of children, adolescents, and their parents, the multiple risk factors for suicide (Jacobsen et al. 1994). Clinicians should be trained to enhance their skills for evaluating suicide risk in children and adolescents. Particular skill is required in interviewing children and adolescents who may be resistant to discussing their suicidal or symptomatic conditions, who may not be truthful, or who may be psychotic or learning disabled and thus not able to communicate logically (Jacobsen et al. 1994). History from parents is helpful, especially to validate or identify suicide risk factors. However, children's reports, compared with parental reports, tend to yield more symptoms of internalizing problems, such as suicidal ideation or suicidal acts, and symptoms of psychiatric disorders, such as depression and anxiety (Pfeffer et al. 1993).

Treatment of Suicidal Children and Adolescents

In general, treatment strategies for suicidal children and adolescents are based on interventions to decrease risk factors for suicide. Thus, such treatments principally focus on treating mood disorders. Few strategies are specific to treatment of suicidal children and adolescents. Furthermore, the efficacy of such treatments to prevent suicide or suicidal acts has not been established for children and adolescents.

Treatments that have been used for suicidal children and adolescents include psychopharmacological agents and psychotherapy. Types of clinical services in which such treatments are administered include pediatric and psychiatric emergency settings and psychiatric outpatient, day treatment, and inpatient settings. A coordinated network of treatment services is required to provide comprehensive suicide prevention services.

Suicidal children and adolescents often are initially admitted for medical or psychiatric care to emergency services. In these settings, the main aspects of treatment involve treatment of the immediate physical effects of the suicidal act and triage to follow-up medical and psychiatric care. It is essential that emergency service staff be trained to be sensitive to the emotional and practical needs of suicidal children, adolescents, and their parents. Addressing these needs in a clear and sensitive manner can increase compliance with treatment planning (American Academy of Child and Adolescent Psychiatry 2001).

Several important guidelines should be followed before discharging suicidal children and adolescents from an emergency service (American Academy of Child and Adolescent Psychiatry 2001). First, the clinician must discuss with the parents or primary caregivers of suicidal youths the importance of removing firearms from the home and of making firearms and other lethal methods inaccessible to suicidal children and adolescents (Brent et al. 1991). This task is often difficult because it has been suggested that family compliance with relinquishing firearms tends to be limited (Brent et al. 2000). Therefore, before discharging suicidal children and adolescents from emergency services, the clinician must obtain parental agreement that they will safely secure any firearms in the home and make them inaccessible to their children.

Second, prior to discharge from an emergency service, the clinician must evaluate the degree and quality of social support suicidal children and adolescents may receive from the family or others. Such supportive individuals must be capable of recognizing whether a suicidal crisis occurs and whether suicidal risk has increased. Such individuals must be able to ensure that suicidal children and adolescents can be brought to treatment facilities if a suicidal crisis occurs.

Third, prior to discharge from an emergency service, the clinician must verify with the parents or caregivers the history provided by suicidal children and adolescents. This may limit the possibility of underrecognizing the degree of suicidal risk.

Fourth, prior to discharge from an emergency service, the clinician must ensure that a follow-up treatment appointment is scheduled. Such appointments should be scheduled so that suicidal children and adolescents are seen in treatment settings soon after the emergency service discharge. The location and cost of the follow-up facility should be considered. If the location is not accessible or the cost of a follow-up visit is prohibitive for the family, compliance will not be possible.

Psychiatric hospitalization is indicated if 1) there are limitations to treatment compliance on the part of suicidal children or adolescents or their parents or caregivers, 2) high degrees of unpredictability produced by impulsive or psychotic behaviors of suicidal children and adolescents occur, and 3) there is minimal consistent social support in the home. A clear plan for continued psychiatric treatment should be made before discharge from psychiatric inpatient services.

Relatively few psychotherapeutic techniques have been developed or evaluated that are specific for suicidal children and adolescents. Methods that have been developed for adults and that have been developed for specific suicide risk factors have been modified and are being evaluated for children and adolescents who may be at risk for suicidal behavior. Most treatments focus on decreasing symptoms of psychopathological risk factors, such as mood disorders. Three methods of psychotherapies have been applied to children and adolescents at elevated risk for suicidal behavior. These include dialectical behavior therapy, interpersonal psychotherapy, and cognitive-behavioral therapy (American Academy of Child and Adolescent Psychiatry 2001).

Dialectical behavior therapy is the only psychotherapeutic treatment that has been developed specifically for suicidal individuals, especially those with borderline personality disorder. Other treatments, such as interpersonal psychotherapy and cognitive-behavioral therapy, are primarily intended to treat depression in children and adolescents. They may be helpful in suicide prevention efforts because they reduce symptoms of depression, a significant risk factor for childhood and adolescent suicide.

Notably, suicidal children and adolescents frequently experience extensive family conflicts. Therefore, family-focused treatment approaches should be considered in the treatment planning of suicidal children and adolescents. Efforts to increase treatment compliance of adolescents after suicide attempts must focus on individual and family factors and service delivery barriers (Spirito et al. 2002).

Psychopharmacological treatment of suicidal children and adolescents also has not been empirically studied. Methods of medication treatment involve goals of decreasing psychiatric symptoms that are significantly associated with suicidal behavior, such as mood disorders. Specifically, in the treatment of suicidal children and adolescents, antidepressants have been used to decrease symptoms of major depressive disorder (Emslie and Mayes 2001). Mood stabilizers and atypical antipsychotic medications have been used to decrease symptoms of aggression, impulsivity, and psychotic thinking, and of bipolar disorder and schizophrenia, among suicidal children and adolescents. These medications have not been empirically studied for treatment of suicidal children and adolescents. However, in empirical studies of adults, suicidal behaviors were reduced when clozapine was used to treat suicidal schizophrenic adults (Meltzer et al. 2003) and when lithium was used to treat suicidal adults with bipolar disorder (Tondo et al. 1997). Discontinuation of lithium is associated with a ninefold increase in suicide among adults with bipolar disorder (Tondo et al. 1997).

Empirical studies to identify effective medications to decrease risk among suicidal children and adolescents are an essential aspect of developing effective suicide prevention strategies.

Considerations for Prevention of Suicide Among Children and Adolescents

Strategies for suicide prevention involve varied techniques. Among those that may be most effective are to identify those at high risk, as noted earlier. In addition, these identification techniques may be beneficial to apply when children and adolescents have been exposed to or know a peer who has committed suicide. Prevention of clusters of suicide is an important goal. Media presentations of fictional or real suicidal deaths may increase incidence of adolescent suicide (American Academy of Child and Adolescent Psychiatry 2001). Guidelines for the media about methods of presenting suicidal behavior may be useful to prevent future youth suicide. Although hot line services are available, they have not been proven effective in reducing sui-

cidal risk among children and adolescents (American Academy of Child and Adolescent Psychiatry 2001).

Children and adolescents whose parent or sibling committed suicide may be at high risk for suicide. Prospective follow-up of such youths may be a significant suicide prevention technique for this population. In this way, risk for suicidal behavior may be identified and intervention offered to reduce suicide risk.

Finally, new research is essential to integrate current knowledge of suicide risk factors and treatment strategies for childhood and adolescent suicidal behavior with greater understanding of etiological factors. Application of new treatment methods may be derived from these essential endeavors.

Conclusion

Advances have been made in understanding risk factors for childhood and adolescent suicide. This knowledge of the significance of prior suicide attempts, presence of mood and substance abuse disorders, history of cumulative family and other life event stresses, and biological indicators of suicide risk has provided direction in developing treatment and prevention strategies. Among these strategies are identification of those at risk, treatment with psychotherapeutic techniques and psychopharmacological agents, and application of approaches of lethal method restriction through decreasing accessibility to firearms. Education of the general public and of clinicians and professionals who are involved with children and adolescents is essential in youth suicide prevention efforts. At the same time, research is essential to develop therapeutic strategies that effectively reduce suicide risk among children and adolescents.

References

Ambrosini PJ, Metz C, Arora RC, et al: Platelet imipramine binding in depressed children. J Am Acad Child Adolesc Psychiatry 31:298–305, 1992

American Academy of Child and Adolescent Psychiatry: Practice parameter for the assessment and treatment of children and adolescents with suicidal behavior. J Am Acad Child Adolesc Psychiatry 40 (7 suppl):24S–51S, 2001

Andrews JA, Lewinsohn PM: Suicidal attempts among older adolescents: prevalence and co-occurrence with psychiatric disorders. J Am Acad Child Adolesc Psychiatry 4:655–662, 1992

Arias E, Anderson RN, Kung HC, et al: Deaths: final data for 2001. Natl Vital Stat Rep 52(3):1–115, 2003

Beautrais AL: Risk factors for suicide and attempted suicide among young people. Aust N Z J Psychiatry 34:420–436, 2000

Beck AT, Steer RA, Kovacs M, et al: Hopelessness and eventual suicide: a 10-year prospective study of patients hospitalized with suicidal ideation. Am J Psychiatry 142:559–563, 1985

Brent DA, Perper JA, Goldstein CE, et al: Risk factors for adolescent suicide: a comparison of adolescent suicide victims with suicidal inpatients. Arch Gen Psychiatry 45:581–588, 1988

Brent DA, Perper JA, Allman CJ, et al: The presence and accessibility of firearms in the homes of adolescent suicides: a case-control study. JAMA 266:2989–2995, 1991

Brent DA, Perper JA, Moritz G, et al: Psychiatric risk factors for adolescent suicide: a case-control study. J Am Acad Child Adolesc Psychiatry 32:521–529, 1993a

Brent DA, Perper JA, Moritz G, et al: Psychiatric sequelae to the loss of an adolescent peer to suicide. J Am Acad Child Adolesc Psychiatry 32:509–517, 1993b

Brent DA, Johnson BA, Perper J, et al: Personality disorder, personality traits, impulsive violence, and completed suicide in adolescence. J Am Acad Child Adolesc Psychiatry 33:1080–1086, 1994

Brent DA, Bridge J, Johnson BA, et al: Suicidal behavior runs in families: a controlled family study of adolescent suicide victims. Arch Gen Psychiatry 53:1145–1152, 1996

Brent DA, Baugher M, Bridge J, et al: Age- and sex-related risk factors for adolescent suicide. J Am Acad Child Adolesc Psychiatry 38:1497–1505, 1999

Brent DA, Baugher M, Birmaher B, et al: Compliance with recommendations to remove firearms in families participating in a clinical trial for adolescent depression. J Am Acad Child Adolesc Psychiatry 39:1220–1226, 2000

Brown J, Cohen P, Johnson JG, et al: Childhood abuse and neglect: specificity of effects on adolescent and young adult depression and suicidality. J Am Acad Child Adolesc Psychiatry 38:1490–1496, 1999

Caspi A, Sugden K, Moffitt TE, et al: Influence of life stress on depression: moderation by a polymorphism in the 5-HTT gene. Science 301:386–389, 2003

Dahl RE, Puig-Antich J, Ryan ND, et al: EEG sleep in adolescents with major depression: the role of suicidality and inpatient status. J Affect Disord 19:63–75, 1990

Du L, Bakish D, Lapierre YD, et al: Association of polymorphism of serotonin 2A receptor gene with suicidal ideation in major depressive disorder. Am J Med Genet 96:56–60, 2000

Emslie GJ, Mayes TL: Mood disorders in children and adolescents: psychopharmacological treatment. Biol Psychiatry 49:1082–1090, 2001

Fergusson DM, Horwood J, Beautris AL: Is sexual orientation related to mental health problems and suicidality in young people? Arch Gen Psychiatry 56:876–880, 1999

Gardner P, Hudson BL: Advance report of final mortality statistics, 1993. Mon Vital Stat Rep 44 (7 suppl), 1996

Gould MS, Fisher P, Parides M, et al: Psychosocial risk factors of child and adolescent completed suicide. Arch Gen Psychiatry 53:1155–1162, 1996

Greenhill L, Waslick B, Parides M, et al: Biological studies in suicidal adolescent inpatients. Scientific Proceedings of the Annual Meeting of the American Academy of Child and Adolescent Psychiatry 11:124, 1995

Heim C, Nemeroff CB: The role of childhood trauma in the neurobiology of mood and anxiety disorders: preclinical and clinical studies. Biol Psychiatry 49:1023–1039, 2001

Jacobsen LK, Rabinowitz I, Popper MS, et al: Interviewing prepubertal children about suicidal ideation and behavior. J Am Acad Child Adolesc Psychiatry 33:439–452, 1994

Johnson JG, Cohen P, Skodol AE, et al: Personality disorders in adolescence and risk of major mental disorders and suicidality during adulthood. Arch Gen Psychiatry 56:805–811, 1999

Johnson JG, Cohen P, Gould MS, et al: Childhood adversities, interpersonal difficulties, and risk for suicide attempts during late adolescence and early adulthood. Arch Gen Psychiatry 59:741–749, 2002

Kamali M, Oquendo MA, Mann JJ: Understanding the neurobiology of suicidal behavior. Depress Anxiety 14:164–176, 2001

Kann L, Kinchen SA, Williams BI, et al: Youth Risk Behavior Surveillance—United States, 1999. J Sch Health 70:271–285, 2000

Mann JJ, Arango V: Abnormalities of brain structure and function in mood disorders, in The Neurobiology of Mental Illness. Edited by Charney DS, Nestler EJ, Bunny BS. New York, Oxford University Press, 1999, pp 285–393

Meltzer JY, Alphs L, Green AL, et al: Clozapine treatment for suicidality in schizophrenia: International Suicide Prevention Trial (InterSePT). Arch Gen Psychiatry 60:82–91, 2003

Olfson M, Shaffer D, Marcus SC, et al: Relationship between antidepressant medication treatment and suicide in adolescents. Arch Gen Psychiatry 60:978–982, 2003

Pandey GN, Dwivedi Y, Rizavi HS, et al: Higher expression of serotonin 5-HT$_{2A}$ receptors in the postmortem brains of teenage suicide victims. Am J Psychiatry 159:419–429, 2002

Pfeffer CR, Stokes P, Shindledecker R: Suicidal behavior and hypothalamic-pituitary-adrenal cortical axis indices in child psychiatric inpatients. Biol Psychiatry 29:909–917, 1991

Pfeffer CR, Klerman GL, Hurt SW, et al: Suicidal children grow up: rates and psychosocial risk factors of suicide attempts during follow-up. J Am Acad Child Adolesc Psychiatry 32:106–113, 1993

Pfeffer CR, Normandin L, Kakuma T: Suicidal children grow up: suicidal behavior and psychiatric disorders among relatives. J Am Acad Child Adolesc Psychiatry 33:1087–1097, 1994

Pfeffer CR, McBride A, Anderson GM, et al: Peripheral serotonin measures in prepubertal psychiatric inpatients and normal children: associations with suicidal behavior and its risk factors. Biol Psychiatry 44:568–577, 1998a

Pfeffer CR, Normandin L, Kakuma T: Suicidal children grow up: relations between family psychopathology and adolescents' lifetime suicidal behavior. J Nerv Ment Dis 186:269–275, 1998b

Pfeffer CR, Jiang H, Kakuma R: Child-Adolescent Suicidal Potential Index (CASPI): a screen for risk for early onset suicidal behavior. Psychol Assess 12:304–318, 2000

Remafedi G, French S, Story M, et al: The relationship between suicide risk and sexual orientation: results of a population-based study. Am J Public Health 88:57–60, 1998

Shaffer D: Worsening suicide rate in black teenagers. Am J Psychiatry 151:1810–1812, 1994

Shaffer D, Gould MS, Fisher P, et al: Psychiatric diagnosis in child and adolescent suicide. Arch Gen Psychiatry 53:339–348, 1996

Spirito A, Boergers J, Donaldson D, et al: An intervention trial to improve adherence to community treatment by adolescents after a suicide attempt. J Am Acad Child Adolesc Psychiatry 41:435–442, 2002

Strober M, Lampert C, Schmidt S, et al: The course of major depressive disorder in adolescents, I: recovery and risk of manic switching in a follow-up of psychotic and nonpsychotic subtypes. J Am Acad Child Adolesc Psychiatry 32:34–42, 1993

Tondo L, Jamison KR, Baldessarini RJ: Effect of lithium maintenance on suicidal behavior in major mood disorders. Ann N Y Acad Sci 836:339–351, 1997

U.S. Public Health Service. The Surgeon General's Call to Action to Prevent Suicide. Washington, DC, U.S. Department of Health and Human Services, 1999

Weissman MM, Wolk S, Wickramaratne P, et al: Children with prepubertal-onset major depressive disorder and anxiety grown up. Arch Gen Psychiatry 56:794–801, 1999

Zalsman G, Frisch A, Bromberg M, et al: Family based association study of serotonin transporter promoter in suicidal adolescents: no association with suicidality but possible role in violence traits. Am J Med Genet 105:239–245, 2001a

Zalsman G, Frisch A, King RA, et al: Case control and family based studies of tryptophan hydroxylase gene A218C polymorphism and suicidality in adolescents. Am J Med Genet 105:451–457, 2001b

31

Medication Combination and Augmentation Strategies in the Treatment of Major Depression

PIERRE BLIER, M.D., PH.D.

APPROXIMATELY TWO-THIRDS of depressed patients will experience various degrees of improvement to a first antidepressant drug trial. The response criterion, generally accepted to be a 50% improvement, is, however, no longer the standard used to assess the effectiveness of antidepressant treatments ("New Federal Guidelines" 1993; Nierenberg and DeCecco 2001). This change is largely based on the observation that patients who have responded to their therapeutic regimen but still show significant residual symptoms have a higher relapse rate than do patients treated to remission (Judd et al. 2000; Paykel et al. 1995). When the remission criterion is used, the success rate of any antidepressant drug is less than 50% in placebo-controlled trials (Thase 2003; Thase et al. 2001). Consequently, more than half of the depressed patients will require additional measures after a first drug treatment (Figure 31–1).

The available options for additional measures consist of medication substitution, drug combination, and augmentation. A *medication substitution* consists of switching an antidepressant drug for another of the same or different class, with or without a washout period. Classically, the *combination* strategy entails keeping the first drug and

adding a second agent that is also a recognized antidepressant monotherapy. The *augmentation*, or *potentiation*, approach consists of adding a second agent that is not an established monotherapy for depression. In this chapter, I make no distinction between combination and augmentation because the difference is largely semantic; both strategies consist of combining two pharmacological agents with different mechanisms of action to increase the symptomatic benefit. Furthermore, on the basis of a few randomized, controlled trials, no evidence indicates that these two strategies differ in their effectiveness. The concomitant use of two medications is thus referred to as *augmentation strategies*, and the emphasis is placed on the neuronal target(s) of the different drugs.

This chapter is not an exhaustive review of all the augmentation strategies ever reported. Rather, I concentrate on the major commonly used approaches and emphasize their biological targets. Even for these selected strategies, I do not describe and analyze details of every single report but rather focus on the main findings, with the caveat that many publications in this area are based on open-label designs and on how to use the strategies safely and effectively.

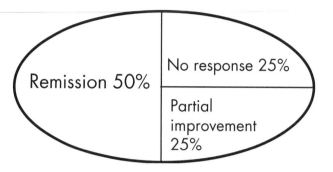

FIGURE 31–1. **Approximate outcome of depressed patients treated with a first antidepressant drug given at an adequate dose for a sufficient time.**

Remission rates in placebo-controlled studies are generally between 35% and 45% but are on the order of 50%–60% when active drugs are used as sole comparators in double-blind studies.

Targets for Antidepressant Strategies

The antidepressant response achieved with currently marketed drugs relies on the enhancement of either serotonin (5-hydroxytryptamine; 5-HT) or norepinephrine transmission and to some extent on the dopamine system. This is best exemplified by the depletion studies of serotonin and catecholamines in patients with treatment-responsive depression. Basically, a significant proportion of the patients who respond to a selective serotonin reuptake inhibitor (SSRI) will experience, typically within a few hours, a return of depressive symptoms with a dietary depletion of tryptophan, the amino acid precursor for serotonin (Booij et al. 2002; Delgado et al. 1990, 1999). Of note, even patients who respond to monoamine oxidase inhibitors (MAOIs), which enhance brain levels of serotonin, norepinephrine, and dopamine, also will relapse with this challenge (Delgado et al. 1990). In contrast, patients with a favorable response to a norepinephrine reuptake inhibitor experience a return of symptoms with the inhibition of dopamine and norepinephrine synthesis (Miller et al. 1996).

However, transmission of each of these systems can be enhanced in multiple ways. These approaches may lead to differential effects in various brain structures and even different side effects. For instance, when serotonin availability is increased with an SSRI, about 20% of patients will experience nausea to various degrees. When MAOIs are used, which raise serotonin and dopamine levels, nausea is uncommon. Yet, increased dopamine type 2 receptor activation with apomorphine can lead to problematic nausea (Martinez et al. 2003).

Another example of the differential synaptic effects of agents that act on these specific neurotransmission systems is illustrated by the prolactin-enhancing effect of serotonin agents. Tryptophan stimulates prolactin release, which is blocked by 5-HT_{1A} antagonists, whereas the effect of the serotonin releaser/reuptake blocker fenfluramine on prolactin is blocked by a 5-HT_2 antagonist (Goodall et al. 1993; Park and Cowen 1995). Consequently, use of two serotonin agents may alter serotonin transmission through different mechanisms even within the same brain neurocircuitry. It is therefore conceivable that targeting two different neuronal elements on the same types of neurons may lead to a much greater effect on that specific neurotransmission than does either agent when used alone. For instance, it is well known that norepinephrine reuptake inhibitors enhance the synaptic availability of norepinephrine (about twofold), whereas α_2-adrenergic antagonists may have a more modest effect. However, their combined use leads to a more than fivefold increase in the levels of norepinephrine (Dennis et al. 1987; Sacchetti et al. 1999).

Augmentation strategies should, therefore, be attempted with this framework in mind because targeting various neuronal elements will not produce the same synaptic alterations of a neurotransmitter. Figure 31–2 illustrates the sites of action of some antidepressants on the serotonin system, as well as those of some augmentation strategies. There can be at the very least a summation, if not a potentiation, of effects, as described earlier, whereby the net action of both drugs when used together is greater than the sum of each.

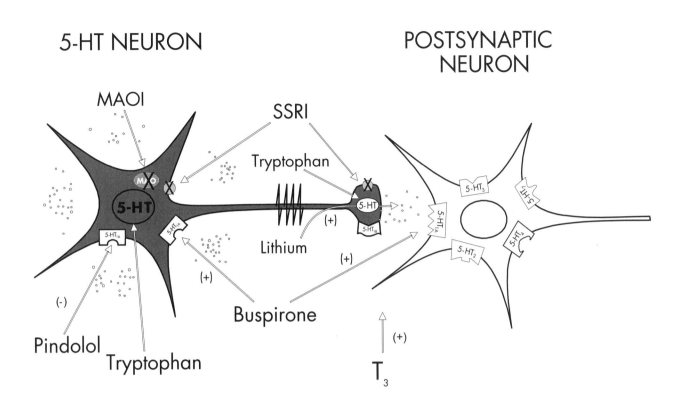

FIGURE 31–2.   **Diagram of the serotonin (5-hydroxytryptamine; 5-HT) system with its various elements controlling its function.**

Only the postsynaptic 5-HT receptors for which an electrophysiological response has been characterized are depicted. The 5-HT$_{1A}$ autoreceptors on the 5-HT cell body exert an inhibitory action on the firing activity of the neurons. The 5-HT$_{1B}$ autoreceptors on the terminals also exert an inhibitory action on 5-HT release. The signs (+) and (−) represent, respectively, an activation and a blockade. The circles on the 5-HT neuron represent the high-affinity reuptake transporters, and the X's represent their inhibition by the SSRI. MAOI=monoamine oxidase inhibitor; SSRI=selective serotonin reuptake inhibitor; T$_3$=triiodothyronine.

Switching Versus Augmenting a First Antidepressant Drug

Switching consists of replacing one antidepressant drug with another. It has the advantage of continuing mono-therapy, thereby avoiding drug interactions, potentially enhancing adherence, and minimizing cost. Switching from an SSRI to a dual serotonin and norepinephrine reuptake inhibitor (e.g., venlafaxine, duloxetine, or mil-nacipran) can be considered to be an augmentation strat-egy from a mechanistic viewpoint. Indeed, at moderate to high doses, venlafaxine acts on both reuptake systems in depressed patients (Debonnel et al. 1998). Such a switch can be carried out without a washout period because both the SSRI and the dual-action agent inhibit serotonin reuptake.

A true switch strategy carries several disadvantages (Table 31–1). In particular, a small beneficial action ob-tained with the first drug may be lost on its discontinua-tion. In addition, if the first drug has a short half-life, there may be discontinuation symptoms, which would re-quire a gradual reduction of the drug. Moreover, an im-mediate substitution can place patients in a drug combi-nation situation between the elimination of the first agent and the achievement of steady-state level of the other drug. This may even lead to a transient response because drug combinations, as discussed later, sometimes produce a rapid response. The best example of such a situation would be a switch from fluoxetine, in which it may take up to 5 weeks for the drug to be eliminated.

Another factor to consider before opting for switching rather than augmentation is time to response or remission. Figure 31–3 illustrates theoretical time courses for both

TABLE 31–1. Drawbacks associated with switching medications when facing an unsatisfactory response to a given drug

Possible loss of a partial response

Discontinuation phenomena

Negative psychological aspect of the washout period

Long duration of a second trial: 6–8 weeks

strategies. A first antidepressant drug trial carried out at an optimal pace (i.e., an increase in dose after 2 and 4 weeks in the absence of significant improvement) would require about 6 weeks. A second trial with the substitution strategy, in which a washout period is used, would require an additional 8 weeks. In contrast, if the augmentation strategy were chosen, two or three drug combinations could be sequentially attempted within the same period, depending on the agents used. Even if drug substitution were of equal effectiveness to any drug combination, the probability of achieving a response or remission would be greater with the augmentation approach within the subsequent 8-week time frame. Furthermore, if a patient did not respond to the second drug in the switching paradigm, he or she would still be depressed after 14 weeks of treatment and would have endured some side effects without beneficial actions, thus perhaps adding to the burden of depression.

The time elapsing before a satisfactory outcome is achieved is a crucial factor in the treatment of depression for two main reasons. First, it appears that the longer an episode is allowed to continue, the lower the probability of achieving remission (Keller et al. 1992). This may be related to the atrophy of certain brain structures with ongoing depression (Sheline et al. 1999). Second, the patient's distress and hopelessness may grow with repeated treatment failures, all the more so if each attempt takes about 2 months. This may decrease compliance and possibly increase the risk for suicide.

Choosing the Second Agent for Augmentation

The first step in choosing a drug for the augmentation approach is to identify possible medical contraindications of the agents that are contemplated. An absolute contraindication would be the concomitant use of a potent serotonin reuptake inhibitor (i.e., clomipramine or any of the SSRIs) and an irreversible MAOI. In the early 1990s, the underestimation of the long elimination of fluoxetine and its active metabolite norfluoxetine led to fatalities

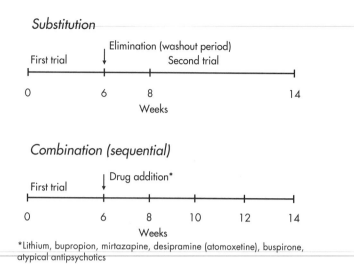

FIGURE 31–3. Approximate time courses necessary to carry out a medication substitution and sequential augmentation strategies.

In the lower time line, the first antidepressant drug is maintained, and the other agents are added one at a time. Two weeks would be a minimal time of treatment before determining whether the strategy is producing any beneficial action. In the presence of a detectable amelioration, the strategy should be continued and optimized if necessary.

when irreversible MAOIs were prematurely introduced (Sternbach 1991). This combination of drugs neutralizes the two inactivation pathways for serotonin and leads to an excessive accumulation of this neurotransmitter, thereby producing a serotonin syndrome.

However, several safe drug combinations target the serotonin system to produce pharmacodynamic actions and possibly a therapeutic response (Figure 31–2). In the process, serotonergic side effects (nausea, increased anxiety, and agitation) may be triggered, as can be the case even with SSRIs used alone. These effects are not life-threatening like the serotonin syndrome and can be easily managed by dose reduction or the cessation of one of the two drugs. It is noteworthy that such a potentially lethal drug interaction should not occur when a norepinephrine reuptake inhibitor is used with an MAOI. In fact, the combination of such drugs was reported to be effective in treatment-resistant cases (Schmauss et al. 1988). The relative safety of the latter approach is likely a result of the presence of alternative metabolic inactivation pathways for norepinephrine, such as catechol-O-methyltransferase. Such a drug combination even protects the patients from hypertensive crises produced by the ingestion of tyramine in the presence of an MAOI. Indeed, the norepinephrine reuptake inhibitor would prevent the entry of tyramine into norepinephrine terminals that normally would produce the calcium-independent release of norepinephrine, leading to the peak of blood pressure. Nevertheless, such a combination does require careful monitoring of the patients and should be considered only after failures of more commonly used strategies.

Another absolute contraindication would be using the β-adrenergic/5-HT$_{1A}$ antagonist pindolol in patients with asthma because it could trigger a bronchospasm unresponsive to bronchodilating noradrenergic agents. With respect to relative contraindications, the addition of lithium may not be a wise choice in patients with a thyroid condition or renal insufficiency.

As a second consideration, one may opt for a second drug with a property that would help treat a problematic symptom of the depression or even a concomitant medical condition. If the patient has marked insomnia, for instance, one could use mirtazapine because of its beneficial action on sleep architecture (Nutt 2002). The presence of psychotic symptoms would be an obvious indication for adding an atypical antipsychotic. Finally, the dopamine type 2 (D$_2$) receptor agonist pramipexole may be helpful for treating depression in parkinsonian patients, in patients with restless legs syndrome, and in patients with elevated prolactin because this drug is also effective in these disorders (Corrigan et al. 2000; Happe and Trenkwalder 2004; Sporn et al. 2000).

Beyond these first two guidelines, no additional firm recommendations exist for drug selection. Furthermore, there is no predictor of response for augmentation strategies, just as is the case when initiating a first antidepressant drug trial. For instance, a clinician may not want to use bupropion in patients with marked anxiety because it is generally considered an activating drug. However, Rush et al. (2001) observed an equal response with the SSRI sertraline and bupropion in a double-blind monotherapy study in depressed patients with moderate to marked anxiety. At this point, one may choose a strategy with the most evidence for efficacy (i.e., one or more controlled studies, beyond case series and/or open-label studies). In this respect, lithium addition is by far the best-documented augmentation strategy (Bauer et al. 2003). It is effective not only in patients with depression resistant to tricyclics and MAOIs but also in patients resistant to SSRIs (Baumann et al. 1996; Fava et al. 1994; Katona et al. 1995). However, clinicians have shied away from this effective approach in the last few years, possibly because of the availability of other antidepressant drugs that do not require plasma level monitoring. In addition, once remission has been maintained for an adequate period of

time using two antidepressants, clinicians have a choice of which medication to discontinue first. In contrast, lithium addition does not offer this possibility because lithium is not effective on its own for relapse/recurrence prevention in unipolar depression.

The presence of a pharmacokinetic interaction should not be a deterrent for choosing a drug for treatment-resistant depression. For instance, when adding a tricyclic norepinephrine reuptake blocker, such as desipramine or nortriptyline, to paroxetine or fluoxetine, the usual doses of the tricyclic must be decreased by three- to fourfold (Table 31–2) (Nelson et al. 2004). This is because these two SSRIs at therapeutic doses completely inactivate the cytochrome P450 2D6 (CYP2D6) enzyme that metabolizes tricyclics (Harvey and Preskorn 1996a, 1996b). Administering tricyclics with these two SSRIs even removes uncertainty about the doses to be used. Indeed, there is always the risk of prescribing a standard dose of a tricyclic to a poor 2D6 metabolizer and producing an intoxication in the 7% of Caucasians or up to 19% of the black population who lack this enzymatic activity (Bradford et al. 1998). In contrast, the use of paroxetine or fluoxetine transforms all normal metabolizers into slow metabolizers and does not further decrease the metabolism of the tricyclics in slow metabolizers. The half-life of desipramine is about 18 hours in a normal metabolizer, and it is about 50 hours both in slow metabolizers and in the presence of paroxetine, regardless of whether the patient is a slow metabolizer (Brosen et al. 1993).

Effect of Selective Serotonin Reuptake Inhibitors on the Serotonergic System in Treatment Resistance

SSRIs have become the first line of treatment for major depression in many countries. Consequently, most patients failing a first antidepressant trial now find themselves in an SSRI-treatment-failure group. SSRIs initially decrease the firing rate of serotonin neurons as a result of the blockade of serotonin transporters on their cell bodies. This attenuation of firing is mediated by the excess activation of 5-HT$_{1A}$ autoreceptors (see Figure 31–4). At the other end of the neuron, the synaptic availability of serotonin is not increased in a sustained fashion because despite the inhibition of serotonin transporters on serotonin terminals contributing to enhancing serotonin availability, the main driving force for releasing serotonin, the flow of electrical impulses, is decreased. As the treatment is prolonged, 5-HT$_{1A}$ autoreceptors desensitize and allow

TABLE 31-2.　Approximate doses of agents used to augment a first antidepressant drug

Agent	Dose[a]	Reported to be effective when combined with
Lithium[b]	600–900 mg at bedtime	All antidepressants
Buspirone	10–15 mg three times a day	SSRIs
Triiodothyronine[b]	25–50 µg/day	Tricyclics
Desipramine[b]	50–125 mg/day	SSRIs
Atomoxetine	18–80 mg/day	SSRIs
Bupropion	150–300 mg/day	SSRIs, SNRIs, mirtazapine
Mirtazapine[b]	15–45 mg/day	SSRIs, SNRIs, bupropion
Olanzapine[b]	5–15 mg/day	SSRIs, SNRIs
Risperidone	0.5–2 mg/day	SSRIs
Pramipexole	0.25–1 mg three times a day	SSRIs
Pindolol[b]	2.5 mg three times a day	SSRIs

Note. SSRIs=selective serotonin reuptake inhibitors; SNRIs = serotonin-norepinephrine reuptake inhibitors.

[a]These doses may need to be diminished by half, or more, when treating elderly patients.

[b]Strategies for which at least one randomized, double-blind study supports efficacy.

a full recovery of firing of serotonin neurons with ongoing reuptake inhibition (Blier and de Montigny 1983; Jolas et al. 1994). In addition, terminal 5-HT$_{1B/D}$ autoreceptors also desensitize and permit more serotonin to be released per action potential reaching the terminals (Chaput et al. 1986, 1991). Because this process occurs in the presence of serotonin reuptake inhibition, serotonin transmission is then markedly enhanced at postsynaptic serotonin receptors (Haddjeri et al. 1998). The 5-HT$_{1A}$ receptors in the hippocampus do not desensitize after long-term SSRI treatment, which allows a net increase in transmission (see Figure 31–4).

It is thus conceivable that in patients whose symptoms do not respond to an SSRI, such adaptive changes do not occur. Alternatively, the level of increased serotonin transmission achieved with the SSRI may not be sufficient to produce a clinical response or remission. Finally, it is also possible that by enhancing serotonin transmission, SSRIs cause a dampening of the function of another neurotrans-

mitter system that plays an important role in the antidepressant response. Indeed, serotonin neurons send inhibitory projections to norepinephrine neurons of the locus coeruleus (Haddjeri et al. 1997) (Figure 31–5). Therefore, when serotonin transmission is enhanced in that pathway by long-term SSRI treatment, the spontaneous firing activity of norepinephrine neurons decreases markedly (Szabo et al. 2000) (Figure 31–6). Because this system may exert a crucial role in the antidepressant response, it is conceivable that a lack of clinical response by long-term SSRI treatment also may result from a dampening of the norepinephrine tone. In fact, these drugs sometimes leave patients with persistent fatigue or anergia. This is reminiscent of the clinical effect of the α_2-adrenergic agonist clonidine, which also suppresses norepinephrine neuronal firing, when used for the treatment of hypertension. It then may be useful to use norepinephrine-enhancing strategies in patients with SSRI-resistant depression.

Augmentation and Combination Strategies

Norepinephrine Reuptake Inhibitors: Addition to Selective Serotonin Reuptake Inhibitor Regimen

Most tricyclic antidepressants are weak serotonin reuptake inhibitors (Hyttel 1982). The best clinical evidence in support of this assertion is the observation that all SSRIs are effective for treatment of obsessive-compulsive disorder, but only clomipramine among all tricyclics is active in this condition; clomipramine is the most potent serotonin reuptake inhibitor in that family of drugs (Goodman 1999). Combining serotonin and norepinephrine reuptake inhibition thus represents rational pharmacotherapy. As mentioned earlier, the simplest way to achieve this combination with fewer side effects than with clomipramine is to do an immediate switch from an SSRI to an intermediate dose of venlafaxine. Indeed, this dual reuptake inhibitor has been reported to double the remission rate of that achieved with the SSRI paroxetine (42% vs. 20%) in a 4-week double-blind design in a group of mostly patients with SSRI-resistant depression (Poirier and Boyer 1999). With this substitution, patients do not risk having discontinuation symptoms because venlafaxine is also a potent serotonin reuptake inhibitor, it will achieve steady-state level within 3 days, and it will likely start inhibiting norepinephrine reuptake at 150 mg/day. In the absence of any significant response, the dose can be increased by 75 mg every week. The daily dose then can be titrated up to 375 mg according to side effects and response (although the label for the extended-release formulation recommends only up to

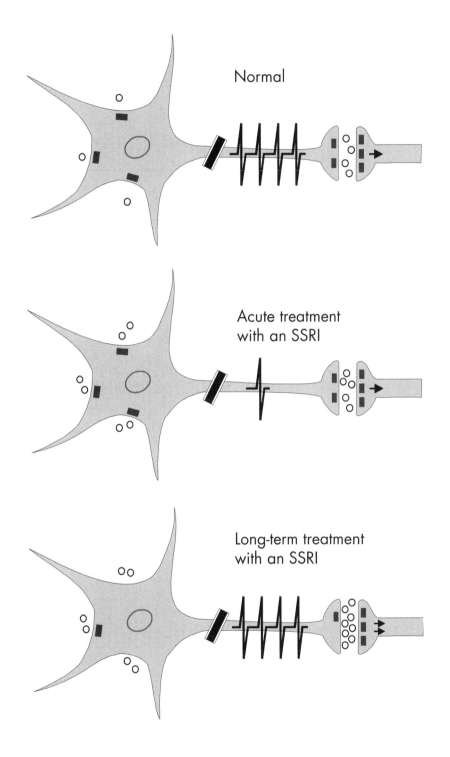

FIGURE 31–4.   Effect of sustained serotonin (5-HT) reuptake inhibition on 5-HT transmission.

The black rectangles on the neurons represent 5-HT receptors: at the cell body level, 5-HT$_{1A}$ autoreceptors; on the terminals, 5-HT$_1$ autoreceptors; and on the postsynaptic neuron, 5-HT$_{1A}$ receptors. The disappearance of some of these receptors represents their functional desensitization during sustained selective serotonin reuptake inhibitor (SSRI) administration. The firing frequency of 5-HT neurons is represented by the number of action potentials on their axon. The arrows within the postsynaptic boutons represent the intensity of serotonin transmission.

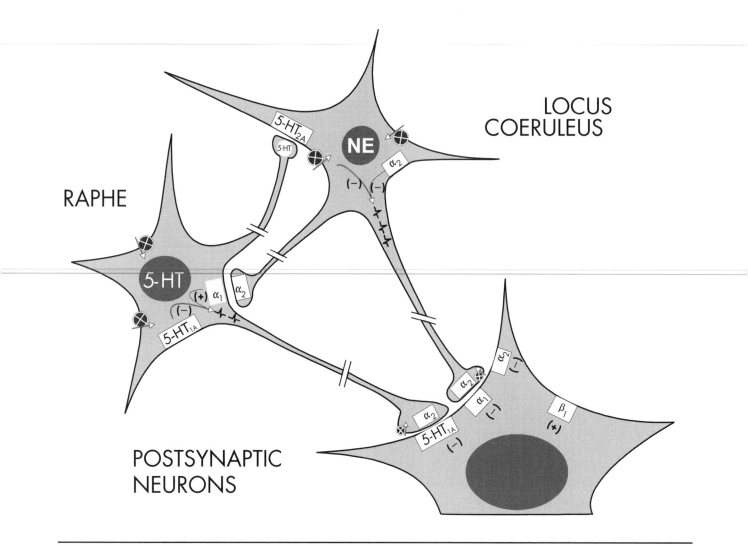

FIGURE 31–5.   Diagram of the reciprocal interactions of the serotonin (5-HT) and norepinephrine (NE) neurons.

The general actions of the various receptors on neuronal function are indicated by the (+) and (−) signs, which represent excitatory and inhibitory influences, respectively. 5-HT neurons in the raphe nuclei exert an inhibitory action on locus coeruleus NE neurons. The cogwheels with arrows pointing toward the inside of the cell bodies and terminals represent reuptake transporters. The 5-HT$_{2A}$ receptor positioned on the NE neuron is actually an excitatory receptor located on an inhibitory γ-aminobutyric acid (GABA) interneuron to the NE neuron.
Source.   Szabo and Blier 2001.

225 mg/day). This immediate substitution may not be as well tolerated if patients have been taking a high dose of fluoxetine because this SSRI and its active metabolite norfluoxetine are slowly eliminated over about 1 month.

Even though venlafaxine likely exerts a significant degree of norepinephrine reuptake inhibition at 225–375 mg/day (Debonnel et al. 1998), it may not be as potent on this transporter as the tricyclics or other nontricyclic agents, such as reboxetine and atomoxetine (Dostert et al. 1994; Zerbe et al. 1985). Consequently, adding desipramine, reboxetine, or atomoxetine to an SSRI still

may be a worthwhile strategy in a patient with a history of failed venlafaxine treatment. The doses of tricyclics to be used with different SSRIs have been discussed earlier (see section "Choosing the Second Agent for Augmentation"). It is nevertheless important that 150 mg/day of sertraline, 40 mg/day of citalopram, and 20 mg/day of escitalopram do inhibit to a moderate degree CYP2D6 (Belpaire et al. 1998; Kurtz et al. 1997; "Lexapro product monograph" 2005). The usual monotherapy doses of antidepressants that are substrates of this cytochrome should therefore be halved when used with the latter SSRIs.

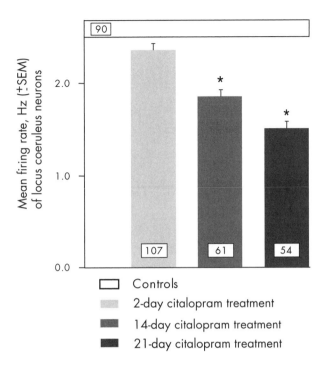

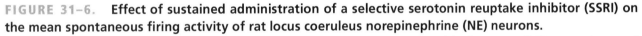

FIGURE 31-6. **Effect of sustained administration of a selective serotonin reuptake inhibitor (SSRI) on the mean spontaneous firing activity of rat locus coeruleus norepinephrine (NE) neurons.**

The horizontal bar (top) represents the range (mean±standard error of the mean [SEM]) of the firing rate of NE neurons in control rats. The drug was administered by an osmotic minipump implanted subcutaneously.
*$P<0.05$.

Now that the selective norepinephrine reuptake inhibitor atomoxetine is available in many countries for the treatment of attention-deficit disorder, this drug represents a safer choice over the tricyclics to potently inhibit the norepinephrine reuptake process because it is not toxic in overdosage. This drug, however, is also a substrate for CYP2D6 (Belle et al. 2002). Consequently, the treatment should be initiated at low doses (18–25 mg/day) in adults when it is combined with SSRIs, especially paroxetine or fluoxetine. Atomoxetine then may be titrated according to side effects and response. Reboxetine, another nontricyclic norepinephrine reuptake inhibitor, should be initiated at 2 mg twice a day and titrated up to 4 mg twice a day according to tolerability and response. Because this drug is metabolized by CYP3A4, the only situation in which doses lower than those mentioned above should be used is if it is prescribed with nefazodone, or other potent CYP3A4 inhibitors.

Lithium

In animal experiments, plasma lithium levels as low as 0.4 mEq/L enhance serotonin release in some brain structures involved in mediating depressive symptoms (Blier et al. 1987). In the clinic, adding lithium to an ongoing SSRI treatment in one evening dose of 600–900 mg usually will achieve this level and produce an antidepressant response with a delay of a few days to about 2 weeks (Bauer et al. 2003; de Montigny et al. 1981, 1983). Studies monitoring lithium plasma levels in patients with treatment-resistant depression indicate that levels between 0.5 and 0.8 mEq/L may produce an optimum response (Stein and Bernadt 1993). It is useful to ensure that the proper lithium level has been achieved after 1 week.

Lithium addition has been reported to be effective with virtually every class of antidepressant drugs, at least in open-label studies if not in controlled trials. In a head-to-head comparison, lithium and electroconvulsive shocks administered twice a week in patients with tricyclic-resistant severe depression produced the same improvement after 21 days (Dinan and Barry 1989). Given that all major classes of antidepressant treatments increase serotonin transmission, it is thus conceivable that lithium may be acting by potentiating serotonin transmission (Haddjeri et al. 1998, 2000) (see Figure 31–2). Obviously, its effect on second-messenger systems also may be contributing to its potentiating effect. Depressed patients need not have bipolar illness to respond to lithium augmentation. Another misconception is that patients need to have a partial response to their antidepressant drug for lithium to work. From the very first studies, it was observed that patients with no response at all could have a strong response to lithium addition (de Montigny et al. 1981, 1983).

Buspirone

Buspirone, a 5-HT$_{1A}$ agonist, has been reported to be effective in several case series of SSRI-resistant depression, even in patients in whom electroconvulsive shocks had failed (Bouwer and Stein 1997; Dimitriou and Dimitriou 1998; Joffe and Schuller 1993). Presumably, this drug increases serotonin transmission selectively at postsynaptic 5-HT$_{1A}$ receptors because the prior SSRI treatment may have desensitized the 5-HT$_{1A}$ autoreceptors (see Figure 31–2). This drug—when initiated at 20 mg/day in fractionated doses—is usually very well tolerated in SSRI-treated patients because patients have already developed a tolerance to serotonergic side effects. Total daily doses of 30–40 mg have classically been used in such studies. Buspirone may occasionally reverse sexual dysfunctions produced by SSRIs (Landen et al. 1999).

Note that two placebo-controlled studies failed to show unequivocally the beneficial action of buspirone in patients with SSRI-resistant depression. In the first trial, the severity cutoff score for including patients in the study was quite low, which may have contributed to increasing the placebo response (Landen et al. 1998). In the second study, patients had a greater improvement after 1 week of treatment in the buspirone group, but at the end of the 6-week trial, only the more severely ill patients responded more favorably (Appelberg et al. 2001).

Triiodothyronine

The addition of triiodothyronine (T$_3$; 25–50 μg/day) is a strategy that is seldom used now possibly because it has not yet been reported to be effective for SSRI-resistant depression and with other newly developed antidepressants. The published data showing some efficacy are mostly with tricyclics. It also may increase anxiety and create or worsen insomnia. The suggestion that the strategy may be more effective in women than in men also may contribute to the dilution of the effect size (Aronson et al. 1996; Joffe et al. 1993). Recent results obtained in laboratory animals indicate that T$_3$ addition to antidepressant drugs increases serotonin release in certain brain structures (Gur et al. 1999). Therefore, this approach also may be considered to act in part as serotonin-enhancing agents (see Figure 31–2).

Bupropion

The addition of bupropion is one of the most popular strategies in the United States, although double-blind studies to confirm its effectiveness are still lacking (Mischoulon et al. 2000). Nevertheless, it is safe to use with SSRIs, dual reuptake inhibitors, and mirtazapine, and it is well tolerated at an initial dose of 150 mg, which is effective by itself in monotherapy. Given that bupropion is metabolized by CYP2B6 and that inhibiting properties of various antidepressants at this isoenzyme are not known, it would be prudent in most patients not to go above 300 mg/day (Kirchheiner et al. 2003). This would avoid reaching plasma levels that could be in the range of those producing epileptic activity (Davidson 1989).

Bupropion can be considered as acting primarily on norepinephrine neurons but also on serotonin neurons (Cooper et al. 1994; Dong and Blier 2001). The drug should not be primarily considered as a dopaminergic reuptake blocker. Indeed, three recent positron emission tomography studies have shown that in usual clinical regimens, bupropion occupies only about 20% of dopamine transporters in the brain (Kugaya et al. 2003; Learned-Coughlin et al. 2003; Meyer et al. 2002). Furthermore, it does not alter the firing rate of rat dopamine neurons, which would be expected from a dopamine reuptake blocker (Dong and Blier 2001). Bupropion is a norepinephrine releaser, which initially decreases norepinephrine neuronal firing through an excess activation of the norepinephrine cell body autoreceptors. Because it also increases norepinephrine release on serotonin neurons, it drives up the firing rate of serotonin neurons in a sustained fashion. With treatment prolongation, the firing rate of norepinephrine neurons gradually recovers, and these neurons discharge more in a burst-firing mode, which contributes to increased norepinephrine release (Janssen and Blier 2003). Consequently, bupropion can be considered an agent that increases both serotonin and norepinephrine transmission but not via reuptake inhibition. Therefore, the drug may be expected to have a beneficial action when added to SSRIs and possibly even a greater one when combined with a dual reuptake inhibitor such as venlafaxine.

Given the norepinephrine-releasing action of bupropion, this strategy would appear more conservative than using psychostimulants, such as methylphenidate (10–40 mg/day). Indeed, psychostimulants may have abuse potential in some individuals, may worsen insomnia and anxiety, and do not have sustained intrinsic antidepressant activity as does bupropion. In contrast, several lines of evidence indicate that modafinil might not be considered as a psychostimulant per se. Emerging data suggest that addition of this drug, at doses of 100–400 mg/day, to the therapeutic regimen of depressed patients with incomplete responses has beneficial actions on fatigue and sleepiness (DeBattista et al. 2003; Fava et al. 2005).

α_2-Adrenergic Antagonists

Positive results have been reported in double-blind studies with α_2-adrenergic antagonists when the two antidepressant drugs mianserin and mirtazapine, and yohimbine, were used in combination with SSRIs (Cappiello et al. 1995; Carpenter et al. 2002; Maes et al. 1999). The two antidepressant agents are structurally very similar and mainly differ in that mianserin has a higher affinity for α_1-adrenergic receptors than does mirtazapine (Kelder et al. 1997). Interestingly, these drugs are racemic mixtures with their (–) enantiomers being selective for the α_2-adrenergic receptors present on serotonin terminals and their (+) enantiomers selective for the α_2-adrenergic receptors present on norepinephrine terminals. These drugs, therefore, have the capacity to increase the function of both norepinephrine and serotonin terminals through their antagonism of these presynaptic receptors (Haddjeri et al. 1996).

Blocking α_2-adrenergic autoreceptors on the cell body of norepinephrine neurons increases the firing activity of norepinephrine neurons in the locus coeruleus (Figure 31–5). This enhanced function of norepinephrine neurons is likely partially offset by the unaffected activity of the norepinephrine reuptake transporters. In the case of mirtazapine, the increased norepinephrine release in the rat dorsal raphe nucleus produces a transient increase in the firing of serotonin neurons, which becomes sustained after 3 weeks of administration (Haddjeri et al. 1996, 1997). Again, this enhanced function of serotonin neurons may be partially offset by serotonin reuptake transporters, which are not affected by mirtazapine. It would appear that the antidepressant action of mirtazapine would depend on an enhancement of both serotonin and norepinephrine transmission because its therapeutic effect can be reversed by both serotonin and norepinephrine synthesis inhibition in improved depressed patients (Delgado et al. 2002). The beneficial action of mianserin and mirtazapine in patients with SSRI-resistant depression thus may stem from counteracting the dampening action of the SSRIs on the firing rate of norepinephrine neurons described earlier.

It is important to note that these drugs also may exert their beneficial action in SSRI-resistant depression through their potent 5-HT$_2$ receptor antagonism. Indeed, it was reported that the combination of serotonin reuptake inhibition and 5-HT$_{2A}$ receptor antagonism acutely in-

creases norepinephrine release in the rat frontal cortex and in the locus coeruleus (Szabo and Blier 2002; Hatanaka et al. 1997). Initially, the firing rate of norepinephrine neurons is dampened, but it recovers gradually to normal after 3 weeks in the presence of a drug that selectively exerts these two actions. The exact basis for this increased norepinephrine produced by the interference of two serotonin neuronal elements remains to be elucidated.

Nefazodone

Some reports have described a beneficial action of adding nefazodone in patients with SSRI-resistant depression patients (Sajatovic 1999). This effect is unlikely to result from additional serotonin reuptake inhibition by nefazodone given its extremely weak activity in blocking this transporter site. In contrast, nefazodone is a potent 5-HT$_2$ receptor antagonist. It is thus conceivable that this strategy could be acting through an increase in norepinephrine release, with the caveat that its action on this process may not be as sustained as that of mirtazapine given its very short elimination half-life.

Atypical Antipsychotics: Addition to Selective Serotonin Reuptake Inhibitor Regimen

Increasing evidence now indicates that the addition of atypical antipsychotics to the regimen of depressed patients not responding to an SSRI may produce a rapid and consistent antidepressant response. Double-blind studies support the marked beneficial effect of olanzapine addition, and open-label designs also indicate a similar effect of risperidone augmentation (Corya et al. 2003; Gharabawi et al. 2004; Ostroff and Nelson 1999; Shelton et al. 2001; Tohen et al. 2003).

Such a positive response to the addition of an atypical antipsychotic does not rely on the presence of psychotic symptoms to manifest itself. Because it is widely accepted that typical antipsychotics are not useful adjuncts in the management of treatment-resistant unipolar depression without psychotic features, the atypical antipsychotics must not exert this action via the antagonism of D$_2$ receptors that is common to all antipsychotics. Microdialysis studies examining the levels of extracellular serotonin, norepinephrine, and dopamine following the administration of fluoxetine and olanzapine have shown that these drugs markedly enhance the synaptic availability of these three neurotransmitters (Koch et al. 2004). The exact basis for this phenomenon remains to be elucidated, but by comparing the neurochemical profile of olanzapine and risperidone at various receptor sites, it would seem that the antagonism of 5-HT$_{2A}$ receptors in the presence of serotonin reuptake inhibition is a likely candidate. As described earlier, the combination of these two actions leads to increased norepinephrine release. Given the pivotal role that the norepinephrine system can play in the antidepressant response, the latter action could contribute to a significant extent to the therapeutic action of this strategy. Furthermore, given that SSRIs can decrease the norepinephrine tone in the central nervous system (Seager et al. 2004; Szabo et al. 2000), based on the attenuation of norepinephrine neuronal firing in rats receiving SSRIs (Figure 31–6) and the decrease of the main metabolite of norepinephrine in the cerebrospinal fluid of patients taking an SSRI (Copland et al. 1997), an increased norepinephrine availability by the combination of an atypical antipsychotic plus an SSRI appears to be a very plausible explanation for the beneficial action of this drug combination.

Dopamine Type 2 Receptor Agonists

It may seem paradoxical that augmentation studies in which the dopaminergic agonists bromocriptine, pergolide, and pramipexole were used have produced positive results in open-label design given that atypical antipsychotics are also effective adjuvants (Inoue et al. 1996; Izumi et al. 2000; Lattanzi et al. 2002). As explained earlier, however, the antidepressant efficacy of the atypical antipsychotics is not likely to result from their D$_2$ receptor antagonism. Pramipexole increases dopaminergic transmission at D$_2$ and D$_3$ receptors, which, in turn, increases the firing activity of serotonin neurons in the dorsal raphe (Haj-Damane 2001). The antidepressant activity of pramipexole used by itself in a placebo-controlled trial gives credence to this approach (Corrigan et al. 2000). Although taking pramipexole may be somewhat cumbersome because it has to be used on a thrice-daily basis, it will not impair sexual function and may even help reverse an SSRI-induced dysfunction (Sporn et al. 2000). In addition, it may help simplify the therapeutic regimen of patients with Parkinson's disease. In treatment-resistant depression, it can be prescribed at 0.125 mg three times a day and doubled every week, according to side effects and response, up to 3–4 mg/day, its effective regimen as monotherapy in depression.

Combining Antidepressants and Other Agents From Treatment Initiation

Although depressed patients have likely been ill for weeks, if not months or years, when they consult, there may be a state of urgency. Therefore, drug combination from treatment initiation may be considered in the hope of achieving earlier relief. There is no consensus on what a rapid onset of action is, but some studies suggest that within a standard antidepressant drug trial, a superior outcome may be achieved with drug combination. Although initiating treatment with two drugs is somewhat unconventional for depression, combination treatment is the norm for some medical illnesses. For example, asthma is treated at the outset with inhaled β$_2$-adrenergic agonists and steroids. In the treatment of depression, a benzodiazepine receptor ligand in combination with an antidepressant to improve sleep and decrease anxiety is commonly prescribed. Therefore, the prescription of two antidepressants at treatment initiation may not seem that unusual from that perspective.

Positive results when two medications are used from treatment onset have been reported in double-blind studies: fluoxetine and mianserin (Maes et al. 1999), fluoxetine and desipramine (Nelson et al. 2004), fluoxetine and olanzapine (Shelton et al. 2001; Tohen et al. 2003), paroxetine and mirtazapine (Debonnel et al. 2000), and SSRIs and pindolol (for a review, see Blier 2003). Although controversy exists regarding the efficacy of pindolol addition in SSRI-resistant patients, 8 of 10 double-blind studies have reported an acceleration of the antidepressant response. This action of pindolol is believed to result from prevention of an initial suppression of firing of serotonin neurons on SSRI initiation (see Figure 31–4).

How Long Should Effective Combined Pharmacotherapies Be Used?

On achieving remission, the next concern becomes the duration of the treatment. Clear guidelines are available for treatment with a single agent. No such recommendations exist for combined treatments because this issue has not been thoroughly studied. Only a few studies have examined this problem. For instance, lithium cessation immediately after achieving remission or after a short-term treatment has produced about a 50% relapse rate in two studies (Bauer et al. 2000; de Montigny et al. 1983). Ongoing studies are examining this issue with antidepressant drugs and thus far are yielding results similar to those obtained with lithium cessation (Blier et al. 2004; Gharabawi et al. 2004). Thus, it would be prudent to continue the combined therapies for about 6 months before considering tapering off one of the two drugs. It is wise to err on the side of safety because no data are available on the rate of resistance following reintroduction of the prior drug regimen. Such observations have been reported for single agents, such as tricyclics and lithium, in mood disorders and should constitute sufficient evidence for clinicians to avoid early discontinuation of drug combinations after achieving the desired end point.

Conclusion

Numerous strategies are now available to treat depression that does not respond or remit to a first antidepressant drug. Although the number of possibilities may be limited by consideration of undesired side effects, several options remain to produce full recovery. When taking charge of treatment-resistant patients, it is imperative to reassure them that a treatment that will not fail them can be found. Indeed, after the clinician makes a proper diagnosis, he or she must tell the patient that medications, when taken adequately, fail them and not the opposite. The uncertainty about which strategy will bring about the desired improvement, however, needs to be emphasized. Such clear and supportive explanations generally enhance compliance with the treatment plan. When compliant patients do not achieve remission with sequential and rational drug combinations, clinicians should always consider complicating issues precluding a favorable outcome. These may include alcohol abuse, illicit drug use, unresolved psychosocial issues, and undiagnosed medical illnesses.

Although new treatment strategies are still eagerly awaited, the vast majority of depressed patients can be brought to remission with the present pharmacopoeia. Novel strategies, even if not superior in terms of effectiveness to the current medications, will help increase the possibilities of treatment approaches to improve outcome and comfort. Given the heterogeneity of depression, it is most unlikely that a single drug will ever be able to treat all patients with this syndrome. Therefore, the basic principles of drug management covered in this chapter must always be retained, albeit modified and improved with new developments in this field. For instance, research into predictors of response may help shorten the time necessary to achieve remission. All in all, the burden of depression can be markedly attenuated with rational site-directed pharmacotherapy.

References

Appelberg BG, Syvalahti EK, Koskinen TE, et al: Patients with severe depression may benefit from buspirone augmentation of selective serotonin reuptake inhibitors: results from a placebo-controlled, randomized, double-blind, placebo wash-in study. J Clin Psychiatry 62:448–452, 2001

Aronson R, Offman HJ, Joffe RT, et al: Triiodothyronine augmentation in the treatment of refractory depression: a meta-analysis. Arch Gen Psychiatry 53:842–848, 1996

Bauer M, Bschor T, Kunz D, et al: Double-blind, placebo-controlled trial of the use of lithium to augment antidepressant medication in continuation treatment of unipolar major depression. Am J Psychiatry 157:1429–1435, 2000

Bauer M, Fortsthoff A, Baethge C, et al: Lithium augmentation therapy in refractory depression—update 2002. Eur Arch Psychiatry Clin Neurosci 253:132–139, 2003

Baumann P, Nil R, Souche A, et al: A double-blind, placebo-controlled study of citalopram with and without lithium in the treatment of therapy-resistant depressive patients: a clinical, pharmacokinetic, and pharmacogenetic investigation. J Clin Psychopharmacol 16:307–314, 1996

Belle DJ, Ernest CS, Sauer JM, et al: Effect of potent CYP2D6 inhibition by paroxetine on atomoxetine pharmacokinetics. J Clin Pharmacol 42:1219–1227, 2002

Belpaire FM, Wijnant P, Temmerman A, et al: The oxidative metabolism of metoprolol in human liver microsomes: inhibition by the selective serotonin reuptake inhibitors. Eur J Clin Pharmacol 54:261–264, 1998

Blier P: The pharmacology of putative early-onset antidepressant strategies. Eur Neuropsychopharmacol 13:57–66, 2003

Blier P, de Montigny C: Electrophysiological investigations on the effect of repeated zimelidine administration on serotonergic neurotransmission in the rat. J Neurosci 3:1270–1278, 1983

Blier P, de Montigny C, Tardif D: Short-term lithium treatment enhances responsiveness of postsynaptic 5-HT1A receptors without altering 5-HT autoreceptor sensitivity: an electrophysiological study in the rat brain. Synapse 1:225–232, 1987

Blier P, Ward HE, Jacobs W, et al: Combining two antidepressants from treatment start: a preliminary analysis (NR357), in 2004 New Research Program and Abstracts, American Psychiatric Association 157th Annual Meeting, New York, NY, May 1–6, 2004. Washington, DC, American Psychiatric Association, 2004, p 157

Booij L, Van der Does W, Benkelfat C, et al: Predictors of mood response to acute tryptophan depletion: a reanalysis. Neuropsychopharmacology 27:852–861, 2002

Bouwer C, Stein DJ: Buspirone is an effective augmenting agent of serotonin selective re-uptake inhibitors in severe treatment-refractory depression. S Afr Med J 87 (4 suppl):534–537, 540, 1997

Bradford LD, Gaedigk A, Leeder JS: High frequency of CYP2D6 poor and "intermediate" metabolizers in black populations: a review and preliminary data. Psychopharmacol Bull 34:797–804, 1998

Brosen K, Hansen JG, Nielsen KK, et al: Inhibition by paroxetine of desipramine metabolism in extensive but not in poor metabolizers of sparteine. Eur J Clin Pharmacol 44:349–355, 1993

Cappiello A, McDougle CJ, Malison RT, et al: Yohimbine augmentation of fluvoxamine in refractory depression: a single-blind study. Biol Psychiatry 38:765–767, 1995

Carpenter LL, Yasmin S, Price LH: A double-blind, placebo-controlled study of antidepressant augmentation with mirtazapine. Biol Psychiatry 51:182–188, 2002

Chaput Y, de Montigny C, Blier P: Effects of a selective 5-HT re-uptake blocker, citalopram, on the sensitivity of 5-HT autoreceptors: electrophysiological studies in the rat brain. Naunyn Schmiedebergs Arch Pharmacol 333:342–348, 1986

Chaput Y, de Montigny C, Blier P: Presynaptic and postsynaptic modifications of the serotonin system by long-term administration of antidepressant treatment: an in vivo electrophysiologic study in the rat. Neuropsychopharmacology 5:219–229, 1991

Cooper BR, Wang CM, Cox RF, et al: Evidence that the acute behavioral and electrophysiological effects of bupropion (Wellbutrin) are mediated by a noradrenergic mechanism. Neuropsychopharmacology 11:133–141, 1994

Coplan JD, Papp LA, Pine D, et al: Clinical improvement with fluoxetine therapy and noradrenergic function in patients with panic disorder. Arch Gen Psychiatry 54:643–648, 1997

Corrigan MH, Denahan AQ, Wright CE, et al: Comparison of pramipexole, fluoxetine, and placebo in patients with major depression. Depress Anxiety 11:58–65, 2000

Corya SA, Andersen SW, Detke HC, et al: Long-term antidepressant efficacy and safety of olanzapine/fluoxetine combination: a 76-week open-label study. J Clin Psychiatry 64:1349–1356, 2003

Davidson J: Seizures and bupropion: a review. J Clin Psychiatry 50:256–261, 1989

DeBattista C, Doghramji K, Menza MA, et al: Adjunct modafinil for the short-term treatment of fatigue and sleepiness in patients with major depressive disorder: a preliminary double-blind, placebo-controlled study. J Clin Psychiatry 64:1057–1064, 2003

Debonnel G, Blier P, St-André É, et al: Comparison of the effect of low and high doses of venlafaxine on serotonin and norepinephrine reuptake processes in patients with major depression and healthy volunteers (abstract). Int J Neuropsychopharmacol 1 (suppl 1):17, 1998

Debonnel G, Gobbi G, Turcotte J, et al: Effects of mirtazapine, paroxetine and their combination: a double-blind study in major depression (abstract). Eur Neuropsychopharmacol 10 (suppl 3):S252, 2000

Delgado PL, Charney DS, Price LH, et al: Serotonin function and the mechanism of antidepressant action: reversal of antidepressant-induced remission by rapid depletion of plasma tryptophan. Arch Gen Psychiatry 47:411–418, 1990

Delgado PL, Miller HL, Salomon RM, et al: Tryptophan-depletion challenge in depressed patients treated with desipramine or fluoxetine: implications for the role of serotonin in the mechanism of antidepressant action. Biol Psychiatry 46:212–220, 1999

Delgado PL, Moreno FA, Onate L, et al: Sequential catecholamine and serotonin depletion in mirtazapine treated depressed patients. Int J Neuropsychopharmacol 5:63–66, 2002

de Montigny C, Grunberg F, Mayer A, et al: Lithium induces rapid relief of depression in tricyclic antidepressant drug non-responders. Br J Psychiatry 138:252–256, 1981

de Montigny C, Cournoyer G, Morissette R, et al: Lithium carbonate addition in tricyclic antidepressant-resistant unipolar depression: correlations with the neurobiologic actions of tricyclic antidepressant drugs and lithium ion on the serotonin system. Arch Gen Psychiatry 40:1327–1334, 1983

Dennis T, L'Heureux R, Carter C, et al: Presynaptic alpha-2 adrenoceptors play a major role in the effects of idazoxan on cortical noradrenaline release (as measured by in vivo dialysis) in the rat. J Pharmacol Exp Ther 241:642–649, 1987

Dimitriou EC, Dimitriou CE: Buspirone augmentation of antidepressant therapy. J Clin Psychopharmacol 18:465–469, 1998

Dinan TG, Barry S: A comparison of electroconvulsive therapy with a combined lithium and tricyclic combination among depressed tricyclic nonresponders. Acta Psychiatr Scand 80:97–100, 1989

Dong J, Blier P: Modification of norepinephrine and serotonin, but not dopamine neuron firing by sustained bupropion treatment. Psychopharmacology 155:52–57, 2001

Dostert P, Castelli MG, Cicioni P, et al: Reboxetine prevents the tranylcypromine-induced increase in tyramine levels in rat heart. J Neural Transm Suppl 41:149–153, 1994

Fava M, Rosenbaum JF, McGrath PJ, et al: Lithium and tricyclic augmentation of fluoxetine treatment for resistant major depression: a double-blind, controlled study. Am J Psychiatry 151:1372–1374, 1994

Fava M, Thase ME, DeBattista C: A multicenter, placebo-controlled study of modafinil augmentation in partial responders to selective serotonin reuptake inhibitors with persistent fatigue and sleepiness. J Clin Psychiatry 66:85–93, 2005

Gharabawi G, Mahmoud R, Bossie C, et al: Augmentation with risperidone in resistant depression (arise-rd): maintenance of remission in a double-blind placebo-controlled trial (abstract). Int J Neuropsychopharmacol 7:S163, 2004

Goodall EM, Cowen PJ, Franklin M, et al: Ritanserin attenuates anorectic, endocrine and thermic response to d-fenfluramine in human volunteers. Psychopharmacology 112:461–466, 1993

Goodman WK: Obsessive-compulsive disorder: diagnosis and treatment. J Clin Psychiatry 60 (suppl 18):27–32, 1999

Gur E, Lerer B, Newman ME: Chronic clomipramine and triiodothyronine increase serotonin levels in rat frontal cortex in vivo: relationship to serotonin autoreceptor activity. J Pharmacol Exp Ther 388:81–87, 1999

Haddjeri N, Blier P, de Montigny C: Effect of the alpha-2 adrenoceptor antagonist mirtazapine on the 5-hydroxytryptamine system in the rat brain. J Pharmacol Exp Ther 277:861–871, 1996

Haddjeri N, de Montigny C, Blier P: Modulation of the firing activity of noradrenergic neurons in the rat locus coeruleus by the 5-hydroxytryptamine system. Br J Pharmacol 120:865–875, 1997

Haddjeri N, Blier P, de Montigny C: Long-term antidepressant treatments result in a tonic activation of forebrain 5-HT1A receptors. J Neurosci 18:10150–10156, 1998

Haddjeri N, Szabo ST, de Montigny C, et al: Increased tonic activation of rat forebrain 5-HT (1A) receptors by lithium addition to antidepressant treatments. Neuropsychopharmacology 22:346–356, 2000

Haj-Dahmane S: D2-like dopamine receptor activation excites rat dorsal raphe 5-HT neurons in vitro. Eur J Neurosci 14:125–134, 2001

Happe S, Trenkwalder C: Role of dopamine receptor agonists in the treatment of restless legs syndrome. CNS Drugs 18:27–36, 2004

Harvey AT, Preskorn SH: Cytochrome P450 enzymes: interpretation of their interactions with selective serotonin reuptake inhibitors, part I. J Clin Psychopharmacol 16:273–285, 1996a

Harvey AT, Preskorn SH: Cytochrome P450 enzymes: interpretation of their interactions with selective serotonin reuptake inhibitors, part II. J Clin Psychopharmacol 16:345–355, 1996b

Hatanaka K, Yatsugi S, Yamaguchi T: Effect of acute treatment with YM992 on extracellular norepinephrine levels in the rat frontal cortex. Eur J Pharmacol 395:31–36, 2000

Hyttel J: Citalopram: pharmacological profile of a specific serotonin uptake inhibitor with antidepressant activity. Prog Neuropsychopharmacol Biol Psychiatry 6:277–295, 1982

Inoue T, Tsuchiya K, Miura J, et al: Bromocriptine treatment of tricyclic and heterocyclic antidepressant-resistant depression. Biol Psychiatry 40:151–153, 1996

Izumi T, Inoue T, Kitagawa N, et al: Open pergolide treatment of tricyclic and heterocyclic antidepressant-resistant depression. J Affect Disord 61:127–132, 2000

Janssen S, Blier P: Effects of prolonged bupropion treatment on the firing activity of norepinephrine and serotonin neurons (abstract). Biol Psychiatry 53:51S, 2003

Joffe RT, Schuller DR: An open study of buspirone augmentation of serotonin reuptake inhibitors in refractory depression. J Clin Psychiatry 54:269–271, 1993

Joffe RT, Singer W, Levitt AJ, et al: A placebo-controlled comparison of lithium and triiodothyronine augmentation of tricyclic antidepressants in unipolar refractory depression. Arch Gen Psychiatry 50:387–393, 1993

Jolas T, Haj-Dahmane S, Kidd EJ, et al: Central pre- and postsynaptic 5-HT1A receptors in rats treated chronically with a novel antidepressant, cericlamine. J Pharmacol Exp Ther 268:1432–1443, 1994

Judd LL, Paulus MJ, Schettler PJ, et al: Does incomplete recovery from first lifetime major depressive episode herald a chronic course of illness? Am J Psychiatry 157:1501–1504, 2000

Katona CL, Abou-Saleh MT, Harrison DA, et al: Placebo-controlled trial of lithium augmentation of fluoxetine and lofepramine. Br J Psychiatry 166:80–86, 1995

Kelder J, Funke C, De Boer T, et al: A comparison of the physiochemical and biological properties of mirtazapine and mianserin. J Pharm Pharmacol 49:403–411, 1997

Keller MB, Lavori PW, Mueller TI, et al: Time to recovery, chronicity, and levels of psychophathology in major depression: a 5-year prospective follow-up of 431 subjects. Arch Gen Psychiatry 49:809–816, 1992

Kirchheiner J, Klein C, Meineke I, et al: Bupropion and 4-OH-bupropion pharmacokinetics in relation to genetic polymorphisms in CYP2B6. Pharmacogenetics 13:619–626, 2003

Koch S, Perry KW, Bymaster FP: Brain region and dose effects of an olanzapine/fluoxetine combination on extracellular monoamine concentrations in the rat. Neuropharmacology 46:232–242, 2004

Kugaya A, Seneca NM, Snyder PJ, et al: Changes in human in vivo serotonin and dopamine transporter availabilities during chronic antidepressant administration. Neuropsychopharmacology 28:413–420, 2003

Kurtz DL, Bergstrom RF, Goldberg MJ, et al: The effect of sertraline on the pharmacokinetics of desipramine and imipramine. Clin Pharmacol Ther 62:145–156, 1997

Landen M, Bjorling G, Agren H, et al: A randomized, double-blind, placebo-controlled trial of buspirone in combination with an SSRI in patients with treatment-refractory depression. J Clin Psychiatry 59:664–668, 1998

Landen M, Eriksson E, Agren H, et al: Effect of buspirone on sexual dysfunction in depressed patients treated with selective serotonin reuptake inhibitors. J Clin Psychopharmacol 19:268–271, 1999

Lattanzi L, Dell'Osso L, Cassano P, et al: Pramipexole in treatment-resistant depression: a 16-week naturalistic study. Bipolar Disord 4:307–314, 2002

Learned-Coughlin SM, Bergstrom M, Savitcheva I, et al: In vivo activity of bupropion at the human dopamine transporter as measured by positron emission tomography. Biol Psychiatry 54:800–805, 2003

Lexapro Web site. Available at: http://www.lexapro.com. New York, NY, Forest Pharmaceuticals, 2005

Maes M, Libbrecht I, van Hunsel F, et al: Pindolol and mianserin augment the antidepressant activity of fluoxetine in hospitalized major depressed patients, including those with treatment resistance. J Clin Psychopharmacol 19:177–182, 1999

Martinez R, Puigvert A, Pomerol JM, et al: Clinical experience with apomorphine hydrochloride: the first 107 patients. J Urol 170 (6 pt 1):2352–2355, 2003

Meyer JH, Goulding VS, Wilson AA, et al: Bupropion occupancy of the dopamine transporter is low during clinical treatment. Psychopharmacology (Berl) 163:102–105, 2002

Miller HL, Delgado PL, Salomon RM, et al: Clinical and biochemical effects of catecholamine depletion on antidepressant-induced remission of depression. Arch Gen Psychiatry 53:117–128, 1996

Mischoulon D, Nierenberg AA, Kizilbash L, et al: Strategies for managing depression refractory to selective serotonin reuptake inhibitor treatment: a survey of clinicians. Can J Psychiatry 45:476–481, 2000

Nelson JC, Mazure CM, Jatlow PI, et al: Combining norepinephrine and serotonin reuptake inhibition mechanisms for treatment. Biol Psychiatry 55:296–300, 2004

New federal guidelines seek to help primary care providers recognize and treat depression. Agency for Health Care Policy and Research (AHCPR) of the Department of Human Services. Hosp Community Psychiatry 44:598, 1993

Nierenberg AA, DeCecco LM: Definitions of antidepressant treatment response, remission, nonresponse, partial response, and other relevant outcomes: a focus on treatment-resistant depression. J Clin Psychiatry 62 (suppl 16):5–9, 2001

Nutt DJ: Tolerability and safety aspects of mirtazapine. Hum Psychopharmacol 17 (suppl 1):S37–S41, 2002

Ostroff RB, Nelson JC: Risperidone augmentation of selective serotonin reuptake inhibitors in major depression. J Clin Psychiatry 60:256–259, 1999

Park SB, Cowen PJ: Effect of pindolol on the prolactin response to d-fenfluramine. Psychopharmacology 118:471–474, 1995

Paykel ES, Ramana R, Cooper Z, et al: Residual symptoms after partial remission: an important outcome in depression. Psychol Med 25:1171–1180, 1995

Poirier MF, Boyer P: Venlafaxine and paroxetine in treatment-resistant depression: double-blind, randomized comparison. Br J Psychiatry 175:12–16, 1999

Rush AJ, Trivedi MH, Carmody TJ, et al: Response in relation to baseline anxiety levels in major depressive disorder treated with bupropion sustained release of sertraline. Neuropsychopharmacology 25:131–138, 2001

Sacchetti G, Bernini M, Bianchetti A, et al: Studies on the acute and chronic effects of reboxetine on extracellular noradrenaline and other monoamines in the rat brain. Br J Pharmacol 128:1332–1338, 1999

Sajatovic M, DiGiovanni S, Fuller M, et al: Nefazodone therapy in patients with treatment-resistant or treatment-intolerant depression and high psychiatric comorbidity. Clin Ther 21:733–740, 1999

Schmauss M, Kampfhammer HP, Meyr P, et al: Combined MAO-inhibitor and tri- (tetra) cyclic antidepressant in therapy resistant depression. Prog Neuropsychopharmacol Biol Psychiatry 12:523–532, 1988

Seager MA, Huff KD, Barth VN, et al: Fluoxetine administration potentiates the effect of olanzapine on locus coeruleus neuronal activity. Biol Psychiatry 55:1103–1109, 2004

Sheline YI, Sanghavi M, Mintun MA, et al: Depression duration but not age predicts hippocampal volume loss in medically healthy women with recurrent major depression. J Neurosci 19:5034–5043, 1999

Shelton RC, Tollefson GD, Tohen M, et al: A novel augmentation strategy for treating resistant major depression. Am J Psychiatry 158:131–134, 2001

Sporn J, Ghaemi SN, Sambur MR, et al: Pramipexole augmentation in the treatment of unipolar and bipolar depression: a retrospective chart review. Ann Clin Psychiatry 12:137–140, 2000

Stein G, Bernadt M: Lithium augmentation therapy in tricyclic-resistant depression: a controlled trial using lithium in low and normal doses. Br J Psychiatry 162:634–640, 1993

Sternbach H: The serotonin syndrome. Am J Psychiatry 148:705–713, 1991

Szabo ST, Blier P: Functional and pharmacological characterization of the modulatory role of serotonin on the firing activity of locus coeruleus norepinephrine neurons. Brain Res 922:9–20, 2001

Szabo ST, Blier P: Effects of serotonin (5-hydroxytryptamine, 5-HT) reuptake inhibition plus 5-HT (2A) receptor antagonism on the firing activity of norepinephrine neurons. J Pharmacol Exp Ther 302:983–991, 2002

Szabo ST, de Montigny C, Blier P: Progressive attenuation of the firing activity of locus coeruleus noradrenergic neurons by sustained administration of selective serotonin reuptake inhibitors. Int J Neuropsychopharmacol 3:1–11, 2000

Thase ME: Achieving remission and managing relapse in depression. J Clin Psychiatry 64 (suppl 18):3–7, 2003

Tohen M, Vieta E, Calabrese J, et al: Efficacy of olanzapine and olanzapine-fluoxetine combination in the treatment of bipolar I depression. Arch Gen Psychiatry 60:1079–1088, 2003 [published erratum appears in 61:176, 2004]

Zerbe RL, Row H, Enas GG, et al: Clinical pharmacology of tomoxetine, a potential antidepressant. J Pharmacol Exp Ther 232:139–143, 1985

PART 7

Subtypes of Mood Disorders

SECTION EDITOR: ALAN F. SCHATZBERG, M.D.

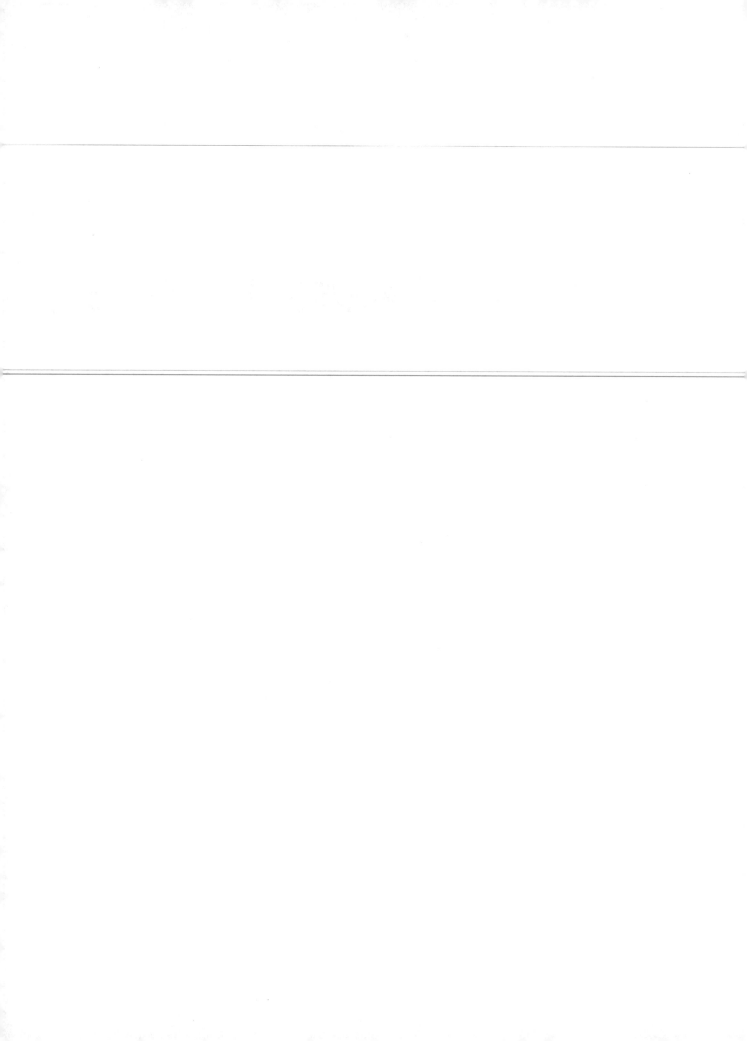

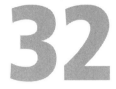

CHAPTER

32

Seasonal Affective Disorder

JOSHUA Z. ROSENTHAL, M.D.

NORMAN E. ROSENTHAL, M.D.

SEASONAL AFFECTIVE DISORDER (SAD) was initially described by Rosenthal et al. (1984) as a condition in which patients experience recurrent depressions in autumn and winter, alternating with nondepressed periods in spring and summer. Subsequently, an opposite form of SAD was described in which depressions typically occur in spring and summer, alternating with nondepressed periods in fall and winter (Boyce and Parker 1988; Wehr et al. 1987a). In this chapter, we use the term *SAD* to refer to the condition of winter depressions and *summer SAD* to describe its polar opposite. These basic definitions were later incorporated into DSM-III-R (American Psychiatric Association 1987), and then into DSM-IV and DSM-IV-TR (American Psychiatric Association 1994, 2000), as the phrase "with seasonal pattern," which can be used to modify any form of recurrent mood disorder. Following the description of SAD, there has been renewed interest in seasonal influences on a variety of human behaviors. We refer to this tendency of seasonal variability in behavior as *seasonality*. In this chapter, we summarize the history of SAD and seasonality and describe the clinical and demographic features, prevalence, treatment, and pathophysiology of SAD.

History of Seasonality and Seasonal Affective Disorder

The idea that seasons could influence illness goes back to Hippocrates (1923–1931), who wrote, "it is chiefly the changes of seasons which produce diseases." He also noted that "of constitutions some are well or ill adapted to summer, others are well or ill adapted to winter." These two threads—the seasons as a general influence on disease and as a recurrent pathogenic influence on particular vulnerable individuals—are evident both in ancient writings and in those of nineteenth-century psychiatrists such as Pinel and Esquirol (Wehr 1989).

Seasonal influences on suicide and suicide attempts, as well as episodes of depression and mania, have been thoroughly explored in the twentieth century (Rosenthal et al. 1983). The peak incidence of suicide in spring and summer is one of the most consistent epidemiological findings in the suicide literature (Altamura et al. 1999) and has been reported in both the Northern and the Southern Hemispheres (Gaedeken 1911). This observation has been variously attributed to seasonal changes in social behavior by some researchers, such as Durkheim (1951), and to meteorological factors, such as change in temperature, by others, such as Morselli (1881). There is some consensus that depressive episodes are most likely to begin in spring and fall and mania in summer (Rosenthal et al. 1983).

Although isolated cases of what in retrospect appears to have been SAD were reported for many years, it was in the mid-1980s that the condition was first described as a syndrome with specific clinical and demographic features, a predictable clinical course, and a response to a particular form of treatment—namely, light therapy. The DSM-III-R architects were confronted with the question of how to classify a disorder that could overlap with other recognized conditions, such as bipolar disorder. Their conclusion, to develop an adjectival modifier, has the advantage of flexibility insofar as it can be used for any recurrent mood disorder and can apply to both winter and summer varieties of the condition. Its disadvantage is in not conferring on individuals with a classical picture of SAD a specific diagnosis, which is useful both in a clinical setting and for research purposes.

The criteria for SAD, as outlined by Rosenthal et al. (1984) and subsequently by the DSM-III-R and DSM-IV committees, are shown in Table 32–1. All three sets of criteria include elements that refer to 1) a recurrent pattern of winter depression, 2) nondepressed periods in spring and summer, and 3) some degree of severity with regard to the winter depressions. Although there may be debate about the particulars of these criteria, they are in concept all reasonable. Included in all three sets of criteria is a fourth element, which, in the light of clinical experience, appears less useful; that is, there should be no recurrent psychosocial variable that might account for the regular seasonal pattern of symptoms. Since SAD was originally described, numerous scholarly articles have appeared on the subject, as well as many useful books, to which the interested reader is directed (Lam 1998; Partonen and Magnusson 2001; Rosenthal et al. 1993a, 1993b).

Clinical and Demographic Features

Seasonal Affective Disorder

By now, SAD has been described on four continents (North America, Europe, Asia, and Australia) (Eagles et al. 1998; Han et al. 2000; Morrissey 1996; Rosen et al. 1990; Saarijarvi et al. 1999), and there are anecdotal reports of the condition from South America (H.M. Calil, personal communication, 2003). The clinical and demographic features of SAD obtained from groups in different parts of the world show a remarkably consistent picture.

SAD most commonly begins in the 20s, and the peak time for presentation to research programs usually has been the late 30s and early 40s, by which age many cycles of winter depression have occurred. With the growing awareness of SAD, one might predict that the condition will be recognized earlier and that the latency between onset and first treatment will diminish. It is important to recognize that the onset of SAD is not always clear cut. Many patients with SAD report that they had endured winter difficulties for years before their symptoms met criteria for major depression. After several such episodes, symptoms may cross this threshold for various reasons, including stress at work or in relationships or diminished social supports, for example, after leaving home. The first year of college is therefore a time of special risk for patients with SAD.

Most SAD patients meet criteria for major depressive disorder (MDD), recurrent, with a minority meeting criteria for bipolar II disorder and a very few for bipolar I disorder. In the early years of SAD research, higher bipolar II disorder figures were reported because at that time, the criteria for hypomania were far more lenient. Current hypomania criteria require some degree of dysfunction as a result of the hypomanic state. Relatively few SAD patients have trouble during spring and summer by virtue of their mood states. Rather, many experience exhilaration, increased energy, decreased need for sleep, and greater productivity and creativity during the summer. These behavioral changes do not generally require treatment and subside on their own accord at the approach of autumn.

Symptoms of SAD may begin as early as late August or as late as January or February. In general, however, in the temperate regions, symptoms begin in October or November and last an average of 5 months. The timing of symptoms may vary with climatic conditions—notably, cloud cover and snow. Dark days tend to bring on symptoms in some SAD patients regardless of time of year, whereas the light reflected off snow tends to mitigate symptoms.

Most patients with SAD have reverse vegetative symptoms (overeating, carbohydrate craving, weight gain, lethargy, and oversleeping), whereas a minority have a vegetative presentation more typical of melancholic depression (Rosenthal et al. 1984). It is common for patients to report increased levels of pain when their moods are depressed in the winter (Dilsaver and Jaeckle 1990; Eagles et al. 2002; Schlager et al. 1995). Many women with SAD complain of premenstrual mood changes, which are often worse in the winter months (Praschak-Rieder et al. 2001). One characteristic symptom of SAD is that symptoms improve when patients are closer to the equator (Rosenthal et al. 1984).

In addition to their vegetative symptoms, SAD patients report the ordinary mood changes seen in depression, including sadness, anxiety, and irritability. These

TABLE 32–1. Diagnostic criteria for seasonal affective disorder (SAD) versus seasonal pattern specifier for mood disorders

Original SAD criteria (Rosenthal et al. 1984)	DSM-III-R criteria for major depression, with seasonal pattern (American Psychiatric Association 1987)	DSM-IV-TR criteria for major depression, with seasonal pattern (American Psychiatric Association 1994, 2000)[a]
A history of major affective disorder, according to Research Diagnostic Criteria (Spitzer et al. 1978)	A history of major affective disorder, according to DSM-III-R criteria	There has been a regular temporal relationship between the onset of major depressive episodes in bipolar I or bipolar II disorder or major depressive disorder, and a particular time of the year (e.g., regular appearance of the major depressive episode in the fall or winter) [Criterion A]
	Onset and full remission of each depressive episode, which occur within specific 60-day periods of each other	Full remissions (or a change from depression to mania or hypomania) also occur at a characteristic time of the year (e.g., depression disappears in the spring) [Criterion B]
At least 2 consecutive previous years in which the depressions developed during fall or winter and remitted by the following spring or summer	At least three previous winter depressive episodes (two of which were consecutive)	In the last 2 years, two major depressive episodes have occurred that demonstrate the temporal seasonal relationships defined in Criteria A and B, and no nonseasonal major depressive episodes have occurred during that same period
Absence of any other Axis I DSM-III psychiatric disorder	Seasonal episodes of mood disturbance outnumbered any nonseasonal episodes of mood disturbance that may have occurred by more than three to one	Seasonal major depressive episodes (as described above) substantially outnumber the nonseasonal major depressive episodes that may have occurred over the individual's lifetime
Absence of any clear-cut seasonally changing psychological variables that would account for the seasonal variability in mood and behavior	Absence of any clear-cut seasonally changing psychosocial variables that would account for the seasonal variability in mood and behavior	**Note:** Do not include cases in which there is an obvious effect of seasonal-related psychosocial stressors (e.g., regularly being unemployed every winter).

[a]The criteria for major depression, with seasonal pattern, are identical in DSM-IV and DSM-IV-TR.

Source. DSM-III-R criteria adapted from American Psychiatric Association: *Diagnostic and Statistical Manual of Mental Disorders,* 3rd Edition, Revised. Washington, DC, American Psychiatric Association, 1987, p. 224. Used with permission. DSM-IV-TR criteria reprinted, with format alterations, from American Psychiatric Association: *Diagnostic and Statistical Manual of Mental Disorders,* 4th Edition, Text Revision. Washington, DC, American Psychiatric Association, 2000, p. 427. Used with permission.

symptoms can be quite severe. For example, a recent study found that SAD patients were more symptomatic than nonseasonal depressed patients admitted to an inpatient unit after a suicide attempt (Pendse et al. 2003). In addition, one survey showed that 6%–35% of SAD patients required hospitalization for their winter depressions at some point in their illness (Oren and Rosenthal 1992).

The sequence of development of SAD symptoms is of some interest because the earliest symptoms may be neurovegetative, rather than mood changes, which often occur relatively late in the season (Young et al. 1991). For this reason, many SAD patients present to primary care physicians with physical complaints (Eagles et al. 2002), and if SAD is not part of the differential diagnosis of lack of energy, overeating, and weight gain, the correct diagnosis, and its treatment, can easily be missed.

Subsyndromal Seasonal Affective Disorder and Summer Seasonal Affective Disorder

In researching SAD, it became clear early on that some affected individuals fail to meet full syndromal criteria yet have problems as a result of the changing seasons. They may experience changes in sleeping and eating typical of SAD: decreased productivity or creativity and a diminished sense of well-being. Although these changes might not be severe enough to induce people to seek medical help, such subsyndromal SAD patients also can benefit from treatment with bright environmental light like those with the full-fledged syndrome (Kasper et al. 1989).

The description of the winter form of SAD was soon followed by descriptions of a summer version of the disorder (Wehr et al. 1987a). In contrast to the winter form, patients with summer SAD tend to report more agitation and more typical vegetative symptoms: decreased appetite, weight loss, and insomnia. In addition, they are more likely than their winter counterparts to have suicidal ideas. That may correspond to the observation that suicide tends to peak in the spring and summer months. Patients with summer SAD are more likely to attribute their symptoms to the heat of summer, as opposed to patients with winter SAD, who are more likely to attribute their symptoms to the dark days of winter than to cold weather. It cannot be assumed, however, that heat is the trigger for all summer SAD symptoms. In at least one summer SAD patient, we observed an association between increased light levels (e.g., following a snowstorm) and increased depression.

Thus far, no special treatments have been found that tap into the clue provided by the summer seasonality of this disorder. To date, no systematic studies have been performed to evaluate the possible therapeutic effects of cold or dark environments on summer SAD. Anecdotally, however, some patients with summer SAD have reported improved mood when they travel north in the summer, take cold baths, or keep the air conditioning set on high. Likewise, wearing dark glasses may be helpful for people with summer SAD. For the most part, however, summer SAD is best treated with antidepressant medications. The predictable recurrence of the depressions allows the treating physician to start antidepressants early, thereby preempting or reversing symptoms.

Comorbidity and Seasonal Affective Disorder

Surveys suggest that SAD may exist in conjunction with other psychiatric disorders. Thus, approximately 45% of the patients with SAD have a lifetime risk for an anxiety disorder (Levitt et al. 1993), and 23%–58% have a risk for a comorbid Axis II disorder, depending on the different methodologies used (Reichborn-Kennerud et al. 1994, 1997). Women with adult attention-deficit/hyperactivity disorder have a 10%–20% rate of SAD, depending on the diagnostic criteria used (Levitan et al. 1999). The overeating that occurs in SAD resembles in some ways the behaviors of patients with eating disorders. Patients with eating disorders, particularly bulimia nervosa, have higher scores on the Global Seasonality Scale (GSS) than do control subjects without eating disorders (Brewerton et al. 1994; Hardin et al. 1991; Lam et al. 1996a; Yamatsuji et al. 2003). Between 42% and 69% of bulimic patients satisfy criteria for SAD, according to the Seasonal Pattern Assessment Questionnaire (SPAQ) (Lam et al. 1996a; Levitan et al. 1994; Yamatsuji et al. 2003), and bingeing and purging behavior varied seasonally in a 4-year retrospective study of bulimic patients (Blouin et al. 1992). Compared with matched control subjects, SAD patients scored higher on the Eating Disorders Inventory, a self-rating questionnaire that assesses abnormal eating attitudes and behaviors (Berman et al. 1993). In a small, controlled study of patients with seasonal bulimia, bright light therapy was superior to dim light control in improving winter mood and in improvement on eating outcome measures (Lam et al. 1994).

Prevalence of Seasonal Affective Disorder and Seasonality

In considering the prevalence of SAD and seasonality, several issues must be taken into account. First, how should prevalence be measured in population studies? Second, how can the results of such studies be validated?

Finally, what is the relation between prevalence and the criteria for SAD existing at the time of the study?

The criteria for SAD have changed markedly over the relatively short time in which the disease has been recognized (see Table 32–1). The criteria of Rosenthal et al. are the most inclusive, the DSM-III-R criteria are the least inclusive, and the DSM-IV criteria occupy a middle zone. The stricter the criteria, the less prevalent the condition will appear to be. It could be argued that greater strictness has a value in producing more homogeneous or severely affected groups of patients. However, greater rigor may serve to eliminate clear-cut cases of SAD from being diagnosed or counted in epidemiological studies. In addition, no scientific evidence shows that the stricter criteria are more valid or useful than the more inclusive ones. On the contrary, consider the criterion in DSM-IV, for example, that requires that a patient must have two major depressive episodes in the 2 years prior to presentation. Such a criterion would exclude a patient with a long-standing history of recurrent winter depressions who might have skipped a winter depressive episode in the past 2 years perhaps for a very good reason, such as the use of medications or relocation to a sunny climate. Prevalence studies of SAD have straddled the different definitions, which complicates comparisons across studies.

The main screening instrument that has been used in epidemiological studies of SAD is the SPAQ, which has been translated into many different languages and used worldwide in at least 27 studies. One key element of the questionnaire is the GSS score, which is derived from scoring the six items on Question 12 of the SPAQ: sleep length, social activity, mood, weight, appetite, and energy level. Each item can receive from 0 to 4 on a Likert scale. The sum of these scores, the GSS score, thus can range from 0 to 24. The GSS has been used, in conjunction with other elements of the SPAQ, for case-finding purposes in population studies. The items on the GSS have been shown to have a high internal consistency (Magnusson et al. 1997), and the SPAQ as a whole appears to have good test-retest reliability over a period of months to years (Hardin et al. 1991; Raheja et al. 1996).

At least 29 epidemiological studies in adults have used the SPAQ. Despite methodological differences across studies, certain general trends emerged. In particular, a clear association exists (at least in the United States) between prevalence of SAD and latitude. For example, respondents in Sarasota, Florida (23° N), showed a prevalence of only 1.4%, and those in Nashua, New Hampshire (42° N), showed a prevalence of 9.7% (Rosen et al. 1990). The overall correlation between latitude and SAD prevalence in Europe is weaker than in the United States (Mersch et al. 1999), owing perhaps to variables such as climate,

methodology, and genetic factors. Studies of people living or born in Iceland, for example, show a lower than expected prevalence of SAD, given their prolonged exposure to darkness in winter, and may suggest that this population is genetically resistant to SAD on the whole (Magnusson and Axelsson 1993; Magnusson and Stefansson 1993).

A few studies have estimated the prevalence of SAD with diagnostic criteria other than the SPAQ. The two largest studies of this kind estimated the prevalence of SAD in the general population to be much lower than in previous studies that used the SPAQ. On the basis of DSM-III-R criteria, the estimated prevalence of major depression with a seasonal pattern was found to be approximately 2.9% in Canada (Levitt et al. 2000) and 0.4% in the United States (Blazer et al. 1998). This latter estimate was increased to 1% when combining rates of both major and minor depression with a seasonal pattern. Another way of estimating the prevalence of SAD in selected samples is by examining the proportion of patients with MDD who meet criteria for this subcategory. Examined in this way, SAD has been estimated to represent between 11% and 38% of the patients with recurrent MDD in several countries (Faedda et al. 1993; Garvey et al. 1988; Kasper and Kamo 1990; Srivastava and Sharma 1998; Williams and Schmidt 1993).

Seasonal Affective Disorder Across the Age Spectrum

SAD appears to be fairly common in adolescents. A survey of 1,458 adolescents in Finland (60–67° N) found high rates of seasonal symptoms (60%–90%), such as changes in energy level, social activity, sleep, and mood, in fall and winter (Sourander et al. 1999). Adolescents living farther north were more likely to experience seasonal distress than were those living farther south. One study of middle and high school children in Maryland by Swedo et al. (1995) found an SAD prevalence rate of about 3%, suggesting that an estimated 1 million United States children and adolescents may be affected by the condition. The researchers observed a sharp rise in prevalence of SAD in girls after puberty, which has its counterpart at the opposite end of the reproductive cycle. Kasper et al. (1989) found that women in their reproductive years have higher GSS scores than do men of similar ages, a difference that disappears in the 40s and 50s. Together, these findings suggest that the cyclical secretion of female sex hormones may influence the brain's sensitivity to environmental light deprivation. Some evidence also indicates that SAD prevalence for both genders declines later in life (Booker and Hellekson 1992; Eagles et al. 1999; Hegde and Woodson 1996; Rosen et al. 1990).

Treatment of Seasonal Affective Disorder

It is best to treat SAD, like other mood disorders, with a variety of interventions. The clinician seeks to blend these interventions together and customize them for each patient. In clinical practice, clinicians routinely use psychotherapy while monitoring light therapy and medications in order to achieve the best effect. On the other hand, scientists attempting to explore the therapeutic value of different treatment modalities seek to isolate these modalities to avoid confounding influences. It is important, however, to be aware that in practice these elements are rarely applied in isolation. The best-studied treatment for SAD is light therapy, which is effective, safe, and well tolerated. We begin our treatment discussion with light therapy because in clinical practice, it is frequently the first treatment modality to be used.

Light Therapy

In contemplating the use of light therapy, several factors must be considered. How depressed is the patient? What is the time of year? What are the patient's daily habits: the time of sleep onset and waking; the amount of time in the morning before the patient has to leave home; the patient's work setup? What is the patient's financial status (light fixtures can be quite costly)? When is the patient likely to be able to use the light box? All of these questions will prove relevant to the clinical recommendations.

For instance, if a patient presents in the autumn with mild symptoms of SAD, it may be appropriate to start with a short duration of light therapy (about 10–15 minutes in the morning) and gradually increase the duration as the season deepens. On the other hand, if a patient presents with severe symptoms in mid-winter, it may be best to start with much more light therapy (about 45 minutes in the morning and 20 minutes in the evening), monitor symptoms closely, and adjust treatment accordingly.

If a patient has time in the morning before work, it may be best to undertake light therapy before leaving home. If someone needs to be at work early, it might be best to wait until arriving at the office to undertake light therapy. The latter suggestion requires careful exploration because a light box in the office is an open acknowledgment of a seasonal problem, which may not be acceptable or politic in some work settings.

The size of the light box is another issue that merits discussion. Smaller light boxes are popular because they are cheaper, take up less space on a desktop, and are less cumber-

some. However, less light is emitted from a smaller surface area. Most light therapy research has been performed with light fixtures of a certain size (approximately 18×24 inches). No data show that smaller light boxes work as well. Although these smaller light boxes are advertised as emitting the same amount of light as the larger boxes, one would expect them to influence a smaller area of the retina. In addition, movements of the head from side to side or to and fro can make a large difference in the amount of light received, and the smaller the light box, the more these movements are likely to affect the therapeutic benefits of the light.

To give light therapy the best chance of working, the clinician must explore and discuss all these points with the patient in an attempt to make treatment feasible and convenient. Light therapy is most likely to be user-friendly if the treating clinician is knowledgeable and comfortable with the modality. For more suggestions about how to make light treatment work, the interested reader is referred elsewhere (Rosenthal et al. 1993b).

History of Light Therapy for SAD

Light therapy has been used for more than a century in the treatment of numerous conditions. Niels Finsen received the Nobel Prize for his work on the beneficial effects of ultraviolet light on tuberculosis of the skin, and many other therapeutic uses for ultraviolet light have been advocated.

Before the modern era of SAD, at least two striking examples of visible light were used to treat winter symptoms, which sound quite similar to those of SAD. In the first instance, Antarctic explorer Frederick Cook, observing that his men had symptoms resembling those of SAD, exposed them to the light of an open fire with good results (Cameron 1974). In the second instance, German physician Helmut Marx (1946) used bright artificial light to successfully treat the symptoms in four men who had become depressed during a winter trip to the Arctic.

The modern era of light therapy for SAD was ushered in by the treatment of a scientist, Herb Kern, who had observed seasonal depressions in himself for 15 years before he presented to the National Institute of Mental Health (NIMH) (Lewy et al. 1982). His winter depression responded to treatment with bright environmental light. The following year, Rosenthal et al. (1984) recruited the first cohort of SAD patients and treated nine of them with light treatments of different intensities in a crossover study. Since then, about 60 controlled studies of different types of light therapy have been performed, most of them showing favorable effects of treatment.

One pervasive issue in research on the efficacy of light therapy has been controlling for the placebo effect, something that is particularly difficult when dealing with a transparent intervention. To control for the placebo effect, researchers have used light sources of different intensity or color, treatments administered at different times of day or for different durations, and, most recently, negative ion generators, some of which were calibrated to emit rather small amounts of ions. The overarching conclusion is that light therapy appears to work by specific mechanisms other than merely the placebo effect (Golden et al. 2005).

Parameters of Importance for the Efficacy of Light Therapy

Intensity of light was the first parameter to be studied in the treatment of SAD. This line of work was inspired by the finding that bright light (2,500 lux) was a more potent suppressor of human nocturnal melatonin secretion than ordinary room light (Lewy et al. 1980). This intensity of light (2,500 lux) was the first to be tested in treating SAD, and it proved superior to control treatments with intensities ranging from 100 to 400 lux (Rosenthal et al. 1988b). J.S. Terman et al. (1990) first showed 10,000 lux to be superior to 2,500 lux, and this higher intensity has become the treatment standard. Still higher intensities of light have not been systematically tested and cannot be recommended at this time. A meta-analysis of 39 studies of light therapy in which different light intensities were used found a dose–response effect of light for typical but not atypical symptoms of SAD (Lee and Chan 1999).

Clinical experience suggests that the longer the duration of light therapy, the stronger the treatment effect. To date, however, duration rarely has been manipulated systematically in research studies. To obtain the best treatment results, duration should be modified just as one might modify dosage of an antidepressant; the patient's response and side-effect profile should be used as a guide to increasing or decreasing length of treatment. Optimal duration will depend on the individual, the time of year, and the weather. Some people feel light-deprived during a spell of cloudy weather regardless of season. Although winter is the peak time for light use, some people use lights during other seasons as well.

A great deal of research has focused on the importance of timing of light therapy. Lewy et al. (1987) first suggested that light therapy is most potent when administered in the morning. Several individual studies and meta-analyses have now confirmed this (Golden et al. 2005; Lee et al. 1997a; M. Terman et al. 1989; Thompson et al. 1999). In these meta-analyses, the difference in efficacy between morning and evening light emerged most clearly when remission rates were considered, as opposed to re-

ductions in depression scores. Terman and colleagues have found that those who are more alert and active in the morning benefit from light therapy administered earlier in the day compared with those who are most alert and active in the evening. These researchers have developed an algorithm by which it is possible to compute the most likely optimal time for treatment for a particular individual on the basis of that person's tendency to be an "owl" or a "lark." (For more information, see Center for Environmental Therapeutics Web site, http://www.cet.org.) In many instances, however, the optimal time turns out to be too early for the patient's comfort. Nevertheless, it provides a useful ideal.

Although morning light treatments are optimal in general, meta-analyses have shown that light treatment in the evening is superior to placebo interventions (M. Terman et al. 1989; Thompson et al. 1999). In addition, one meta-analysis showed that light treatment in both morning and evening was superior to treatment at other times of day (Lee and Chan 1999). This is consistent with clinical experience, which suggests that many patients benefit by supplementing the effects of morning light with additional light in the late afternoon or early evening.

In one early study, Wehr et al. (1987b) set out to determine whether light therapy was mediated via the eyes or the skin. They found light exposure to the eyes to be superior to light exposure to the skin. We do not yet know which photoreceptors or photopigments are responsible for mediating the antidepressant effects of light therapy. Some clue to the pigment comes from the observation that green light is superior to red light exposure (Lee et al. 1997b; Oren et al. 1991). Little is known, however, about the mechanisms by which light rays are transduced into nerve signals that result in antidepressant effects. Although many studies have used full-spectrum fluorescent light (i.e., the color spectrum of sunlight) as a treatment source, no evidence shows that this is superior to ordinary white fluorescent light.

Side Effects of Light Therapy

The most common short-term side effects of light therapy are headache, eyestrain, nausea, and jumpiness or agitation. The jumpiness and agitation (Kogan and Guilford 1998; Labbate et al. 1994; M. Terman and Terman 1999) resemble the hypomanic symptoms that some SAD patients experience during the summer (Depue et al. 1989). All of these side effects usually can be successfully treated by reducing light exposure (e.g., by decreasing duration of treatment or asking the subject to sit a bit farther from the light box). The development of side effects also can be minimized by starting treatment gradually and building up to full dose over a week or two, much as one might titrate up the dosage of an antidepressant. Two follow-up studies also addressed possible long-term effects of light treatment on the eyes. Neither Schwartz et al. (1996) nor Gallin et al. (1995) found any ill effects of continued treatments with light therapy after an average of 8.8 and 2–5 years, respectively.

Light Fixtures

Therapeutic light fixtures usually contain the following specific elements: fluorescent light tubes encased in a metal frame behind a plastic diffusing screen, which contains an ultraviolet filter. Although it is possible for people to build their own light boxes, most patients prefer to purchase ready-made units, which are provided by several commercial companies. The fluorescent bulbs are preferable to incandescent ones because they spread the light over a larger surface area, which is safer for the eyes. It is important not to stare directly at incandescent lights because their sharp point sources can damage the retina. It is even dangerous to stare directly at fluorescent bulbs for prolonged periods; hence the diffusing screen. Finally, the ultraviolet filter is valuable because it has been shown that even with such filters in place, a substantial amount of ultraviolet light escapes through the screen, which could potentially be harmful to the eyes (Oren et al. 1990) (see preceding section, "Side Effects of Light Therapy").

An alternative type of light therapy unit, the light visor, allows light to be delivered to patients while they are moving around. This caplike device contains light sources in the visor, which shine light into the eyes. Although one would expect that light administered this way would be effective in reversing the symptoms of SAD, researchers have been unable to show a dose–response curve for light visor treatments of different intensities (Joffe et al. 1993; Rosenthal et al. 1993a; Teicher at al. 1995). Nevertheless, a couple of studies showed the devices to be equally effective to light boxes in both treatment (Stewart et al. 1990) and prevention (Meesters et al. 1999) of symptoms. In summary, although some patients report beneficial effects of the light visor, its specific efficacy has not been fully established in controlled studies.

Dawn Simulation

One way to administer light in the early morning hours is by providing a dawn pulse, the simulation of a summer dawn. Various dawn simulators have been designed to do just this. One model connects to a bedside lamp and can be programmed to turn the lamp on at a particular time, such as 5:30 A.M., and slowly increase the light intensity to full power over a predetermined interval (say 45 minutes). Controlled studies that used such devices (Avery et al. 1993,

1994, 2001) and one meta-analysis (Golden et al. 2005) found dawn simulators to be effective. The efficacy of this treatment, considering that the light used is far dimmer than 2,500 lux and is presented to the closed eyelids, bears testimony to the sensitivity of the eyes in the predawn hours. It is unclear whether dawn simulation is as effective as regular light therapy in reversing the symptoms of SAD, with head-to-head studies of the two treatments yielding mixed results (Avery et al. 1992, 2001; Lingjaerde et al. 1998). In practice, dawn simulators are generally used in conjunction with light therapy fixtures. Dawn simulators may help SAD patients wake up and get out of bed (Avery et al. 2002)—a process that can be a major ordeal in the winter—and can therefore make it easier for a patient to find time for light therapy in the morning. If a patient is unable to afford a dawn simulator, a simple timer attached to a bedside lamp can provide a handy and less costly alternative.

Prediction of Response to Light Therapy

In most instances, light therapy in the treatment of SAD has an effect within 2–4 days (Rosenthal et al. 1984), earlier than the antidepressant effects of medications in the treatment of nonseasonal depression. The effect may increase over the following days, and some have suggested that a full effect may occur only after 2–4 weeks of treatment (Bauer et al. 1994; Eastman et al. 1998; Labbate et al. 1995). In general, however, a consistent effect can be seen within a week provided the duration, timing, and intensity are adequate. Many people report an almost immediate activating and mood-enhancing effect of light exposure, and sometimes this effect can be seen during a consultation in which the patient is exposed to bright light. Atypical vegetative symptoms of SAD are among the best predictors of outcome of light therapy (Krauchi et al. 1993; Lam et al. 1994; Oren et al. 1992; M. Terman et al. 1996).

Natural Light

Although it has been little studied, clinical experience confirms the intuitive notion that increasing environmental light naturalistically can be useful. One small study did in fact report a 50% remission rate after a 1-week regimen of outdoor morning light exposure for 1 hour (Wirz-Justice et al. 1996). The results of this study could have been confounded by the beneficial effects of exercise; nonetheless, it makes sense empirically to recommend such outdoor walks to SAD patients, particularly in the morning. Patients also should be encouraged to have plenty of light indoors and to have at least one bright room in the house. White walls and light carpets will reflect more light and create a brighter ambience. In fact, one SAD clinic in Stockholm, Sweden, administers light therapy by means of indirect lighting in a room with white walls and white drapes over the furniture. Patients are asked to wear white gowns to ensure that the maximum amount of light is reflected off surfaces (St. Goran's Hospital, Stockholm, personal communication).

Pharmacotherapy

Although light therapy is effective, it is often not sufficient. Many SAD patients do not respond fully to this treatment, whereas others find it inconvenient and cumbersome. Clearly, other forms of treatment are needed. As in other forms of depression, medications often are the easiest and most convenient form of treatment. What is the evidence that they are of use in SAD? Several studies of antidepressant medications suggested that patients with SAD respond to selective serotonin reuptake inhibitors (Lam et al. 1995; Moscovitch et al. 2004; Ruhrmann et al. 1998). Most of these studies had small sample sizes and a lack of control treatments. The largest controlled treatment study, involving sertraline, yielded a small but statistically significant effect (Moscovitch et al. 2004). Nevertheless, clinical experience suggests that antidepressants can be very helpful in the treatment of winter depressive symptoms. Antidepressants can be used in combination with light therapy, which may allow the patient to take smaller doses and experience correspondingly fewer side effects.

Medication dosages need to be titrated according to the season, increased as the winter deepens, and decreased at the approach of spring. If antidepressants are not tapered after winter passes, this can result in hypomanic symptoms or other side effects, such as fatigue, that were not apparent during the winter but emerge later. Presumably, seasonal changes in brain chemistry present a moving target for antidepressant action, and the astute clinician should be aware of such movement and be ready to make dosage changes up or down in response to it.

Two large controlled studies found that initiating the antidepressant bupropion XL (150–300 mg/day) in advance of the development of winter symptoms prevented the emergence of winter depression in some patients (Rosenthal et al. 2003). For some people, this strategy may prove preferable to light therapy both because of its ease of administration and because it gets a jump start on the winter to minimize time spent experiencing symptoms.

Psychotherapy

Little systematic research has been done on the effects of psychotherapy in the treatment of SAD. One preliminary study by Rohan et al. (2003) suggested that cognitive-behavioral therapy (CBT) might be as effective as light therapy in reversing the symptoms of winter depression. These

researchers further suggested that CBT, particularly in combination with light therapy, might have significant prophylactic benefits over light therapy alone.

In practice, dealing with the patient in an empathic and therapeutic manner has great value. As in the treatment of many other psychiatric conditions, the relationship between clinician and patient can be a crucial element in producing a response. Helping the patient understand the seasonal nature of the condition is extremely useful. Even sophisticated patients can forget the connection between mood, light, and season in the midst of a depression. Behavioral adjustments that seek to minimize stresses in winter and delay controllable stress to spring and summer can be quite useful. It makes clinical sense to challenge cognitive distortions and help patients to reframe these more usefully. It seems likely that psychotherapy will work best when combined with light therapy and/or medications rather than when used in isolation.

Other Forms of Therapy

Several other types of intervention show evidence of benefit. Aerobic exercise has been shown to be useful for patients with subsyndromal SAD symptoms, alone or in combination with light therapy (Leppamaki et al. 2002; Partonen et al. 1998). Because exercise appears to have antidepressant effects in other forms of depression, it is a safe bet to recommend it for SAD patients as well. It is easy to combine exercise with light therapy, for example, by using a stationery bicycle in front of a light box or walking briskly outdoors.

Two studies have shown that exposure to high-density negative ions may be therapeutic (M. Terman and Terman 1995; M. Terman et al. 1998). These findings should probably be replicated before a negative ion generator can be widely recommended.

Winter vacations in sunny climates are often experienced as helpful, although it is important to initiate light therapy on returning to avoid a precipitous mood drop. Some patients with severe cases of SAD have actually chosen to relocate to sunnier locations to good effect. Clearly, relocation is a complex life decision, requiring careful consideration of many different factors.

Preliminary evidence suggests that vitamin D_3 may be of some value in reversing winter depressive symptoms (Gloth et al. 1999).

Course of Seasonal Affective Disorder After Treatment

Several groups have questioned what happens to SAD patients in the years following diagnosis and initial treatment. In follow-up studies performed at intervals ranging from 2 to 8.8 years, researchers found that about a third of patients (22%–42%) continued to show symptoms of SAD. Overall, a similar proportion showed a more complicated pattern of subsequent depressions, which were not strictly seasonal, raising the possibility that treatment changes the temporal pattern of recurrence. In a somewhat smaller proportion (14%–27%), symptoms appeared to have remitted. It is difficult to know quite what to make of these figures because there are, of course, no control groups of untreated SAD patients. Clinical impressions suggest that patients are greatly helped by treatment and that even when winter depressions do recur, they are milder and more quickly detected and successfully treated. Certainly, patients appear to benefit by recognizing the seasonal nature of their illness and learning about the available treatment approaches that can alleviate their symptoms. These observations suggest that untreated, SAD would continue to result in considerable morbidity year after year.

Pathophysiology of Seasonal Affective Disorder and Mechanisms of Action of Light Therapy

Insofar as the symptoms of SAD develop when the amount of ambient light declines, it is reasonable to suspect that the physiological processes that underlie the development of SAD symptoms are somehow related to the effects of declining light on the brain. Conversely, these processes are likely reversed by exposure to more light. We therefore deal with these interconnected processes together.

Research into these processes has centered mainly on the following areas of interest: 1) patterns of melatonin secretion; 2) circadian rhythms; 3) brain neurotransmitter systems, particularly serotonin, norepinephrine, and dopamine; 4) visual sensitivity; and 5) other areas of interest. For the sake of organization, we deal with these areas separately, but they are obviously interconnected. For example, the timing of nocturnal melatonin secretion is a marker of the circadian system (Lewy et al. 1988). Brain neurotransmitter systems influence one another, and melatonin is secreted in response to a β-adrenergic receptor on the pineal gland (Cone et al. 2003). If SAD patients have abnormalities in visual sensitivity, these might well influence patterns of brain neurotransmitter secretion. In addition, different people might develop SAD by different mechanisms, and light therapy might work in different ways to repair the underlying deficit.

Seasonal Affective Disorder, Melatonin Secretion, and the Photoperiod

Seasonal rhythms in animals are entrained by environmental time cues, particularly the length of daylight (photoperiod) (Immelman 1973). Melatonin is of widespread importance as a transducer of seasonal rhythms in animals (Tamarkin et al. 1985), and environmental light has been shown to exert its effect on melatonin via neural connections from the retina through a series of pathways in the central nervous system to the pineal gland, which secretes melatonin (Moore 1978). The possibility that melatonin secretion might somehow be involved in the symptoms of SAD was inherent in the earliest research on the condition (Rosenthal et al. 1984). The discovery that human melatonin secretion could be suppressed by bright light (Lewy et al. 1980) suggested that environmental light and changes in the photoperiod might have other nonvisual effects in humans as well. It was logical, therefore, to explore the possibility that melatonin might be important in understanding the symptoms of SAD: that manipulations of the photoperiod and suppression or modification of melatonin by exposure to bright light at particular times of day might be instrumental in the antidepressant effects of light therapy.

The NIMH group undertook several studies to test the so-called melatonin hypothesis. First, they extended the photoperiod of SAD patients with light therapy administered in the morning and the evening, and after inducing remission, they administered melatonin orally to patients while receiving light therapy (Rosenthal et al. 1986). Patients reported some return of atypical depressive symptoms following melatonin administration, which partially supported a role for melatonin in the pathogenesis of SAD.

Second, these researchers compared the effects of two patterns of light treatment: early morning plus evening treatment versus treatments timed more closely together around the middle of the day (Wehr et al. 1986). Animal experiments that used such "skeleton photoperiods" found that the former pattern has the same effect as a long photoperiod, resulting in melatonin suppression, whereas the latter pattern has the effect of a short photoperiod, resulting in no change in melatonin secretion (Hoffman 1981). The NIMH group found that the two patterns had similar antidepressant efficacy and concluded that this argued against the melatonin hypothesis (Wehr et al. 1986). In retrospect, the conclusion might have been premature because the study had certain limitations, including its relatively small sample size.

Finally, the researchers studied the effects of the long-acting β-adrenergic blocking agent atenolol on the symptoms of SAD. They administered atenolol or placebo in the evening and found no difference between the two interventions, even though atenolol blocked melatonin secretion (Rosenthal et al. 1988a). Later, Schlager (1994) treated SAD with the short-acting β-adrenergic blocking agent propranolol in the morning. After observing a therapeutic response, these researchers undertook a double-blind study in which they discontinued propranolol in some of the patients and switched the others to placebo. They found that the propranolol-treated patients maintained their remissions to a greater degree than did the placebo-treated subjects. Schlager et al. (1996) presented a follow-up study in which SAD patients received either propranolol or placebo in a double-blind, controlled study and found the active treatment to be superior. These promising studies bear following up not only for what they can tell us about the role of melatonin in SAD but also because of their therapeutic implications.

In summary, the possible role of melatonin in the pathogenesis of SAD remains unresolved at this time.

Circadian Rhythms, Seasonal Affective Disorder, and Light Therapy

Lewy et al. (1984) first suggested that abnormal circadian rhythms might be key to the development of SAD. Because many SAD patients have difficulty waking in the morning, these researchers suggested that this might reflect a delay in their circadian rhythms (Lewy et al. 1985). They used a circadian rhythm marker called the "dim light melatonin onset" and found that morning light treatment shifted the dim light melatonin onset earlier and that evening light treatment shifted it later, which correlated with the mood improvement they found after morning light treatment and the lack of improvement after evening light treatment (Lewy et al. 1987). These observations were the basis of this group's "phase shift hypothesis" (Lewy et al. 1988), according to which the symptoms of SAD were due to phase-delayed circadian rhythms, and the beneficial effects of light were due to restoration of these rhythms to their normal phase position.

The part of the phase response theory that is best substantiated in the literature is, as we noted earlier, that the morning hours are generally the best time for light therapy. However, morning light therapy may be best because the eyes are in general more sensitive in the early morning hours.

Other aspects of the phase shift hypothesis are less well founded. First, contrary to Lewy's findings, most subsequent studies have found evening light therapy to be therapeutic (Lee et al. 1997a; M. Terman et al. 1989;

Thompson et al. 1999). Because evening light therapy almost certainly would delay, rather than advance, circadian rhythms, according to our understanding of the human circadian system, this would argue against the phase shift hypothesis.

In various experiments, Lewy et al. (1988) compared dim light melatonin onset measurements in SAD patients and control subjects and, after pooling the results of their studies, found no significant difference overall between groups. They suggested that there may be subgroups of SAD patients, some phase delayed and others phase advanced, which would result in no difference on average between patients and control subjects. Although this may indeed be correct, differences between subjects with regard to dim light melatonin onset may simply reflect the ordinary variability within the population.

The phase shift hypothesis would be supported by evidence that light therapy is efficacious in proportion to its phase-shifting effects. The best example of such evidence comes from the work of J.S. Terman et al. (2001), who found that the degree of efficacy of morning light therapy was directly correlated with the degree to which treatment phase advanced dim light melatonin onset measurements. However, other studies have failed to show a similar correlation between degree of phase shift and response to light (Eastman et al. 1993; Thalen et al. 1995; Thompson et al. 1997).

More recently, Lewy's group conducted a study during the winters of 1999–2002; they administered small doses of melatonin (0.3 mg) to SAD patients at times of day calculated to shift circadian rhythms in a therapeutic direction (Lewy et al. 2003). Melatonin did appear to have an antidepressant effect. Although initial data from the early parts of the study suggested that this effect was in proportion to the degree of phase advance (Lewy et al. 2000), this correlation is less clear from the most recent data (Lewy et al. 2003). It is too early to say whether these studies support the phase shift hypothesis.

The most comprehensive study of melatonin profiles in SAD was conducted by Wehr et al. (2001). These researchers monitored plasma melatonin levels from the afternoon through the night to the following morning in SAD patients and healthy control subjects maintained in conditions of continuous dim light. They found no delay in dim light melatonin onset in SAD patients compared with control subjects. On the contrary, the major circadian difference was seen in the melatonin *offset*, which shifted across seasons, occurring slightly later in SAD patients in winter relative to their summer profiles. This difference was not seen in control subjects (Wehr et al. 2001). These data could be interpreted to support a phase shift (delay) in SAD patients as measured by melatonin *offset* rather than onset. They also could support the melatonin hypothesis of light therapy (i.e., light therapy works best in the morning because it may suppress morning melatonin secretion, which is abnormally extended in SAD patients, thereby correcting the abnormality).

To complicate matters, Wehr et al. (1995) found that human circadian rhythms (including the rhythm of melatonin secretion) appear to be governed by two oscillators, one that tracks dusk and is responsible for timing of evening rhythms (such as onset of melatonin secretion) and one that tracks dawn and is responsible for the timing of late-night rhythms (such as offset of melatonin secretion). If these data are correct, it is less meaningful to talk of phase advance or delay of the circadian system as a whole than of the dawn or dusk oscillator.

In summary, Lewy and his group are still working on the phase shift hypothesis, which continues to be modified according to the results of new experiments.

Seasonal Affective Disorder and Neurotransmitter-Associated Hypotheses

Numerous studies suggest involvement of serotonergic pathways in seasonal rhythms, in the effects of light, and in the pathogenesis of SAD. These include the observations that 1) hypothalamic serotonin levels in postmortem specimens decline to their nadir in winter (Carlsson et al. 1980); 2) turnover of serotonin in the brains of healthy subjects, as measured by jugular venous concentrations, is lowest in winter and correlated with levels of exposure to sunlight on the day of the measurement (Lambert et al. 2002); 3) positron emission tomography data show that SAD patients have a reduced availability of serotonin transporters in the thalamus-hypothalamus compared with control subjects (Willeit et al. 2000); 4) tryptophan depletion, which reduces brain serotonin synthesis, reverses the effects of light therapy (Lam et al. 1996b; Neumeister et al. 1997, 1998a); 5) *m*-chlorophenylpiperazine (m-CPP), a serotonin agonist, produces different behavioral effects in SAD patients than in control subjects (Levitan et al. 1994; Jacobsen et al. 1994; Schwartz et al. 1997); and 6) these effects are normalized in summer and following light therapy (Jacobsen et al. 1994; Joseph-Vanderpool et al. 1993; Schwartz et al. 1997).

Further evidence in support of serotonin's involvement in the pathophysiology of SAD is that serotonergic agents are effective in treating SAD symptoms. Administration of tryptophan has improved symptoms when used as an adjunct to light therapy (Lam et al. 1997) or on its own (Ghadirian et al. 1998; McGrath et al. 1990). Other serotonergic agents, such as *d*-fenfluramine (O'Rourke et al. 1989), metergoline (Turner et al. 2002), and, of most

clinical relevance, sertraline (Moscovitch et al. 2004) and fluoxetine (Lam et al. 1995), also have produced positive results in SAD.

The importance of hypothalamic serotonin transmission in modulating satiety and feeding behaviors also may shed light on the role of this neurotransmitter in SAD. Carbohydrate intake in animals has been shown to raise the brain's production of serotonin by increasing its uptake of tryptophan (Fernstrom and Wurtman 1971). By a complex behavioral-biochemical feedback loop, patients might crave and consume large amounts of carbohydrate-rich foods in an attempt to regulate their brain serotonin transmission (Wurtman 1988). Interestingly, depressed SAD patients become activated by carbohydrate-rich meals, which tend to sedate healthy control subjects (Rosenthal et al. 1989). Carbohydrate intake decreases in summer or after light therapy (Krauchi et al. 1990; Rosenthal et al. 1987). A history of increased carbohydrate intake is a good predictor of response to light therapy (Krauchi et al. 1993). Relative to control subjects, SAD patients appear to have a higher sweet taste threshold in the winter than in the summer (Arbisi et al. 1996). Thus, SAD symptoms, carbohydrate craving, and serotonergic transmission appear to be connected in some meaningful way.

Neumeister et al. (1998b), however, found that light therapy does not exert its beneficial effects exclusively via serotonergic pathways. Noradrenergic pathways also appear to be involved. In a crossover study, these researchers compared the effects of tryptophan depletion, which lowers brain serotonin transmission, with α-methyl-*p*-tyrosine, which lowers brain catecholamine transmission. They found that both techniques reversed the effects of light therapy to a similar degree.

Further evidence for the role of norepinephrine in SAD comes from an open trial of the norepinephrine reuptake inhibitor reboxetine. Over 6 weeks of treatment, 11 of 16 SAD patients (69%) reported improvement in symptoms, with 9 of the 11 responding within the first week (Hilger et al. 2001). Baseline plasma levels of norepinephrine (but not cerebrospinal fluid levels of norepinephrine metabolites) have been inversely correlated with level of depression in SAD patients (Rudorfer et al. 1993; Skwerer et al. 1988).

Depue and others (1989) have suggested that SAD patients may have abnormalities in brain dopamine transmission, which may be responsible for their deficits in behavioral engagement (Krauss et al. 1992). Consistent with this theory are findings of abnormal eye blink rates (Depue et al. 1988), serum prolactin levels (Depue et al. 1990; Oren et al. 1996), and thermoregulatory responses in SAD patients (Arbisi et al. 1989, 1994) because all of these functions are mediated, at least in part, by dopamine. Some evidence indicates that light therapy might reverse these abnormalities (Arbisi et al. 1989; Depue et al. 1988).

Perhaps the best piece of evidence supporting the role of dopaminergic pathways in the pathophysiology of SAD is the ability of bupropion, a dopaminergic (and noradrenergic) agent, to prevent the onset of winter depression (Rosenthal et al. 2003). Finally, a brain imaging study that used single photon emission computed tomography found that 11 SAD patients had reduced availability of striatal dopamine transporter binding sites when depressed in winter, compared with 11 healthy age- and gender-matched control subjects (Neumeister et al. 2001).

Seasonal Affective Disorder and the Eyes

What makes only some people susceptible to the declining light levels that occur in autumn and winter? One possibility is that these vulnerable individuals somehow may not process environmental light normally. As Wehr and colleagues (1987b) have shown, the antidepressant effects of light are probably mediated via the eyes rather than the skin. In addition, photoperiodically mediated seasonal rhythms in animals are regulated through the eyes rather than the skin. For these reasons, it is logical to explore the possibility that a clue to the origins of SAD may reside, at least for some people, in the eyes themselves. This theory is supported by the report on plasma melatonin profiles in SAD patients and control subjects mentioned earlier (see section "Circadian Rhythms, Seasonal Affective Disorder, and Light Therapy"); SAD patients show seasonal changes in melatonin profiles, whereas control subjects do not. One explanation for this difference is that ordinary indoor lighting may be biologically active for healthy control subjects but not for SAD patients, whose eyes may be subsensitive in certain respects. If SAD patients are unable to perceive light normally, what is the nature of the abnormality? That question has been addressed by several researchers.

The most interesting data come from electroretinography (ERG) studies. This test measures electrical potential generated by the retina in response to light stimuli. Lam and colleagues (1992) exposed dark-adapted SAD patients and control subjects to a single intensity of light to elicit a mixed rod and cone response. They found that the female, but not the male, SAD patients were subsensitive to these stimuli. In two separate ERG studies that used lower intensities of light to target rods specifically, Hébert and colleagues also found that patients with SAD (Hébert et al. 2004) and subsyndromal SAD (Hébert et al. 2002) were subsensitive to visual stimuli, an abnormality that was corrected in the latter study during the summer.

Hébert et al. pointed out that these abnormalities may reflect an excess of dopamine in the retina because dopamine suppresses the sensitivity of rods.

An excess of dopamine in the retina may explain another eye-related finding in SAD. J.S. Terman and Terman (1999) measured dark adaptation in patients and control subjects and found that SAD patients had *increased* sensitivity to light in the portion of the curve that reflects cone functioning. In contrast to its effects on the rods, retinal dopamine facilitates cone sensitivity.

Genetics Findings in Seasonal Affective Disorder

Family history studies suggest that SAD may be familial (Lam et al. 1989), and many patients report SAD in their family members. These latter observations are, of course, crude. More sophisticated studies of seasonality have been performed with heritability models in twin populations and have found significant heritability (Jang et al. 1997; Madden et al. 1996).

More recently, researchers have turned their attention to a search for candidate genes, particularly those involving the serotonin system, in SAD patients. One promising candidate has been the serotonin transporter-linked promoter region (5-HTTLPR) polymorphism, in which one version, the short S allele, appears to be more common than the long L version in patients with neuroticism and depression than in the normal population (Collier et al. 1996). In a pooled analysis of 464 patients and 414 control subjects from different studies, no association could be established between SAD patients and the S allele (Johansson et al. 2003). More consistent in the literature is an association between higher seasonality in the general population, as assessed by the GSS, and either the S allele (Sher et al. 2000) or the S/S phenotype (Johansson et al. 2003). A few other studies have been done to investigate associations between SAD and serotonin genetic variation, with mixed results.

Other Psychobiological Areas of Interest in Seasonal Affective Disorder

As with other forms of mood disorder, researchers have investigated neuroendocrine systems in SAD, particularly the hypothalamic-pituitary-adrenal (HPA) axis and thyroid functioning. No evidence to date indicates that overactivity of the HPA axis occurs in SAD, as has been described in nonseasonal depression, particularly of the melancholic type (Rubin 1989). However, abnormal hormonal responses (e.g., for corticotropin, cortisol, or prolactin) have been documented in SAD patients in response to infusions of both corticotropin (Joseph-Vanderpool et al. 1991) and various neurotransmitter agonists (Garcia-Borreguero et al. 1995; Schwartz et al. 1997). HPA axis responses to m-CPP are inconsistent and cannot be woven into a simple theory at this time.

All studies of thyroid function in SAD are limited to those subjects who are prescreened for relatively normal thyroid function. Nevertheless, Sher et al. (1999) did find slightly but significantly lower thyroxine levels in SAD patients compared with control subjects. Coiro et al. (1994) found that peak thyrotropin response to thyrotropin-releasing hormone was lower in SAD patients in both winter and summer. Light therapy suppressed thyrotropin secretion in one study (Skwerer et al. 1988) and thyrotropin-releasing hormone secretion in another (Oren et al. 1996). In summary, reduced thyroid functioning is suggested in SAD, although the findings probably have been minimized by criteria for patient selection.

Various electroencephalogram changes have been observed in sleep architecture in patients with SAD before and after light therapy. The NIMH group reported that SAD patients showed the following: 1) increased sleep length and decreased delta sleep (Anderson et al. 1994; Rosenthal et al. 1984; Skwerer et al. 1988); 2) normal rapid eye movement (REM) sleep latency (Anderson et al. 1994; Skwerer et al. 1988); and 3) increased REM sleep density (both summer and winter), REM sleep time, and REM sleep percentage (Skwerer et al. 1988). Light therapy appears to normalize some of these sleep changes in SAD patients.

Several neuroimaging studies in SAD patients and control subjects have been performed to date, which have resulted in diverse findings. At present, it is difficult to tie all these findings together into a coherent story. For a more complete picture of neuroimaging in SAD, the interested reader is referred elsewhere (Vasile et al. 1997).

Conclusion

In the two decades since SAD in its pure form was first described, it has emerged more and more clearly as a condition with a specific clinical profile, course, treatment response pattern, and psychobiology. Nevertheless, it also shares both clinical and biological features with nonseasonal depression. Some have suggested that patients with SAD may have two separate vulnerabilities, one for depression and one for seasonality (Lam et al. 2001).

Seasonality also can be seen in the population as a whole and appears to be heritable to a significant degree. In clinical practice, seasonality can be seen cutting across

other syndromes. In these instances, it might be worth using light therapy, which may be beneficial, for example, in bulimic patients (Lam et al. 1994). Although the research criteria for SAD are strictly followed to obtain homogeneous populations, clinicians should not feel constrained to the same degree; otherwise, they may risk missing the opportunity to help patients with more mixed clinical pictures. Indeed, the value of light therapy may extend well beyond the confines of SAD. According to a recent meta-analysis, light therapy may even benefit patients with nonseasonal depressions (Golden et al. 2005).

Rapid advances in genetics, neuroimaging, and other technological areas can be expected to further our understanding of SAD and its treatment. In the meantime, the informed clinician can do a great deal to help SAD patients feel well all year long.

References

Altamura C, VanGastel A, Pioli R, et al: Seasonal and circadian rhythms in suicide in Cagliari, Italy. J Affect Disord 53:77–85, 1999

American Psychiatric Association: Diagnostic and Statistical Manual of Mental Disorders, 3rd Edition, Revised. Washington, DC, American Psychiatric Association, 1987

American Psychiatric Association: Diagnostic and Statistical Manual of Mental Disorders, 4th Edition. Washington, DC, American Psychiatric Association, 1994

American Psychiatric Association: Diagnostic and Statistical Manual of Mental Disorders, 4th Edition, Text Revision. Washington, DC, American Psychiatric Association, 2000

Anderson JL, Rosen LN, Mendelson WB, et al: Sleep in fall/winter seasonal affective disorder: effects of light and changing seasons. J Psychosom Res 38:323–337, 1994

Arbisi PA, Depue RA, Spoont MR, et al: Thermoregulatory response to thermal challenge in seasonal affective disorder: a preliminary report. Psychiatry Res 28:323–334, 1989

Arbisi PA, Depue RA, Krauss S, et al: Heat-loss response to a thermal challenge in seasonal affective disorder. Psychiatry Res 52:199–214, 1994

Arbisi PA, Levine AS, Nerenberg J, et al: Seasonal alteration in taste detection and recognition threshold in seasonal affective disorder: the proximate source of carbohydrate craving. Psychiatry Res 59:171–182, 1996

Avery D, Bolte MA, Millet M: Bright dawn simulation compared with bright morning light in the treatment of winter depression. Acta Psychiatr Scand 85:430–434, 1992

Avery DH, Bolte MA, Dager SR, et al: Dawn simulation treatment of winter depression: a controlled study. Am J Psychiatry 150:113–117, 1993

Avery DH, Bolte MA, Wolfson K, et al: Dawn simulation compared with a dim red signal in the treatment of winter depression. Biol Psychiatry 36:180–188, 1994

Avery DH, Eder DN, Bolte MA, et al: Dawn simulation and bright light in the treatment of SAD: a controlled study. Biol Psychiatry 50:205–216, 2001

Avery DH, Kouri ME, Monaghan K, et al: Is dawn simulation effective in ameliorating the difficulty awakening in seasonal affective disorder associated with hypersomnia? J Affect Disord 69:231–236, 2002

Bauer MS, Kurtz JW, Rubin LB, et al: Mood and behavioral effects of four-week light treatment in winter depressives and controls. J Psychiatr Res 28:135–145, 1994

Berman K, Lam RW, Goldner EM: Eating attitudes in seasonal affective disorder and bulimia nervosa. J Affect Disord 29:219–225, 1993

Blazer DG, Kessler RC, Swartz MS: Epidemiology of recurrent major and minor depression with a seasonal pattern: the National Comorbidity Survey. Br J Psychiatry 172:164–167, 1998

Blouin A, Blouin J, Aubin P, et al: Seasonal patterns of bulimia nervosa. Am J Psychiatry 149:73–81, 1992

Booker JM, Hellekson CJ: Prevalence of seasonal affective disorder in Alaska. Am J Psychiatry 149:1176–1182, 1992

Boyce P, Parker G: Seasonal affective disorder in the southern hemisphere. Am J Psychiatry 145:96–99, 1988

Brewerton TD, Krahn DD, Hardin TA, et al: Findings from the Seasonal Pattern Assessment Questionnaire in patients with eating disorders and control subjects: effects of diagnosis and location. Psychiatry Res 52:71–84, 1994

Cameron I: Antarctica: The Last Continent. Boston, MA, Little, Brown, 1974

Carlsson A, Svennerholm L, Winblad B: Seasonal and circadian monoamine variations in human brains examined post mortem. Acta Psychiatr Scand Suppl 280:75–85, 1980

Coiro V, Volpi R, Marchesi C, et al: Lack of seasonal variation in abnormal TSH secretion in patients with seasonal affective disorder. Biol Psychiatry 35:36–41, 1994

Collier DA, Stober G, Li T, et al: A novel functional polymorphism within the promoter of the serotonin transporter gene: possible role in susceptibility to affective disorders. Mol Psychiatry 1:453–460, 1996

Cone RD, Low MJ, Elmquist JK, et al: Neuroendocrinology, in Williams Textbook of Endocrinology, 10th Edition. Edited by Larsen PR, Kronenberg HM, Melmed S, et al. Philadelphia, PA, WB Saunders, 2003, pp 81–176

Depue RA, Iacono WG, Muir R, et al: Effect of phototherapy on spontaneous eye blink rate in subjects with seasonal affective disorder. Am J Psychiatry 145:1457–1459, 1988

Depue RA, Arbisi P, Spoont MR, et al: Dopamine functioning in the behavioral facilitation system and seasonal variation in behavior: normal population and clinical studies, in Seasonal Affective Disorders and Phototherapy. Edited by Rosenthal NE, Blehar MC. New York, Guilford, 1989, pp 230–259

Depue RA, Arbisi P, Krauss S, et al: Seasonal independence of low prolactin concentration and high spontaneous eye blink rates in unipolar and bipolar II seasonal affective disorder. Arch Gen Psychiatry 47:356–364, 1990

Dilsaver SC, Jaeckle RS: Winter depression responds to an open trial of tranylcypromine. J Clin Psychiatry 51:326–329, 1990

Durkheim E: Suicide: A Study in Sociology. New York, Free Press, 1951

Eagles JM, Naji SA, Gray DA, et al: Seasonal affective disorder among primary care consulters in January: prevalence and month by month consultation patterns. J Affect Disord 49:1–8, 1998

Eagles JM, Wileman SM, Cameron IM, et al: Seasonal affective disorder among primary care attenders and a community sample in Aberdeen. Br J Psychiatry 175:472–475, 1999

Eagles JM, Howie FL, Cameron IM, et al: Use of health care services in seasonal affective disorder. Br J Psychiatry 180:449–454, 2002

Eastman CI, Gallo LC, Lahmeyer HW, et al: The circadian rhythm of temperature during light treatment for winter depression. Biol Psychiatry 34:210–220, 1993

Eastman CI, Young MA, Fogg LF, et al: Bright light treatment of winter depression: a placebo-controlled trial. Arch Gen Psychiatry 55:883–889, 1998

Faedda GL, Tondo L, Teicher MH, et al: Seasonal mood disorders: patterns of seasonal recurrence in mania and depression. Arch Gen Psychiatry 50:17–23, 1993

Fernstrom JD, Wurtman RJ: Brain serotonin content: increase following ingestion of carbohydrate diet. Science 174:1023–1025, 1971

Gaedeken P: Über die psychophysiologische Bedeutung der atmosphärischen Verhaltnisse, insbesondere des Lichts. Zeitschrift für Psychotherapie III:129, 1911

Gallin PF, Terman M, Reme CE, et al: Ophthalmologic examination of patients with seasonal affective disorder, before and after bright light therapy. Am J Ophthalmol 199:202–210, 1995

Garcia-Borreguero D, Jacobsen FM, Murphy DL, et al: Hormonal responses to the administration of m-chlorophenylpiperazine in patients with seasonal affective disorder and controls. Biol Psychiatry 37:740–749, 1995

Garvey MJ, Wesner R, Goes M: Comparison of seasonal and nonseasonal affective disorders. Am J Psychiatry 145:100–102, 1988

Ghadirian AM, Murphy BE, Gendron MJ: Efficacy of light versus tryptophan therapy in seasonal affective disorder. J Affect Disord 50:23–27, 1998

Gloth FM 3rd, Alam W, Hollis B: Vitamin D vs broad spectrum phototherapy in the treatment of seasonal affective disorder. J Nutr Health Aging 3:5–7, 1999

Golden RN, Gaynes BN, Ekstrom RD, et al: The efficacy of light therapy in the treatment of mood disorders: a review and meta-analysis of the evidence. Am J Psychiatry 162:656–662, 2005

Han L, Wang K, Du Z, et al: Seasonal variations in mood and behavior among Chinese medical students. Am J Psychiatry 157:133–135, 2000

Hardin TA, Wehr TA, Brewerton T, et al: Evaluation of seasonality in six clinical populations and two normal populations. J Psychiatr Res 25:75–87, 1991

Hébert M, Dumont M, Lachapelle P: Electrophysiological evidence suggesting a seasonal modulation of retinal sensitivity in subsyndromal winter depression. J Affect Disord 68:191–202, 2002

Hébert M, Beattie CW, Tam EM, et al: Electroretinography in patients with winter seasonal affective disorder. Psychiatry Res 127:27–34, 2004

Hegde AL, Woodson H: Prevalence of seasonal changes in mood and behavior during the winter months in central Texas. Psychiatry Res 62:265–271, 1996

Hilger E, Willeit M, Praschak-Rieder N, et al: Reboxetine in seasonal affective disorder: an open trial. Eur Neuropsychopharmacol 11:1–5, 2001

Hippocrates: Works of Hippocrates. Cambridge, MA, Harvard University Press, 1923–1931

Hoffman K: Photoperiodism in vertebrates, in Handbook of Behavioral Neurobiology, Vol 4: Biological Rhythms. Edited by Aschoff J. New York, Plenum, 1981, pp 449–473

Immelman K: Role of the environment in reproduction as source of "predictive" information, in Breeding Biology of Birds. Edited by Farner DS. Washington, DC, National Academy of Sciences, 1973, pp 121–147

Jacobsen FM, Mueller EA, Rosenthal NE, et al: Behavioral responses to intravenous meta-chlorophenylpiperazine in patients with seasonal affective disorder and control subjects before and after phototherapy. Psychiatry Res 52:181–197, 1994

Jang KL, Lam RW, Livesley WJ, et al: Gender differences in the heritability of seasonal mood change. Psychiatry Res 70:145–154, 1997

Joffe RT, Moul DE, Lam RW, et al: Light visor treatment for seasonal affective disorder: a multicenter study. Psychiatry Res 46:29–39, 1993

Johansson C, Willeit M, Levitan R, et al: The serotonin transporter promoter repeat length polymorphism, seasonal affective disorder and seasonality. Psychol Med 33:785–792, 2003

Joseph-Vanderpool JR, Rosenthal NE, Chrousos GP, et al: Abnormal pituitary-adrenal responses to corticotropin-releasing hormone in patients with seasonal affective disorder: clinical and pathophysiological implications. J Clin Endocrinol Metab 72:1382–1387, 1991

Joseph-Vanderpool JR, Jacobsen FM, Murphy DL, et al: Seasonal variation in behavioral responses to m-CPP in patients with seasonal affective disorder and controls. Biol Psychiatry 33:496–504, 1993

Kasper S, Kamo T: Seasonality in major depressed inpatients. J Affect Disord 19:243–248, 1990

Kasper S, Wehr TA, Bartko JJ, et al: Epidemiological findings of seasonal changes in mood and behavior: a telephone survey of Montgomery County, Maryland. Arch Gen Psychiatry 46:823–833, 1989

Kogan AO, Guilford PM: Side effects of short-term 10,000-lux light therapy. Am J Psychiatry 155:293–294, 1998

Krauchi K, Wirz-Justice A, Graw P, et al: The relationship of affective state to dietary preference: winter depression and light therapy as a model. J Affect Disord 20:43–53, 1990

Krauchi K, Wirz-Justice A, Graw P: High intake of sweets late in the day predicts a rapid and persistent response to light therapy in winter depression. Psychiatry Res 46:107–117, 1993

Krauss SS, Depue RA, Arbisi PA, et al: Behavioral engagement level, variability, and diurnal rhythm as a function of bright light in bipolar II seasonal affective disorder: an exploratory study. Psychiatry Res 43:147–160, 1992

Labbate LA, Lafer B, Thibault A, et al: Side effects induced by bright light treatment for seasonal affective disorder. J Clin Psychiatry 55:189–191, 1994

Labbate LA, Lafer B, Thibault A, et al: Influence of phototherapy treatment duration for seasonal affective disorder: outcome at one vs. two weeks. Biol Psychiatry 38:747–750, 1995

Lam RW (ed): Seasonal Affective Disorder and Beyond: Light Treatment of SAD and Non-SAD Conditions. Washington, DC, American Psychiatric Press, 1998

Lam RW, Buchanan A, Remick RA: Seasonal affective disorder: a Canadian sample. Ann Clin Psychiatry 1:241–245, 1989

Lam RW, Beattie CW, Buchanan A, et al: Electroretinography in seasonal affective disorder. Psychiatry Res 43:55–63, 1992

Lam RW, Goldner EM, Solyom L, et al: A controlled study of light therapy for bulimia nervosa. Am J Psychiatry 151:744–750, 1994

Lam RW, Gorman CP, Michalon M, et al: Multicenter, placebo-controlled study of fluoxetine in seasonal affective disorder. Am J Psychiatry 152:1765–1770, 1995

Lam RW, Goldner EM, Grewal A: Seasonality of symptoms in anorexia and bulimia nervosa. Int J Eat Disord 19:35–44, 1996a

Lam RW, Zis AP, Grewal A, et al: Effects of rapid tryptophan depletion in patients with seasonal affective disorder in remission after light therapy. Arch Gen Psychiatry 53:41–44, 1996b

Lam RW, Levitan RD, Tam EM, et al: L-tryptophan augmentation of light therapy in patients with seasonal affective disorder. Can J Psychiatry 42:303–306, 1997

Lam RW, Tam EM, Yatham LN, et al: Seasonal depression: the dual vulnerability hypothesis revisited. J Affect Disord 63:123–132, 2001

Lambert GW, Reid C, Kaye DM, et al: Effect of sunlight and season on serotonin turnover in the brain. Lancet 360(9348):1840–1842, 2002

Lee TM, Chan CC: Dose-response relationship of phototherapy for seasonal affective disorder: a meta-analysis. Acta Psychiatr Scand 99:315–323, 1999

Lee TM, Blashko CA, Janzen HL, et al: Pathophysiological mechanism of seasonal affective disorder. J Affect Disord 46:25–38, 1997a

Lee TM, Chan CC, Paterson JG, et al: Spectral properties of phototherapy for seasonal affective disorder: a meta-analysis. Acta Psychiatr Scand 96:117–121, 1997b

Leppamaki S, Partonen T, Lonnqvist J: Bright-light exposure combined with physical exercise elevates mood. J Affect Disord 72:139–144, 2002

Levitan RD, Kaplan AS, Levitt AJ, et al: Seasonal fluctuations in mood and eating behavior in bulimia nervosa. Int J Eat Disord 16:295–299, 1994

Levitan RD, Jain UR, Katzman MA: Seasonal affective symptoms in adults with residual attention-deficit hyperactivity disorder. Compr Psychiatry 40:261–267, 1999

Levitt AJ, Joffe RT, Brecher D, et al: Anxiety disorders and anxiety symptoms in a clinic sample of seasonal and nonseasonal depressives. J Affect Disord 28:51–56, 1993

Levitt AJ, Boyle MH, Joffe RT, et al: Estimated prevalence of the seasonal subtype of major depression in a Canadian community sample. Can J Psychiatry 45:650–654, 2000

Lewy AJ, Wehr TA, Goodwin FK, et al: Light suppresses melatonin secretion in humans. Science 210(4475):1267–1269, 1980

Lewy AJ, Kern HA, Rosenthal NE, et al: Bright artificial light treatment of a manic-depressive patient with a seasonal mood cycle. Am J Psychiatry 139:1496–1498, 1982

Lewy AJ, Sack RA, Singer CL: Assessment and treatment of chronobiologic disorders using plasma melatonin levels and bright light exposure: the clock-gate model and the phase response curve. Psychopharmacol Bull 20:561–565, 1984

Lewy AJ, Sack RL, Singer CM: Immediate and delayed effects of bright light on human melatonin production: shifting "dawn" and "dusk" shifts the dim light melatonin onset (DLMO). Ann N Y Acad Sci 453:253–259, 1985

Lewy AJ, Sack RL, Miller RS, et al: Antidepressant and circadian phase-shifting effects of light. Science 235:352–354, 1987

Lewy AJ, Sack RL, Singer CM, et al: Winter depression and the phase-shift hypothesis for bright light's therapeutic effects: history, theory, and experimental evidence. J Biol Rhythms 3:121–134, 1988

Lewy AJ, Bauer VK, Bish HA, et al: Antidepressant response correlates with the phase advance in winter depression. Abstracts of the 12th Annual Meeting, Evanston, IL, May 2000. San Francisco, CA, Society for Light Treatment and Biological Rhythms, 2000, p 22

Lewy AJ, Lefler BJ, Hasler BP, et al: Plasma DLMO10 zeitgeber time 14: the therapeutic window for phase-delayed winter depressives treated with melatonin. Chronobiol Int 20:1215–1217, 2003

Lingjaerde O, Foreland AR, Dankertsen J: Dawn simulation vs. lightbox treatment in winter depression: a comparative study. Acta Psychiatr Scand 98:73–80, 1998

Madden PA, Heath AC, Rosenthal NE, et al: Seasonal changes in mood and behavior: the role of genetic factors. Arch Gen Psychiatry 53:47–55, 1996

Magnusson A, Axelsson J: The prevalence of seasonal affective disorder is low among descendants of Icelandic emigrants in Canada. Arch Gen Psychiatry 50:947–951, 1993

Magnusson A, Stefansson JG: Prevalence of seasonal affective disorder in Iceland. Arch Gen Psychiatry 50:941–946, 1993

Magnusson A, Friis S, Opjordsmoen S: Internal consistency of the Seasonal Pattern Assessment Questionnaire (SPAQ). J Affect Disord 42:113–116, 1997

Marx H: "Hypophysäre Insuffizienz" bei Lichtmangel. Klin Wochenschr 24/25:18–21, 1946

McGrath RE, Buckwald B, Resnick EV: The effect of L-tryptophan on seasonal affective disorder. J Clin Psychiatry 51:162–163, 1990

Meesters Y, Beersma DG, Bouhuys AL, et al: Prophylactic treatment of seasonal affective disorder (SAD) by using light visors: bright white or infrared light? Biol Psychiatry 46:239–246, 1999

Mersch PP, Middendorp HM, Bouhuys AL, et al: The prevalence of seasonal affective disorder in The Netherlands: a prospective and retrospective study of seasonal mood variation in the general population. Biol Psychiatry 45:1013–1022, 1999

Moore RY: Neural control of pineal function in mammals and birds. J Neural Transm Suppl 13:47–58, 1978

Morrissey SA, Raggatt PT, James B, et al: Seasonal affective disorder: some epidemiological findings from a tropical climate. Aust N Z J Psychiatry 30:579–586, 1996

Morselli E: Suicide: An Essay on Comparative Statistics. London, Kegan Paul, 1881

Moscovitch A, Blashko CA, Eagles JM, et al: A placebo-controlled study of sertraline in the treatment of outpatients with seasonal affective disorder. Psychopharmacology (Berl) 171:390–397, 2004

Neumeister A, Praschak-Rieder N, Hesselmann B, et al: Effects of tryptophan depletion on drug-free patients with seasonal affective disorder during a stable response to bright light therapy. Arch Gen Psychiatry 54:133–138, 1997

Neumeister A, Praschak-Rieder N, Hesselmann B, et al: Effects of tryptophan depletion in fully remitted patients with seasonal affective disorder during summer. Psychol Med 28:257–264, 1998a

Neumeister A, Turner EH, Matthews JR, et al: Effects of tryptophan depletion vs catecholamine depletion in patients with seasonal affective disorder in remission with light therapy. Arch Gen Psychiatry 55:524–530, 1998b

Neumeister A, Willeit M, Praschak-Rieder N, et al: Dopamine transporter availability in symptomatic depressed patients with seasonal affective disorder and healthy controls. Psychol Med 31:1467–1473, 2001

O'Rourke D, Wurtman JJ, Wurtman RJ, et al: Treatment of seasonal depression with d-fenfluramine. J Clin Psychiatry 50:343–347, 1989

Oren DA, Rosenthal NE: Seasonal affective disorders, in Handbook of Affective Disorders. Edited by Paykel ES. New York, Guilford, 1992, pp 551–567

Oren DA, Rosenthal FS, Rosenthal NE, et al: Exposure to ultraviolet B radiation during phototherapy. Am J Psychiatry 147:675–676, 1990

Oren DA, Brainard GC, Johnston SH, et al: Treatment of seasonal affective disorder with green light and red light. Am J Psychiatry 148:509–511, 1991

Oren DA, Jacobsen FM, Wehr TA, et al: Predictors of response to phototherapy in seasonal affective disorder. Compr Psychiatry 33:111–114, 1992

Oren DA, Levendosky AA, Kasper S, et al: Circadian profiles of cortisol, prolactin, and thyrotropin in seasonal affective disorder. Biol Psychiatry 39:157–170, 1996

Partonen T, Magnusson A (eds): Seasonal Affective Disorder: Practice and Research. New York, Oxford University Press, 2001

Partonen T, Leppamaki S, Hurme J, et al: Randomized trial of physical exercise alone or combined with bright light on mood and health-related quality of life. Psychol Med 28:1359–1364, 1998

Pendse BP, Ojehagen A, Engstrom G, et al: Social characteristics of seasonal affective disorder patients: comparison with suicide attempters with non-seasonal major depression and other mood disorder patients. Eur Psychiatry 18:36–39, 2003

Praschak-Rieder N, Willeit M, Neumeister A, et al: Prevalence of premenstrual dysphoric disorder in female patients with seasonal affective disorder. J Affect Disord 63:239–242, 2001

Raheja SK, King EA, Thompson C: The Seasonal Pattern Assessment Questionnaire for identifying seasonal affective disorders. J Affect Disord 41:193–199, 1996

Reichborn-Kjennerud T, Lingjaerde O, Dahl AA: Personality disorders in patients with winter depression. Acta Psychiatr Scand 90:413–419, 1994

Reichborn-Kjennerud T, Lingjaerde O, Dahl AA: DSM-III-R personality disorders in seasonal affective disorder: change associated with depression. Compr Psychiatry 38:43–48, 1997

Rohan KJ, Tierney Lindsey K, Roecklein KA, et al: Cognitive-Behavioral and Light Treatments for Seasonal Affective Disorder: Interim Analyses From a Controlled Randomized Clinical Trial. Bethesda, MD, Uniformed Services University of the Health Sciences, 2003

Rosen LN, Targum SD, Terman M, et al: Prevalence of seasonal affective disorder at four latitudes. Psychiatry Res 31:131–144, 1990

Rosenthal NE, Sack DA, Wehr TA: Seasonal variation in affective disorders, in Circadian Rhythms in Psychiatry. Edited by Wehr TA, Goodwin FK. Pacific Grove, CA, Boxwood Press, 1983, pp 185–201

Rosenthal NE, Sack DA, Gillin JC, et al: Seasonal affective disorder: a description of the syndrome and preliminary findings with light therapy. Arch Gen Psychiatry 41:72–80, 1984

Rosenthal NE, Carpenter CJ, James SP, et al: Seasonal affective disorder in children and adolescents. Am J Psychiatry 143:356–358, 1986

Rosenthal NE, Genhart M, Jacobsen FM, et al: Disturbances of appetite and weight regulation in seasonal affective disorder. Ann N Y Acad Sci 499:216–230, 1987

Rosenthal NE, Jacobsen FM, Sack DA, et al: Atenolol in seasonal affective disorder: a test of the melatonin hypothesis. Am J Psychiatry 145:52–56, 1988a

Rosenthal NE, Sack DA, Skwerer RG, et al: Phototherapy for seasonal affective disorder. J Biol Rhythms 3:101–120, 1988b

Rosenthal NE, Genhart MJ, Caballero B, et al: Psychobiological effects of carbohydrate- and protein-rich meals in patients with seasonal affective disorder and normal controls. Biol Psychiatry 25:1029–1040, 1989

Rosenthal NE, Moul DE, Hellekson CJ, et al: A multicenter study of the light visor for seasonal affective disorder: no difference in efficacy found between two different intensities. Neuropsychopharmacology 8:151–160, 1993a

Rosenthal NE, Sack DA, Wehr TA: Winter Blues. New York, Guilford, 1993b

Rosenthal NE, Modell JG, Harriett A, et al: Wellbutrin XL for the prevention of seasonal depressive episodes. Paper presented at the 42nd meeting of the American College of Neuropsychopharmacology, San Juan, Puerto Rico, December 2003

Rubin RT: Pharmacoendocrinology of major depression. Eur Arch Psychiatry Neurol Sci 238:259–267, 1989

Rudorfer MV, Skwerer RG, Rosenthal NE: Biogenic amines in seasonal affective disorder: effects of light therapy. Psychiatry Res 46:19–28, 1993

Ruhrmann S, Kasper S, Hawellek B, et al: Effects of fluoxetine versus bright light in the treatment of seasonal affective disorder. Psychol Med 28:923–933, 1998

Saarijarvi S, Lauerma H, Helenius H, et al: Seasonal affective disorders among rural Finns and Lapps. Acta Psychiatr Scand 99:95–101, 1999

Schlager DS: Early morning administration of short-acting beta blockers for treatment of winter depression. Am J Psychiatry 151:1383–1385, 1994

Schlager D, Froom J, Jaffe A: Winter depression and functional impairment among ambulatory primary care patients. Compr Psychiatry 36:18–24, 1995

Schlager D, Norman C, Brown G: Early-morning short-acting beta-adrenergic blockers for treatment of winter depression: a replication. Abstracts of the 8th Annual Meeting, Bethesda, MD, June 1996. San Francisco, CA, Society for Light Treatment and Biological Rhythms, 1996, p 15

Schwartz PJ, Brown C, Wehr TA, et al: Winter seasonal affective disorder: a follow-up study of the first 59 patients of the National Institute of Mental Health Seasonal Studies Program. Am J Psychiatry 153:1028–1036, 1996

Schwartz PJ, Murphy DL, Wehr TA, et al: Effects of meta-chlorophenylpiperazine infusions in patients with seasonal affective disorder and healthy control subjects: diurnal responses and nocturnal regulatory mechanisms. Arch Gen Psychiatry 54:375–385, 1997

Sher L, Rosenthal NE, Wehr TA: Free thyroxine and thyroid-stimulating hormone levels in patients with seasonal affective disorder and matched controls. J Affect Disord 56:195–199, 1999

Sher L, Greenberg BD, Murphy DL, et al: Pleiotropy of the serotonin transporter gene for seasonality and neuroticism. Psychiatr Genet 10:125–130, 2000

Skwerer RG, Jacobsen FM, Duncan CC, et al: Neurobiology of seasonal affective disorder and phototherapy. J Biol Rhythms 3:135–154, 1988

Sourander A, Koskelainen M, Helenius H: Mood, latitude, and seasonality among adolescents. J Am Acad Child Adolesc Psychiatry 38:1271–1276, 1999

Spitzer RL, Endicott J, Robins E: Research Diagnostic Criteria: rationale and reliability. Arch Gen Psychiatry 35:773–782, 1978

Srivastava S, Sharma M: Seasonal affective disorder: report from India (latitude 26 degrees 45′N). J Affect Disord 49:145–150, 1998

Stewart KT, Gaddy JR, Benson DM, et al: Treatment of winter depression with a portable, head-mounted phototherapy device. Prog Neuropsychopharmacol Biol Psychiatry 14:569–578, 1990

Swedo SE, Pleeter JD, Richter DM, et al: Rates of seasonal affective disorder in children and adolescents. Am J Psychiatry 152:1016–1019, 1995

Tamarkin L, Baird CJ, Almeida OF: Melatonin: a coordinating signal for mammalian reproduction? Science 227(4688): 714–720, 1985

Teicher MH, Glod CA, Oren DA, et al: The phototherapy light visor: more to it than meets the eye. Am J Psychiatry 152:1197–1202, 1995

Terman JS, Terman M: Photopic and scotopic light detection in patients with seasonal affective disorder and control subjects. Biol Psychiatry 46:1642–1648, 1999

Terman JS, Terman M, Schlager D, et al: Efficacy of brief, intense light exposure for treatment of winter depression. Psychopharmacol Bull 26:3–11, 1990

Terman JS, Terman M, Lo ES, et al: Circadian time of morning light administration and therapeutic response in winter depression. Arch Gen Psychiatry 58:69–75, 2001

Terman M, Terman JS: Treatment of seasonal affective disorder with a high-output negative ionizer. J Altern Complement Med 1:87–92, 1995

Terman M, Terman JS: Bright light therapy: side effects and benefits across the symptom spectrum. J Clin Psychiatry 60:799–808; quiz 809, 1999

Terman M, Terman JS, Quitkin FM, et al: Light therapy for seasonal affective disorder: a review of efficacy. Neuropsychopharmacology 2:1–22, 1989

Terman M, Amira L, Terman JS, et al: Predictors of response and nonresponse to light treatment for winter depression. Am J Psychiatry 153:1423–1429, 1996

Terman M, Terman JS, Ross DC: A controlled trial of timed bright light and negative air ionization for treatment of winter depression. Arch Gen Psychiatry 55:875–882, 1998

Thalen BE, Kjellman BF, Morkrid L, et al: Melatonin in light treatment of patients with seasonal and nonseasonal depression. Acta Psychiatr Scand 92:274–284, 1995

Thompson C, Childs PA, Martin NJ, et al: Effects of morning phototherapy on circadian markers in seasonal affective disorder. Br J Psychiatry 170:431–435, 1997

Thompson C, Rodin I, Birtwhistle J: Light therapy for seasonal and non-seasonal affective disorder: a Cochrane meta-analysis. Abstracts of the 11th Annual Meeting, Alexandria, VA, May 1999. San Francisco, CA, Society for Light Treatment and Biological Rhythms, 1999, p 11

Turner EH, Schwartz PJ, Lowe CH, et al: Double-blind, placebo-controlled study of single-dose metergoline in depressed patients with seasonal affective disorder. J Clin Psychopharmacol 22:216–220, 2002

Vasile RG, Sachs G, Anderson JL, et al: Changes in regional cerebral blood flow following light treatment for seasonal affective disorder: responders versus nonresponders. Biol Psychiatry 42:1000–1005, 1997

Wehr TA: Seasonal affective disorders: a historical overview, in Seasonal Affective Disorders and Phototherapy. Edited by Rosenthal NE, Blehar MC. New York, Guilford, 1989, pp 11–32

Wehr TA, Jacobsen FM, Sack DA, et al: Phototherapy of seasonal affective disorder: time of day and suppression of melatonin are not critical for antidepressant effects. Arch Gen Psychiatry 43:870–875, 1986

Wehr TA, Sack DA, Rosenthal NE, et al: Seasonal affective disorder with summer depression and winter hypomania. Am J Psychiatry 144:1602–1603, 1987a

Wehr TA, Skwerer RG, Jacobsen FM, et al: Eye versus skin phototherapy of seasonal affective disorder. Am J Psychiatry 144:753–757, 1987b

Wehr TA, Schwartz PJ, Turner EH, et al: Bimodal patterns of human melatonin secretion consistent with a two-oscillator model of regulation. Neurosci Lett 194:105–108, 1995

Wehr TA, Duncan WC Jr, Sher L, et al: A circadian signal of change of season in patients with seasonal affective disorder. Arch Gen Psychiatry 58:1108–1114, 2001

Willeit M, Praschak-Rieder N, Neumeister A, et al: [123I]-Beta-CIT SPECT imaging shows reduced brain serotonin transporter availability in drug-free depressed patients with seasonal affective disorder. Biol Psychiatry 47:482–489, 2000

Williams RJ, Schmidt GG: Frequency of seasonal affective disorder among individuals seeking treatment at a northern Canadian mental health center. Psychiatry Res 46:41–45, 1993

Wirz-Justice A, Graw P, Krauchi K, et al: "Natural" light treatment of seasonal affective disorder. J Affect Disord 37:109–120, 1996

Wurtman RJ: Effects of their nutrient precursors on the synthesis and release of serotonin, the catecholamines, and acetylcholine: implications for behavioral disorders. Clin Neuropharmacol 11 (suppl 1):S187–S193, 1988

Yamatsuji M, Yamashita T, Arii I, et al: Seasonal variations in eating disorder subtypes in Japan. Int J Eat Disord 33:71–77, 2003

Young MA, Watel LG, Lahmeyer HW, et al: The temporal onset of individual symptoms in winter depression: differentiating underlying mechanisms. J Affect Disord 22:191–197, 1991

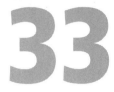

CHAPTER

33

Atypical Depression, Dysthymia, and Cyclothymia

JONATHAN W. STEWART, M.D.

FREDERIC M. QUITKIN, M.D., D.M.Sc.

CARRIE DAVIES, B.S.

THE DSM-IV-TR (American Psychiatric Association 2000) criteria for major depression and mania are arbitrary. Thus, patients with less persistent symptoms or fewer symptoms also have significant morbidity, and the same treatments are as effective as for more severe affective illness. Also, little evidence indicates that the less intense and less severe forms of mood disorder reflect different pathophysiology. The current importance of these forms, rather, lies in the need for clinicians to recognize patients with less symptomatology because their illnesses are treatable, and treatment may lessen such patients' considerable psychosocial disability. In this chapter, we discuss depression with atypical features, dysthymia, and cyclothymia. Depression with atypical features bridges the distinction between major and nonmajor depression and illustrates the artificiality of major and nonmajor distinctions. As with atypical features, true distinctions may cut across the DSM-IV-TR mood categories.

Depression With Atypical Features

DSM-IV-TR Definition

"Atypical features" is a modifier for both major depression and dysthymia. During a depressive episode, there must be distinct reactivity of mood plus at least two of four associated features. In addition, melancholic or catatonic features cannot also be present. The associated features include significant degrees of excessive appetite or increased eating and weight, excessive sleep, leaden paralysis, and a pathological sensitivity to interpersonal rejection. The vegetative associated features must occur on most days during the most recent 2 weeks (for major depression) or the most recent 2 years (for dysthymic disorder) and cannot be attributable to other factors. Leaden paralysis is an intense feeling of heaviness, not just the lack of energy most depressed patients experience, and is to be distinguished from poor motivation. Rejection sensitivity requires a lifelong pattern of functional impairment in response to perceived rejection, not necessarily limited to periods of depressed mood. Evidence of impairment can come from social, vocational, or social spheres and can include excessive missed work, frequent job or romantic partner changes, stormy relationships, and avoidance of jobs and/or relationships. These impairments must be in response to perceived rejection, must not be attributable to other causes (such as physical illness, lack of interest, or partner's moodiness), and must be characteristic.

Epidemiology

Epidemiological studies suggest that 0.7%–4.0% of the general population experience depression with atypical features during their lifetimes. Horwath et al. (1992b) reanalyzed Epidemiologic Catchment Area (ECA) data from five United States communities and reported that 0.7% had major depression with atypical features, or 16% of depressed subjects. These are likely low estimates because Horwath et al. required both overeating and oversleeping, whereas subjects with either or even neither could still meet DSM-IV (American Psychiatric Association 1994) criteria for atypical features. Applying latent class analysis to 14 symptoms of major depression, Kendler et al. (1996) determined that 3.9% of the female twins in the state of Virginia had atypical depression, and Sullivan et al. (1998) reported that 4.0% of the National Comorbidity Survey (NCS) sample had depression with atypical features. Both groups reported that overeating and oversleeping were particularly found in only one (Kendler et al. 1996) or two (Sullivan et al. 1998) of the computer-generated groupings of subjects. Matza et al. (2003) reanalyzed the NCS data and labeled patients who reported both hyperphagia and hypersomnia as having atypical depression, which accounted for 4% of the total and 36% of the depressed sample. Thus, as with Horwath and colleagues' (1992b) presumed low estimate, how representative the Kendler et al. (1996), Sullivan et al. (1998), and Matza et al. (2003) findings are of depression with atypical symptoms is open to question. Only Angst et al. (2002) assessed full DSM-IV criteria for atypical features in an epidemiological sample and reported that among a population-based sample of 19- to 20-year-olds in Zurich, Switzerland, 2.8% developed depression with atypical features during 10-year follow-up.

Prevalence of atypical depression in clinical populations is, of course, more common, ranging from 22% (Posternak and Zimmerman 2002) to 36% (Zisook et al. 1993) of depressed patients presenting for treatment.

Thus, in both general and clinical populations, depression with atypical features appears to be quite common, belying the term *atypical*, which persists on a historical basis.

Demographics

Most studies report the usual 2:1 female-to-male ratio among depressed patients with atypical features (e.g., Asnis et al. 1995; Benazzi 2002; Davidson et al. 1982; Levitan et al. 1997b; Perugi et al. 1998). However, other studies—particularly epidemiological as opposed to clinical studies—do not always support this gender split (e.g., Horwath et al. 1992b). Depressed patients with atypical features are as educated as other depressed patients but less likely to be ever or currently married (Perugi et al. 1998; Stewart et al. 1993). Horwath et al. (1992b) did not find racial/ethnic differences between depressed ECA subjects with and without atypical features.

Comorbid Disorders

The original description by West and Dally (1959) included prominent symptoms of anxiety, and Davidson et al. (1982) posited an anxious subtype. Indeed, increased rates of various anxiety disorders in depressed patients with atypical features have been reported, including panic disorder (Horwath et al. 1992b), social phobia (Alpert et al. 1997; Angst et al. 2002; Perugi et al. 1998), generalized anxiety disorder (Angst et al. 2002), and hypochondriasis or somatization (Horwath et al. 1992b; Posternak and Zimmerman 2002). However, Sullivan et al. (1998) did not find increased anxiety in the NCS sample, and Kendler et al. (1996) found decreased anxiety in depressed twins with atypical features relative to typical depressed subjects. From a practical standpoint, Quitkin et al. (1990) were unable to show that concomitant anxiety affected treatment. Whether comorbidity with anxiety disorders is more than definitional and has implications for making treatment decisions remains to be clarified.

High rates of bipolar disorder have been reported among depressed patients with atypical features (summarized by Angst et al. 2002). Others have not found increased bipolarity in clinical (Stewart et al. 1993) or epidemiological populations (Horwath et al. 1992b; Kendler et al. 1996; Sullivan et al. 1998). Of note is that Perugi et al. (1998), Benazzi (2002), and Angst et al. (2002) used a broad definition of bipolar disorder. Whether depression with atypical features should alert the clinician to the likely presence of bipolar disorder may rest on whether "soft" bipolar features indicate a bipolar diathesis.

The other disorder that is sometimes found to have increased comorbidity with depression with atypical features is drug or alcohol abuse or dependence. Horwath et al. (1992b), for example, found drug abuse to occur more than twice as often in depressed ECA subjects who also had atypical features as in other depressed subjects (29% vs. 12%, P<0.001). Angst et al. (2002), however, did not find differences between atypical and nonatypical depression in substance abuse or dependence in his sample of Zurich young adults, nor did Sullivan et al. (1998) in the NCS sample or Posternak and Zimmerman (2002) in a clinical population. If a connection exists between substance abuse and depression with atypical features, it could rest on either the chronicity of this disorder or its possible relation to bipolar disorder because both are associated with increased rates of substance abuse.

Increased rates of personality disorders, including avoidant personality, histrionic personality, and borderline personality, have been reported among depressed patients with atypical features (Perugi et al. 1998). The chronicity of depression with atypical features (Angst et al. 2002; McGinn et al. 1996; Stewart et al. 1993), plus one of its defining criteria being a character trait (pathological rejection sensitivity), may result in overlap with personality disorders being partly definitional. Until definitive etiological data are described, it seems most practical for nosology to retain depression with atypical features among the mood disorders because its treatment appears to mimic that effective for depressive disorders.

Biology

The hypothalamic-pituitary-adrenal (HPA) axis, sleep and other physiology, and psychophysiology of depression with atypical features have been studied. Lack of the biological findings of melancholia, or findings in between those for melancholia and for nondepressed control subjects, would be consistent with atypical depression representing a milder form of the illness. Alternatively, findings different from those for melancholia, or showing controls to lie between the two depressed groups, would argue that they are different disorders.

The HPA axis has been extensively studied in depressive disorders. Patients with melancholia or psychotic depression have elevated resting cortisol levels (Carroll et al. 1976; Sachar 1975), early release of cortisol from dexamethasone suppression (Carroll 1982; Sachar et al. 1985), blunted stimulation of cortisol by dextroamphetamine (Sachar et al. 1981) and desipramine (Asnis et al. 1985), and elevated corticotropin-releasing hormone in cerebrospinal fluid (Gold et al. 1995). Gold et al. (1995) summarized these findings as signaling a failure of negative feedback inhibition by cortisol at the level of the hypothalamus or higher. Because depression with atypical fea-

tures has vegetative features opposite to those of melancholia, Gold et al. further hypothesized that depression with atypical features should be characterized by a hypoactive HPA axis, a conjecture largely supported by the literature. For example, Anisman et al. (1999) showed low unstimulated cortisol levels in depressed patients with atypical features, and Levitan et al. (1997a) found low plasma cortisol in depressed patients with hypersomnia and bulimia. Furthermore, increased cortisol sensitivity to pharmacological challenges has been reported by Asnis et al. (1995) with desipramine. Finally, Geracioti et al. (1997) reported decreased cerebrospinal fluid corticotropin-releasing hormone levels relative to control subjects in 10 patients with major depression, most of whom had atypical symptoms, and Levitan et al. (2002) showed that women with atypical depression hypersuppress cortisol in response to dexamethasone. Thus, five studies provide evidence of a hypoactive HPA axis supersensitive to negative feedback and stimulation in depressed patients with atypical features, the opposite of the hyperactive HPA axis commonly noted in melancholia.

Depressed patients with melancholia have abnormal laterality on auditory (Bruder et al. 1989) and visual (Bruder et al. 2002) perceptual processing—favoring the left hemisphere and differing significantly from that in both control subjects and patients with atypical depression. In the visual test, depressed patients with atypical features favored their left brains significantly less than control subjects. Thus, depression with atypical features may identify brains that behave differently from the brains of both control subjects and depressed patients with melancholic features.

Finally, Quitkin et al. (1985) showed that depressed patients with atypical features have either normal sleep or only minimal abnormalities, whereas Harrison et al. (1984) showed that depressed patients with melancholic features but not those with atypical features excreted abnormally low amounts of tyramine following an oral tyramine load. In general, depressed patients with atypical features do not share the biological abnormalities typical of melancholia and sometimes (e.g., HPA axis, perceptual processing) show abnormalities opposite to those of melancholia.

Course of Illness

Follow-back studies have reported that depression with atypical features has earlier onset (e.g., Angst et al. 2002; Benazzi 2002; Horwath et al. 1992b; Stewart et al. 1993) and a more chronic course (Angst et al. 2002; McGinn et al. 1996; Stewart et al. 1993) than does melancholia. Repeated episodes of illness are likely to have vegetative symptoms similar to an index depressive episode (Angst et al. 2002; Kendler et al. 1996), suggesting stability of the illness over time.

Family and Genetic Studies

Perugi et al. (1998) reported increased bipolarity in relatives of depressed patients with atypical features. Stewart et al. (1993) found increased depression and chronic depression in the families of depressed probands with atypical features but decreased severe and episodic depression relative to depressed patients with melancholic features. Stewart et al. (1993) did not find an increased rate of bipolar illness, but Perugi et al. used a looser definition of bipolarity than did Stewart et al. Kendler et al. (1996), in a study of female twins, found significant concordant symptomatology if both twins were depressed. Together, these findings suggest familial, and perhaps genetic, transmission.

Treatment

Atypical depression was originally described as specifically responsive to monoamine oxidase inhibitors (MAOIs) (West and Dally 1959), an observation confirmed by subsequent double-blind studies (summarized by Stewart et al. 1993). Newer antidepressants have been suggested as effective for depression with atypical features (Goodnick and Extein 1989; Pande et al. 1996; Reimherr et al. 1984), but the studies were small, open-label, and not placebo-controlled or did not find statistical differences. Only two studies showed that newer agents were effective in randomized, placebo-controlled studies. In the first study, 62% (18 of 29) responded to gepirone, an unmarketed medication, and 20% (6 of 30) responded to placebo ($\chi^2 = 9.14$, df=1, $P < 0.002$; McGrath et al. 1994). In the second study, fluoxetine (50% responding) was superior to placebo (25% responding) (McGrath et al. 2000). Neither study compared the newer agent with an MAOI, so their relative efficacies remain unclear. Also, the fluoxetine study included a group treated with imipramine, to which 50% also responded; thus, fluoxetine did not show the superior efficacy relative to imipramine that characterizes MAOIs. The role of newer antidepressants in the treatment of depression with atypical features remains to be clarified.

Two studies reported that psychotherapy had efficacy for depressed patients with atypical features (Jarrett et al. 1999; Stewart et al. 1998). Finally, two nontraditional treatments have shown efficacy: Davidson et al. (2003) found that chromium was more effective than placebo, and Bouwer et al. (2000) reported that prednisone was helpful in five of six hypocortisolemic patients who had treatment-refractory major depression with atypical features.

Future Directions

In summary, depressed patients with atypical features have an illness that is stable over time; appears to be familial and perhaps genetic; and, relative to melancholia, has earlier onset, a more chronic course, and a different biology. Together, these findings argue that atypical depression is a different disorder (Angst et al. 2002; Stewart et al. 1993), although Parker et al. (2002) has presented data suggesting that the DSM-IV-TR category is problematic.

One problem with the concept of atypical depression is that some symptoms respond to a treatment (i.e., imipramine) that is effective for melancholia, and some do not. One possibility is that the DSM-IV-TR criteria for atypical features identify a heterogeneous group, with some having the same illness as melancholia and others having a different disorder. In support of heterogeneity, Stewart et al. (2002) showed that atypical patients who had either onset after age 20 or episodic illness had a robust imipramine response, unlike those with early-onset (before age 20) and very chronic (no spontaneous well-being since onset) depressive illness who responded to imipramine no more often than to placebo. Similarly, patients with atypical depression with either later onset or a less chronic illness showed preference for left hemisphere perceptual processing (Stewart et al. 2003), a characteristic of depression with melancholic features (Bruder et al. 1989, 2002). The group with chronic, early-onset depression had decreased left hemisphere processing relative to control subjects (Stewart et al. 2003). Finally, patients with later-onset, less chronic depression with atypical features had significantly increased baseline and postdexamethasone cortisol; the early-onset, very chronically ill group had abnormally low cortisol levels (Stewart et al. 2005). Thus, DSM-IV-TR criteria for depression with atypical features define a heterogeneous group consisting of at least two subgroups. One group is identified by the relatively late onset (after age 20) of a nonchronic illness course, imipramine responsivity, preference for left hemisphere perceptual processing, and hypercortisolemia, thus resembling depressed patients with melancholic features. A second group has early onset, a very chronic illness course, no response to tricyclic antidepressants, decreased preference for left hemisphere perceptual processing, and possibly hypocortisolemia. These findings argue that the DSM-IV-TR criteria for depression with atypical features should require early onset and a very chronic illness course in order to identify a more homogeneous patient group.

Dysthymic Disorder

DSM-IV-TR Definition

Dysthymic disorder is a chronic, nonbipolar, nonpsychotic disorder requiring at least 2 years (1 year in children) of dysphoric mood more days than not plus at least two of six major depressive–like symptoms, including sleep disturbance, appetite change, poor energy or fatigue, difficulty concentrating or making decisions, feelings of hopelessness, and low self-esteem. The symptoms cannot meet criteria for major depression during the first 2 years. These arbitrary criteria define a nosological convenience rather than a validated distinct disorder. Dysthymic disorder's utility lies in identifying a treatable group of dysphoric, dysfunctional patients without major depressive disorder.

Epidemiology

Published prevalence rates of dysthymic disorder range from 0.9% to 20.6% (summarized by Waintraub and Guelfi 1998). However, most epidemiological studies report rates between 2% and 4% (Angst and Wicki 1991; Canino et al. 1987; Faravelli and Incerpi 1985; Weissman et al. 1988). Weissman et al. (1988) found no association between dysthymia and ethnicity or employment status, but dysthymic patients were less likely to be married, and younger (i.e., younger than 45) dysthymic patients had lower income.

Demographics

Dysthymia has the 2:1 preponderance of females (Kessler et al. 1994; Weissman et al. 1993) found for major depression (Weissman et al. 1984). Devanand et al. (1994) did not find a female preponderance in elderly dysthymic patients coming to a psychiatric clinic; however, Kirby et al. (1999) did not confirm this finding in a random sample of medical clinic patients—68% of the elderly dysthymic patients were female.

Comorbid Disorders

Dysthymic disorder is frequently comorbid with major depression. Over a lifetime, estimates of comorbid major depression range from -39% to 76% (Kovacs et al. 1994; Weissman et al. 1988). Amore and Jori (2001) reported that 67% of a clinical sample with dysthymic disorder had a current (38%) or past history (29%) of comorbid major depression. Markowitz et al. (1992) similarly found that 68% of the patients with dysthymia had current or past

histories of major depression. In a 9-year follow-up of 55 dysthymic patients ages 8–14 years, Kovacs et al. (1994) reported that 76% developed a major depressive episode.

Dysthymia is also often comorbid with anxiety and substance use disorders. For example, Weissman et al. (1988) reported that 46% of the ECA subjects with dysthymic disorder also met criteria for one or more anxiety disorders, whereas Markowitz et al. (1992) found that 26% of 34 dysthymic patients presenting for treatment also had panic disorder, and 24% had a history of substance abuse. Masi et al. (2003) found that among 100 consecutive child and adolescent outpatients with dysthymia, 59% also met criteria for generalized anxiety disorder, 28% for simple phobia, 18% for separation anxiety, 13% for social phobia, and 10% for panic disorder. In contrast, only 22% of the 55 dysthymic children in the Kovacs et al. (1994) study had a comorbid anxiety disorder.

Our own analyses of the NCS data found that relative to patients without a depressive diagnosis, dysthymic patients have increased alcohol abuse or dependence (36% vs. 22%; $\chi^2 = 42.95$, df=1, $P < 0.001$), drug abuse or dependence (21% vs. 10%, $\chi^2 = 44.44$, df=1, $P < 0.001$), simple phobia (27% vs. 10%, $\chi^2 = 107.03$, df=1, $P < 0.001$), panic disorder (13% vs. 3%, $\chi^2 = 107.68$, df=1, $P < 0.001$), and social phobia (30% vs. 12%, $\chi^2 = 100.21$, df=1, $P < 0.001$) (V. Agosti, unpublished analyses from the public access NCS data, June 2004). Shankman and Klein (2002) followed up 86 patients with dysthymic disorder for 5 years and reported that those who also had a comorbid anxiety disorder recovered about half as often as did those without comorbid anxiety (31% vs. 61%). Thus, despite Kovacs and colleagues' (1994) dissenting report, comorbid anxiety appears to be common in dysthymia and adversely affects outcome.

Among the elderly, rates of comorbidity with other Axis I disorders, including major depression, are relatively low in both clinical (Devanand et al. 1994) and epidemiological (Kirby et al. 1999) samples, accounting for fewer than 20% of patients. Thus, dysthymic disorder in the elderly may be a different disorder. Another argument is that Devanand et al. (1994) found few elderly patients with early-onset dysthymia.

Axis II disorders co-occur with dysthymic disorder in as many as 60% of patients, including 24% with borderline, 14% with histrionic, 16% with avoidant, and 10% with self-defeating personality disorder (Pepper et al. 1995). Rates of comorbid personality disorders did not differ between those with and without comorbid major depression. Whether associations between dysthymic disorder and Axis II disorder result from anything more than partially overlapping criteria is an open question.

Biology

Pathophysiology has been less well studied in dysthymia than in major depression. We review studies of sleep electroencephalograms (EEGs), the HPA axis, brain imaging, and immune function and focus on whether major depression's abnormalities also occur in dysthymic disorder.

Patients with dysthymic disorder have abnormalities in sleep architecture similar to those reported for major depression (Gillin et al. 1979) and especially melancholia (Quitkin et al. 1985). For example, poor sleep efficiency, increased sleep latency, increased awakenings, increased total rapid eye movement (REM) sleep, and increased Stage I sleep also have been reported in patients with dysthymic disorder (Saletu-Zyhlarz et al. 2001). Others have reported shortened REM period latency in patients with dysthymic disorder (Akiskal et al. 1984; Berger et al. 1983; Hauri and Sateia 1984). Thus, other than Arriaga and associates' (1990) inability to find shortened REM period latency in patients with dysthymic disorder, most studies found dysthymic disorder to have the same sleep EEG abnormalities as are found in major depression.

The HPA axis has been investigated in multiple ways in patients with dysthymic disorder. Catalán et al. (1998), for example, reported elevated baseline cortisol levels in 10 patients with dysthymic disorder, relative to control subjects, and the dysthymic patients did not differ from 26 patients with major depression. Leake et al. (1989) also found that 7 dysthymic patients had baseline cortisol levels similar to those in 10 patients with major depression, and both groups had significantly higher levels than control subjects. Ravindran et al. (1996), however, did not find elevated baseline cortisol or corticotropin in 72 patients with dysthymic disorder.

Multiple reports on the dexamethasone suppression test had varying results. Howland and Thase (1991) summarized the studies up to 1991 as finding normal postdexamethasone cortisol levels in patients with dysthymia, the composite of 10 studies showing that 14% of dysthymic patients (33 of 243) had abnormal postdexamethasone cortisol levels, compared with 6% of control subjects (4 of 72) and 59% of patients with major depression (131 of 221). Since Howland and Thase's (1991) review, Szádóczky et al. (1994) showed dexamethasone escape in 22% of 53 patients with early-onset dysthymia compared with 9% of 22 patients with late-onset dysthymia. Both groups, however, suppressed significantly less often than 105 patients with major depression, 46% of whom showed dexamethasone nonsuppression. Rihmer and Szádóczky (1993) also reported increased nonsuppression (23%) in dysthymic patients, but it is not clear that these were different patients from the somewhat larger group

on which Szádóczky et al. (1994) reported. In contrast, Ravindran et al. (1994) found that only 7% of dysthymic patients (2 of 30) failed to suppress cortisol following dexamethasone.

Other suggestions of possible HPA axis abnormalities in dysthymic disorder include a blunted cortisol response to ipsapirone, a serotonin type 1A ($5-HT_{1A}$) receptor partial agonist (Riedel et al. 2002); relative cortisol nonsuppression following hydrocortisone (Gispen-de Wied et al. 1998); and increased baseline corticotropin-releasing hormone in patients with dysthymic and major depressive disorder relative to control subjects (Catalán et al. 1998).

One magnetic resonance imaging study showed a smaller corpus callosum size in young, unmedicated depressed patients (mostly dysthymic patients) than in control subjects (Lyoo et al. 2002). This finding is consistent with reports of decreased frontal lobe function (MacFall et al. 2001) and/or asymmetry (Diego et al. 2001) in patients with major depression, although normal (Husain et al. 1991) or larger (Wu et al. 1993) corpus callosum sizes have been reported. Schlatter et al. (2001) reported that relative to 15 control subjects, 12 dysthymic patients and 10 patients with major depression had elevated interleukin-1β and interleukin-6, but the two depressed groups did not differ.

Taken together, most biological studies of dysthymic disorder show abnormalities similar to those seen in major depression, but some show less common abnormality or no difference from control subjects. These findings are consistent with two hypotheses of depressive illness. If depression exists on a continuum, with dysthymic disorder a milder form, then some investigations should fail to differentiate dysthymic disorder from major depressive disorder and others should find less frequent abnormalities in dysthymic disorder or fail to distinguish patients with dysthymic disorder from control subjects. Alternatively, if dysthymic disorder and major depressive disorder are both heterogeneous, including patients with the same pathophysiologies in differing proportions, then varied findings should also occur.

Course of Illness

Over time, dysthymia shows varying degrees of affective psychopathology. For example, Horwath et al. (1992a) and Judd et al. (1997) reported significantly increased risk for future major depressive disorder in 1-year follow-up of ECA patients with dysthymic disorder. Angst and Wicki (1991) reinterviewed 16 subjects with dysthymic disorder 2 years later, reporting varying degrees of depressive symptoms from complete remission to development of major depression. Klein et al. (2000) followed up 125 depressed outpatients and reported that at 5-year follow-up, relative to patients with index major depression, those with index dysthymic disorder had higher follow-up Hamilton Rating Scale for Depression scores, more suicide attempts, and more frequent hospitalization. Furthermore, only half of the patients with dysthymia had recovered at 4 years. The instability of diagnosis over time is consistent with a dimensional view of depressive illness varying over time from no symptoms to subsyndromal symptoms to full syndromal symptoms without clear distinctions.

Treatment

Extensive review of the pharmacological treatment of dysthymic disorder (Brunello et al. 1999; Howland 1991) concluded that antidepressant medications are approximately as effective for dysthymic disorder as for major depression. In addition to medication, Weissman (1997) suggested the efficacy of interpersonal psychotherapy, and Keller et al. (2000) showed the utility of the cognitive-behavioral analysis system of psychotherapy. Thus, treatments effective for major depression often also help dysthymic disorder. Unfortunately, these patients too often go unnoticed (Howland 1993; Weissman et al. 1988), and their symptoms are often untreated or undertreated (Haykal and Akiskal 1999; Shelton et al. 1997), yet they use a disproportionate amount of health services (Howland 1993; Weissman et al. 1988).

Functioning

Zlotnick et al. (2000) showed that NCS subjects with dysthymia have significant impairment in interpersonal functioning relative to nondepressed individuals and similar to that in patients with major depression. Because dysthymia is chronic, its associated burden of psychosocial impairment is extensive (Wells et al. 1989) and disproportionate to its prevalence (Johnson et al. 1992).

Future Trends

Dysthymia is a nosological label of convenience rather than a true disorder. Thus, few data differentiate it from major depression. Both disorders appear etiologically heterogeneous; the same underlying disorders are represented within both, perhaps in different proportions. Future nosological systems will likely replace dysthymic disorder with etiologically distinct categories.

We propose three candidates for possibly etiologically distinct categories within dysthymia. Dysthymia with atypical features might best be disentangled from other types of dysthymia and combined with major depression with atypical features. Another possibly distinct group is dysthymia in the elderly, as argued by Devanand et al. (1994). Dysthymia in this group generally has late onset and may not be more likely in females (Devanand et al. 1994), infrequently has comorbid disorders (Devanand et al. 1994; Kirby et al. 1999), and may not share major depression's HPA abnormalities (Szádóczky et al. 1994). Finally, some patients with dysthymia have biological abnormalities similar to those in depressed patients with melancholic features.

Thus, a diagnosis of dysthymia probably identifies a biologically and etiologically heterogeneous group of patients whose degree of symptomatology can be expected to wax and wane over time. Its recognition is important, however, because treatment ameliorates its accompanying dysfunction.

Cyclothymic Disorder

DSM-IV-TR Definition

Cyclothymic disorder is characterized by at least 2 years of numerous (undefined) mood swings, including periods with hypomanic symptoms alternating with nonmajor dysphoria with days to weeks of normal mood in between, but euthymia cannot last more than 2 months. During the first 2 years, there cannot be symptoms sufficient to meet criteria for major depression, mania, or a mixed episode. Another disorder, such as a psychotic disorder or substance abuse, cannot be considered to better account for the symptoms, and there must be significant distress about the condition or impairment attributable to it. As with dysthymic disorder, criteria for cyclothymic disorder are arbitrary and lack empirical data demonstrating that they define an illness etiologically different from other bipolar disorders, but its recognition and treatment may help lessen the disability it entails.

Few studies used DSM-IV criteria but rather included patients with hypomanic symptoms without careful assessment of whether each DSM-IV criterion also was met. Thus, it is unclear how applicable the cited literature is.

Epidemiology

Depending on the criteria used, from 0.3% to 6.0% of the population have cyclothymia. Estimates at the low end include those by Lewinsohn et al. (1995), who reported cyclothymia in 0.3% of 15- to 21-year-olds; Weissman and Myers (1978), who found 0.4% in an epidemiological sample from New Haven, Connecticut; and Faravelli et al. (1990), who diagnosed cyclothymia in 0.4% of 1,000 randomly selected Italian primary health care users. High rates were reported by Angst et al. (2003), who found that 12% of Zurich, Switzerland, 20-year-olds have minor bipolar disorder (i.e., submajor depressive symptoms plus hypomania or hypomanic symptoms); Depue et al. (1981), who found that 6% of nonpatient college students had cyclothymic symptoms; and Eckblad and Chapman (1986), who reported recurrent hypomania in 6% of college students. Carlson and Kashani (1988) found that 1.5% of a community sample of adolescents had cyclothymia. Judd and Akiskal (2003) reanalyzed the ECA data and reported that 5.1% of this sample had two or more hypomanic symptoms without meeting criteria for mania or hypomania, usually because the episode duration is too short. Thus, diagnosable cyclothymic disorder may occur in 0.3% or 0.4% of the population, and perhaps as many as 1.5% of teenagers, but in addition, between 5% and 10% may have some hypomanic symptoms without meeting full syndromal criteria.

Demographics

As with bipolar I and bipolar II disorders, epidemiological samples suggest that males and females may be equally likely to develop cyclothymic disorder. For example, Judd and Akiskal (2003) reported that women made up 52% of the ECA subjects who reported hypomanic symptoms. Lewinsohn et al. (1995) reported that females accounted for 57% of their 15- to 21-year-olds who had hypomanic symptoms without bipolar II disorder. Unlike epidemiological studies, females predominate in clinical samples. Thus, Akiskal (1979) reported that 62% of cyclothymic patients were females, and Howland and Thase (1993) concluded that clinical populations of cyclothymic patients are "mostly female." Whether females are more likely to enter treatment or whether the common comorbid substance abuse shifts males out of general psychiatric clinics is unclear. Ethnic differences were not found in adolescents (Lewinsohn et al. 1995), college students (Depue et al. 1981), or a clinical sample (Akiskal et al. 1979).

Comorbid Disorders

Comorbid mood disorder and affective symptoms are common in subjects with hypomanic symptoms or cyclothymia. For example, in 2- to 3-year follow-up, 35% of the cyclothymic patients developed frank mood episodes (i.e., mania, hypomania, or major depression) (Akiskal et al. 1977), compared with 4% of a control group without mood disorder. In addition, patients with cyclothymia were more likely to develop hypomania when given antidepressants (44% vs. 0%), a rate comparable to that observed in frank bipolar disorder (38%) (Akiskal et al. 1977).

Medical and other psychiatric disorders are also common. Thus, relative to nonbipolar subjects, patients with bipolar symptoms have increased anxiety disorders (30% vs. 6%), panic attacks (18% vs. 4%), migraine (24% vs. 11%), asthma (17% vs. 10%), and allergies (42% vs. 29%) (Calabrese et al. 2003). Also reported have been increased rates of separation anxiety, panic, obsessive-compulsive, and overanxious disorders; attention-deficit/hyperactivity disorder; conduct and oppositional defiant disorders; and major depression and submajor dysphoria (Lewinsohn et al. 1995; Perugi et al. 2003), as well as bulimia, borderline personality, and dependent personality (Perugi et al. 2003) and drug and alcohol abuse (Akiskal et al. 1979; Gawin and Ellinwood 1988; Lewinsohn et al. 1995; Mirin et al. 1991; Perugi et al. 2003). Comorbid personality disorders occur in 29% of bipolar patients (George et al. 2003) and predict negative outcome in follow-up (Bieling et al. 2003). Thus, cyclothymia, or even mild hypomanic symptoms, is often accompanied by other disorders, including medical disorders, such as allergies, asthma, and migraine headaches.

Biology

Relatively little has been published on the possible biological profile of cyclothymia. Depue et al. (1985) reported cortisol hypersecretion in 15 cyclothymic college students compared with 10 students who scored low on a screening questionnaire. Akiskal et al. (1979) reported a dramatic decline in REM period latency in a single cyclothymic patient—from 170 minutes when hypomanic to 35 minutes when he had switched to a depressive state, suggesting that this one patient had melancholia-like sleep physiology. Finally, subjects with nonclinical cyclothymia had reduced skin conductance (Lenhart 1985) relative to students without evidence of cyclothymia, similar to patients with major depression (Donat and McCullough 1983). Thus, the few biological variables that differentiate cyclothymic patients from control subjects are similar to those observed in patients with major depression. It is not surprising, then, that patients diagnosed with cyclothymia often provide histories of major depression or go on to develop major depression later (Akiskal et al. 1977; Kwapil et al. 2000).

Course of Illness

During 2- to 3-year follow-up, 6% of patients with cyclothymia develop mania (Akiskal et al. 1977), whereas 25% have at least one major depressive episode (Akiskal et al. 1977), and 16% develop hypomania (Akiskal et al. 1979). Half of cyclothymic patients report episodic drug and/or alcohol abuse (Akiskal et al. 1977). Major depression has onset at about age 20 when superimposed on cyclothymia, about 20 years earlier than onset of unipolar depression (Akiskal et al. 1979). Furthermore, the cyclothymic children of a bipolar parent are more vulnerable to having manic or hypomanic episodes than are their noncyclothymic siblings (Akiskal et al. 1985), and behavioral and mood difficulties predate diagnosable mania by about 10 years (Egeland et al. 2000), suggesting that mania and hypomania evolve out of a cyclothymic substrate (Akiskal et al. 2003). Kwapil et al. (2000) reported that during 4-year follow-up, cyclothymic college students were at significantly increased risk for developing mania or hypomania, major depression, substance abuse, and psychotic episodes and had lower levels of social adjustment compared with students without cyclothymia. Thus, cyclothymic adolescents have increased risk of more severe psychiatric disorders and poor psychosocial outcome.

Family and Genetic Studies

Childhood mood lability, distractibility, and easy excitement may represent prodromal symptoms of more serious mood disorder. Children of parents with bipolar I disorder more frequently had these symptoms than did children of parents without bipolar disorder (Egeland et al. 2003). Even among children without a bipolar parent, those considered labile, distractible, and excitable invariably had a more distant relative (e.g., aunt) with bipolar disorder. Although these children did not receive the diagnosis of cyclothymic disorder, the descriptive resemblance suggests that cyclothymia may be familially related to bipolar disorder.

Cassano et al. (1992) showed that among patients with major depression, those with hyperthymic temperament had increased rates of bipolar illness in their families relative to patients with major depression without hyperthymic temperament and similar to the families of patients with cyclothymia and bipolar II disorder. Thus, even without cyclothymic mood swings or diagnosable hypomania, patients with increased mood and energy below that required for hypomania still may have a familial disorder that belongs in the bipolar spectrum. Similarly, Akiskal et al. (1979) reported that 30% of the patients with cyclothymia have first-degree relatives with bipolar illness, a rate similar to patients with bipolar I and II disorder, 26% of whom report bipolar relatives.

The genetics of bipolar disorder are unclear. However, because cyclothymia occurs at increased rates in bipolar families and may presage frank bipolar illness, genetic linkage is more difficult to establish if such family members are not considered cases.

Treatment

Akiskal (1983; Akiskal et al. 2003) considers cyclothymia a prodrome of more severe bipolar pathology and therefore recommends treatment with mood stabilizers, such as lithium or valproate (Akiskal 1994). For example, 60% of patients with cyclothymia respond to lithium, compared with 20% of patients with nonaffective personality disorders (Akiskal et al. 1979), and Rosier et al. (1974) reported excellent prophylactic effects of lithium in cyclothymic patients. Jacobsen (1993) reported that 65% of cyclothymic patients stopped cycling while taking valproate, a rate similar to the 70% response to valproic acid reported by Semadeni (1976). For the depression that cyclothymic patients experience, standard antidepressants appear useful, although we did not find placebo-controlled trials. In short, patients with cyclothymia appear to respond well to the treatments used for other patients with mood disorders. The presence of cyclothymia as a dysfunctional disorder that presages more severe disorders indicates the need for aggressive use of mood stabilizers and antidepressants.

Functioning

Cyclothymia is associated with significant impairment. Judd and Akiskal (2003), for example, showed that ECA subjects who had hypomanic symptoms without meeting criteria for hypomania or mania had increased marital disruption, health service utilization, suicidal behavior, and need for welfare and disability benefits compared with a no disorder group. Similarly, Calabrese et al. (2003) reported increased difficulties with work-related performance, social and leisure activities, and social and family interactions in a group considered by questionnaire to be at risk for bipolar disorder. Fichtner et al. (1989) reported that among 126 inpatients followed up for 2–6 years, those with baseline cyclothymic features had significantly worse global functioning during follow-up than did patients without cyclothymic history. Even among more severe disorders, patients with premorbid cyclothymia function worse. Poor psychosocial functioning associated with cyclothymia or similar symptoms also has been reported by Lewinsohn et al. (1995) in prospectively followed up adolescents, by Klein and Depue (1984) in nonpatient college students, and by Klein et al. (1985) and Egeland et al. (2003) in children of bipolar parents.

Even in patients who do not warrant a diagnosis of bipolar illness, subsyndromal hypomanic symptoms disrupt life in multiple spheres, including school, work, interpersonal relationships, and health care utilization. Clinicians should therefore note and treat hypomanic symptoms, even if they are subsyndromal.

Future Directions

Several issues seem clear. One is that the term *cyclothymia* has been used differently by various nosological systems and authors. However, whatever the definition used, cyclothymia and subsyndromal hypomanic symptoms are associated with high risk for both familial and personal major depression, hypomania, and mania. Thus, variously defined subsyndromal mood lability identifies a group best considered to lie within the bipolar spectrum. Furthermore, the presence of mood lability should alert the clinician, the patient, and the patient's family to the likelihood of future major depressive episodes, hypomania, and mania in both the patient and his or her offspring, as well as the presence of other disorders, including substance abuse and anxiety disorders. Presence of cyclothymia should influence treatment decisions, particularly early intervention with mood stabilizers and possibly avoidance of antidepressants without concurrent mood stabilizers. For research, and especially for genetic studies, because cyclothymia appears to be the field in which major mood disorders grow, inclusion of family members with cyclothymia among bipolar affected cases may improve the likelihood of detecting biological abnormalities, including genetic transmission of bipolar illness.

References

Akiskal HS: Diagnosis and classification of affective disorders: new insights from clinical and laboratory approaches. Psychiatr Dev 1:123–160, 1983

Akiskal HS: Dysthymic and cyclothymic depressions: therapeutic considerations. J Clin Psychiatry 55 (suppl, April):46–52, 1994

Akiskal HS, Djenderedjian AH, Rosenthal RH, et al: Cyclothymic disorder: validating criteria for inclusion in the bipolar affective group. Am J Psychiatry 134:1227–1233, 1977

Akiskal HS, Khani MK, Scott-Strauss A: Cyclothymic temperamental disorders. Psychiatr Clin North Am 2:527–554, 1979

Akiskal HS, Lemmi H, Dickson H, et al: Chronic depressions, part 2: sleep EEG differentiation of primary dysthymic disorders from anxious depressions. J Affect Disord 6:287–295, 1984

Akiskal HS, Downs J, Jordan P, et al: Affective disorders in referred children and younger siblings of manic-depressives: mode of onset and prospective course. Arch Gen Psychiatry 42:996–1003, 1985

Akiskal HS, Hantouche EG, Allilaire JF: Bipolar II with and without cyclothymic temperament: "dark" and "sunny" expressions of soft bipolarity. J Affect Disord 73:49–57, 2003

Alpert JE, Uebelacker LA, McLean NE, et al: Social phobia, avoidant personality disorder and atypical depression: co-occurrence and clinical implications. Psychol Med 27:627–633, 1997

American Psychiatric Association: Diagnostic and Statistical Manual of Mental Disorders, 4th Edition. Washington, DC, American Psychiatric Association, 1994

American Psychiatric Association: Diagnostic and Statistical Manual of Mental Disorders, 4th Edition, Text Revision. Washington, DC, American Psychiatric Association, 2000

Amore M, Jori MC (on behalf of AMISERT investigators): Faster response on amisulpride 50 mg versus sertraline 50–100 mg in patients with dysthymia or double depression: a randomized, double-blind, parallel group study. Int Clin Psychopharmacol 16:317–324, 2001

Angst J, Wicki W: The Zurich study, XI: is dysthymia a separate form of depression? Results of the Zurich cohort study. Eur Arch Psychiatry Clin Neurosci 240:349–354, 1991

Angst J, Gamma A, Sellaro R, et al: Toward validation of atypical depression in the community: results of the Zurich cohort study. J Affect Disord 72:125–138, 2002

Angst J, Gamma A, Benazzi F, et al: Toward a re-definition of subthreshold bipolarity: epidemiology and proposed criteria for bipolar-II, minor bipolar disorders and hypomania. J Affect Disord 73:133–146, 2003

Anisman H, Ravindran AV, Griffiths J, et al: Endocrine and cytokine correlates of major depression and dysthymia with typical or atypical features. Mol Psychiatry 4:182–188, 1999

Arriaga F, Rosado P, Paiva T: The sleep of dysthymic patients: a comparison with normal controls. Biol Psychiatry 27:649–656, 1990

Asnis GM, Halbreich U, Rabinovich H, et al: The cortisol response to desipramine in endogenous depressives and normal controls: preliminary findings. Psychiatry Res 14:225–233, 1985

Asnis GM, McGinn LK, Sanderson WC: Atypical depression: clinical aspects and noradrenergic function. Am J Psychiatry 152:31–36, 1995

Benazzi F: Psychomotor changes in melancholic and atypical depression: unipolar and bipolar-II subtypes. Psychiatry Res 112:211–220, 2002

Berger M, Lund R, Bronisch T, et al: REM latency in neurotic and endogenous depression and the cholinergic REM induction test. Psychiatry Res 10:113–123, 1983

Bieling PJ, MacQueen GM, Marriot MJ, et al: Longitudinal outcome in patients with bipolar disorder assessed by life-charting is influenced by DSM-IV personality disorder symptoms. Bipolar Disord 5:14–21, 2003

Bouwer C, Claassen J, Dinan TG, et al: Prednisone augmentation in treatment-resistant depression with fatigue and hypocortisolaemia: a case series. Depress Anxiety 12:44–50, 2000

Bruder GE, Quitkin FM, Stewart JW, et al: Cerebral laterality and depression: differences in perceptual asymmetry among diagnostic subtypes. J Abnorm Psychol 98:177–186, 1989

Bruder GE, Stewart JW, McGrath PJ, et al: Atypical depression: enhanced right hemispheric dominance for perceiving emotional chimeric faces. J Abnorm Psychol 111:446–454, 2002

Brunello N, Akiskal H, Boyer P, et al: Dysthymia: clinical picture, extent of overlap with chronic fatigue syndrome, neuropharmacological considerations, and new therapeutic vistas. J Affect Disord 52:275–290, 1999

Calabrese JR, Hirschfeld RM, Reed M, et al: Impact of bipolar disorder on a U.S. community sample. J Clin Psychiatry 64:425–432, 2003

Canino GJ, Bird HR, Shrout PE, et al: The prevalence of specific psychiatric disorders in Puerto Rico. Arch Gen Psychiatry 44:727–735, 1987

Carlson GA, Kashani JH: Manic symptoms in a non-referred adolescent population. J Affect Disord 15:219–226, 1988

Carroll BJ: The dexamethasone suppression test for melancholia. Br J Psychiatry 140:292–304, 1982

Carroll BJ, Curtis GC, Mendels J: Cerebrospinal fluid and plasma free cortisol concentrations in depression. Psychol Med 6:235–244, 1976

Cassano GB, Akiskal HS, Savino M, et al: Proposed subtypes of bipolar II and related disorders: with hypomanic episodes (or cyclothymia) and with hyperthymic temperament. J Affect Disord 17:127–140, 1992

Catalán R, Gallart JM, Castellanos JM, et al: Plasma corticotropin-releasing factor in depressive disorders. Biol Psychiatry 44:15–20, 1998

Davidson JRT, Miller RD, Turnbull CD, et al: Atypical depression. Arch Gen Psychiatry 39:527–534, 1982

Davidson JRT, Abraham K, Connor KM, et al: Effectiveness of chromium in atypical depression: a placebo-controlled trial. Biol Psychiatry 53:261–264, 2003

Depue RA, Slater JF, Wolfstetter-Kausch H, et al: A behavioral paradigm for identifying persons at risk for bipolar depressive disorder: a conceptual framework and five validation studies. J Abnorm Psychol 90:381–437, 1981

Depue RA, Kleiman RM, Davis P, et al: The behavioral high-risk paradigm and bipolar affective disorder, VIII: serum free cortisol in nonpatient cyclothymic subjects selected by the General Behavior Inventory. Am J Psychiatry 142:175–181, 1985

Devanand DP, Nobler MS, Singer T, et al: Is dysthymia a different disorder in the elderly? Am J Psychiatry 151:1592–1599, 1994

Diego MA, Field T, Hernandez-Reif M: CES-D depression scores are correlated with frontal EEG alpha asymmetry. Depress Anxiety 13:32–37, 2001

Donat DC, McCullough JP: Psychophysiological discriminants of depression at rest and in response to stress. J Clin Psychol 39:315–320, 1983

Eckblad M, Chapman LJ: Development and validation of a scale for hypomanic personality. J Abnorm Psychol 95:214–222, 1986

Egeland JA, Hostetter AM, Pauls DL, et al: Prodromal symptoms before onset of manic-depressive disorder suggested by first hospital admission histories. J Am Acad Child Adolesc Psychiatry 39:1245–1252, 2000

Egeland JA, Shaw JA, Endicott J, et al: Prospective study of prodromal features for bipolarity in well Amish children. J Am Acad Child Adolesc Psychiatry 42:786–796, 2003

Faravelli C, Incerpi G: Epidemiology of affective disorders in Florence. Acta Psychiatr Scand 72:331–333, 1985

Faravelli C, Guerrini Degl'Innocenti B, Aiazzi L, et al: Epidemiology of mood disorders: a community survey in Florence. J Affect Disord 20:135–141, 1990

Fichtner CG, Grossman LS, Harrow M, et al: Cyclothymic mood swings in the course of affective disorders and schizophrenia. Am J Psychiatry 146:1149–1154, 1989

Gawin FH, Ellinwood EH Jr: Cocaine and other stimulants: actions, abuse and treatment. N Engl J Med 318:1173–1182, 1988

George EL, Miklowitz DJ, Richards JA, et al: The comorbidity of bipolar disorder and Axis II personality disorders: prevalence and clinical correlates. Bipolar Disord 5:115–122, 2003

Geracioti TD Jr, Loosen PT, Orth DN: Low cerebrospinal fluid corticotropin-releasing hormone concentrations in eucortisolemic depression. Biol Psychiatry 42:166–174, 1997

Gillin JC, Duncan W, Pettigrew KD, et al: Successful separation of depressed, normal, and insomniac subjects by EEG sleep data. Arch Gen Psychiatry 36:85–90, 1979

Gispen-de Wied CC, Jansen LM, Wynne HJ, et al: Differential effects of hydrocortisone and dexamethasone on cortisol suppression in a child psychiatric population. Psychoneuroendocrinology 23:295–306, 1998

Gold PW, Licinio J, Wong ML, et al: Corticotropin releasing hormone in pathophysiology of melancholic and atypical depression and in the mechanism of action of antidepressant drugs. Ann N Y Acad Sci 771:716–729, 1995

Goodnick PJ, Extein I: Bupropion and fluoxetine in depressive subtypes. Ann Clin Psychiatry 1:119–122, 1989

Harrison WM, Cooper TB, Stewart JW, et al: The tyramine challenge test as a marker for melancholia. Arch Gen Psychiatry 41:681–685, 1984

Hauri P, Sateia MJ: REM sleep in dysthymic disorders. Sleep Res 13:119, 1984

Haykal RF, Akiskal HS: The long-term outcome of dysthymia in private practice: clinical features, temperament, and the art of management. J Clin Psychiatry 60:508–518, 1999

Horwath E, Johnson J, Klerman GL, et al: Depressive symptoms as relative and attributable risk factors for first-onset major depression. Arch Gen Psychiatry 49:817–823, 1992a

Horwath E, Johnson J, Weissman MM, et al: The validity of major depression with atypical features based on a community study. J Affect Disord 26:117–126, 1992b

Howland RH: Pharmacotherapy of dysthymia: a review. J Clin Psychopharmacol 11:83–92, 1991

Howland RH: General health, health care utilization, and medical comorbidity in dysthymia. Int J Psychiatry Med 23:211–238, 1993

Howland RH, Thase ME: Biological studies of dysthymia. Biol Psychiatry 30:283–304, 1991

Howland RH, Thase ME: A comprehensive review of cyclothymic disorder. J Nerv Ment Dis 181:485–493, 1993

Husain MM, Figiel GS, Lurie SN, et al: MRI of corpus callosum and septum pellucidum in depression. Biol Psychiatry 29:300–301, 1991

Jacobsen FM: Low-dose valproate: a new treatment for cyclothymia, mild rapid cycling disorders, and premenstrual syndrome. J Clin Psychiatry 54:229–234, 1993

Jarrett RB, Schaffer M, McIntire D, et al: Treatment of atypical depression with cognitive therapy or phenelzine: a double-blind, placebo-controlled trial. Arch Gen Psychiatry 56:431–437, 1999

Johnson J, Weissman MM, Klerman GL: Service utilization and social morbidity associated with depressive symptoms in the community. JAMA 267:1478–1483, 1992

Judd LL, Akiskal HS: The prevalence and disability of bipolar spectrum disorders in the US population: re-analysis of the ECA database taking into account subthreshold cases. J Affect Disord 73:123–131, 2003

Judd LL, Akiskal HS, Paulus MP: The role and clinical significance of subsyndromal depressive symptoms (SDS) in unipolar major depressive disorder. J Affect Disord 45:5–18, 1997

Keller MB, McCullough JP, Klein DN, et al: A comparison of nefazodone, the cognitive behavioral-analysis system of psychotherapy, and their combination for the treatment of chronic depression. N Engl J Med 342:1462–1470, 2000

Kendler KS, Eaves LJ, Walters EE, et al: The identification and validation of distinct depressive syndromes in a population-based sample of female twins. Arch Gen Psychiatry 53:391–399, 1996

Kessler R, McGonagle K, Zhao S, et al: Lifetime and 12-month prevalence of DSM-III-R psychiatric disorders in the United States: results from the National Comorbidity Survey. Arch Gen Psychiatry 51:8–19, 1994

Kirby M, Bruce I, Coakley D, et al: Dysthymia among the community-dwelling elderly. Int J Geriatr Psychiatry 14:440–445, 1999

Klein DN, Depue RA: Continued impairment in persons at risk for bipolar affective disorder: results of a 19-month follow-up study. J Abnorm Psychol 93:345–347, 1984

Klein DN, Depue RA, Slater JF: Cyclothymia in the adolescent offspring of parents with bipolar affective disorder. J Abnorm Psychol 94:115–127, 1985

Klein DN, Schwartz JE, Rose S, et al: Five-year course and outcome of dysthymic disorder: a prospective, naturalistic follow-up study. Am J Psychiatry 157:931–939, 2000

Kovacs M, Akiskal HS, Gatsonis C, et al: Childhood onset of dysthymic disorder: clinical features and prospective naturalistic outcome. Arch Gen Psychiatry 51:365–374, 1994

Kwapil TR, Miller MB, Zinser MC, et al: A longitudinal study of high scorers on the hypomanic personality scale. J Abnorm Psychol 109:222–226, 2000

Leake A, Griffiths HW, Ferrier IN: Plasma N-POMC, ACTH and cortisol following hCRH administration in major depression and dysthymia. J Affect Disord 17:57–64, 1989

Lenhart RE: Lowered skin conductance in a subsyndromal high-risk depressive sample: response amplitudes versus tonic levels. J Abnorm Psychol 94:649–652, 1985

Levitan RD, Kaplan AS, Brown BM, et al: Low plasma cortisol in bulimia nervosa patients with reversed neurovegetative symptoms of depression. Biol Psychiatry 41:366–368, 1997a

Levitan RD, Lesage A, Parikh SV, et al: Reversed neurovegetative symptoms of depression: a community study of Ontario. Am J Psychiatry 154:934–940, 1997b

Levitan RD, Vaccarino FJ, Brown GM, et al: Low-dose dexamethasone challenge in women with atypical major depression: pilot study. J Psychiatry Neurosci 27:47–51, 2002

Lewinsohn PM, Klein DN, Seeley JR: Bipolar disorders in a community sample of older adolescents: prevalence, phenomenology, comorbidity, and course. J Am Acad Child Adolesc Psychiatry 34:454–463, 1995

Lyoo IK, Kwon JS, Lee SJ, et al: Decrease in genu of the corpus callosum in medication-naïve, early onset dysthymia and depressive personality disorder. Biol Psychiatry 52:1134–1143, 2002

MacFall JR, Payne ME, Provenzale JE, et al: Medial orbital frontal lesions in late-onset depression. Biol Psychiatry 49:803–806, 2001

Markowitz JC, Moran ME, Kocsis JH, et al: Prevalence and comorbidity of dysthymic disorder among psychiatric outpatients. J Affect Disord 24:63–71, 1992

Masi G, Millepiedi S, Mucci M, et al: Phenomenology and comorbidity of dysthymic disorder in 100 consecutively referred children and adolescents: beyond DSM-IV. Can J Psychiatry 48:99–105, 2003

Matza LS, Revick DA, Davidson JR, et al: Depression with atypical features in the National Comorbidity Survey: classification, description, and consequences. Arch Gen Psychiatry 60:817–826, 2003

McGinn LK, Asnis GM, Rubinson E: Biological and clinical validation of atypical depression. Psychiatry Res 60:191–198, 1996

McGrath PJ, Stewart JW, Quitkin FM, et al: Gepirone treatment of atypical depression: preliminary evidence of serotonergic involvement. J Clin Psychopharmacol 14:347–352, 1994

McGrath PJ, Stewart JW, Janal MN, et al: A placebo-controlled study of fluoxetine versus imipramine in the acute treatment of atypical depression. Am J Psychiatry 157:344–350, 2000

Mirin SM, Weiss RD, Griffin ML, et al: Psychopathology in drug abusers and their families. Compr Psychiatry 32:36–51, 1991

Pande AC, Birkett M, Fechner-Bates S, et al: Fluoxetine versus phenelzine in atypical depression. Biol Psychiatry 40:1017–1020, 1996

Parker G, Roy K, Michell P, et al: Atypical depression: a reappraisal. Am J Psychiatry 159:1470–1479, 2002

Pepper CM, Klein DN, Anderson RL, et al: DSM-III-R Axis II comorbidity in dysthymia and major depression. Am J Psychiatry 152:239–247, 1995

Perugi G, Akiskal HS, Lattanzi L, et al: The high prevalence of "soft" bipolar (II) features in atypical depression. Compr Psychiatry 39:63–71, 1998

Perugi G, Toni C, Travierso MC, et al: The role of cyclothymia in atypical depression: toward a data-based reconceptualization of the borderline-bipolar II connection. J Affect Disord 73:87–98, 2003

Posternak MA, Zimmerman M: Partial validation of the atypical features subtype of major depressive disorder. Arch Gen Psychiatry 59:70–76, 2002

Quitkin FM, Rabkin G, Stewart JW, et al: Sleep of atypical depressives. J Affect Disord 8:61–67, 1985

Quitkin FM, McGrath PJ, Stewart JW, et al: Atypical depression, panic attacks, and response to imipramine and phenelzine: a replication. Arch Gen Psychiatry 47:935–941, 1990

Ravindran AV, Bialik RJ, Lapierre YD: Primary early onset dysthymia, biochemical correlates of the therapeutic response to fluoxetine, I: platelet monoamine oxidase and the dexamethasone suppression test. J Affect Disord 31:111–117, 1994

Ravindran AV, Griffiths J, Merali Z, et al: Primary dysthymia: a study of several psychosocial, endocrine and immune correlates. J Affect Disord 40:73–84, 1996

Reimherr FW, Wood DR, Byerley B, et al: Characteristics of responders to fluoxetine. Psychopharmacol Bull 20:70–72, 1984

Riedel WJ, Klaassen T, Griez E, et al: Dissociable hormonal, cognitive and mood responses to neuroendocrine challenge: evidence for receptor-specific serotonergic dysregulation in depressed mood. Neuropsychopharmacology 26:358–367, 2002

Rihmer Z, Szádóczky E: Dexamethasone suppression test and TRH-TSH test in subaffective dysthymia and character-spectrum disorder. J Affect Disord 28:287–291, 1993

Rosier YA, Broussolle P, Fontany M: [Lithium gluconate: systematic and factorial analysis of 104 cases which have been studied for 2 and one-half to 3 years in patients regularly observed and showing periodic cyclothymia or dysthymia] (French). Ann Med Psychol (Paris) 1:389–397, 1974

Sachar EJ: Twenty-four-hour cortisol secretory patterns in depressed and manic patients. Prog Brain Res 42:81–91, 1975

Sachar EJ, Halbreich U, Asnis GM, et al: Paradoxical cortisol responses to dextroamphetamine in endogenous depression. Arch Gen Psychiatry 38:1113–1117, 1981

Sachar EJ, Puig-Antich J, Ryan ND, et al: Three tests of cortisol secretion in adult endogenous depressives. Acta Psychiatr Scand 71:1–8, 1985

Saletu-Zyhlarz GM, Abu-Bakr MH, Anderer P, et al: Insomnia related to dysthymia: polysomnographic and psychometric comparison with normal controls and acute therapeutic trials with trazodone. Neuropsychobiology 44:139–149, 2001

Schlatter J, Ortuño F, Cervera-Enguix S: Differences in interleukins' patterns between dysthymia and major depression. Eur Psychiatry 16:317–319, 2001

Semadeni GW: [Clinical study of the normothymic effect of dipropylacetamide]. Acta Psychiatr Belg 76:458–466, 1976

Shankman SA, Klein DN: The impact of comorbid anxiety disorders on the course of dysthymic disorder: a 5-year prospective longitudinal study. J Affect Disord 70:211–217, 2002

Shelton RC, Davidson J, Yonkers KA, et al: The undertreatment of dysthymia. J Clin Psychiatry 58:59–65, 1997

Stewart JW, McGrath PJ, Rabkin JG, et al: Atypical depression: a valid clinical entity? Psychiatr Clin North Am 16:479–495, 1993

Stewart JW, Garfinkel R, Nunes EV, et al: Atypical features and treatment response in the National Institute of Mental Health Treatment of Depression Collaborative Research Program. J Clin Psychopharmacol 18:429–434, 1998

Stewart JW, McGrath PJ, Quitkin FM: Do age of onset and course of illness predict different treatment outcome among DSM IV depressive disorders with atypical features? Neuropsychopharmacology 26:237–245, 2002

Stewart JW, Bruder GE, McGrath PJ, et al: Do age of onset and course of illness define biologically distinct groups within atypical depression? J Abnorm Psychol 112:253–262, 2003

Stewart JW, Quitkin FM, McGrath PJ, et al: Defining the boundaries of atypical depression: evidence from the HPA axis supports course of illness distinctions. J Affect Disord 86:161–167, 2005

Sullivan PF, Kessler RC, Kendler KS: Latent class analysis of lifetime depressive symptoms in the National Comorbidity Survey. Am J Psychiatry 155:1398–1406, 1998

Szádóczky E, Fazekas I, Rihmer Z, et al: The role of psychosocial and biological variables in separating chronic and non-chronic major depression and early late-onset dysthymia. J Affect Disord 32:1–11, 1994

Waintraub L, Guelfi JD: Nosological validity of dysthymia, part 1: historical, epidemiological and clinical data. Eur Psychiatry 13:173–180, 1998

Weissman MM: Interpersonal psychotherapy: current status. Keio Journal of Medicine 46:105–110, 1997

Weissman MM, Myers JK: Affective disorders in a US urban community: the use of research diagnostic criteria in an epidemiological survey. Arch Gen Psychiatry 35:1304–1311, 1978

Weissman MM, Leaf PJ, Holzer CE III, et al: The epidemiology of depression: an update on sex differences in rates. J Affect Disord 7:179–188, 1984

Weissman MM, Leaf PJ, Bruce ML, et al: The epidemiology of dysthymia in five communities: rates, risks, comorbidity, and treatment. Am J Psychiatry 145:815–819, 1988

Weissman MM, Bland R, Joyce PR, et al: Sex differences in rates of depression: cross-national perspectives. J Affect Disord 29:77–84, 1993

Wells KB, Stewart A, Hays RD, et al: The functioning and well-being of depressed patients: results from the Medical Outcomes Study. JAMA 262:914–919, 1989

West ED, Dally PJ: Effects of iproniazid in depressive syndromes. BMJ 1:1491–1494, 1959

Wu JC, Buchsbaum MS, Johnson JC, et al: Magnetic resonance and positron emission tomography imaging of the corpus callosum: size, shape and metabolic rate in unipolar depression. J Affect Disord 28:15–25, 1993

Zisook S, Shuchter SR, Gallagher T, et al: Atypical depression in an outpatient psychiatric population. Depression 1:268–274, 1993

Zlotnick C, Kohn R, Keitner G, et al: The relationship between quality of interpersonal relationships and major depressive disorder: findings from the National Comorbidity Survey. J Affect Disord 59:205–215, 2000

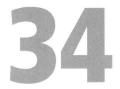

Psychotic Depression

BENJAMIN H. FLORES, M.D.
ALAN F. SCHATZBERG, M.D.

IN DSM-IV-TR (American Psychiatric Association 2000), psychotic depression is classified as a major depressive disorder, severe with psychotic features. This classification requires the usual criteria for a major depressive episode with the additional symptoms of hallucinations or delusions, which can be either mood-congruent or mood-incongruent. Data continue to emerge that support psychotic depression as a distinct clinical entity when compared with nonpsychotic depression. This distinction is based on statistically significant differences in presenting features, biology, familial transmission, course, and response to treatment between unipolar major depression with psychotic features and nonpsychotic major depression.

Epidemiology

In a sample of nearly 19,000 subjects across five European countries, nearly 20% of those who fulfilled criteria for major depression reported psychotic features (Ohayon and Schatzberg 2002). In this latter study, unipolar major depression with psychotic features was found to affect 4 in 1,000 individuals (Ohayon and Schatzberg 2002). Cross-sectional and 1-year prospective data from the Epidemiological Catchment Area study indicated that 14% of the

patients with major depression were classified as having psychotic features (Johnson et al. 1991). In a study of consecutively admitted depressed patients, approximately 25% were psychotically depressed (Coryell et al. 1984).

Genetics and Family History

Psychotic major depression is associated with a 10% concordance rate (Cardno et al. 1999), and specific patterns of familial transmission have been noted. A family history of schizophrenia has been reported to be more typically associated with psychotic depression as compared with nonpsychotic depression (Coryell et al. 1984). First-degree relatives of those with psychotic major depression also have been shown to have a greater likelihood of both major depression and psychotic major depression as compared with first-degree relatives of subjects with nonpsychotic major depression (Leckman et al. 1984; S. Simpson et al. 1999). A higher rate of bipolar disorder also has been reported among first-degree relatives of subjects with psychotic major depression as compared with first-degree relatives of subjects with nonpsychotic major depression (Schatzberg and Rothschild 1992; Weissman et al. 1988).

Interestingly, subjects with major depressive disorder, severe with mood-incongruent psychotic features, appear to have family histories more similar to those reported for patients with schizophrenia (Coryell et al. 1982, 1985). Furthermore, data have suggested a trend toward a much lower risk for family history of affective illness among subjects with major depressive disorder, severe with mood-incongruent psychotic features, as compared with those with mood-congruent psychotic features (Maj et al. 1991). In contrast, subjects with major depressive disorder, severe with mood-congruent psychotic features, have been found to have family histories more consistent with those found among patients with nonpsychotic major depressive disorder and significantly different from those found in schizophrenic patients (Coryell et al. 1982).

Symptomatology

Differences Between Psychotic and Nonpsychotic Major Depression in Symptomatology and Comorbidity

Subjects with psychotic major depression have been reported to experience more severe depressive symptoms when compared with subjects with nonpsychotic major depression (Coryell et al. 1985). Psychotic major depression has been associated with younger age at onset than nonpsychotic major depression (Black et al. 1992).

Psychotic major depression in patients older than 50 years is associated with both longer duration of illness and lower comorbidity as compared with psychotic major depression in patients younger than 50 years (Benazzi 1999b). Among patients with a major depressive episode older than 50 years, psychotic major depression is associated with significantly greater severity, lower comorbidity, greater likelihood of diagnosis of bipolar I disorder, and lower likelihood of unipolar disorder as compared with nonpsychotic major depression (Benazzi 1999b).

Bipolar and unipolar disorder with psychotic features have been reported to show no significant differences in age, gender, duration of illness, severity, recurrences, chronicity, comorbidity, hallucinations, and delusions (Benazzi 1999a).

Symptoms Highly Correlated With Psychotic Major Depression

A retrospective study of patients with major depression found that subjects with psychotic major depression were more ruminative, had more feelings of guilt, and showed more psychomotor agitation (Charney and Nelson 1981). Overall, feelings of worthlessness, guilt, and suicidal ideation have been found to be highly associated with symp-

toms of psychosis in psychotic depression (Ohayon and Schatzberg 2002). In a study of patients with major depression, psychotic major depression was found to be most commonly associated with psychomotor disturbance, feeling sinful and guilty, feeling deserving of punishment, constipation, terminal insomnia, appetite and weight loss, and loss of pleasure and interest (Parker et al. 1995). In fact, both of these latter studies suggested that the presence of these highly associated nonpsychotic features may be indicative of the diagnosis of psychotic major depression in the absence of psychosis being elicited or acknowledged (Ohayon and Schatzberg 2002; Parker et al. 1995).

Psychotic Features

Psychotic depression appears to show a high rate of stability of diagnosis on follow-up (Schwartz et al. 2000), with the form and content of delusional thinking being consistent across recurrent episodes (Charney and Nelson 1981). According to DSM-IV-TR, in psychotic major depressive disorder, the psychotic features are classified as either mood-congruent or mood-incongruent. Interestingly, a study of patients hospitalized for a diagnosis of psychotic major depression found that 50%–60% of the subjects experienced both mood-congruent and mood-incongruent psychotic features (Burch et al. 1994). In addition, this latter study reported that approximately half of the subjects with mood-incongruent features experienced at least one mood-congruent symptom (Burch et al. 1994). Also, approximately two-thirds of the patients with mood-congruent features experienced at least one mood-incongruent symptom (Burch et al. 1994). Thus, it has been suggested that the subclassification of major depressive disorder, severe with psychotic features, into mood-congruent and mood-incongruent may be an artificial one because features of both are commonly encountered together (Burch et al. 1994).

The presence of psychotic features in major depression has been associated with greater levels of both morbidity and impairment in insight as compared with those with nonpsychotic major depression.

For example, compared with nonpsychotic depression, patients with psychotic depression are more likely to have been ill for a longer time and to have experienced more episodes of depression (Leyton et al. 1995). Analysis of data from the Netherlands Mental Health Survey and Incidence Study (NEMESIS) found that patients with psychotic major depression had the greatest levels of physical, psychological, and social functioning impairment among all levels of severity of depression, including severe, nonpsychotic depression (Kruijshaar et al. 2003).

Furthermore, when the Scale to Assess Unawareness of Mental Disorders was used to compare various psychotic disorders, subjects with psychotic depression showed a lack of insight into the presence of symptoms such as hallucinations, delusions, and thought disorder comparable to that of patients with schizophrenia, schizoaffective disorder, and bipolar disorder (Pini et al. 2001).

Neuropsychological Impairments

Patients with psychotic major depression have been shown to have a pattern of neuropsychological dysfunction that is distinct from that of nonpsychotic major depression (Belanoff et al. 2001b; Fleming et al. 2004; Hill et al. 2004; Jeste et al. 1996; Schatzberg et al. 2000). Subjects with psychotic major depression have been shown to perform significantly more poorly on measures of visual memory and visual-spatial perception as compared with subjects with nonpsychotic major depression (Hill et al. 2004). Significantly greater impairment on measures of psychomotor speed, motor skills, attention, and learning also has been reported in elderly subjects with psychotic major depression as compared with those with nonpsychotic major depression (Jeste et al. 1996). Subjects with psychotic depression have been shown to have significantly greater impairment on tests of attention, response inhibition, and verbal declarative memory as compared with patients with nonpsychotic depression (Schatzberg et al. 2000). In addition, subjects with psychotic major depression have been found to show a significantly greater impairment in verbal recognition memory as compared with subjects with nonpsychotic major depression (Belanoff et al. 2001b). Overall, the most consistently reported deficits in cognitive performance that have been associated with psychotic major depression as compared with nonpsychotic major depression occur on measures of verbal memory, executive functioning, and psychomotor speed (Fleming et al. 2004).

Interestingly, the pattern of neuropsychological dysfunction among subjects with psychotic major depression appears to be similar to that seen in schizophrenia (Hill et al. 2004; Jeste et al. 1996). In a study of first-episode, antipsychotic-naïve patients, both those with psychotic depression and those with schizophrenia showed a similar pattern of neuropsychological impairment on measures of verbal memory, visual memory, motor skills, and visual-spatial abilities (Hill et al. 2004). This latter study, however, found a degree of impairment for subjects with psychotic major depression that was less severe than was found among schizophrenic subjects (Hill et al. 2004). In contrast, another study comparing neuropsychological performance in elderly subjects with schizophrenia and elderly subjects with psychotic major depression reported comparable degrees of neuropsychological impairment for both groups (Jeste et al. 1996).

Comorbidity

Panic disorder, obsessive-compulsive disorder, and social phobia may be commonly comorbid with affective psychoses, such as psychotic depression (Cassano et al. 1999). In a study of first-admission psychotic patients, more than 50% and 35% of male and female subjects with psychotic depression, respectively, fulfilled criteria for at least one substance use disorder (Rabinowitz et al. 1998). In addition, subjects with psychotic depression have been found to have a higher rate of Cluster A personality disorders and lower levels of education as compared with subjects with nonpsychotic depression (Serretti et al. 1999).

Pathogenesis

Psychotic depression is more frequently and consistently associated with biological abnormalities as compared with nonpsychotic depression. For instance, negative life events are less likely to be associated with psychotic depression than with nonpsychotic depression (Kohn et al. 2001).

Neurophysiology

Psychotic major depression is associated with significantly increased wakefulness, decreased rapid eye movement (REM) sleep percentage, decreased REM activity, and decreased sleep-onset REM latencies as compared with nonpsychotic major depression (Thase et al. 1986).

Abnormalities of the P300 component of event-related potentials have been suggested as clinical correlates of psychotic depression. For instance, although prolonged P300 latency has been associated with clinical depression, decreased P300 amplitude has been correlated with paranoid ideation in psychotic major depression (Karaaslan et al. 2003). In addition, it also has been shown that P300 abnormalities, both prolonged latency and decreased amplitude, resolve with successful drug treatment of psychotic major depression (Karaaslan et al. 2003).

Neuroendocrinology

Psychotic major depression is consistently and commonly associated with more severe abnormalities of the hypothalamic-pituitary-adrenocortical axis when compared with nonpsychotic major depression (Coryell et al. 1984). We hypothesized years ago that increased cortisol activity could enhance mesolimbic dopamine and could explain the development of psychosis in psychotic major depression (Schatzberg et al. 1985). For instance, significantly higher plasma dopamine levels have been reported among subjects with psychotic major depression compared with subjects with nonpsychotic major depression (Rothschild et al. 1987). Similarly, significantly higher plasma dopamine levels have been reported among subjects with psychotic major depression compared with patients with nonpsychotic major depression in response to a 1-mg dose of dexamethasone (Rothschild et al. 1987). More recently, Lupien and colleagues (1995) have reported that metyrapone, a glucocorticoid synthesis blocker, results in increases in plasma homovanillic acid, a dopamine metabolite, in healthy control subjects, suggesting that cortisol may result in decreased dopamine activity. Thus, the earlier effects of dexamethasone on plasma dopamine may reflect a rebound effect of rising corticotropin-releasing hormone on dopamine. In rats, we have reported that corticosterone decreases prefrontal dopamine metabolism, an effect that could account for the prefrontal cognitive deficits seen in the disorder (Lindley et al. 1999, 2002). Indeed, in squirrel monkeys, we have observed that cortisol results in prefrontal cognitive defects similar to those seen with dopamine depletion (Lyons et al. 2000).

In addition, the mean plasma activity of dopamine β-hydroxylase, the enzyme that converts dopamine to norepinephrine, has been reported to be significantly lower among patients with psychotic major depression as compared with subjects with nonpsychotic major depression (Cubells et al. 2002). However, no association between specific dopamine β-hydroxylase alleles and psychotic major depression has been shown (Cubells et al. 2002).

Subjects with psychotic major depression have been found to have significantly elevated cortisol levels after administration of dexamethasone as compared with subjects with nonpsychotic major depression and control subjects (Maes et al. 1989; Rothschild et al. 1982; Schatzberg et al. 1983). A positive dexamethasone suppression test result has been reported to be a statistically significant correlate of psychotic depression (Vythilingam et al. 2003). Subjects with psychotic major depression have been shown to have a significantly higher rate of positive dexamethasone suppression test results compared with subjects with nonpsychotic major depression (J.C. Nelson and Davis 1997; Rihmer et al. 1984). Predexamethasone studies of cortisol (e.g., urinary free cortisol) have reported it to be significantly elevated in patients with psychotic major depression (Anton 1987; W.H. Nelson et al. 1984).

In a study assessing 24-hour cortisol and corticotrophin secretion, nonpsychotic major depression was most associated with reduced amplitude of cortisol secretion relative to control subjects (Posener et al. 2000). In contrast, this latter study found that subjects with psychotic major depression had significantly increased corticotropin secretion compared with control subjects (Posener et al. 2000). In a study assessing patterns of afternoon cortisol secretion among depressed and healthy subjects, subjects with psychotic major depression were found to have significantly higher mean and a nonlinear pattern of cortisol levels throughout the afternoon (Belanoff et al. 2001b). Most recently, we have reported elevated nocturnal cortisol levels in patients with psychotic depression (Flores et al., in review).

Neuroimaging

A computed tomographic study of depressed subjects found significantly larger ventricle-to-brain ratios and inferior parietal brain atrophy among subjects with psychotic depression that were associated with nonsuppression on the dexamethasone suppression test and greater impairment on cognitive testing (Rothschild et al. 1989).

A single photon emission computed tomography study of subjects with major depression compared with healthy control subjects found that those with psychotic major depression had significantly decreased regional cerebral blood flow in both the left subgenual anterior cingulate cortex and the right inferior frontal cortex as compared with those with nonpsychotic major depression (Skaf et al. 2002).

Magnetic resonance imaging studies of late-life depression have reported significant atrophy in specific brain regions. In one study, S. Simpson et al. (1999) found the strongest correlates of psychotic features to be with diencephalic atrophy, reticular activating system lesions, brain stem atrophy, and left-sided frontotemporal atrophy. Similarly, Kim et al. (1999) reported prefrontal atrophy in elderly patients with psychotic depression. Of interest, in a review of studies examining cognitive deficits in psychotic depression, we noted that the most commonly reported areas of impairment corresponded to cognitive domains thought to be mediated by frontal and medial temporal brain regions (Fleming et al. 2004).

Treatment

Various data have been put forth supporting the efficacy of electroconvulsive therapy (ECT) and combination antidepressant and antipsychotic therapies in the treatment of psychotic major depression. Most studies clearly indicate that ECT and combination antidepressant and antipsychotic interventions are superior to antidepressant therapy alone in the treatment of psychotic major depression. Psychotic major depression has, in general, also been associated with a lower placebo response rate when compared with nonpsychotic major depression. Furthermore, ECT appears to be more likely to be effective in psychotic major depression than in nonpsychotic major depression.

Placebo Response

Generally, data examining placebo response in psychotic major depression have been derived from single-blind, run-in studies. Spiker and Kupfer (1988) reviewed placebo response rates in psychotic major depression versus nonpsychotic major depression and found response rates of 0% and 13.3%, respectively. A recent controlled comparison of olanzapine, fluoxetine, and placebo reported higher placebo response rates (approximately 28%) in a parallel, non-placebo washout design (Rothschild et al. 2004).

Antidepressant Monotherapy

Glassman et al. (1977), in their classic study on imipramine blood levels and response in hospitalized depressed patients, noted that patients with psychotic major depression had poor responses to imipramine monotherapy. Two early retrospective studies of patients with major depression (Brown et al. 1982; Charney and Nelson 1981) reported that in contrast to patients with nonpsychotic depression, subjects with psychotic depression had a poor response to antidepressant monotherapy but had a good response to either combination antidepressant and antipsychotic therapy or ECT. These observations were followed by a prospective comparison study of 35 patients with psychotic depression who received amitriptyline, perphenazine, or the combination (Spiker et al. 1986). In this latter study, combination therapy was found to be significantly more effective than either component alone. A 6-week study of imipramine, dosed to a target blood level of 200–300 µg/L, in the treatment of major depression found a response rate of 69% and 44%, respectively, for subjects with psychotic depression and those with nonpsychotic depression (Bruijn et al. 2001).

More recent antidepressant studies have concentrated on the selective serotonin reuptake inhibitors (SSRIs). An 8-week open-label study of patients with major depression treated with sertraline monotherapy found a significantly lower likelihood of achieving 50% reduction or complete remission of symptoms among patients with psychotic major depression as compared with nonpsy-

chotic major depression (G.M. Simpson et al. 2003). In this study, psychosis was found to be a predictor of response independent of degree of depression and general psychopathology.

In contrast, a 6-week study of patients with psychotic depression found a response rate of 84% for open-label fluvoxamine monotherapy (Gatti et al. 1996). Similarly, a 6-week prospective, randomized, double-blind study of subjects with psychotic major depression treated with either venlafaxine or fluvoxamine monotherapy found response rates of 58% and 79%, respectively (Zanardi et al. 2000). A 6-week double-blind study of subjects with psychotic major depression found response rates of 75% and 46% for sertraline and paroxetine monotherapy, respectively (Zanardi et al. 1996). Overall, however, these data do not agree with the general United States experience, and questions have been raised as to the consistency in diagnoses between Europe and the United States.

Combination Antidepressant and Antipsychotic Therapy

The early study of Spiker et al. (1985b) reported response rates of approximately 78%, 41%, and 19%, respectively, for amitriptyline plus perphenazine, amitriptyline alone, and perphenazine alone.

Similarly, a response rate of 73% was reported for patients with psychotic depression treated for 5 weeks with fluoxetine plus perphenazine (Rothschild et al. 1993a). It is notable that this latter study found an overall lower likelihood of side effects with this combination as compared with the combination of a tricyclic antidepressant and an antipsychotic (Rothschild et al. 1993a).

A 6-week study comparing the efficacy of haloperidol and amitriptyline with that of risperidone monotherapy found the former to be significantly superior in the treatment of psychotic depression on measures of depression and the Brief Psychiatric Rating Scale (BPRS) (Muller-Schneider et al. 1998).

Olanzapine may be an effective adjunctive therapy and monotherapy intervention in the treatment of psychotic major depression because of its antipsychotic and potential antidepressant properties (E.B. Nelson et al. 2001; Rothschild et al. 1999). An open-label study of patients with psychotic major depressive disorder treated with olanzapine combined with fluoxetine found an overall response rate of 55.6% and a remission rate of 40.7% at 6 weeks (Matthews et al. 2002). However, a report on combined data from two parallel 8-week double-blind studies of patients with major depression with psychotic features reported response rates of 63.6% for those treated with a combination of olanzapine and fluoxetine,

34.9% for olanzapine monotherapy, and 28.0% for placebo treatment (Rothschild et al. 2004). Interestingly, when this single analysis was divided into two studies, one of the two trials failed to show statistically significant superiority for the combination of olanzapine and fluoxetine (Rothschild et al. 2004).

Electroconvulsive Therapy

In a study of 55 consecutively admitted inpatients with major depression, ECT was associated with significantly greater likelihood of achieving a 50% reduction in symptoms (92% vs. 55%) and complete remission (57% vs. 24%) of symptoms among patients with psychotic depression than among patients with nonpsychotic depression (Birkenhager et al. 2003). Similarly, a study of 37 patients with psychotic depression found a response rate of 86% for ECT (Spiker et al. 1985a).

Treatment-Refractory Psychotic Depression

Among patients with psychotic depression refractory to combined antidepressant and antipsychotic therapy, lithium has been reported as an effective augmentation strategy (J.C. Nelson and Mazure 1986; Price et al. 1983). In an open-label study of six patients with psychotic depression refractory to combination therapy, lithium augmentation resulted in significant improvement in symptoms in three subjects and a more gradual improvement in two (Price et al. 1983). In contrast, another study reported lithium augmentation to be effective in 8 of 9 patients with bipolar, but in only 3 of 12 with unipolar, refractory psychotic depression (J.C. Nelson and Mazure 1986).

Adequacy and Duration of Treatment

Data have suggested that psychotic major depression is often inadequately treated. In a study of 187 depressed patients referred for ECT, only 4% of the subjects with psychotic major depression had received at least one adequate antidepressant and antipsychotic medication trial, and 47% of the subjects with psychotic major depression either had received no antipsychotic medication or had received antipsychotic treatment for less than 3 weeks (Mulsant et al. 1997). In contrast, this latter study reported that more than 50% of the subjects with nonpsychotic major depression had received at least one adequate medication trial (Mulsant et al. 1997). On the basis of the above data, it has been suggested that several of the patients classified as treatment-refractory depressed, especially among those referred for ECT, were actually subjects with unidentified psychosis who also had been

prescribed inadequate pharmacotherapy (Fink 2003a, 2003b). These latter concerns underscore the importance of both distinguishing psychotic depression from nonpsychotic depression and improving the diagnostic criteria by which this condition is defined.

The findings of a recent study that followed up patients with psychotic depression for 11 months after discontinuation of both antidepressant and antipsychotic therapy suggested that antipsychotic therapy should be continued for at least 4 months after remission of psychosis symptoms (Rothschild and Duval 2003). In this latter study, 73% of the subjects with psychotic depression who initially responded to combination fluoxetine and perphenazine therapy remained remitted at study end and after discontinuation of the antipsychotic at 4 months and discontinuation of the antidepressant at 12 months (Rothschild and Duval 2003).

Novel Strategies

Amoxapine has been suggested as a potential monotherapy in the treatment of psychotic depression because of its combined antidepressant and antipsychotic properties. A double-blind study comparing amoxapine monotherapy with amitriptyline combined with perphenazine in the treatment of psychotic depression found overall comparable improvements in depression and psychosis but significantly fewer extrapyramidal side effects among those receiving amoxapine (Anton and Burch 1990).

Recent studies have suggested that glucocorticoid receptor antagonists may be useful in the treatment of psychotic depression. In a 4-day double-blind, placebo-controlled, crossover study, five subjects with psychotic depression treated with the glucocorticoid receptor antagonist mifepristone, 600 mg/day, had greater improvement in BPRS, Hamilton Rating Scale for Depression (21-item; Ham-D-21), and Clinical Global Impression Scale scores while receiving the active drug (Belanoff et al. 2001a). Interestingly, this latter study found that at the conclusion of the 9-day study, four of the five patients were no longer psychotic, and all subjectively noted improved cognitive abilities (Belanoff et al. 2001a).

Another study that compared the efficacy of 50 mg, 600 mg, or 1,200 mg of mifepristone for 7 days in subjects with psychotic major depression found that 13 of 19 individuals (68.4%) in the latter two groups showed at least a 30% decline in BPRS score, 12 of 19 (63.2%) showed a 50% decrease in BPRS positive symptoms subscale score, and 8 of 19 (42.1%) had a 50% decline in Ham-D-21 score (Belanoff et al. 2002). In contrast, among those in the 50-mg group, 4 of 11 (36.4%) showed at least a 30% decline in BPRS score, 3 of 11 (27.3%) had a 50% decrease in BPRS positive symptoms subscale score, and 2 of 11 (18.2%) had a 50% decline in Ham-D-21 score (Belanoff et al. 2002).

Recently, we found that in 30 patients randomly assigned to receive mifepristone or placebo, significantly more mifepristone-treated patients showed a 50% reduction in BPRS positive symptoms than those given placebo (B.H. Flores H. Kenna, J. Keller, et al.: "Clinical and Biological Effects of Mifepristone Treatment for Psychotic Depression," unpublished data, May 2005).

Course and Follow-Up

In a study examining diagnostic predictors among 45 inpatients with major depression, psychotic features were found to predict an unfavorable course (Maier et al. 1989). According to 1-year prospective data from the Epidemiological Catchment Area study, psychotic major depression when compared with nonpsychotic major depression was associated with an overall more severe course, increased risk of relapse, persistence of symptoms over 1 year, suicide attempts, hospitalization, comorbid psychiatric diagnoses, and greater impairment in psychosocial functioning (Johnson et al. 1991). Similarly, a study of patients with either psychotic major depression or nonpsychotic major depression, assessed at 1 year after discharge from inpatient treatment, found that those with psychotic major depression had an overall poorer clinical course, a greater likelihood of depression lasting longer than 9 months, and a greater likelihood of being in a depressive episode at follow-up (Robinson and Spiker 1985). We reported that at 1-year follow-up, patients with psychotic major depression had significantly poorer psychosocial function than did patients with nonpsychotic major depression (Rothschild et al. 1993b). In this study, the two groups did not differ on measures of depression or psychosis at follow-up.

In a study examining the risk of relapse of symptoms in subjects with psychotic depression treated with fluoxetine and perphenazine, it was reported that patients who had signs of relapse after discontinuation of antipsychotic therapy at 4 months were more likely to have had a longer duration of the current episode, to have had a history of more frequent episodes, and to be younger (Rothschild and Duval 2003).

Despite an initial response rate of 80%–90% to acute treatment with ECT, patients with psychotic depression are found to have a high relapse rate (50%) at 1-year follow-up (Spiker et al. 1985a).

A 2-year follow-up study of patients with major depression found significantly greater levels of psychosocial impairment both in the 5 years preceding study entry and at the 6-month follow-up among subjects with psychotic major depression than among subjects with nonpsychotic major depression (Coryell et al. 1987). Interestingly, this latter study also reported that at 2-year follow-up, the significant differences in psychosocial impairment between psychotic major depression and nonpsychotic major depression had resolved (Coryell et al. 1987).

A 40-year follow-up study of patients with psychotic depression found that mood-incongruent psychotic features were associated with a long-term outcome intermediate between nonpsychotic depression and schizophrenia (Coryell and Tsuang 1985). In contrast, subjects with major depression with mood-congruent psychotic features in this latter study had a long-term outcome that was similar to that of subjects with nonpsychotic depression (Coryell and Tsuang 1985). However, an 8-year follow-up of patients with psychotic depression found the prognosis of those with mood-incongruent psychotic features to be comparable to the prognosis of those with mood-congruent psychotic features (Tsuang and Coryell 1993).

In a study of patients with major depression followed up for up to 15 years after hospital admission, those with psychotic features, as compared with those without psychotic features, had a twofold greater mortality rate (41% vs. 20%) (Vythilingam et al. 2003).

In a study of patients admitted for a first episode of psychotic depression, nearly one in eight developed symptoms of mania or hypomania within 2 years after discharge (DelBello et al. 2003). Interestingly, this latter study also found that antidepressant treatment was associated with a significantly reduced risk of developing a manic or hypomanic episode (DelBello et al. 2003).

Suicide

Elevated suicide risk was first reported in a retrospective study at New York State Psychiatric Institute (Roose et al. 1983). This risk also has been reported by others. For example, psychotic depression was associated with a greater lifetime risk of suicide attempts as compared with schizophrenia—42.4% and 27.3%, respectively (Radomsky et al. 1999). Furthermore, a violent means of suicide appears to be more commonly associated with psychotic major depression as compared with nonpsychotic major depression (Isometsa et al. 1994). A retrospective study of 45 inpatients with a diagnosis of psychotic depression found delusions of persecution and guilt to be significantly associated with a greater likelihood of making a medically serious suicide attempt (Miller and Chabrier 1987, 1988). In contrast, psychotic depression with delusions of bodily disease, damage, and malfunction has been found to be associated with a significantly lower likelihood of medically serious suicide attempt (Miller and Chabrier 1987). Although these data point to increased risk of suicide in psychotic depression, the Collaborative Depression Study failed to find an increased rate at 5-year follow-up (Fawcett et al. 1987).

Conclusion

Psychotic depression is a relatively common psychiatric condition that affects up to 20% of patients with major depression. Psychotic depression appears distinct from nonpsychotic depression on the basis of noted differences in family psychiatric histories, with an increased risk of schizophrenia, bipolar affective disorder, and unipolar depression reported. Psychotic depression is also differentiated from nonpsychotic depression by the greater severity of depressive symptoms. Psychotic depression is more commonly associated with feelings of guilt, worthlessness, and suicidal ideation in addition to, and highly correlated with, symptoms of psychosis. Psychotic depression also has been found to be characterized by a specific pattern of neuropsychological impairment that appears to overlap with that observed in schizophrenia. Psychotic depression distinguishes itself from nonpsychotic depression because of differences in neurophysiology, neuroendocrinology, and neuroimaging findings.

Psychotic depression is generally associated with low placebo response rate and poor response to antidepressant monotherapy, although recent data have raised questions about the validity of these findings. Data thus far best support efficacy for the combination of an antidepressant and an antipsychotic or ECT in the treatment of psychotic depression. Data are limited on the utility of lithium augmentation in treatment-refractory psychotic depression. Recent findings suggest the possible utility of glucocorticoid receptor antagonists in the treatment of psychotic depression.

In addition, studies have shown that psychotic depression is associated with a greater risk of relapse, suicide, mortality, and poor long-term psychosocial functioning as compared with nonpsychotic depression. Unfortunately, data also have been put forth suggesting that psychotic depression may be frequently underdiagnosed and undertreated. Such findings greatly underscore the importance of both distinguishing psychotic depression from nonpsychotic depression and improving the diagnostic criteria for and treatment of this condition.

In summary, data support psychotic depression as a distinct clinical entity from nonpsychotic depression. This distinction is based on statistically significant differences in presenting features, biology, familial transmission, course, and response to treatment between psychotic depression and nonpsychotic depression.

References

American Psychiatric Association: Diagnostic and Statistical Manual of Mental Disorders, 4th Edition, Text Revision. Washington, DC, American Psychiatric Association, 2000

Anton RF: Urinary free cortisol in psychotic depression. Biol Psychiatry 22:24–34, 1987

Anton RF, Burch EA: Amoxapine versus amitriptyline combined with perphenazine in the treatment of psychotic depression. Am J Psychiatry 147:1203–1208, 1990

Belanoff JK, Flores BH, Kalehzan M, et al: Rapid reversal of psychotic depression using mifepristone. J Clin Psychopharmacol 21:516–521, 2001a

Belanoff JK, Kalehzan M, Sund B, et al: Cortisol activity and cognitive changes in psychotic major depression. Am J Psychiatry 158:1612–1616, 2001b

Belanoff JK, Rothschild AJ, Cassidy F, et al: An open label trial of C-1073 (mifepristone) for psychotic major depression. Biol Psychiatry 52:386–392, 2002

Benazzi F: Bipolar versus unipolar psychotic outpatient depression. J Affect Disord 55:63–66, 1999a

Benazzi F: Psychotic late-life depression: a 376-case study. Int Psychogeriatr 11:325–332, 1999b

Birkenhager TK, Pluijms EM, Lucius SAP: ECT response in delusional versus non-delusional depressed inpatients. J Affect Disord 74:191–195, 2003

Black DW, Winokur G, Nasrallah A, et al: Psychotic symptoms and age of onset in affective disorders. Psychopathology 25:19–22, 1992

Brown RP, Frances A, Kocsis JH, et al: Psychotic versus nonpsychotic depression: comparison of treatment response. J Nerv Ment Dis 170:635–637, 1982

Bruijn JA, Moleman P, Mulder PGH, et al: Treatment of mood-congruent psychotic depression with imipramine. J Affect Disord 66:165–174, 2001

Burch EA, Anton RF, Carson WH: Mood congruent and incongruent psychotic depressions: are they the same? J Affect Disord 31:275–280, 1994

Cardno AG, Marshall EJ, Coid B, et al: Heritability estimates for psychotic disorders. Arch Gen Psychiatry 56:162–168, 1999

Cassano GB, Pini S, Saettoni M, et al: Multiple anxiety disorder comorbidity in patients with mood spectrum disorders with psychotic features. Am J Psychiatry 156:474–476, 1999

Charney DS, Nelson JC: Delusional and nondelusional unipolar depression: further evidence for distinct subtypes. Am J Psychiatry 138:328–333, 1981

Coryell W, Tsuang MT: Major depression with mood-congruent or mood-incongruent psychotic features: outcome after 40 years. Am J Psychiatry 142:479–482, 1985

Coryell W, Tsuang MT, McDaniel J: Psychotic features in major depression: is mood congruence important? J Affect Disord 4:227–236, 1982

Coryell W, Pfohl B, Zimmerman M: The clinical and neuroendocrine features of psychotic depression. J Nerv Ment Dis 172:521–528, 1984

Coryell W, Endicott J, Keller M, et al: Phenomenology and family history in DSM-III psychotic depression. J Affect Disord 9:13–18, 1985

Coryell W, Endicott J, Keller M: The importance of psychotic features to major depression: course and outcome during a 2-year follow-up. Acta Psychiatr Scand 75:78–85, 1987

Cubells JF, Price LH, Meyers BS, et al: Genotype-controlled analysis of plasma dopamine B-hydroxylase activity in psychotic major depression. Biol Psychiatry 51:358–364, 2002

DelBello MP, Carlson GA, Tohen M, et al: Rates and predictors of developing a manic or hypomanic episode 1 to 2 years following a first hospitalization for major depression with psychotic features. J Child Adolesc Psychopharmacol 13:173–185, 2003

Fawcett J, Scheftner W, Clark D, et al: Clinical predictors of suicide in patients with major affective disorders: a controlled prospective study. Am J Psychiatry 144:35–40, 1987

Fink M: Electroconvulsive therapy update: recognizing and treating psychotic depression. J Clin Psychiatry 64:232–234, 2003a

Fink M: Separating psychotic depression from nonpsychotic depression is essential to effective treatment. J Affect Disord 76:1–3, 2003b

Fleming SK, Blasey C, Schatzberg AF: Neuropsychological correlates of psychotic features in depressive disorders: a review and meta-analysis. J Psychiatr Res 38:27–35, 2004

Gatti F, Bellini L, Gasperini M, et al: Fluvoxamine alone in the treatment of delusional depression. Am J Psychiatry 153:414–416, 1996

Glassman AH, Perez JM, Shostak M, et al: Clinical implications of imipramine plasma levels for depressive illness. Arch Gen Psychiatry 34:197–204, 1977

Hill SK, Keshavan MS, Thase ME, et al: Neuropsychological dysfunction in antipsychotic naïve first-episode unipolar psychotic depression. Am J Psychiatry 161:996–1003, 2004

Isometsa E, Henriksson M, Aro H, et al: Suicide in psychotic major depression. J Affect Disord 31:187–191, 1994

Jeste DV, Heaton SC, Paulsen JS, et al: Clinical and neuropsychological comparison of psychotic depression with nonpsychotic depression and schizophrenia. Am J Psychiatry 153:490–496, 1996

Johnson J, Horwath E, Weissman MM: The validity of major depression with psychotic features based on a community study. Arch Gen Psychiatry 48:1075–1081, 1991

Karaaslan F, Gonul AS, Oguz A, et al: P300 changes in major depressive disorders with and without psychotic features. J Affect Disord 73:283–287, 2003

Kim DK, Kim BL, Sohn SE, et al: Candidate neuroanatomic substrates of psychosis in old-aged depression. Prog Neuropsychopharmacol Biol Psychiatry 23:793–807, 1999

Kohn Y, Zislin J, Agid O, et al: Increased prevalence of negative life events in subtypes of major depressive disorder. Compr Psychiatry 42:57–63, 2001

Kruijshaar ME, Hoeymans N, Bijl RV, et al: Levels of disability in major depression findings from the Netherlands Mental Health Survey and Incidence Study (NEMESIS). J Affect Disord 77:53–64, 2003

Leckman JF, Weissman MM, Prusoff BA, et al: Subtypes of depression: family study perspective. Arch Gen Psychiatry 41:833–838, 1984

Leyton M, Corin E, Martial J, et al: Psychotic symptoms and vulnerability to recurrent major depression. J Affect Disord 33:107–115, 1995

Lindley SE, Bengoechea TG, Schatzberg AF, et al: Glucocorticoid effects on mesotelencephalic dopamine neurotransmission. Neuropsychopharmacology 21:399–407, 1999

Lindley SE, Bengoechea TG, Wong DL, et al: Mesotelencephalic dopamine neurochemical responses to glucocorticoid administration and adrenalectomy in Fischer 344 and Lewis rats. Brain Res 958:414–422, 2002

Lupien S, Richter R, Risch SG, et al: Time course of the corticosteroid-dopaminergic interaction during metyrapone and dexamethasone administration. Psychiatry Res 58:23–35, 1995

Lyons DM, Lopez JM, Yang C, et al: Stress-level cortisol treatment impairs inhibitory control of behavior in monkeys. J Neurosci 20:7816–7821, 2000

Maes M, Minner B, Suy E: The influence of dexamethasone levels on the predictive value of the DST for unipolar major depression and the relationships between post-dexamethasone cortisol and ACTH levels. J Affect Disord 17:39–46, 1989

Maier W, Philipp M, Schlegel S, et al: Diagnostic determinants of response to treatment with tricyclic antidepressants: a polydiagnostic approach. Psychiatry Res 30:83–93, 1989

Maj M, Starace F, Pirozzi R: A family study of DSM-III-R schizoaffective disorder, depressive type, compared with schizophrenia and psychotic and nonpsychotic major depression. Am J Psychiatry 148:612–616, 1991

Matthews JD, Bottonari KA, Polania LM, et al: An open study of olanzapine and fluoxetine for psychotic major depressive disorder: interim analyses. J Clin Psychiatry 63:1164–1170, 2002

Miller F, Chabrier LA: The relation of delusional content in psychotic depression to life-threatening behavior. Suicide Life Threat Behav 17:13–17, 1987

Miller FT, Chabrier LA: Suicide attempts correlate with delusional content in major depression. Psychopathology 21:34–37, 1988

Muller-Schneider F, Muller MJ, Hillbert A, et al: Risperidone versus haloperidol and amitriptyline in the treatment of patients with a combined psychotic and depressive syndrome. J Clin Psychopharmacol 18:111–120, 1998

Mulsant B, Haskett RF, Prudic J, et al: Low use of neuroleptic drugs in the treatment of psychotic major depression. Am J Psychiatry 154:559–561, 1997

Nelson EB, Rielage E, Welge JA, et al: An open trial of olanzapine in the treatment of patients with psychotic depression. Ann Clin Psychiatry 13:147–151, 2001

Nelson JC, Davis JM: DST studies in psychotic depression: a meta analysis. Am J Psychiatry 154:1497–1503, 1997

Nelson JC, Mazure CM: Lithium augmentation in psychotic depression refractory to combined drug treatment. Am J Psychiatry 143:363–366, 1986

Nelson WH, Khan A, Orr WW: Delusional depression: phenomenology, neuroendocrine function, and tricyclic antidepressant response. J Affect Disord 6:297–306, 1984

Ohayon MM, Schatzberg AF: Prevalence of depressive episodes with psychotic features in the general population. Am J Psychiatry 159:1855–1861, 2002

Parker G, Hadzi-Pavlovic D, Brodaty H, et al: Subtyping depression, II: clinical distinction of psychotic depression and nonpsychotic melancholia. Psychol Med 25:825–832, 1995

Pini S, Cassano GB, Dell'Osso L, et al: Insight into illness in schizophrenia, schizoaffective disorder, and mood disorders with psychotic features. Am J Psychiatry 158:122–125, 2001

Posener JA, DeBattista C, Williams GH, et al: 24-Hour monitoring of cortisol and corticotrophin secretion in psychotic and nonpsychotic major depression. Arch Gen Psychiatry 57:755–760, 2000

Price LH, Conwell Y, Nelson JC: Lithium augmentation of combined neuroleptic-tricyclic treatment in delusional depression. Am J Psychiatry 140:318–322, 1983

Rabinowitz J, Bromet EJ, Lavelle J, et al: Prevalence and severity of substance use disorders and onset of psychosis in first-admission psychotic patients. Psychol Med 28:1411–1419, 1998

Radomsky ED, Haas GL, Mann JJ, et al: Suicidal behavior in patients with schizophrenia and other psychotic disorders. Am J Psychiatry 156:1590–1595, 1999

Rihmer Z, Arato M, Szadoczky E, et al: The dexamethasone suppression test in psychotic versus nonpsychotic endogenous depression. Br J Psychiatry 145:508–511, 1984

Robinson DG, Spiker DG: Delusional depression: a one year follow-up. J Affect Disord 9:79–83, 1985

Roose SP, Glassman AH, Walsh BT, et al: Depression, delusions, and suicide. Am J Psychiatry 140:1159–1162, 1983

Rothschild AJ, Duval SE: How long should patients with psychotic depression stay on the antipsychotic medication? J Clin Psychiatry 64:390–396, 2003

Rothschild AJ, Schatzberg AF, Rosenbaum AH, et al: The dexamethasone suppression test as a discriminator among subtypes of psychotic patients. Br J Psychiatry 141:471–474, 1982

Rothschild AJ, Schatzberg AF, Langlais PJ, et al: Psychotic and nonpsychotic depressions, I: comparison of plasma catecholamines and cortisol measures. Psychiatry Res 20:143–153, 1987

Rothschild AJ, Benes F, Hebben N, et al: Relationships between brain CT scan findings and cortisol in psychotic and nonpsychotic depressed patients. Biol Psychiatry 26:565–575, 1989

Rothschild AJ, Samson JA, Bessette MP, et al: Efficacy of the combination of fluoxetine and perphenazine in the treatment of psychotic depression. J Clin Psychiatry 54:338–342, 1993a

Rothschild AJ, Samson JA, Bond TC, et al: Hypothalamic-pituitary-adrenal axis activity and 1-year outcome in depression. Biol Psychiatry 34:392–400, 1993b

Rothschild AJ, Bates KS, Boehringer KL, et al: Olanzapine response in psychotic depression. J Clin Psychiatry 60:116–118, 1999

Rothschild AJ, Williamson DJ, Tohen MF, et al: A double-blind, randomized study of olanzapine and olanzapine/fluoxetine combination for major depression with psychotic features. J Clin Psychopharmacol 24:365–373, 2004

Schatzberg AF, Rothschild AJ: Psychotic (delusional) major depression: should it be included as a distinct syndrome in DSM-IV? Am J Psychiatry 149:733–745, 1992

Schatzberg AF, Rothschild AJ, Stahl JB, et al: The dexamethasone suppression test: identification of subtypes of depression. Am J Psychiatry 140:88–91, 1983

Schatzberg AF, Rothschild AJ, Langlais PJ, et al: A corticosteroid/dopamine hypothesis for psychotic depression and related states. J Psychiatr Res 19:57–64, 1985

Schatzberg AF, Posener JA, DeBattista C, et al: Neuropsychological deficits in psychotic versus nonpsychotic major depression and no mental illness. Am J Psychiatry 157:1095–1100, 2000

Schwartz JE, Fennig S, Tanenberg-Karant M, et al: Congruence of diagnoses 2 years after a first admission diagnosis of psychosis. Arch Gen Psychiatry 57:593–600, 2000

Serretti A, Lattuada E, Cusin C, et al: Clinical and demographic features of psychotic and nonpsychotic depression. Compr Psychiatry 40:358–362, 1999

Simpson GM, Sheshai EL, Rady A, et al: Sertraline as monotherapy in the treatment of psychotic and nonpsychotic depression. J Clin Psychiatry 64:959–965, 2003

Simpson S, Baldwin RC, Jackson A, et al: The differentiation of DSM-IV psychotic depression in later life from nonpsychotic depression: comparisons of brain changes measured by multispectral analysis of magnetic resonance brain images, neuropsychological findings, and clinical features. Biol Psychiatry 45:193–204, 1999

Skaf CR, Yamada A, Garrido GE, et al: Psychotic symptoms in major depressive disorder are associated with reduced regional cerebral blood flow in the subgenual anterior cingulate cortex: a voxel-based single photon emission computed tomography (SPECT) study. J Affect Disord 68:295–305, 2002

Spiker DG, Kupfer DJ: Placebo response rates in psychotic and nonpsychotic depression. J Affect Disord 14:21–23, 1988

Spiker DG, Stein J, Rich CL: Delusional depression and electroconvulsive therapy: one year later. Convuls Ther 1:167–172, 1985a

Spiker DG, Weiss JC, Dealy RS, et al: The pharmacological treatment of delusional depression. Am J Psychiatry 142:430–436, 1985b

Spiker DG, Perel JM, Hanin I, et al: The pharmacological treatment of delusional depression: part II. J Clin Psychopharmacol 6:339–342, 1986b

Thase ME, Kupfer DJ, Ulrich RF: Electroencephalographic sleep in psychotic depression: a valid subtype? Arch Gen Psychiatry 43:886–893, 1986

Tsuang D, Coryell W: An 8-year follow-up of patients with DSM-III-R psychotic depression, schizoaffective disorder, and schizophrenia. Am J Psychiatry 150:1182–1188, 1993

Vythilingam M, Chen J, Bremner JD, et al: Psychotic depression and mortality. Am J Psychiatry 160:574–576, 2003

Weissman MM, Warner V, John K, et al: Delusional depression and bipolar spectrum: evidence for a possible association from a family study of children. Neuropsychopharmacology 1:257–264, 1988

Zanardi R, Franchini L, Gasperini M, et al: Double-blind controlled trial of sertraline versus paroxetine in the treatment of delusional depression. Am J Psychiatry 153:1631–1633, 1996

Zanardi R, Franchini L, Serretti A, et al: Venlafaxine versus fluvoxamine in the treatment of delusional depression: a pilot double-blind controlled study. J Clin Psychiatry 61:26–29, 2000

35

Pediatric Mood Disorders

GRAHAM J. EMSLIE, M.D.

TARYN L. MAYES, M.S.

BETH D. KENNARD, PSY.D.

JENNIFER L. HUGHES, B.A.

MOOD DISORDERS are serious conditions that cause significant morbidity and mortality in children and adolescents. As recently as 30–40 years ago, mood disorders before adulthood were considered rare (Anthony and Scott 1960; Douvan and Adelson 1966). However, research over the past two decades has clearly shown that children and adolescents can experience both depression and mania (Birmaher et al. 1996b; Carlson and Kashani 1988b; Lewinsohn et al. 1995; Ryan et al. 1987). Despite increasing awareness of mood disorders in children and adolescents, these disorders remain underdiagnosed and undertreated (Coyle et al. 2003).

Mood disorders are categorized by DSM-IV-TR (American Psychiatric Association 2000a) into depressive disorders, bipolar disorders, mood disorder due to a general medical condition, and substance-induced mood disorder. In this chapter, we focus on the features that are specific to the pediatric age group. We review the symptomatology, epidemiology, pathogenesis, pharmacotherapy, and psychotherapy of pediatric mood disorders.

Depressive Disorders

Symptomatology

Assessment

Although the criteria for pediatric depression are the same as those for adult depression, the assessment and diagnostic process for pediatric depression is quite different. Children and adolescents do not generally seek treatment for themselves; rather, they are brought in for assessment and treatment by a concerned caregiver, via a school referral, or by juvenile authorities.

Clinicians use multiple informants when diagnosing depressive disorders in youths. Caregivers and children frequently do not agree on the presence of symptoms (Jensen et al. 1999). Children and adolescents tend to report more accurately on the internalizing symptoms of the disorder, whereas caregivers report on the more behavioral, externalizing symptoms (Herjanic and Reich

1997; Hope et al. 1999). Mesman and Koot (2000) found that teachers are also more likely to report internalizing symptoms than are caregivers. Children also have trouble reporting frequency and duration of symptoms, so parent reports are needed to establish onset dates and course of illness. Thus, with the variety of information obtained and the disparity often found between reports, clinical acumen is needed to synthesize all of the information obtained.

A blend of clinician-rated and parent and self-report rating scales is often useful to assess the level of depression in children and adolescents. Both diagnostic and severity measures are available for the pediatric age group. Scales vary in length, ranging from quite long, semistructured interviews designed to ascertain a wide variety of diagnoses to short, unstructured interviews specific to depression. Myers and Winters (2002a, 2002b) provide detailed information about commonly used assessment and severity scales for this population.

One important aspect of early-onset depression is the high familial aggregation of depression, alcoholism, anxiety, and other psychiatric diagnoses in first- and second-degree relatives (Biederman et al. 1991; Brumback et al. 1977), with a positive family history of mood disorders in 50%–80% of patients. Evaluation of children and adolescents with mood disorders will include a detailed biological family history, including first-, second-, and third-degree relatives. Also, the current mental state of the caregiver is significant because the child's treatment outcome may be affected by parental disorders. The effect of parental depression on the parents' ability to report depression accurately in their children has received little study. Parents may not identify the disorder in themselves (Beardslee et al. 1998) and may benefit from a referral for assessment and treatment of mood disorders in themselves.

Symptoms

Depressive disorders are categorized the same across the life span. DSM-IV-TR includes diagnoses of major depressive disorder (MDD), dysthymic disorder, depressive disorder not otherwise specified, and adjustment disorder with depressed mood. Both pediatric and adult depressive disorders involve essentially the same symptoms for diagnosis, including depressed or irritable mood, anhedonia, sleep and appetite disturbance, feelings of worthlessness or guilt, psychomotor disturbance, decreased concentration, decreased energy, and suicidal ideation. One possible exception is the symptom of irritability. Children may present with irritable mood without explicit sadness.

Age-related differences in depressive symptoms are difficult to detect, if they do indeed exist, because of the problems in accurately eliciting symptoms from children and adolescents. Kovacs (1996) has pointed out that most empirical evidence indicates only less hypersomnia, more appetite and weight changes, and delusions in younger depressed patients as compared with adolescents. Luby et al. (2003) concluded that depressed preschool children show fewer "masked" symptoms (e.g., sleep problems, appetite changes) and more typical symptoms (e.g., anhedonia, sadness/irritability).

Limited research is available on cultural differences in depression presentation. Stewart and colleagues (2002) found symptomatological similarities and differences between Hong Kong and Canadian high school students. Both groups reported similar levels of depressed mood, anhedonia, and sleep changes; however, more Canadian youths reported irritability, whereas Hong Kong youths reported more weight and appetite changes, fatigue, psychomotor changes, guilt, concentration difficulties, and suicidal ideation (Stewart et al. 2002). Cultural differences in symptomatology could be related to cultural mediators, such as support systems within the culture or demands placed on the individual by the culture (Stewart et al. 1999).

Regardless of age, gender, and race, depressive symptoms in pediatric patients tend to be more contextual in nature than in adult depression (Hammen et al. 1992). Psychosocial factors contribute to the development and maintenance of the disorders. Alternatively, depression itself leads to increased psychosocial problems. Therefore, determining the precursors and consequences of the disorder is important but can be difficult to separate. For example, bereaved children commonly report symptoms of grief, but R.A. Weller et al. (1991) noted that family history of depression was associated with the development of MDD in the bereaved children.

In summary, the assessment process for identifying depression in children and adolescents often requires substantial clinical acumen to determine 1) current symptoms, 2) attribution of symptoms, 3) psychosocial difficulties (both precursors and consequences), 4) primary disorder requiring treatment, 5) secondary or comorbid disorders, and 6) best course of treatment.

Suicide and Depression

Focus on teenaged suicide has been increasing as a result of public media attention on teenaged suicide attempts and completions. Suicide is the third leading cause of death in adolescents ages 15–19, leading to 2,000 deaths annually (National Center for Health Statistics 2001). As one of the nine criteria for depression, suicidal behavior occurs relatively frequently in youth depression. Likewise, suicidal youth often present with a mood disorder. Several reports indicated that 40%–80% of adolescent suicide attempters met diagnostic criteria for depression at the time of the attempt (Beautrais 2000; Fergusson and Lynskey 1995; Fergusson et al. 2000; Gould et al. 1998; Lewinsohn et al. 1996; Reinherz et al. 1995). In a study by Shaffer and colleagues (1996), 40% of the adolescent suicide completers had a mood disorder, compared with 0.05% of age-, sex-, and ethnic-matched control subjects. Brent et al. (1993) also found that most suicide victims had a primary affective disorder (P<0.0001). In evaluating and treating depression in youths, clinicians will likely encounter youths with suicidal thoughts or behaviors. Assessing the level of severity of the thoughts and the danger the patient may be to himself or herself is an essential component of the evaluation and treatment plan. Similarly, youths who present with suicidal thoughts or attempts as the primary complaint will need assessment for depression, as well as for other mood and psychiatric disorders.

Associated Features

Aside from the DSM-IV-TR criteria, depression presents with a variety of common features. Depressed children have been shown to have negative cognitions, including increased cognitive distortions, negative attributions, hopelessness, and low self-esteem (Asarnow and Bates 1988; Garber and Hilsman 1992; Garber et al. 1993; Marton and Kutcher 1995). There is debate in the literature as to whether these cognitions are state or trait (Garber and Hilsman 1992); however, most studies have found that negative cognitions are related to mood state and change with improvement in mood (Asarnow and Bates 1988; Gotlib et al. 1993; McCauley et al. 1988; Tems et al. 1993). Whether negative cognitions are precursors to the depressive episode or a consequence of the episode remains unclear. Evidence exists that dysfunctional thinking is a strong predictor of recurrent depression (Lewinsohn et al. 1999) and that continued cognitive distortions following treatment may be predictive of shorter time to return of depression (Beevers et al. 2003). Thus, cognitive symptoms may be of particular importance in assessing the residual symptoms after treatment.

Certain psychosocial difficulties are also common features of depression (Table 35–1). When compared with nondepressed control subjects, children with MDD experience increased school difficulties (P<0.0001), including problems with behavior, attitude, and academic achievement (Puig-Antich et al. 1993). School difficulties gener-

TABLE 35–1. Long-term psychosocial difficulties of pediatric depression

Deficit	Reference
Impaired academic functioning or educational underachievement	Aronen and Soininen 2000; Bardone et al. 1996; Fergusson and Woodward 2002; Geller et al. 2001; Rao et al. 1999a
Impaired occupational functioning or increased unemployment	Aronen and Soininen 2000; Fergusson and Woodward 2002; Geller et al. 2001; Lewinsohn et al. 2003; Weissman et al. 1999
Social difficulties or poor peer relationships	Aronen and Soininen 2000; Devine et al. 1994; Fombonne et al. 2001a; Garber et al. 1988; Geller et al. 2001; Kandel and Davies 1986; Lewinsohn et al. 2003; Rao et al. 1995; Reinherz et al. 1999; Weissman et al. 1999
Poor family relationships	Geller et al. 2001; Lewinsohn et al. 2003
Lowered life satisfaction; decreased self-esteem	Aronen and Soininen 2000; Devine et al. 1994; Geller et al. 2001; Lewinsohn et al. 2003; Rao et al. 1995; Reinherz et al. 1999
Increased treatment use later in life	Harrington et al. 1990; Lewinsohn et al. 2003; Weissman et al. 1999
Increased incidence of suicide attempts and completion	Fergusson and Woodward 2002; Fombonne et al. 2001a; Harrington et al. 1990; Kovacs et al. 1993; Rao et al. 1993; Reinherz et al. 1999; Weissman et al. 1999
Reduced global functioning	Ferdinand et al. 1999; Lewinsohn et al. 2003; Rao et al. 1995; Reinherz et al. 1999; Weissman et al. 1999

ally improve as the depression improves. Studies also indicate significant social impairment in clinically depressed children (Hamilton et al. 1997; Hops et al. 1990; Puig-Antich et al. 1985a, 1985b). Puig-Antich et al. (1993) reported that children with MDD have greater impairment than do nondepressed control subjects on measures of social skills and peer relationships (P<0.001).

Depressed children and adolescents also have poorer family relationships (Hops et al. 1990; Kashani et al. 1988; Puig-Antich et al. 1985a, 1985b, 1993), including poor relationships with mother, father, and siblings (*P*<0.05 when compared with control subjects; Flament et al. 2001). Strober et al. (1993) found that some of these psychosocial impairments, such as poor peer and family relationships, continue even after remission of the depressive episode. Because early-onset depression may be more contextual in nature, it remains unclear if psychosocial difficulties are precursors to depression or consequences of the disorder. Although the relation between cause and effect must continue to be evaluated, treatment of both is needed. That is, the depressive episode is treated, but the concurring difficulties (i.e., family conflict, poor school performance) are also addressed during treatment.

Comorbidity

The diagnosis of a mood disorder is often obscured by the presence of other comorbid psychiatric diagnoses, as well as general medical disorders. Various medical conditions are associated with high rates of depression. In pediatric populations, these include diabetes mellitus, asthma, and neurological conditions (e.g., epilepsy). Certain medical disorders can present as depressive symptoms (e.g., hypothyroidism and systemic lupus). Conversely, depression is more common in chronic medical conditions, such as diabetes and asthma (for review of depression and diabetes, see Grey et al. 2002; Vila et al. 1999, 2000). Medications also can induce depression (e.g., isotretinoin). Controversy has developed over whether isotretinoin, which is used to treat recalcitrant nodular acne, can cause depression (for review, see O'Donnell 2003). Studies also have identified high rates of psychiatric disorders in children and adolescents with various neurological conditions (Cantwell and Baker 1980), including brain injury (Robinson and Starkstein 1990; Robinson et al. 1988; Starkstein et al. 1990), epilepsy (Barraclough 1981; Ring and Trimble 1993; Robertson 1989; Rutter et al. 1976), migraine (Ling et al. 1970), and learning disabilities (Brumback and Weinberg 1990; Emslie et al. 1995; Livingston 1985; Weinberg et al. 1973; Weinberg and Rehmet 1983).

Concurrent psychiatric disorders occur frequently with depression. Puig-Antich and colleagues (1989, p. 414) said that comorbidity is an "intrinsic characteristic of children with major affective illness." Anxiety disorders and disruptive behavior disorders are the most frequent comorbid conditions in children and adolescents. Emslie and colleagues (1997a) found that in a sample of 96 depressed children and adolescents, 56% had comorbid anxiety disorder, 30% had comorbid attention-deficit/hyperactivity disorder (ADHD), 30% had a comorbid oppositional or conduct disorder, and 35% had comorbid dysthymia. Other reports of pediatric depression confirm high rates of anxiety (Axelson and Birmaher 2001; Lewinsohn et al. 1991), behavior disorders (Kovacs et al. 1988; Lewinsohn et al. 1991), and dysthymia (Kovacs et al. 1984b, 1997). Several of the symptoms of these disorders overlap, so evaluating each diagnosis is essential. Similar rates of comorbid disorders were found in 230 children and adolescents with MDD evaluated by Emslie and colleagues (unpublished data). The depressed outpatients were enrolled in one of two National Institute of Mental Health (NIMH)–sponsored studies conducted 1991–1995 (*N*=130) and 2000–2005 (*N*=100) (see Table 35–2).

Substance abuse is often a feature of adolescent depression, with rates from 25% to 48% (Deykin et al. 1992; Greenbaum et al. 1991; Rao et al. 1999b; Rohde et al. 1996). The development of a substance use disorder tends to follow the onset of the psychiatric disorder (Rohde et al. 1996). Rao et al. (1999b) found that those depressed adolescents who went on to develop substance use disorder had greater psychosocial impairment prior to the onset of the substance use disorder.

In addition to causing increased impairment, comorbid psychiatric disorders can affect treatment outcomes in children and adolescents. Hughes et al. (1990) found that children with concurrent depression and anxiety disorder had a higher drug response rate compared with those with comorbid conduct or oppositional defiant disorders (57% vs. 33%). Subjects with comorbid conduct or oppositional defiant disorders had a higher placebo response rate (67% vs. 20%). Rohde et al. (2001) found that overall lifetime comorbid diagnoses were unrelated to outcome of cognitive-behavioral therapy (CBT), but those with comorbid depression and substance abuse disorders recovered more slowly, and those with comorbid depression and anxiety disorder showed the greatest improvement. Brent et al. (1999) found that adolescents with double depression sought more outside treatment when involved in a clinical trial, suggesting that these cases are more severe and may require multiple treatment modalities.

Course of Illness

More than 90% of children and adolescents recover from an initial episode of MDD within 1–2 years of onset (Emslie et al. 1997b; Kovacs et al. 1984a; McCauley et al. 1993; Strober et al. 1993), even with minimal treatment (Keller et al. 1991; Kovacs et al. 1984a). Kovacs et al. (1984a), in a longitudinal investigation of depressed 8- to 13-year-olds, found that the recovery rate was signifi-

TABLE 35–2. Comorbidity in a recent sample of children and adolescents with major depression

| | | Comorbidity, n (%) | | | |
| | | Males (n=127) | | Females (n=103) | |
Comorbid diagnosis	Total	≤12 y (n=74)	≥13 y (n=53)	≤12 y (n=53)	≥13 y (n=50)
None (major depressive disorder only)**	64	19 (26)	15 (28)	9 (17)	21 (42)
Dysthymic disorder	75	24 (32)	20 (38)	20 (38)	11 (22)
ADHD***	76	36 (49)	17 (32)	17 (32)	6 (12)
Anxiety*	77	26 (35)	10 (19)	23 (43)	18 (36)
Behavioral	48	18 (24)	13 (25)	10 (19)	7 (14)
Other	8	3 (4)	3 (6)	0 (0)	2 (4)

Note. ADHD=attention-deficit/hyperactivity disorder.
*$P<0.05$ (older vs. younger boys; older boys vs. older girls); $P<0.01$ (older boys vs. younger girls).
**$P≤0.005$ (older vs. younger females).
***$P<0.0001$ (younger boys vs. older girls).
Source. Ongoing trial by Emslie and coworkers, "Childhood Depression: Remission and Relapse," and completed trial by Emslie and coworkers, "Childhood Depression: Biological Correlates" (both supported by National Institute of Mental Health grant MH39188).

cantly better for MDD than for depressive disorder; children with MDD experienced a peak in recovery around 15–18 months, with maximal recovery rate occurring at 1.5 years, whereas the median time to recovery in children with depressive disorder was 3.5 years. The rate of remission was independent of gender, although an earlier age at onset predicted a more lengthy recovery.

Depending on length of follow-up, recurrence rates are 40%–72% in depressed youths followed for 1–8 years (Emslie et al. 1997b, 1998; Garber et al. 1988; Kovacs et al. 1984b; McCauley et al. 1993; Rao et al. 1995). These rates are based on naturalistic follow-up studies, which do not take into account whether patients are taking medication at the time of the recurrence or the length of time medication had been taken prior to the recurrence. Factors contributing to recurrence of depression include comorbidity (Birmaher et al. 2000; Brent et al. 1999; Kovacs et al. 1984b; Vostanis et al. 1998), severity of depression (Birmaher et al. 2000; Emslie et al. 1997b), hopelessness (Birmaher et al. 2000), low self-esteem at baseline and follow-up (Vostanis et al. 1998), family dysfunction (Asarnow et al. 1994; Brent et al. 1999; Goodyer et al. 1997; Lewinsohn et al. 1990), stress and life events (Garber et al. 1992; Goodyer et al. 1997; Williamson et al. 1998), and suicidality at baseline (Emslie et al. 2001a). In a recent longitudinal study investigating recurrence of MDD during adulthood (ages 19–23 years) in formerly treated depressed adolescents, Lewinsohn et al. (2001) found that recurrence was predicted by multiple episodes of depression, family history of recurrence of major depression,

borderline personality disorder symptoms, and increased conflict with parents (for females only).

A diagnosis of depression in children and adolescents increases the risk for subsequent depressive episodes in adulthood (for review, see Birmaher et al. 1996b). Long-term studies report high risk for later-life depression in 60%–70% of those who received diagnoses in childhood (Fergusson and Woodward 2002; Fombonne et al. 2001b; Harrington et al. 1990; Kovacs et al. 1984a). Depressive episodes in childhood also can be an early indication of bipolar disorder. Rao et al. (1995) found that 19% of depressed adolescents eventually presented with new-onset bipolar disorder. Geller et al. (2001) reported that 49% of their sample of adults who had prepubertal MDD later presented with bipolar I disorder; other studies also found similar rates of later development of bipolar disorder (20%–40%) (Garber et al. 1988; Geller et al. 1994; Kovacs and Gatsonis 1989; Strober and Carlson 1982; Strober et al. 1993). Birmaher and colleagues (1996b) reviewed risk factors for the development of bipolar disorder from pediatric-onset depression, which include depression accompanied by psychomotor retardation or psychotic features, a family history of bipolar disorder or several mood disorders, pharmacologically induced hypomania, atypical depression, seasonal affective disorder, protracted depressive episodes, mood lability, comorbid substance abuse, and high rates of psychosocial problems.

Finally, depression in adolescents is also highly correlated with later nicotine dependence (Bardone et al. 1998;

Fergusson and Woodward 2002; Kandel and Davies 1986), substance abuse or dependence (Fergusson and Woodward 2002; Geller et al. 2001), increased medical problems (Bardone et al. 1998), and poorer overall physical well-being (Lewinsohn et al. 2003). Reducing the psychosocial impairments within the episode, shortening the episode, and preventing relapse and recurrence in pediatric depression are essential to reduce subsequent difficulties across the life span.

Epidemiology

Major mood disorders often begin in early life (for review of epidemiology, see Kessler et al. 2001). Epidemiological studies that used clinical interviews reported MDD rates from 4% (Whitaker et al. 1990) to 6% (Shaffer et al. 1996) and even as high as 25% (Lewinsohn et al. 1998). In the National Comorbidity Survey, Kessler et al. (1994) found prevalence rates of 14% in adolescents. Epidemiological studies of dysthymia have found rates from 0.6% to 8.0% in children and adolescents (Kashani et al. 1987; Lewinsohn et al. 1993, 1994). Rates of depression are similar in males and females during childhood (Fleming and Offord 1990; Kashani et al. 1987; Lewinsohn et al. 1995; Nolen-Hoeksema et al. 1991); however, in adolescents, depression becomes more prevalent in females (Angold et al. 1998; Wade et al. 2002), with females twice as likely to have depression when compared with males. This gender difference remains consistent throughout adulthood and holds true across cultures as well (Wade et al. 2002).

Depressive disorders differ within and among cultures. In a study of 3,294 United States high school students of mixed ethnic background, Emslie et al. (1990b) found that self-reported depressive symptoms were greatest among Hispanic females (22.4%) and lowest among white males (7.9%). Overall, African Americans and Hispanics had more self-reported depressive symptomatology than did whites ($P<0.01$). Interestingly, white adults are more likely to seek treatment for depression than are other racial groups (Cooper et al. 2003).

Studies of pediatric depression throughout the world are limited; however, several studies have found that prevalence rates are similar to those in the United States. Canals (1997) suggested that these similar rates of depression in Europe and the United States could be the result of psychosocial similarities across cultures and culture-independent risk factors for depression, such as biological factors. Stewart and colleagues (2002) reported similar rates of depression among adolescents in Hong Kong and the United States (Hong Kong: 2.2%; United States: 2.2%). Polaino-Lorente and Domenech (1993) found that in a sample of 9-year-olds in Spain, 1.8% met criteria for major depression. The rate in Spanish adolescents ranges from 1.4% in males to 3.3% in females (Canals et al. 1997). In French adolescents, the prevalence of depression has been reported as 4.4% (Bailly et al. 1992).

Pathogenesis

The pathogenesis of depression in children and adolescents is generally believed to be the same as that in adults. That is, depression is the same disorder across the life span with essentially the same phenomenology, pathophysiology, and treatment response, with developmental variations present.

Depression results from variable degrees of innate susceptibility and environmental factors resulting in either frank illness or increasing vulnerability to later episodes of depression. Environmental factors are also potentially protective. Of interest is a recent finding that a dysfunctional polymorphism in the serotonin transporter gene (*5-HTT*) moderates the influence of stressful life events on depression. Individuals with one or two copies of the short allele of the *5-HTT* promoter polymorphism had more depressive symptoms, diagnoses of depression, and suicidality in relation to stressful life events than did those with an individual homozygote for the long allele (Caspi et al. 2003).

Studying biological, pathophysiological, and environmental factors associated with depression shows that the adolescent age group is important for several reasons. To study the reasons for gender differences and problems with depression, adolescence becomes a particularly important age period to explore given that before adolescence, the prevalence is similar between boys and girls.

Given the earlier stages of illness in children and adolescents, it is likely that biological abnormalities identified are more central to the illness as opposed to consequences of prolonged depression. For example, hypercortisolemia is a feature of depression in adults ("The Dexamethasone Suppression Test" 1987; Stokes and Sikes 1987), but it is not seen in children and adolescents (Birmaher et al. 1996a), except possibly around sleep onset. However, challenge tests (e.g., dexamethasone suppression test) have been reported to have abnormal results in children and adolescents as well as in adults.

One of the most consistent findings related to the hypothalamic-pituitary-adrenal (HPA) axis is the finding of a blunted growth hormone (GH) response to GH-releasing hormone (GHRH). This finding has been reported in depressed children compared with control subjects (Ryan et al. 1994), remitted depressed children (Dahl et al. 2000), and children at high risk for MDD (Birmaher et al. 2000).

Interest in HPA axis abnormalities is also increasing in the role of stress response; Kaufman et al. (1997) noted more HPA axis problems in depressed, abused children compared with depressed, nonabused children and nondepressed control subjects.

Developmental biological differences may obscure biological findings that are characteristically seen in adults. For example, depressed adults show several specific sleep polysomnographic findings (i.e., sleep continuity disturbances): decreased slow-wave sleep (Stage III and IV non–rapid eye movement [NREM] sleep), decreased REM latency (time from sleep onset to first REM period), and increased REM sleep density. Sleep continuity disturbance appears less pronounced in depressed children and adolescents, and no studies have identified slow-wave sleep deficits (Dahl et al. 1990, 1991; Emslie et al. 1990a, 1994; Goetz et al. 1987; Kutcher et al. 1991; Lahmeyer et al. 1983; Puig-Antich et al. 1982). Given that even depressed children and adolescents have less insomnia than do adults and have substantially more slow-wave sleep, subtle differences in sleep architecture are likely obscured by the developmental differences in sleep between children and adults. Even the REM sleep phenomena are most evident in a more controlled environment (e.g., depressed inpatients; Dahl et al. 1990; Emslie et al. 1990a, 1994). More sensitive measures of sleep architecture (e.g., microanalysis, computer score sleep; Armitage et al. 2002) and challenge tests may be needed to identify specific abnormalities associated with depression in pediatric patients.

Sleep architecture disturbances also have been identified in at-risk adult populations (Giles et al. 1998) and adolescent females (Morehouse et al. 2002). Also, shortened REM latency in adults predicted response to treatment and probability of relapse (Giles et al. 1987; Rush et al. 1989). Similarly, sleep latency predicted relapse in a naturalistic follow-up of depressed children and adolescents (Emslie et al. 2001a).

Future areas of research into the pathophysiology of depression in children and adolescents will likely continue to examine relations between stress, genetic vulnerability, and developmental factors. Clearly, with the development of functional magnetic resonance imaging (MRI), interest will increase in functional imaging in both depressed and remitted individuals at different developmental stages. Preliminary data suggest similarities to adults, including neurobiological abnormalities in dorsolateral prefrontal cortex with spectroscopy (Farchione et al. 2002; Steingard et al. 2000) and MRI (Nolan et al. 2002; Steingard et al. 1996).

In summary, investigations of the pathophysiology of depression in children and adolescents support the con-

cept of similarities in depression across the life span. Studying children and adolescents is also likely to contribute to a greater understanding of depression across the life span.

Pharmacotherapy

Acute Treatment

Until quite recently, data about effectiveness of antidepressant medication treatment was limited in the pediatric age group, despite widespread prescribing practices (Zito et al. 2003). Guidelines or algorithms for treatment provide clinicians with a reasoned, scientific-based approach to pharmacological management that synthesizes available data and expert clinical consensus. Thus, The Texas Children's Medication Algorithm Project (CMAP) developed a medication algorithm for MDD to be studied at the Texas Department of Mental Health and Mental Retardation Services (Hughes et al. 1999). The resulting algorithm for MDD is shown in Figure 35–1. The design is based on providing initial strategies of single medications with favorable side-effect profiles, high safety, and low toxicity. Treatment progresses to the next strategy because of either inadequate symptom improvement or medication intolerance.

However, before initiating medication treatment, several factors must be considered, including course of illness, severity, and psychosocial factors. In addition, the family must be involved in the decision process of medication treatment. Once a decision is made to initiate medication, determining which antidepressant to use is the next step. Table 35–3 provides a list of factors to consider when deciding which medication to use.

Because of the lack of established efficacy of tricyclic antidepressants in this population, combined with the growing research supporting the efficacy and safety of the newer selective serotonin reuptake inhibitors (SSRIs), SSRIs are considered the first line of treatment for early-onset depression. Studies of SSRIs have been promising, with four of these medications now showing positive response in children and/or adolescents. Dosing is similar to that for adults (Table 35–4). To date, only fluoxetine has a U.S. Food and Drug Administration (FDA) indication for treatment of pediatric depression. The approval was based on two positive trials (Emslie et al. 1997a, 2002). Other SSRIs with positive trials include paroxetine (Keller et al. 2001), sertraline (Wagner et al. 2003), and citalopram (Wagner et al. 2004).

The first study to show that an antidepressant medication treatment was superior to placebo in treating early-onset depression was by Emslie et al. (1997a). In this study of 96 children and adolescents (ages 8–18) with

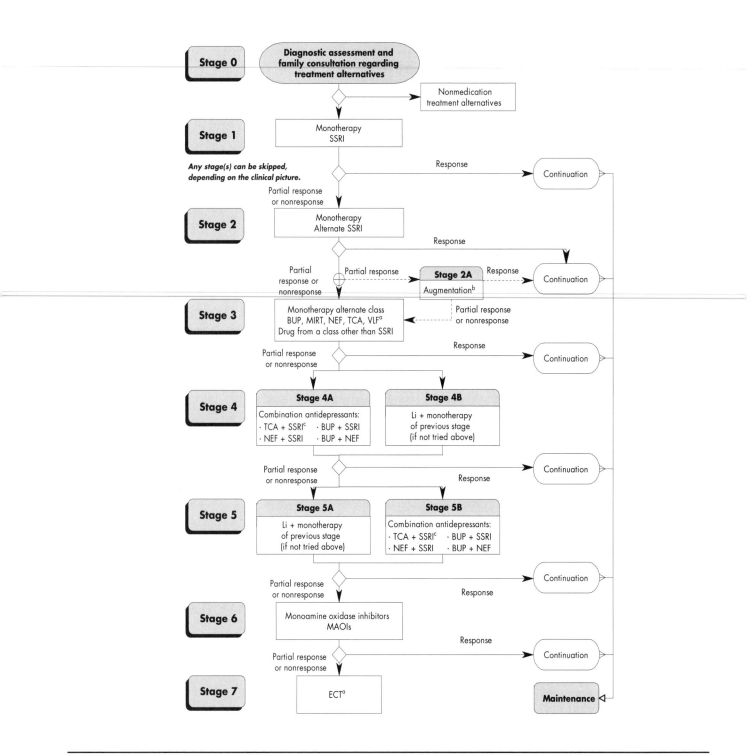

FIGURE 35–1.   Strategies for the treatment of childhood major depression.

Note.   SSRI=selective serotonin reuptake inhibitor; BUP=bupropion; MIRT=mirtazapine; NEF=nefazodone; TCA=tricyclic anti-depressant; VLF=venlafaxine; Li=lithium; ECT=electroconvulsive therapy.
[a]Consider TCA or VLF.
[b]With Li or buspirone.
[c]Most studied combination in adults.
[d]ECT not allowed in Texas in children 16 years or younger.
Source.   Adapted from Hughes et al (1999). The Children's Medication Algorithm Project algorithms are in the public domain and may be reproduced without permission.

TABLE 35–3. Guidelines for choosing medication

Medications with fewer side effects and established efficacy in controlled trials are first-line treatment.

Medication is selected to prevent certain side effects (e.g., an overweight child would not be started on medications commonly known for causing significant weight gain).

Consider also:

Previous response to a medication

Previous tolerability of a medication

Other family members' response to a medication

Physician preference

Patient and family preference

Cost

TABLE 35–4. Selective serotonin reuptake inhibitors in children and adolescents

Medication	Pediatric dose (mg)	How supplied
Citalopram	10–40 q am	20-, 40-mg tablets
Escitalopram	5–20 q am	5-, 10-, 20-mg tablets
Fluoxetine	10–40 q am	10-, 20-mg capsules and concentrate
Fluvoxamine	25–150 twice a day	25-, 50-, 100-mg tablets
Paroxetine	10–40 q am	10-, 20-, 30-mg tablets
Sertraline	25–200 q am	25-, 50-, 100-mg tablets

MDD, 56% of those randomly assigned to fluoxetine and 33% of those randomly assigned to placebo were considered much or very much improved after 8 weeks of treatment (Emslie et al. 1997a). In a study replicating the findings by Emslie et al., 219 children and adolescents (ages 8–17) with MDD were randomly assigned to 9 weeks of treatment in a multisite study of fluoxetine versus placebo. As in the initial study, 52% and 37%, respectively, were considered much or very much improved (Emslie et al. 2002).

In another large multisite, industry-funded study, 275 adolescents (ages 12–18) with MDD were randomly assigned to paroxetine, imipramine, or placebo for an 8-week acute trial. Paroxetine was superior in efficacy to placebo (66% vs. 48%), but imipramine (52%) was not; efficacy was defined as an end-point Clinical Global Impression (CGI) Scale improvement rated as "much" or "very much" improved (Keller et al. 2001). Outcomes based on Ham-D scores ≤8 were similar: 63% paroxetine, 50% imipramine, and 46% placebo (paroxetine vs. placebo, $P=0.02$). However, in the primary outcomes (Ham-D ≤8 or 50% decrease on Ham-D; change in Ham-D total score), there was no significant difference between the groups. This study was important in two ways. It provided additional support for the efficacy of SSRIs in the treatment of adolescent MDD and reinforced the suggestion that tricyclic antidepressants are not effective in depressed children and adolescents as a group but may have a role in specific individuals. Two other double-blind trials of paroxetine in pediatric depression have had negative results (Emslie et al. 2004a, 2004b; Milin et al. 1999)).

Two multisite studies of sertraline versus placebo were conducted and combined a priori for outcome analyses.

A total of 376 children and adolescents (ages 6–17) with MDD were randomly assigned to 10 weeks of sertraline ($n=189$) or placebo ($n=187$). Response was defined with two measures. First, on the basis of a 40% decrease in the Children's Depression Rating Scale—Revised (CDRS-R; Poznanski et al. 1984) score at the end of the study, with the last observation carried forward, 69% of the sertraline-treated subjects and 59% of the placebo-treated subjects were considered responders ($P=0.05$). Second, on the basis of a CGI Scale rating of "much" or "very much" improved, 63% of the sertraline-treated subjects and 53% of the placebo-treated subjects were considered responders ($P=0.05$). Although only a 10% difference was found between active medicine and placebo, because of the large number of subjects in this trial, the difference was statistically significant (Wagner et al. 2003).

Finally, Wagner et al. (2004) reported on an 8-week multisite, double-blind, placebo-controlled study of citalopram in 174 children and adolescents (ages 7–17) with MDD. Following a 1-week placebo run-in, subjects were randomly assigned to citalopram (20–40 mg/day; $n=89$) or placebo ($n=85$). Citalopram showed significant improvement over placebo as early as week 1 ($F=6.58$, $P<0.05$), and this improvement persisted throughout the study. Additionally, more citalopram-treated subjects than placebo-treated subjects met the defined response criterion of a CDRS-R score of 28 or less (36% vs. 24%, $P<0.05$). Although these response rates appear quite low, the defined response criterion is typically used in studies as the remission criterion (e.g., "well"). The rates of remission are similar to those in other studies (Emslie et al. 1997a, 2002). No differences were found in CGI Scale improvement ratings of 1 or 2 ("much" or "very much" improved) between citalopram and placebo (47% vs. 45%) or mean CGI Scale severity scores (4.4 vs. 4.3).

Another trial of citalopram, which included adolescent inpatients and outpatients, showed no difference between active treatment and placebo. The design of the study is unknown, which makes it difficult to evaluate the outcome. However, because inpatients were included, it is likely that the depression severity was substantially higher in this trial (Medicines and Healthcare Products Regulatory Agency 2003).

Trials of other newer antidepressants, such as nefazodone, venlafaxine, and mirtazapine, recently have been completed. Results of nefazodone and venlafaxine have been presented; results from mirtazapine have not yet been published. Preliminary results of nefazodone in adolescents appear positive (Emslie et al. 2002). Venlafaxine did not show any significant improvement over placebo in two studies of children and adolescents. However, when the studies were combined, adolescents (but not children) showed greater improvement with venlafaxine than with placebo (Emslie et al. 2004b). Although data from the mirtazapine trials are not available, the FDA report stated that the results were negative.

One important point regarding the above-mentioned trials is the difference between response and remission. *Response* is significant improvement in symptoms, whereas *remission* suggests "wellness" or being symptom-free. The range of response of these trials was 55%–60%, but remission was substantially lower. Table 35–5 shows the response and remission rates of the trials discussed in this subsection.

Recently, controversies about SSRIs have surfaced. The recent controversy was initially sparked by a review of paroxetine data by the Medicines and Healthcare Products Regulatory Agency, the drug regulatory agency in the United Kingdom. In December 2003, the Medicines and Healthcare Products Regulatory Agency's Committee on Safety of Medicines and its Expert Working Group on SSRIs advised that the balance of the risks and benefits for the treatment of MDD in patients younger than 18 years was judged to be unfavorable for sertraline, citalopram, paroxetine, and escitalopram and unassessable for fluvoxamine. The FDA conducted a reanalysis of all suicide-related events occurring in 24 randomized, controlled pediatric antidepressant trials. It was determined that the average risk of suicidal events (including suicidal behaviors and suicidal ideation) in patients receiving antidepressants was 4%, twice the placebo risk of 2%. Thus, the FDA issued a black box warning describing an increased risk of suicidality for all current and future antidepressants used in those under the age of 18. The warning recommends close observation of all patients for clinical worsening, suicidality, or unusual changes in behavior. Families and caregivers should be advised of the need for close observation and communication with the prescriber. The warning further suggests that patients should be seen weekly for the first month of treatment, then every other week for a month, and again after 12 weeks of treatment. It is important to note that no completed suicides have been reported in any of the randomized, controlled trials of these medications in children and adolescents. Interestingly, Gould et al. (2003) recently found that the rate of youth suicide has decreased in the past decade and suggested that this could be a result of the increase in the prescription of antidepressants in youths.

TABLE 35–5.   Pharmacotherapy trials in children and adolescents

Medication	Duration (weeks)	Ages (years)	N	Response rates	Reference
Citalopram	8	7–17	174 (89 citalopram, 85 placebo)	Significant improvement beginning at week 1	Wagner et al. 2004
Fluoxetine	8	8–18	96 (48 fluoxetine, 48 placebo)	56% vs. 33% (P=0.02)	Emslie et al. 1997a
Fluoxetine	9	8–17	219 (109 fluoxetine, 110 placebo)	52% vs. 37% (P=0.03)	Emslie et al. 2002
Paroxetine	8	12–18	275 (93 paroxetine, 95 imipramine, 87 placebo)	63% vs. 50% vs. 46% (P=0.02)	Keller et al. 2001
Sertraline (two studies)	10	6–17	376 (189 sertraline, 187 placebo)	69% vs. 59% (P=0.05)	Wagner et al. 2003

Although SSRIs are under scrutiny, these medications continue to be used in the pediatric population and, as a group, remain the pharmacological treatment of choice for depression in this age group because untreated depression is equally or even more dangerous for these youngsters. The inconsistencies among trials are likely a result of methodological differences in the studies rather than differences between the individual SSRIs. At this point, however, only fluoxetine has had two or more positive trials and has been approved for the treatment of depression in the pediatric population. Despite the inconsistencies in the trials, SSRIs are still considered the first line of medication treatment in this population because they have shown some positive efficacy, have relatively low side-effect profiles, and are safe in overdose.

Treatment-Resistant Depression

The goal of acute treatment is symptom remission, not just symptom improvement. As mentioned, results of symptom remission were not as consistent, ranging from 31% to 63% for active medication. Remission may take up to 12 weeks of acute treatment (Emslie et al. 1998). No specific data are available in children and adolescents; however, partial remission increases risk for relapse in adults, which suggests that treatment should be lengthened beyond 8 weeks.

To date, no empirical evidence exists for managing treatment-resistant depression in children and adolescents. The medication algorithm (Figure 35–1) indicates that the clinician should switch to an alternative SSRI or a serotonin-norepinephrine reuptake inhibitor such as mirtazapine, nefazodone, or venlafaxine. Although these medications are often used in clinical practice as initial treatments or second-line medications, no data have been published yet to establish their safety and efficacy in children and adolescents with depression. Regardless of the treatment, once remission is achieved, the patient enters the continuation and maintenance phases of treatment.

The length of continuation treatment has not received much attention in this population because acute trials have begun showing efficacy only recently. Thus, clinicians look to adult data, which suggest continuation treatment for 6–9 months following remission (for review, see Montgomery 1994). Only one medication continuation trial in pediatric depression has been conducted. Forty children and adolescents whose symptoms had responded to fluoxetine, 20–60 mg, during a 19-week double-blind, placebo-controlled study were rerandomized to either continue fluoxetine or switch to placebo for an additional 36 weeks (Emslie et al. 2001b). Relapse was defined as a CDRS-R score greater than 40 with a history of

2 weeks of clinical deterioration or physician perception. Fewer fluoxetine subjects (34%) than placebo subjects (60%) met criteria for relapse (not significant). Furthermore, time to relapse was shorter for placebo subjects than for fluoxetine subjects (71.2 ± 9.5 days vs. 180.7 ± 17.0 days, $P=0.046$). The findings in this study were similar to those in adult studies. Thus, in the one continuation trial of depressed children and adolescents reported to date, fluoxetine appeared to be a safe and effective treatment for reducing relapse.

Psychotherapy

Specific psychotherapies, primarily CBT and interpersonal therapy (IPT), are effective treatments for early-onset depression, specifically in adolescents (for review, see Compton et al. 2004; Curry 2001; Reinecke et al. 1998). These psychotherapies originated for the treatment of adults and therefore must be modified to meet the child's or adolescent's developmental stage and increase family member involvement (Wilkes and Rush 1988). Many believe that prepubertal children are not eligible for therapies such as CBT because of their limited verbal abilities and abstract thinking. However, studies of CBT in depressed children have suggested positive response (Butler et al. 1980; Kahn et al. 1990; Stark et al. 1987; Vostanis et al. 1996; Weisz et al. 1997). Generally, CBT and IPT are considered to be individual treatments; however, some modifications may include group treatments and family education sessions.

CBT

CBT, which is the most commonly used and the most widely studied specific therapy for child and adolescent depression, is generally time-limited and focused on identifying thought and behavior patterns that contribute to the child's depressed mood. The goal of CBT is for the therapist and adolescent to collaboratively increase their understanding of how the adolescent's thoughts and behavior influence his or her emotions. (See Table 35–6 for common components of CBT.) Several studies have reported the effectiveness of child and adolescent CBT (see Curry 2001; Reinecke et al. 1998) (see also Weersing and Brent, Chapter 26, in this volume). For example, a study by Brent et al. (1997) compared CBT, systematic-behavioral family therapy, and individual nondirective supportive therapy and found rates of remission to be 60%, 37%, and 39%, respectively. A meta-analysis of six controlled CBT studies in depressed adolescents yielded a reasonably strong overall posttreatment effect size of 1.02, whereas the overall effect size at follow-up was 0.61 (Reinecke et al. 1998).

TABLE 35–6.   Empirically effective components of acute cognitive-behavioral therapy trials

Component	Reference
Noticing and correcting automatic thoughts, assumptions, and beliefs (adapted from Beck's treatment model)	Brent et al. (1997); Butler et al. (1980); Clarke et al. (1999); Vostanis et al. (1996); Wood et al. (1996)
Use of self-control and coping skills	Kahn et al. (1990); Lewinsohn et al. (1990); Reynolds and Coats (1986); Rossello and Bernal (1999); Stark et al. (1987); Vostanis et al. (1996)
Use of problem-solving skills (i.e., recognizing problems and solutions and evaluating outcomes)	Butler et al. (1980); Lerner and Clum (1990); Liddle and Spence (1990); Stark et al. (1987); Vostanis et al. (1996); Wood et al. (1996)
Use of cognitive-behavioral model of psychoeducation	Kahn et al. (1990); Rossello and Bernal (1999)
Use of homework	Kahn et al. (1990); Lewinsohn et al. (1990); Reynolds and Coats (1986); Weisz et al. (1997)
Role-play	Butler et al. (1980); Kahn et al. (1990); Weisz et al. (1997)
Parent group	Clarke et al. (1999); Lewinsohn et al. (1990)
Goal-setting	Stark et al. (1987)

Group CBT for adolescents also has been found to be effective. Clarke et al. (1999) reported on adolescents randomly assigned to adolescent group CBT, adolescent group CBT plus a parent group, or a wait-list control for 8 weeks. The two CBT groups were not different; however, 66.7% of the subjects assigned to either CBT group improved, compared with only 48.1% of the wait-list control subjects. Group CBT has been extensively studied and appears to be effective in both depressed and at-risk adolescents (Clark et al. 1999; Kahn et al. 1990; Lewinsohn et al. 1990, 1996; Reynolds and Coats 1986).

IPT

The premise of IPT is that depression—regardless of symptom patterns, severity, biological vulnerability, or personality—occurs in an interpersonal context and within the framework of one of four problem areas: grief, interpersonal role disputes, role transitions, or interpersonal deficits or issues with single-parent families (in adolescents). Thus, the goal of IPT when treating depression is to understand current relationships and renegotiate interpersonal problems occurring at the onset of depressive symptoms.

IPT has shown effectiveness in the treatment of depressive symptoms in adolescents. In a study of clinical-referred depressed adolescents, IPT was more effective than clinical monitoring for depressive symptom reduction and social functioning improvement (Mufson et al. 1999). Similarly, in a 12-week open study of IPT for 25 moderately to severely depressed adolescents, 84%

met criteria for remission by the end of the treatment (Santor and Kusumakar 2001).

IPT also has been shown to be effective in Puerto Rican populations and was believed to have consonance with Puerto Rican cultural values (Rossello and Bernal 1999). IPT and CBT were compared with wait-list control in the treatment of adolescent depression. Seventy-one adolescents, ages 13–18, were randomly assigned to IPT, CBT, or wait list. IPT and CBT were found to reduce depressive symptoms significantly when compared with the wait-list condition. IPT was superior to the wait-list condition in increasing self-esteem and social adaptation. Clinical significance tests suggested that 82% of the adolescents receiving IPT and 59% of those receiving CBT were considered responders (Children's Depression Inventory score ≤17) after treatment (Rossello and Bernal 1999). Both treatments were superior to the wait list at the end of 12 weeks of acute treatment and at 3-month follow-up.

Continuation Psychotherapy

Acute-phase treatment with CBT and IPT is effective in the short term but may not have lasting effects for some youths. Naturalistic follow-up studies in children and adolescents showed no difference between these specific therapies and control groups during follow-up periods up to 2 years later (Birmaher et al. 2000; Lewinsohn et al. 1990; Vostanis et al. 1998; Wood et al. 1996). However, a 1-year naturalistic follow-up by Mufson and Fairbanks (1996) found that adolescents who received IPT continued to report few depressive symptoms. However, the study was limited by lack of a control group and a small sample size, resulting in limited conclusions about the long-term effectiveness of IPT (Mufson and Fairbanks 1996).

To our knowledge, only two studies have evaluated continuation CBT in youths. Clarke et al. (1999) reported inconclusive findings regarding the efficacy of continuation-phase treatment after adding booster sessions to acute-phase CBT. After 8 weeks of acute-phase treatment (group CBT, group CBT plus a parent group, or wait-list control), patients were followed up for 24 months. All patients were randomly assigned to 1) assessments quarterly, 2) assessments quarterly plus booster sessions, or 3) annual assessments. Booster sessions did not reduce relapse; however, booster treatment did accelerate remission in patients with depression at the end of the acute phase. One limitation of this study was that the booster sessions were only quarterly, which may be insufficient to prevent relapse.

Kroll et al. (1996), in a pilot study of continuation-phase CBT, found that 6 months of continuation-phase CBT significantly lowered relapse rates compared with historical control subjects (6% rate vs. 50% rate). In the acute phase of treatment, 33 subjects (ages 9–17) received five to eight sessions of CBT. Twenty patients remitted, with an average time to remission of 10 weeks. Seventeen patients went on to participate in the continuation-phase CBT treatment. The CBT continuation-phase treatment sessions were biweekly to monthly for 6 months. After 6 months, only 1 subject in the continuation phase relapsed, compared with 6 control subjects. However, this was not a randomized, controlled trial. The study was limited by a relatively small sample size and by the use of a historical control group for comparisons.

Other Psychotherapies

Recently, dialectical behavior therapy (DBT), a treatment shown to be effective in reducing the rate of self-harm or parasuicidal behavior in adult women, has been adapted for use with adolescents. Family treatments also have received recent attention and have shown promise in the treatment of early-onset depression (Diamond et al. 2002; Fristad et al. 1998).

DBT.   DBT is an empirically supported psychotherapy that has been adapted for use with adolescent populations, particularly those with suicidal ideation and/or borderline personality features (Rathus and Miller 2002). The focus of this treatment for adolescents is primarily on affect regulation, problem solving, improving communication, and maintaining a balance between acceptance

and change. A multifamily group is a component of this treatment with adolescents.

In adult women, DBT was found to significantly reduce anger, suicide attempts, parasuicidal acts, and the number of inpatient psychiatric days. It also has been shown to improve social adjustment, treatment compliance, and dropout rates (Linehan et al. 1991). The improvement in dropout rates is potentially important for adolescent populations because 77% of adolescent suicide attempters do not attend or fail to complete treatment (Trautman et al. 1993).

The efficacy of DBT was shown in a group of 27 suicidal adolescents ages 14–19 years who had diagnoses of borderline personality disorder or borderline features. The adolescents completed pre- and posttreatment evaluations and had significant reductions in borderline personality disorder symptoms in four common problem areas (confusion about self, impulsivity, emotional instability, and interpersonal problems). The most helpful DBT skills were identified as mindfulness and distress tolerance (Miller et al. 2000).

Family therapy.   Family factors appear to play a role in relapse or depression maintenance in children and adolescents (Gillham et al. 2000). Some studies point to the importance of family intervention in adolescents with mood disorders. Lewinsohn et al. (1990) reported that those adolescents whose parents attended the group parenting course on depression showed greater reduction in depressive symptoms (as rated by parents). In addition, Kolko et al. (2000) found that those adolescents who had participated in family treatment had significantly improved parent–child relationships at a 2-year follow-up.

Family therapies for mood disorders in children and adolescents are in the early development phase but show promise. Diamond and colleagues (Diamond and Siqueland 1995; Diamond et al. 2002) introduced a model of treatment that included reducing maladaptive interactions between family members or between these families and external systems of care. Harrington and colleagues (1998) presented an in-home problem-solving treatment with adolescents who had suicidal behaviors (poison ingestion). They found that in adolescents who were both suicidal and depressed, this approach was effective in reducing suicidal ideation compared with a group receiving treatment as usual.

Fristad et al. (1998), in a pilot study of nine children and adolescents, found that multifamily psychoeducational group therapy (a six-session treatment program) may improve the family climate in children with mood disorders immediately after the treatment and at 4-month follow-up.

Finally, Beardslee and colleagues (1997) examined

family cognitive restructuring treatment for the depressed offspring of depressed parents. This preventive family treatment resulted in improved family communication and increased closeness in the family. In addition, preliminary evidence for improved child outcomes (i.e., higher global functioning) was reported.

Integrating Pharmacotherapy and Psychotherapy

Until recently, no controlled trials of combination medication and psychotherapy have been reported. However, new research into this area is under way. A recent collaborative contract with the NIMH to compare medication treatment (with fluoxetine), CBT, combination treatment, and placebo recently has been completed (Treatment for Adolescents With Depression Study Team 2003). Four hundred thirty-nine adolescents were randomly assigned to 12 weeks of fluoxetine alone, CBT alone, combination fluoxetine plus CBT, or placebo. On the basis of CGI Scale improvement ratings of 1 or 2 ("much" or "very much" improved), response was greatest in the combination treatment group (71%), followed by fluoxetine alone (61%), CBT alone (43%), and placebo (35%). Combination treatment and fluoxetine alone were significantly better than placebo ($P=0.001$ for both), but CBT alone was not ($P=0.196$). Combination treatment and fluoxetine alone were not significantly different ($P=0.106$), but both combination treatment and fluoxetine were superior to CBT alone ($P=0.001$ and $P=0.011$, respectively). This study further confirmed the effectiveness of SSRI medication over placebo and indicated that combination treatment may be the best option for treating adolescent depression (Treatment for Adolescents With Depression Study Team 2004). In addition, an ongoing study of treatment-resistant depression in adolescents is examining combination treatment. In this study, adolescents who did not show adequate response to treatment with an SSRI were randomly assigned to receive alternative medication only (alternative SSRI or venlafaxine) or an alternative medication plus CBT. This study is scheduled for completion by summer 2007.

To date, no guidelines for single modality treatment versus combination treatments have been established for early-onset depression. The American Psychiatric Association practice guidelines for adults state that combination treatment is needed if an individual has significant psychosocial problems, a history of partial response to pharmacotherapy or psychotherapy alone, or poor adherence to a single mode of treatment (American Psychiatric Association 2000b). Combination treatment serves to enhance the magnitude of response to treatment and to enhance the probability of response; two treatments are more powerful than one, and if one form of treatment does not help, the other one probably will. The breadth of response also tends to be better when combination treatment is used. Medication often works quickly to reduce symptoms of depression, but the rate of failure is also higher with medication alone. Combination therapy in pediatric depression serves to enhance the acceptability of treatment.

Bipolar Disorders

Symptomatology

Bipolar disorder, according to DSM-IV-TR, is divided into bipolar I disorder, bipolar II disorder, bipolar disorder not otherwise specified, and cyclothymic disorder. Secondary bipolar disorder could result from a known medical condition or substance-induced mania (e.g., antidepressant use). The distinction between bipolar disorder and depression is based on the presence of symptoms of mania either in a mixed state with depression or as a discrete episode of mania.

Lively debate continues around the phenomenology of bipolar disorder in children and adolescents, but generally more consent than disagreement is found (Biederman 2003; Fristad et al. 1995). Although the general consensus is that bipolar disorder in youths may be more common than previously thought, the disorder remains difficult to diagnose. Bipolar I disorder (full criteria for mania with or without episodes of depression) and bipolar II disorder (major depressive episodes with at least one hypomanic episode) are clearly diagnosable in children, although diagnostic certainty declines with decreasing age of the child. Recent attempts have been made to better describe children who would generally fall into a category of bipolar disorder not otherwise specified because many prepubertal children present with severe symptoms not clearly characterized by bipolar I or II disorder.

There is general agreement that preadolescent-onset bipolar disorder often presents very early, is characterized by rapid mood shifts with substantial irritability, and has a high rate of comorbidity with ADHD (Biederman et al. 2000; Carlson et al. 2003; Geller et al. 2000). Many children have severe affective disturbance (e.g., extreme irritability and agitation, high levels of aggression and impulse control disorders, and frequent mood lability), but despite clear symptoms of mania and/or depression, many of these youths when assessed prior to 1990 did not receive a diagnosis of affective disorder (Akiskal et al. 1985). Several reports in the mid-1980s began recognizing that this symptom presentation may be a form of early-onset bipolar disorder (Akiskal et al. 1985; Carlson 1984; De-Long and Nieman 1983; R.A. Weller et al. 1986). Current consensus is that many prepubertal children with bipolar disorder likely present with this presentation. In addition, bipolar children commonly present with a mixed and dysphoric picture, with these same intense periods of irritability and mood lability rather than classic euphoria (Geller et al. 1995). This clinical picture of periods of mania or hypomania interspersed with periods of dysphoria is characteristic of a presentation common in adult bipolar patients, called *dysphoric mania* (Post et al. 1989).

In addition to the differing symptom presentation compared with classic adult mania, prepubertal mania appears to be less acute and episodic and more chronic and continuous. Fewer well-defined episodes occur in preadolescent-onset bipolar disorder (Biederman et al. 2000; Tillman and Geller 2003). Geller et al. (1995) found that in a group of 25 bipolar children and adolescents, "complex" cycling patterns characterized by brief manic periods lasting 4 or more hours occurred in 81% of these patients.

DSM-IV-TR specifies a subtype of bipolar disorder as "with rapid cycling," meaning that an individual must have had "four or more mood episodes during the previous 12 months" (American Psychiatric Association 2000a, p. 427). Dunner et al. (1976) were the first to identify rapid cycling in patients with bipolar disorder, and Geller et al. (1998b) found that 83.3% of the individuals with pediatric-onset bipolar disorder experienced cycling. Kramlinger and Post (1996) identified two other cycling patterns associated with bipolar disorder: ultrarapid (mood disturbances that cycle within weeks or a few days) and ultradian (marked and abrupt mood changes that cycle in less than 24 hours). Geller et al. (1998b) found that in a sample of 60 subjects with prepubertal-onset bipolar disorder, 8.3% presented with ultrarapid cycling, and 75% presented with ultradian cycling. Those with ultradian cycling experienced, on average, four cycles per day (Geller et al. 1998b). These factors contribute to the difficulties in diagnosing very-early-onset bipolar disorder in children, yet many clinicians and researchers agree that the population is severely impaired and warrants treatment.

Contrary to the disparate clinical presentation in younger children, adolescent-onset bipolar disorder often presents with more typical discrete episodes of mania and depression (Carlson et al. 2003). DSM-IV-TR criteria for a manic episode include a "distinct period" of abnormally elevated, expansive, or irritable mood for at least 1 week (4 days for hypomania), accompanied by at least three of

the following symptoms: extremely inflated self-esteem or grandiosity, decreased need for sleep, increased talking or pressured speech, flight of ideas or racing thoughts, distractibility, increased goal-directed activity or psychomotor agitation, and excessive involvement in pleasurable activities with a high potential for serious consequences (American Psychiatric Association 2000a, p. 362). The manic phase must be a change from previous functioning and must cause impairment. Teenagers are more likely to present with these more classic signs. However, developmental differences still may exist, requiring adequate diagnosis by clinicians to avoid under- or overdiagnosis of bipolar disorder (Geller et al. 2002). Examples of specific manifestations of child and adolescent mania are listed in Table 35–7. Geller and colleagues (2002) also provided excellent guidelines for recognizing varying levels of symptom manifestation in early-onset bipolar disorder.

One significant difficulty in diagnosing bipolar disorder is the overlap with symptoms of ADHD. As is detailed in the section on comorbidity later in this chapter, concurrent bipolar disorder and ADHD is common in children and adolescents. Many of the symptoms also overlap, such as irritable mood, accelerated speech, distractibility, and increased energy. Hypersexuality, daredevil acts, and uninhibited people-seeking are partially overlapping symptoms. Symptoms that are clearly manic, with no overlap with ADHD, are elated mood, grandiosity, flight of ideas and racing thoughts, and a decreased need for sleep. The nonoverlapping features are the most clinically useful determinants of bipolar disorder (Geller et al. 2002).

Thus, mania is often difficult to diagnose in the pediatric population, particularly in prepubertal children because the pediatric presentation of the disorder does not mimic the classic adult presentation. The disorder in children is often further complicated by a high frequency of parental bipolar illness, which impairs the parent's ability to recognize problems in or seek treatment for the child (Geller 1996). However, the disorder is a diagnosable condition in this population, and in fact, there is more agreement among experts about the condition (and its presentation) than disagreement.

Associated Features

Like depression and other psychiatric disorders, bipolar disorder causes substantial psychosocial difficulties. It is associated with school difficulties, suicide attempts, sexual promiscuity, and substance abuse, often leading to legal difficulties and hospitalizations (Akiskal et al. 1985; Carlson and Kelly 1998; Geller and Luby 1997; Lewinsohn et al. 1995; Strober et al. 1995). Furthermore, Geller et al. (2000) reported increased difficulties in school, poorer

TABLE 35–7.   Manic symptoms in children and adolescents

DSM-IV-TR criteria	Child symptoms	Adolescent symptoms
Elevated or expansive mood	Inappropriate silliness, constant singing, and excessive happiness (more than the situation warrants)	Excessive silliness or unrealistic optimism with no insight related to the inappropriateness of the moods
Irritable mood	Marked belligerence, high irritability with frequent, intense "anger outbursts"	Extremely oppositional, belligerence, short, curt, or hostile in tone
Inflated self-esteem or grandiosity	Thoughts of having "super powers" (e.g., "I am Superman; nothing can kill me or stop me.")	"I can speak 13 different languages and have solved the problem of world peace."
Decreased need for sleep	Refusing to go to bed before 1:00 or 2:00 A.M. and sleeping only 3 or 4 hours a night	Staying up all night and then "crashing" for short periods during the day
More talkative than usual	Blurting out answers during class repeatedly and appearing to "know it all"; unintelligible or difficult to follow	Very rapid and pressured speech to the point at which it is continuous and at times difficult to understand
Flight of ideas or racing thoughts	"I have so many great ideas that I can't keep them straight" or "get them out fast enough."	Racing thoughts sometimes will be evident in pressured speech; rhyming of words and taking great pleasure in being able "to think faster than others"
Distractibility, short attention span	May report inability to pay attention in class because his or her thoughts are moving along too fast.	May report inability to pay attention in class because his or her thoughts are moving along too fast.
Increase in goal-directed activity	Restlessness, motor-driven behavior, and shifting from activity to activity rapidly	Hyperactive but able to complete the multiple projects before moving on to another project
Excessive involvement in pleasurable activities that have a high potential for painful consequences	Hypersexual behavior and inappropriately touching peers or adults in an attempt to engage them in sex	Displaying a marked increase in reckless, thrill-seeking behavior (e.g., promiscuous behavior, binge drinking, shopping sprees)

peer relationships, and poorer family functioning in bipolar children compared with children with ADHD.

High familial aggregation of bipolar disorder also has been noted; many children and adolescents with bipolar disorder diagnoses have at least one first-degree relative with a mood disorder (Geller 1996; Gershon 1988; Strober et al. 1988). High rates of parental bipolar disorder often lead to underdiagnosis in children and adolescents because many of the bipolar parents have not received diagnoses themselves (Geller 1996).

Comorbidity

Like pediatric depression, comorbidity is common in early-onset bipolar disorder. The most common comorbid diagnosis in this population is ADHD. Wozniak et al. (1995) reported that of 262 consecutively referred children to a pediatric psychopharmacology clinic, 16% met DSM-III-R (American Psychiatric Association 1987) criteria for mania, and 98% of these bipolar children also

met criteria for ADHD. Geller and colleagues (2002) also found high rates of comorbid ADHD (87%), with higher rates among males (98%) than females (69%) (P<0.001). In differentiating between bipolar disorder and ADHD, clinicians should remember that elevated mood, irritability, grandiosity, and a decreased need for sleep are symptoms of only bipolar disorder; these are not present in ADHD (Geller et al. 2002). In addition, ADHD, which must have an onset before age 7 years, is primarily a disorder of behavior, not mood.

Conduct disorder is also common in bipolar disorder, in part because of the intense irritability and aggression common in prepubertal bipolar disorder. Kovacs and Pollock (1995) found a 69% rate of conduct disorder among 26 bipolar children and adolescents as well as a worse clinical course than in those bipolar patients without conduct disorder. Kutcher and colleagues (1989) reported conduct disorder in 42% of youths hospitalized for mania. However, bipolar disorder often is misdiagnosed as conduct disorder. During a manic or hypomanic episode, an adolescent's reckless, antisocial behavior may be mistakenly viewed as indicative of conduct disorder, leaving the bipolar disorder undiagnosed and possibly untreated. Therefore, it is important to keep in mind that conduct disorder is a more "predatory" type of disorder, whereas bipolar disorder is a disorder of mood.

Course of Illness

Bipolar disorder is a chronic disorder that often includes complex cycling patterns in children and adolescents (Geller et al. 1995). Geller and Luby (1997) found that prepubertal- and young adolescent–onset bipolar disorder manifests as an initial major depressive episode, with a rapid-cycling or mixed-episode type that is chronic and continuous. These investigators found that functioning was poor between these episodes. However, with older adolescent- and adult-onset bipolar disorder, the initial episode presented as mania, with a discrete episode type with sudden onsets and noticeable offsets. These episodes lasted for weeks, but functioning was improved between episodes.

Relatively few longitudinal studies of pediatric-onset bipolar disorder can be found in the literature. Strober et al. (1995) followed up 54 adolescents with bipolar I disorder every 6 months for 5 years, into adulthood. All had received treatment with mood stabilizers. The mean time to recovery for adolescents with an index episode of depression was 26 weeks, for adolescents with an index episode of mania was 9 weeks, and for adolescents with an initial mixed episode was 11 weeks. By the 5-year follow-up, however, 44% had one or more relapses, with multiple relapses being most common (60%) in subjects with mixed or cycling episodes at intake. Strober et al., however, failed to find any significant predictors of relapse. Also, by the 5-year follow-up, 20% had made at least one medically significant suicide attempt (Strober et al. 1995).

Coryell and colleagues (1998) followed up adult patients with bipolar disorder for 15 years and found that 20% of the patients showed bipolar symptoms throughout the whole study; a subgroup of individuals with bipolar disorder have a considerably adverse long-term outcome (Coryell et al. 1998). Coryell and colleagues (1998) also failed to find any predictors of relapse, except for lower functioning in the 5 years prior to baseline assessment and the increased presence of depressive symptoms in the first 2 years after baseline assessment.

Calabrese et al. (2003) found that adults with bipolar disorder experience more social and family difficulties, increased work impairment, and more criminal arrests than do other United States adults. They also have more physical problems, such as anxiety, panic attacks, migraines, and asthma attacks (Calabrese et al. 2003). Because bipolar disorder is a lifelong illness, children and adolescents will have an increased likelihood of experiencing these same problems.

Epidemiology

Bipolar disorder is not as prevalent as depression. Most reports suggest that the prevalence of early-onset bipolar disorder is approximately 1% (Keller and Baker 1991). More children tend to have significant symptoms but do not meet full diagnostic criteria for the disorder. Up to 12% of children and adolescents claim maniclike symptoms (subthreshold) that cause significant impairment at home, at school, or with peers (Carlson and Kashani 1988a; Kessler and Walters 1998; Lewinsohn et al. 1995); however, parents did not always agree with the child's statement of pathology (Carlson and Kashani 1988b). However, Wozniak and colleagues (1995) found that 16% of 262 consecutively referred children met criteria for mania when assessed.

Lewinsohn and colleagues (1995) found that 1% of adolescents have bipolar disorder. To date, no epidemiological studies have been done to confirm bipolar disorder in children (Angold et al. 2002; Costello et al. 1988, 1996, 2002). Adult epidemiological studies report that 0.4%–1.6% of the population have bipolar disorders (American Psychiatric Association 2000a), and 0.5% of adults with bipolar disorder report that their age at onset was during childhood (Loranger and Levine 1978). Some experts claim that bipolar disorder is much more prevalent in children and has been underdiagnosed (Geller and Luby 1997; E.B. Weller et al. 1995). Others, in both the United States (Biederman et al. 1998; Carlson 1998) and Europe (Harrington and Myatt 2003), express doubt that bipolar disorder is any more prevalent. Many, in fact, state that bipolar disorder cannot be diagnosed before age 10 (Carlson et al. 2003). The difficulty in determining prevalence stems in part from the difficulty in assessment and diagnosis of this complicated disorder (Coyle et al. 2003).

Pathogenesis

Limited information is available on the pathophysiology of bipolar disorder specific to children and adolescents. However, family aggregation and genetic transmission of bipolar disorder have been clearly documented through family twin and adoption studies. However, these studies support the concept that earlier age at onset confers a greater familiar risk of bipolar disorder (for review, see Faraone et al. 2003).

Of interest is the relation between ADHD and bipolar

disorder in early-onset bipolar disorder (Biederman et al. 1996). Leibenluft and colleagues (2003) suggested that the association between earlier-onset bipolar disorder and ADHD and the presence of high rates of irritability and rapid-cycling mood disturbances are important areas of research focus for better understanding of pediatric bipolar disorder. This expands the understanding of the pathophysiology of bipolar disorder to encompass not only mood lability but also executive function deficit and reward mechanism (for review, see Leibenluft et al. 2003).

Separating the consequences of the effect of the illness or prolonged medication treatments on neurocognitive development is difficult in adults. Chang et al. (2003) suggested that studying the offspring of adults with bipolar disorder may "present phenomenological, temperamental and biological clues to early presentation of bipolar disorder" (p. 945). Bipolar offspring are at high risk for development of bipolar disorder (DelBello and Geller 2001). Early intervention may prevent full expression of bipolar disorder in children.

In summary, recent advances in our understanding of the phenomenology of bipolar disorder have set the stage for defining areas of research that potentially will substantially increase our understanding of the pathophysiology of bipolar disorder in children, adolescents, and adults.

Pharmacotherapy

The treatment of pediatric-onset bipolar disorder most often begins with pharmacotherapy; however, most of the literature on medication in bipolar children and adolescents consists of open trials and case studies. Limited controlled data are available in this age group.

Acute Treatment

Three classes of medications are most commonly used to treat bipolar disorder, whether adult-onset or pediatric-onset: mood stabilizers, anticonvulsants, and atypical antipsychotics. Lithium, a mood stabilizer, has been the most studied medication in this population. Most open trials reported improvement in 50%–60% of the subjects. In an open trial of lithium, Kafantaris et al. (2003) found a 63% response rate to lithium; however, only 26% achieved remission of manic symptoms within 4 weeks. Only one placebo-controlled trial has been reported in pediatric bipolar disorder. In a 6-week double-blind, placebo-controlled trial of lithium for bipolar disorder and substance abuse, Geller and colleagues (1998a) reported a significant difference between lithium (46.2% response rate) and placebo (8.3% response rate), with lithium treatment leading to greater improvement in both disorders.

Divalproex and carbamazepine are two commonly used anticonvulsants in the treatment of bipolar disorder. Open trials of divalproex reported positive responses ranging from 61% to 87% of pediatric subjects (Papatheodorou et al. 1995; Wagner et al. 2002). Although there have been no open trials of carbamazepine, case reports have confirmed its use in adolescent bipolar disorder. Only one trial has compared the efficacy of these medications against one another. Kowatch et al. (2000) compared lithium, divalproex, and carbamazepine for the treatment of bipolar disorder in children and adolescents. The response rate, defined as a 50% or more increase in the Young Mania Rating Scale (YMRS) score, was found to be 53% for divalproex, 38% for lithium, and 38% for carbamazepine after 6 weeks of treatment (P=0.60).

Finally, atypical antipsychotics such as olanzapine and risperidone also have been examined in open-label trials. An open-label study of olanzapine for pediatric bipolar disorder yielded an overall response rate of 61%, measured by a greater than 30% decline in the mean YMRS score (Frazier et al. 2001). Frazier and colleagues (1999) also conducted a retrospective chart review of risperidone and found that out of 28 individuals treated, 82% showed improvement in both manic and aggressive symptoms. However, these patients were not treated solely with risperidone; concomitant medications, including mood stabilizers, anti-ADHD treatments, other antipsychotics, and lorazepam, were used in 96% of the patients. In open treatment of 11 children and adolescents with bipolar disorder, risperidone was shown to have a 73% response rate (Schreier 1998). These trials were all quite small, and the criteria used for diagnosis were not consistent across trials. Yet there appears to be at least some suggestion that these medications may reduce symptoms of mania.

One important issue in bipolar disorder, both adult and pediatric, is compliance with treatment (Geller and Luby 1997). Strober et al. (1990) studied an 18-month continuation treatment with lithium in 37 patients. They found only a 37% relapse rate in those patients believed to be compliant with the medication but a 92% relapse rate in those who were noncompliant. Because compliance is clearly an issue with this disorder and noncompliance significantly affects treatment outcome, education about the disorder and medications is essential.

Treatment-Resistant Bipolar Disorder

As noted earlier, even in open trial studies, bipolar disorder medications are effective in only a little more than half of the population. In many cases, additional treatment is necessary. In the extension phase of the Kowatch et al. (2003) study, 58% of the patients had to be given a second mood stabilizer and either an antipsychotic drug, an antidepressant, or a stimulant; 80% showed improvement with this combination therapy. Similarly, in an open study of 90 subjects (ages 5–17) with bipolar I or II disorder, combination lithium and divalproex significantly improved symptoms of mania, depression, and global functioning ($P<0.0001$) by the end of 8 weeks of treatment and the end of the study (Findling et al. 2003). However, only 47% met a priori criteria for remission (minimal symptoms of mania and depression for at least 4 weeks, clinically stable, and no evidence of mood cycling). DelBello et al. (2002) examined the effectiveness of topiramate as an adjunctive treatment in pediatric bipolar disorder. In this retrospective chart review, they found 23 patients who had received combination therapy with topiramate. Separate CGI Scale ratings were made for mania and overall bipolar illness; consequently, the response rate for mania was 73% and for overall illness was 62% (DelBello et al. 2002). Chang and Ketter (2000) studied the success of olanzapine as an adjunctive treatment in three patients and found improvement in all; however, Soutullo et al. (1999) found only a 71% response rate with a slightly larger sample size ($n=7$). Finally, Ryback et al. (1997) examined the effectiveness of gabapentin as an adjunctive treatment in 18 patients; they found that in 88.9% of the patients, the drug helped to stop the cycling, and in 33% of the patients, the drug actually improved mood. Clearly, augmenting the initial medication may improve outcome in patients with bipolar disorder.

Psychotherapy

Specific psychotherapy, such as CBT or IPT, as a single-modality treatment is not suggested for treating bipolar disorder because of the severity of the illness. However, the use of adjunctive psychotherapy to medication treatment in the management of bipolar disorder is critical (Craighead and Miklowitz 2000). Similar to the course of schizophrenia, bipolar disorder has a high rate of relapse, a significant rate of residual symptoms posttreatment, and precipitation of episodes by psychosocial stressors. In addition, because the first line of treatment is pharmacotherapy, the need to manage nonadherence is important. These factors can be effectively treated with psychosocial interventions, including psychotherapy. In the adult bipolar population, three psychotherapies have shown positive outcomes (Sachs et al. 2003): CBT (Cochran 1984; Otto et al. 2003), family-focused therapy (Miklowitz et al. 2003), and IPT with a social rhythm component (Frank et al. 2000).

Psychotherapy in Adults With Bipolar Disorder

Psychosocial treatment studies of children and adolescents with bipolar disorder are limited. We begin with a brief review of the psychosocial studies that have been done in the adult bipolar population.

CBT. Evidence indicates that CBT is an effective adjunctive treatment strategy for bipolar disorder in adults (Otto et al. 2003). In a controlled trial, Cochran (1984) treated adult bipolar disorder with lithium and brief CBT and found better medication adherence and fewer relapse episodes related to nonadherence compared with patients receiving lithium alone. Similarly, Lam et al. (2000) randomly assigned a sample of 25 bipolar patients to either treatment as usual or treatment as usual combined with individual CBT. They found that the group who received CBT had a lower rate of manic, hypomanic, and depressed episodes than did the control group at 6- and 12-month follow-up.

IPT. Frank et al. (1997) showed a positive effect for IPT combined with social rhythm therapy (regulation of daily routines and sleep cycles) and psychoeducation (IPSRT). IPSRT has been found to be effective in maintaining stability in daily routines and lowering depressive symptoms in this population. However, it is unclear whether it can reduce the recurrence rate of mania (Frank et al. 2000).

Family-focused therapy. Family-focused therapy is a family psychosocial intervention that provides education about the illness, teaches methods for coping with the illness, and trains families on good communication and problem-solving skills (Miklowitz and Goldstein 1990). Family-focused therapy developed out of the schizophrenia studies, which found that psychoeducational treatment for the families of schizophrenic patients was successful in reducing relapse rates and improving psychosocial function (Falloon and Pederson 1985). Several empirical trials have shown family-focused therapy to be an effective intervention for reducing relapse rates in bipolar adults (Miklowitz et al. 2000; Rea et al. 2003). In addition, family-focused therapy and pharmacotherapy in a 2-year outcome study were determined to be more effective in reducing mood symptoms and increasing medication adherence than were medication and crisis management (Miklowitz et al. 2003).

Other family intervention studies provide similar support for a family, psychoeducational approach. Medication alone was compared with medication combined with psychoeducational marital intervention in an 11-month treatment study. Medication adherence was better in the experimental group along with improvement in global functioning (Clarkin et al. 1998). Similar results supporting family intervention in bipolar disorder also have been reported (Clarkin et al. 1990; Miklowitz and Goldstein 1990).

Psychosocial Interventions in Pediatric Bipolar Patients

Current efforts are under way to adapt family-focused therapy to an adolescent population (Taylor et al. 2003). The available empirical support for psychosocial treatments of pediatric bipolar disorder is limited, however. Most of the work in this population has been in the area of family psychoeducational treatment. Fristad and colleagues (1998) have developed a multifamily group psychoeducational treatment, which provides education to families about bipolar illness, an opportunity for group discussion, and a skill component for parents and separately for children. Parents and children have separate curricula, and the format has been expanded from the original 6 weeks to 8 weeks (Fristad et al. 2003). Multifamily psychoeducational group treatment has been shown to increase social support from families and peers of bipolar children and to improve family communication skills as compared with wait-list control subjects. Fristad and colleagues (2003) are currently adapting the multifamily format to individual family format to allow the treatment to be provided more easily by practitioners who are not in clinic settings. Further research into the role of adjunctive psychotherapy treatments for children and adolescents with mania is needed.

Conclusion

Mood disorders are serious disorders in the pediatric population, causing significant morbidity and mortality. Although mood disorders are now more recognized and acknowledged in the pediatric population, they remain underdiagnosed and therefore undertreated in children and adolescents. The diagnostic process differs slightly from adult evaluations, in that multiple informants (e.g., child, parents, teachers, and other caregivers) are needed to gather adequate clinical information to establish symptoms, severity, and course of illness, which will guide treatment decisions. The disorders are complicated and frequently present with a multitude of comorbid psychiatric conditions.

At present, specific psychotherapies such as CBT and IPT and certain antidepressants known as SSRIs (e.g., fluoxetine) are the only treatments that have shown efficacy in depressed youths. Only fluoxetine has received an indication from the FDA for treating pediatric depression. Yet even these treatments are beneficial to only about 65% of youths. Research in treatments for bipolar disorder is even less consistent, with many bipolar children and adolescents requiring multiple medications. Further-

more, long-term benefits of these treatments remain unknown because limited research has been conducted in the continuation and maintenance treatment of mood disorders in children and adolescents.

In summary, many significant advances have been made in pediatric mood disorders. Yet much remains unknown. Additional research into treatments, including new medications and specific therapies, relapse prevention treatments, and predictors of response (e.g., which youths will respond to which treatments), will lead to further advancement of the treatment of pediatric mood disorders.

References

Akiskal HS, Downs J, Jordan P, et al: Affective disorders in referred children and young siblings of manic-depressives. Arch Gen Psychiatry 42:996–1003, 1985

American Psychiatric Association: Diagnostic and Statistical Manual of Mental Disorders, 3rd Edition, Revised. Washington, DC, American Psychiatric Association, 1987

American Psychiatric Association: Diagnostic and Statistical Manual of Mental Disorders, 4th Edition, Text Revision. Washington, DC, American Psychiatric Association, 20000a

American Psychiatric Association: Practice guideline for the treatment of patients with major depressive disorder (revision). American Psychiatric Association. Am J Psychiatry 157 (4 suppl):1–45, 2000b

Angold A, Costello EJ, Worthman CM: Puberty and depression: the roles of age, pubertal status and pubertal timing. Psychol Med 28:51–61, 1998

Angold A, Erkanli A, Farmer E, et al: Psychiatric disorder, impairment, and service use in rural African American and white youth. Arch Gen Psychiatry 59:893–901, 2002

Anthony J, Scott P: Manic depressive psychosis in childhood. J Child Psychol Psychiatry 1:52–72, 1960

Armitage R, Hoffman RF, Emslie GJ, et al: Sleep microarchitecture as a predictor of recurrence in children and adolescents with depression. Int J Neuropsychopharmacol 5:217–228, 2002

Aronen ET, Soininen M: Childhood depressive symptoms predict psychiatric problems in young adults. Can J Psychiatry 45:465–470, 2000

Asarnow JR, Bates S: Depression in child psychiatric inpatients: cognitive and attributional patterns. J Abnorm Child Psychol 16:601–615, 1988

Asarnow JR, Tompson M, Hamilton EB, et al: Family expressed emotion, childhood-onset depression, and childhood-onset schizophrenia spectrum disorders: is expressed emotion a nonspecific correlate of child psychopathology or a specific risk factor for depression? J Abnorm Child Psychol 22:129–146, 1994

Axelson DA, Birmaher B: Relation between anxiety and depressive disorders in childhood and adolescence. Depress Anxiety 14:67–78, 2001

Bailly D, Beuscart R, Collinet C, et al: Sex differences in the manifestations of depression in young people: a study of French high school students, I: prevalence and clinical data. Eur Child Adolesc Psychiatry 1:135–145, 1992

Bardone AM, Moffitt TE, Caspi A, et al: Adult mental health and social outcomes of adolescent girls with depression and conduct disorder. Dev Psychopathol 8:811–829, 1996

Bardone AM, Moffitt TE, Caspi A, et al: Adult physical health outcomes of adolescent girls with conduct disorder, depression, and anxiety. J Am Acad Child Adolesc Psychiatry 37:594–601, 1998

Barraclough B: Suicide and epilepsy, in Epilepsy and Psychiatry. Edited by Reynolds EH, Trimble MR. Edinburgh, UK, Churchill Livingstone, 1981, pp 72–76

Beardslee WR, Wright EJ, Salt P, et al: Examination of children's responses to two preventive intervention strategies over time. J Am Acad Child Adolesc Psychiatry 36:196–204, 1997

Beardslee WR, Versage EM, Gladstone TR: Children of affectively ill parents: a review of the past 10 years. J Am Acad Child Adolesc Psychiatry 37:1134–1141, 1998

Beautrais AL: Risk factors for suicide and attempted suicide among young people. Aust N Z J Psychiatry 34:420–436, 2000

Beevers CG, Keitner GI, Ryan CE, et al: Cognitive predictors of symptom return following depression treatment. J Abnorm Psychol 112:488–496, 2003

Biederman J: Pediatric bipolar disorder coming of age. Biol Psychiatry 53:931–934, 2003

Biederman J, Faraone SV, Keenan K, et al: Evidence of familial association between attention deficit disorder and major affective disorders. Arch Gen Psychiatry 48:633–642, 1991

Biederman J, Faraone SV, Mick E, et al: Attention-deficit hyperactivity disorder and juvenile mania: an overlooked comorbidity? J Am Acad Child Adolesc Psychiatry 35:997–1008, 1996

Biederman J, Klein RG, Pine DS, et al: Resolved: mania is mistaken for ADHD in prepubertal children. J Am Acad Child Adolesc Psychiatry 37:1091–1096, 1998

Biederman J, Mick E, Faraone SV, et al: Pediatric mania: a developmental subtype of bipolar disorder? Biol Psychiatry 48:458–466, 2000

Birmaher B, Dahl RE, Perel J, et al: Corticotropin-releasing hormone challenge in prepubertal major depression. Biol Psychiatry 39:267–277, 1996a

Birmaher B, Ryan N, Williamson DE, et al: Childhood and adolescent depression: a review of the past 10 years, part I. J Am Acad Child Adolesc Psychiatry 35:1427–1439, 1996b

Birmaher B, Brent DA, Kolko D, et al: Clinical outcome after short-term psychotherapy for adolescents with major depressive disorder. Arch Gen Psychiatry 57:29–36, 2000

Brent DA, Kolko DJ, Wartella ME, et al: Adolescent psychiatric inpatients' risk of suicide attempt at 6-month follow-up. J Am Acad Child Adolesc Psychiatry 32:95–105, 1993

Brent DA, Holder D, Kolko D, et al: A clinical psychotherapy trial for adolescent depression comparing cognitive, family, and supportive therapy. Arch Gen Psychiatry 54:877–885, 1997

Brent DA, Kolko DJ, Birmaher B, et al: A clinical trial for adolescent depression: predictors of additional treatment in the acute and follow-up phases of the trial. J Am Acad Child Adolesc Psychiatry 38:263–270, 1999

Brumback RA, Weinberg WA: Pediatric behavioral neurology: an update on the neurologic aspects of depression, hyperactivity, and learning disabilities. Neurol Clin 8:677–703, 1990 [published erratum appears in 9:viii, 1991]

Brumback RA, Dietz-Schmidt SG, Weinberg WA: Depression in children referred to an educational diagnostic center: diagnosis and treatment and analysis of criteria and literature review. Dis Nerv Syst 38:529–535, 1977

Butler L, Mietzitis S, Friedman R, et al: The effect of two school-based intervention programs on depressive symptoms in preadolescents. Am Educ Res J 17:111–119, 1980

Calabrese JR, Hirschfeld RM, Reed M, et al: Impact of bipolar disorder on a U.S. community sample. J Clin Psychiatry 64:425–432, 2003

Canals J: Prevalence of depression in Europe. J Am Acad Child Adolesc Psychiatry 36:1325–1326, 1997

Canals J, Domenech E, Carbajo G, et al: Prevalence of DSM-III-R and ICD-10 psychiatric disorders in a Spanish population of 18-year-olds. Acta Psychiatr Scand 96:287–294, 1997

Cantwell D, Baker L: Academic failures in children with communication disorders. J Am Acad Child Psychiatry 19:579–591, 1980

Carlson GA: Classification issues of bipolar disorder in childhood. Psychiatr Dev 2:273–285, 1984

Carlson GA: Mania and ADHD: comorbidity or confusion. J Affect Disord 51:177–187, 1998

Carlson GA, Kashani JH: Manic symptoms in a non-referred adolescent population. J Affect Disord 15:219–226, 1988a

Carlson GA, Kashani JH: Phenomenology of major depression from childhood through adulthood. Am J Psychiatry 145:1222–1225, 1988b

Carlson GA, Kelly KL: Manic symptoms in psychiatrically hospitalized children—what do they mean? J Affect Disord 51:123–135, 1998

Carlson GA, Jensen PS, Findling RL, et al: Methodological issues and controversies in clinical trials with child and adolescent patients with bipolar disorder: report of a consensus conference. J Child Adolesc Psychopharmacol 13:13–27, 2003

Caspi A, Sugden K, Moffitt TE, et al: Influence of life stress on depression: moderation by a polymorphism in the 5-HTT gene. Science 301:386–389, 2003

Chang KD, Ketter TA: Mood stabilizer augmentation with olanzapine in acutely manic children. J Child Adolesc Psychopharmacol 10:45–49, 2000

Chang KD, Steiner H, Dienes K, et al: Bipolar offspring: a window into bipolar disorder evolution. Biol Psychiatry 53:945–951, 2003

Clarke GN, Rohde P, Lewinsohn PM, et al: Cognitive-behavioral treatment of adolescent depression: efficacy of acute group treatment and booster sessions. J Am Acad Child Adolesc Psychiatry 38:272–279, 1999

Clarkin JF, Glick I, Haas GL, et al: A randomized clinical trial of inpatient family intervention, V: results for affective disorders. J Affect Disord 18:17–28, 1990

Clarkin JF, Carpenter D, Hull J, et al: Effects of psychoeducational intervention for married patients with bipolar disorder and their spouses. Biol Psychiatry 53:1000–1008, 1998

Cochran SD: Preventing medical noncompliance in the outpatient treatment of bipolar affective disorders. J Consult Clin Psychol 52:873–878, 1984

Compton SN, March JS, Brent D, et al: Cognitive-behavioral psychotherapy for anxiety and depressive disorders in children and adolescents: an evidence-based medicine review. J Am Acad Child Adolesc Psychiatry 43:930–959, 2004

Cooper LA, Gonzales JJ, Gallo JJ, et al: The acceptability of treatment for depression among African-American, Hispanic, and white primary care patients. Med Care 41:479–489, 2003

Coryell W, Turvey C, Endicott J, et al: Bipolar I affective disorder: predictors of outcome after 15 years. J Affect Disord 50:109–116, 1998

Costello EJ, Costello AJ, Edelbrock C, et al: Psychiatric disorders in pediatric primary care: prevalence and risk factors. Arch Gen Psychiatry 45:1107–1116, 1988

Costello EJ, Angold A, Burns BJ, et al: The Great Smoky Mountains Study of Youth goals, design, methods, and the prevalence of DSM-III-R disorders. Arch Gen Psychiatry 53:1129–1136, 1996

Costello EJ, Pine DS, Hammen C, et al: Development and natural history of mood disorders. Biol Psychiatry 52:529–542, 2002

Coyle JT, Pine DS, Charney DS, et al: Depression and Bipolar Support Alliance consensus statement on the unmet needs in diagnosis and treatment of mood disorders in children and adolescents. J Am Acad Child Adolesc Psychiatry 42:1494–1503, 2003

Craighead WE, Miklowitz DJ: Psychosocial interventions for bipolar disorder. J Clin Psychiatry 61 (suppl 13):58–64, 2000

Curry JF: Specific psychotherapies for childhood and adolescent depression. Biol Psychiatry 49:1091–1100, 2001

Dahl RE, Puig-Antich J, Ryan N, et al: EEG sleep in adolescents with major depression: the role of suicidality and inpatient status. J Affect Disord 19:63–75, 1990

Dahl RE, Ryan ND, Birmaher B, et al: Electroencephalographic sleep measures in prepubertal depression. Psychiatry Res 38:201–214, 1991

Dahl RE, Birmaher B, Williamson DE, et al: Low growth hormone response to growth hormone-releasing hormone in child depression. Biol Psychiatry 48:981–988, 2000

DelBello MP, Geller B: Review of studies of child and adolescent offspring of bipolar parents. Bipolar Disord 3:325–334, 2001

DelBello MP, Kowatch RA, Warner J, et al: Adjunctive topiramate treatment for pediatric bipolar disorder: a retrospective chart review. J Child Adolesc Psychopharmacol 12:323–330, 2002

DeLong GR, Nieman GW: Lithium-induced behavior changes in children with symptoms suggesting manic-depressive illness. Psychopharmacol Bull 19:258–265, 1983

Devine D, Kempton T, Forehand R: Adolescent depressed mood and young adult functioning: a longitudinal study. J Abnorm Child Psychol 22:629–640, 1994

Deykin EY, Buka SL, Zeena TH: Depressive illness among chemically dependent adolescents. Am J Psychiatry 149:1341–1347, 1992

The dexamethasone suppression test: an overview of its current status in psychiatry. APA Task Force on Laboratory Tests in Psychiatry. Am J Psychiatry 144:1253–1262, 1987

Diamond G, Siqueland L: Family therapy for the treatment of depressed adolescents. Psychotherapy: Theory, Research, Practice, Training 32:77–90, 1995

Diamond GS, Reis BF, Diamond GM, et al: Attachment-based family therapy for depressed adolescents: a treatment development study. J Am Acad Child Adolesc Psychiatry 41:1190–1196, 2002

Douvan EA, Adelson J: The Adolescent Experience. New York, Wiley, 1966

Dunner DL, Fleiss JL, Fieve RR: The course of development of mania in patients with recurrent depression. Am J Psychiatry 133:905–908, 1976

Emslie GJ, Rush AJ, Weinberg WA, et al: Children with major depression show reduced rapid eye movement latencies. Arch Gen Psychiatry 47:119–124, 1990a

Emslie GJ, Weinberg WA, Rush AJ, et al: Depressive symptoms by self-report in adolescence: phase I of the development of a questionnaire for depression by self-report. J Child Neurol 5:114–121, 1990b

Emslie GJ, Rush AJ, Weinberg WA, et al: Sleep EEG features of adolescents with major depression. Biol Psychiatry 36:573–581, 1994

Emslie GJ, Kennard BD, Kowatch RA: Affective disorders in children: diagnosis and management. J Child Neurol 10 (suppl 1):S42–S49, 1995

Emslie GJ, Rush AJ, Weinberg WA, et al: A double-blind, randomized, placebo-controlled trial of fluoxetine in children and adolescents with depression. Arch Gen Psychiatry 54:1031–1037, 1997a

Emslie GJ, Rush AJ, Weinberg WA, et al: Recurrence of major depressive disorder in hospitalized children and adolescents. J Am Acad Child Adolesc Psychiatry 36:785–792, 1997b

Emslie GJ, Rush AJ, Weinberg WA, et al: Fluoxetine in child and adolescent depression: acute and maintenance treatment. Depress Anxiety 7:32–39, 1998

Emslie GJ, Armitage R, Weinberg WA, et al: Sleep polysomnography as a predictor of recurrence in children and adolescents with major depressive disorder. Int J Neuropsychopharmacol 4:159–168, 2001a

Emslie GJ, Heiligenstein JH, Hoog SL, et al: Fluoxetine for maintenance of recovery from depression in children and adolescents: a placebo-controlled, randomized clinical trial. Paper presented at the 154th meeting of the American Psychiatric Association, New Orleans, LA, May 5–10, 2001b

Emslie GJ, Heiligenstein JH, Wagner KD, et al: Fluoxetine for acute treatment of depression in children and adolescents: a placebo-controlled, randomized clinical trial. J Am Acad Child Adolesc Psychiatry 41:1205–1215, 2002

Emslie GJ, Findling R, Yeung P, et al: Venlafaxine XR in pediatric patients with major depressive disorder. Paper presented at the American Academy of Child and Adolescent Psychiatry 51st annual meeting, Washington, DC, October 2004a

Emslie G, Wagner K, Kutcher S, et al: Paroxetine treatment in children and adolescents with major depressive disorder. Paper presented at the American Academy of Child and Adolescent Psychiatry 51st annual meeting, Washington, DC, October 2004b

Falloon IR, Pederson J: Family management in the prevention of morbidity of schizophrenia: the adjustment of the family unit. Br J Psychiatry 147:156–163, 1985

Faraone SV, Glatt SJ, Tsuang MT: The genetics of pediatriconset bipolar disorder. Biol Psychiatry 53:970–977, 2003

Farchione TR, Moore GJ, Rosenberg DR: Proton magnetic resonance spectroscopic imaging in pediatric major depression. Biol Psychiatry 52:86–92, 2002

Ferdinand RF, Stijnen T, Verhulst FC, et al: Associations between behavioural and emotional problems in adolescence and maladjustment in young adulthood. J Adolesc 22:123–136, 1999

Fergusson DM, Lynskey MT: Suicide attempts and suicidal ideation in a birth cohort of 16-year-old New Zealanders. J Am Acad Child Adolesc Psychiatry 34:1308–1317, 1995

Fergusson DM, Woodward LJ: Mental health, educational, and social role outcomes of adolescents with depression. Arch Gen Psychiatry 59:225–231, 2002

Fergusson DM, Woodward LJ, Horwood LJ: Risk factors and life processes associated with the onset of suicidal behavior during adolescence and early adulthood. Psychol Med 30:23–39, 2000

Findling RL, McNamara NK, Gracious BL, et al: Combination lithium and divalproex sodium in pediatric bipolarity. J Am Acad Child Adolesc Psychiatry 42:895–901, 2003

Flament MF, Cohen D, Choquet M, et al: Phenomenology, psychosocial correlates, and treatment seeking in major depression and dysthymia of adolescence. J Am Acad Child Adolesc Psychiatry 40:1070–1078, 2001

Fleming JE, Offord DR: Epidemiology of child depressive disorders: a critical review. J Am Acad Child Adolesc Psychiatry 29:571–580, 1990

Fombonne E, Wostear G, Cooper V, et al: The Maudsley long-term follow-up of child and adolescent depression, 2: suicidality, criminality and social dysfunction in adulthood. Br J Psychiatry 179:218–223, 2001a

Fombonne E, Wostear G, Harrington R, et al: The Maudsley long-term follow-up of child and adolescent depression, 1: psychiatric outcomes in adulthood. Br J Psychiatry 179:210–217, 2001b

Frank E, Hlastala S, Ritenour A, et al: Inducing lifestyle regularity in recovering bipolar disorder patients: results from the maintenance therapies in bipolar disorder protocol. Biol Psychiatry 41:1165–1173, 1997

Frank E, Swartz HA, Kupfer DJ: Interpersonal and social rhythm therapy: managing the chaos of bipolar disorder. Biol Psychiatry 48:593–604, 2000

Frazier JA, Meyer MC, Biederman J, et al: Risperidone treatment for juvenile bipolar disorder: a retrospective chart review. J Am Acad Child Adolesc Psychiatry 38:960–965, 1999

Frazier JA, Biederman J, Tohen M, et al: A prospective open-label treatment trial of olanzapine monotherapy in children and adolescents with bipolar disorder. J Child Adolesc Psychopharmacol 11:239–250, 2001

Fristad MA, Weller EB, Weller RA: Bipolar disorder in children: misdiagnosis, under diagnosis, and future directions. J Am Acad Child Adolesc Psychiatry 34:709–714, 1995

Fristad MA, Gavazzi SM, Soldano KW: Multi-family psycho-education groups for childhood mood disorders: a program description and preliminary efficacy data. Contemporary Family Therapy 20:385–402, 1998

Fristad MA, Gavazzi SM, Mackinaw-Koons B: Family psycho-education: an adjunctive intervention for children with bipolar disorder. Biol Psychiatry 53:1000–1008, 2003

Garber J, Hilsman R: Cognitions, stress, and depression in children and adolescents. Child Adolesc Psychiatr Clin N Am 1:129–167, 1992

Garber J, Kriss MR, Koch M, et al: Recurrent depression in adolescents: a follow-up study. J Am Acad Child Adolesc Psychiatry 27:49–54, 1988

Garber J, Weiss B, Shanley N: Cognitions, depressive symptoms, and development in adolescents. J Abnorm Psychol 102:47–57, 1993

Geller B: The high prevalence of bipolar parents among prepubertal mood-disordered children necessitates appropriate questions to establish bipolarity. Curr Opin Psychiatry 9:239–240, 1996

Geller B, Luby J: Child and adolescent bipolar disorder: a review of the past 10 years. J Am Acad Child Adolesc Psychiatry 36:1168–1176, 1997

Geller B, Fox LW, Clark KA: Rate and predictors of prepubertal bipolarity during follow-up of 6- to 12-year-old depressed children. J Am Acad Child Adolesc Psychiatry 33:461–468, 1994

Geller B, Sun K, Zimerman B, et al: Complex and rapid-cycling in bipolar children and adolescents: a preliminary study. J Affect Disord 34:259–268, 1995

Geller B, Cooper TB, Sun K, et al: Double-blind and placebo-controlled study of lithium for adolescent bipolar disorders with secondary substance dependency. J Am Acad Child Adolesc Psychiatry 37:171–178, 1998a

Geller B, Williams M, Zimerman B, et al: Prepubertal and early adolescent bipolarity differentiate from ADHD by manic symptoms, grandiose delusions, ultra-rapid or ultradian cycling. J Affect Disord 51:81–91, 1998b

Geller B, Bolhofner K, Craney JL, et al: Psychosocial functioning in a prepubertal and early adolescent bipolar disorder phenotype. J Am Acad Child Adolesc Psychiatry 39:1543–1548, 2000

Geller B, Zimerman B, Williams M, et al: Adult psychosocial outcome of prepubertal major depressive disorder. J Am Acad Child Adolesc Psychiatry 40:673–677, 2001

Geller B, Zimerman B, Williams M, et al: DSM-IV mania symptoms in prepubertal and early adolescent bipolar disorder phenotype compared to attention-deficit hyperactive and normal controls. J Child Adolesc Psychopharmacol 12:11–25, 2002

Gershon ES: Genetics, in Manic-Depressive Illness. Edited by Goodwin FK, Jamison KR. New York, Oxford University Press, 1988, pp 373–401

Giles DE, Jarrett RB, Roffwarg HP, et al: Reduced rapid eye movement latency: a predictor of recurrence in depression. Neuropsychopharmacology 1:33–39, 1987

Giles DE, Kupfer DJ, Rush AJ, et al: Controlled comparison of electrophysiological sleep in families of probands with unipolar depression. Am J Psychiatry 155:192–199, 1998

Gillham JE, Shatte AJ, Freres DR: Preventing depression: a review of cognitive-behavioral and family interventions. Appl Prev Psychol 9:63–88, 2000

Goetz RR, Puig-Antich J, Ryan N, et al: Electroencephalographic sleep of adolescents with major depression and normal controls. Arch Gen Psychiatry 44:61–68, 1987

Goodyer IM, Herbert J, Tamplin A, et al: Short-term outcome of major depression, II: life events, family dysfunction, and friendship difficulties as predictors of persistent disorder. J Am Acad Child Adolesc Psychiatry 36:474–480, 1997

Gotlib IH, Lewinsohn PM, Seeley JR, et al: Negative cognitions and attributional style in depressed adolescents: an examination of stability and specificity. J Abnorm Psychol 102:607–615, 1993

Gould MS, King RA, Greenwald S, et al: Psychopathology associated with suicidal ideation and attempts among children and adolescents. J Am Acad Child Adolesc Psychiatry 37:915–923, 1998

Gould MS, Greenberg T, Velting DM, et al: Youth suicide risk and preventive interventions: a review of the past 10 years. J Am Acad Child Adolesc Psychiatry 42:386–405, 2003

Greenbaum PE, Prange ME, Friedman RM, et al: Substance abuse prevalence and comorbidity with other psychiatric disorders among adolescents with severe emotional disturbances. J Am Acad Child Adolesc Psychiatry 30:575–585, 1991

Grey M, Whittemore R, Tamborlane W: Depression in type I diabetes in children: natural history and correlates. J Psychosom Res 53:907–911, 2002

Hamilton EB, Asarnow JR, Tompson MC: Social, academic, and behavioral competence of depressed children: relationship to diagnostic status and family interaction style. J Youth Adolesc 26:77–87, 1997

Hammen C, Davila J, Brown G, et al: Psychiatric history and stress: predictors of severity of unipolar depression. J Abnorm Psychol 101:45–52, 1992

Harrington R, Myatt T: Is preadolescent mania the same condition as adult mania? A British perspective. Biol Psychiatry 53:961–969, 2003

Harrington R, Fudge H, Rutter M, et al: Adult outcomes of childhood and adolescent depression, I: psychiatric status. Arch Gen Psychiatry 47:465–473, 1990

Harrington R, Kerfoot M, Dyer E, et al: Randomized trial of a home-based family intervention for children who have deliberately poisoned themselves. J Am Acad Child Adolesc Psychiatry 37:512–518, 1998

Herjanic B, Reich W: Development of a structured psychiatric interview for children: agreement between child and parent on individual symptoms. J Abnorm Child Psychol 10:307–324, 1997

Hope TL, Adams C, Reynolds L, et al: Parent vs. self-report: contributions toward diagnosis of adolescent psychopathology. Journal of Psychopathology and Behavioral Assessment 21:349–363, 1999

Hops H, Lewinsohn PM, Andrews JA, et al: Psychosocial correlates of depressive symptomatology among high school students. J Clin Child Psychol 19:211–220, 1990

Hughes CW, Preskorn SH, Weller EB, et al: The effect of concomitant disorders in childhood depression on predicting treatment response. Psychopharmacol Bull 26:235–238, 1990

Hughes CW, Emslie GJ, Crismon ML, et al: The Texas Children's Medication Algorithm Project: report of the Texas Consensus Conference Panel on medication treatment of childhood major depressive disorder. J Am Acad Child Adolesc Psychiatry 38:1442–1454, 1999

Jensen PS, Rubio-Stipec M, Canino G, et al: Parent and child contributions to diagnosis of mental disorder: are both informants always necessary? J Am Acad Child Adolesc Psychiatry 38:1569–1579, 1999

Kafantaris V, Coletti DJ, Dicker R, et al: Lithium treatment of acute mania in adolescents: a large open trial. J Am Acad Child Adolesc Psychiatry 42:1038–1045, 2003

Kahn JS, Kehle TJ, Jenson WR, et al: Comparison of cognitive-behavioral, relaxation, and self-modeling interventions for depression among middle-school students. School Psych Rev 19:196–211, 1990

Kandel DB, Davies M: Adult sequelae of adolescent depressive symptoms. Arch Gen Psychiatry 43:255–262, 1986

Kashani JH, Beck NC, Hoeper EW, et al: Psychiatric disorders in a community sample of adolescents. Am J Psychiatry 144:584–589, 1987

Kashani JH, Burbach DJ, Rosenberg DR: Perception of family conflict resolution and depressive symptomatology in adolescents. J Am Acad Child Adolesc Psychiatry 27:42–48, 1988

Kaufman J, Birmaher B, Perel J, et al: The corticotropin-releasing hormone challenge in depressed abused, depressed nonabused, and normal control children. Biol Psychiatry 42:669–679, 1997

Keller MB, Baker L: Bipolar disorder: epidemiology, course, diagnosis, and treatment. Bull Menninger Clin 55:172–181, 1991

Keller MB, Lavori PW, Beardslee WR, et al: Depression in children and adolescents: new data on "undertreatment" and a literature review on the efficacy of available treatments. J Affect Disord 21:163–171, 1991

Keller MB, Ryan N, Strober M, et al: Efficacy of paroxetine in the treatment of adolescent major depression: a randomized, controlled trial. J Am Acad Child Adolesc Psychiatry 40:762–772, 2001

Kessler RC, Walters EE: Epidemiology of DSM-III-R major depression and minor depression among adolescents and young adults in the National Comorbidity Survey. Depress Anxiety 7:3–14, 1998

Kessler RC, McGonagle KA, Zhao S, et al: Lifetime and 12-month prevalence of DSM-III-R psychiatric disorders in the United States: results from the National Comorbidity Study. Arch Gen Psychiatry 51:8–19, 1994

Kessler RC, Avenevoli S, Merikangas R: Mood disorders in children and adolescents: an epidemiologic perspective. Biol Psychiatry 49:1002–1014, 2001

Kolko DJ, Brent DA, Baugher M, et al: Cognitive and family therapies for adolescent depression: treatment specificity, mediation, and moderation. J Consult Clin Psychol 68:603–614, 2000

Kovacs M: Presentation and course of major depressive disorder during childhood and later years of the life span. J Am Acad Child Adolesc Psychiatry 35:705–715, 1996

Kovacs M, Gatsonis C: Stability and change in childhood-onset depressive disorders: longitudinal course as a diagnostic validator, in The Validity of Psychiatric Diagnosis. Edited by Robins LN, Barrett JE. New York, Raven, 1989, pp 57–75

Kovacs M, Pollock M: Bipolar disorder and comorbid conduct disorder in childhood and adolescence. J Am Acad Child Adolesc Psychiatry 34:715–723, 1995

Kovacs M, Feinberg TL, Crouse-Novak MA, et al: Depressive disorders in childhood, I: a longitudinal prospective study of characteristics and recovery. Arch Gen Psychiatry 41:229–237, 1984a

Kovacs M, Feinberg TL, Crouse-Novak MA, et al: Depressive disorders in childhood, II: a longitudinal study of the risk for a subsequent major depression. Arch Gen Psychiatry 41:643–649, 1984b

Kovacs M, Paulauskas SL, Gatsonis C, et al: Depressive disorders in childhood, III: a longitudinal study of comorbidity with and risk for conduct disorders. J Affect Disord 15:205–217, 1988

Kovacs M, Goldston D, Gatsonis C: Suicidal behaviors and childhood-onset depressive disorders: a longitudinal investigation. J Am Acad Child Adolesc Psychiatry 32:8–20, 1993

Kovacs M, Devlin B, Pollock M, et al: A controlled family history study of childhood-onset depressive disorder. Arch Gen Psychiatry 54:613–623, 1997

Kowatch RA, Suppes T, Carmody T, et al: Effect size of lithium, divalproex sodium, and carbamazepine in children and adolescents with bipolar disorder. J Am Acad Child Adolesc Psychiatry 39:713–720, 2000

Kowatch RA, Sethuraman G, Hume JH, et al: Combination pharmacotherapy in children and adolescents with bipolar disorder. Biol Psychiatry 53:978–984, 2003

Kramlinger KG, Post R: Ultra-rapid and ultradian cycling in bipolar affective illness. Br J Psychiatry 168:314–323, 1996

Kroll L, Harrington R, Jayson D, et al: Pilot study of continuation cognitive-behavioral therapy for major depression in adolescent psychiatric patients J Am Acad Child Adolesc Psychiatry 35:1156–1161, 1996

Kutcher SP, Marton P, Korenblum M: Relationship between psychiatric illness and conduct disorder in adolescents. Can J Psychiatry 34:526–529, 1989

Kutcher S, Malkin D, Silverberg J, et al: Nocturnal cortisol, thyroid stimulating hormone, and growth hormone secretory profiles in depressed adolescents. J Am Acad Child Adolesc Psychiatry 30:407–414, 1991

Lahmeyer HW, Poznanski EO, Bellur SN: EEG sleep in depressed adolescents. Am J Psychiatry 140:1150–1153, 1983

Lam DH, Bright J, Jones S, et al: Cognitive therapy for bipolar illness—a pilot study of relapse prevention. Cognit Ther Res 24:503–520, 2000

Leibenluft E, Charney DS, Pine DS: Researching the pathophysiology of pediatric bipolar disorder. Biol Psychiatry 53:1009–1020, 2003

Lerner MS, Clum GA: Treatment of suicide ideators: a problem-solving approach. Behav Ther 21:403–411, 1990

Lewinsohn PM, Clarke GN, Hops H, et al: Cognitive-behavioral treatment for depressed adolescents. Behav Ther 21:385–401, 1990

Lewinsohn PM, Rohde P, Seeley JR, et al: Comorbidity of unipolar depression, I: major depression with dysthymia. J Abnorm Psychol 100:205–213, 1991

Lewinsohn PM, Hops H, Roberts RE, et al: Adolescent psychopathology, I: prevalence and incidence of depression and other DSM-III-R disorders in high school students. J Abnorm Psychol 102:135–144, 1993

Lewinsohn PM, Clarke GN, Seeley JR, et al: Major depression in community adolescents: age at onset, episode duration, and time to recurrence. J Am Acad Child Adolesc Psychiatry 33:809–818, 1994

Lewinsohn PM, Klein DN, Seeley JR: Bipolar disorders in a community sample of older adolescents: prevalence, phenomenology, comorbidity, and course. J Am Acad Child Adolesc Psychiatry 34:454–463, 1995

Lewinsohn PM, Rohde P, Seeley JR: Adolescent suicidal ideation and attempts: prevalence, risk factors, and clinical implications. Clinical Psychology Science Practices 3:25–46, 1996

Lewinsohn PM, Rohde P, Seeley JR: Major depressive disorder in older adolescents: prevalence, risk factors, and clinical implications. Clin Psychol Rev 18:765–794, 1998

Lewinsohn PM, Allen NB, Seeley JR, et al: First onset versus recurrence of depression: differential processes of psychosocial risk. J Abnorm Psychol 108:483–489, 1999

Lewinsohn PM, Joiner TE Jr, Rohde P: Evaluation of cognitive diathesis-stress models in predicting major depressive disorder in adolescents. J Abnorm Psychol 110:203–215, 2001

Lewinsohn PM, Rohde P, Gotlib IH, et al: Psychosocial functioning of young adults who have experienced and recovered from major depressive disorder during adolescence. J Abnorm Psychol 112:353–363, 2003

Liddle B, Spence SH: Cognitive-behaviour therapy with depressed primary school children: a cautionary note. Behavioural Psychotherapy 18:85–102, 1990

Linehan MM, Armstrong HE, Suarez A, et al: Cognitive-behavioral treatment of chronically parasuicidal borderline patients. Arch Gen Psychiatry 48:1060–1064, 1991

Ling W, Oftedal G, Weinberg WA: Depressive illness in childhood presenting as severe headache. Am J Dis Child 120:122–124, 1970

Livingston R: Depressive illness and learning difficulties: research needs and practical implications. J Learn Disabil 18:518–520, 1985

Loranger AW, Levine PM: Age at onset of bipolar affective illness. Arch Gen Psychiatry 35:1345–1348, 1978

Luby J, Heffelfinger AK, Mrakotsky C, et al: The clinical picture of depression in preschool children. J Am Acad Child Adolesc Psychiatry 42:340–348, 2003

Marton P, Kutcher S: The prevalence of cognitive distortion in depressed adolescents. J Psychiatry Neurosci 20:33–38, 1995

McCauley E, Mitchell JR, Burke PM, et al: Cognitive attributes of depression in children and adolescents. J Consult Clin Psychol 56:903–908, 1988

McCauley E, Myers K, Mitchell J, et al: Depression in young people: initial presentation and clinical course. J Am Acad Child Adolesc Psychiatry 32:714–722, 1993

Medicines and Healthcare Products Regulatory Agency: News in 2003. Available at: http://www.mhra.gov.uk/news/2003.htm. December 2003

Mesman J, Koot HM: Child-reported depression and anxiety in preadolescence, I: associations with parent- and teacher-reported problems. J Am Acad Child Adolesc Psychiatry 39:1371–1378, 2000

Miklowitz DJ, Goldstein MJ: Behavioral family treatment for patients with bipolar affective disorder. Behav Modif 14:457–489, 1990

Miklowitz DJ, Simoneau TL, George EL, et al: Family focused treatment of bipolar disorder: 1-year effects of a psychoeducational program in conjunction with pharmacotherapy. Biol Psychiatry 48:582–592, 2000

Miklowitz DJ, George EL, Richards JA, et al: A randomized study of family focused psychoeducation and pharmacotherapy in the outpatient management of bipolar disorder. Arch Gen Psychiatry 60:904–912, 2003

Milin RP, Simeon J, Spenst W: Double-blind study of paroxetine in adolescents with unipolar major depression. Paper presented at the American Academy of Child and Adolescent Psychiatry 46th annual meeting, Chicago, IL, October 1999

Miller AL, Wyman SE, Huppert JD, et al: Analysis of behavioral skills utilized by suicidal adolescents receiving dialectical behavioral therapy. Cognitive and Behavioral Practice 7:183–187, 2000

Montgomery SA: Antidepressants in long-term treatment. Annu Rev Med 45:447–457, 1994

Morehouse RL, Kusumakar V, Kutcher SP, et al: Temporal coherence in ultradian sleep EEG rhythms in a never-depressed, high-risk cohort of female adolescents. Biol Psychiatry 51:446–456, 2002

Mufson L, Fairbanks J: Interpersonal psychotherapy for depressed adolescents: a one-year naturalistic follow-up study. J Am Acad Child Adolesc Psychiatry 35:1145–1155, 1996

Mufson L, Weissman MM, Moreau D, et al: Efficacy of interpersonal psychotherapy for depressed adolescents. Arch Gen Psychiatry 56:573–579, 1999

Myers K, Winters NC: Ten-year review of rating scales, I: overview of scale functioning, psychometric properties, and selection. J Am Acad Child Adolesc Psychiatry 41:114–122, 2002a

Myers K, Winters NC: Ten-year review of rating scales, II: scales for internalizing disorders. J Am Acad Child Adolesc Psychiatry 41:634–659, 2002b

National Center for Health Statistics: Death Rates for 72 Selected Causes, by 5-Year Groups, Race and Sex: United States, 1979–1997. Hyattsville, MD, National Center for Health Statistics, 2001, pp 4485–4490

Nolan CL, Moore GJ, Madden R, et al: Prefrontal cortical volume in childhood-onset major depression: preliminary findings. Arch Gen Psychiatry 59:173–179, 2002

Nolen-Hoeksema S, Girgus JS, Seligman ME: Sex differences in depression and explanatory style in children. J Youth Adolesc 20:233–245, 1991

O'Donnell J: Overview of existing research and information linking isotretinoin (Accutane), depression, psychosis, and suicide. Am J Ther 10:148–159, 2003

Otto MW, Reilly Harrington N, Sachs G: Psychoeducational and cognitive-behavioral strategies in the management of bipolar disorder. J Affect Disord 73:171–181, 2003

Papatheodorou G, Kutcher S, Katic M, et al: The efficacy and safety of divalproex sodium in the treatment of acute mania in adolescents and young adults: an open clinical trial. J Clin Psychopharmacol 15:110–116, 1995

Polaino-Lorente A, Domenech E: Prevalence of childhood depression: results of the first study in Spain. J Child Psychol Psychiatry 34:1007–1017, 1993

Post RM, Rubinow DR, Uhde TW, et al: Dysphoric mania: clinical and biological correlates. Arch Gen Psychiatry 46:353–358, 1989

Poznanski EO, Grossman JA, Buchsbaum Y, et al: Preliminary studies of the reliability and validity of the Children's Depression Rating Scale. J Am Acad Child Psychiatry 23:191–197, 1984

Puig-Antich J, Goetz R, Hanlon C, et al: Sleep architecture and REM sleep measures in pre-pubertal major depressives. Arch Gen Psychiatry 40:932–939, 1982

Puig-Antich J, Lukens E, Davies M, et al: Psychosocial functioning in prepubertal major depressive disorders, I: interpersonal relationships during the depressive episode. Arch Gen Psychiatry 42:500–507, 1985a

Puig-Antich J, Lukens E, Davies M, et al: Psychosocial functioning in prepubertal major depressive disorders, II: interpersonal relationships after sustained recovery from affective episode. J Affect Disord 42:511–517, 1985b

Puig-Antich J, Goetz D, Davies M, et al: A controlled family history study of prepubertal major depressive disorder. Arch Gen Psychiatry 46:406–418, 1989

Puig-Antich J, Kaufman J, Ryan N, et al: The psychosocial functioning and family environment of depressed adolescents. J Am Acad Child Adolesc Psychiatry 32:244–253, 1993

Rao U, Weissman MM, Martin JA, et al: Childhood depression and risk of suicide: a preliminary report of a longitudinal study. J Am Acad Child Adolesc Psychiatry 32:21–27, 1993

Rao U, Neal RD, Birmaher B, et al: Unipolar depression in adolescents: clinical outcome in adulthood. J Am Acad Child Adolesc Psychiatry 34:566–578, 1995

Rao U, Hammen C, Daley S: Continuity of depression during the transition to adulthood: a 5-year longitudinal study of young women. J Am Acad Child Adolesc Psychiatry 38:908–915, 1999a

Rao U, Ryan ND, Dahl RE, et al: Factors associated with the development of substance use disorder in depressed adolescents. J Am Acad Child Adolesc Psychiatry 38:1109–1117, 1999b

Rathus JH, Miller AL: Dialectical behavior therapy adapted for suicidal adolescents. Suicide Life Threat Behav 32:146–157, 2002

Rea MM, Miklowitz DJ, Tompson MC, et al: Family focused treatment versus individual treatment for bipolar disorder: results of a randomized clinical trial. J Consult Clin Psychol 71:482–492, 2003

Reinecke MA, Ryan NE, DuBois DL: Cognitive-behavioral therapy of depression and depressive symptoms during adolescence: a review and meta-analysis. J Am Acad Child Adolesc Psychiatry 37:26–34, 1998

Reinherz HZ, Giaconia RM, Silverman AB, et al: Early psychological risks for adolescent suicidal ideation and attempts. J Am Acad Child Adolesc Psychiatry 34:599–611, 1995

Reinherz HZ, Giaconia RM, Hauf AMC, et al: Major depression in the transition to adulthood: risks and impairments. J Abnorm Psychol 108:500–510, 1999

Reynolds WM, Coats KI: A comparison of cognitive-behavioral therapy and relaxation training for the treatment of depression in adolescents. J Consult Clin Psychol 54:653–660, 1986

Ring HA, Trimble MR: Depression in epilepsy, in Depression in Neurological Disease. Edited by Starkstein SE, Robinson RG. Baltimore, MD, Johns Hopkins University Press, 1993, pp 63–83

Robertson MM: The organic contribution to depressive illness in patients with epilepsy. J Epilepsy 2:189–230, 1989

Robinson RG, Starkstein SE: Current research in affective disorders following stroke. J Neuropsychiatry Clin Neurosci 2:1–14, 1990

Robinson RG, Boston JD, Starkstein SE, et al: Comparison of mania and depression after brain injury: casual factors. Am J Psychiatry 145:172–178, 1988

Rohde P, Lewinsohn PM, Seeley JR: Psychiatric comorbidity with problematic alcohol use in high school students. J Am Acad Child Adolesc Psychiatry 35:101–109, 1996

Rohde P, Clarke GN, Lewinsohn PM, et al: Impact of comorbidity on a cognitive-behavioral group treatment for adolescent depression. J Am Acad Child Adolesc Psychiatry 40:795–802, 2001

Rossello J, Bernal G: The efficacy of cognitive-behavioral and interpersonal treatments for depression in Puerto Rican adolescents. J Consult Clin Psychol 67:734–745, 1999

Rush AJ, Giles DE, Jarrett RB, et al: Reduced REM latency predicts response to tricyclic medication in depressed outpatients. Biol Psychiatry 26:61–72, 1989

Rutter M, Tizard J, Yule W, et al: Research report: Isle of Wight Studies, 1964–1974. Psychol Med 6:313–332, 1976

Ryan ND, Puig-Antich J, Ambrosini PJ, et al: The clinical picture of major depression in children and adolescents. Arch Gen Psychiatry 44:854–861, 1987

Ryan N, Dahl RE, Birmaher B, et al: Stimulatory tests of growth hormone secretion in prepubertal major depression: depressed versus normal children. J Am Acad Child Adolesc Psychiatry 33:824–833, 1994

Ryback RS, Brodsky L, Munasifi F: Gabapentin in bipolar disorder (letter). J Neuropsychiatry Clin Neurosci 9:301, 1997

Sachs GS, Thase ME, Otto MW, et al: Rationale, design, and methods of the systematic treatment enhancement program for bipolar disorder (STEP-BD). Biol Psychiatry 53:1028–1042, 2003

Santor DA, Kusumakar V: Open trial of interpersonal therapy in adolescents with moderate to severe major depression: effectiveness of novice IPT therapists. J Am Acad Child Adolesc Psychiatry 40:236–240, 2001

Schreier HA: Risperidone for young children with mood disorders and aggressive behavior. J Child Adolesc Psychopharmacol 8:49–59, 1998

Shaffer D, Gould MS, Fisher P, et al: Psychiatric diagnosis in child and adolescent suicide. Arch Gen Psychiatry 53:339–348, 1996

Soutullo CA, Sorter MT, Foster KD, et al: Olanzapine in the treatment of adolescent acute mania: a report of seven cases. J Affect Disord 53:279–283, 1999

Stark KD, Reynolds WM, Kaslow NJ: A comparison of the relative efficacy of self-control therapy and a behavioral problem-solving therapy for depression in children. J Abnorm Child Psychol 15:91–113, 1987

Starkstein SE, Cohen BS, Federoff P, et al: Relationship between anxiety disorders and depressive disorders in patients with cerebrovascular injury. Arch Gen Psychiatry 47:246–251, 1990

Steingard RJ, Renshaw PF, Yurgelun-Todd DA, et al: Structured abnormalities in brain magnetic resonance images of depressed children. J Am Acad Child Adolesc Psychiatry 35:307–311, 1996

Steingard RJ, Yurgelun-Todd DA, Hennen J, et al: Increased orbitofrontal cortex levels of choline in depressed adolescents as detected by in vivo proton magnetic resonance spectroscopy. Biol Psychiatry 48:1053–1061, 2000

Stewart SM, Betson CL, Lam TH, et al: The correlates of depressed mood in adolescents in Hong Kong. J Adolesc Health 25:27–34, 1999

Stewart SM, Lewinsohn PM, Lee PW, et al: Symptom patterns in depression and "subthreshold" depression among adolescents in Hong Kong and the United States. J Cross Cult Psychol 33:559–576, 2002

Stokes PE, Sikes CR: Hypothalamic-pituitary-adrenal axis in affective disorders, in Psychopharmacology: The Third Generation of Progress. Edited by Meltzer HY. New York, Raven, 1987, pp 589–608

Strober M, Carlson G: Bipolar illness in adolescents with major depression: clinical, genetic, and psychopharmacologic predictors in a three- to four-year prospective follow-up investigation. Arch Gen Psychiatry 39:549–555, 1982

Strober M, Morrell W, Burroughs J, et al: A family study of bipolar I disorder in adolescence. J Affect Disord 15:255–268, 1988

Strober M, Morrell W, Lampert C, et al: Relapse following discontinuation of lithium maintenance therapy in adolescents with bipolar illness: a naturalistic study. Am J Psychiatry 147:457–461, 1990

Strober M, Lampert C, Schmidt-Lackner S, et al: The course of major depressive disorder in adolescents, I: recovery and risk of manic switching in a follow-up of psychotic and nonpsychotic subtypes. J Am Acad Child Adolesc Psychiatry 32:34–42, 1993

Strober M, Schmidt-Lackner S, Freeman R, et al: Recovery and relapse in adolescents with bipolar affective illness: a five-year naturalistic, prospective follow-up. J Am Acad Child Adolesc Psychiatry 34:724–731, 1995

Taylor DO, Miklowitz DJ, George EL, et al: Modifying focused family therapy for adolescents with bipolar disorder. Paper presented at the 5th International Conference on Bipolar Disorder, Pittsburgh, PA, June 12–14, 2003

Tems CL, Stewart SM, Skinner JR, et al: Cognitive distortions in depressed children and adolescents: are they state dependent or traitlike? J Clin Child Psychol 22:316–326, 1993

Tillman R, Geller B: Definitions of rapid, ultrarapid, and ultradian cycling and of episode duration in pediatric and adult bipolar disorders: a proposal to distinguish episodes from cycles. J Child Adolesc Psychopharmacol 13:267–271, 2003

Trautman P, Stewart N, Morishima A: Are adolescent suicide attempters non-compliant with outpatient care? J Am Acad Child Adolesc Psychiatry 32:89–94, 1993

Treatment for Adolescents With Depression Study Team: Treatment for Adolescents With Depression Study (TADS): rationale, design, and methods. J Am Acad Child Adolesc Psychiatry 42:531–542, 2003

Treatment for Adolescents With Depression Study Team: The Treatment for Adolescents With Depression Study (TADS): Stage I outcomes. JAMA 292:307–820, 2004

Vila G, Nollet-Clemencon C, Vera M, et al: Prevalence of DSM-IV disorders in children and adolescents with asthma versus diabetes. Can J Psychiatry 44:562–569, 1999

Vila G, Nollet-Clemencon C, de Blic J, et al: Prevalence of DSM IV anxiety and affective disorders in a pediatric population of asthmatic children and adolescents. J Affect Disord 58:223–231, 2000

Vostanis P, Feehan C, Grattan EF, et al: A randomised controlled out-patient trial of cognitive-behavioural treatment for children and adolescents with depression: 9-month follow-up. J Affect Disord 40:105–116, 1996

Vostanis P, Feehan C, Grattan E: Two-year outcome of children treated for depression. Eur Child Adolesc Psychiatry 7:12–18, 1998

Wade TJ, Cairney J, Pevalin DJ: Emergence of gender differences in depression during adolescence: National Panel results from three countries. J Am Acad Child Adolesc Psychiatry 41:190–198, 2002

Wagner KD, Weller EB, Carlson GA, et al: An open-label trial of divalproex in children and adolescents with bipolar disorder. J Am Acad Child Adolesc Psychiatry 41:1224–1230, 2002

Wagner KD, Ambrosini PJ, Rynn M, et al: Efficacy of sertraline in the treatment of children and adolescents with major depressive disorder. JAMA 290:1033–1041, 2003

Wagner KD, Robb AS, Findling RL, et al: A randomized, placebo-controlled trial of citalopram for the treatment of major depression in children and adolescents. Am J Psychiatry 161:1079–1083, 2004

Weinberg WA, Rehmet A: Childhood affective disorder and school problems, in Affective Disorders in Childhood and Adolescence: An Update. Edited by Cantwell DP, Carlson GA. Jamaica, NY, Spectrum Publications, 1983, pp 109–128

Weinberg WA, Rutman J, Sullivan L, et al: Depression in children referred to an educational diagnostic center: diagnosis and treatment: preliminary report. J Pediatr 83:1065–1072, 1973

Weissman MM, Wolk S, Goldstein RB, et al: Depressed adolescents grown up. JAMA 281:1707–1713, 1999

Weisz JR, Thurber CA, Sweeney L, et al: Brief treatment of mild-to-moderate child depression using primary and secondary control enhancement training. J Consult Clin Psychol 65:703–707, 1997

Weller EB, Weller RA, Fristad MA: Bipolar disorder in children: misdiagnosis, underdiagnosis, and future directions. J Am Acad Child Adolesc Psychiatry 34:709–714, 1995

Weller RA, Weller EB, Tucker SG, et al: Mania in prepubertal children: has it been underdiagnosed? J Affect Disord 11:151–154, 1986

Weller RA, Weller EB, Fristad MA, et al: Depression in recently bereaved prepubertal children. Am J Psychiatry 148:1536–1540, 1991

Whitaker A, Johnson J, Shaffer D, et al: Uncommon troubles in young people: prevalence estimates of selected psychiatric disorders in a nonreferred adolescent population. Arch Gen Psychiatry 47:487–496, 1990

Wilkes TC, Rush AJ: Adaptations of cognitive therapy for depressed adolescents. J Am Acad Child Adolesc Psychiatry 27:381–386, 1988

Williamson DE, Birmaher B, Frank E, et al: Nature of life events and difficulties in depressed adolescents. J Am Acad Child Adolesc Psychiatry 37:1049–1057, 1998

Wood A, Harrington R, Moore A: Controlled trial of a brief cognitive-behavioural intervention in adolescent patients with depressive disorders. J Child Psychol Psychiatry 37:737–746, 1996

Wozniak J, Biederman J, Kiely K, et al: Mania-like symptoms suggestive of childhood-onset bipolar disorder in clinically referred children. J Am Acad Child Adolesc Psychiatry 34:867–876, 1995

Zito JM, Safer DJ, DosReis S, et al: Psychotropic practice patterns for youth: a 10-year perspective. Arch Pediatr Adolesc Med 157:17–25, 2003

CHAPTER

36

Geriatric Mood Disorders

STEVEN P. ROOSE, M.D.

D. P. DEVANAND, M.D.

DEMOGRAPHIC DATA make a compelling case that we are living in an aging society. By the year 2030, more than 70 million people in the United States will be older than 65 years, and the "old-old," people older than 85 years, will be the most rapidly growing segment of the population. The aging of society is not restricted to just one country or one continent; the rate of increase in the proportion of the population older than 65 will be equaled, if not exceeded, in Africa, Asia, and South America compared with the United States and Europe. Consequently, illnesses such as depression that are prevalent and cause significant morbidity and mortality in the elderly will become increasingly prominent.

Clinical observations and systematic studies suggest that patients with late-life depression are different in many important dimensions from younger adult patients with depression. Conceptually, the critical question is whether these differences result primarily from age-associated physiological changes and a high prevalence of comorbid medical conditions (differences in young vs. old patients) or whether late-life depression is a disease entity distinct in its presentation, etiology, course, and treatment response from the illness afflicting younger adults (differences in early-onset vs. late-life depressive illness). In this chapter, we review data on the phenomenology, psychobiology, and treatment of late-life major depression and dysthymia and highlight differences compared with younger adults.

Influence of Age on Illness Presentation and the Problem of Diagnosis

The physiological changes associated with aging may significantly influence the phenomenology and course of depressive illness. Changes in brain structure and function may, in part, explain the increased frequency of the melancholic and delusional subtype of depressive episode in late life compared with younger adult samples. Regional brain dysfunction, especially in the prefrontal areas, is associated with instability of temperament, vulnerability to and intensification of the experience of distress, and a degrading of coping mechanisms. Such alterations in an individual's psychic capacities may result in increased social isolation, loss of independence, and related behaviors that can precipitate, intensify, or prolong a depressive episode. Another example of how age may alter the nature of depression in late life is the effect of ischemic vascular disease. Magnetic resonance imaging (MRI) studies have found a high rate of structural abnormalities compatible with cerebrovascular disease, especially among patients with late-onset depressive illness (Steffens and Krishnan 1998). These lesions have been associated with symptoms of cognitive impairment, a decreased and slower response to antidepressant medication, and a deteriorating course of illness.

Other differences in the presentation of late-life depression appear to be a function of social context rather than brain structure. For example, functional impairment as a symptom of depression is expressed differently throughout the life cycle. Depression-associated dysfunction in childhood can present as poor performance in school or antisocial behavior, in young adults as dissatisfaction in work or love, and in older patients as hypochondriasis and increased use of medical resources.

The age-associated changes in the presentation of depression undoubtedly contribute to the problem of underdiagnosis and inadequate treatment of late-life depression in both medical and psychiatric settings. Some older patients report fewer affective symptoms and present predominantly with cognitive somatic symptoms (e.g., apathy, sleep disturbance, appetite loss, fatigue, and pain). In fact, this type of late-life depressed patient may never complain of, or indeed may deny, the experience of depressed mood. This presentation of late-life depression has been referred to as "depression without sadness" (Gallo and Rabins 1999). If a physician considers depressed mood to be the sine qua non of a major depressive episode, then depression will be omitted from the differential diagnosis of the older patient presenting with nonspecific somatic complaints.

Major Depression

Epidemiology

Further complicating the issue of diagnosis are epidemiological studies indicating that among the elderly, milder subthreshold depressive syndromes may be more common than major depression. Epidemiological studies of late-life samples generally have reported a lower than expected rate of current major depression with a range from 1% to 3% (Beekman et al. 1999; Blazer et al. 1987). However, the rate of major depression changes significantly depending on the setting. Studies of patients in medical clinics reported rates of 10% for major depression; for nonpsychiatric hospital inpatients, the rate increases to 15%–25%, and it is even higher in nursing homes (Parmelee et al. 1989). These studies primarily used assessment instruments and diagnostic criteria that were developed for and/or validated in a younger population, and it is not known whether the adoption of age-adjusted diagnostic criteria would produce significantly different results.

Pathogenesis

The term *late-life depression* may represent a heterogeneous group of disorders that differ in etiology, pathophysiology, and prognosis, some of which may be distinct from the depressive disorder experienced by younger adults.

One example of heterogeneity is the distinction between the late-life patient with recurrent major depressive illness with onset of the first episode early in life and the older patient with first onset of major depressive illness after age 60. The hypothesis that early-onset (before age 50 or 60) and late-onset depression may be, despite similarities, distinct entities is suggested by data from epidemiological, brain imaging, treatment, and long-term outcome studies. Patients with late-onset depression have a lower rate of family history of depression and a greater frequency of MRI abnormalities compatible with ischemic cerebrovascular disease and, possibly, the development of dementia (O'Brien et al. 1998).

Another example of a form of late-life depression that represents an etiologically distinct subtype is poststroke depression. Stroke occurs most commonly in late life and is frequently followed by a depressive syndrome. However, patients with poststroke depression may have a different response pattern to antidepressant medications than do patients with late-life depressive syndromes not associated with a vascular event (Robinson and Price 1982).

Thus, late-life depression is most probably a collection of disorders that presents with a mosaic of symptoms. Heterogeneity in the phenomenology, etiology, treatment response, and course of late-life depression can obfuscate accurate diagnosis and optimal treatment.

Treatment of Late-Life Depression With Antidepressant Medication

The pharmacological treatment of late-life depression has been based on three beliefs: 1) older patients do not respond at the same rate or as consistently as younger patients; 2) older patients take longer to respond to antidepressant medication, and therefore a 12-week trial is mandatory; and 3) older patients have a higher rate of side effects and adverse events. Although these beliefs appear to be strongly held by many clinicians, only recently have there been a sufficient number of methodologically rigorous randomized, controlled trials of antidepressants in late-life depression to test them.

Moderators and mediators influence response to antidepressants, and variability in results of randomized, controlled trials of antidepressants in late-life depression may be caused by heterogeneity in the patient cohorts or variation in study design (Kraemer et al. 2002). The moderators that have been suggested as significant for late-life depression, some unique to this age group, include

- Late onset (first episode after age 60) (Figiel et al. 1991)
- Subtype (e.g., melancholic or delusional) (Glassman and Roose 1981; Roose et al. 1994)
- Severity (D.F. Klein and Ross 1993)
- Medical burden (Caine et al. 1994)
- Social support (George et al. 1989)
- Abnormalities on MRI scans indicating vascular disease (Hickie et al. 1995)
- A pattern of neurocognitive abnormalities labeled *executive dysfunction* (Alexopoulos et al. 2000)

Unfortunately, even though most of these moderators are easily established in the course of a routine clinical evaluation and only the acquisition of imaging and neuropsychological data is intrusive, expensive, and time consuming, most clinical trials either do not document these moderators or do not analyze outcome with the use of moderators as covariates.

In geriatric antidepressant clinical trials, the study design mediators of treatment response are the same as for trials in younger adult patients—namely, randomization, placebo versus comparator control, dose, duration, and criteria for response and remission. In particular, the effect of a placebo control group and the optimal duration of treatment both have been recently revisited.

Placebo- Versus Comparator-Controlled Trials

In the posttricyclic era of antidepressants, only four placebo-controlled trials of antidepressant treatment in patients with late-life depression have been done (Roose et al. 2002; Schneider et al. 2003; Tollefson and Holzman 1993) (A.F. Schatzberg and S.P. Roose, "A Double-blind, Placebo-controlled Study of Venlafaxine and Fluoxetine in Geriatric Outpatients With Major Depression," unpublished manuscript, 2005). Two of these trials had negative results (i.e., medication did not show a statistical difference from placebo), although across the four studies, the response rates to medication were similar.

Although placebo-controlled trials are the gold standard to establish the efficacy of medication, several issues have been raised about the generalizability of the results of these trials to the clinical situation (Roose et al. 2002). The first issue is whether patients received interventions in addition to standard clinical management and placebo. Surely, a placebo-controlled trial is not a comparison of medication and "doing nothing." Rather, in randomized, controlled trials, various nonspecific psychosocial supports accompany the administration of placebo and med-

ication. For example, relative to clinical care in the community, randomized, controlled trials differ in the frequency and duration of physician visits, provision of free medication and medical workup, intensive interaction with study staff during and between visits, provision of social service support, and so forth. Few randomized, controlled trials or naturalistic studies have systematically assessed the extent and nature of "extrastudy" psychosocial support that may have significant effects on therapeutic outcomes, especially in the elderly who are often socially isolated and with limited financial resources. Variation in the availability of social supports delivered outside the boundaries of the study design may be a critical component in the phenomena of significant site variability in therapeutic outcome in multicenter studies.

Moreover, the ethical concerns inherent in a placebo-controlled trial have prompted internal review boards to require frequent and extensive assessment of enrolled patients. It is not surprising that the response rate in the placebo cell of controlled trials has been steadily increasing over the past 20 years. Unfortunately, it is unlikely that in the current research climate an internal review board would approve a study design in which a comparison of medication to placebo mirrored standard clinical practice in as many respects as possible, including the frequency and duration of visits and the type and extent of psychosocial support provided.

A second issue is whether results of placebo-controlled trials delimit the response and remission rates observed when treating late-life major depression in clinical practice. In addition to the four placebo-controlled trials, six recent comparator trials had rigorous study designs (Bondareff et al. 2000; Mulsant et al. 2001b; Navarro et al. 2001; Nelson et al. 1999; Newhouse et al. 2000; Schatzberg et al. 2002). Compared with the placebo-controlled trials, the comparator trials consistently reported greater effect sizes and higher response and remission rates.

Traditionally, the higher response rates observed in comparator or even open trials are considered inflated beyond the "true" effect of the antidepressant and attributed to physician and patient expectation bias (i.e., all parties know that the patient is receiving an active treatment, and consequently, expectations are increased that improvement will occur). What has not been sufficiently considered is that response rates in placebo-controlled trials may be systematically suppressed. Older patients may find it disconcerting, or even humiliating, to respond to a placebo, believing that they will be labeled as hypochondriacal. Many patients with late-life depression may believe, perhaps unconsciously, that it is acceptable to be a medication nonresponder but not a placebo responder. This would induce patients to report minimal improvement to protect against an embarrassing outcome.

In summary, many of the procedures of placebo-controlled trials are radically different from standard practice, and the results may have limited bearing on clinical practice. In contrast, comparator or even open trials of antidepressants may more truly approach the response and remission rates that can be expected in clinical practice.

Duration of Treatment

A guiding principle in the treatment of late-life depression is that older patients take longer to respond to antidepressant treatment compared with younger patients. It is believed that the physiological effects of aging and the more treatment-resistant nature of mood disorders over time account for this observation, although a plausible alternative is that a prolonged time to response in the elderly may result from slower dose escalation of medication. The "start low and go slow" approach to antidepressant medication reflects the belief that older patients are more sensitive to the side effects of medication, and consequently, a lower starting dose and slower dose escalation of antidepressant medication would improve tolerability. However, little evidence indicates that the "start low and go slow" strategy increases tolerability of either the tricyclic antidepressants (TCAs) or the selective serotonin reuptake inhibitors (SSRIs) in the elderly, and this approach can obviously delay response or result in inadequate dosing (Roose et al. 1986).

Regardless of the reasons underlying the belief that patients with late-life depression take longer to respond to antidepressant treatment than do younger patients, the most significant clinical consequence is the dictum that for the treatment of late-life depression, 12 weeks is the minimum duration necessary for an adequate antidepressant trial (Young and Meyers 1992). However, do all patients require a complete 12-week trial before being declared nonresponders? An affirmative answer implies that patients with late-life depression may be not simply slow responders but late responders (i.e., a patient who is still quite ill at week 11 may improve dramatically and meet remission criteria by week 12).

The data relevant to the issue of long trials and late response in the elderly are actually quite limited and somewhat contradictory. Georgotas et al. (1989) reported that extending a nortriptyline trial from 7 to 9 weeks resulted in an increase in the response rate from 54% to 62%. However, only four patients were slow responders to nortriptyline, and the slow responders had low plasma levels of nortriptyline in the early weeks of the trial and responded after the dose was increased. Nonetheless, the results of this study are frequently cited as strong evidence that longer treatment trials in late-life depression are necessary.

The results of other studies are consistent with the hypothesis that a low starting dose and slow dose escalation result in a slower response to TCAs in older patients. Studies in which patients reached a therapeutic plasma level of TCA (either imipramine, nortriptyline, or desipramine) after 2 weeks of treatment reported that 90% of all responders reached that degree of improvement after 4 weeks of treatment (Roose et al. 1986).

Supporting the argument for longer treatment trials in older depressed patients are the results of two 12-week randomized, controlled trials of SSRIs in late-life depression (Bondareff et al. 2000; Newhouse et al. 2000). The studies compared sertraline with fluoxetine and sertraline with nortriptyline; both reported an increase in response rates at week 12 compared with week 8. Hypothetically, patients who did not meet response criteria by week 8 but did so by week 12 represent two different groups: 1) patients who were close to response criteria by week 8 and crossed the threshold by week 12 and 2) patients who had little or no significant symptom reduction by week 8 but then improved dramatically over the next 4 weeks to meet response criteria at week 12 (so-called late responders). If the higher response rate at week 12 resulted primarily from patients in the second group, then it would imply that all patients deserve a 12-week trial, even those who have no significant improvement by week 8. However, if the new responders at week 12 had already shown significant improvement by week 8, then it would imply that an extended treatment trial primarily benefits patients significantly well on their way to remission.

Related to trial duration are the clinically vital issues of time to response and early identification of nonresponders. Analyses of the same 12-week trials, one comparing sertraline with fluoxetine and the other comparing sertraline with nortriptyline, address these issues (Sackeim and Roose 2002).

In the first study, 236 patients were randomly assigned to fluoxetine or sertraline, and in the second study, 210 patients were randomly assigned to treatment with either sertraline or nortriptyline for 12 weeks. The patients who completed the 12-week trials did not differ in demographic or clinical features nor did the groups differ in rates of response or remission. Therefore, the patients who completed the trials in the four groups were combined for the purpose of enhancing sample size with respect to other analyses.

For the total sample of patients who completed the 12-week trials ($N=304$), the remission rate (defined as a 24-item Hamilton Rating Scale for Depression [Ham-D] final score ≤ 10) was 59%, and for a final Ham-D score of 6 or less, the remission rate was 34%. The median time to onset of sustained remission was 4 weeks. However, 36% of the patients who achieved sustained remission required

8 or more weeks to do so. If the remission criterion were a final Ham-D score of 6 or less, then the time to sustained remission was 8 weeks, with 29% reaching this criterion only in week 12. Thus, not surprisingly but often overlooked, time to remission is dependent on the remission criteria, which makes it difficult to compare studies with respect to this finding. Nonetheless, the results of these analyses, which are the most extensive to date, do not support the belief that patients with late-life depression are less responsive to antidepressant medication or take longer to respond than younger patients.

With respect to the early identification of nonresponders, when the remission criterion of a final Ham-D score of 10 or less was used, there is strong predictive power (i.e., by week 6, if a patient did not achieve a 30% reduction from baseline Ham-D score, then he or she had only a 22% chance of being in remission at the end of the study).

The most important implication of these data is that clinicians no longer have to mandate a 12-week trial of antidepressant medication to all depressed patients older than 60. Rather, they can make informed decisions about changing or continuing treatment at the 4- and 6-week time points on the basis of the probability that given the patient's improvement to date, he or she will or will not meet remission criteria by week 12.

Antidepressant Medication

Randomized, controlled trials can have significant differences in study design. The review of antidepressants that follows does not attempt to be inclusive of all studies. The intent is to illustrate the effect of antidepressant medication by considering the most methodologically rigorous clinical trials.

TCAs. Many placebo-controlled and comparator trials of TCAs for the treatment of late-life depression have been done. However, none of the placebo-controlled trials of TCAs used plasma level measurements to ensure optimal TCA treatment. Furthermore, the SSRI manufacturers who supported the studies comparing SSRIs with TCAs had no desire to compare their new SSRI compound against optimal tricyclic treatment. Nonetheless, the results of these studies established that tricyclics are an effective treatment for depression in geriatric patients. Nortriptyline has emerged as the TCA of choice to treat late-life depression because nortriptyline induces less orthostatic hypotension than do other TCAs (Roose et al. 1981). However, no placebo-controlled trials of nortriptyline in late-life depression have been done; thus, the effectiveness of this medication is inferred from two open trials and three randomized, comparator trials, all of which used plasma level measurements.

In an open 6-week study, 101 depressed patients were given nortriptyline, reaching a dose of 75 mg/day by the end of week 1 (Flint and Rifat 1996). Subsequently, the dose was adjusted if necessary to achieve a plasma level within the "therapeutic window" of 50–150 ng/mL. When the criterion of a final Ham-D score of 10 or less was used, 60% of the intent-to-treat sample and 75% of those who completed the study were in remission at the end of the trial. A second open 6-week trial of nortriptyline at a therapeutic plasma level included 42 depressed patients with ischemic heart disease (Roose et al. 1994). With remission defined as a final Ham-D score of 8 or less, the intent-to-treat remission rate was 67%, the completer remission rate was 82%, and the dropout rate was 19%.

Three studies compared nortriptyline with an SSRI—two studies compared a therapeutic plasma level of nortriptyline with that of paroxetine (Mulsant et al. 2001b; Nelson et al. 1999), and one study compared flexible-dose nortriptyline with sertraline. In the first study, which compared paroxetine with a therapeutic plasma level of nortriptyline, 116 patients (mean age=72) were entered into a 12-week trial. Remission was defined as a final Ham-D score of 10 or less; the intent-to-treat remission rate was 57% for the nortriptyline group and 55% for the paroxetine group. The dropout rate in the nortriptyline group was significantly higher than in the paroxetine group (33% vs. 16%, P=0.04). The second nortriptyline-paroxetine comparison study included 81 depressed patients with ischemic heart disease and was only 6 weeks in duration. The remission criterion was a final Ham-D score of 8 or less; in the intent-to-treat analysis, 63% of the nortriptyline group and 61% of paroxetine group were remitters. As in the previous study, the dropout rate for nortriptyline (35%) was significantly higher than the dropout rate for paroxetine (10%). The 12-week study comparing sertraline with flexible-dose nortriptyline included 210 patients (Bondareff et al. 2000). This study reported only response rates defined as a 50% reduction from baseline Ham-D score; the response rate for nortriptyline was 41% and for sertraline was 52%.

Side effects and safety. Despite the effectiveness of TCAs, their use in the late-life population is limited by their anticholinergic and cardiac effects (Roose and Glassman 1989). The anticholinergic effects of tricyclics result in dry mouth, constipation, and blurred vision, and more important, the older patient is particularly susceptible to urinary retention and confusional states (Pollock 1999).

In addition to causing an increased heart rate and orthostatic hypotension, the tricyclics have type 1A antiarrhythmic activity similar to that of moricizine and quinidine. Consequently, patients with ischemic heart disease are considered to be at increased risk for sudden cardiovascular death if they are given a TCA (Glassman et al. 1993). Given the prevalence of ischemic heart disease in both men and women older than 60, the use of tricyclics in this population, although not contraindicated, requires an informed calculation of the risk-benefit ratio.

SSRIs. The SSRIs are the most prescribed class of antidepressants for late-life depression even though clinical trials data are quite limited. As in the treatment of other disorders, the SSRIs appear to have equivalent efficacy and comparable side-effect profiles when used in older patients, but there are differences in pharmacokinetics and potential for drug-drug interactions.

Fluoxetine. Two studies of fluoxetine in late-life depression had a placebo-control cell. In a 6-week trial, fluoxetine 20 mg/day was compared with placebo in 671 patients (Tollefson and Holman 1993). Remission was defined as a Ham-D score of 7 or less after 4 weeks; the intent-to-treat analysis remission rate was 23% for fluoxetine and 13% for placebo; in the completer analysis, the remission rate was 27% for fluoxetine and 16% for placebo. (The other placebo-controlled trial is discussed in the subsection on venlafaxine later in this chapter.) In a 12-week comparator trial, 225 patients were randomly assigned to either fluoxetine 20–40 mg/day or sertraline 50–100 mg/day (Newhouse et al. 2000). The intent-to-treat remission rate was 46% for fluoxetine and 45% for sertraline; and the remission rate for those who completed the trial was 60% for fluoxetine and 59% for sertraline; the dropout rate was 33% for fluoxetine and 32% for sertraline. An 8-week open trial of 20 mg/day of fluoxetine included 308 depressed patients (Mesters et al. 1992). Remission was defined as a final Ham-D score of 10 or less; the intent-to-treat remission rate was 35%, the completer remission rate was 50%, and the dropout rate was 29%.

Sertraline. One placebo-controlled trial of sertraline in late-life depression has been done. This 8-week study included 716 patients who were randomly assigned to flexible-dose sertraline 50–100 mg or placebo (Schneider et al. 2003). Remission was defined as a final Ham-D score of 10 or less; the intent-to-treat remission rate was 29% for sertraline compared with 23% for placebo ($P<0.05$). The 29% sertraline remission rate found in the placebo-controlled trial stands in comparison to the 52% and 45% remission rates in the two randomized, controlled comparator trials previously described: nortriptyline versus

sertraline and fluoxetine versus sertraline, respectively (Bondareff et al. 2000; Newhouse et al. 2000).

Paroxetine. In addition to the two previously described comparator trials that compared a therapeutic plasma level of nortriptyline with that of paroxetine (in which the intent-to-treat remission rates for final 24-item Ham-D scores ≤10 and ≤8 were 55% and 61%, respectively), a third recently completed trial compared mirtazapine with paroxetine (described in the "Mirtazapine" subsection later in this chapter).

Citalopram. Only two studies of citalopram for the treatment of late-life depression in patients without dementia or significant cognitive impairment exist. The first was a single-blind comparison between citalopram and a therapeutic plasma level of nortriptyline, and the second was a recently completed comparison of citalopram and placebo in depressed patients older than 75. In a 12-week clinical trial, 58 patients were randomly assigned to treatment with citalopram 30–40 mg/day or nortriptyline with the dose adjusted to produce a therapeutic plasma level (Navarro et al. 2001). The intent-to-treat remission rate, defined as a final Ham-D score less than 7, was 69% for citalopram and 93% for nortriptyline. In this study, the remission rates for both medications were strikingly high in comparison to other trials. The reason for this result (e.g., differences in patient population or study design) is not obviously apparent.

The citalopram–placebo trial is unique in the literature because it is the only study to focus on treatment of depression in the "old-old" (Roose et al. 2004). In an 8-week trial, 174 patients (mean age=80) were randomly assigned to treatment with either citalopram 20–40 mg/day or placebo. The intent-to-treat response rate (50% reduction from baseline Ham-D) was 41% in the citalopram group compared with 39% in the placebo group.

Side-effect profiles in geriatric patients. The SSRIs have the same side-effect profile in older patients as in younger patients (e.g., nausea, insomnia, and sexual dysfunction). Discontinuation rates for SSRIs in late-life samples are not statistically different from discontinuation rates in younger depressed patients.

In contrast to the TCAs, the SSRIs are relatively benign in overdose. With respect to cardiac effects, several studies of SSRIs have been done in patients with ischemic heart disease, with congestive heart failure, and immediately post–myocardial infarction (Glassman et al. 2002; Roose et al. 1997, 1998). The SSRIs have a relatively benign cardiovascular profile. There is no evidence of a clinically significant effect on blood pressure, heart rate, cardiac conduction, or cardiac rhythm. In a placebo-controlled trial of sertraline in depressed patients post–myocardial infarction, the patients who received sertraline had significantly fewer major cardiovascular events than did the patients who received placebo (Glassman 2002).

Other antidepressants.

Venlafaxine. One study of venlafaxine has been done in a geriatric population: an 8-week three-cell study of 204 depressed patients that compared venlafaxine 75–225 mg/day, fluoxetine 20–60 mg/day, and placebo (A.F. Schatzberg and S.P. Roose, "A Double-blind, Placebo-controlled Study of Venlafaxine and Fluoxetine in Geriatric Outpatients With Major Depression," unpublished manuscript, 2005). Remission was defined as a final Ham-D score of 8 or less; the intent-to-treat remission rate was 42% for venlafaxine, 29% for fluoxetine, and 38% for placebo (no statistically significant differences). Significantly more patients who received venlafaxine (27%) and fluoxetine (19%) discontinued study participation because of side effects compared with those who received placebo (9%) (*P*<0.05).

Mirtazapine. In an 8-week trial that included 255 patients, mirtazapine 30–45 mg/day was compared with paroxetine 30–40 mg/day (Schatzberg et al. 2002). Remission was defined as a final Ham-D score of 7 or less; the intent-to-treat remission rate for mirtazapine (38%) was not statistically different from that for paroxetine (28%). The discontinuation as a result of adverse events was similar in both groups: 33% for mirtazapine and 29% for paroxetine.

Bupropion. The only data available on bupropion in a geriatric population come from a 6-week trial that included 100 patients and compared bupropion 100–300 mg with paroxetine 10–40 mg (Weihs et al. 2002). In the intent-to-treat analysis, the response rate (defined as 50% reduction from baseline Ham-D score) was 71% in the bupropion group compared with 77% in the paroxetine group, and the discontinuation rate was 17% in the bupropion group and 15% in the paroxetine group.

Dysthymic Disorder and Other Subthreshold Depressions

The classification of subthreshold depression (defined as less severe than major depression) in the elderly remains the subject of ongoing debate. Geiselmann and Bauer (2000) classified subthreshold depression in the elderly as a quantitatively minor variant of depression, or a depression-like state with fewer symptoms or with less continuity, and as a qualitatively different condition from major depression, with fewer suicidal thoughts or feelings of guilt or worthlessness but accompanied by prominent worries about health and weariness of living. Although this conceptualization is useful, empirical data and validation studies to support these assertions are generally lacking.

In contrast to the low prevalence of major depression, studies report a 13%–35% prevalence of "clinically significant" depressive symptoms in late-life samples (Blazer and Williams 1980; Koenig et al. 1988; Weissman et al. 1988). Subsyndromal and mild, chronic depressive disorders may be even more difficult for the clinician to recognize, especially if he or she does not have a high index of suspicion for mood disorder. Moreover, even if a mild to moderately severe depressive syndrome is diagnosed, especially in the setting of serious medical illness, clinicians often may take a pseudoempathic approach, in which the depression is considered a "normal reaction" to serious or debilitating illness. In particular, younger clinicians may believe that depressive symptoms are "normal" in older patients, even in the absence of a comorbid condition, especially because negative or stressful life events, such as retirement, death of family members and lifelong friends, and medical illness and infirmity, are common in late life. The consequence of these commonly held beliefs is that even when diagnosed, mild or moderate depression often goes untreated in this population.

Among the subthreshold depressive syndromes, dysthymic disorder has been the most studied. Some of the other categories (e.g., minor depression) remain controversial entities, and fewer data are available. Dysthymic disorder in the elderly is the focus in this part of the chapter, with reference to relevant published research on minor depression and other subthreshold depressive disorders in the elderly. Dysthymic disorder denotes chronic depression of moderate severity with fewer symptoms than major depressive disorder (MDD), and it affects approximately 2%–4% of adults (Gwirtsman et al. 1997).

Epidemiology

In the Epidemiologic Catchment Area study of five United States communities, the prevalence of DSM-III (American Psychiatric Association 1980) dysthymic disorder was 3.1% in the adult population (Weissman et al. 1988). In the elderly subgroup, the prevalence of dysthymic disorder was 1.5%. Blazer et al. (1988) found that 27% of the community-residing elderly individuals reported depressive symptoms: 19% mild dysphoria, 4% symptomatic depression, 2% dysthymia, 1% mixed anxiety–depressive disorder, and 1% major depression. In the Cache County epidemiological study of 4,559 elderly subjects, the prevalence of MDD was high, whereas the prevalence of dysthymic disorder was barely 1% (Steffens et al. 2000). In that study, the low prevalence of dysthymic disorder may have been related to the use of a narrow definition of dysthymic disorder requiring two of four symptoms preselected from the DSM-IV (American Psychiatric Association 1994) diagnostic criteria list of six symptoms, and two of these four symptoms were neurovegetative symptoms that are not common in elderly patients with dysthymic disorder (Devanand et al. 2005; Oxman et al. 2000). Also, the sample was almost exclusively Mormon, raising questions about generalizability. In contrast to this report, in most published epidemiological studies, the prevalence of dysthymic disorder in the elderly is higher, ranging from 2% to 7% (Carta et al. 1995; Fichter et al. 1995; Stefansson et al. 1991). The studies to date support the view that severe depressive disorders may decrease in old age and that milder forms, including dysthymic disorder, may become more prevalent (Ernst and Angst 1995).

Clinical Features

Most elderly patients with dysthymic disorder have a late age at onset, typically after 50 years, with limited comorbid Axis I and II disorders (Devanand et al. 1994, 2004). In contrast, young adults with dysthymic disorder commonly have onset of dysthymia before age 21 years, with a high rate of comorbid Axis I and II disorders (Keller et al. 1995; Kirby et al. 1999; D.N. Klein et al. 1998). In young adults, dysthymic disorder is often associated with personality disorders, and in the elderly, it is associated with health problems and life losses (Bellino et al. 2001).

These findings raise the intriguing question of what happens to young adults with dysthymic disorder as they grow older. Possibilities include progression to recurrent or chronic major depression, remission from depressive illness, or death due to suicide. The long-term studies needed to clarify the course of dysthymic disorder from young adulthood to old age have not yet been conducted. Data on young adults with dysthymic disorder followed up for a few years suggest that most have a persistent, chronic illness (D.N. Klein et al. 2000). In community samples, chronicity appears to characterize elderly subjects with dysthymic disorder as well (Pulska et al. 1998).

Symptoms and Diagnosis of Geriatric Dysthymic Disorder

In DSM-III, the types of symptoms selected to make the diagnosis of dysthymic disorder were arbitrary, as was the minimum 2-year duration criterion (Kocsis and Francis 1987). Subsequently, an effort was made to identify the characteristic symptom profile in dysthymic disorder in adults. In the DSM-IV Mood disorders field trial of 524 depressed adults, double depression (dysthymic disorder plus MDD) was common: 62% of patients with dysthymic disorder had concurrent MDD, and 79% had lifetime MDD (Keller et al. 1995). In dysthymic disorder, cognitive and social or motivational symptoms, not neurovegetative symptoms, were common. These data led to the "Alternative Research Criterion B for Dysthymic Disorder" (nine symptoms; see DSM-IV Appendix B, "Criteria Sets and Axes Provided for Further Study"), which excluded neurovegetative symptoms.

The few studies on the symptoms manifested by elderly patients with dysthymic disorder indicate predominant amotivational (e.g., loss of interest, lack of energy) and cognitive (e.g., hopelessness, worthlessness) symptoms, whereas neurovegetative symptoms are less common (Devanand et al. 2005; Oxman et al. 2000). Oxman et al. (2000) evaluated 216 patients with dysthymic disorder in the age groups 18–59 years and older than 60 years in primary care settings. Younger patients were more likely to have symptoms of worthlessness, guilt, feeling trapped, feeling blue, feeling lonely, blaming the self, decreased sexual interest, and overeating. However, age at onset was not systematically evaluated, and elderly dysthymic patients with early onset may be more similar to young dysthymic patients than to patients with late-onset dysthymia. The results from a range of studies in both young adults and elderly patients with dysthymic disorder suggest that the symptoms listed under the "Alternative Research Criterion B for Dysthymic Disorder" may be more valid than the main symptom criteria for the DSM-IV diagnosis of dysthymic disorder.

Gender, Age at Onset, and Psychiatric Comorbidity

The preponderance of females with adult depression appears to diminish and perhaps disappear in late-life depression, particularly in subthreshold depressive disorders (Angst et al. 2002; Devanand et al. 2004; Heikkinen et al. 2002). The high prevalence of comorbid Axis I and II disorders in young adults with dysthymic disorder is particularly prominent in patients with early onset, as defined in DSM-IV-TR; that is, onset before age 21 years (American Psychiatric Association 2000; D.N. Klein et al. 2000). Most adults with dysthymic disorder report onset before age 21 years, whereas only 10%–20% of elderly dysthymic patients report an onset before age 21 years (Devanand et al. 1994, 2004).

Antecedent adverse life events are commonly reported

by depressed patients in all age groups. In the elderly, as in young adults, the characteristic feature of depressed patients is that they perceive life events as having a much greater effect on them than do healthy control subjects (Devanand et al. 2002). This difference from healthy control subjects applies particularly to elderly patients with major depression and, to a lesser degree, dysthymic disorder (Devanand et al. 2002).

In an outpatient series of 211 elderly patients with MDD and 159 patients with dysthymic disorder, the combined late-onset (onset at age 60 years or older) sample had a higher rate of cardiovascular disease, lower rate of anxiety disorder, and lower rate of family history of mood disorder compared with early-onset patients (Devanand et al. 2004). Patients with late-onset dysthymic disorder were more likely to have cardiovascular disease than were patients with early-onset dysthymic disorder, but the rate of cardiovascular disease did not differ between patients with late- and early-onset MDD. Prevalence of anxiety disorders did not differ between the early- and late-onset MDD groups but was more common in the early-onset compared with the late-onset dysthymic disorder group. Late-onset dysthymic disorder did not differ from late-onset MDD in the rates of cardiovascular disease, anxiety disorders, and family history of mood disorder.

These results support the view that in the elderly, late-onset dysthymic disorder is typically different from early-onset dysthymic disorder. Cerebrovascular disease may play a role in the etiology of late-onset dysthymic disorder. The similarities between late-onset dysthymic disorder and late-onset MDD suggest that these disoders in many elderly depressed patients form a single condition along a continuum.

Family History

Across subtypes of dysthymic disorder, some evidence indicates that dysthymia may run "true" in the families of patients with dysthymic disorder (D.N. Klein et al. 1995). In early-onset (before age 21 years) patients, dysthymia may have a stronger familial association with personality disorders than with major depression (D.N. Klein et al. 1995). As is the case with MDD, elderly patients with late-onset (onset in middle to old age) dysthymic disorder typically do not have high familial loading for mood disorder, indicating that genetic etiology is not a likely explanation for late-onset depressive illness (Devanand et al. 2004).

Course of Illness

In a 12-year follow-up study of adults with depressive disorders, diagnostic criteria for minor depression and dys-

thymia were met frequently during the course of recurrent MDD, suggesting that diagnoses shifted over time during long-term follow-up (Judd et al. 1996). In young adults, half of the patients with dysthymic disorder do not recover during 5-year follow-up, and dysthymic disorder is typically a chronic condition with a protracted course and high risk of relapse (D.N. Klein et al. 2000). In adults with dysthymic disorder, the presence of comorbid anxiety disorder, personality disorders, and chronic stress may be associated with a lower rate of recovery from dysthymic disorder during follow-up (Hayden and Klein 2001).

Limited information is available on the prognosis of clinical samples of elderly patients with subthreshold depression, but extensive epidemiological data have been reported. In an epidemiological study of elderly Finns, survival was lower in both elderly men and women with dysthymic disorder, but this association was largely explained by the high occurrence of somatic diseases and disabilities in these subjects (Pulska et al. 1998). In another study of three Nordic communities followed up for 5 years, the strongest predictors of depressed mood were chronic medical illnesses, feelings of loneliness, and self-ratings of health (Heikkinen et al. 2002). In a 6-year follow-up of Dutch community subjects with late-life depression, symptoms generally persisted, and most patients had a chronic or unfavorable, fluctuating course (Beekman et al. 2002). In a study of 489 community subjects (average age=63 years) with a repeat evaluation up to 4 years after the initial assessment, the average annual incidence of a major depressive episode in the subset with baseline dysthymic disorder was 210 per 1,000 but only 21 per 1,000 for minor depression and 13 per 1,000 for subsyndromal depression (Murphy et al. 2002).

These findings suggest that in the elderly, MDD overlaps with dysthymic disorder but not with other subthreshold depressive syndromes. In the Murphy et al. (2002) study, among subjects without a diagnosis of a depressive disorder at baseline evaluation, the symptoms of "wanting to die" and "feeling worthless" were the most predictive of future depression 4 years later. Therefore, psychological symptoms of self-disparagement may be important indicators of future depressive illness in the elderly.

In 1,920 adults followed up long term in the Baltimore Longitudinal Study on Aging, lifetime prevalence of major depression was 9.8%, dysthymia was 7.3%, and depressive syndrome (broadly defined, including minor depression) was 16%. Double depression (major depression plus dysthymic disorder) had the earliest onset and the worst course (Chen et al. 2000). In a separate report from the same cohort, a history of depressive disorder was associated with an increased risk (relative risk=2.6) for stroke during 13-year follow-up. In another study, dysthymic disorder also was associated with an increased risk for stroke, but the relation was not statistically significant (Larson et al. 2001).

In a psychological autopsy study of 85 completed suicides in Sweden, recurrent major depression and substance use disorder were strong risk factors for suicide (Waern et al. 2002). Dysthymic disorder also posed increased risk for suicide, but this risk was lower than the risk posed by major depression.

In summary, the evidence suggests that dysthymic disorder, which is chronic by definition, usually persists and may worsen over time to reach the level of major depression in the elderly, particularly in the absence of effective treatment. Like major depression, dysthymic disorder appears to be associated with increased cardiovascular and cerebrovascular morbidity and mortality and with some increase in the risk for suicide.

Dysthymic Disorder in Primary Care

Most elderly patients with dysthymic disorder present to a primary care physician and not to a mental health professional (Williams et al. 2000). In a recent study that used the mental component summary of the SF-36 Health Survey (SF-36) rating form in an elderly Medicare fee-for-service sample, the prevalence of either major depression or dysthymia was 25% (McCall et al. 2002). A collaborative care model has been shown to be effective in the treatment of depression in primary care (Unutzer et al. 2002). In an ongoing multicenter study, initial evidence suggested that using a case manager to identify and arrange for treatment of depressed patients helps to improve clinical outcome in the primary care setting (Mulsant et al. 2001a) and that remission rates greater than 80% can be achieved with a rigorous, comprehensive treatment strategy (Thomas et al. 2002).

Social Adjustment, Quality of Life, and Disability

Depressive symptoms are associated with increased service use and social morbidity in the community (Johnson et al. 1992). In young adults, associations are well established among dysthymic disorder, poor social adjustment, and function (Leader and Klein 1996), and subthreshold depressive syndromes are associated with functional impairment across many areas of daily living (Judd et al. 1996). In old age, lack of social support, loneliness, and physical handicap are common in depressed patients (Prince et al. 1997). Subjective and structural dimensions of social support have been shown to protect more

severely depressed elderly patients from the loss of basic maintenance abilities (Hays et al. 2001).

The *Global Burden of Disease* report of the World Health Organization (1996) identified unipolar depression as the world's leading cause of disability, accounting for 10.7% of all disability and being responsible for more than 1 in 10 years lived with disability. In a study of 11,242 medical outpatients, current depression was associated with physical, social, and role impairment; poor perceived current health; and greater bodily pain (Wells et al. 1989). In a Finnish survey (6- to 12-year follow-up), dysthymic disorder in the elderly was associated with higher mortality, mainly because of physical illness and disability (Pulska et al. 1998). In various clinical trials in young adults and the elderly, the disability and poor general and social functioning associated with MDD and dysthymic disorder improved significantly with successful antidepressant (Devanand et al. 2005; Kocsis et al. 1988a, 1997; Mazumdar et al. 1996; Stewart et al. 1988) and psychotherapy treatment (Mazumdar et al. 1996).

From these reports, it is clear that depressive disorders across the life span are associated with poor social adjustment and general functioning. In elderly depressed patients, assessing a broad spectrum of functions is important because few experience major disabilities, but many report problems in social activities. The elderly have considerable disability as a result of depressive illness, and interventions directed at improving depressive symptoms also should aim at improving function and quality of life.

Pathogenesis

In young adults, subgroups of patients with dysthymic disorder have been shown to have abnormalities in plasma and urinary metabolites of catecholamines and lower platelet monoamine oxidase activity, but these findings are not consistent (Ravindran et al. 1994a, 1994b). Interleukin-1B levels in patients with dysthymic disorder have been shown to be elevated before and after sertraline treatment, suggesting that this immunological abnormality is a trait and not a state phenomenon (Anisman et al. 1999). Dysthymic disorder has been shown to be associated with elevated levels of circulating natural killer cells but without increase in corticotropin or norepinephrine (Ravindran et al. 1996).

In a small clinical series, Seidman et al. (2002) reported that testosterone levels were lower in elderly men with dysthymic disorder compared with healthy male control subjects, with no significant differences between elderly men with major depression and healthy control subjects. Indirect evidence shows that women with major depression who are receiving estrogen may have a superior response to antidepressants (Schneider et al. 1997), but this issue has not been studied in elderly patients with dysthymic disorder.

As described earlier in the section on major depression ("Influence of Age on Illness Presentation and the Problem of Diagnosis"), hyperintensities on MRI scan are two- to fivefold greater in patients with late-life major depression than in nondepressed control subjects (Boone et al. 1992; Christiansen et al. 1994) and are more frequent in patients with late- than in patients with early-onset major depression (Dahabra et al. 1998; Fujikawa et al. 1994; Krishnan et al. 1993, 1997; Lesser et al. 1996; O'Brien et al. 1998), with a few contradictory reports (Greenwald et al. 1996; Iidaka et al. 1996). In most MRI studies in late-life major depression, hyperintensities have been found across a wide spectrum of severity, suggesting that they also may occur frequently in elderly patients with late-onset dysthymic disorder.

Most patients with dysthymic disorder have a late age of onset. Therefore, many elderly patients with dysthymic disorder are likely to have cerebrovascular disease and hyperintensities, which also commonly occur in late-onset major depression (Alexopoulos et al. 1997; Steffens and Krishnan 1998). Cardiovascular disease has been shown to be common in elderly patients with dysthymic disorder (Devanand et al. 2004), but systematic studies of cerebrovascular disease are lacking in elderly patients with dysthymic disorder.

In geriatric major depression, hyperintensities and executive dysfunction may predict poor antidepressant response (Alexopoulos et al. 2002; Hickie et al. 1997) and a shorter time to relapse (O'Brien et al. 1998). An important issue that needs to be considered in the evaluation of cognitive impairment in patients with depressive disorders, both MDD and dysthymic disorder, is the well-established finding that increased severity of depression is associated with greater cognitive impairment (Elderkin-Thompson et al. 2003).

A structural MRI study in geriatric patients found that the degree of hippocampal atrophy in patients with minor depression was intermediate between that in patients with major depression and that in control subjects (Kumar et al. 1998). Hippocampal atrophy may characterize late-onset major depression (Sheline 2000; Sheline et al. 1999), and this may explain the memory loss that sometimes accompanies depression in the elderly. One possibility is that persistently high levels of corticosteroids in major depression (as exemplified by an abnormal dexamethasone suppression test result) lead to hippocampal damage and atrophy (Sheline 2000; Sheline et al. 1999).

Although evidence indicates that cerebrovascular disease, cerebral atrophy (global and regionally specific), and executive function deficits characterize geriatric major depression, particularly in patients with late-onset depression, and that these factors may be associated with poor treatment response and prognosis, such information is lacking in elderly patients with dysthymic disorder and minor depression.

Treatment

In the 1990s, the greatest increase in antidepressant prescribing in the United States was for depressive disorders of mild to moderate severity (Olfson et al. 1998). However, these disorders continue to be undertreated in young adults (Shelton et al. 1997) and in the elderly (Devanand et al. 2005; Williams et al. 2000).

Antidepressant Medication

Several studies in young adults showed that antidepressant medications were moderately efficacious in the treatment of dysthymic disorder, both in patients with primary dysthymic disorder (no antecedent Axis I or II diagnoses) and in patients with double depression (Boyer et al. 1999; de Lima et al. 1999; Hellerstein et al. 1993; Kocsis et al. 1988b; Lecrubier et al. 1997; Smeraldi 1998; Versiani et al. 1997). Studies comparing an SSRI with placebo in adults with dysthymic disorder have shown an advantage for the SSRI (Hellerstein et al. 1993; Ravindran et al. 2000; Vanelle et al. 1997). In a double-masked study of 416 (310 completers) young adult outpatients with primary dysthymic disorder, intent-to-treat response rates were 64% to imipramine, 59% to sertraline, and 44% to placebo (Thase et al. 1996). Similar results were seen in a broader sample that included patients with chronic MDD (Keller et al. 2000). Venlafaxine also may be an effective treatment in adults with dysthymic disorder, but placebo-controlled trials are lacking (Ballus et al. 2000; Dunner et al. 1997; Ravindran et al. 1998).

In contrast to the data in young adults, a paucity of controlled data exists on the treatment of dysthymic disorder in elderly patients. The only published randomized, double-masked, placebo-controlled treatment study was conducted in primary care, and it found a small but significant advantage for paroxetine over problem-solving therapy or placebo on the Hopkins Symptom Checklist–90. However, response rates (40%–51%) did not differ significantly among the three conditions (Williams et al. 2000). An initial open pilot trial of fluoxetine in elderly patients with dysthymic disorder found moderate efficacy with relatively few side effects (Nobler et al. 1996). However, a subsequent double-masked, placebo-controlled study of 91 outpatients did not find significant superiority for fluoxetine over placebo; response rates were 27.3% for fluoxetine and 19.6% for placebo in intent-to-treat analyses and 37.5% for fluoxetine and 23.1% for placebo in completer analyses (Devanand et al. 2005). A recent pilot open treatment trial showed that citalopram was effective in elderly men with minor depression (Kasckow et al. 2002), but placebo-controlled trials are lacking in elderly patients with minor depression. Interestingly, placebo-controlled trials of SSRIs in elderly patients with major depression also have generally found small to no advantages for active medication over placebo (Gottfries 1996; Nyth et al. 1992; Schatzberg and Cantillon 2000; Schneider et al. 2003; Tollefson and Holman 1993).

Psychotherapy

Group therapy may have some utility in adults with dysthymic disorder, particularly when used in conjunction with antidepressant medication treatment (Hellerstein et al. 2001; Ravindran et al. 1999). In a study of 26 married women who received doxepin, marital therapy, placebo, or minimal contact, both active treatments appeared to reduce depressive symptoms, but marital therapy had a superior effect on marital intimacy (Waring et al. 1988). In a nonblind study that compared sertraline (50–200 mg/day) with 10 sessions of interpersonal therapy (IPT) and with sertraline plus IPT in a primary care adult sample, response rates (40% improvement in symptoms) were 60.2% for sertraline, 46.6% for IPT, and 57.5% for combined treatment (Browne et al. 2002). The response rates would have been lower if standard response criteria of 50% rather than 40% improvement in symptoms were used.

In the only study that compared an antidepressant, placebo, and psychotherapy in elderly patients with dysthymic disorder, problem-solving therapy was not superior to placebo or paroxetine treatment (Williams et al. 2000). Of note, large intersite differences in response rates to problem-solving therapy were seen, emphasizing the difficulty in standardizing psychotherapy in treatment trials in elderly patients.

Overall, psychotherapy of several types has shown limited efficacy in depressed patients, but this remains to be shown in controlled studies of elderly patients with dysthymic disorder and other subthreshold depressive syndromes.

Treatment of Nonresponders

In a large-scale study of adults with chronic depression, half the patients who did not respond to sertraline responded to imipramine, and half the patients who did not respond to imipramine responded to sertraline

(Thase et al. 2002). In elderly patients, major depression that does not respond to one antidepressant medication usually responds to subsequent trials of alternative antidepressant medications (Flint and Rifat 1996). In elderly patients with dysthymic disorder, if symptoms have not responded to one class of antidepressant medications, switching to a different class of medications may prove to be an effective strategy. Clinically, the choice of medication should be based more on potential side effects than on putative differences in efficacy that have been small in magnitude across studies.

Continuation Treatment

After acute response to antidepressant treatment, adults with dysthymic disorder invariably maintain their improvement if medication is continued for extended periods (Hellerstein et al. 1996; Koran et al. 2001). Conversely, adults with dysthymic disorder commonly relapse if the antidepressant medication is discontinued (Bogetto et al. 2002; Kocsis et al. 1995) but recover if the antidepressant medication is reinstituted (Friedman et al. 1995).

In a small sample of elderly patients with dysthymic disorder, 6 of 12 patients relapsed within 6 months of discontinuation of fluoxetine after clinical response was achieved (Devanand et al. 1997). In an elderly community sample with mild to moderate depression that included a broad range of subjects, 113 responders to open treatment with sertraline were randomly assigned after a short continuation phase to sertraline or placebo (Wilson et al. 2003). No difference in relapse rates was found between the two groups, but several methodological limitations make it difficult to draw firm conclusions. With the caveat that adequate clinical research studies are still lacking, it appears that antidepressant medications should be continued for at least a year, perhaps longer, after clinical response is achieved in elderly patients with dysthymic disorder.

Antipsychotic Medication

In European studies, atypical antipsychotic medications have been shown to be efficacious in treating dysthymic disorder in adults. Amisulpride, which is available in Europe, is a presynaptic dopamine-blocking antipsychotic at low doses and a postsynaptic blocker at higher doses, and it does not act in the striatum. In a trial of 323 patients with dysthymic disorder, both amisulpride and amineptine (approved as an antidepressant in some European countries) were superior to placebo (Boyer et al. 1999). In another study of 313 outpatients with dysthymic disorder, including double depression, amisulpride 50 mg/day, was compared with sertraline, 50–100 mg/day

(Amore and Jori 2001). Response rates after 8 weeks of treatment were 82% in the amisulpride group and 69% in the sertraline group. Patients taking amisulpride showed shorter time to response, and tolerability was good. No data are available on the use of atypical antipsychotics in elderly patients with dysthymic disorder, but these results suggest that this class of medication merits investigation in the elderly.

Conclusion

Dysthymic disorder affects 2%–4% of the elderly population and leads to disability and poor quality of life. Both epidemiological and clinical studies show that dysthymic disorder in the elderly is typically different from dysthymic disorder in young adults. Dysthymic disorder in the elderly is predominantly of the late-onset type with onset typically after age 40 years, and it is associated with few comorbid Axis I or II disorders. This suggests that most elderly patients with dysthymic disorder are not young patients with dysthymic disorder who simply grew older.

For both young adults and elderly patients, the symptoms listed under the alternative research criterion B for dysthymic disorder in DSM-IV Appendix B, which emphasize motivational and cognitive/ideational symptoms, may be more valid than the symptom criteria that are listed under the main DSM-IV-TR diagnostic criteria for dysthymic disorder, which emphasize neurovegetative symptoms. In elderly patients with dysthymic disorder, obsessive-compulsive and avoidant personality disorders are the most common personality disorders, as in elderly patients with MDD. Patients with onset of dysthymia in middle to old age typically do not have comorbid anxiety disorders or high familial loading for mood disorder, indicating that genetic etiology is not a likely explanation for late-onset dysthymia.

Depressive disorders across the life span are associated with poor social adjustment and general functioning. In addition, elderly patients endure considerable disability as a result of depressive illness, and interventions directed at improving depressive symptoms also should aim at improving function and quality of life.

Considerable evidence indicates that cerebrovascular disease, cerebral atrophy (global and regionally specific), and executive function deficits characterize geriatric major depression, particularly in patients with late-onset depression. These features appear to be associated with poor treatment response and prognosis. A similar profile may occur in elderly patients with late-onset dysthymic disorder, in whom a high rate of cardiovascular disease has been reported.

There are limited data on the treatment of dysthymic disorder in elderly patients, and virtually no data exist on the treatment of minor depression in elderly patients. A randomized, double-blind, placebo-controlled treatment study in elderly patients with dysthymic disorder conducted in primary care found minimal advantage for paroxetine over problem-solving therapy or placebo. Results from a recent study showed minimal advantages for fluoxetine over placebo in elderly outpatients with dysthymic disorder, and response rates were low in both groups. Therefore, despite general progress in antidepressant therapeutics, no treatment with proven efficacy exists for geriatric dysthymic disorder, and we know even less about the efficacy of treatment in geriatric minor depression. Psychotherapy of various types has shown limited efficacy in elderly patients with major depression, but this remains to be shown in controlled studies in elderly patients with dysthymic disorder and other subthreshold depressive disorders.

References

Alexopoulos GS, Meyers BS, Young RC, et al: "Vascular depression" hypothesis. Arch Gen Psychiatry 54:915–922, 1997

Alexopoulos GS, Meyers BS, Young RC, et al: Executive dysfunction and risk for relapse and recurrence of geriatric depression. Arch Gen Psychiatry 57:285–290, 2000

Alexopoulos GS, Kiosses DN, Choi SJ, et al: Frontal white matter microstructure and treatment response of late-life depression: a preliminary study. Am J Psychiatry 159:1929–1932, 2002

American Psychiatric Association: Diagnostic and Statistical Manual of Mental Disorders, 3rd Edition. Washington, DC, American Psychiatric Association, 1980

American Psychiatric Association: Diagnostic and Statistical Manual of Mental Disorders, 4th Edition. Washington, DC, American Psychiatric Association, 1994

American Psychiatric Association: Diagnostic and Statistical Manual of Mental Disorders, 4th Edition, Text Revision. Washington, DC, American Psychiatric Association, 2000

Amore M, Jori MC: Faster response on amisulpride 50 mg versus sertraline 50–100 mg in patients with dysthymia or double depression: a randomized, double-blind, parallel group study. Int Clin Psychopharmacol 16:317–324, 2001

Angst J, Gamma A, Gastpar M, et al: Depression Research in European Society Study: Gender differences in depression: epidemiological findings from the European DEPRES I and II studies. Eur Arch Psychiatry Clin Neurosci 252:201–209, 2002

Anisman H, Ravindran AV, Griffiths J, et al: Interleukin-1 beta production in dysthymia before and after pharmacotherapy. Biol Psychiatry 46:1649–1655, 1999

Ballus C, Quiros G, De Flores T, et al: The efficacy and tolerability of venlafaxine and paroxetine in outpatients with depressive disorder or dysthymia. Int Clin Psychopharmacol 15:43–48, 2000

Beekman A, Copeland J, Prince M: Review of community prevalence of depression in later life. Br J Psychiatry 174:307–311, 1999

Beekman AT, Geerlings SW, Deeg DJ, et al: The natural history of late-life depression: a 6-year prospective study in the community. Arch Gen Psychiatry 59:605–611, 2002

Bellino S, Patria L, Ziero S, et al: Clinical features of dysthymia and age: a clinical investigation. Psychiatry Res 103:219–228, 2001

Blazer D, Williams C: The epidemiology of dysphoria and depression in an elderly population. Am J Psychiatry 137:439–444, 1980

Blazer D, Hughes D, George L: The epidemiology of depression in an elderly community population. Gerontologist 27:281–287, 1987

Blazer D, Swartz M, Woodbury M, et al: Depressive symptoms and depressive diagnoses in a community population. Arch Gen Psychiatry 45:1078–1084, 1988

Bogetto F, Bellino S, Revello RB, et al: Discontinuation syndrome in dysthymic patients treated with selective serotonin reuptake inhibitors: a clinical investigation. CNS Drugs 16:273–283, 2002

Bondareff W, Alpert M, Friedhoff AJ, et al: Comparison of sertraline and nortriptyline in the treatment of major depressive disorder in late-life. Am J Psychiatry 157:729–736, 2000

Boone KB, Miller BL, Lesser IM, et al: Neuropsychological correlates of white-matter lesions in healthy elderly subjects. Arch Neurol 49:549–554, 1992

Boyer P, Lecrubier Y, Stalla-Bourdillon A, et al: Amisulpride versus amineptine and placebo for the treatment of dysthymia. Neuropsychobiology 39:25–32, 1999

Browne G, Steiner M, Roberts J, et al: Sertraline and/or interpersonal psychotherapy for patients with dysthymic disorder in primary care: 6-month comparison with longitudinal 2-year follow-up of effectiveness and costs. J Affect Disord 68:317–330, 2002

Caine ED, Lyness JM, King DA, et al: Clinical and etiological heterogeneity of mood disorders in elderly patients, in Diagnosis and Treatment of Depression in Late Life. Edited by Schneider LS, Reynolds CF III, Lebowitz BD, et al. Washington, DC, American Psychiatric Press, 1994, pp 21–54

Carta MG, Carpiniello B, Kovess V, et al: Lifetime prevalence of major depression and dysthymia: results of a community survey in Sardinia. Eur Neuropsychopharmacol 5 (suppl):103–107, 1995

Chen L, Eaton WW, Gallo JJ, et al: Understanding the heterogeneity of depression through the triad of symptoms, course and risk factors: a longitudinal, population-based study. J Affect Disord 59:1–11, 2000

Christiansen P, Larsson HB, Thomsen C, et al: Age dependent white matter lesions and brain volume changes in healthy volunteers. Acta Radiol 35:117–122, 1994

Dahabra S, Ashton CH, Bahrainian M, et al: Structural and functional abnormalities in elderly patients clinically recovered from early and late-onset depression. Biol Psychiatry 44:34–46, 1998

de Lima MS, Hotoph M, Wessely S: The efficacy of drug treatments for dysthymia: a systematic review and meta-analysis. Psychol Med 29:1273–1289, 1999

Devanand DP, Nobler MS, Singer T, et al: Is dysthymia a different disorder in the elderly? Am J Psychiatry 151:1592–1599, 1994

Devanand DP, Kim MK, Nobler MS: Fluoxetine discontinuation in elderly dysthymic patients. Am J Geriatr Psychiatry 5:83–87, 1997

Devanand DP, Kim MK, Paykina N, et al: Adverse life events in elderly patients with major depression or dysthymic disorder and in healthy-control subjects. Am J Geriatr Psychiatry 10:265–274, 2002

Devanand DP, Adorno E, Cheng J, et al: Late onset dysthymic disorder and major depression differ from early onset dysthymic disorder and major depression in elderly outpatients. J Affect Disord 78:259–267, 2004

Devanand DP, Nobler MS, Cheng J, et al: Randomized, double-blind, placebo-controlled trial of fluoxetine treatment for elderly patients with dysthymic disorder. Am J Geriatr Psychiatry 13:59–68, 2005

Dunner DL, Hendrickson HE, Bea C, et al: Venlafaxine in dysthymic disorder. J Clin Psychiatry 58:528–531, 1997

Elderkin-Thompson V, Kumar A, Bilker WB, et al: Neuropsychological deficits among patients with late-onset minor and major depression. Arch Clin Neuropsychol 18:529–549, 2003

Ernst C, Angst J: Depression in old age: is there a real decrease in prevalence? A review. Eur Arch Psychiatry Clin Neurosci 245:272–287, 1995

Fichter MM, Bruce ML, Schroppel H, et al: Cognitive impairment and depression in the oldest old in a German and in U.S. communities. Eur Arch Psychiatry Clin Neurosci 245:319–325, 1995

Figiel GS, Krishnan KRR, Doraiswamy PM, et al: Subcortical hyperintensities on brain magnetic resonance imaging: a comparison between late age onset and early onset elderly depressed subjects. Neurobiol Aging 26:245–247, 1991

Flint AJ, Rifat SL: The effect of sequential antidepressant treatment on geriatric depression. J Affect Disord 36:95–105, 1996

Friedman RA, Mitchell J, Kocsis JH: Retreatment for relapse following desipramine discontinuation in dysthymia. Am J Psychiatry 152:926–928, 1995

Fujikawa T, Yamawaki S, Touhouda Y: Background factors and clinical symptoms of major depression with silent cerebral infarction. Stroke 25:798–801, 1994

Gallo JJ, Rabins PV: Depression without sadness: alternative presentations of depression in late life. Am Fam Physician 60:820–826, 1999

Geiselmann B, Bauer M: Subthreshold depression in the elderly: qualitative or quantitative distinction? Compr Psychiatry 41 (2 suppl 1):32–38, 2000

George LK, Blazer DG, Hughes DC, et al: Social support and the outcomes of major depression. Br J Psychiatry 154:478–485, 1989

Georgotas A, McCue RE, Cooper TBN, et al: Factors affecting the delay of antidepressant effect in responders to nortriptyline and phenelzine. Psychiatry Res 28:1–9, 1989

Glassman AH, Roose SP: Delusional depression: a distinct clinical entity? Arch Gen Psychiatry 38:424–427, 1981

Glassman AH, Roose SP, Bigger JT Jr: The safety of tricyclic antidepressants in cardiac patients—risk/benefit reconsidered. JAMA 269:20, 2673–2675, 1993

Glassman AH, O'Connor CM, Califf RM, et al: Sertraline treatment of major depression in patients with acute MI or unstable angina. JAMA 288:701–709, 2002

Gottfries CG: Scandinavian experience with citalopram in the elderly. Int Clin Psychopharmacol 11:41–44, 1996

Greenwald BS, Kramer-Ginsberg E, Krishnan RR, et al: MRI signal hyperintensities in geriatric depression. Am J Psychiatry 153:1212–1215, 1996

Gwirtsman HE, Blehar MC, McCullough JP, et al: Standardized assessment of dysthymia: report of a National Institute of Mental Health conference. Psychopharmacol Bull 33:3–11, 1997

Hayden EP, Klein DN: Outcome of dysthymic disorder at 5-year follow-up: the effect of familial psychopathology, early adversity, personality, comorbidity, and chronic stress. Am J Psychiatry 158:1864–1870, 2001

Hays JC, Steffens DC, Flint EP, et al: Does social support buffer functional decline in elderly patients with unipolar depression? Am J Psychiatry 158:1850–1855, 2001

Heikkinen RL, Berg S, Avlund K, et al: Depressed mood: changes during a five-year follow-up in 75-year-old men and women in three Nordic localities. Aging Clin Exp Res 14 (3 suppl):16–28, 2002

Hellerstein DJ, Yanowitch P, Rosenthal J, et al: A randomized double-blind study of fluoxetine versus placebo in the treatment of dysthymia. Am J Psychiatry 150:1169–1175, 1993

Hellerstein DJ, Samstag LW, Cantillon M, et al: Follow-up assessment of medication-treated dysthymia. Biol Psychiatry 20:427–442, 1996

Hellerstein DJ, Little SA, Samstag LW, et al: Adding group psychotherapy to medication treatment in dysthymia: a randomized prospective pilot study. J Psychother Pract Res 10:93–103, 2001

Hickie I, Scott E, Mitchell P, et al: Subcortical hyperintensities on magnetic resonance imaging: clinical correlates and prognostic significance in patients with severe depression. Biol Psychiatry 37:151–160, 1995

Hickie I, Scott E, Wilhelm K, et al: Subcortical hyperintensities on magnetic resonance imaging in patients with severe depression—a longitudinal evaluation. Biol Psychiatry 42:367–374, 1997

Iidaka T, Nakajima T, Kawamoto K, et al: Signal hyperintensities on brain magnetic resonance imaging in elderly depressed patients. Eur Neurol 36:293–299, 1996

Johnson J, Weissman MM, Klerman GL: Service utilization and social morbidity associated with depressive symptoms in the community. JAMA 267:1478–1483, 1992

Judd LL, Paulus MP, Wells KB, et al: Socioeconomic burden of subsyndromal depressive symptoms and major depression in a sample of the general population. Am J Psychiatry 153:1411–1417, 1996

Kasckow JW, Welge J, Carroll BT, et al: Citalopram treatment of minor depression in elderly men: an open pilot study. Am J Geriatr Psychiatry 10:344–347, 2002

Keller MB, Klein DN, Hirschfeld RMA, et al: Results of the DSM-IV mood disorders field trial. Am J Psychiatry 152:843–849, 1995

Kirby M, Bruce I, Coakley D, et al: Dysthymia among the community-dwelling elderly. Int J Geriatr Psychiatry 14:440–445, 1999

Klein DF, Ross DC: Reanalysis of the National Institute of Mental Health Treatment of Depression Collaborative Research Program General Effectiveness Report. Neuropsychopharmacology 8:241–251, 1993

Klein DN, Riso LP, Donaldson SK, et al: Family study of early onset dysthymia: mood and personality disorders in relatives of outpatients with dysthymia and episodic major depression and normal controls. Arch Gen Psychiatry 52:487–496, 1995

Klein DN, Norden KA, Ferro T, et al: Thirty-month naturalistic follow-up study of early onset dysthymic disorder: course, diagnostic stability, and prediction of outcome. J Abnorm Psychol 107:338–348, 1998

Klein DN, Schwartz JE, Rose S, et al: Five-year course and outcome of dysthymic disorder: a prospective, naturalistic follow-up study. Am J Psychiatry 157:931–939, 2000

Kocsis JH, Francis AJ: A critical discussion of DSM-III dysthymic disorder. Am J Psychiatry 144:1534–1542, 1987

Kocsis JH, Frances AJ, Voss C, et al: Imipramine and social-vocational adjustment in chronic depression. Am J Psychiatry 145:997–999, 1988a

Kocsis JH, Frances AJ, Voss C, et al: Imipramine treatment for chronic depression. Arch Gen Psychiatry 45:253–257, 1988b

Kocsis JH, Friedman RA, Markowitz JC, et al: Stability of remission during tricyclic antidepressant continuation therapy for dysthymia. Psychopharmacol Bull 31:213–216, 1995

Kocsis JH, Zisook S, Davidson J, et al: Double-blind comparison of sertraline, imipramine, and placebo in the treatment of dysthymia: psychosocial outcomes. Am J Psychiatry 154:390–395, 1997

Koenig H, Meador K, Cohen H, et al: Depression in elderly hospitalized patients with medical illness. Arch Intern Med 148:1929–1936, 1988

Koran LM, Gelenberg AJ, Kornstein SG, et al: Sertraline versus imipramine to prevent relapse in chronic depression. J Affect Disord 65:27–36, 2001

Kraemer HC, Wilson GT, Fairburn CG, et al: Mediators and moderators of treatment effects in randomized clinical trials. Arch Gen Psychiatry 59:877–883, 2002

Krishnan KR, McDonald WM, Doraiswamy PM, et al: Neuroanatomical substrates of depression in the elderly. Eur Arch Psychiatry Clin Neurosci 243:41–46, 1993

Krishnan KR, Hays JC, Blazer DG: MRI-defined vascular depression. Am J Psychiatry 154:497–501, 1997

Kumar A, Jin Z, Bilker W, et al: Late-onset minor and major depression: early evidence for common neuroanatomical substrates detected by using MRI. Proc Natl Acad Sci U S A 95:7654–7658, 1998

Larson SL, Owens PL, Ford D, et al: Depressive disorder, dysthymia, and risk of stroke: thirteen-year follow-up from the Baltimore Epidemiologic Catchment Area study. Stroke 32:1979–1983, 2001

Leader JB, Klein DN: Social adjustment in dysthymia, double depression and episodic major depression. J Affect Disord 37:91–101, 1996

Lecrubier Y, Boyer P, Turjanski S, et al: Amisulpride versus imipramine and placebo in dysthymia and major depression. J Affect Disord 43:95–103, 1997

Lesser IM, Boone KB, Mehringer CM, et al: Cognition and white matter hyperintensities in older depressed patients. Am J Psychiatry 153:1280–1287, 1996

Mazumdar S, Reynolds CF, Houck PR, et al: Quality of life in elderly patients with recurrent major depression: a factor analysis of the General Life Functioning Scale. Psychiatry Res 63:183–190, 1996

McCall NT, Parks P, Smith K, et al: The prevalence of major depression or dysthymia among aged Medicare fee-for-service beneficiaries. Int J Geriatr Psychiatry 17:557–565, 2002

Mesters P, Ansseau M, Brasseur R, et al: An open multicentre study to evaluate the efficacy and tolerance of fluoxetine 20 mg in depressed ambulatory patients. Acta Psychiatr Belg 92:232–245, 1992

Mulsant BH, Alexopoulos GS, Reynolds CF 3rd, et al: Pharmacological treatment of depression in older primary care patients: the PROSPECT algorithm. Int J Geriatr Psychiatry 16:585–592, 2001a

Mulsant BH, Pollock BG, Nebes R, et al: A twelve-week, double-blind, randomized comparison of nortriptyline and paroxetine in older depressed inpatients and outpatients. Am J Geriatr Psychiatry 9:406–414, 2001b

Murphy JM, Nierenberg AA, Laird NM, et al: Incidence of major depression: prediction from subthreshold categories in the Stirling County Study. J Affect Disord 68:251–259, 2002

Navarro V, Gasto C, Torres X, et al: Citalopram versus nortriptyline in late-life depression: a 12-week randomized single-blind study. Acta Psychiatr Scand 103:435–440, 2001

Nelson JC, Kennedy JS, Pollock BG, et al: Treatment of major depression with nortriptyline and paroxetine in patients with ischemic heart disease. Am J Psychiatry 156:1024–1028, 1999

Newhouse PA, Krishnan KRR, Doraiswami PM, et al: A double blind comparison of sertraline and fluoxetine in depressed elderly outpatients. J Clin Psychiatry 61:559–568, 2000

Nobler MS, Devanand DP, Kim MK, et al: Fluoxetine treatment of dysthymia in the elderly. J Clin Psychiatry 57:254–256, 1996

Nyth AL, Gottfries CG, Lyby K, et al: A controlled multicenter clinical study of citalopram and placebo in elderly depressed patients with and without concomitant dementia. Acta Psychiatr Scand 86:138–145, 1992

O'Brien J, Ames D, Chiu E, et al: Severe deep white matter lesions and outcome in elderly patients with major depressive disorder: follow up study. BMJ 317:982–984, 1998

Olfson M, Marcus SC, Pincus HA, et al: Antidepressant prescribing practices of outpatient psychiatrists. Arch Gen Psychiatry 55:310–316, 1998

Oxman TE, Barrett JE, Sengupta A, et al: The relationship of aging and dysthymia in primary care. Am J Geriatr Psychiatry 8:318–326, 2000

Parmelee PA, Katz IR, Lawton MP: Depression among institutionalized aged: assessment and prevalence estimation. J Gerontol 44:M22–M29, 1989

Pollock BG: Adverse reactions of antidepressants in elderly patients. J Clin Psychiatry 60 (suppl 20):4–8, 1999

Prince MJ, Harwood RH, Blizard RA, et al: Impairment, disability and handicap as risk factors for depression in old age. The Gospel Oak Project V. Psychol Med 27:311–321, 1997

Pulska T, Pahkala K, Laippala P, et al: Survival of elderly Finns suffering from dysthymic disorder: a community study. Soc Psychiatry Psychiatr Epidemiol 33:319–325, 1998

Ravindran AV, Bialik RJ, Brown GM, et al: Primary onset dysthymia, biochemical correlates of the therapeutic response to fluoxetine, II: urinary metabolites of serotonin, norepinephrine, epinephrine, and melatonin. J Affect Disord 31:119–123, 1994a

Ravindran AV, Bialik RJ, Lapierre YD: Primary early onset dysthymia, biochemical correlates of the therapeutic response to fluoxetine, I: platelet monoamine oxidase and the dexamethasone suppression test. J Affect Disord 31:111–117, 1994b

Ravindran AV, Griffiths J, Merali Z, et al: Primary dysthymia: a study of several psychosocial, endocrine and immune correlates. J Affect Disord 40:73–84, 1996

Ravindran AV, Charbonneau Y, Zaharia MD, et al: Efficacy and tolerability of venlafaxine in the treatment of primary dysthymia. J Psychiatry Neurosci 23:288–292, 1998

Ravindran AV, Anisman H, Merali Z, et al: Treatment of primary dysthymia with group cognitive therapy and pharmacotherapy: clinical symptoms and functional impairments. Am J Psychiatry 156:1608–1617, 1999

Ravindran AV, Guelfi JD, Lane RM, et al: Treatment of dysthymia with sertraline: a double-blind, placebo-controlled trial in dysthymic patients without major depression. J Clin Psychiatry 61:821–827, 2000

Robinson RG, Price TR: Post-stroke depressive disorders: a follow-up study of 103 outpatients. Stroke 13:635–641, 1982

Roose SP, Glassman AH, Siris SG, et al: Comparison of imipramine and nortriptyline induced orthostatic hypotension: a meaningful difference. J Clin Psychopharmacol 1:316–319, 1981

Roose SP, Glassman AH, Walsh BT: Tricyclic antidepressants: plasma level measurements and clinical outcome. Clin Neuropharmacol 9:263–264, 1986

Roose SP, Glassman AH, Attia E, et al: Comparative efficacy of the selective serotonin reuptake inhibitors and the tricyclics in the treatment of melancholia. Am J Psychiatry 151:1735–1739, 1994

Roose SP, Laghrissi-Thode F, Kennedy JS, et al: A comparison of paroxetine to nortriptyline in depressed patients with ischemic heart disease. JAMA 279:287–291, 1997

Roose SP, Glassman AH, Attia E, et al: Cardiovascular effects of fluoxetine in depressed patients with heart disease. Am J Psychiatry 155:660–665, 1998

Roose SP, Sackeim HA, Krishnan KR, et al; Old-Old Depression Study Group: Antidepressant pharmacotherapy in the treatment of depression in the very old: a randomized, placebo-controlled trial. Am J Psychiatry 161:2050–2059, 2004

Sackeim H, Roose S: How long should antidepressant trials be in geriatric depression? Paper presented at the 155th annual meeting of the American Psychiatric Association, Philadelphia, PA, May 18–23, 2002

Schatzberg A, Cantillon M: Antidepressant early response and remission with venlafaxine or fluoxetine in depressed geriatric outpatients. Paper presented at the meeting of the European College of Neuropsychopharmacology, Nice, France, June 2000

Schatzberg AF, Kremer C, Rodrigues HE, et al: Double-blind, randomized comparison of mirtazapine and paroxetine in elderly depressed patients. Am J Geriatr Psychiatry 10:541–550, 2002

Schneider LS, Small GW, Hamilton SH, et al: Estrogen replacement and response to fluoxetine in a multicenter geriatric depression trial. Fluoxetine Collaborative Study Group. Am J Geriatr Psychiatry 5:97–106, 1997

Schneider LS, Nelson JC, Clary CM, et al: An 8-week multicenter, parallel-group, double-blind, placebo-controlled study of sertraline in elderly outpatients with major depression. Am J Psychiatry 160:1277–1285, 2003

Seidman SN, Araujo AB, Roose SP, et al: Low testosterone levels in elderly men with dysthymic disorder. Am J Psychiatry 159:456–459, 2002

Sheline YI: 3D MRI studies of neuroanatomic changes in unipolar major depression: the role of stress and medical comorbidity. Biol Psychiatry 48:791–800, 2000

Sheline YI, Sanghavi M, Mintun MA, et al: Depression duration but not age predicts hippocampal volume loss in medically healthy women with recurrent major depression. J Neurosci 19:5034–5043, 1999

Shelton RC, Davidson J, Yonkers KA, et al: The undertreatment of dysthymia. J Clin Psychiatry 58:59–65, 1997

Smeraldi E: Amisulpride versus fluoxetine in patients with dysthymia or major depression in partial remission: a double-blind, comparative study. J Affect Disord 48:47–56, 1998

Stefansson JG, Lindal E, Bjornsson JK, et al: Lifetime prevalence of specific mental disorders among people born in Iceland in 1931. Acta Psychiatr Scand 84:142–149, 1991

Steffens DC, Krishnan KR: Structural neuroimaging and mood disorders: recent findings, implications for classification, and future directions. Biol Psychiatry 43:705–712, 1998

Steffens DC, Skoog I, Norton MC, et al: Prevalence of depression and its treatment in an elderly population: the Cache County study. Arch Gen Psychiatry 57:601–607, 2000

Stewart JW, Quitkin FM, McGrath PJ, et al: Social functioning in chronic depression: effect of 6 weeks of antidepressant treatment. Psychiatry Res 25:213–222, 1988

Thase ME, Fava M, Halbreich U, et al: A placebo-controlled, randomized clinical trial comparing sertraline and imipramine for the treatment of dysthymia. Arch Gen Psychiatry 53:777–784, 1996

Thase ME, Rush AJ, Howland RH, et al: Double-blind switch study of imipramine or sertraline treatment of antidepressant-resistant chronic depression. Arch Gen Psychiatry 59:233–239, 2002

Thomas L, Mulsant BH, Solano FX, et al: Response speed and rate of remission in primary and specialty care of elderly patients with depression. Am J Geriatr Psychiatry 10:583–591, 2002

Tollefson GD, Holman SL: Analysis of the Hamilton Depression Rating Scale factors from a double-blind, placebo-controlled trial of fluoxetine in geriatric major depression. Int Clin Psychopharmacol 8:253–259, 1993

Unutzer J, Katon W, Callahan CM, et al: Collaborative care management of late-life depression in the primary care setting: a randomized controlled trial. JAMA 288:2836–2845, 2002

Vanelle J, Attar-Levy D, Poirier M, et al: Controlled efficacy study of fluoxetine in dysthymia. Br J Psychiatry 170:345–350, 1997

Versiani M, Amrein R, Stabl M: Moclobemide and imipramine in chronic depression (dysthymia): an international double-blind, placebo-controlled trial. International Collaborative Study Group. Int Clin Psychopharmacol 12:183–193, 1997

Waern M, Runeson BS, Allebeck P, et al: Mental disorder in elderly suicides: a case-control study. Am J Psychiatry 159:450–455, 2002

Waring EM, Chamberlaine CH, McCrank EW, et al: Dysthymia: a randomized study of cognitive marital therapy and antidepressants. Can J Psychiatry 33:96–99, 1988

Weihs KL, Settle EC Jr, Batey SR, et al: Bupropion sustained release versus paroxetine for the treatment of depression in the elderly. J Clin Psychiatry 61:196–202, 2002

Weissman MM, Leaf PJ, Bruce ML, et al: The epidemiology of dysthymia in five communities: rates risks, comorbidity, and treatment. Am J Psychiatry 145:815–819, 1988

Wells KB, Stewart A, Hays RD, et al: The functioning and well-being of depressed patients. JAMA 262:914–919, 1989

Williams JW Jr, Barrett J, Oxman T, et al: Treatment of dysthymia and minor depression in primary care: a randomized controlled trial in older adults. JAMA 284:1519–1526, 2000

Wilson KC, Mottram PG, Ashworth L, et al: Older community residents with depression: long-term treatment with sertraline: randomised, double-blind, placebo-controlled study. Br J Psychiatry 182:492–497, 2003

World Health Organization: The Global Burden of Disease: A Comprehensive Assessment of Mortality and Disability From Diseases, Injuries, and Risk Factors in 1990 and Projected to 2020. Edited by Murray CJ, Lopez AD. 1996

Young RC, Meyers BS: Psychopharmacology, in Comprehensive Review of Geriatric Psychiatry. Edited by Sadavoy J, Lazarus LW, Jarvik LF. Washington, DC, American Psychiatric Press, 1992, pp 435–467

PART 8

Additional Perspective on Mood Disorders

SECTION EDITOR: DAVID J. KUPFER, M.D.

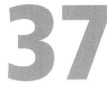

Depression in Primary Care

SUSAN BENTLEY, D.O.

WAYNE J. KATON, M.D.

EFFECTIVE TREATMENT OF depression in primary care settings presents unique challenges. Multiple factors contribute to the complex nature of major depression in the primary care population. Depressive symptoms are often intertwined with social stressors, medical symptoms, and chronic medical illness, resulting in competing priorities for attention by primary care physicians (Klinkman et al. 1997; Rost et al. 2000). Primary care physicians' training in diagnosis and management of depression is highly variable. Family practitioners are more likely to prefer treating depression with medication or counseling compared with internists or obstetricians-gynecologists (Gallo et al. 2002). Also, major problems in the system of primary care influence the diagnosis and management of depressive illness and its effect on the practice of general medicine, including brief, infrequent visits and dependence on the physician exclusively for all components of disease management. Primary care providers also perceive that they have more difficulty contacting psychiatrists for consultations or referrals compared with other medical specialists. The artificial barriers created by "carved out" behavioral mental health insurance programs have further distanced primary care and mental health providers.

In this chapter, we review the epidemiology of depression in primary care; the comorbidity of depression with medical illness; the effect of depression on symptom burden, functioning, and medical utilization and costs; the association of depression with adverse health risk behaviors (e.g., obesity, smoking, and sedentary lifestyle) and lack of adherence to medical regimens; differences between patients with depression in primary and tertiary care; and the lack of quality treatment for depression and barriers to quality treatment in primary care. We also review evidenced-based research models that have been shown to improve quality of care and outcomes of depression in primary care studies.

Epidemiology

Community samples have shown a 2%–4% 1-month prevalence of major depression. This prevalence increases to 5%–10% for patients in primary care clinics and to 10%–15% for primary care patients with chronic medical illnesses such as diabetes and heart disease. Dysthymic disorder occurs in 3%–6% of primary care patients and is highly prevalent in elderly patients with chronic medical illness (Unützer et al. 2001).

Most community residents with depression are seen exclusively in primary care settings, not by mental health specialists, over a 1-year period. Approximately 90% of primary care patients with depression have one or more visits to a primary care physician over a 12-month period, whereas fewer than one-third see a mental health professional (Kessler et al. 1994). Primary care has been described as the "de facto" mental health service by Regier et al. (1993) on the basis of findings from the National Institute of Mental Health Epidemiologic Catchment Area Program, which highlighted the need for more accurate recognition and effective treatment of depressive disorders in this setting of care.

The course of depressive illness in primary care has been described as "more like asthma than appendicitis" (Klinkman 1997) because patients with major depressive disorder usually have a relapsing and remitting or chronic course. The Epidemiologic Catchment Area Study found that 20% of the community patients with major depression diagnoses were still depressed 1 year after their initial interview (Sargeant et al. 1990). One-year longitudinal studies in both psychiatric and primary care patients (Lin et al. 1998) found a 20%–35% rate of chronicity and a 30% relapse rate among patients who initially recovered from major depression.

Identifying clinical characteristics of depressed patients that are associated with increased risk of relapse can help focus relapse prevention strategies. Lin and colleagues (1998) found that in primary care patients who initially recovered from a depressive episode, the three major risk factors associated with relapse were 1) persistence of subthreshold depressive symptoms, 2) history of two or more major depressive episodes, and 3) chronic mood symptoms that lasted for more than 2 years. Patients with two risk factors were three times more likely to relapse compared with patients with no risk factors. The severity of the initial depressive episode and high neuroticism levels also have been shown to independently predict disease persistence in longitudinal primary care studies (Katon et al. 1993). Many, but not all, primary care studies have shown that severity of comorbid medical illness predicts persistence of depression (Schulberg et al. 1998).

Almost three-quarters of the patients with lifetime major depression have been found to meet criteria for at least one other DSM-IV-TR (American Psychiatric Association 2000) disorder. The National Comorbidity Study found that patients with major depression had a 59% prevalence of a comorbid anxiety disorder and a 24% prevalence of a substance use disorder (Kessler et al. 2003). Longitudinal studies have shown that most patients with major depression have had one or more anxiety disorders in their teenage or early adult years preceding

development of their mood disorder (Merikangas et al. 2003). Patients with major depression who live in poverty appear to have a higher prevalence of comorbid posttraumatic stress disorder and panic disorder, which may decrease response to acute depression treatments (Mauksch et al. 2001). Comorbid psychiatric disorders such as panic disorder (Felker et al. 2003; Walker et al. 2000) have been associated with decreased response to quality improvement efforts that have been shown to improve outcomes of major depression in primary care settings. Primary care patients with major depression, panic attacks, and flashbacks are more likely to have a higher severity level of depressive symptoms, more impaired health status, worse functional impairment, and a more complicated and persistent history of mental illness when compared with patients who have major depression alone (Felker et al. 2003).

Studies have shown that the incidence of depression is higher in lower-income and less-educated populations (Weich et al. 1997). Patients with lower socioeconomic status also have been shown to have more persistent depressive symptoms (Sherbourne et al. 2001; Weich et al. 1997). A recent study examined a low-income, uninsured population in a rural Colorado primary care clinic and reported an increased prevalence of DSM-IV (American Psychiatric Association 1994) psychiatric illness in these patients compared with more mainstream primary care populations (Mauksch et al. 2001). Of this uninsured primary care population, 51% had symptoms that met DSM-IV criteria for one or more psychiatric diagnoses (Mauksch et al. 2001) compared with approximately 25% in other primary care studies in more representative populations (Spitzer et al. 1999). Olfson and colleagues (2000) also reported a high prevalence of depression, anxiety, and substance abuse associated with decreased function in an urban general medical population of low-income, older, mostly Hispanic adults. These increased depression prevalence rates and diminished health-related quality of life in urban poor may be due to a variety of factors, including being unemployed, living in neighborhoods that are unsafe, and having more adverse health behaviors (e.g., smoking, obesity), with resulting earlier onset of chronic medical illnesses such as diabetes and heart disease.

Depression may lead to unemployment and downward drift into poverty, which may prolong the depressive episode. Depressive symptoms have been associated in longitudinal studies with subsequent unemployment and loss of family income among working young adults. For instance, a recent prospective study of more than 5,000 adults consisting of approximately equal numbers of African Americans, Caucasians, men, and women ages 18–34 years in four United States cities evaluated depressive symptoms and subsequent unemployment. More than 50% of the persons with depressive symptoms (including 21% with substantial depressive symptoms) reported new unemployment during the subsequent 5 years (Whooley et al. 2002). Unemployment also may prolong depression. African Americans at risk for diabetes were longitudinally assessed for depression during a dietary intervention by de Groot et al. (2003). Factors such as unemployment, lack of home ownership, low appraisal of one's economic situation, and low-self esteem were significantly associated with depression at baseline and predicted more adverse depression trajectories over the study time frame. An inference from the study by Whooley and colleagues is that better treatment of depression might help with retention of employment. Schoenbaum and colleagues (2001) have shown that successful quality improvement interventions for depression treatment in primary care clinics that were associated with better depression outcomes compared with usual primary care treatment also were associated with increased job retention.

Major Depression: Overlap With Medical Illness

Given the broad spectrum of conditions seen by the primary care provider, medical comorbidity is an especially important factor in diagnosis and management. Patients with myocardial infarction, cerebrovascular disease, cancer, Parkinson's disease, human immunodeficiency virus (HIV)-related illness, and diabetes mellitus all have higher rates of major depression than do patients without these conditions (Katon 2003a). A recent large community study showed that approximately 4% of the patients with one or more medical conditions compared with 2.8% of the patients without a medical condition met the DSM-IV criteria for major depression (Patten 2001). A recent meta-analysis found that patients with diabetes mellitus had a twofold higher prevalence of major depression compared with those without diabetes (de Groot et al. 2001). In comparison with control populations, patients with HIV infection also have twice the rate of major depression (Ciesla and Roberts 2001).

Major depression has been noted to be especially prevalent in patients with neurological illness. This may be partially a result of the direct effects of the disease process on mood-regulating neurotransmitters. The prevalence of major depression in patients 3–4 months after a stroke was up to 30% in a series of studies reviewed by Whyte and Mulsant (2002). Depressive symptoms occur

in up to half of the patients with Parkinson's disease (McDonald et al. 2003). A recent community survey of patients with multiple sclerosis reported clinically significant depressive symptoms in 41% of the subjects and moderate to severe depression in 29% (Chwastiak et al. 2002). About one-third of the patients with epilepsy have been found to have major depression in population-based studies and up to half of those followed up in tertiary centers (Kanner 2003).

Depression also may increase a patient's risk of developing several chronic medical illnesses. A meta-analysis by Rugulies (2002) and colleagues concluded that major depression earlier in adult life increased the risk for development of coronary heart disease in initially healthy people by about twofold. In the 11 studies reviewed, a stronger effect size was found in clinically depressed patients compared with those with depressive symptoms, suggesting a possible dose-response relation between the severity of depression and coronary heart disease. Several studies also have shown that both major depression and depressive symptoms appear to predict an increased risk for developing diabetes by about twofold (Carnethon et al. 2003; Rugulies 2002).

The interaction between depressive disorders and medical comorbidities is complex. Pain and other aversive symptoms of medical illness may precipitate depression; depression also may decrease a patient's ability to adapt to aversive symptoms (Bair et al. 2003). Functional impairment secondary to complications of medical illness, such as having to stop work or to decrease household responsibilities, may cause depression. Depression itself is associated with increased functional impairment. Clinicians often see a "vicious cycle" of medical illness causing functional impairment, decreased functioning causing depression, and depression worsening the functional impairment (Bruce et al. 1994; Katz 1996; Prince et al. 1998).

Adverse Effect of Depression on Symptom Burden

Multiple medically unexplained symptoms are more common in patients with anxiety and depression than in those without psychiatric illness. Primary care studies have shown that 70%–80% of patients with anxiety and depression present initially with a physical symptom (Bridges and Goldberg 1985; Kirmayer et al. 1993). Primary care studies have supported a relation between an increased number of medical symptoms without identified pathology and an increased likelihood of the patients' symptoms meeting the DSM-IV criteria for a diagnosis of anxiety or depression (Katon et al. 2001a; Kroenke et al. 1997).

Case–control studies of patients with irritable bowel syndrome and inflammatory bowel disease (Walker et al. 1996), chronic fatigue and rheumatoid arthritis (Katon et al. 1991), and fibromyalgia and rheumatoid arthritis (Walker et al. 1997) reported higher rates of lifetime major depressive episodes in the patients with these less clearly defined syndromes. Compared with those with medical illness, these patients with medically unexplained syndromes also have more unexplained medical symptoms in other organ systems (Katon et al. 2001a). For instance, patients with irritable bowel syndrome compared with those with inflammatory bowel disease have not only significantly more gastrointestinal symptoms but also more unexplained symptoms in other organ systems.

Medically ill patients with major depression are likely to experience a higher disease-specific symptom burden than are those patients without depression (Katon 2003a). Patients with medical illness who are not depressed usually adapt over time to their adverse disease symptoms. Comorbid anxiety and depressive disorders interfere with this adaptation process and are associated with heightened awareness and focus on both symptoms of a specific illness and unexplained physical symptoms in other organ systems (Katon 2003a).

Symptom amplification in depression has been seen in several illnesses. In diabetic patients, depressive symptoms were more significantly correlated with nine symptoms traditionally associated with poor glucose control (e.g., polydipsia, polyuria) than with the number of diabetic complications or level of hemoglobin A_1c, a physiological measure of glycemic control (Ciechanowski et al. 2003; Katon et al. 2003b). Patients with hepatitis C and higher depressive symptom severity complained of significantly more impairment from fatigue (the main symptom associated with hepatitis C) compared with less-depressed hepatitis patients, when controlling for severity of pathological liver changes (Dwight et al. 2000). Patients with inflammatory bowel disease and comorbid depressive or anxiety disorders complained of both significantly more gastrointestinal symptoms and more medical symptoms in other organ systems when compared with patients who had inflammatory bowel disease but no psychiatric disorders, after controlling for the severity of bowel disease (Walker et al. 1996). In a prospective study of patients with coronary artery disease, Sullivan and colleagues (2000) reported that baseline levels of anxiety and depression in these patients were significantly associated with more reports of symptomatic chest pain and fatigue 5 years later, after controlling for the number of coronary vessels occluded, ejection fraction at baseline, and cardiac procedures over this period.

Primary care physicians often encounter pain symptoms, and these symptoms often interact with depression. This interaction has been labeled the *depression–pain syndrome* (Lindsay and Wyckoff 1981), which reflects the frequent coexistence, response to similar treatments, and shared biological pathways of these disorders (Blier 2002; Gallagher and Verma 1999). Bair and colleagues (2003) recently conducted an extensive literature review and reported an 18% point prevalence of comorbid major depression and persistent pain in community settings and a 27% prevalence of this comorbidity in primary care clinics. Lifetime prevalence rates of major depression have been reported to be as high as 50% in patients with chronic pain (Bair et al. 2003). Comorbid depression has been shown in patients with chronic pain to be associated with an array of poor outcomes, including more pain complaints, greater pain intensity, and longer duration of pain (Bair et al. 2003). Depressed patients with persistent pain, compared with patients with pain alone, had a worse prognosis with a greater likelihood of persistent pain and nonrecovery than did those without depression (Bair et al. 2003). A bidirectional relation exists between chronic pain and depression. Future episodes of pain (low back pain, chest pain, headache, musculoskeletal complaints) have been shown to be predicted by the presence of major depression, as were poorer adherence to treatment of pain and worse patient satisfaction with care (Bair et al. 2003). Patients with persistent pain also have been shown in a large prospective study to be at higher risk for development of major depression (Gureje et al. 2001).

Adverse Effect of Depression on Function

Major depression is associated with substantial functional impairment in community and primary care populations. More than 95% of the respondents with major depressive disorder from the National Comorbidity Survey Replication (Kessler et al. 2003) reported some degree of role impairment associated with their depression, with 59% reporting severe or very severe impairment. Affective illness is associated with increased sick days from work, work disability, and loss of jobs over time (Miranda et al. 2004; Wells et al. 1989). Berndt et al. (2000) showed that early-onset major depression adversely affects the educational attainment of women.

Patients with major depression and comorbid medical illness have additive functional impairment (Wells et al. 1989). Cross-sectional studies have found that major depression is associated with additive disability in patients with cancer (Breitbart 1995), HIV (Cook et al. 2002), diabetes (Ciechanowski et al. 2000), inflammatory bowel disease (Walker et al. 1996), chronic obstructive pulmonary disease (Felker et al. 2001), and heart disease (Sullivan et al. 1997), after controlling for severity of medical illness. Additive impairment also occurs in work, social, and physical functioning (limited mobility, restricted activity) when pain and depression coexist (Bair et al. 2003).

Depression, coronary heart disease, and cerebrovascular disease each independently predicted functional decline in patients ages 65 and older over a 3-year period (Wang et al. 2002). Unützer and colleagues (2000) compared elderly patients with clinically significant depressive symptoms with patients with one of eight chronic medical illnesses in a study of 2,558 primary care patients. Over the 4-year study period, after adjusting for differences in gender, age, and chronic medical disorders, depressed patients had the third most decrements in quality-adjusted life-years. Patients with chronic medical illness and comorbid depression were shown to have additive decrements in quality-adjusted life-years.

Over time, depression and anxiety are more predictive of functional impairment than is the severity of physical illness. In a longitudinal study of patients with coronary artery disease, depression and anxiety at the time of initial coronary artery disease diagnosis by angiogram were more highly correlated with functional impairment at 1- and 5-year follow-ups than was any physiological measure. The study controlled for vessel occlusion of 70% or more, baseline ejection fraction, and cardiac procedures over time (Sullivan et al. 1997, 2000). Depression and anxiety disorders in patients with recent myocardial infarction predicted poor outcome on all quality-of-life dimensions at 1 year (Mayou et al. 2000).

Depressive symptoms and disability measures change synchronously over time—as depression improves, so do measures of functional impairment (Ormel et al. 1993; Von Korff et al. 1992). Effective treatment of depression has been associated with significant functional improvement in primary care patients in general (Katzelnick et al. 2000; Lin et al. 2000; Unützer et al. 2002) and in patients with comorbid chronic obstructive pulmonary disease (Borson et al. 1992), HIV (Elliott et al. 2002), tinnitus, and hearing impairment (Sullivan et al. 1993).

Effect of Depression on Medical Costs

Patients with depression and anxiety are frequently high utilizers of primary care systems. This may be because depressed patients tend to have multiple medically unexplained symptoms and higher rates of medical comorbidity (Katon et al. 2001a). This increase in medical symptoms in depressed patients may lead to more medical investigations and prescriptions aimed at reducing these symptoms. Simon and colleagues (1995) found that depressive disorder in primary care patients was associated with a 50%–75% increase in 1-year health service costs, after adjusting for comorbid chronic medical illness, when compared with a sample of patients without depression. The higher costs were observed for every category of care (primary care, specialty medical care, inpatient medical care, laboratory, pharmacy). In a large population-based sample of more than 8,500 patients ages 60 and older, Katon and colleagues (2003a) found total ambulatory and inpatient costs to be about 50% higher in depressed compared with nondepressed elderly, after adjusting for chronic medical illness. Like the study by Simon et al. (1995), the cost increases were evident in every component health care expenditure, with only a small percentage due to mental health treatment. Unützer and associates (1997) also found 50% higher health services costs among depressed patients according to data from more than 2,500 Medicare health maintenance organization enrollees. Only 5%–10% of the observed increases in overall health service costs are attributable to depression treatment (antidepressant medication, specialty mental health care, primary care visits with depression diagnoses). The primary effect of depression on health care use is on increased use of general medical services, not on resources directed to the treatment of depression (Simon 2003).

Use of services and subsequent costs of caring for patients with medical illness are also increased by the burden of comorbid depression. Among elderly primary care patients with a diverse range of medical illness, depression makes a significant independent contribution to increased health care use (Unützer et al. 1997). Ciechanowski et al. (2000) examined health care costs of depressed patients with diabetes (most had type 2 diabetes) treated in primary care clinics. For patients in the highest depression tertile, there were 51% higher costs in primary care, 75% higher costs in overall ambulatory care, and 86% higher total health care costs. A recent prospective study of the effect of depression on health care costs in primary care patients with heart failure found treatment costs up to 29% higher for this population compared with those with heart disease alone, after controlling for age, sex, and other medical comorbidities (Sullivan et al. 2002). These increased costs in patients with depression and medical comorbidity may be a result of adverse health habits in the depressed population, decreased ability to adhere to medical recommendations, increased somatization, and possibly the direct negative physiological effects of depression itself.

Association of Depression With Adverse Health Risk Behaviors

The complexity of patients with depression in primary care is heightened by the association of this illness with high-risk behaviors. Major depression has been associated with higher rates of adverse health risk behaviors such as smoking, sedentary lifestyle, overeating, and obesity (Rosal et al. 2001). The increase in these behaviors may explain why major depression earlier in life is associated with a twofold higher incidence of diabetes and heart disease (Katon et al. 2003b).

Adolescents with major depression (particularly females) were found to have an increased risk of developing obesity in their early 20s when compared with nondepressed adolescents in several large longitudinal studies (Goodman and Whitaker 2002; Richardson et al. 2003). In a large prospective study, Patton and colleagues (1998) showed that depressive and anxiety disorders are risk factors for adolescents to initiate smoking through an increased susceptibility to peer pressure. Adults with major depression had significantly higher rates of smoking than did nondepressed responders in the Epidemiologic Catchment Area Study (Glassman et al. 1990). Cigarette smokers in the United States with depression also have been found to be 40% less likely to quit smoking when compared with nondepressed smokers (Anda et al. 1990). When depressed patients attempt to quit smoking, affective symptoms emerge. Patients with a history of major depression have been shown to be at a higher risk for developing a depressive episode when they try to quit smoking than are those without a history of mood disorders (Dierker et al. 2002).

Lack of Adherence to Medical Regimens

Effective treatment of most medical illnesses in primary care settings usually requires a degree of self-management on the part of the patient. Patients with chronic medical conditions frequently need to work in collaboration with their physician on behavioral issues such as dietary changes and adjustment of exercise and physical activity; also, patients must cooperate with their physi-

cians in finding medication regimens with the most optimal therapeutic effects and fewest side effects. Medically ill patients often need to decrease potentially harmful behaviors such as smoking and drinking. Self-monitoring of blood glucose, blood pressure, and somatic symptoms is an integral part of many treatment plans.

Depression has been shown to adversely affect patient self-management in many medical illnesses. DiMatteo and colleagues (2000) conducted a meta-analysis of the effects of anxiety and depression on patient adherence and found that compared with nondepressed patients, the odds are three times greater that depressed patients will be nonadherent with medical treatment recommendations. In patients with heart disease, major depression is associated with lapses in daily aspirin intake (Carney et al. 1995) and in dropout from exercise rehabilitation during recovery from myocardial infarction (Blumenthal et al. 1982). Depressive symptoms in diabetic patients have been associated with poorer diet and more lapses in refills of oral hypoglycemic medications (Ciechanowski et al. 2000). Depression predicts lack of adherence to highly active antiretroviral therapy in patients with HIV (Riera et al. 2002; Spire et al. 2002), as well as lessened likelihood of treatment with highly active antiretroviral therapy by physicians (Cook et al. 2002; Sambamoorthi et al. 2000).

Differences Between Primary Care and Tertiary Care Populations

A growing body of literature on patients with major depression in primary care suggests that these patients have significant differences from patients with depressive illness treated in tertiary care. The Michigan Depression Project found that many patients meeting DSM-IV criteria for a diagnosis of major depressive disorder in primary care had relatively mild depression with little functional impairment compared with those treated in psychiatric settings (Schwenk et al. 1998). These investigators also found that the onset of major depression in family practice patients was usually preceded by a severe life event and that the outcome for patients with unrecognized major depression was comparable to that for patients with detected major depression (Schwenk et al. 1998). The higher initial severity of depression and increased functional impairment in these patients whose affective illness was detected by primary care physicians compared with those whose illness was not detected was probably responsible for these similar outcomes (Coyne et al. 1995). Cooper-Patrick et al. (1994) compared depressed patients receiving care in general medical settings with depressed patients seen in mental health settings. Patients seen in the general medical sector were more likely to be African American, female, and older than 65 years and to have high school or less educational history; they were less likely to be in the highest socioeconomic quartile. These patients had a lower chance of meeting DSM-IV criteria for major depression than did those seen in specialty care. A higher proportion of patients seen in mental health settings had symptoms that met criteria for diagnosis of panic disorder, obsessive-compulsive disorder, or schizophrenia and had a lifetime history of psychiatric hospitalization (Cooper-Patrick et al. 1994). This National Institute of Mental Health/Epidemiologic Catchment Area study suggested that demographic differences in primary care populations may affect a patient's knowledge, attitude toward care, interpretation of symptoms, and treatment preferences regarding depressive illness.

Quality of Diagnosis and Treatment in Primary Care

A decade ago, primary care researchers showed that only one-half of patients with depressive disorders received accurate diagnoses from primary care physicians (Public Health Service Agency for Health Care Policy and Research 1993). In 1994, Wells and colleagues reported that of the 50% of patients with accurate diagnoses of depression, only 25%–50% received guideline-level treatment with pharmacotherapy, and fewer than 10% received evidence-based psychotherapy. Despite advances in the health care system over the intervening years, gaps in the effective diagnosis and treatment of depressive disorders in the primary care setting remain. Young and colleagues (2001) recently conducted a national cross-sectional study of more than 1,600 adults with probable 12-month depressive or anxiety disorder determined by a brief diagnostic interview. They found that over a 1-year period, more than three-quarters of these individuals saw a health care provider, and most visited primary care providers exclusively. Only 30% of the patients received some treatment consistent with guideline-level recommendations for antidepressant medication or psychotherapy. Only 19% of the depressed or anxious patients seen solely in primary care settings received appropriate care. Although rates of outpatient treatment for depression and use of antidepressant medication in primary care have increased over the last 10 years (Olfson et al. 2002a), the duration of treatment has not. Only 25%–50% of primary care patients adhere to antidepressant medication for the duration of guideline-level recommendations (Katon et al. 2001b), with most

patients receiving one to three prescriptions (Simon 2002).

Treatment rates of evidence-based psychotherapy for depression actually may have declined in this managed care era. Olfson and colleagues (2002b) evaluated trends in the rate of psychotherapy use from nationally representative samples gathered for the National Medical Expenditure Survey and Panel. They found a marked increase in the use of psychotropic medications among patients, along with more psychotherapy being provided by physicians, whereas the number of psychotherapy visits per user decreased sharply. Of primary care patients whose major depression is recognized by their physician, only about 40% recover in 4–6 months based on a 50% reduction in depressive symptoms (Katon et al. 1995, 1996).

The Institute of Medicine has developed a nosology that can be used to describe the problems with diagnosis and treatment of depression in primary care (Katon 2003b). *Underuse* of guideline-level treatments is exemplified by the lack of accurate diagnosis in 50% of patients with major depression and nonadherence to guideline-level recommendations for duration of treatment with antidepressants in most patients with depressive disorders. Diagnostic testing for medically unexplained physical symptoms such as headache or abdominal pain is an example of *overuse*. Overuse of medical testing occurs when primary care physicians have heightened concern about somatic symptoms, increased functional impairment, and increased medical testing and costs in patients with depression and unexplained physical symptoms (Katon 2003b). An example of *misuse* of treatment is when patients with adjustment disorders and minor depression are frequently given antidepressants when little evidence shows that these medications are effective in these populations (Katon et al. 1995, 2001b). Studies conducted in the mid-1990s (Katon et al. 1995, 1996) showed that approximately half of the patients started on antidepressant medications by primary care physicians actually met criteria for adjustment disorders or minor depression.

Barriers to Treatment of Depression in Primary Care

Barriers to the effective treatment of depression in primary care settings are encountered on patient, system, and provider levels.

Patient-Level Barriers

The first potential barrier is the patient's unique experience with depression, including his or her understanding of the illness and treatment preferences. Many patients lack knowledge about depression; the options available for treatment; and the cognitive, behavioral, and interpersonal changes they will need to make to care for their illness. Key depressive symptoms may be unrecognized by the patient or may be perceived to be secondary to medical symptoms such as headaches. This lack of knowledge also may affect a patient's response to physicians' screening questions about depression. A patient may conceal or fail to acknowledge his or her symptoms in response to the belief that depression is not a legitimate medical diagnosis requiring treatment (Dew et al. 1988).

A recent study by Nutting and colleagues (2002) showed that primary care physicians believe that barriers to the effective diagnosis and treatment of depression most often arise from factors centered with the patient. The primary care physicians thought that the most challenging barriers to acute-stage care of depression were related to three patient factors: 1) the patient's resistance to the diagnosis and treatment, 2) the patient's noncompliance with visits, and 3) the patient's psychosocial burden of stressors (Nutting et al. 2002).

Patient preferences about treatment of depression also may complicate delivery of effective care. Updated guidelines on the treatment of major depression in primary care from the Agency for Health Care Policy and Research Practice (AHCPR) (Schulberg et al. 1998) indicate that antidepressant pharmacotherapy and depression-specific psychotherapies (interpersonal, cognitive, behavioral, and problem-solving therapies) are efficacious when transferred from psychiatric to primary care settings. Many patients express an initial preference for psychotherapy (Dwight-Johnson et al. 2000), but primary care systems can more easily provide medication. Psychosocial treatments for depression are provided less frequently because of difficulties with referral (i.e., lack of knowledge about effective counselors because of lack of interaction of medical and mental health systems) and because of issues with reimbursement. Lack of parity for insurance coverage for mental health care is a key patient-level barrier to the treatment of depression (Katon 2003b). Patient preferences to receive treatment for depression in general medical rather than mental health care settings also may hinder appropriate care. One-third to one-half of primary care patients will refuse referral to a mental health professional (Orleans et al. 1985). However, interventions that provide on-site mental health services have found more than 90% acceptance of referral (Katon et al. 1995, 1996). Even with the patient's preferences for on-site services, mental health care providers are often not integrated into primary care.

Symptoms associated with depression itself can limit access to treatment on an individual level. The inherent lack of energy and hopelessness of depressive illness may make initiation of treatment and active participation in care difficult. Chronic social stressors can negatively affect self-management by decreasing energy and focus to get effective treatment. The unique stigma (i.e., shame and embarrassment) associated with a diagnosis of depression is another important patient-level barrier to effective treatment that often must be addressed by the primary care physician (Roeloffs et al. 2003).

System-Level Barriers

Primary care medical care systems traditionally have been organized to provide treatment for acute illness but have significant barriers to improving care and outcomes for patients with chronic illness such as depression. One such barrier to effective treatment of depression is infrequent office visits. AHCPR guidelines for acute-phase antidepressant pharmacotherapy recommend that severely depressed patients be seen weekly in follow-up and those with milder illness seen every 10–14 days during the initial 6–8 weeks of treatment (Schulberg et al. 1998). This schedule was thought to improve patient adherence, facilitate dosage adjustment, and permit careful monitoring of symptoms, but it far exceeds routine primary care practice. Several studies provide indirect support for the recommendations that more frequent visits improve clinical outcomes. Schulberg et al. (1996, 1997) found that patients randomly assigned to weekly and twice-monthly visits in a standardized acute-phase pharmacotherapy protocol had significantly better outcomes than did patients provided with usual care. Additional studies have shown that depressed patients in health maintenance organizations who were seen approximately once every 4–6 weeks during acute-phase treatment with pharmacotherapy had poor adherence to antidepressant medication and low recovery rates (Katon et al. 1995, 1996).

Provider-Level Barriers

The organization of primary care practice around the conventional 15-minute office visit is a provider-level barrier to treating depression effectively. This type of scheduling discourages the comprehensive assessment, counseling, treatment planning, and use of telephone contacts that characterize successful chronic illness care (Wagner et al. 1996). The typical brief office visit is associated with lack of adequate time for patient education, activation, and support of behavior changes (exercise, problem-solving, and interpersonal behaviors) that are necessary elements in treating depression. Successful treatment programs for improving the care of chronic illness depend heavily on allied health professionals to conduct the routine assessments and provide most of the counseling and support for patient self-management, whereas most usual primary care practices rely totally on the physician for clinical interventions.

Lack of integration of specialty knowledge is another provider-level barrier to effective treatment of depression in general medical settings. Many primary care physicians have deficiencies in the skill set needed to diagnose and treat depressive illness (Von Korff et al. 2001). Limited decision support is inherent in the cultural and physical separation of primary and specialty care practice.

Organizational-Level Barriers

Many primary care practices lack the electronic technology necessary to identify and track patients with depression. For example, patients who start taking an antidepressant medication are often lost to follow-up. This is due, in part, to a lack of information systems designed to keep track of patients and provide reminders or prompts when follow-up contacts are overdue. Related to this barrier is the lack of agreement on a depression outcome measure by health care systems (Von Korff et al. 2001). Depression outcome measures are well established in research, but health care organizations have not reached a consensus on standardized ways to assess and monitor patient outcomes for depression over time.

Research Interventions to Improve Quality of Care and Outcomes of Depression

Most research on improving quality of care of the prevalent mental disorders has focused on patient-, provider-, and system-level barriers. Initial studies used screening for depression as a means of potentially improving recognition and treatment of mental disorders in primary care. In these studies, patients who screened positive for depression were randomized to usual care or to an intervention in which primary care physicians were provided with the results of depression screening scales. This research has shown that screening for depression alone increases the accuracy of diagnosis and, to a limited extent, improves the provision of guideline-level treatment but has little effect on patient outcomes (Katon and Gonzales 1994).

A second wave of studies focused on improving depression outcomes in primary care by providing enhanced

physician education about guidelines of care and/or specific algorithms for each patient. Five randomized, controlled trials tested interventions consisting of either continuous quality improvement methods targeting improvement of care for patients with depressive disorders or enhanced physician training about the diagnosis and treatment of depression through continuing medical education, academic detailing, and provision of guidelines or specific algorithms of care. None of these trials showed improvement in patient-level outcomes (Brown et al. 2000; Callahan et al. 1994; Goldberg et al. 1998; Rollman et al. 2001; Thompson et al. 2000).

Models that have been successful in improving depression outcomes address important barriers or limitations in the primary care system. These models that have improved patient-level outcomes have two main components: 1) improving organization of the care system so that patients receive enhanced education and proactive follow-up visits, and adherence, symptoms, and side effects are tracked; and 2) integrating specialty knowledge into the general medical setting (Katon 2003b).

Collaborative care interventions were developed to improve the quality of care and outcomes of depression. Collaborative care is a systematic approach that addresses barriers to effective treatment of depression at the patient, provider, and system levels (Von Korff et al. 1997). This model's approach includes 1) a negotiated definition of the clinical problem that both the patient and the physician understand (patient level); 2) joint development of a care plan with goals, targets, and implementation strategies (patient level); 3) support for self-management training and cognitive-behavioral change (provider level); and 4) integration of allied health professionals such as nurses or mental health specialists to provide active sustained follow-up via telephone calls, e-mail, and Web-based monitoring and decision support (system level). Collaborative care interventions that have been tested in randomized, controlled trials fall into three general categories: integration of mental health professionals, integration of care extenders such as nurses, and integration of a mental health team with nurses and master's-level therapists providing additional visits and support with close supervision by a psychiatrist and a primary care physician (Katon et al. 2003b).

A brief model that has been highly successful in improving outcomes of major depression is the collaborative care model that integrated mental health specialists into primary care. This model was initially tested in two large studies of primary care patients who were beginning treatment for depression after being recognized as depressed by their primary care physician (Katon et al. 1995, 1996). In the first collaborative care trial, the depressed patients were randomized to a multifaceted intervention group, in which a psychiatrist worked with the primary care physician, or to a usual care control group, in which the primary care physician provided depression care. In this study, the psychiatrist was integrated into the primary care setting and provided several visits to improve adherence to antidepressant medication, monitor outcomes and side effects, and enhance education and activation (Katon et al. 1995). In the second trial of collaborative care, patients were randomized to a usual care control group or to an intervention group. A psychologist provided enhanced education and activation, counseling to support adherence to pharmacological recommendations, and four to six sessions of cognitive-behavioral treatment to increase the patient's use of adaptive coping skills. The psychologists also reviewed the pharmacological management of their cases with weekly supervision by a psychiatrist and could suggest changes in medication to the primary care physician on the basis of the psychiatrists' recommendations (Katon et al. 1996). Both of these collaborative care interventions were associated with improved satisfaction with care and improved adherence to antidepressant medications. Both also improved depression outcomes, as determined by a 50% or greater reduction in depressive symptoms, from approximately 40% recovery in usual primary care patients to 75% recovery in intervention patients (Katon et al. 1995, 1996).

Collaborative care interventions are also associated with sustained improvement in depressive outcomes in patients with persistent depressive symptoms. Katon and colleagues (2002) recently examined the long-term effects of a stepped collaborative care intervention in a population of primary care patients with persistent depressive symptoms. Patients were recruited if they remained symptomatic 8 weeks after the primary care physician diagnosed major depression and initiated antidepressant treatment. Stepped care provides a framework for managing illness in which care is guided by the patient's response to treatment. The intensity of professional care is augmented for patients who do not achieve an acceptable outcome with lower levels of care (Von Korff 2000). The intervention was multifaceted; collaborative management by a psychiatrist and a primary care physician allowed patient, physician, and process of care to be targeted. The collaborative care intervention was associated with continued improvement in depressive symptoms and antidepressant adherence over a 28-month period. No significant differences in total 28-month ambulatory costs were found between the intervention and the control group.

Recent research also has focused on the use of allied health professionals, such as nurses, to enhance self-management (including treatment adherence) because mental health professionals are not available in many primary care practice settings. The initial interventions that tested the use of these allied health professionals often had limited incorporation of mental health specialty knowledge and specialty decision support on antidepressant medication. Randomized, controlled trials have tested either nursing or case management interventions to improve patient education and activation, monitor symptoms and side effects, attempt to improve antidepressant adherence or referral to psychotherapy, and to facilitate appointments with the primary care physician if the patient remains symptomatic (Hunkeler et al. 2000; Katzelnick et al. 2000; Peveler et al. 1999; Rost et al. 2001; Simon et al. 2000; Wells et al. 2000). These trials varied in the number of visits by the nurse or case manager from 2 visits (Peveler et al. 1999) to 10 visits (Hunkeler et al. 2000). The degree of specialty supervision also was variable; the Katzelnick et al. (2000) study provided the most reliable psychiatric supervision, ad hoc psychiatric consultation for patients who did not improve, and continued monitoring over a 1-year period built into the intervention. Five of these six studies reported significant improvement in depression outcomes for patients in the nurse or case management intervention groups when compared with their control subjects (Hunkeler et al. 2000; Katzelnick et al. 2000; Rost et al. 2001; Simon et al. 2000; Wells et al. 2000). Nurse-delivered interventions were found to improve depression outcomes in the studies that reported the percentage of patients improving 50% or more (Hunkeler et al. 2000; Simon et al. 2000).

A team treatment model for depression in primary care that integrates specialty knowledge with an organized system of care provided by nurses has been demonstrated recently by Unützer and colleagues (2002) in the Improving Mood-Promoting Access to Collaborative Treatment (IMPACT) collaborative care management program for late-life depression to improve depressive outcomes in elderly primary care patients. In this study, more than 1,800 depressed older adults (major depression, dysthymic disorder, or both) from 18 primary care clinics across the United States were enrolled in a randomized trial of a primary care–based collaborative care intervention program (IMPACT) compared with usual care. The IMPACT intervention includes key components of evidence-based models for chronic illness care:

- Collaboration among primary care practitioners, patients, and specialists on a common definition of the problem
- Development of a therapeutic alliance
- Creation of a personalized treatment plan based on patient preferences

- Proactive follow-up and outcomes monitoring by a depression care manager
- Targeted use of specialty consultation
- Use of protocols for stepped care

Intervention patients had access to an IMPACT care manager for up to 12 months. The depression care manager was supervised by a psychiatrist and a primary care expert and offered education, care management, and support of antidepressant management by the patient's primary care physician or brief psychotherapy for depression (problem-solving treatment in primary care).

The IMPACT collaborative care model was significantly more effective than usual care for depression in a wide range of primary care practices. At 12 months, 45% of the intervention patients had a 50% or greater reduction in depressive symptoms from baseline compared with 19% of the usual care group. Intervention patients had significantly more exposure to guideline-level depression treatment, greater satisfaction with depression care, lower depression severity, less functional impairment, and greater quality of life when compared with the control group. This model, with its significant benefits, appears feasible across a broad spectrum of patients and practices. Patient's median household income varied fivefold ($8,400–$40,000 per year), and the proportion of patients with a high school education varied threefold (32%–93%) throughout the eight diverse health care organizations in this national sample. The differences between intervention and usual care patients were equally consistent at the sites that had predominantly patients living below poverty level compared with sites with more middle-class populations (Unützer et al. 2002).

Conclusion

Major depression is as prevalent in primary care as hypertension. Patients with major depression present challenges because their affective symptoms are intertwined with social stressors, physical symptoms, and often chronic medical disorders and adverse health behaviors. Evidence-based models of care have been developed that can markedly improve outcomes of primary care patients with depression.

References

American Psychiatric Association: Diagnostic and Statistical Manual of Mental Disorders, 4th Edition. Washington, DC, American Psychiatric Association, 1994

American Psychiatric Association: Diagnostic and Statistical Manual of Mental Disorders, 4th Edition, Text Revision. Washington, DC, American Psychiatric Association, 2000

Anda RF, Williamson DF, Escobedo LG, et al: Depression and the dynamics of smoking: a national perspective. JAMA 264:1541–1545, 1990

Bair MJ, Robinson RL, Katon W, et al: Depression and pain comorbidity: a literature review. Arch Intern Med 163:2433–2445, 2003

Berndt ER, Koran LM, Finkelstein SN, et al: Lost human capital from early onset chronic depression. Am J Psychiatry 157:940–947, 2000

Blier P: Why treat depression differently from other medical problems? J Psychiatry Neurosci 27:231–232, 2002

Blumenthal JA, Williams RS, Wallace AG, et al: Physiological and psychological variables predict compliance to prescribed exercise therapy in patients recovering from myocardial infarction. Psychosom Med 44:519–527, 1982

Borson S, McDonald GJ, Gayle T, et al: Improvement in mood, physical symptoms, and function with nortriptyline for depression in patients with chronic obstructive pulmonary disease. Psychosomatics 33:190–201, 1992

Breitbart W: Identifying patients at risk for, and treatment of major psychiatric complication of cancer. Support Care Cancer 3:45–60, 1995

Bridges KW, Goldberg DP: Somatic presentation of DSM III psychiatric disorders in primary care. J Psychosom Res 29:563–569, 1985

Brown JB, Shye D, McFarland BH, et al: Controlled trials of CQI and academic detailing to implement a clinical practice guideline for depression. Jt Comm J Qual Improv 26:39–54, 2000

Bruce ML, Seeman TE, Merrill SS, et al: The impact of depressive symptomatology on physical disability: MacArthur Studies of Successful Aging. Am J Public Health 84:1796–1799, 1994

Callahan CM, Hendrie HC, Dittus RS, et al: Improving treatment of late life depression in primary care: a randomized clinical trial. J Am Geriatr Soc 42:839–846, 1994

Carnethon MR, Kinder LS, Fair JM, et al: Symptoms of depression as a risk factor for incident diabetes: findings from the National Health and Nutrition Examination Epidemiologic Follow-up Study, 1971–1992. Am J Epidemiol 158:416–423, 2003

Carney RM, Freedland KE, Eisen SA, et al: Major depression and medication adherence in elderly patients with coronary artery disease. Health Psychol 14:88–90, 1995

Chwastiak L, Ehde DM, Gibbons LE, et al: Depressive symptoms and severity of illness in multiple sclerosis: epidemiologic study of a large community sample. Am J Psychiatry 159:1862–1868, 2002

Ciechanowski PS, Katon WJ, Russo JE: Depression and diabetes: impact of depressive symptoms on adherence, function, and costs. Arch Intern Med 160:3278–3285, 2000

Ciechanowski PS, Katon WJ, Russo JE, et al: The relationship of depressive symptoms to symptom reporting, self-care and glucose control in diabetes. Gen Hosp Psychiatry 25:246–252, 2003

Ciesla JA, Roberts JE: Meta-analysis of the relationship between HIV infection and risk for depressive disorders. Am J Psychiatry 158:725–730, 2001

Cook JA, Cohen MH, Burke J, et al: Effects of depressive symptoms and mental health quality of life on use of highly active antiretroviral therapy among HIV-seropositive women. J Acquir Immune Defic Syndr 30:401–409, 2002

Cooper-Patrick L, Crum RM, Ford DE: Characteristics of patients with major depression who received care in general medical and specialty mental health settings. Med Care 32:15–24, 1994

Coyne JC, Schwenk TL, Fechner-Bates S: Nondetection of depression by primary care physicians reconsidered. Gen Hosp Psychiatry 17:3–12, 1995

de Groot M, Anderson R, Freedland KE, et al: Association of depression and diabetes complications: a meta-analysis. Psychosom Med 63:619–630, 2001

de Groot M, Auslander W, Williams JH, et al: Depression and poverty among African American women at risk for type 2 diabetes. Ann Behav Med 25:172–181, 2003

Dew MA, Dunn LO, Bromet EJ, et al: Factors affecting help-seeking during depression in a community sample. J Affect Disord 14:223–234, 1988

Dierker LC, Avenevoli S, Stolar M, et al: Smoking and depression: an examination of mechanisms of comorbidity. Am J Psychiatry 159:947–953, 2002

DiMatteo MR, Lepper HS, Croghan TW: Depression is a risk factor for noncompliance with medical treatment: meta-analysis of the effects of anxiety and depression on patient adherence. Arch Intern Med 160:2101–2107, 2000

Dwight MM, Kowdley KV, Russo JE, et al: Depression, fatigue, and functional disability in patients with chronic hepatitis C. J Psychosom Res 49:311–317, 2000

Dwight-Johnson M, Sherbourne CD, Liao D, et al: Treatment preferences among depressed primary care patients. Gen Intern Med 15:527–534, 2000

Elliott AJ, Russo J, Roy-Byrne PP: The effect of changes in depression on health related quality of life (HRQoL) in HIV infection. Gen Hosp Psychiatry 24:43–47, 2002

Felker B, Katon W, Hedrick SC, et al: The association between depressive symptoms and health status in patients with chronic pulmonary disease. Gen Hosp Psychiatry 23:56–61, 2001

Felker BL, Hedrick SC, Chaney EF, et al: Identifying depressed patients with a high risk of comorbid anxiety in primary care. Prim Care Companion J Clin Psychiatry 5:104–110, 2003

Gallagher RM, Verma S: Managing pain and comorbid depression: a public health challenge. Semin Clin Neuropsychiatry 4:203–220, 1999

Gallo JJ, Meredith LS, Gonzales J, et al: Do family physicians and internists differ in knowledge, attitudes, and self-reported approaches for depression? Int J Psychiatry Med 32:1–20, 2002

Glassman AH, Helzer JE, Covey LS, et al: Smoking, smoking cessation, and major depression. JAMA 264:1546–1549, 1990

Goldberg HI, Wagner EH, Fihn SD, et al: A randomized controlled trial of CQI teams and academic detailing: can they alter compliance with guidelines? Jt Comm J Qual Improv 24:130–142, 1998

Goodman E, Whitaker RC: A prospective study of the role of depression in the development and persistence of adolescent obesity. Pediatrics 110:497–504, 2002

Gureje O, Simon GE, Von Korff M, et al: A cross-national study of the course of persistent pain in primary care. Pain 92:195–200, 2001

Hunkeler EM, Meresman JF, Hargreaves WA, et al: Efficacy of nurse telehealth care and peer support in augmenting treatment of depression in primary care. Arch Fam Med 9:700–708, 2000

Kanner AM: Depression in epilepsy: prevalence, clinical semiology, pathogenic mechanisms, and treatment. Biol Psychiatry 54:388–398, 2003

Katon WJ: Clinical and health services relationships between major depression, depressive symptoms, and general medical illness. Biol Psychiatry 54:216–226, 2003a

Katon WJ: The Institute of Medicine "Chasm" report: implications for depression collaborative care models. Gen Hosp Psychiatry 25:222–229, 2003b

Katon W, Gonzales J: A review of randomized trials of psychiatric consultation-liaison studies in primary care. Psychosomatics 35:268–278, 1994

Katon WJ, Buchwald DS, Simon GE, et al: Psychiatric illness in patients with chronic fatigue and those with rheumatoid arthritis. J Gen Intern Med 6:277–285, 1991

Katon W, Sullivan M, Russo J, et al: Depressive symptoms and measures of disability: a prospective study. J Affect Disord 27:245–254, 1993

Katon W, Von Korff M, Lin E, et al: Collaborative management to achieve treatment guidelines: impact on depression in primary care. JAMA 273:1026–1031, 1995

Katon W, Robinson P, Von Korff M, et al: A multifaceted intervention to improve treatment of depression in primary care. Arch Gen Psychiatry 53:924–932, 1996

Katon W, Sullivan M, Walker E: Medical symptoms without identified pathology: relationship to psychiatric disorders, childhood and adult trauma, and personality traits. Ann Intern Med 134:917–925, 2001a

Katon W, Von Korff M, Lin E, et al: Rethinking practitioner roles in chronic illness: the specialist, primary care physician, and the practice nurse. Gen Hosp Psychiatry 23:138–144, 2001b

Katon W, Russo J, Von Korff M, et al: Long-term effects of a collaborative care intervention in persistently depressed primary care patients. J Gen Intern Med 17:741–748, 2002

Katon WJ, Lin E, Russo J, et al: Increased medical costs of a population-based sample of depressed elderly patients. Arch Gen Psychiatry 60:897–903, 2003a

Katon W, Von Korff M, Lin E, et al: Improving primary care treatment of depression among patients with diabetes mellitus: the design of the pathways study. Gen Hosp Psychiatry 25:158–168, 2003b

Katz AR: On the inseparability of mental and physical health in aged persons. Am J Geriatr Psychiatry 4:1–16, 1996

Katzelnick DJ, Simon GE, Pearson SD, et al: Randomized trial of a depression management program in high utilizers of medical care. Arch Fam Med 9:345–351, 2000

Kessler RC, McGonagle KA, Zhao S, et al: Lifetime and 12-month prevalence of DSM-III-R psychiatric disorders in the United States: results from the National Comorbidity Survey. Arch Gen Psychiatry 51:8–19, 1994

Kessler R, Berglund P, Demler O, et al: The epidemiology of major depressive disorder: results from the National Comorbidity Survey Replication (NCS-R). JAMA 289:3095–3105, 2003

Kirmayer LJ, Robbins JM, Dworkind M, et al: Somatization and the recognition of depression and anxiety in primary care. Am J Psychiatry 150:734–741, 1993

Klinkman MS: Competing demands in psychosocial care: a model for the identification and treatment of depressive disorders in primary care. Gen Hosp Psychiatry 19:98–111, 1997

Klinkman MS, Schwenk TL, Coyne JC: Depression in primary care—more like asthma than appendicitis: the Michigan Depression Project. Can J Psychiatry 42:966–973, 1997

Kroenke K, Jackson JL, Chamberlin J: Depressive and anxiety disorders in patients presenting with physical complaints: clinical predictors and outcome. Am J Med 3:339–347, 1997

Lin EH, Katon WJ, VonKorff M, et al: Relapse of depression in primary care: rate and clinical predictors. Arch Fam Med 7:443–449, 1998

Lin EH, VonKorff M, Russo J, et al: Can depression treatment in primary care reduce disability? A stepped care approach. Arch Fam Med 9:1052–1058, 2000

Lindsay PG, Wyckoff M: The depression-pain syndrome and its response to antidepressants. Psychosomatics 22:571–573, 576–577, 1981

Mauksch LB, Tucker SM, Katon WJ, et al: Mental illness, functional impairment, and patient preferences for collaborative care in an uninsured, primary care population. J Fam Pract 50:41–47, 2001

Mayou RA, Gill D, Thompson DR, et al: Depression and anxiety as predictors of outcome after myocardial infarction. Psychosom Med 62:212–219, 2000

McDonald WM, Richard IH, DeLong MR: Prevalence, etiology, and treatment of depression in Parkinson's disease. Biol Psychiatry 54:363–375, 2003

Merikangas KR, Zhang H, Avenevoli S, et al: Longitudinal trajectories of depression and anxiety in a prospective community study: the Zurich Cohort Study. Arch Gen Psychiatry 60:993–1000, 2003

Miranda J, Schoenbaum M, Sherbourne C, et al: Effects of primary care depression treatment on minority patients' clinical status and employment. Arch Gen Psychiatry 61:827–834, 2004

Nutting PA, Rost K, Dickinson M, et al: Barriers to initiating depression treatment in primary care practice. J Gen Intern Med 17:103–111, 2002

Olfson M, Shea S, Feder A, et al: Prevalence of anxiety, depression, and substance use disorders in an urban general medical practice. Arch Fam Med 9:876–883, 2000

Olfson M, Marcus SC, Druss B, et al: National trends in the outpatient treatment of depression. JAMA 287:203–209, 2002a

Olfson M, Marcus SC, Druss B, et al: National trends in the use of outpatient psychotherapy. Am J Psychiatry 159:1914–1920, 2002b

Orleans CT, George LK, Houpt JL, et al: How primary care physicians treat psychiatric disorders: a national survey of family practitioners. Am J Psychiatry 142:52–57, 1985

Ormel J, Von Korff M, Van den Brink W, et al: Depression, anxiety, and social disability show synchrony of change in primary care patients. Am J Public Health 83:385–390, 1993

Patten SB: Long-term medical conditions and major depression in a Canadian population study at waves 1 and 2. J Affect Disord 63(1–3):35–41, 2001

Patton GC, Carlin JB, Coffey C, et al: Depression, anxiety, and smoking initiation: a prospective study over 3 years. Am J Public Health 88:1518–1522, 1998

Peveler R, George C, Kinmonth AL, et al: Effect of antidepressant drug counselling and information leaflets on adherence to drug treatment in primary care: randomised controlled trial. BMJ 319:612–615, 1999

Prince MJ, Harwood RH, Thomas A, et al: A prospective population-based cohort study of the effects of disablement and social milieu on the onset and maintenance of late-life depression. The Gospel Oak Project VII. Psychol Med 28:337–350, 1998

Regier DA, Narrow WE, Rae DS, et al: The de facto US mental and addictive disorders service system: Epidemiologic Catchment Area prospective 1-year prevalence rates of disorders and services. Arch Gen Psychiatry 50:85–94, 1993

Richardson LP, Davis R, Poulton R, et al: A longitudinal evaluation of adolescent depression and adult obesity. Arch Pediatr Adolesc Med 157:739–745, 2003

Riera M, La Fuente Ld L, Castanyer B, et al: [Adherence to antiretroviral therapy measured by pill count and drug serum concentrations: variables associated with a bad adherence] (Spanish). Med Clin (Barc) 119:286–292, 2002

Roeloffs C, Sherbourne C, Unützer J, et al: Stigma and depression among primary care patients. Gen Hosp Psychiatry 25:311–315, 2003

Rollman BL, Hanusa BH, Gilbert T, et al: The electronic medical record: a randomized trial of its impact on primary care physicians' initial management of major depression. Arch Intern Med 161:189–197, 2001 [published erratum appears in 161:705, 2001]

Rosal MC, Ockene JK, Ma Y, et al: Behavioral risk factors among members of a health maintenance organization. Prev Med 33:586–594, 2001

Rost K, Nutting P, Smith J, et al: The role of competing demands in the treatment provided primary care patients with major depression. Arch Fam Med 9:150–154, 2000

Rost K, Nutting P, Smith J, et al: Improving depression outcomes in community primary care practice: a randomized trial of the quEST intervention. Quality Enhancement by Strategic Teaming. J Gen Intern Med 16:143–149, 2001

Rugulies R: Depression as a predictor for coronary heart disease: a review and meta-analysis. Am J Prev Med 23:51–61, 2002

Sambamoorthi U, Walkup J, Olfson M, et al: Antidepressant treatment and health services utilization among HIV-infected Medicaid patients diagnosed with depression. J Gen Intern Med 15:311–320, 2000

Sargeant JK, Bruce ML, Florio LP, et al: Factors associated with 1-year outcome of major depression in the community. Arch Gen Psychiatry 47:519–526, 1990

Schoenbaum M, Unützer J, Sherbourne C, et al: Cost-effectiveness of practice-initiated quality improvement for depression: results of a randomized controlled trial. JAMA 286:1325–1330, 2001

Schulberg HC, Block MR, Madonia MJ, et al: Treating major depression in primary care practice: eight-month clinical outcomes. Arch Gen Psychiatry 53:913–919, 1996

Schulberg HC, Block MR, Madonia MJ, et al: The "usual care" of major depression in primary care practice. Arch Fam Med 6:334–339, 1997

Schulberg HC, Katon W, Simon GE, et al: Treating major depression in primary care practice: an update of the Agency for Health Care Policy and Research Practice Guidelines. Arch Gen Psychiatry 55:1121–1127, 1998

Schwenk TL, Klinkman MS, Coyne JC: Depression in the family physician's office: what the psychiatrist needs to know: the Michigan Depression Project. J Clin Psychiatry 59 (suppl 20):94–100, 1998

Sherbourne CD, Dwight-Johnson M, Klap R: Psychological distress, unmet need, and barriers to mental health care for women. Womens Health Issues 11:231–243, 2001

Simon GE: Evidence review: efficacy and effectiveness of antidepressant treatment in primary care. Gen Hosp Psychiatry 24:213–224, 2002

Simon GE: Social and economic burden of mood disorders. Biol Psychiatry 54:208–215, 2003

Simon GE, VonKorff M, Barlow W: Health care costs of primary care patients with recognized depression. Arch Gen Psychiatry 52:850–856, 1995

Simon GE, VonKorff M, Rutter C, et al: Randomised trial of monitoring, feedback, and management of care by telephone to improve treatment of depression in primary care. BMJ 320:550–554, 2000

Spire B, Duran S, Souville M, et al: Adherence to highly active antiretroviral therapies (HAART) in HIV-infected patients: from a predictive to a dynamic approach. Soc Sci Med 54:1481–1496, 2002

Spitzer RL, Kroenke K, Williams JB: Validation and utility of a self-report version of PRIME-MD: the PHQ Primary Care Study. Primary Care Evaluation of Mental Disorders. Patient Health Questionnaire. JAMA 282:1737–1744, 1999

Sullivan M, Katon W, Russo J, et al: A randomized trial of nortriptyline for severe chronic tinnitus: effects on depression, disability, and tinnitus symptoms. Arch Intern Med 153:2251–2259, 1993

Sullivan MD, LaCroix AZ, Baum C, et al: Functional status in coronary artery disease: a one-year prospective study of the role of anxiety and depression. Am J Med 103:348–356, 1997

Sullivan M, Simon G, Spertus J, et al: Depression-related costs in heart failure care. Arch Intern Med 162:1860–1866, 2002

Sullivan MD, LaCroix AZ, Spertus JA, et al: Five-year prospective study of the effects of anxiety and depression in patients with coronary artery disease. Am J Cardiol 86:1135–1138, A6, A9, 2000

Thompson C, Kinmonth AL, Stevens L, et al: Effects of a clinical-practice guideline and practice-based education on detection and outcome of depression in primary care: Hampshire Depression Project randomised controlled trial. Lancet 355:185–191, 2000

Unützer J, Patrick DL, Simon G, et al: Depressive symptoms and the cost of health services in HMO patients aged 65 years and older: a 4-year prospective study. JAMA 277:1618–1623, 1997

Unützer J, Patrick DL, Marmon T, et al: Quality adjusted life years in older adults with depressive symptoms and chronic medical disorders. Int Psychogeriatr 12:15–33, 2000

Unützer J, Katon W, Williams JW Jr, et al: Improving primary care for depression in late life: the design of a multicenter randomized trial. Med Care 39:785–799, 2001

Unützer J, Katon W, Callahan CM, et al: Collaborative care management of late-life depression in the primary care setting: a randomized controlled trial. JAMA 288:2836–2845, 2002

U.S. Department of Health and Human Services, Public Health Service, Agency for Health care Policy and Research: Depression in primary care: detection, diagnosis, and treatment. J Psychosoc Nurs Ment Health Serv 31:19–28, 1993

Von Korff M: Individualized stepped care of chronic illness. Culture and Medicine 172:133–137, 2000

Von Korff M, Ormel J, Katon W, et al: Disability and depression among high utilizers of health care: a longitudinal analysis. Arch Gen Psychiatry 49:91–100, 1992

Von Korff M, Gruman J, Schaefer J, et al: Collaborative management of chronic illness. Ann Intern Med 127:1097–1102, 1997

Von Korff M, Katon W, Unützer J, et al: Improving depression care: barriers, solutions, and research needs. J Fam Pract 50:E1, 2001

Wagner EH, Austin BT, Von Korff M: Organizing care for patients with chronic illness. Milbank Q 74:511–544, 1996

Walker EA, Gelfand MD, Gelfand AN, et al: The relationship of current psychiatric disorder to functional disability and distress in patients with inflammatory bowel disease. Gen Hosp Psychiatry 18:220–229, 1996

Walker EA, Katon WJ, Keegan D, et al: Predictors of physician frustration in the care of patients with rheumatological complaints. Gen Hosp Psychiatry 19:315–323, 1997

Walker EA, Katon WJ, Russo J, et al: Predictors of outcome in a primary care depression trial. J Gen Intern Med 15:859–867, 2000

Wang L, van Belle G, Kukull WB, et al: Predictors of functional change: a longitudinal study of nondemented people aged 65 and older. J Am Geriatr Soc 50:1525–1534, 2002

Weich S, Churchill R, Lewis G, et al: Do socio-economic risk factors predict the incidence and maintenance of psychiatric disorder in primary care? Psychol Med 27:73–80, 1997

Wells KB, Stewart A, Hays RD, et al: The functioning and well-being of depressed patients: results from the Medical Outcomes Study. JAMA 262:914–919, 1989

Wells KB, Katon W, Rogers B, et al: Use of minor tranquilizers and antidepressant medications by depressed outpatients: results from the Medical Outcomes Study. Am J Psychiatry 151:694–700, 1994

Wells KB, Sherbourne C, Schoenbaum M, et al: Impact of disseminating quality improvement programs for depression in managed primary care: a randomized controlled trial. JAMA 283:212–220, 2000

Whooley MA, Kiefe CI, Chesney MA, et al: Depressive symptoms, unemployment, and loss of income: the CARDIA Study. Arch Intern Med 162:2614–2620, 2002

Whyte EM, Mulsant BH: Post stroke depression: epidemiology, pathophysiology, and biological treatment. Biol Psychiatry 52:253–264, 2002

Young AS, Klap R, Sherbourne CD, et al: The quality of care for depressive and anxiety disorders in the United States. Arch Gen Psychiatry 58:55–61, 2001

38

Depression in Medical Illness (Secondary Depression)

ROBERT BOLAND, M.D.

MANY WELL-WRITTEN REVIEWS on depression in medical illness already exist. Most emphasize several points: 1) that depression is more common in medical patients than in the non–medically ill population, 2) that the depression is frequently missed or misattributed to a "normal reaction to illness," 3) that depression is more difficult to treat in this population, but 4) that standard treatments still do help, and 5) that untreated depression will worsen the morbidity and mortality of the medical disease.

Although all these points are likely true, it should not surprise the reader that many of these statements are based more on clinical expertise than on any evidence-based approach. Studies of depression in medical populations—particularly studies with good methodological rigor and large enough sample sizes—are notoriously difficult to do. The populations studied are fragile and often difficult to recruit and retain. Furthermore, the lack of a true gold standard for diagnosing depression in any population renders any statement of prevalence suspect from the start. This difficulty is further reinforced by the wide range of reported prevalence. The standard figures cited are that 5%–10% of primary care patients and 10%–14% of medical inpatients have major depression (Katon and Schulberg 1991; U.S. Department of Health and Human Services 1993). However, figures cited in different studies can vary widely—from 1% to more than 50% of various populations studied—suggesting that these percentiles are more dependent on the methodology of the studies than anything else.

The same criticism can be leveled at many of the other statements listed earlier. However, despite concerns about methodology and study quality, many great minds have devoted themselves to the problem of depression in medical illness and much interesting work has been done. In this chapter, I acknowledge the many limitations of what we know, and question some current wisdom, but the reader should not leave this review with a nihilistic conclusion that nothing is known. I hope the reaction will instead be excitement about the many things we have learned, the developing picture in the field, and the challenges ahead.

This chapter begins with some nosological and diagnostic dilemmas that occur when one considers depression in the setting of medical illness (also called *secondary depression*) as separate from other forms of depression. A discussion of depression in the setting of some specific illnesses follows. I then review data on treatment in various populations and conclude with a consideration of ripe areas for future investigation.

Nosological Dilemmas

The choice to make depressive syndromes that are secondary to a medical disorder distinct from other depressive disorders has its roots in the original distinctions between exogenous and endogenous depression. This distinction can be seen in the first DSM (American Psychiatric Association 1952), which classified all mood disorders as either "organic" or "reactive." The "psychotic/neurotic" distinction in DSM-II (American Psychiatric Association 1968) continued this split. The term *psychotic* as used in DSM-II was defined more broadly than it is now, with a meaning approximately analogous to the term *organic*.

This distinction also dictated treatment, with somatic treatment deemed more appropriate for the psychotic disorders (which would include psychotic depression and bipolar disorder) and all other types of depression held to be more readily treated through psychotherapy.

DSM-III (American Psychiatric Association 1980) caused a major change in this approach to mood disorders. Although the immediate predecessor of DSM-III, the Research Diagnostic Criteria (RDC) (Spitzer et al. 1978), maintained an endogenous/exogenous distinction for mood disorders, this distinction was eliminated by the overall move to the categorical criteria of DSM-III with no causal relationship implied. As a result, the mood disorders were divided on a phenomenological basis into major depressive disorder, bipolar disorder, and the minor mood disorders. However, several subtypes were maintained by DSM-III and continue through the current DSM-IV-TR (American Psychiatric Association 2000). These include the idea of melancholia. DSM-defined melancholia is essentially similar to the original RDC for endogenous depression, but it is now treated as a subtype of major depression, although one that is severe and particularly responsive to somatic treatment. Also broken off from the diagnosis of depression are the diagnoses of adjustment disorder and depression due to a medical condition (or secondary depression). Both can be thought of as the extreme limits of the exogenous/endogenous distinction of mood disorders. Adjustment disorders represent those disturbances of mood that appear purely reactive to an environmental stress, and secondary depression is reserved for those depressions that are of clear biological cause.

One can see the philosophical problems that arise from making such distinctions. Because major depressive disorder no longer carries any etiological distinction, determining where the border should be between adjustment disorder, secondary depression, and major depression is difficult. Similarly, because major depression is presumed to be a biological illness, it is not immediately obvious how it should differ from a depressive syndrome that has a clear biological cause.

Understanding the distinctions between adjustment disorder and major depression is particularly challenging in the medical setting. In theory, if one has a depressive syndrome that is directly caused by a medical disorder, that is secondary depression. However, if one has a depressive syndrome caused by a reaction to the fact of having a medical disorder, that would be adjustment disorder. An additional possibility is that the stress of having a severe medical disorder could cause a "normal" reaction or distress that would not be considered a mental disorder at all. Furthermore, the stress of having a severe medical illness can be significant enough to cause or exacerbate a major depressive disorder. When we try to incorporate all these facts, the nosological dilemmas become overwhelming. DSM-IV-TR guides us by presenting a hierarchy of disease, with major depression superseding an adjustment disorder diagnosis, the presumption being that adjustment disorder is then reserved for those depressive syndromes that are not severe enough to be major depression. However, this does not seem a satisfying distinction. In theory, the diagnosis of adjustment disorder seems to have utility, defining a situation in which the symptoms presented represent an adaptation to a specific stress. However, in practice, without clear diagnosis to guide us through the above dilemmas, adjustment disorder is often used as a "wastebasket diagnosis" (Casey et al. 2001).

Secondary mood disorders present a similar dilemma because the diagnosis implies a particular etiology, making the diagnosis difficult to define within the limits of categorical criteria. Without any biological marker for depression, we must infer causality on the basis of primarily temporal association and a clinical belief about the likelihood of a certain disease causing depression. Because major depression is currently defined in such broad terms—encompassing both agitation and retardation, hyper- and hyporeactivity, and too much and too little emotion—determining a symptom or cluster of symptoms that might suggest secondary depression is difficult. Similarly, many medical disorders can cause symptoms that might overlap with depression, including fatigue, disturbance of sleep and appetite, apathy, and even emotionality (Kim and Choi-Kwon 2000). All of these symptoms can be independent of any depressive disorder, and defining what symptoms or cluster of symptoms can be explained only by comorbid depression can be difficult. Clark and colleagues (1998) suggested that depression in medical patients was best distinguished by the presence of anhedonia, low positive affect, and high physiological arousal. Others have argued for a variety of other cognitive symptoms, such as crying, guilt, suicidal ideation, a sense of failure, or feeling a burden, but these criteria may identify only the most severely depressed (Parker and Kalucy 1999).

Diagnostic Issues

It is frequently reported that depression is underdiagnosed in the medical setting, and it has been estimated that as many as a half of all depressed medical patients are not recognized as such by their primary care physician (Gerber et al. 1989; Lipowski 1992; Perez-Stable et al. 1990). There are various reasons for this, including inadequate training in recognizing depressive symptoms and the fear of jeopardizing reimbursement once a psychiatric diagnosis is made (Rost et al. 1994). Primary care physicians also may misdiagnose these disorders, mistakenly attributing the symptoms of other psychiatric and medical disorders (such as delirium, dementia, and anxiety disorders) to depression (Boland et al. 1996).

The nosological dilemmas discussed in the preceding section are likely a major reason for the underdiagnosis and misdiagnosis of depression in the medical patient. The main issue revolves around how to handle symptoms that can be attributed to either the depression or the primary medical disorder. One can imagine different approaches: an inclusive approach assumes that all depressive symptoms should count toward a depressive diagnosis, regardless of whether alternative explanations for the symptoms exist. Conversely, an exclusive approach would ignore any symptoms that might be otherwise explained. A variant of the exclusive approach, an etiological approach, ignores items if they are thought to be more likely a result of the comorbid medical illness. Finally, a substitutive approach replaces those items that are most likely to be confounded from the diagnostic workup with other symptoms considered less controversial.

Each approach has clear strengths and weaknesses. An inclusive approach will capture the most cases of depression, but at a risk of overinclusion. Note, however, that the current DSM-IV-TR criteria for major depression are conservative, so the risk of overdiagnosis is not as high as it might first seem. The opposite arguments can be made about the exclusive approach, and one can find no a priori reason to assume that potentially overlapping symptoms are not due to depression rather than the primary medical disorder. Although an etiological approach seems to answer this issue, no guidance exists for attributing the overlapping symptoms to one disorder or another, inviting likely bias. The substitutive approach seems a reasonable resolution to this dilemma; however, as in the discussion in the preceding section, no consensus exists about what the substituting symptoms should be.

Attempts to test these different approaches have been mixed. Koenig and colleagues (1997), for example, suggested that a combination of the exclusive and etiological approaches was most sensitive in identifying the most severe cases, but no one approach was clearly superior to another in identifying all cases.

In the research setting, various scales also have been used in an attempt at a standardized approach to diagnosing depression in the medically ill. For example, the Hospital Anxiety and Depression Scale (Zigmond and Snaith 1983) is commonly used, particularly in Europe, but few reports exist of the scale's sensitivity and specificity. Others have tried to identify subsets of questions from common scales that might be adequate for identifying depression in the medically ill. Without a gold standard instrument to serve for comparison, one cannot know what to make of the various reports describing how scales can be whittled down to a few questions. At the extreme is Chochinov and colleagues' (1997) experience diagnosing depression in patients with advanced cancer: the investigators administered the full Schedule for Affective Disorders and Schizophrenia (a semistructured interview based on RDC for depression) (Endicott and Spitzer 1978) and found that it was no better than simply asking the patients whether they were depressed.

With no clear gold standard to guide us, what should the clinician look for when assessing possible secondary depression? Researchers and clinicians alike usually rely on several criteria:

1. *Temporal association*—A depression that begins after, but proximate to, the medical disorder is more suspicious than one that might have preceded the medical illness or occurred much later. This association is more useful if data exist regarding a temporal pattern of occurrence following the onset of an illness.
2. *Atypical symptoms*—If the symptoms of the secondary depression are somehow different from what might be expected for idiopathic depression, this might suggest a unique cause.
3. *Neurophysiological evidence*—The finding of an association between a certain pathological lesion and the onset of depression would be the most convincing evidence. Such research is hampered by the fact that the neurophysiological basis of idiopathic depression is not sufficiently understood, but even associative data would be persuasive.

These criteria, when relevant, are explored in the following section, in which I consider some examples of research on depression in specific disorders. These do not by any means make up a comprehensive list of disorders for which such research exists, but they are good examples of disorders in which researchers have looked for some or all of the above criteria.

Specific Disorders

Neurological Disorders

Poststroke Depression

Investigations into depression following a cerebrovascular accident (CVA), or "poststroke depression," have provided consistent and interesting data about depression in medical illness. It has long been reported that depression is common after a CVA and that this depression produces a level of disability that is much greater than would be expected when compared with other illnesses causing similar disability (Folstein et al. 1977). In addition, poststroke depression is associated with cognitive impairments (both verbal and nonverbal) (Robinson 2003) and increased mortality (Morris et al. 1993).

Among different studies, the prevalence of poststroke depression is highly variable and largely dependent on the methodology of the particular study and the population selected for study. Whyte and Mulsant (2002) reviewed various poststroke depression studies and found that the reported prevalence varied from 6% to 34%, depending on the site and the length of time being investigated. Robinson (2003) pooled data from all available studies on the prevalence of poststroke depression and estimated a prevalence of approximately 19% in hospitalized patients and 23% in outpatients.

The course observed for poststroke depression seems dependent on the study as well. The average duration has been reported at just under a year, with a peak incidence between 3 and 6 months post CVA (Depression Guideline Panel 1993). It has been reported that spontaneous remission of the depression usually occurs within 1–2 years, but poststroke depression of 3 years or more has been reported (Robinson et al. 1987).

The literature on poststroke depression is of particular interest to the study of depression and medical illness. Because CVAs produce relatively discrete lesions that have a clear time of onset and that can be visualized with neuroimaging, researchers have attempted to correlate lesion sites with the onset of depression. As a result, research into the potentially direct effects of a biological injury on depression is more advanced in this area than for most other medical or neurological illnesses. Robinson and colleagues (1984) reported associations between poststroke depression and left anterior and left basal ganglia lesions and lesions close to the frontal pole. Although this information remains correlative and cannot be proof positive of a direct neurological effect on mood, this finding remains one of the more influential arguments for a direct causal relation between any medical illness and de-

pression. It is potentially even more exciting that the depression reported in these disorders is very similar to that reported for idiopathic major depression. Given this, the lesion data may be used for understanding the mechanism of depression overall.

However, caution is warranted for several reasons. First, the fact that the depression reported in poststroke depression is like that seen in idiopathic major depression, although potentially exciting, also can be construed as evidence against a unique secondary disorder. Second, the finding of lesion involvement has not been universally replicated, and a meta-analysis of studies on the subject concluded that no significant relation existed between lesion location and depression (Carson et al. 2000). This meta-analysis, however, may not have been selective enough in its study choice and may not have properly taken into account the role of variables such as personal and family history (Whyte and Mulsant 2002). A subsequent meta-analysis by Robinson (2003) did find an association between depression and lesion location (left frontal and left basal ganglia) during the first 2 months after a stroke.

Even if there is a direct relation between lesion location and depression, the sizes of the reported associations are relatively small. Evidence also exists for the importance of psychosocial factors, such as correlations between the severity of the functional disability (regardless of lesion location) and depressive symptoms (Murphy 1982). Thus, although the data available are potentially exciting, considering poststroke depression as an example of a mood disorder that is directly caused by a medical condition is still likely premature. It is possible, even likely, that some cases are examples of direct causation. However, overall, a multifactorial biopsychosocial explanation for depressive symptoms associated with CVAs—including, but not limited to, direct biological mechanisms—seems most consistent with the literature.

Parkinson's Disease

Depression is thought to be common in Parkinson's disease, and prevalence figures as high as 40% have been reported in some reviews (Cummings 1992). These high figures do not hold up to scrutiny, and studies that used structured criteria have reported lower percentages, sometimes no more than nonneurological control groups (Hantz et al. 1994). Depression can be particularly difficult to diagnose in the setting of Parkinson's disease because the symptoms of major depression and Parkinson's overlap: psychomotor retardation, apathy, and a blunted affect can be interpreted as symptoms of either disorder. Thus, depression can be over- or underdiagnosed in this population, depending on how this overlap is handled.

In cases in which depression does occur, it can be extremely debilitating and may account for more of the disability than do the physical symptoms of Parkinson's disease (Schrag et al. 2000). Some literature also suggests that depression associated with Parkinson's disease presents differently from idiopathic depression (Cummings 1992). Specifically, patients with Parkinson's disease may show fewer of the cognitive symptoms of depression, such as self-denigration, and more comorbidity with anxiety (Menza et al. 1993).

The relation between depression and Parkinson's disease, as with all the disorders discussed in this chapter, is complex as one imagines both reactive and direct causes of depression. Certainly, coping with this debilitating disorder can be seen as a major stress. Similarly, the neuropathology of Parkinson's disease, involving degeneration of neurochemicals and brain areas thought to be involved in depression, makes a plausible case for direct mechanisms. In fact, evidence for direct physiological causes of depression is somewhat more developed in Parkinson's disease than in other disorders. Perhaps most compelling are data that correlate the level of depression with postmortem and imaging studies of disease process (McDonald et al. 2003).

Multiple Sclerosis

The risk of depression appears to be high in multiple sclerosis as well, although as with Parkinson's disease, the overlapping of neurological symptoms makes this risk difficult to detect. Clinically, the demyelination process of multiple sclerosis can be associated with various changes in affect independent of depression, such as pathological laughing or crying; these are assumed to be related to pathology in the frontal lobes.

One study that relied on a self-report survey found that about 40% of the subjects with multiple sclerosis had clinically significant depressive symptoms and that about one-third likely had moderate to severe depression (Chwastiak et al. 2002). This rate seemed to correlate with the severity of disease and with the rapidity of progression of the multiple sclerosis. Although it has been suspected that multiple sclerosis patients with depression would be higher users of health care services, such an association was not found in at least one Canadian study (Patten et al. 2002).

Magnetic resonance imaging (MRI) studies have suggested an association between lesions in the left frontal lobe and depression, a compelling finding given the similar finding in stroke studies. These MRI findings, however, have not been consistent across studies (Berg et al. 2000); other groups, for example, found an association between depression and changes in the right temporal lobe. Some pathological evidence does associate depression with the inflammatory process of multiple sclerosis. For example, one small study found an association between depression and the production of proinflammatory cytokine interferon-γ by autoaggressive T cells in relapsing-remitting multiple sclerosis (Mohr et al. 2001). Although these data are interesting, one should not overvalue the psychobiological contributors because additional studies show the relation between life stress, coping, and depression in patients with multiple sclerosis. Depression can reciprocally affect multiple sclerosis as well in treatment adherence, on performance in cognitive tests that are specific for multiple sclerosis, and in a patient's overall perception of his or her disability (Fruehwald et al. 2001).

Epilepsy

Depression is the most common comorbid psychiatric disorder in patients with epilepsy. Different types of depression may occur, including very brief episodes that occur during a seizure ("ictal depression"); postictal depression, which usually lasts approximately 1 day following a seizure (Kanner 2003); and the more common and more typical interictal episodes of depression. As with many of the other disorders discussed, the estimated prevalence has a wide range: from 6% to 30%. Study results have differed regarding whether the risk for epilepsy is different from that for other neurological disorders. Of great concern, however, are the reports of high rates of suicide in epileptic patients (Gilliam and Kanner 2002). Also of interest is the observation that, at least in one population-based study, episodes of depression occurred proximate to exacerbations of epilepsy (Kanner 2003), suggesting a bidirectional relation between epilepsy and depression. Because norepinephrine and serotonin are implicated in the pathogenesis of both depression and epilepsy, a direct relation between the two is suggested. Although some animal studies support this suggestion, clinical evidence of any direct mechanism is indirect and based on some indication of decreased seizure frequency in patients taking antidepressants (Kanner 2003).

Cancer

It is suggested that up to one-quarter of patients with cancer will develop depression (Croyle and Rowland 2003). The literature on cancer and depression is particularly difficult to summarize because cancer represents a group of diseases, often with different courses and affecting different populations. Taken as a whole, the prevalence of depression varies greatly. When a clinical diagnosis is used, the rate of depression has been reported to vary from 6% to more than 40% (van Heeringen and Zivkov 1996). More rigorous studies that used structured diagnostic interviews reported rates of approximately 5%–10%, much closer to the rate of depression in the general population (Kathol et al. 1990). Certain types of cancers may have higher incidences, although reported ranges vary widely. For example, the prevalence of depression in breast cancer has been reported to be as low as 10% and as high as almost one-third of breast cancer patients (McDaniel et al. 1995). Although one might assume that the distress of being diagnosed with cancer would be sufficient to cause depression in any individual, some groups have proved surprisingly resilient (Moynihan et al. 1998). Thus, as with most medical disorders, one should not assume that depression will be a normal reaction to the disease. Unfortunately, that assumption is often made, and both patients and physicians have a tendency to ignore and neglect depressive symptoms in cancer patients (Croyle and Rowland 2003). This is further complicated by the fact that, even in the most enlightened of circumstances, major depression can be difficult to distinguish from cancer-related symptoms, given the overlap of the two. Both cancer and its treatment can directly cause fatigue, anorexia, weight loss, sleep disturbance, attentional problems, decreased libido, and poor motivation (Raison and Miller 2003). So overlapping are the symptoms that Raison and Miller (2003) suggested a reconceptualization of certain cancer-related behaviors under the designation of "sickness behavior," thus avoiding a preoccupation with questionable distinctions. This behavioral syndrome can encompass "typical" depressive symptoms or be more associated with neurovegetative symptoms such as fatigue and anorexia.

When depression does occur, be it major depression or depressive symptoms, it is usually assumed to be a reaction to the diagnosis, but there can be other causal mechanisms as well. For example, certain cancer treatments, such as the cytokine therapies (e.g., interferon and interleukin) can cause depression, presumably through an inflammatory mechanism (Raison and Miller 2003).

Perhaps the most interesting areas of research on depression and cancer are those that look in the reverse direction: the possibility that depression may have a role in the cause or course of cancer. Studies of depression examine only a subset of the larger relation between stress and cancer, but depression studies have been important in this area because they represent a clear example of a stressed (or distressed) population. Cancer is a potential paradigm for researchers to investigate the effect of stress and depression on the immune system and overall cellular functioning. For cancer cells to accumulate in an individual, several failures in the usual immune and other protective functions of the body must occur. Research exists that bears on a variety of different stages in the propagation of cancer cells. Most of the research examines the relation between depression and immune function, specifically, depression's potential to suppress natural killer cells' ability to clear tumor cells from

the bloodstream. Because depression has been shown to suppress normal natural killer cell function (Herbert and Cohen 1993), theories have suggested that this suppression could be significant enough to cause or worsen cancer (Levy and Wise 1987). Currently, the evidence for this is intriguing but indirect. For example, in a prospective population-based study of more than 4,800 elderly individuals, the investigators found that those with a chronically depressed mood had an 88% increase in cancer risks across the 3.8 years of the study (Penninx et al. 1998). Similar studies suggest that depression also can affect cancer morbidity. For example, one study suggested that cancer patients with depression are 2.6 times more likely to die within the first 19 months of a cancer diagnosis (Stommel et al. 2002). However, we lack any convincing direct evidence of a causal relation, and it remains unclear whether depression can suppress immune function significantly enough to affect cancer development (S. Cohen and Rabin 1998). Other mechanisms have been suggested to explain a link between stress and the damage from cancer, such as damage to DNA, inhibition of DNA repair, effects on apoptosis, and direct effects on somatic mutation. Evidence is insufficient to support any of these theories (Forlenza and Baum 2000).

Heart Disease

Studies suggest that patients with cardiovascular disease are at increased risk for depression. For example, it has been reported that more than two-thirds of patients surviving a myocardial infarction experience some type of depression, whereas one-quarter become severely depressed (Januzzi et al. 2000). High levels of depression have been found in other cardiovascular disease, such as coronary artery disease and congestive heart failure (MacMahon and Lip 2002). The risk of depression may be independent of the severity of disease, and the combination of the two disorders appears to cause more disability than what would be expected by an additive effect (Wells et al. 1992).

Conversely, a reciprocal relation appears to exist as well, and persons with depression are likely to be at increased risk for heart disease. This can be true even for individuals without any previous cardiovascular disease (Wulsin and Singal 2003). Depression also may increase the progression of (Ahern et al. 1990) and mortality (Frasure-Smith et al. 1999) from heart disease. Rugulies (2002), in a review of the subject, estimated that the relative risk of developing cardiovascular disease in the presence of major depression is more than twice that of the nondepressed population.

The mechanism of this effect is not clear. Several mechanisms have been suggested (Joynt et al. 2003). Depression may affect a person's health status, influencing compliance with medications, or other health-related behaviors such as smoking and exercise. The physiological effects of depression could put one at greater cardiovascular risk, either through nervous system activation, cardiac rhythm disturbances, systemic and localized inflammation, or hypercoagulability. Depression and cardiovascular disease also may share an underlying cause, such as stress. As with other disorders, the mechanism of such a relation likely involves multiple factors (Musselman et al. 1996), including depression's effect on rhythmicity, blood pressure, clotting factors, and longer-term factors such as insulin and cholesterol levels. It also may chronically increase the levels of stress hormones, such as cortisol and epinephrine. All these, alone and in combination, are plausible. However, although indirect evidence exists to support all of the above possible links (Joynt et al. 2003), no direct link has been shown, and the relations remain theoretical (Pasic et al. 2003).

Diabetes

Given the long-understood relation between endocrine function and mood, it is understandable that investigators would look to these disorders as another template for better understanding the relation between general medical conditions and mood disorders. Diabetes, in some studies, is thought to double one's risk for depression; these exact figures are difficult to prove, but it does appear that depression is more prevalent in diabetic persons than in the general population (Gavard et al. 1993). Furthermore, the severity of the diabetes also seems to correlate with the risk of depression. The comorbidity of diabetes and depression increases the health care costs of the person beyond that expected from an additive relationship alone. Socioeconomic factors also appear to play a role, and factors such as lower educational status, poor social support, and negative life events are all risk factors for depression in diabetic (type 2) patients (Fisher et al. 2001).

It has been suggested that, unlike disorders such as cancer, the overlap between diabetes and depression is an easier one to distinguish. Lustman and colleagues (1992), for example, reported being able to reliably identify depression in diabetes through the use of an exclusive approach.

Diabetes, itself a complex disease that is multiply determined, can have a potentially reciprocal relation with depression. That is, diabetes can increase one's risk for depression, but depression also may cause diabetes or worsen its course. This is most clear in an indirect sense because diabetes requires a good deal of self-care (which can deteriorate with depression). More direct mechanisms are possible as well, and risk of depression is increased even when controlling for potentially confounding variables such as age, race, gender, socioeconomic

status, education, use of health services, other psychiatric disorders, and body weight (Musselman et al. 2003).

What is the relation between diabetes and depression? One can posit a direct causal mechanism, in which the endocrine (or other) abnormalities also trigger a depressive episode. The same stress hormones that are involved in the regulation of glucose are also likely involved in the regulation of stress and mood (Musselman et al. 2003). Similarly, one can imagine a psychosocial cause, acknowledging the enormous psychological burden of this disease. Talbot and Nouwen (2000) reviewed the available studies that might bear on this question for both type 1 and type 2 diabetes, relying on the criteria for causation suggested in the introduction of this chapter: temporal relations, atypical depressive symptoms, and neurophysiological evidence for a direct association between the two disorders. In the end, they concluded that no one causative theory is more compelling, but more evidence exists for a direct biological cause in type 1 than in type 2 diabetes, and they argued for a biopsychosocial approach to depression and diabetes. As with other illnesses, this lack of a more definitive conclusion results more from the paucity and heterogeneity of the data than from any definitive evidence.

Human Immunodeficiency Virus

Data on human immunodeficiency virus (HIV) and depression are mixed. Prevalence estimates vary widely, and no consensus exists about whether the risk for depression is truly increased in HIV. Many other factors are associated with depression and HIV, including ongoing substance use and preexisting psychiatric pathology. Socioeconomic status represents an important risk factor as well, as does race and ethnicity. For example, one study found that Hispanic HIV-infected women reported more depressive symptoms than white women, who reported more symptoms than African American women (Fleishman and Fogel 1994).

Several studies suggest that persons with HIV may be at increased risk for depression during certain stages in their illness: for example, at the time of HIV infection (Pergami et al. 1994), at the onset of HIV-related symptoms (Belkin et al. 1992), or at the time of acquired immunodeficiency syndrome (AIDS) diagnosis. Thus, understanding the relation between HIV and depression may be more meaningful if one takes into account the longitudinal course of both illnesses.

Ciesla and Roberts (2001), in reviewing published studies on depression and HIV, found no relation between HIV infection and risk for depression in any of the 10 studies identified. However, most of these studies lacked the necessary statistical power to detect anything but a large effect and were unable to control for the many possible intervening variables. Ciesla and Roberts attempted to compensate for these limitations by pooling the data from these 10 studies, and this subsequent meta-analysis did find an almost twofold increased risk of depression in HIV-positive patients over those who were HIV negative. Their meta-analysis lacked sufficient data and power to test the effect of most other potential covariates, such as gender, stage of disease, ongoing substance abuse, or presence of AIDS-related symptoms.

Too few studies examine HIV in women. This is unfortunate because women make up one of the fastest group of new AIDS cases. In a large group of HIV-infected woman, Moore and colleagues (1999) found that these women reported levels of depressive symptomatology significantly above those found in the general population; however, the reported levels were similar to those in a comparison group of demographically similar uninfected women. Severe adverse life events and substance use (injection drug and crack) were strong predictors of depressive symptoms in both groups. In separate longitudinal analyses of this cohort, depression was associated with poorer cognitive performance (R.A. Cohen et al. 2001) and with mortality (Ickovics et al. 2001) in the HIV-infected group.

As with other disorders, HIV provides a model for examining the effects of depression on the immune system, and several investigators have examined whether depression is associated with changes in CD4 cell counts or viral loads. Burack and colleagues (1993) found a significant difference between depressive symptoms and CD4 cell decline in up to 66 months of follow-up, but Lyketsos and colleagues (1993) did not find such an association in a larger sample followed up for 8 years. Leserman and colleagues (2002) studied the relation between depression and HIV in a sample of 96 HIV-infected men followed up for 9 years and found that depression's effect on HIV was more impressive than the reverse relation. Specifically, they found that most patients who were depressed during the study had a history of depression prior to having HIV. CD4[+] cell counts and the presence of AIDS-related symptoms did not predict depression. However, the presence of depressed symptoms did increase the risk for developing AIDS, likely through its effect on HIV risk–related behaviors.

Other Disorders

Any psychiatric textbook lists scores of diseases that can cause depression, and the purpose here is not to present a comprehensive review of all possible combinations but to examine several examples showing the potential relations between medical disorders and depression. It is, however, worth acknowledging a few other disorders that occur frequently and perplex the physicians who treat these patients.

Irritable Bowel Syndrome

Patients with irritable bowel syndrome (IBS) are reported to have a high prevalence of depression. The causal relation between the two disorders is complex, and depression is often reported to precede the onset of IBS. Attempts have been made to correlate IBS, depression, and immune functioning; however, results have largely been equivocal. There may be some evidence for immune suppression in severely depressed patients, but it is not clear from the study whether this was independent of the gastrointestinal pathology (Swiatkowski and Rybakowski 1993).

Tinnitus

Tinnitus is another disorder that is frequently associated with depression, and, as with most of the disorders discussed, the direction of causality appears complex as well. One study found that nortriptyline treatment of the depression associated with tinnitus also improved the tinnitus itself and that improvement in the two conditions was closely associated (Sullivan et al. 1993).

Sleep Apnea

Obstructive sleep apnea is thought to be a highly prevalent and underdiagnosed disorder, which likely affects more than 11 million Americans. It is thought that this disorder can directly cause depressive symptoms. This appears to be more than a mere overlap of symptomatology, in that it is not merely an effect of sleeplessness or fatigue, and patients with sleep apnea are reported to present with the full spectrum of depressive symptoms. Such symptoms apparently improve with treatment of the sleep disorder (National Commission on Sleep Disorders Research 1993).

Thyroid Disease

The relation between thyroid disease and psychiatric disease has been long appreciated (Whybrow et al. 1969), and it has been reported that as many as 15% of the patients who present to a psychiatric facility for depression have at least mild hypothyroidism (Gold et al. 1982). Furthermore, it has been reported that almost one-third of the patients with depression will have a blunted thyrotropin response to thyrotropin-releasing hormone (Dinan 2001). Although treating the hypothyroidism as part of depression treatment is essential, symptoms of depression sometimes persist beyond correction of the thyroid (Cooper et al. 1984) and require specific antidepressant treatment. Similarly, the fatigue that accompanies the depression may not improve with normal antidepressant treatment and may require independent attention (with, for example, stimulant medication) (A.J. Cohen 1993).

Treatment of Depression in Medical Patients

As a last criterion for the uniqueness of secondary depression, one would like to see evidence of a unique response to treatment. The case for secondary depression would be more convincing if this disorder had a different reaction to treatment, compared with idiopathic depression. This is not a necessary condition; one can imagine a case in which the depressive syndrome is a final common pathway regardless of the original etiology and that different types of depression still may have a similar response to standard treatment (e.g., analogous to various psychotic disorders). Furthermore, it is possible that the action of antidepressant medications is nonspecific enough to encompass different depressive disorders, just as antidepressants also treat various anxiety disorders. However, any indications of a unique response, although not required, would be a very persuasive argument for the unique nature of depression in the medical patient.

Most reviews of the subject suggest that medical illness is a negative predictor of treatment response (Reynolds 1992). Unfortunately, very little evidence bears directly on this issue. A systematic review of all antidepressant trials in patients with comorbid medical illness identified only 18 randomized, controlled studies (Gill and Hatcher 2003). None of these studies compared patients with medical illness with those lacking any comorbidity. In practice, most of the statements made about response reflect a comparison of a given response rate to the presumed response rate if the group had iatrogenic depression. However, even this type of inferential data can help shed some light on the nature of treatment response in the depressed medical patient. Some specific information from a review of different disorders follows.

Poststroke Depression

Three placebo-controlled studies of antidepressant treatment have been done in patients who have had a CVA. As a group, they suggested that antidepressants are superior to placebo, and the overall response rate in the studies was about 60%, which put them approximately in the range of response rates in iatrogenic depression. Of most interest are data from Robinson and colleagues (2000), which suggested that a uniqueness of response was evident: patients in the study only responded to the tricyclic antidepressant nortriptyline, and the response to fluoxetine was no better than placebo. If these responses were consistently found, this would be a strong argument for the unique nature of poststroke depression. Not all studies have confirmed this finding,

however; for example, a second study of fluoxetine in poststroke depression did find a significant effect. Whyte and Mulsant (2002) suggested that the differential response may have been an artifact of the study design and of the original subject assignment because the group that eventually received fluoxetine may have been a more resistant group.

The question also has been raised whether antidepressants should be used to prevent poststroke depression. In a recent review of the subject, Anderson et al. (2004) identified 10 studies that bear on the question and concluded that data were inadequate to justify the preventive use of antidepressants. The lack of consensus in the different studies was not surprising: the studies were very heterogeneous in all areas of their design. For example, the time to beginning antidepressant treatment varied across studies from a few hours to 6 months poststroke, and the methods of diagnosing depression and the various treatments used differed greatly across studies.

Cancer

Although a good deal has been written about the need to treat depression in patients with cancer, there are surprisingly few studies of pharmacotherapy for depressed patients with cancer. Of the available randomized, controlled studies, two investigated mianserin (Costa et al. 1985; van Heeringen and Zivkov 1996), a drug that is not available in the United States. One study used the tricyclic antidepressant imipramine (Evans et al. 1988), and a second compared desipramine with fluoxetine (Holland et al. 1998). Among the SSRIs, paroxetine also has been used in a rigorous study (Raison and Nemeroff 2000). Many of the newer drugs have efficacy data from open trials and case studies. In general, studies of the use of antidepressants in this population report that the drugs are relatively safe and effective, although some data suggest that they are less effective for neurovegetative symptoms of depression (Capuron et al. 2002).

The relation between cancer and stress has appeared consistently in the literature, and a good deal of it has focused on the influence of depression on the course of cancer. This focus has been largely encouraged by Spiegel and colleagues (1981), who studied a supportive group intervention for women with metastatic breast cancer. The intervention not only improved quality of life in the intervention group, but in a follow-up study, the mean survival in the intervention group was twice that of the usual care group (Spiegel 2002). Theorists have drawn on research (although it remains unclear) showing depression's detrimental effect on the immune system and a purported overall effect on the body's ability to combat disease. A larger multicenter study was unable to replicate Spiegel's finding regarding survival, but it did find that group therapy had important effects on quality of life, increased improved mood, and decreased pain (Goodwin et al. 2001). Other attempts to replicate the data have been mixed, with some positive results for individual psychotherapy (Kuchler et al. 1999) and a therapeutic home nursing visit (McCorkle et al. 2000); others have not replicated the positive effect of psychotherapy on mood in various groups of cancer patients, including breast cancer (Classen et al. 2001) and testicular cancer (Moynihan et al. 1998). Speculations on these different results included the possibility that some groups are higher functioning to begin with and have more access to supportive care outside the experiment.

Preliminary studies suggest that it may be possible to identify certain cancer populations that are vulnerable to developing depression. For example, Raison and Miller (2003) reported that in their population of cancer patients, those who developed depression with interferon-α treatment were more likely to show increased corticotropin and cortisol production following the first dose of interferon-α, suggesting a stress–reactivity predisposition.

Nevertheless, these clinical investigations have led researchers to wonder whether treating depression could affect the immune system (or other aspects of physiological functioning) in a direct, measurable way. Although some data have suggested that psychological treatment could modulate the immune system, a meta-analysis (Miller and Cohen 2001) of available studies suggested that any effect would be modest and likely overwhelmed by the disease process.

Heart Disease

In the past, clinicians were reluctant to use antidepressants—particularly tricyclic antidepressants—in patients with cardiac disease. This was primarily because of fear of the drugs' effect on cardiac conduction (Roose et al. 1987). With the rise of the selective serotonin reuptake inhibitors (SSRIs), antidepressants have been used more liberally in the setting of acute cardiac disease. However, data on the safety and efficacy of these agents are limited. What data exist suggest that the SSRIs have a very low risk of severe cardiac side effects (Januzzi et al. 2000). Studies of efficacy are largely lacking as well. The largest study to date is the Sertraline Anti-Depressant Heart Attack Randomized Trial (SADHART), which compared sertraline with placebo in more than 350 patients who had major depression after a myocardial infarction or had unstable angina (Glassman et al. 2002). The study did show efficacy for the drug but only in patients with severe or recurrent depression. When patients with mild depression were included in the analysis, sertraline was not more efficacious than placebo. The drug was found safe; in fact, there was a trend toward fewer adverse cardiac effects in the group taking sertraline.

Among the other SSRIs, fluoxetine has been shown to be safe and effective in one open study of elderly patients with depression and cardiac disease, and paroxetine was shown to be safe and effective in a double-blind comparison with nortriptyline (Roose 2003). Among other later-generation antidepressants, only bupropion has been studied in patients with significant cardiac illness (Roose et al. 1991). Generally, bupropion was found to be safe, in that it had no significant effect on heart rate, ejection fraction, or cardiac conduction. However, it did cause an increase in systolic and diastolic blood pressure, which was judged to be statistically, but not clinically, significant, and it caused suppression of ventricular premature depolarization.

As in the discussion of cancer, there has been an interest in whether psychotherapy could improve not only mood disorders but also overall cardiac survival in this population. This improvement seems more likely in the cardiac disease group than in the cancer group because cardiac disease is so frequently linked to stress. However, most of the large-scale cardiac intervention studies have not targeted depression as an outcome and have focused on personality factors such as the type A personality. A review of available studies (Rees et al. 2004) found that psychosocial interventions did not have a significant effect on cardiac mortality. However, any conclusion was limited by the heterogeneity of and methodological flaws in many of the studies. The review did find that psychosocial therapies were effective in reducing depressive symptoms.

Diabetes

To date, no large-scale trials of antidepressant treatment for depressed diabetic patients exist. Among controlled trials, only two medication studies have been done, one with nortriptyline (Lustman et al. 1997a) and one with fluoxetine (Lustman et al. 2000). In addition, one psychotherapy trial compared cognitive-behavioral therapy plus an educational program with the educational program alone (Lustman et al. 1998). All the studies showed good effect in treating depression. Evidence also indicates that treatment of depression in patients with diabetes can improve their diabetic control (Lustman et al. 1997b). Although there has been some concern that antidepressants can cause hyperglycemia (particularly the tricyclic antidepressants), glycemic control generally improves with the use of antidepressants. Psychotherapy, particularly cognitive-behavioral therapy, also has been used in nondepressed diabetic patients to improve diabetes management (Talbot and Nouwen 2000).

Conclusion and Future Directions

Summarizing this varied literature would be difficult. In a sense, any conclusions must mirror the opening statement. The literature on depression in medical illness is beset with many limitations, all of which confine any attempts at grand statements. Even so, the opening contentions of this chapter—1) that depression is more common in medical patients than in the non–medically ill population, 2) that the depression is frequently missed or misattributed to a "normal reaction to illness," 3) that depression is more difficult to treat in this population, but 4) that standard treatments still do help, and 5) that untreated depression will worsen the morbidity and mortality of the medical disease—all still seem reasonable conclusions to take from this review.

An additional conclusion can be drawn as well. To a degree, some literature on depression in medical illness reflects an overall trend toward the medicalization of psychiatry—an attempt to stress the biological underpinnings of psychiatric disease. However, a larger reading of the literature suggests that one oversimplifies only at one's own peril. Although it is tempting to see evidence of biological causes as proof of a "purely" biological depression, such interpretations do not account for the whole of the literature. As with psychiatry overall, depression due to medical illness is best understood within the framework of the biopsychosocial model. Whether one is approaching depressed medical patients from the research bench or the clinical bedside, the approach is likely to be most satisfying, and the treatment most successful, if it allows for this larger perspective.

In considering areas for future research, it is clear that almost all the topics discussed are in need of better and larger studies. The following specific questions require further study:

- **What is the true prevalence of depression in various medical illnesses?** The wide range of prevalence figures cited for the various diseases attests to the fact that the gold standard studies are yet to be done. One might contest the need for devoting large resources necessary to evaluate depression in the medical setting with rigorous epidemiological techniques, particularly because all seem to agree that depression is common in this setting. However, despite informal agreement, the treatment of depression in the medical setting is not receiving the attention that other potential medical risk factors routinely receive. As long as we are hindered by weak data, some will continue to believe that this area is too "soft" to deserve the same efforts as, for instance, the prevention of hypertension in cardiovascular disease.

- **How is it best to diagnose depression in the medical setting?** Most of the illnesses covered lack standardized approaches to identifying symptoms of depression in the setting of possible overlapping symptoms. It can be argued that there is little point in pursuing further epidemiological work until valid and reliable instruments are tested in the various medical disorders. Because we continue to lack a gold standard test for idiopathic depression, this can be a challenge; however, we have seen examples (e.g., in Parkinson's disease) in which psychometrically sound approaches can be devised.

- **What is the nature of the relationship between depression and various medical illnesses?** Clearly, impressive work in teasing out the intricacies of the relation between depression and medical illness already has occurred, such as in the areas of poststroke depression and Parkinson's disease. However, the work to date invites as many questions as it answers, and more work needs to be done. This is likely to be a particularly fruitful area because it will teach us more about the nature of depression itself.

- **How can we best treat depression in the medical setting?** Most of the examples discussed lack any large-scale treatment studies. In the clinical setting, most treatments of these disorders continue with the assumption that the treatment should be similar to that for idiopathic depression. However, as discussed in this chapter, evidence shows both nonresponse and differential response in different settings. In addition, different symptoms may respond to different treatments: some may respond better to pharmacotherapy, and others may respond better to psychotherapy. As we have seen in the treatment of major depression, useful efficacy data can be derived only with large-scale studies, and these are clearly needed for the various medical comorbidities discussed.

References

Ahern DK, Gorkin L, Anderson JL, et al: Biobehavioral variables and mortality or cardiac arrest in the Cardiac Arrhythmia Pilot Study. Am J Cardiol 66:59–62, 1990

American Psychiatric Association: Diagnostic and Statistical Manual: Mental Disorders. Washington, DC, American Psychiatric Association, 1952

American Psychiatric Association: Diagnostic and Statistical Manual of Mental Disorders, 2nd Edition. Washington, DC, American Psychiatric Association, 1968

American Psychiatric Association: Diagnostic and Statistical Manual of Mental Disorders, 3rd Edition. Washington, DC, American Psychiatric Association, 1980

American Psychiatric Association: Diagnostic and Statistical Manual of Mental Disorders, 4th Edition, Text Revision. Washington, DC, American Psychiatric Association, 2000

Anderson CS, Hackett ML, House AO: Interventions for preventing depression after stroke (Cochrane Review), in The Cochrane Library, Vol 3. Chichester, UK, Wiley, 2004

Belkin GS, Fleishman JA, Stein MD, et al: Physical symptoms and depressive symptoms among individuals with HIV infection. Psychosomatics 33:416–427, 1992

Berg D, Supprian T, Thomae J, et al: Lesion pattern in patients with multiple sclerosis and depression. Mult Scler 6:156–162, 2000

Boland RJ, Diaz S, Lamdan RM, et al: Overdiagnosis of depression in the general hospital. Gen Hosp Psychiatry 18:28–35, 1996

Burack JH, Barrett DC, Stall RD, et al: Depressive symptoms and CD4 lymphocyte decline among HIV-infected men. JAMA 270:2568–2573, 1993

Capuron L, Gumnick JF, Musselman DL, et al: Neurobehavioral effects of interferon-alpha in cancer patients: phenomenology and paroxetine responsiveness of symptom dimensions. Neuropsychopharmacology 26:643–652, 2002

Carson A, MacHale S, Allen K, et al: Depression after stroke and lesion location: a systematic review. Lancet 356:122–126, 2000

Casey P, Dowrick C, Wilkinson G: Adjustment disorders: fault line in the psychiatric glossary. Br J Psychiatry 179:479–481, 2001

Chochinov HM, Wilson KG, Enns M, et al: "Are you depressed?" Screening for depression in the terminally ill. Am J Psychiatry 154:674–676, 1997

Chwastiak L, Ehde DM, Gibbons LE, et al: Depressive symptoms and severity of illness in multiple sclerosis: epidemiologic study of a large community sample. Am J Psychiatry 159:1862–1868, 2002

Ciesla JA, Roberts JE: Meta-analysis of the relationship between HIV infection and risk for depressive disorders. Am J Psychiatry 158:725–730, 2001

Clark DA, Cook A, Snow D: Depressive symptom differences in hospitalized, medically ill, depressed psychiatric inpatients and nonmedical controls. J Abnorm Psychol 107:38–48, 1998

Classen C, Butler LD, Koopman C, et al: Supportive-expressive group therapy and distress in patients with metastatic breast cancer: a randomized clinical intervention trial. Arch Gen Psychiatry 58:494–501, 2001

Cohen AJ: Treatment of anergic depression in Hashimoto's thyroiditis with fluoxetine and d-amphetamine. Depression 1:110–114, 1993

Cohen RA, Boland R, Paul R, et al: Neurocognitive performance enhanced by highly active antiretroviral therapy in HIV-infected women. AIDS 15:341–345, 2001

Cohen S, Rabin BS: Psychologic stress, immunity, and cancer. J Natl Cancer Inst 90:3–4, 1998

Cooper DS, Halpern R, Wood LC, et al. L-Thyroxine therapy in subclinical hypothyroidism. Ann Intern Med 101:18–24, 1984

Costa E, Mogos I, Toma T: Efficacy and safety of mianserin in the treatment of depression of women with cancer. Acta Psychiatr Scand 72:85–92, 1985

Croyle RT, Rowland JH: Mood disorders and cancer: a National Cancer Institute perspective. Biol Psychiatry 54:191–194, 2003

Cummings JL: Depression and Parkinson's disease: a review. Am J Psychiatry 149:443–454, 1992

Depression Guideline Panel: Clinical Practice Guideline, Number 5. Depression in Primary Care, Vol 1: Detection and Diagnosis (AHCPR Publ No 93-0551). Rockville, MD, Agency for Health Care Policy and Research, 1993

Dinan TG: Psychoneuroendocrinology of mood disorders. Curr Opin Psychiatry 14:51–55, 2001

Endicott J, Spitzer RL: A diagnostic interview: the Schedule for Affective Disorders and Schizophrenia. Arch Gen Psychiatry 35:837–844, 1978

Evans DL, McCartney CF, Haggerty JJ: Treatment of depression in cancer patients is associated with better life adaptation. Psychosom Med 50:72–76, 1988

Fisher L, Chesla CA, Mullan JT, et al: Contributors to depression in Latino and European-American patients with type 2 diabetes. Diabetes Care 24:1751–1757, 2001

Fleishman JA, Fogel B: Coping and depressive symptoms among people with AIDS. Health Psychol 13:156–169, 1994

Folstein M, Maiberger R, McHugh P: Mood disorder as a specific complication of stroke. J Neurol Neurosurg Psychiatry 40:1018–1020, 1977

Forlenza MJ, Baum A: Psychosocial influences on cancer progression: alternative cellular and molecular mechanisms. Curr Opin Psychiatry 13:639–645, 2000

Frasure-Smith N, Lesperance F, Juneau M, et al: Gender, depression, and one-year prognosis after myocardial infarction. Psychosom Med 61:26–37, 1999

Fruehwald S, Loeffler-Stastka H, Eher R, et al: Depression and quality of life in multiple sclerosis. Acta Neurol Scand 104:257–261, 2001

Gavard JA, Lustman PJ, Clouse RE: Prevalence of depression in adults with diabetes. Diabetes Care 16:1167–1178, 1993

Gerber PD, Barrett J, Barrett J, et al: Recognition of depression by internists in primary care: a comparison of internist and "gold standard" psychiatric assessment. J Gen Intern Med 4:7–13, 1989

Gill D, Hatcher S: Antidepressants for depression in medical illness (Cochrane Review), in The Cochrane Library, Vol 3. Chichester, UK, Wiley, 2003

Gilliam F, Kanner AM: Treatment of depressive disorders in epilepsy patients. Epilepsy Behav 3 (5 suppl):2–9, 2002

Glassman AH, O'Connor CM, Califf RM, et al: Sertraline treatment of major depression in patients with acute MI or unstable angina (the SADHART trial). JAMA 288:701–709, 2002

Gold MS, Pottash AC, Extein I: Symptomless autoimmune thyroiditis in depression. Psychiatry Res 6:261–269, 1982

Goodwin PJ, Leszcz M, Ennis M, et al: The effect of group psychosocial support on survival in metastatic breast cancer. N Engl J Med 345:1719–1726, 2001

Hantz P, Caradoc-Davies G, Caradoc-Davies T, et al: Depression in Parkinson's disease. Am J Psychiatry 151:1010–1014, 1994

Herbert TB, Cohen S: Stress and immunity in humans: a meta-analytic review. Psychosom Med 55:364–379, 1993

Holland JC, Romano SJ, Heiligenstein JH, et al: A controlled trial of fluoxetine and desipramine in depressed women with advanced cancer. Psychooncology 7:291–300, 1998

Ickovics JR, Hamburger ME, Vlahov D, et al: Mortality, CD4 cell count decline, and depressive symptoms among HIV-seropositive women: longitudinal analysis from the HIV epidemiology research study. JAMA 285:1466–1474, 2001

Januzzi JL, Stern TA, Pasternak RC, et al: The influence of anxiety and depression on outcomes of patients with coronary artery disease. Arch Intern Med 160:1913–1921, 2000

Joynt KE, Whellan DJ, O'Connor CM: Depression and cardiovascular disease: mechanisms of interaction. Biol Psychiatry 54:248–261, 2003

Kanner AM: Depression in epilepsy: prevalence, clinical semiology, pathogenic mechanisms, and treatment. Biol Psychiatry 54:388–398, 2003

Kathol RG, Mutgi A, Williams J, et al: Diagnosis of major depression in cancer according to four sets of criteria. Am J Psychiatry 147:1021–1024, 1990

Katon W, Schulberg H: Epidemiology of depression in primary care. Gen Hosp Psychiatry 14:237–247, 1991

Kim JS, Choi-Kwon S: Post stroke depression and emotional incontinence. Neurology 54:1805–1810, 2000

Koenig HG, George LK, Peterson BL, et al: Depression in medically ill hospitalized older adults: prevalence, characteristics, and course of symptoms according to six diagnostic schemes. Am J Psychiatry 154:1376–1383, 1997

Kuchler T, Henne-Bruns D, Rappat S, et al: Impact of psychotherapeutic support on gastrointestinal cancer patients undergoing surgery: survival results of a trial. Hepatogastroenterology 46:322–335, 1999

Leserman J, Petitto JM, Gu H, et al: Progression to AIDS, a clinical AIDS condition, and mortality: psychosocial and physiological predictors. Psychol Med 32:1059–1073, 2002

Levy SM, Wise BD: Psychosocial risk factors, natural immunity, and cancer progression. Current Psychology Research and Reviews 6:229–243, 1987

Lipowski ZJ: Is the education of primary care physicians adequate? Gen Hosp Psychiatry 14:361–362, 1992

Lustman PJ, Griffith LS, Gavard JA, et al: Depression in adults with diabetes. Diabetes Care 15:1631–1639, 1992

Lustman PJ, Griffith LS, Clouse RE, et al: Effects of nortriptyline on depression and glucose regulation in diabetes: results of a doubleblind, placebo-controlled trial. Psychosom Med 59:241–250, 1997a

Lustman PJ, Griffith LS, Freedland KE, et al: The course of major depression in diabetics. Gen Hosp Psychiatry 19:138–143, 1997b

Lustman PJ, Griffith LS, Freedland KE, et al: Cognitive behavior therapy for depression in type 2 diabetes mellitus: a randomized, controlled trial. Ann Intern Med 129:613–621, 1998

Lustman PJ, Freedland KE, Griffith LS, et al: Fluoxetine for depression in diabetes: a randomized, doubleblind, placebo-controlled trial. Diabetes Care 23:618–623, 2000

Lyketsos CG, Hoover DR, Guccione M, et al: Depressive symptoms as predictors of medical outcomes in HIV infection. JAMA 270:2563–2567, 1993

MacMahon KMA, Lip GYH: Psychological factors in heart failure: a review of the literature. Arch Intern Med 162:509–516, 2002

McCorkle R, Strumpf NE, Nuamah IF, et al: A specialized home care intervention improves survival among older post-surgical cancer patients. J Am Geriatr Soc 48:1707–1713, 2000

McDaniel JS, Musselman DL, Porter MR, et al: Depression in patients with cancer: diagnosis, biology, and treatment. Arch Gen Psychiatry 52:89–99, 1995

McDonald WM, Richard IH, DeLong MR: Prevalence, etiology, and treatment of depression in Parkinson's disease. Biol Psychiatry 54:363–375, 2003

Menza MA, Robertson-Hoffman DE, Bonapace AS: Parkinson's disease and anxiety: comorbidity with depression. Biol Psychiatry 34:465–470, 1993

Miller GE, Cohen S: Psychological interventions and the immune system: a meta-analytic review and critique. Health Psychol 20:47–53, 2001

Mohr DC, Goodkin DE, Islar J, et al: Treatment of depression is associated with suppression of nonspecific and antigen-specific T(H)1 responses in multiple sclerosis. Arch Neurol 58:1081–1086, 2001

Moore J, Schuman P, Schoenbaum E, et al: Severe adverse life events and depressive symptoms among women with, or at risk for, HIV infection in four cities in the United States of America. AIDS 13:2459–2468, 1999

Morris PLP, Robinson RG, Andrezejewski P, et al: Association of depression with 10-year poststroke mortality. Am J Psychiatry 150:124–129, 1993

Moynihan C, Bliss JM, Davidson J, et al: Evaluation of adjuvant psychological therapy in patients with testicular cancer: randomized controlled trial. BMJ 316:429–435, 1998

Murphy E: Social origins of depression in old age. Br J Psychiatry 141:134–142, 1982

Musselman DL, Tomer A, Manatunga AK, et al: Exaggerated platelet activity in major depression. Am J Psychiatry 153:1313–1317, 1996

Musselman DL, Betan E, Larsen H, et al: Relationship of depression to diabetes types 1 and 2: epidemiology, biology, and treatment. Biol Psychiatry 54:317–329, 2003

National Commission on Sleep Disorders Research: Wake up America: A National Sleep Alert, Executive Summary and Report. Bethesda, MD, U.S. Department of Health and Human Services, 1993

Parker G, Kalucy M: Depression comorbid with physical illness. Curr Opin Psychiatry 12:87–92, 1999

Pasic J, Levy W, Sullivan M: Cytokines in depression and heart failure. Psychosom Med 65:181–193, 2003

Patten SB, Jacobs P, Petcu R, et al: Major depressive disorder and health care costs in multiple sclerosis. Int J Psychiatry Med 32:167–178, 2002

Penninx BW, Guralnik JM, Pahor M, et al: Chronically depressed mood and cancer risk in older persons. J Natl Cancer Inst 90:1888–1893, 1998

Perez-Stable EJ, Miranda J, Ying Y: Depression in medical outpatients. Arch Intern Med 150:1083–1088, 1990

Pergami A, Gala C, Burgess A, et al: Heterosexuals and HIV disease: a controlled investigation into the psychosocial factors associated with psychiatric morbidity. J Psychosom Res 38:305–313, 1994

Raison CL, Miller AH: Depression in cancer: new developments regarding diagnosis and treatment. Biol Psychiatry 54:283–294, 2003

Raison CL, Nemeroff CB: Cancer and depression: prevalence, diagnosis, and treatment. Home Health Care Consultant 7:34–41, 2000

Rees K, Bennett P, West R, et al: Psychological interventions for coronary heart disease (Cochrane Review), in The Cochrane Library, Vol 2. Chichester, UK, Wiley, 2004

Reynolds CF: Treatment of depression in special populations. J Clin Psychiatry 53 (9 suppl):45–53, 1992

Robinson R: Poststroke depression: prevalence, diagnosis, treatment, and disease progression. Biol Psychiatry 54:376–387, 2003

Robinson R, Kubos K, Starr L, et al: Mood disorders in stroke patients: importance of location of lesion. Brain 107:81–93, 1984

Robinson R, Bolduc P, Price T: Two-year longitudinal study of poststroke mood disorders: diagnosis and outcome at one and two years. Stroke 18:837–843, 1987

Robinson R, Schultz S, Castillo C: Nortriptyline versus fluoxetine in the treatment of depression and in short-term recovery after stroke: a placebo-controlled, double-blind study. Am J Psychiatry 157:351–359, 2000

Roose SP: Treatment of depression in patients with heart disease. Biol Psychiatry 54:262–268, 2003

Roose SP, Glassman AH, Giardina EG, et al: Tricyclic antidepressants in depressed patients with cardiac conduction disease. Arch Gen Psychiatry 44:273–275, 1987

Roose SP, Dalack GW, Glassman AH, et al: Cardiovascular effects of bupropion in depressed patients with heart disease. Am J Psychiatry 148:512–516, 1991

Rost K, Smith R, Matthew DB, et al: The deliberate misdiagnosis of major depression in primary care. Arch Fam Med 3:333–337, 1994

Rugulies R: Depression as a predictor for coronary heart disease: a review and meta-analysis. Am J Prev Med 23:51–61, 2002

Schrag A, Jahanshahi M, Quin N: What contributes to quality of life in patients with Parkinson's disease. J Neurol Neurosurg Psychiatry 69:308–312, 2000

Spiegel D: Effects of psychotherapy on cancer survival. Nat Rev Cancer 2:383–389, 2002

Spiegel D, Bloom JR, Yalom I: Group support for patients with metastatic cancer: a randomized outcome study. Arch Gen Psychiatry 38:527–533, 1981

Spitzer RL, Endicott J, Robins E: Research Diagnostic Criteria: rationale and reliability. Arch Gen Psychiatry 35:773–782, 1978

Stommel M, Given BA, Given CW: Depression and functional status as predictors of death among cancer patients. Cancer 94:2719–2727, 2002

Sullivan M, Katon W, Russo J, et al: A randomized trial of nortriptyline for severe chronic tinnitus. Arch Intern Med 153:2251–2259, 1993

Swiatkowski M, Rybakowski JK: Depression and T lymphocytes in patients with irritable bowel syndrome. J Affect Disord 28:199–202, 1993

Talbot F, Nouwen A: A review of the relationship between depression and diabetes in adults: is there a link? Diabetes Care 23:1556–1562, 2000

U.S. Department of Health and Human Services: Depression in Primary Care (AHCPR Publ No 93-0550). Rockville, MD, Agency for Health Care Policy and Research, 1993

van Heeringen K, Zivkov M: Pharmacological treatment of depression in cancer patients: a placebo-controlled study of mianserin. Br J Psychiatry 169:440–443, 1996

Wells KB, Burnam MA, Rogers W, et al: The course of depression in adult outpatients: results from the Medical Outcomes Study. Arch Gen Psychiatry 49:788–794, 1992

Whybrow PC, Prange AJ, Treadway CR: Mental changes accompanying thyroid gland dysfunction. Arch Gen Psychiatry 20:48–63, 1969

Whyte EM, Mulsant BH: Post stroke depression: epidemiology, pathophysiology, and biological treatment. Biol Psychiatry 52:253–264, 2002

Wulsin LR, Singal BM: Do depressive symptoms increase the risk for the onset of coronary disease? A systematic quantitative review. Psychosom Med 65:201–210, 2003

Zigmond AS, Snaith RP: The Hospital Anxiety and Depression Scale. Acta Psychiatr Scand 61:361–370, 1983

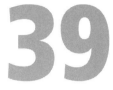

Mood Disorders and Substance Use

EDWARD NUNES, M.D.

ERIC RUBIN, M.D., PH.D.

KENNETH CARPENTER, PH.D.

DEBORAH HASIN, PH.D.

THE USE OF ADDICTIVE SUBSTANCES has been ubiquitous in human cultures since the dawn of civilization and remains almost universal across a wide variety of contemporary cultures, especially when one considers caffeine and nicotine in addition to alcohol and harder drugs. Substance use disorders, including abuse and dependence, are among the most common mental disorders in the general population (Grant et al. 2004). Furthermore, the presence of a mood disorder at least doubles the odds of having a substance use disorder in general population surveys in which this issue has been examined (Grant 1995; Grant and Harford 1995; Grant et al. 2004; Kessler et al. 1994; Regier et al. 1990). This strong and consistent association raises the question of what the relation may be between these two sets of disorders.

Substance use disorders are in some respects the best-understood mental disorders in terms of pathophysiology and neuropharmacology. What addictive substances have in common, and what sets them apart from all other drugs and compounds, is that they target brain reward circuitry centered around mesolimbic and mesocortical dopamine fibers (Gardner 1997). The understanding of drugs as positive reinforcers and their effects on and relation to the brain reward circuitry have led to a rich array of animal models (Johanson and Schuster 1981; Robbins and Everitt 2002), which, arguably, come closer to modeling the actual human disorder than do animal models of other common psychiatric disorders. The addictive substances all affect mood and have euphorigenic effects during intoxication and often dysphorigenic effects during withdrawal, suggesting relations at the

This work was supported in part by grants P50 DA09236, R01 DA12271, R01 DA08950, and K02 DA00288 from the National Institute on Drug Abuse and K05 AA00161 from the National Institute on Alcohol Abuse and Alcoholism. The authors are grateful to Carrie Davies, Richard Malkin, and Valerie Richmond for assistance in preparation of the manuscript and to Eve Vagg and Rachel Yarmolinsky for assistance with illustration.

level of brain circuitry between mood and substance use. Thus, we would argue that any effort to understand mood disorders is incomplete without a consideration of substance use and substance use disorders. Not only are substance use disorders prevalent among mood disorder patients, presenting a significant clinical problem, but also insights into the pathophysiology of addiction may be useful in further developing our understanding of mood disorders, and vice versa.

In this chapter, we review the pathophysiology and phenomenology of substance use disorders and the epidemiological evidence regarding their co-occurrence with mood disorders. We then discuss various lines of evidence (longitudinal and family genetic studies, behavioral and neurobiological studies, and treatment studies) relevant to understanding the potential relations between mood and substance use disorders. We conclude the chapter with sections on clinical evaluation and treatment.

Overview of Pathophysiology of Substance Use Disorders

The brain reward system was first suggested in the 1950s when it was found that electrical stimulation of sites corresponding to the median forebrain was highly positively reinforcing. Animals would work for direct stimulation of these regions. Subsequently, the circuitry has been described in some detail, as reviewed by Gardner (1997). Figure 39–1 shows Gardner's summary of brain reward circuitry, adapted for this text to highlight points of overlap with regions thought to be involved in mood regulation. The core of the system consists of mesolimbic and mesocortical dopamine fibers that originate in the ventral tegmental area in the brain stem. These fibers course rostrally to an array of targets, including the nucleus accumbens (a portion of the ventral striatum), the amygdala, and the frontal cortex. These targets of the brain stem dopaminergic projection sit within frontal and limbic circuitry that mediates executive cognitive functioning, as well as emotional and motivational functioning (Heimer 2003). The involvement of these same frontal and limbic circuits in the regulation of mood (Drevets 2000) (see Mayberg, Chapter 13, in this volume) provides an ample neurobiological substrate for interactions between the effects of abused substances and long-term mood regulation.

Microiontophoretic studies have documented that substances of abuse, although having a wide variety of pharmacological actions and pharmacological effects, have in common that they enhance the release of dopamine from the mesolimbic and mesocortical fibers in their target areas. Stimulants, such as cocaine and amphetamines, act directly on dopaminergic synapses. Other drugs, such as nicotine,

opiates, and cannabis, act through systems that impinge on and modulate the physiology of the dopamine release. Each of those substances has diverse pharmacological effects related to their unique pharmacology. For example, alcohol is a tranquilizer, used in diverse social settings as a social lubricant. Stimulants, such as cocaine, nicotine, and caffeine, have been used throughout history to promote productivity.

Several animal models have been developed that have enhanced our understanding of the pathophysiology of addictive disorders (Johanson and Schuster 1981; Robbins and Everitt 2002). Important findings from such models include 1) drugs addictive for humans are likely to be self-administered by laboratory animals, functioning in a behaviorally lawful way as positive reinforcers; 2) different genetic strains of animals vary in their propensity to administer different drugs; and 3) animals will work hard to obtain doses of drugs and, in some instances, will tolerate substantial aversive stimuli in order to receive doses of drugs.

A particularly useful model for understanding the mechanism of addiction has been the model of brain stimulation reward (Gardner 1997). In this model, a microelectrode is situated within the brain reward system of an animal, and the animal is allowed to work (e.g., press a lever) for electrical stimulation at that site. The stimulation strength is then gradually reduced until a threshold is reached at which the animal will no longer work for stimulation. This is called the threshold for brain stimulation reward. It has been found that acute doses of addictive drugs lower the brain stimulation threshold—that is, they appear to sensitize the brain reward system to the effects of electrical stimulation. However, chronic administration of addictive drugs has the opposite effect—namely, to raise the threshold for brain stimulation reward. This finding appears to model the state of tolerance that occurs in response to most addictive drugs (i.e., larger doses are needed over time to achieve the same effects). Tolerance is likely transduced via neuronal intracellular adaptations at the levels of second messengers and gene expression (Nestler 1993). Tolerance is also consistent with a state of anhedonia, in which the brain reward system becomes less responsive to natural reinforcers, such as food and social interaction. This common ground between drug tolerance and anhedonia within the brain reward system suggests a possible fundamental relation with mood disorders, in which anhedonia is a core symptom.

Phenomenology of Substance-Related Disorders

The major substance-related disorders include intoxication, withdrawal, abuse, and dependence. General psychiatrists

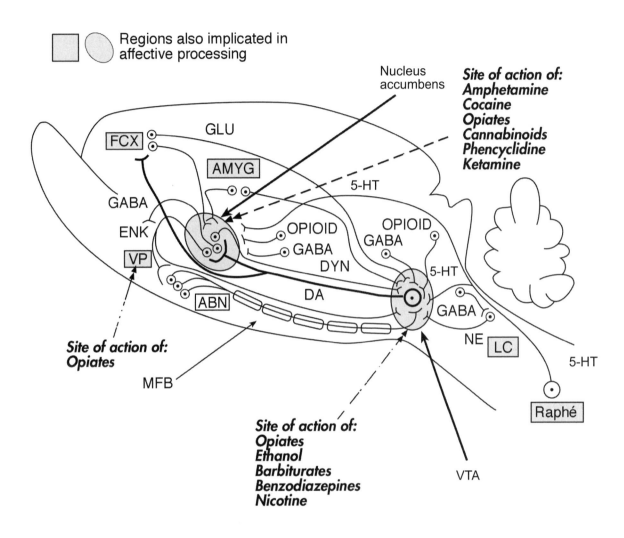

FIGURE 39–1.   Presumed neural substrate for interactions between substance abuse and mood regulation.
Illustration shows anatomical pathways and regional neurotransmitter mechanisms involved in brain reward and in effects of abused drugs. The core of the system comprises two components: myelinated fibers of the median forebrain bundle (MFB), which provide input to dopaminergic (DA) cells in the ventral tegmental area (VTA), and axons of the VTA cells (indicated with bold line) that ascend to the nucleus accumbens (mesolimbic fibers), frontal cortex (FCX) (mesocortical fibers), and other targets not detailed. Sites at which various addictive substances are thought to act on the brain reward system are indicated. Data on drug effects are derived primarily from invasive studies in laboratory animals and hence are presented on a cartoon of the rat brain, although the essential features have been verified in primate studies. Shaded regions (ovals and boxes) indicate structures whose homologues in the human are likely involved in the regulation of emotion and affect. Data regarding brain mechanisms for human mood regulation derive primarily from functional imaging studies in humans during induced mood states or in clinical mood disorders (see Drevets 2000 and Mayberg, Chapter 13, in this volume).
ABN=anterior bed nuclei of median forebrain bundle; AMYG=amygdala; DYN=dynorphin; ENK=enkephalin; GABA=γ-aminobutyric acid; GLU=glutamate; 5-HT=serotonin; LC=locus coeruleus; NE=norepinephrine; OPIOID=endogenous opioid peptide systems; VP=ventral pallidum.
Source.   Modified from Gardner 1997.

should be familiar with the various intoxication and withdrawal syndromes produced by addictive substances. These syndromes, well summarized in DSM-IV-TR (American Psychiatric Association 2000), include several symptoms that overlap phenotypically with mood disorder, including manic-level euphoria, depression, anxiety, appetite disturbances, sleep disturbances, excess energy, and lack of energy. Familiarity with such effects is important in making the differential diagnosis between a mood disorder and intoxication or withdrawal. To some extent, the intoxication syndromes can be viewed as mimicking hypomania, whereas the withdrawal states mimic depressive or anxiety symptoms. This overlap in symptoms again suggests fundamental common ground between the pathophysiology of substance use and mood disorders and invites inquiry into how substance intoxication and withdrawal states might serve as models of mood disorders.

Substance abuse and dependence represent chronic, maladaptive patterns of the use of substances. The DSM-IV-TR criteria are shown in Table 39–1. As can be seen in the table, criteria for substance dependence fall into three broad categories: 1) physiological symptoms (tolerance and withdrawal), 2) loss of control, and 3) psychosocial impairment. Substance use disorders are highly comorbid—that is, a history of one such disorder substantially increases the risk of having others (Grant 1995; Grant and Harford 1995; Grant et al. 2004; Kessler et al. 1994; Regier et al. 1990).

Substance dependence has a typical natural history, with onset in the early- to mid-teenage years. It may remit as young individuals make the transition into adulthood, with its occupational and family responsibilities. However, among some, substance dependence has a chronic, relapsing course. These individuals are most likely to enter treatment, and contrary to popular belief, many effective treatments for drug dependence are available (see later sections of this chapter). However, onset can occur at any age, even among the elderly population.

Several well-established risk factors exist for the development of substance dependence, including availability of substances, without which use and dependence cannot occur. Other risk factors include family history of substance dependence, which reflects a moderate degree of genetic influence; childhood externalizing disorders, such as conduct disorder; and childhood temperamental features, including aggressiveness, impulsivity, and inattention. Adverse events in childhood, such as parental loss (Kendler et al. 2002) or being physically or sexually abused (Kendler et al. 2000), have been implicated as risk factors as well. Animal studies also suggest a role for stress as a risk factor for the development of substance abuse and dependence. The role of stress and trauma in the eti-

ology of both substance use disorders and mood disorders represents another point of common ground between the two sets of disorders.

The diagnostic category of substance abuse has undergone change across different versions of the DSM criteria. DSM-IV-TR conceptualizes substance abuse as a distinct category representing a repeated pattern of use that results in dangerous or life-threatening consequences (most often, driving after drinking too much) (Hasin and Paykin 1999) or severe psychosocial impairment. A common assumption about alcohol abuse is that it is a prodromal condition to dependence. However, longitudinal studies of substance abuse indicate that it often resolves without recurrence or development into dependence (Grant et al. 2001; Hasin et al. 1997; Schuckit et al. 2000), as opposed to dependence, which is more likely to have a chronic, relapsing course. Furthermore, many individuals with dependence do not also meet criteria for abuse, especially women and minorities (Hasin and Grant 2004). Nonetheless, substance abuse is important to distinguish because of its serious and potentially life-threatening consequences, including motor vehicle accidents and violent deaths.

Comorbidity of Mood Disorders and Substance Use Disorders

Clinical Samples and Issues in Diagnostic Assessment

With the introduction of contemporary psychiatric diagnostic criteria, prevalence studies of mood disorders among patients in treatment for substance use disorder began to appear in the literature (for a review, see Hasin et al. 2004). These studies included alcohol-, opiate-, and cocaine-dependent samples. Lifetime rates of major depression in several early studies were in the 30%–50% range, whereas current rates ranged from 10% to 30%. Because the rates were high, concerns were raised that this result actually represented diagnostic confusion with symptoms of intoxication or withdrawal rather than true mood disorders (Schuckit 1986).

In an effort to avoid such misdiagnosis, some early investigators focused on *primary depression*, defined as depression whose lifetime onset predated the onset of the substance use disorder. Studies that used this definition found lower lifetime rates of primary depression, in the range of 10%–20% (Hasin and Nunes 1998). However, the natural history of major depression indicates a later lifetime onset than the onset of substance use disorders. Hence, basing the diagnosis entirely on initial lifetime

---

TABLE 39–1.   DSM-IV-TR criteria for substance abuse and substance dependence

Substance Abuse

A. A maladaptive pattern of substance use leading to clinically significant impairment or distress, as manifested by one (or more) of the following, occurring within a 12-month period:

(1) recurrent substance use resulting in a failure to fulfill major role obligations at work, school, or home (e.g., repeated absences or poor work performance related to substance use; substance-related absences, suspensions, or expulsions from school; neglect of children or household)

(2) recurrent substance use in situations in which it is physically hazardous (e.g., driving an automobile or operating a machine when impaired by substance use)

(3) recurrent substance-related legal problems (e.g., arrests for substance-related disorderly conduct)

(4) continued substance use despite having persistent or recurrent social or interpersonal problems caused or exacerbated by the effects of the substance (e.g., arguments with spouse about consequences of intoxication, physical fights)

B. The symptoms have never met the criteria for substance dependence for this class of substance.

Substance Dependence

A maladaptive pattern of substance use, leading to clinically significant impairment or distress, as manifested by three (or more) of the following, occurring at any time in the same 12-month period:

Physiological symptoms

(1) tolerance, as defined by either of the following:

(a) a need for markedly increased amounts of the substance to achieve intoxication or desired effect

(b) markedly diminished effect with continued use of the same amount of the substance

(2) withdrawal, as manifested by either of the following:

(a) the characteristic withdrawal syndrome for the substance (see specific criteria for substance withdrawal in DSM-IV-TR)

(b) the same (or a closely related) substance is taken to relieve or avoid withdrawal symptoms

Loss of control

(3) the substance is often taken in larger amounts or over a longer period than was intended

(4) there is a persistent desire or unsuccessful efforts to cut down or control substance use

(5) a great deal of time is spent in activities necessary to obtain the substance

Impairment

(6) important social, occupational, or recreational activities are given up or reduced because of substance use

(7) the substance use is continued despite knowledge of having a persistent or recurrent physical or psychological problem that is likely to have been caused or exacerbated by the substance

Source.   Adapted from American Psychiatric Association: *Diagnostic and Statistical Manual of Mental Disorders, 4th Edition, Text Revision.* Washington, DC, American Psychiatric Association, 2000, pp. 197–199. Used with permission. Division of dependence criteria into physiological symptoms, loss of control, and impairment is our addition.

---

onset may cause true depressions among substance abusers to be overlooked. The DSM-IV-TR category of substance-induced mood disorder provides an updated way to address this diagnostic challenge without relying on the order of lifetime onset. In DSM-IV-TR, substance-induced mood disorders are those occurring among substance abusers whose symptoms clearly exceed the expected intoxication and withdrawal symptoms of the drugs being used. The DSM-IV-TR substance-induced category provides recog-

nition of the potential clinical importance of mood disorders among individuals who abuse alcohol or drugs.

Another criticism of these data is that the elevated rates of depression may be a manifestation of Berkson's bias or the clinician's illusion (Cohen and Cohen 1984), whereby patients with multiple disorders are more likely to seek treatment, so that the elevated rate of comorbidity is an artifact of treatment-seeking rather than a reflection of a true relation between the two disorders.

The importance of identifying depressive disorders among substance abusers is highlighted by the relatively consistent finding that a mood disorder, particularly major depression, predicts poor prognosis and treatment outcome among substance-dependent patients. In a recent review (Hasin et al. 2004), prospective studies of the effect of depression on the course of substance dependence were divided into two groups: 1) studies that used mood symptom scales and 2) studies that diagnosed mood disorders with standardized diagnostic criteria and structured interviews. Mood disorders identified by diagnostic criteria (e.g., Greenfield et al. 1998; Hasin et al. 2002) consistently predicted poor outcome of the substance use disorders, whereas the prognostic effect of low mood assessed by symptom scales was much less consistent. Similarly, a lifetime diagnosis of major depression among nicotine-dependent patients reduces the likelihood of sustained smoking cessation (Glassman 1993). Thus, the accumulated evidence indicates that the occurrence of depression in substance-dependent patients is a significant clinical problem and supports the importance of careful clinical diagnosis.

Data on the occurrence of bipolar illness with substance dependence emerge mainly from studies of patients hospitalized or admitted to psychiatric treatment with a primary diagnosis of bipolar illness. Prevalence rates of bipolar illness in substance-dependent patients have been relatively low and variable (for a review, see Hasin et al. 2004), reflecting both the relatively low prevalence of bipolar disorder in the general population and confusion about how to distinguish symptoms of bipolar illness from euphoria, impulsivity, and poor judgment related to substance intoxication. However, studies among samples of bipolar disorder patients suggested that substance abuse and dependence, particularly alcohol and cocaine dependence, are highly prevalent among patients with bipolar disorder and are associated with treatment resistance.

General Population Surveys

The Epidemiologic Catchment Area (ECA) study (Regier et al. 1990), the National Comorbidity Survey (NCS) (Kessler et al. 1994), and the National Longitudinal Alcohol Epidemiologic Survey (NLAES) (Grant 1995; Grant and Harford 1995) were three studies undertaken with the aim of determining the prevalence of psychiatric disorders in large samples representative of the general population. A major advantage of these studies in terms of evaluating comorbidity is that they avoided the concern about Berkson's bias because the samples were not treatment-seeking. A potential for diagnostic confusion

remains; however, in each study, the structured interviewing methods used included features that attempted to help interviewers distinguish true mood disorders from substance-related toxicity or withdrawal effects.

The prevalence of substance use disorders and mood disorders in these studies is presented in Table 39–2, and the odds ratios that represent the degree of association between substance and mood disorders are presented in Table 39–3. (Recall that an odds ratio of 1.0 represents no association; odds ratios greater than 1.0 indicate association, generally considered of a meaningful magnitude when the odds ratio is 2.0 or greater.) As can be seen from the tables, rates of disorders vary across surveys, likely reflecting differences in diagnostic methodology. However, the odds ratios, reflecting degree of association between mood disorders and substance use disorders, are relatively consistent across studies. The data suggest that the presence of a substance use disorder at least doubles the odds of major depression, and the associations of substance use disorders and bipolar disorders are even larger. The associations are also generally larger for current disorders than for lifetime disorders, but they are similar for men and women. Similar findings are emerging from the National Epidemiologic Survey of Alcohol and Related Disorders (Grant et al. 2004), a recently completed large-scale community survey. In summary, the data from these community surveys confirm that the high rate of co-occurrence between mood and substance use disorders is not simply an artifact of treatment-seeking but, instead, reflects some fundamental relations between these syndromes.

Relations Between Mood and Substance Use Disorders

Types of Relations

As has been previously elucidated (Meyer 1986), several types of relations between two comorbid syndromes are theoretically possible. These are summarized in Table 39–4, along with the types of evidence that would support each relation. Mood disorders may function as a causal risk factor for substance abuse or dependence. One mechanism for this could be self-medication (Khantzian 1985), whereby a patient with a mood disorder takes addictive substances in an effort to elevate or control his or her mood. For example, regular drug or alcohol use might be initiated or maintained in an effort to relieve the low mood, low energy, or insomnia associated with depression. Alcohol might be abused in an effort to control excessive energy during mania. However, evidence for such mecha-

TABLE 39–2. Prevalence (% of sample) with substance use disorders in community surveys

	ECA[a]	NCS[b]	NLAES[c]
Lifetime			
Any substance use disorder	16.7	26.6	—
Alcohol dependence	7.9	14.1	13.3
Alcohol abuse only	5.6	9.4	4.9
Drug dependence	3.5	7.5	2.9
Drug abuse only	2.6	4.4	3.1
Current[d]			
Any substance use disorder	6.1	11.3	—
Alcohol dependence	2.8	7.2	4.4
Alcohol abuse only	1.9	2.5	3.0
Drug dependence	1.2	2.8	0.5
Drug abuse only	0.9	0.8	1.1

Note. ECA=Epidemiologic Catchment Area study; NCS=National Comorbidity Survey; NLAES=National Longitudinal Alcohol Epidemiologic Survey.
[a]ECA data are from Regier et al. 1990.
[b]NCS data are from Kessler et al. 1994.
[c]NLAES data are from Grant 1995 and Grant and Harford 1995.
[d]Current disorders are past 6 months for ECA and past year for NCS and NLAES.

nisms has been inconsistent (Aharonovich et al. 2001). Also, the pathophysiology of mood disorders might predispose a patient to substance abuse disorders at a neurochemical level. Conversely, substance abuse or dependence could function as a causal risk factor for mood disorders. Substance abuse might trigger the onset of mood disorders or promote dysregulation in neural systems that regulate mood. In some instances, substance abuse may be a consequence of the impulsivity and poor judgment of bipolar illness, which resolves once mania resolves (Schuckit 1986). Toxic effects of substances may be mistaken for the symptoms of a depressive disorder, resulting in diagnostic confusion (Schuckit 1986). However, a study of a national sample of former drinkers, most of them abstinent for many years, refuted this as a full explanation (Hasin and Grant 2002). In this study, a history of past, remitted DSM-IV (American Psychiatric Association 1994) alcohol dependence increased the risk of current major depression fourfold when use of other drugs and nicotine was controlled. In this study, even the most protracted withdrawal would have had time to resolve, suggesting that some other factor was causing the associa-

tion between alcohol dependence and major depression.

Mood and addictive disorders might share common underlying risk factors. Several analyses of twin studies have suggested common genetic liabilities (Fu et al. 2002; Kendler et al. 1993a, 1993b), predisposing individuals to both sets of disorders. Life events and social stress are environmental risk factors that have been associated with both mood disorders and addictive disorders (Dohrenwend et al. 1992).

Finally, in some individuals, mood disorders and substance use disorders may be independent but co-occur by chance. However, this cannot explain the substantial rates of co-occurrence (see Table 39–2). However, even if the initial occurrence of the two disorders is independent, they may become associated within an individual over time (Meyer 1986). One mechanism for this could be classical conditioning, whereby external environmental stimuli or internal sensations become conditioned cues that trigger drug use behavior. Of particular interest here, unpleasant moods, particularly anger and sadness, have been shown to function as conditioned cues that trigger craving for opiates in opiate-dependent patients (Childress et al. 1994). This association could gradually amplify a link between depression and substance use.

In the following sections, we review various types of evidence that bear on the relation between mood and substance use disorders, including longitudinal studies, family and genetic studies, behavioral and neurobiological evidence, and treatment studies of co-occurring mood and substance use disorders.

Longitudinal Studies

Longitudinal studies that follow up cohorts of individuals from childhood into adolescence and adulthood seeking to uncover risk factors for substance dependence (J.S. Brook et al. 1990; Kellam et al. 1983; Martin et al. 1994; Moss et al. 1994) consistently identify childhood externalizing disorders, such as conduct disorder, as strong risk factors but also identify an anxious-depressive temperament in early childhood as a risk factor. Striking evidence has emerged more recently that early-onset nicotine (Breslau et al. 1993) and marijuana use (D.W. Brook et al. 2002; Fergusson et al. 2002; Patton et al. 2002) increase the subsequent risk for anxiety and depressive disorders. Taken together, these studies suggest a potentially complex bidirectional relation between mood and substance use disorders during development.

In adults, some studies have suggested that cannabis abuse increases subsequent risk for depression (Bovasso 2001; Kuo et al. 2001). Various longitudinal studies have found that a current mood disorder increases the risk for

TABLE 39–3.   Increased risk (odds ratios) for substance use disorders (abuse or dependence) among individuals with mood disorders (or vice versa) in community surveys

	ECA[a]		NCS[a]		NLAES[b]	
	Alcohol	**Drug**	**Alcohol**	**Drug**	**Alcohol**	**Drug**
Lifetime						
Major depression	1.9	3.5	1.9	2.4	3.6	5.2
Dysthymia	2.0	3.2	2.1	2.3		
Bipolar disorder (mania)	4.6	7.4	4.9	4.9		
Current[c]						
Major depression	2.7	3.4	2.6	3.0	3.7	7.2
Dysthymia	1.7	2.0	1.8	4.3		
Bipolar disorder (mania)	3.8	3.2	5.6	5.7		

Note. ECA=Epidemiologic Catchment Area study; NCS=National Comorbidity Survey; NLAES=National Longitudinal Alcohol Epidemiologic Survey.
[a]Data for ECA and NCS are from Kessler 1995. ECA odds ratios calculated on the subsample of participants younger than age 55 years for comparability with the NCS sample.
[b]Data from NLAES are from Grant 1995 and Grant and Harford 1995.
[c]Current disorders are past 6 months for ECA and NCS and past year for NLAES.

poor course and outcome of substance use disorders (for review, see Hasin et al. 2004). For example, a history of major depressive disorder reduces the odds of successfully quitting smoking (Glassman 1993) and increases the risk of relapse to alcohol or drug dependence (Greenfield et al. 1998; Hasin et al. 1996, 2002). Similarly, psychiatric disorders, including depression, have been found to be associated with worse prognosis in samples of opiate- (Rounsaville et al. 1986b), alcohol- (Rounsaville et al. 1987), and cocaine-dependent patients (K.M. Carroll et al. 1993), and substance abuse worsens prognosis in bipolar disorder (Sonne and Brady 1999).

Conversely, among opiate-dependent patients, depression has been found to be transient over long-term follow-up, suggesting that some depressions in this population represent either responses to substance toxicity and withdrawal or responses to psychosocial stress, to which this population is particularly subject (DeLeon et al. 1973; Rounsaville et al. 1986a). Similarly, among alcohol-dependent (S.A. Brown et al. 1995; Liappas et al. 2002) and cocaine-dependent patients (Satel et al. 1991; Weddington et al. 1990), it has been shown that most mood symptoms resolve after detoxification and a brief period of abstinence, again suggesting that these symptoms represent toxic or withdrawal effects. These latter findings relate mainly to depressive symptoms rather than to depressive disorders, which have more clear adverse prognostic effects (Hasin et al. 2004).

In summary, the longitudinal studies, taken together, suggest a complex bidirectional relation between the two sets of disorders—mood disorders may function as a risk factor for substance use disorders, and, conversely, substance use disorders function as a risk factor for mood disorders.

Family and Genetic Studies

Early family studies (Winokur and Coryell 1992) suggested that depressive disorders could be divided into two types: pure depressive disorder and depression spectrum disorder, the latter including a mixture of depression, alcoholism, and other comorbid disorders that appear to aggregate in some families. Family studies have found increased rates of depression among families with alcohol (Schuckit 1986) or drug dependence (Rounsaville et al. 1991), but the pattern suggests various interpretations, including that the disorders aggregate in families but are causally independent. Such a pattern could result from assortative mating, the increased likelihood of individuals with one condition to marry and have children with individuals who have the other disorder.

Adoption studies (Goodwin 1979; Sigvardsson et al. 1996) provided the initial basis for the genetic study of alcoholism by clarifying that among those adopted away at a very early age, alcoholism among the biological but not the adoptive parents predicted alcoholism in the adoptee.

TABLE 39–4.   Potential relations between mood and substance use disorders

Relation	Supporting evidence
Mood disorder is a causal risk factor for substance abuse or dependence (e.g., self-medication).	• Mood disorder precedes onset of substance use disorder (chronologically primary) • Mood disorder associated with greater severity, worse outcome of substance use disorder • Treatment of mood disorder improves substance abuse
Substance abuse or dependence is a causal risk factor for mood disorder.	• Substance use disorder precedes onset of mood disorder (chronologically secondary) • Substance use associated with greater severity, worse prognosis for mood disorder (e.g., in bipolar illness) • Treatment of substance abuse improves mood disorder
Substance toxicity or withdrawal mimics symptoms of mood disorder (i.e., diagnostic confusion).	• Mood symptoms resolve with abstinence
Mood and substance use disorders share common risk factors.	• Twin studies show common genetic factors predisposing to both sets of disorders • Role of stress as risk factor for both
Mood and substance use disorders occur together but are independent disorders.	• Both sets of disorders are common and will co-occur by chance
Mood and substance use disorders become linked over time.	• Co-occurrence associated with greater severity and worse outcome, suggesting interaction • Moods as conditioned cues triggering craving and drug-seeking behavior

However, attempts in adoption studies to identify a subtype of alcohol dependence partially defined by accompanying depressive or anxious traits (Cloninger 1987) were not supported in subsequent research (Babor et al. 1992). Some twin studies (Kendler et al. 1993a, 1993b) have suggested patterns consistent with common genetic risk factors that underlie both substance use disorders and major depression. Other studies suggested that genetic factors for internalizing disorders (including depression) and externalizing disorders (including substance dependence) are largely distinct (Kendler et al. 2003). One study suggested that the common genetic risk may be mediated by antisocial personality traits (Fu et al. 2002), consistent with a typology of alcohol dependence proposed by Babor et al. (1992). These issues may be resolved more clearly when specific genetic polymorphisms are studied.

Identifying specific genes involved in the risk for complex disorders such as substance dependence and major depression has been a challenge, but the progress in understanding the genetic etiology of alcohol dependence is advancing rapidly. Because γ-aminobutyric acid (GABA) transmission mediates several effects of alcohol, GABA receptor genes have been investigated in several studies.

Whole-genome surveys (Long et al. 1998; Reich et al. 1998) implicated the *GABRB1* gene on chromosome 4, as did a study that used brain oscillations measured by electroencephalogram (EEG-β), a trait associated with alcoholism (Porjesz et al. 2002). A study of single nucleotide polymorphisms in the four genes of chromosome 4 that encode subunits of the GABA$_A$ receptor found strong evidence that variation in the *GABRA2* gene influenced both alcohol dependence and EEG-β (Edenberg et al. 2004). Studies designed to generate a similar line of research for major depression (Holmans et al. 2004; Levinson et al. 2003) are now under way. A linkage study of an "either/or" phenotype (alcohol dependence or major depression) in alcoholic probands and their relatives suggested linkage in an area of chromosome 1 that also has been implicated in linkage studies of affective disorders (Nurnberger et al. 2001).

Perspectives From Behavioral Science

Behavioral models of substance use and depression emphasize the role of environmental contingencies (e.g., reinforcement and punishment) in both disorders. Drug dependence is associated with significant psychosocial deficits (e.g., unemployment, lower education) that restrict access to alternative nondrug positive reinforcement and increase the rate of negative life events, both of which increase the probability of substance use and depressive disorders (Dohrenwend et al. 1992; Kessler 1997). Human and animal laboratory studies indicated that the presence of alternative nondrug reinforcers reduced the probability of drug use across a wide range of substances (M.E. Carroll 1996; Hart et al. 2000), and clinical interventions that increased the accessibility of alternative nondrug reinforcement reduced both drug use (Iguchi et al. 1997) and depressive symptoms (Jacobson et al. 1996; Lewinsohn and Graf 1973).

Although the amount of positive reinforcement and punishment in the environment can be an important link between depression and drug dependence, the two disorders also may be linked by changes in the hedonic value of previous reinforcers. As noted earlier, addictive substances function as positive reinforcers, and models of both classical and operant conditioning afford powerful explanatory schemes for these disorders. As also noted earlier, during development of tolerance to an addictive drug, the hedonic value of that drug, as well as of all natural reinforcers, is gradually reduced, as reflected in the model of altered brain stimulation reward thresholds (Gardner 1997). The addictive substance engages the brain reward system so powerfully that the system is rendered less responsive to natural reinforcers, producing an anhedonic state, a state that also could be viewed as a model of depression.

Behavioral formulations of depression also have featured the loss of reinforcer effectiveness as a central factor (Costello 1972). Experimental studies show that individuals with depressive disorders have a blunted response to pleasurable stimuli compared with nondepressed people (Berenbaum and Oltmanns 1992; Sloan et al. 2001). Corresponding animal models, such as the forced swim test, are useful in predicting the efficacy of antidepressant medications. The inability to escape aversive conditions is a model of psychological stress, and similar stress that has been modeled in animals has been found to increase the propensity of animals to self-administer various drugs (Goeders 2003). Thus, similarities between behavioral models of mood disorders and behavioral models of addiction emerge with respect to environmental contingencies (e.g., positive reinforcement), response to stress, and status of the brain reward system. Pathophysiological models of depression have tended to focus on neurochemical deficits (e.g., serotonin system deficits) (Malone and Mann 1993) or corticotropin-releasing factor excess (Nemeroff 1992). The notion of depression as a disorder

of the brain reward system has received less attention but is an implication of the comorbidity of mood and substance use disorders that may represent a promising direction for future research (see Naranjo et al. 2001).

Neurobiological Commonalities

A comprehensive review by Markou et al. (1998) examined the evidence on derangements in a wide variety of neurochemical and neurohumoral systems, including serotonin and corticotropin-releasing factor, in depressed and substance-dependent populations. The review found substantial concordance—that is, derangements that tended to point in the same direction in both sets of disorders. Such findings strengthen the argument for a pathophysiological common ground.

Brain imaging offers another framework to elucidate neuroanatomical and neurochemical relations between substance use disorders and other psychiatric disorders (Volkow 2001). Broadly speaking, human brain imaging studies support the notion of an overlap in the brain pathways that are involved in the symptomatic expression of substance dependence and depression (see Figure 39–1). Such outlining of shared circuitry, without necessarily specifying particular neurotransmitter abnormalities within the circuitry, is an important first step in establishing neurobiological commonality between substance use and mood disorders. Much of this transmitter-neutral information comes from positron emission tomography (PET) or single photon emission computed tomography (SPECT) studies of regional neural metabolism or cerebral blood flow, procedures that show regional patterns of neurophysiological activity. Such functional and structural imaging studies have identified deficits in the frontal lobes in association with various forms of substance dependence (Goldstein and Volkow 2002). Frontal deficits also have been implicated in depressive disorders (Drevets 2000) (see Mayberg, Chapter 13, in this volume). Overall, the human functional imaging data implicate frontal-striatal-limbic circuitry in executive, motivational, and emotional functioning of both humans and laboratory animals (Heimer 2003). Common deficits in these systems observed in mood and substance use disorders suggest pathophysiological common ground as well as ways in which understanding the pathophysiology of both disorders might be enhanced.

Less consensus emerges from the sparser literature on brain imaging studies of specific transmitter systems implicated in human substance use and mood disorders. Availability of striatal D_2 dopamine receptors has been reduced in association with substance use disorders (Goldstein and Volkow 2002). The notion of a "dopamine hypothesis" for depression remains controversial (Naranjo et al. 2001).

Other neurochemical commonalities between the pathophysiology of substance abuse and mood disorders are emerging from imaging studies. Zubieta et al. (2003) reported involvement of the μ-opioid system, an important site of action in opiate addiction, in human mood regulation. During induced sadness, μ-opioid transmission was decreased in the anterior cingulate cortex, ventral pallidum, amygdala, and inferior temporal cortex. These regions, plus the hypothalamus and insular cortex, showed a correlation between the degree of experienced depressed mood and μ-opioid activity.

Another area of active study is focused on GABA and glutamate, the dominant inhibitory and excitatory transmitters, respectively, involved in cortical-subcortical interactions in both mood regulation and drug abuse. Many recent reports on these transmitters in animal models of drug dependence, often based on invasive procedures such as microdialysis or intracerebral infusion of transmitter agonists or antagonists, have been published (Bardo 1998; Cousins et al. 2002; Gerasimov et al. 1999). At the same time, noninvasive imaging studies in humans, particularly those that used magnetic resonance imaging (MRI), indicated a shared feature of decreased cortical GABA in both substance abuse and mood disorders (Hetherington et al. 2000; Sanacora et al. 2000).

Rapid advances currently being made in MRI and other imaging modalities will undoubtedly identify further neurochemical bases for interactions between substance use disorders and mood disorders. Finally, the power of functional imaging to detect neural bases for such interactions can be enhanced by increasing the diagnostic rigor used to characterize affective states during imaging of drug users and by comparing groups with mood disorder alone, substance dependence alone, and a combination of both disorders (Rubin et al. 2003).

Treatment Studies of Co-occurring Mood and Substance Use Disorders

In unipolar depression, several reports of clinical trials have accumulated in the literature that examined the treatment of depression with antidepressant medications in substance-dependent populations, including treatment-seeking alcoholic patients, opiate-addicted patients, and cocaine-dependent patients. A recent meta-analysis (Nunes and Levin 2004) identified 14 studies that used rigorous diagnostic criteria to identify unipolar depressive disorders in samples of treatment-seeking substance-dependent patients. These studies had small to moderate sample sizes, in the range of 30–130 patients, which speaks to the difficulty of recruiting for a clinical trial

patients with two major concurrent disorders. Nevertheless, more than half of the studies reported significant or trend antidepressant effects (i.e., antidepressant medication was effective in treating depressive symptoms among these substance-dependent patients). Among studies with an effect size on depressive outcome of at least 0.5, a significant effect of medication on self-reported substance abuse outcome also was found. This suggests that when medication was effective in treating depression, it also was helpful in treating substance abuse. This pattern is suggestive of a causal relation in which mood disorders are functioning as risk factors for substance abuse such that mood improvement helps reduce substance abuse.

However, some cautionary notes arise regardng this meta-analysis. Rates of sustained abstinence were low in most of the studies reviewed and differed little between medication and placebo groups. Thus, treatment of depression is far from a panacea in such dually diagnosed patients, concurrent efforts to treat the substance use disorders directly are also needed, and the influence of depression on addictions is modest from an etiological standpoint. Many of the studies had high placebo response rates, and high placebo response was associated with a failure to detect medication–placebo differences. Such high placebo response rates may reflect the difficulty in implementing diagnostic methods that can successfully select true depressive disorders, as opposed to transient mood syndromes resulting from substance toxicity or stress. Interestingly, larger effect sizes were associated with studies that required a period of abstinence prior to diagnosis of depression, an association that is consistent with the classic recommendation that a period of abstinence is necessary for an accurate mood disorder diagnosis (Brady et al. 1999; Schuckit 1986). High placebo response and lack of medication–placebo differences also were associated with provision of manual-guided psychotherapies to trial participants. This suggests both the promise of such psychotherapeutic approaches as treatments for dual diagnoses and the limitations that such treatments impose as design features on the ability to detect medication effects.

Fewer randomized trials of bipolar illness have been done. A small placebo-controlled trial in adolescents with substance abuse and bipolar illness found lithium superior to placebo in improving both mood and substance use outcome (Geller et al. 1998). Carbamazepine was studied in a placebo-controlled trial in cocaine-dependent patients with or without a lifetime history of mood disorder, many in the bipolar spectrum (Brady et al. 2002). The study found trends toward a favorable effect of carbamazepine on cocaine use outcome among patients with a history of mood disorders. Similar to the findings from the meta-analysis regarding unipolar depression (Nunes and Levin 2004), these studies suggest the utility of treatment for bipolar spectrum illness in influencing the outcome of comorbid substance abuse and support a model in which the bipolar illness functions as a causal risk factor promoting substance abuse.

Clinical Approach to Co-occurring Mood and Substance Use Disorders

Evaluation of Substance Use in Patients With Mood Disorders

In view of their prevalence and prognostic implications, a careful screening and diagnostic assessment for substance use disorders is an essential element of the clinical history and evaluation of any patient with a mood disorder. Although screening instruments exist and may be useful (Levin et al. 2004), the most important tool is a careful clinical history that seeks evidence of substance use, abuse, or dependence, according to DSM-IV-TR criteria. Practice with the Structured Clinical Interview for DSM-IV (SCID) or similar structured instruments can be useful training in how to ask about these symptoms. It is important to inquire about substance use and abuse in an accepting and nonjudgmental fashion because substance use disorders are still stigmatized, and patients may be defensive and motivated to conceal or minimize the extent of substance use. Gentle inquiry with an accepting stance is often sufficient to overcome this. Biological testing using urine toxicology or breath-alcohol levels is often advisable if concealment is suspected.

As part of the evaluation process, it is important to anticipate potential intoxication and withdrawal symptoms, which can confuse the diagnostic picture. Also, if the patient is abstinent, withdrawal symptoms may emerge and need to be treated. Withdrawal symptoms are often benign and can be treated in an office setting. However, alcohol and sedative-hypnotic withdrawal can be quite serious or even life threatening, and opiate withdrawal is extremely unpleasant and almost invariably leads to relapse unless treated aggressively.

Evaluation of Mood Disorders in Patients With Substance Use Disorders

The essential problem is that of distinguishing true mood disorders from mood symptoms that represent substance toxicity or withdrawal. No sure method exists for solving this problem, as reflected in the results of the meta-analysis discussed earlier in the "Treatment Studies of Co-occurring Mood and Substance Use Disorders" section (Nunes and Levin 2004), which showed that despite efforts at careful

clinical diagnosis, high placebo response rates, consistent with the selection of transient mood disturbances, were a problem in some of the trials. Various approaches have been developed to address this problem (Nunes et al. 2004), many of which are integrated in the DSM-IV-TR constructs of primary and substance-induced depression.

In brief, a DSM-IV-TR primary syndrome is one that has been shown to occur independently of substance abuse over time; that is, during abstinence from substances. A substance-induced mood syndrome is one that has never occurred independent of substance use but in which the symptoms are in excess of what would be expected given the toxic and withdrawal effects of the substances alone. Substance use disorders often have an early onset and a chronic course, making it difficult to find a period of abstinence in the history during which to inquire about mood disorders. The substance-induced category recognizes that depression in this setting still may be clinically significant. Both primary and substance-induced depression are to be distinguished from usual, expected toxic or withdrawal effects of substances.

The DSM-IV-TR criteria for primary depression are straightforward and can be determined by taking a careful parallel history of mood and substance problems over the lifetime, but DSM-IV-TR is less clear on specific criteria for substance-induced mood disorder, leaving this to the clinician's judgment. The Psychiatric Research Interview for Substance and Mental Disorders (PRISM) is a structured clinical interview that provides a reliable method for diagnosing primary and substance-induced depression among substance-dependent patients. Predictive validity has been established in that both PRISM-identified primary and substance-induced depressions have been shown to have adverse prognostic effects among substance-dependent patients (Hasin et al. 2002). Clinicians might be encouraged to practice interviewing with the PRISM as a way of developing interviewing skills with dual diagnosis patients. Other historical features to look for include severity or chronicity of depressive symptoms, suicidality, and other comorbid disorders such as anxiety or personality syndromes (Nunes et al. 2004). Such features would suggest that the mood syndrome is in excess of what would be expected from routine toxic or withdrawal symptoms from substances. The surest method of diagnosing a mood disorder is to have the patient become abstinent for a period of time before making a final evaluation. Thus, all such patients should be encouraged to make an attempt to achieve abstinence. However, hospitalization is less of an option in the current health care system, and then clinicians often will have a patient who is actively using substances and has a mood syndrome that needs diagnostic assessment and treatment planning.

Treatment of Substance Abuse in Patients With Mood Disorders

Complete coverage of the treatment of substance use disorders is well beyond the scope of this chapter. Excellent textbooks exist (e.g., Galanter and Kleber 2004). Nonetheless, substance use or abuse is likely to worsen mood symptoms, which may resolve if abstinence is achieved, and substance abuse increases suicide risk (Aharonovich et al. 2002; Levy and Deykin 1989; Murphy et al. 1992). Therefore, treatment of substance use disorders should be a high priority from the outset in mood disorder patients presenting with substance abuse. We believe that all clinicians should be familiar with the basic tools for treating substance use disorders.

Psychosocial and Behavioral Methods

Several psychosocial and behavioral methods are likely to be particularly useful to general clinicians and those working with patients with mood disorders. Even simple advice from a physician to quit substance use can be an effective intervention (Fleming et al. 1997). For patients with ambivalence or resistance to giving up drugs or alcohol (which is to be expected), motivational interviewing is a useful tool that shows substantial evidence of efficacy (Miller and Rollnick 2002). Motivational interviewing shifts the clinician away from an authoritarian stance and toward an empathic and collaborative approach, seeking to elicit the patient's own point of view, concerns about substances, and reasons for quitting.

Self-help groups, such as Alcoholics Anonymous, have a strong tradition, and most communities have active groups of this type. Evidence suggests that referral to 12-step groups is effective (Project MATCH Research Group 1997), and it is useful for clinicians to be familiar with their principles and procedures to encourage patients to participate (Emrick and Tonigan 2004).

Other useful techniques include cognitive-behavioral relapse prevention, which is based on social learning theory and seeks to help patients to see the connections between events within themselves and their environment that trigger substance use (K.M. Carroll et al. 2004), and the use of positive reinforcement with voucher incentives (Higgins et al. 1993; Silverman et al. 1996).

Pharmacotherapy

For nicotine, alcohol, and opiate dependence, a general psychiatrist should be familiar with and relatively comfortable in using several effective medication treatments. As a general rule, such medications are more effective when used in concert with some form of psychosocial intervention.

Nicotine dependence is very common among psychiatric patients and can be effectively treated with nicotine-replacement products, including nicotine-containing chewing gum and nicotine patches (Hughes et al. 1996), which are available over the counter. Patients should be encouraged to set a quit date on which they will apply the nicotine patch and chew nicotine gum at times when they experience craving for a cigarette. If patients fail to quit or relapse to smoking, it is best to praise their effort and suggest that they try again. This positive, encouraging approach is important in the treatment of any substance dependence. Furthermore, in the case of nicotine dependence, the statistics suggest that any single quit attempt has a low likelihood of success, but patients who try to quit repeatedly are likely to succeed eventually. Noradrenergic antidepressant medications, including bupropion (Hurt et al. 1997) and nortriptyline (Hall et al. 1998), are also effective for smoking cessation; they should be started several weeks before the determined quit date and can be used in concert with nicotine replacement. Interestingly, these medications may work by reducing the dysphoric symptoms that often follow smoking cessation (Hall et al. 1998). The typical recommendation would be to discontinue the antidepressant several months after successful quitting, although evidence now shows that continuation of the medication has a role in preventing relapse (Hays et al. 2001). It is also important to be aware that major depression may emerge after a successful quit attempt (Glassman 1993).

Detoxification from alcohol is usually benign and can be treated supportively or with a tapering schedule of a long-acting benzodiazepine such as chlordiazepoxide. For prevention of alcohol relapse, disulfiram is a clinical tool that is rarely used, even though it can be extremely effective if its daily ingestion is monitored by a significant other (Schuckit and Tapert 2004). Disulfiram impairs the metabolism of acetaldehyde, a toxic by-product of alcohol metabolism, such that any drinking produces an unpleasant reaction. The opiate antagonist naltrexone is also modestly effective for alcohol dependence (Kranzler and Van Kirk 2001), particularly in combination with relapse prevention therapy. Again, involvement of a significant other to monitor the medication is likely to be helpful. Interestingly, naltrexone may act by blunting the reinforcing effects of alcohol or may interfere with the role of moods, both positive and negative, in triggering drinking behavior (Kranzler et al. 2004).

For opiate dependence, methadone maintenance is a powerful treatment (Schottenfeld 2004), although it is for the most part little known and poorly understood by general clinicians. Methadone is an orally bioavailable, long-acting opiate agonist that terminates opiate withdrawal and, when given at sufficiently high doses over a prolonged period, induces tolerance and blockade of the effects of other opiates. By law, methadone maintenance can be administered only by specially licensed clinics. Buprenorphine, a long-acting partial opiate agonist, is an alternative to methadone maintenance and can be prescribed by any physician who has taken a brief training course and received certification. It is hoped that this will increase the involvement of general physicians in treatment of opiate dependence and attract more opiate-dependent patients into treatment. The opiate antagonist naltrexone is an effective maintenance treatment for opiate dependence as long as patients take it; drawbacks include that it requires detoxification from opiates before it can be safety started (otherwise it precipitates withdrawal), and compliance is usually poor (O'Brien and Kampman 2004). Recent efforts to improve compliance and effectiveness by combining naltrexone with various psychosocial and behavioral techniques show promise (Rothenberg et al. 2002). In addition, formulation of naltrexone into long-lasting depot injections may markedly increase the effectiveness of this treatment in the future (Comer et al. 2002).

Treatment of Mood Disorders in Patients With Substance Use Disorders

Depression

The evidence on treatment of depression among substance-dependent patients, reviewed earlier in this chapter in the section "Treatment Studies of Co-Occurring Mood and Substance Use Disorders" (Nunes and Levin 2004), suggests that depressive syndromes, carefully diagnosed by clinical history according to standard diagnostic criteria, respond to antidepressant medications. The placebo response rates reported were often high, reflecting either diagnostic confusion and poor selection of patients or favorable effects of concurrent psychotherapy. Some of the largest antidepressant effects were seen in studies that required a period of abstinence from substances prior to diagnosis of depression. In view of this evidence, the most prudent clinical approach is to start by encouraging abstinence and offer psychosocial methods or pharmacotherapy to help initiate abstinence. After a period of treatment for the substance use disorder and an effort to achieve abstinence, if the depression persists, then it should be treated with either antidepressant medication or specific psychotherapy. It is important not to delay treatment of depression beyond a reasonable period, even if abstinence is not achieved, because such depression may have adverse prognostic effects (Hasin et al. 2002) and risk of suicide

(Aharonovich et al. 2002; Levy and Deykin 1989; Murphy et al. 1992). Finally, the evidence from clinical trials suggests that treatment of depression, even in the setting of active substance abuse, can be effective (Nunes and Levin 2004).

Although tricyclic antidepressants show more evidence of efficacy among the published clinical trials (Nunes and Levin 2004), selective serotonin reuptake inhibitors (SSRIs) have shown efficacy in several trials (Cornelius et al. 1997; Roy 1998). SSRIs can be recommended as the first treatment of choice in dually diagnosed patients because of the good tolerability and low toxicity of these agents. If an SSRI fails, then antidepressant agents with alternative mechanisms should be considered. Agents with antianxiety or soporific effects (e.g., tricyclic antidepressants or trazodone) should be considered, particularly for patients with substantial anxiety or insomnia as components of their depression. As always, the potential risks of combining therapeutic medications with substances of abuse need to be weighed. More research is needed on the use of psychotherapeutic techniques that have been designed specifically for the treatment of depression. Preliminary research suggests that cognitive-behavioral therapy for depression was useful in reducing alcohol abuse in a dually diagnosed sample of patients (R.A. Brown et al. 1997).

Bipolar Disorder

As noted earlier, few systematic placebo-controlled trials of treatment of bipolar illness have been done among substance-dependent patients (Brady and Malcolm 2004). Small controlled trials suggest that both lithium (Geller et al. 1998) and the anticonvulsant carbamazepine (Brady et al. 2002) are effective among such patients. Concurrent specific treatment for substance use disorders is important, and an integrative group therapy approach has shown promise in this regard (Weiss et al. 2000).

Future Directions

The comorbidity of mood and substance use disorders has been a long-standing source of controversy for the field. Clinicians at one time were polarized into camps, either viewing substance abuse as the predominant force among comorbid patients, with mood symptoms representing mainly toxic effects, or viewing the mood disturbance as predominant and substance abuse as a response to it, as in self-medication. Research from recent decades, reviewed here, suggests a multiplicity of possible relationships between mood and substance use disorders (see

Table 39–4), the high prevalence of comorbidity clinically, and potential common ground at the neurobiological level. A challenge for the future will be to design more research that seeks to translate findings and insights back and forth across basic and clinical disciplines and across disorders, and it is hoped that this chapter has stimulated interest in the potential of this approach.

At the clinical level, clinicians, services, and treatment systems remain, in many instances, polarized into those that provide care for mood and other psychiatric disorders and those that provide care for addictions, and the availability of treatment for mood disorders in substance abuse treatment settings remains uneven (Petrakis et al. 2003). The challenge here is to place evaluation and treatment of substance use, as well as of mood disorders, among the core skills of psychiatrists and allied mental health professionals and to design more integrated systems of care.

References

Aharonovich E, Nguyen HT, Nunes EV: Anger and depressive states among treatment-seeking drug abusers: testing the psychopharmacological specificity hypothesis. Am J Addict 10:327–334, 2001

Aharonovich E, Liu X, Nunes E, et al: Suicide attempts in substance abusers: effects of major depression in relation to substance use disorders. Am J Psychiatry 159:1600–1602, 2002

American Psychiatric Association: Diagnostic and Statistical Manual of Mental Disorders, 4th Edition. Washington, DC, American Psychiatric Association, 1994

American Psychiatric Association: Diagnostic and Statistical Manual of Mental Disorders, 4th Edition, Text Revision. Washington, DC, American Psychiatric Association, 2000

Babor TF, Hoffman M, Delboca FK, et al: Types of alcoholics, I: evidence for an empirically derived typology based on indicators of vulnerability and severity. Arch Gen Psychiatry 49:599–608, 1992

Bardo MT: Neuropharmacological mechanisms of drug reward: beyond dopamine in the nucleus accumbens. Crit Rev Neurobiol 12:37–67, 1998

Berenbaum H, Oltmanns TE: Emotional experience and expression in schizophrenia and depression. J Abnorm Psychol 101:37–44, 1992

Bovasso GB: Cannabis abuse as a risk factor for depressive symptoms. Am J Psychiatry 158:2033–2037, 2001

Brady KT, Malcolm RJ: Substance use disorders and co-occurring Axis I psychiatric disorders, in The American Psychiatric Publishing Textbook of Substance Abuse Treatment, 3rd Edition. Edited by Galanter M, Kleber HD. Arlington, VA, American Psychiatric Publishing, 2004, pp 529–537

Brady KT, Halligan P, Malcolm RJ: Dual diagnosis, in The American Psychiatric Press Textbook of Substance Abuse Treatment, 2nd Edition. Edited by Galanter M, Kleber HD. Washington, DC, American Psychiatric Press, 1999, pp 475–483

Brady KT, Sonne SC, Malcolm RJ, et al: Carbamazepine in the treatment of cocaine dependence: subtyping by affective disorder. Exp Clin Psychopharmacol 10:276–285, 2002

Breslau N, Kilbey MM, Andreski P: Nicotine dependence and major depression: new evidence from a prospective investigation. Arch Gen Psychiatry 50:31–35, 1993

Brook DW, Brook JS, Zhang C, et al: Drug use and the risk of major depressive disorder, alcohol dependence and substance use disorders. Arch Gen Psychiatry 59:1039–1044, 2002

Brook JS, Brook DW, Gordon AS, et al: The psychosocial etiology of adolescent drug use: a family interactional approach. Genet Soc Gen Psychol Monogr 116:111–267, 1990

Brown RA, Evans DM, Miller IW, et al: Cognitive-behavioral treatment for depression in alcoholism. J Consult Clin Psychol 65:715–726, 1997

Brown SA, Inaba RK, Gillin JC, et al: Alcoholism and affective disorder: clinical course of depressive symptoms. Am J Psychiatry 152:45–52, 1995

Carroll KM, Power ME, Bryant K, et al: One-year follow-up status of treatment-seeking cocaine abusers: psychopathology and dependence severity as predictors of outcome. J Nerv Ment Dis 181:71–79, 1993

Carroll KM, Ball SA, Martino S: Cognitive, behavioral, and motivational therapies, in The American Psychiatric Publishing Textbook of Substance Abuse Treatment, 3rd Edition. Edited by Galanter M, Kleber HD. Arlington, VA, American Psychiatric Publishing, 2004, pp 365–376

Carroll ME: Reducing drug abuse by enriching the environment with alternative reinforcers, in Advances in Behavioral Economics: Substance Use and Abuse, Vol 3. Edited by Green L, Kagel JH. Norwood, NJ, Ablex Publishing, 1996, pp 37–68

Childress AR, Ehrman R, McLellan AT, et al: Can induced moods trigger drug-related responses in opiate abuse patients? J Subst Abuse Treat 11:17–23, 1994

Cloninger CR: Neurogenetic adaptive mechanisms in alcoholism. Science 236:410–416, 1987

Cohen P, Cohen J: The clinician's illusion. Arch Gen Psychiatry 41:1178–1182, 1984

Comer SD, Collins ED, Kleber HD, et al: Depot naltrexone: long-lasting antagonism of the effects of heroin in humans. Psychopharmacology 159:351–360, 2002

Cornelius JR, Salloum IM, Ehler JG, et al: Fluoxetine in depressed alcoholics: a double-blind, placebo-controlled trial. Arch Gen Psychiatry 54:700–705, 1997

Costello CG: Depression: loss of reinforcers or loss of reinforcer effectiveness? Behav Ther 3:240–247, 1972

Cousins MS, Roberts DC, de Wit H: GABA(B) receptor agonists for the treatment of drug addiction: a review of recent findings. Drug Alcohol Depend 65:209–220, 2002

DeLeon G, Skodol A, Rosenthal MS: Phoenix House: changes in psychopathological signs of resident addicts. Arch Gen Psychiatry 28:131–135, 1973

Dohrenwend BP, Levav I, Shrout PE, et al: Socioeconomic status and psychiatric disorders: the causation-selection issue. Science 255:946–952, 1992

Drevets WC: Neuroimaging studies of mood disorders. Biol Psychiatry 48:813–829, 2000

Edenberg HJ, Dick DM, Xuei X, et al: Variations in GABRA2, encoding the alpha 2 subunit of the GABA(A) receptor, are associated with alcohol dependence and with brain oscillations. Am J Hum Genet 74:705–714, 2004

Emrick CD, Tonigan JS: Alcoholics Anonymous and other 12-step groups, in The American Psychiatric Publishing Textbook of Substance Abuse Treatment, 3rd Edition. Edited by Galanter M, Kleber HD. Arlington, VA, American Psychiatric Publishing, 2004, pp 433–443

Fergusson DM, Horwood LJ, Swain-Campbell N: Cannabis use and psychosocial adjustment in adolescence and young adulthood. Addiction 97:1123–1135, 2002

Fleming MF, Barry KL, Manwell LB, et al: Brief physician advice for problem alcohol drinkers: a randomized controlled trial in community-based primary care practices. JAMA 277:1039–1045, 1997

Fu Q, Heath AC, Bucholz KK, et al: Shared genetic risk of major depression, alcohol dependence, and marijuana dependence: contribution of antisocial personality disorder in men. Arch Gen Psychiatry 59:1125–1132, 2002

Galanter M, Kleber HD (eds): The American Psychiatric Publishing Textbook of Substance Abuse Treatment, 3rd Edition. Arlington, VA, American Psychiatric Publishing, 2004

Gardner EL: Brain reward mechanisms, in Substance Abuse: A Comprehensive Textbook. Edited by Lowinson JH, Ruiz P, Millman RB, et al. Baltimore, MD, Williams & Wilkins, 1997, pp 51–85

Geller B, Cooper TB, Sun K, et al: Double-blind and placebo-controlled study of lithium for adolescent bipolar disorders with secondary substance dependency. J Am Acad Child Adolesc Psychiatry 37:171–178, 1998

Gerasimov MR, Ashby CR Jr, Gardner EL, et al: Gamma-vinyl GABA inhibits methamphetamine, heroin, or ethanol-induced increases in nucleus accumbens dopamine. Synapse 34:11–19, 1999

Glassman AH: Cigarette smoking: implications for psychiatric illness. Am J Psychiatry 150:546–553, 1993

Goeders NE: The impact of stress on addiction. Eur Neuropsychopharmacol 13:435–441, 2003

Goldstein RZ, Volkow ND: Drug addiction and its underlying neurobiological basis: neuroimaging evidence for the involvement of the frontal cortex. Am J Psychiatry 159:1642–1652, 2002

Goodwin DW: Alcoholism and heredity. Arch Gen Psychiatry 36:57–61, 1979

Grant BF: Comorbidity between DSM-IV drug use disorders and major depression: results of a national survey. J Subst Abuse 7:481–497, 1995

Grant BF, Harford TC: Comorbidity between DSM-IV alcohol use disorders and major depression: results of a national survey. Drug Alcohol Depend 39:197–206, 1995

Grant BF, Stinson FS, Harford TC: Age at onset of alcohol use and DSM-IV alcohol abuse and dependence: a 12-year follow-up. J Subst Abuse 13:493–504, 2001

Grant BF, Stinson FS, Dawson DA, et al: Prevalence and co-occurrence of substance use disorders and independent mood and anxiety disorders: results from the National Epidemiologic Survey on Alcohol and Related Conditions (NESARC). Arch Gen Psychiatry 61:807–816, 2004

Greenfield SF, Weiss RD, Muenz LR, et al: The effect of depression on return to drinking: a prospective study. Arch Gen Psychiatry 55:259–265, 1998

Hall SM, Reus VI, Munoz RF, et al: Nortriptyline and cognitive-behavioral therapy in the treatment of cigarette smoking. Arch Gen Psychiatry 55:683–690, 1998

Hart CL, Haney M, Foltin RW, et al: Alternative reinforcers differentially modify cocaine self-administration by humans. Behav Pharmacol 11:87–91, 2000

Hasin DS, Grant BF: Major depression in 6,050 former drinkers: association with past alcohol dependence. Arch Gen Psychiatry 59:794–800, 2002

Hasin DS, Grant BF: The co-occurrence of DSM-IV alcohol abuse in DSM-IV alcohol dependence: NESARC results on heterogeneity that differs by population subgroup. Arch Gen Psychiatry 61:891–896, 2004

Hasin D, Paykin A: DSM-IV alcohol abuse: investigation in a sample of at-risk drinkers in the community. J Stud Alcohol 60:180–187, 1999

Hasin D, Tsai W, Endicott J, et al: The effects of major depression on alcoholism: five year course. Am J Addict 5:144–155, 1996

Hasin D, Van Rossem R, McCloud S, et al: Differentiating DSM-IV alcohol dependence and abuse by course: community heavy drinkers. J Subst Abuse 9:127–135, 1997

Hasin D, Liu X, Nunes E, et al: Effects of major depression on remission and relapse of substance dependence. Arch Gen Psychiatry 59:375–380, 2002

Hasin D, Nunes E, Meydan J: Comorbidity of alcohol, drug and psychiatric disorders: epidemiology, in Dual Diagnosis and Treatment: Substance Abuse and Comorbid Disorders, 2nd Edition. Edited by Kranzler HR, Tinsley JA. New York, Marcel Dekker, 2004, pp 1–34

Hays JT, Hurt RD, Rigotti NA, et al: Sustained-release bupropion for pharmacologic relapse prevention after smoking cessation: a randomized, controlled trial. Ann Intern Med 135:423–433, 2001

Heimer L: A new anatomical framework for neuropsychiatric disorders and drug abuse. Am J Psychiatry 160:1726–1739, 2003

Hetherington HP, Pan JW, Telang F, et al: Reduced brain GABA levels in cocaine abusers (abstract no. 523). Paper presented at the Proceedings of the International Society of Magnetic Resonance Medicine, Denver, CO, April 3–7, 2000

Higgins ST, Budney AJ, Bickel WK, et al: Achieving cocaine abstinence with a behavioral approach. Am J Psychiatry 150:763–769, 1993

Holmans P, Zubenko GS, Crowe RR, et al: Genomewide significant linkage to recurrent, early onset major depressive disorder on chromosome 15q. Am J Hum Genet 74:1154–1167, 2004

Hughes JR, Fiester S, Goldstein M, et al: American Psychiatric Association practice guideline for the treatment of patients with nicotine dependence. Am J Psychiatry 153 (suppl 10):S1–S31, 1996

Hurt RD, Sachs DP, Glover ED, et al: A comparison of sustained-release bupropion and placebo for smoking cessation. N Engl J Med 337:1195–1202, 1997

Iguchi MY, Belding MA, Morral AR, et al: Reinforcing operants other than abstinence in drug abuse treatment: an effective alternative for reducing drug use. J Consult Clin Psychol 65:421–428, 1997

Jacobson NS, Dobson K, Truax PA, et al: A component analysis of cognitive-behavioral treatment for depression. J Consult Clin Psychol 64:295–304, 1996

Johanson CE, Schuster CR: Animal models of drug self-administration, in Advances in Substance Abuse, Vol 2. Edited by Mello NK. Greenwich, CT, JAI Press, 1981, pp 219–297

Kellam SG, Brown CH, Rubin BR, et al: Paths leading to teenage psychiatric symptoms and substance use: developmental epidemiological studies in Woodlawn, in Childhood Psychopathology and Development. Edited by Guze SB, Earls FJ, Barrett JE. New York, Raven, 1983, pp 17–51

Kendler KS, Heath AC, Neale MC, et al: Alcoholism and major depression in women: a twin study of the causes of comorbidity. Arch Gen Psychiatry 50:690–698, 1993a

Kendler KS, Neale MC, MacLean CJ, et al: Smoking and major depression: a causal analysis. Arch Gen Psychiatry 50:36–43, 1993b

Kendler KS, Bulik CM, Silberg J, et al: Childhood sexual abuse and adult psychiatric and substance use disorders in women. Arch Gen Psychiatry 57:953–959, 2000

Kendler KS, Sheth K, Gardner CO, et al: Childhood parental loss and risk for first-onset of major depression and alcohol dependence: the time-decay of risk and sex differences. Psychol Med 32:1187–1194, 2002

Kendler KS, Prescott CA, Myers JK, et al: The structure of genetic and environmental risk factors for common psychiatric and substance use disorders in men and women. Arch Gen Psychiatry 60:929–937, 2003

Kessler RC: Epidemiology of psychiatric comorbidity, in Textbook in Psychiatric Epidemiology. Edited by Tsuang MT, Tohen M, Zahner GEP. New York, Wiley, 1995, pp 179–197

Kessler RC: The effects of stressful life events on depression. Annu Rev Psychol 48:191–214, 1997

Kessler R, McGonagle K, Zhao S, et al: Lifetime and 12-month prevalence of DSM-III-R psychiatric disorders in the United States: results from the National Comorbidity Survey. Arch Gen Psychiatry 51:8–19, 1994

Khantzian EJ: The self-medication hypothesis of addictive disorders: focus on heroin and cocaine dependence. Am J Psychiatry 142:1259–1264, 1985

Kranzler HR, Van Kirk J: Efficacy of naltrexone and acamprosate for alcoholism treatment: a meta-analysis. Alcohol Clin Exp Res 25:1335–1341, 2001

Kranzler HR, Armeli S, Feinn R, et al: Targeted naltrexone treatment moderates the relations between mood and drinking behavior among problem drinkers. J Consult Clin Psychol 72:317–327, 2004

Kuo WH, Gallo JJ, Tien AY: Incidence of suicide ideation and attempts in adults: the 13-year follow-up of a community sample in Baltimore, Maryland. Psychol Med 31:1181–1191, 2001

Levin FR, Gunderson EW, Levounis P: Medical education, in The American Psychiatric Publishing Textbook of Substance Abuse Treatment, 3rd Edition. Edited by Galanter M, Kleber HD. Arlington, VA, American Psychiatric Publishing, 2004, pp 597–609

Levinson DF, Zubenko GS, Crowe RR, et al: Genetics of recurrent early onset depression (GenRED): design and preliminary clinical characteristics of a repository sample for genetic linkage studies. Am J Med Genet 119B:118–130, 2003

Levy JC, Deykin EY: Suicidality, depression, and substance abuse in adolescence. Am J Psychiatry 146:1462–1467, 1989

Lewinsohn PM, Graf M: Pleasant activities and depression. J Consult Clin Psychol 41:261–268, 1973

Liappas J, Paparrigopoulos E, Tzavellas G, et al: Impact of alcohol detoxification on anxiety and depressive symptoms. Drug Alcohol Depend 68:215–220, 2002

Long JC, Knowler WC, Hanson R, et al: Evidence for genetic linkage to alcohol dependence on chromosomes 4 and 11 from an autosome-wide scan in an American Indian population. Am J Med Genet 81:216–221, 1998

Malone K, Mann JJ: Serotonin and depression, in Biology of Depressive Disorders, Part A: A Systems Perspectives. Edited by Mann JJ, Kupfer DJ. New York, Plenum, 1993, pp 29–49

Markou A, Kosten TR, Koob GF: Neurobiologic similarities in depression and drug dependence: a self-medication hypothesis. Neuropsychopharmacology 18:135–174, 1998

Martin CS, Earleywine M, Blackson TC, et al: Aggressivity, inattention, hyperactivity, and impulsivity in boys at high and low risk for substance abuse. J Abnorm Child Psychol 22:177–203, 1994

Meyer RE: How to understand the relationship between psychopathology and addictive disorders: another example of the chicken and the egg, in Psychopathology and Addictive Disorders. Edited by Meyer RE. New York, Guilford, 1986, pp 3–16

Miller WR, Rollnick S: Motivational Interviewing: Preparing People for Change, 2nd Edition. New York, Guilford, 2002

Moss HB, Majumder PP, Vanyukov M: Familial resemblance for psychoactive substance use disorders: behavioral profile of high risk boys. Addict Behav 19:199–208, 1994

Murphy GE, Wetzel RD, Robins E, et al: Multiple risk factors predict suicide in alcoholism. Arch Gen Psychiatry 49:459–463, 1992

Naranjo CA, Tremblay LK, Busto U: The role of the brain reward system in depression. Prog Neuropsychopharmacol Biol Psychiatry 25:781–823, 2001

Nemeroff CB: New vistas in neuropeptide research in neuropsychiatry: focus on corticotropin-releasing factor. Neuropsychopharmacology 6:69–75, 1992

Nestler EJ: Cellular responses to chronic treatment with drugs of abuse. Crit Rev Neurobiol 7:23–39, 1993

Nunes EV, Levin FR: Treatment of depression in patients with alcohol or drug dependence: a meta-analysis. JAMA 291:1887–1896, 2004

Nunes E, Hasin D, Blanco C: Substance abuse and psychiatric co-morbidity: overview of diagnostic methods, diagnostic criteria, structured and semi-structured interviews, and biological markers, in Dual Diagnosis and Treatment: Substance Abuse and Comorbid Disorders, 2nd Edition. Edited by Kranzler HR, Tinsley JA. New York, Marcel Dekker, 2004, pp 61–101

Nurnberger JI, Foroud T, Flury L, et al: Evidence for a locus on chromosome 1 that influences vulnerability to alcoholism and affective disorder. Am J Psychiatry 158:718–724, 2001

O'Brien CP, Kampman KM: Opioids: antagonists and partial agonists, in The American Psychiatric Publishing Textbook of Substance Abuse Treatment, 3rd Edition. Edited by Galanter M, Kleber HD. Arlington, VA, American Psychiatric Publishing, 2004, pp 305–319

Patton GC, Coffey C, Carlin JB, et al: Cannabis use and mental health in young people: cohort study. BMJ 325:1195–1198, 2002

Petrakis IL, Leslie D, Rosenheck R: The use of antidepressants in alcohol dependent veterans. J Clin Psychiatry 64:865–870, 2003

Porjesz B, Almasy L, Edenberg HJ, et al: Linkage disequilibrium between the beta frequency of the human EEG and a GABAA receptor gene locus. Proc Natl Acad Sci U S A 99:3729–3733, 2002

Project MATCH Research Group: Matching alcoholism treatments to client heterogeneity: Project MATCH posttreatment drinking outcomes. J Stud Alcohol 58:7–29, 1997

Regier DA, Farmer ME, Rae DS, et al: Comorbidity of mental disorders with alcohol and other drug abuse: results from the Epidemiological Catchment Area (ECA) study. JAMA 264:2511–2518, 1990

Reich T, Edenberg HJ, Goate A, et al: Genome-wide search for genes affecting the risk for alcohol dependence. Am J Med Genet 81:207–215, 1998

Robbins TW, Everitt BJ: Limbic-striatal memory systems and drug addiction. Neurobiol Learn Mem 78:625–636, 2002

Rothenberg JL, Sullivan MA, Church SH, et al: Behavioral naltrexone therapy: an integrated treatment for opiate dependence. J Subst Abuse Treat 23:351–360, 2002

Rounsaville BJ, Kosten TR, Kleber HD: Long-term changes in current psychiatric diagnoses of treated opiate addicts. Compr Psychiatry 27:480–498, 1986a

Rounsaville BJ, Kosten TR, Weissman MM, et al: Prognostic significance of psychopathology in treated opiate addicts: a 2.5 year follow-up study. Arch Gen Psychiatry 43:739–745, 1986b

Rounsaville BJ, Dolinsky ZS, Babor TF, et al: Psychopathology as a predictor of treatment outcome in alcoholics. Arch Gen Psychiatry 44:505–513, 1987

Rounsaville BJ, Kosten TR, Weisman MM, et al: Psychiatric disorders in relatives of probands with opiate addiction. Arch Gen Psychiatry 48:33ñ42, 1991

Roy A: Placebo-controlled study of sertraline in depressed recently abstinent alcoholics. Biol Psychiatry 44:633–637, 1998

Rubin E, Nunes E, Koetitz R, et al: Brain metabolism in early cocaine abstinence: relationship to drug use and mood. Abstract presented at the 65th annual meeting of the College on Problems of Drug Dependence, Bal Harbour, FL, June 2003

Sanacora G, Mason GF, Krystal JH: Impairment of GABAergic transmission in depression: new insights from neuroimaging studies. Crit Rev Neurobiol 14:23–45, 2000

Satel SL, Price LH, Palumbo JM, et al: Clinical phenomenology and neurobiology of cocaine abstinence: a prospective inpatient study. Am J Psychiatry 148:1712–1716, 1991

Schottenfeld RS: Opioids: maintenance treatment, in The American Psychiatric Publishing Textbook of Substance Abuse Treatment, 3rd Edition. Edited by Galanter M, Kleber HD. Arlington, VA, American Psychiatric Publishing, 2004, pp 291–304

Schuckit MA: Genetic and clinical implications of alcoholics and affective disorder. Am J Psychiatry 143:140–147, 1986

Schuckit MA, Tapert S: Alcohol, in The American Psychiatric Publishing Textbook of Substance Abuse Treatment, 3rd Edition. Edited by Galanter M, Kleber HD. Arlington, VA, American Psychiatric Publishing, 2004, pp 151–166

Schuckit MA, Smith TL, Landi NA: The 5-year clinical course of high-functioning men with DSM-IV alcohol abuse or dependence. Am J Psychiatry 157:2028–2035, 2000

Sigvardsson S, Bohman M, Cloninger CR: Replication of the Stockholm Adoption Study of alcoholism: confirmatory cross-fostering analysis. Arch Gen Psychiatry 53:681–687, 1996

Silverman K, Higgins ST, Brooner RK, et al: Sustained cocaine abstinence in methadone maintenance patients through voucher-based reinforcement therapy. Arch Gen Psychiatry 53:409–415, 1996

Sloan DM, Strauss ME, Wisner KL: Diminished response to pleasant stimuli by depressed women. J Abnorm Psychol 110:488–493, 2001

Sonne SC, Brady KT: Substance abuse and bipolar comorbidity. Psychiatr Clin North Am 22:609–627, 1999

Volkow ND: Drug abuse and mental illness: progress in understanding comorbidity. Am J Psychiatry 158:1181–1183, 2001

Weddington WW, Brown BS, Haertzen CA, et al: Changes in mood, craving, and sleep during short-term abstinence reported by male cocaine addicts: a controlled, residential study. Arch Gen Psychiatry 47:861–868, 1990

Weiss RD, Griffin ML, Greenfield SF, et al: Group therapy for patients with bipolar disorder and substance dependence: results of a pilot study. J Clin Psychiatry 61:361–367, 2000

Winokur G, Coryell W: Familial subtypes of unipolar depression: a prospective study of familial pure depressive disease compared to depression spectrum disease. Biol Psychiatry 32:1012–1018, 1992

Zubieta JK, Ketter TA, Bueller JA, et al: Regulation of human affective responses by anterior cingulate and limbic mu-opioid neurotransmission. Arch Gen Psychiatry 60:1145–1153, 2003

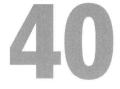

Depression and Personality

SHIRLEY YEN, PH.D.

MEGHAN E. McDEVITT-MURPHY, PH.D.

M. TRACIE SHEA, PH.D.

THE RELEVANCE OF PERSONALITY to depression is apparent in the long history and sizable literature devoted to this topic. Examples include theories implicating personality in the etiology of depression, various attempts to define meaningful subtypes of depression, and more simply, attempts to determine the effect of personality on the course and treatment response in depression. The term *personality* is broad, and the literature relevant to the current chapter covers a wide range of different conceptualizations of personality, including traits and disorders. The earliest attention to personality in depression was focused on certain traits that were observed as common in individuals with depression. Subsequent to the introduction of Axis II in DSM-III (American Psychiatric Association 1980), attention to the personality disorders and their relevance to depressed patients has been more prominent. Consistent findings of high rates of comorbidity between personality disorders and depressive disorders underscore the importance of understanding the relation between these disorders and the implications of personality psychopathology for the prognosis and treatment of depression.

We begin this chapter with an overview of assessment issues and available measures of personality traits and disor-

ders, followed by a summary of findings on the rates of personality disorders in depressed samples. Next, we address the various ways in which the relation between personality psychopathology and depression has been conceptualized, including the most prominent personality dimensions that have been postulated and studied in connection with depression. We then summarize findings on the prognostic importance of personality disorders in outcome of treatment for depression. Finally, we discuss treatment approaches and strategies for depression with co-occurring personality disorders and specific issues in establishing rapport and maintaining safety in the clinical care of these patients.

Relation Between Personality and Depression: Assessment and Prevalence

There is an inherent paradox in the assessment of personality disorders, as Widiger (1993) aptly pointed out: namely, that "the assessment is based in large part on self-descriptions by persons who are characterized in part by distorted, inaccurate perceptions and presentations of themselves" (p. 101). The task of diagnosing personality disorder in the presence of depression is particularly complicated because of the potential for additional response distortion caused by the thought patterns characteristic of depression; patients tend to rate their personality as more pathological when depressed than when not depressed (O'Boyle and Self 1990). A critical task in assessing personality disorder is establishing the course of symptoms over time and determining whether personality disorder symptoms are pervasive and persistent, that is, occurring across situations and throughout adulthood. Furthermore, they should be independent of the fluctuations of extreme stress, medical conditions that may affect personality, or Axis I disorders, particularly major depressive disorder, in which traits are exclusionary for some personality features (e.g., loss of interest in sex during depressive episodes should not be considered for the schizoid personality disorder trait of little interest in having sexual experiences).

Because of the particular challenges of assessing personality disorders, such as poor insight, ego-syntonicity, and potential response biases, clinicians should take advantage of behavioral observations occurring naturalistically. The patient's behavior while interacting with the clinician and staff, as well as with significant others, offers a rich source of data for making a personality disorder diagnosis.

Various standardized self-report and interview instruments exist to assess personality traits and disorders. (See Kaye and Shea [2002] for a detailed review of these instruments.) Table 40–1 presents information on several of the most commonly used instruments. Self-report instruments refer to those completed by respondents in questionnaire format and are relatively easy to administer (i.e., not time-intensive for the clinician). However, self-report measures tend to be oversensitive and have only moderate psychometric reliability (Widiger and Frances 1987). Furthermore, it is difficult to discern whether endorsed symptoms are more characteristic of an Axis I disorder or personality disorder pathology. Semistructured interviews are designed to be administered by a trained and experienced clinician. These diagnostic interviews, although labor-intensive, offer the clinician the opportunity to use follow-up questions or prompts and thus more accurately judge a symptom's presence or absence. In structured or semistructured interviews, the solicitation of examples is of utmost importance. When questioning patients about personality disorder criteria, each affirmative response should be followed by a request for examples so that the clinician can judge the degree to which the behavior is characteristic of a given diagnosis (or should be excluded

because it is better accounted for by an Axis I disorder). Assessment instruments also vary with regard to source of information, organizational structure (e.g., by diagnosis vs. content), and whether they provide categorical or continuous scores. Depending on the goal of the assessment, these factors are important to consider because interviews can be lengthy.

When the administration of standardized assessment instruments is not possible because of time or logistical constraints, personality disorder must be diagnosed via a standard clinical interview. This is the most frequent method of personality disorder assessment in clinical settings. Ideally, a "LEAD" standard (longitudual, expert, all data), in which all available data, including intake assessments, past records, data from informants, observational data from inpatient stays, and response to treatment, would be used in diagnosing personality disorders (Perry 1992).

The development and psychometric validation of semistructured clinical interviews enable studies to estimate the prevalence of personality disorders. A review of studies found that the prevalence of DSM-III-defined personality disorders was estimated to be between 6% and 9% of the general population (Corruble et al. 1996). Furthermore, an estimated 20%–50% of inpatients and 50%–85% of outpatients with a current major depressive disorder have an associated personality disorder, with the Cluster B disorders of borderline (10%–30%), histrionic (2%–20%), and antisocial (0%–10%) being most predominant. In a large-scale epidemiologic study, the prevalence of 7 of the 10 DSM-IV personality disorders was assessed. It was estimated that approximately 15% of adults in the United States has at least one personality disorder (Grant et al. 2004). A study using ICD-10 personality disorder criteria estimated that approximately 6.5% of the adult population in Australia has one or more personality disorders (Jackson and Burgess 2000). Rates across studies are highly variable, partially because of variations in methodology such as the use of different diagnostic criteria (DSM-III, DSM-III-R, DSM-IV [American Psychiatric Association 1980, 1987, 1994]; ICD-9, ICD-10 [World Health Organization 1977, 1992]) and assessment instruments.

These same methodological limitations extend to studies estimating the prevalence of personality disorders among those with lifetime (as opposed to current) major depression and the prevalence of current or lifetime major depression among patients with personality disorders have not been widely examined. A study of first-degree relatives of a predominantly patient sample reported that among individuals with a lifetime diagnosis of major depression, 13% met criteria for schizotypal personality dis-

TABLE 40–1. Self-report and interview assessment instruments for Axis II disorders

Instrument	Authors	Time to administer (min)	Categorical or dimensional	DSM-IV-TR correspondent?
Self-Report Instruments				
Millon Clinical Multiaxial Inventory—III	Millon et al. (1994)	30	Both	Yes
Personality Diagnostic Questionnaire—4+	Hyler (1994)	20–30	Categorical	Yes
Schedule for Nonadaptive and Adaptive Personality	Clark (1993)	45	Both	Yes, also includes scales measuring non-DSM traits
NEO Personality Inventory—Revised	Costa and McCrae (1992)	30–45	Dimensional	No, scales measure five-factor model traits
Personality Assessment Inventory	Morey (1991)	45–60	Dimensional	In part[a]
Interviews				
Diagnostic Interview for DSM-IV Personality Disorders	Zanarini et al. (1996)	90	Categorical	Yes
International Personality Disorder Examination	Loranger (1999)	90	Both	Yes[b]
Personality Disorder Interview—IV	Widiger et al. (1995)	90–120	Both	Yes
Structured Clinical Interview for DSM-IV Axis II Personality Disorders	First et al. (1996)	60	Categorical	Yes
Structured Interview for DSM-IV Personality	Pfohl et al. (1997)	90	Categorical	Yes

Note. DSM-IV-TR=*Diagnostic and Statistical Manual of Mental Disorders*, 4th Edition, Text Revision (American Psychiatric Association 2000).
[a]The Personality Assessment Inventory includes several scales relevant to DSM-IV-TR Axis I disorders and two scales relevant to Axis II disorders (borderline and antisocial personality disorders).
[b]An ICD-10 (World Health Organization 1992) version of the International Personality Disorder Examination also exists.

order, 10% for histrionic personality disorder, 9% for passive-aggressive personality disorder, 8% for antisocial personality disorder, and 7% for borderline and avoidant personality disorders each, with the remaining personality disorders diagnosed at a rate of less than 5% (Zimmerman and Coryell 1989). In this same study, the lifetime prevalence of major depression among individuals with no personality disorders was found to be 9%; among those who had a diagnosis of personality disorder, the lifetime prevalence rate of major depression ranged between 0% (schizoid personality disorder) and 80% (avoidant personality disorder) (Zimmerman and Coryell 1989). Other personality disorders associated with a high lifetime prevalence rate of major depression include schizotypal (65%), borderline (61%), histrionic (46%), passive-aggressive (38%), antisocial (35%), obsessive-compulsive (31%), paranoid (29%), and dependent (29%) (Zimmerman and Coryell 1989). An examination of inpatients with unipolar and bipolar affective disorders using DSM-IV personality disorder criteria found the most frequently co-occurring disorders among unipolar inpatients to be borderline (32%), dependent (25%), and obsessive-compulsive (14%). Among inpatients with bipolar disorder, the most frequently diagnosed personality disorders were borderline (41%), narcissistic (21%), and dependent (13%) (Schiavone et al. 2004). A recent study that used ICD personality disorder criteria found a personality disorder comorbidity rate of 22% among those who also met criteria for a major depressive disorder, recruited from a community sample (Casey et al. 2004). In general, personality disorders are highly comorbid with one another and with Axis I disorders, which has raised questions as to the validity of current diagnostic constructs and criteria.

Relation Between Personality and Depression: Conceptualization and Empirical Findings

The nature of the personality–depression relation has been understood from quite different perspectives. Several models have been articulated to explain the associations (Klein et al. 1993). Some of these models focus on causal or etiological associations; for example, one view, referred to as the *vulnerability model*, is that certain personality traits or disorders represent a predisposition, or vulnerability, to developing depression. Furthermore, certain types of life events, such as losses or failures, are hypothesized as more likely to precipitate depression in such individuals. This model assumes that the disorders are distinct but causally related through conditions of one that increase risk for another. A similar model, the *complication* or *scar model*, also assumes that depressive and personality disorders are distinct but that one condition develops as a result or complication of another. For example, a severe or prolonged episode of depression can lead to interpersonal dependency. The difference is that the scar model emphasizes the persistence of the second condition even after recovery from the initial disorder. The *spectrum model* suggests that personality and depression are distinct but arise from the same original causes. A closely related view, referred to as the *subclinical model*, sees the personality features as manifestations of a mood disorder rather than as distinct phenomena. For example, the negative dysphoric affect of borderline personality disorder may be understood as a manifestation of a chronic mood disorder, or the affect lability may be understood as a manifestation of an underlying bipolar disorder. In summary, these models are useful in illuminating the various ways in which personality and depression may be linked, but much conceptual overlap among them exists because they are not mutually exclusive, and it is very difficult to test these models empirically (Klein et al. 1993).

One prospective study that has examined the relation between selected personality disorders and Axis I disorders has identified a significant longitudinal association between borderline personality disorder and major depressive disorder, in that changes in the status for these disorders are closely linked in time (Shea et al. 2004). Furthermore, among individuals with major depressive disorder, those with comorbid schizotypal, borderline, and

avoidant personality disorders had a significantly longer time to remission compared with depressed individuals without personality disorders (Grilo et al. 2005). These results provide support for the notion of shared dimensions of psychopathology between major depressive disorder and borderline personality disorder (Shea et al. 2004). However, methodological limitations preclude the determination of the exact mechanism of etiological association.

One specific spectrum model involves four crosscutting dimensions, each with a psychobiological basis, that span Axis I and personality disorders (Siever and Davis 1991). The *cognitive and perceptual organization dimension* is characterized by disorganized and psychotic-like symptoms that may be seen in schizophrenia or Cluster A personality disorders such as schizotypal personality disorder. Evidence for this hypothesis comes from attention and information-processing tests that have shown similar abnormalities in schizophrenic and schizotypal personality disorder patients (Siever 1985). The *impulsivity and aggression dimension* is hypothesized to be genetically transmitted and related to reductions in serotonergic activity (Coccaro et al. 1989). Characteristic traits can be seen in impulsive disorders of both Axis I disorders (e.g., substance use disorders) and Axis II disorders (e.g., Cluster B personality disorders). The *affective instability dimension* is also speculated to be genetically transmitted but has greater associations with abnormalities in cholinergic and catecholaminergic functioning (Siever 1985). Characterized by transient affective shifts, disturbances in this dimension can be seen in major mood disorders and Cluster B disorders, particularly borderline personality disorder. In fact, some have speculated that Cluster B personality disorders (particularly borderline personality disorder) represent subsyndromal disturbances in affect regulation, which reflect an underlying diathesis to bipolar disorder (Akiskal 1994). Finally, the *anxiety and inhibition dimension* is characterized by autonomic arousal, fearfulness, and inhibition and can be seen in the anxiety disorders and Cluster C personality disorders, particularly avoidant personality disorder. This heuristic approach offers an alternative framework, supported by evidence from biological and genetic studies, from which to understand the interactions between personality traits or disorders and depression.

Dimensional models of personality traits and their relation to depression also have been the focus of theoretical and empirical investigation (Table 40–2). Starting with Kraepelin, several writers described a "depressive personality," characterized by features such as persistent gloominess, seriousness, proneness to guilt and self-reproach, and low self-confidence. The traits were described as becoming apparent by late adolescence or early adulthood and persisting throughout the person's lifetime (Kraepe-

TABLE 40–2. Personality traits and depression

Personality trait	Description	Relevant models
Depressive temperament	Gloomy, serious, guilt-ridden, self-reproaching, low self-confidence	Spectrum and subclinical
Depressive character	Helpless, dependent, guilty, self-deprecating	Vulnerability
Sociotropy or interpersonal dependency; reward dependence	Uses interpersonal relationships to maintain self-esteem	Vulnerability
Autonomy or self-criticism	Uses achievement and goals to maintain self-esteem	Vulnerability
Neuroticism or negative affectivity	Stable propensity to experience range of negative affects (e.g., dysphoria, anxiety, guilt, hostility, self-dissatisfaction)	Vulnerability Spectrum and subclinical
Introversion or low positive affectivity	Stable propensity toward low positive affect, low energy, low affiliation, low dominance	Vulnerability Spectrum and subclinical

lin 1921). In Kraepelin's view, these traits were manifestations of inherited temperament and formed the basis from which more severe episodes of depression arose. Schneider (1958) described a depressive type of personality with similar features but placed greater emphasis on the role of developmental and environmental factors in their origin. Psychoanalytic theorists described similar depressive types (depressive character), but, like Schneider, they emphasized the importance of early developmental influences related to disturbed relationships.

Other theorists have described personality types that are vulnerable to depression because of maladaptive mechanisms for maintaining self-esteem. Psychoanalytic and cognitive-behavioral theories have independently proposed very similar personality traits linked to corresponding types of depression. Interpersonal dependency (Blatt et al. 1976; Hirschfeld et al. 1977) is similar to the construct of sociotropy (Beck 1983). Both refer to a tendency to achieve or maintain self-esteem through interpersonal relationships, resulting in an increased vulnerability to depression when such relationships are lost or fail. Autonomy (Beck 1983), self-criticism (Blatt et al. 1976), and dominant-goal personalities (Arieti and Bemporad 1980) all refer to the tendency to establish or maintain self-esteem by achievements. Failure to meet the excessively high internal standards leads to self-criticism and depression.

Neuroticism and introversion or extraversion, derived from factor analytic studies beginning with Eysenck's work (Eysenck 1990), have been studied extensively in relation to depression. More recent refinement and modification of these two robust dimensions have led to similar dimensions called *negative affectivity* and *positive affectivity*,

respectively (Clark and Watson 1991). Both are described as stable and heritable temperamental traits. The essence of negative emotionality or neuroticism is sensitivity to negative stimuli and the propensity to experience a broad range of negative mood states, including not only depression and dysphoria but also anxiety, guilt, hostility, and self-dissatisfaction. In addition, high levels of negative affectivity or neuroticism are characterized by negative cognitions, low self-esteem, and life dissatisfaction (Clark et al. 1994). This dimension is clearly very similar to the depressive personality types described earlier. Positive affectivity or extraversion refers to the propensity to experience positive mood states, as well as energy, affiliation, and dominance. The low end of this dimension captures the absence of positive affect (i.e., introversion). Both of these dimensions are understood as stable traits, but they also have a state component. That is, levels of the mood states may increase and decrease at different times, relative to the characteristic level for an individual. High levels of negative affectivity or neuroticism have been associated not only with depressive disorders but also with anxiety disorders. Low levels of positive affectivity or extraversion (low energy and activity levels, withdrawal, decreased cognitive capacity, anhedonia, depressed mood) may have a more specific association with depression (Clark et al. 1994).

Another dimensional model (Cloninger 1986, 1987) proposes a basic set of heritable traits (novelty-seeking, harm avoidance, and reward dependence), each associated with a different neurobiological system. Of these, reward dependence is most closely related to depressive symptoms. A high level of this trait is characterized by a strong need for praise and approval of others and strong sensitivity to social cues or rejection—clearly overlapping with the interpersonal dependency or sociotropy construct described earlier in this section.

Of all of the personality dimensions examined in relation to depression, negative affectivity or neuroticism has shown the strongest and most consistent empirical support. The other traits (e.g., depressive personality; interpersonal dependency or sociotropy; self-criticism; reward dependence) likely reflect components of the negative affectivity or neuroticism construct. Prospective studies with assessments prior to the first onset of depression have shown negative affectivity or neuroticism to be a significant predictor of depression, suggesting this dimension represents a vulnerability to depression. Other studies have reported that negative affectivity or neuroticism predicts a more chronic course of depression and a poorer overall outcome (Hirschfeld et al. 1986). Research also has suggested that the significant association between negative affectivity or neuroticism and major depression is a result of genetic factors that predispose to both neuroticism and depression (Kendler et al. 1993).

Another interpretation of the "vulnerability" findings is that negative affectivity or neuroticism is simply a subsyndromal manifestation of depression rather than a distinct personality trait (Hirschfeld et al. 1989). Recently, dimensional approaches to the classification of depression, in which the disorder would be represented on a continuum as opposed to discrete categories, have been under consideration (First et al. 2002). A similar ongoing debate has been occurring with regard to personality disorders, in which the distinctions between normal personality functioning and personality disorders and among specific disorders are often unclear. For example, borderline personality disorder can be understood as extreme variants of angry hostility, impulsivity, and other traits that are often evident in the nonpsychiatric population (First et al. 2002). Furthermore, given the centrality and commonality of affective styles and temperament to both personality and depression, the meaningfulness of making conceptual distinctions between mood and personality disorders has been questioned (Klein et al. 1993).

Influence of Personality Disorders on Outcome of Treatment for Depression

The association between depressive disorders and personality traits or disorders also can be seen in treatment outcome studies. In examining the relation between per-

sonality disorders and depression, the predominant conclusion among empirical studies as well as clinically based reviews is that having a comorbid personality disorder is a negative prognostic factor in the course and outcome of major depression. For example, personality disorders have been found to predict the development of depression (Alnaes and Torgersen 1997) as well as relapse to depression (Hart et al. 2001; Ilardi et al. 1997). Furthermore, having a comorbid personality disorder can have a negative effect on the treatment of depression (Shea et al. 1990). High levels of personality pathology predict higher rates of depression recurrence and a shorter time to recurrence during the maintenance phase of treatment (Cyranowski et al. 2004), and less severe personality dysfunction predicts early recovery among persons with less severe depression (Meyers et al. 2002). Although few studies have examined whether and how personality traits affect depressive symptomatology and vice versa, relatively more studies have focused on examining the effect of personality disorder on treatment efficacy for depression. Nevertheless, there continues to be a general lack of consensus as to whether having a personality disorder negatively affects somatic and psychosocial treatment for depression. Earlier studies and reviews seemed to suggest that having a personality disorder diagnosis had a negative, nonspecific effect on the treatment of depression. However, more recent studies and reviews have presented mixed findings. Some have suggested that studies that implement more rigorous controls do not find that personality traits or disorders have a negative effect on treatment of depression (Mulder et al. 2003), whereas others have noted that the design of rigorously controlled studies may in fact neutralize some of the potentially detrimental effects of personality disorders (e.g., such studies have more stringent inclusion and exclusion criteria, and they may remove early dropouts from analyses) (Reich 2003). The following is a brief synopsis of such studies based on type of treatment.

Psychotherapy

Earlier studies of psychosocial treatment outcome generally found worse outcomes among depressed patients with personality disorders compared with depressed patients without personality disorders (Shea et al. 1992). In the National Institute of Mental Health Treatment of Depression Collaborative Research Program, patients with personality disorders did not have different mean depression scores at termination but did have significantly less improvement on measures of social and global functioning compared with depressed patients without personality disorders (Shea et al. 1990). This pattern of worse outcome was present in all treatment conditions, with the exception of cognitive-behavioral therapy. Additionally, Hardy and colleagues (1995) reported that patients with Cluster C personality disorders did not respond differently from those without personality disorders after 1 year of cognitive-behavioral therapy. In contrast, the same study found that Cluster C patients receiving psychodynamic interpersonal therapy improved less than did those without a Cluster C personality disorder (Hardy et al. 1995). Therefore, these earlier studies suggested that, in findings similar to those for somatic treatments, depressed patients with comorbid personality disorders show a less favorable response to short-term psychotherapy, although this also may vary depending on the type of therapy and the specific personality disorder.

Relative to the field of research on pharmacotherapy, there has been very little focus on psychotherapy outcome for depressed patients with comorbid personality disorders. Although many medication trials have been conducted without adjunctive psychotherapy for the treatment of depression, most studies of psychotherapy involve adjunctive pharmacotherapy. One study that examined combined psychotherapy and antidepressant treatment in a sample of depressive outpatients found that those with personality disorders were slower responders to treatment (Frank et al. 1987; Pilkonis and Frank 1988). The personality disorders most represented were avoidant, compulsive, and dependent; more severe disorders were excluded on the basis of study exclusion criteria. One possible explanation for the different rates of response is that those without personality disorders had a more rapid response to the tricyclic medication, whereas those with personality disorders were responding primarily to the interpersonal therapy (Frank et al. 1987; Pilkonis and Frank 1988). In a 6-month randomized clinical trial of antidepressants alone and combined with psychotherapy, Kool et al. (2003) reported that combined therapy was more effective than pharmacotherapy for depressed patients with personality disorders, but it was not more effective than pharmacotherapy alone for depressed patients without personality disorders. Even though it remains unclear whether personality disorders have a negative effect on treatment efficacy, these results do reaffirm the recommendation that a combination of antidepressant medication and psychotherapy is the best treatment for depressed patients with comorbid personality disorders.

Somatic Treatments

An early review that examined studies published from 1981 to 1991 reported that in all six studies that examined response to antidepressant treatment, depressed patients with personality disorders had a poorer response to antidepressant medication than did those without a personality disorder (Shea et al. 1992). Most of these studies were naturalistic treatment studies or were based on chart reviews. More recently, with the advent of new drug treatments, some randomized, controlled studies have examined the efficacy of pharmacological interventions for treatment of depression while also ascertaining the effect of personality disorders. One study of chronic major depression (i.e., double depression) in which subjects were randomized to either sertraline or imipramine found that personality disorder comorbidity did not appear to diminish symptomatic response to acute treatment (Russell et al. 2003). However, potential subjects with severe personality disorders, such as borderline and antisocial personality disorders, were excluded from the study, and Cluster C disorders were most frequently represented in the sample.

Among other studies, specific interactions between Axis I disorders and comorbid personality traits or disorders have been observed. A recent randomized, controlled treatment study reported that depressed patients with comorbid Cluster B personality disorders had a relatively poor response to nortriptyline compared with fluoxetine (Joyce et al. 2003; Mulder et al. 2003). The investigators also found that in comparing depressed patients with comorbid borderline personality disorder, other personality disorders, and no personality disorder, those with other personality disorders had consistently worse outcomes (Joyce et al. 2003). In fact, depressed patients with borderline personality disorder were found to have a good outcome at 6 months and were even comparable to those with no personality disorders on measures of depressive symptoms and social functioning. This finding is contrary to what would be predicted given the numerous empirical studies reporting a worse prognostic outcome associated with borderline personality disorder compared with other personality disorders. The specific drug type by personality disorder interaction may be an indicator that the underlying mechanisms of borderline personality disorder and major depressive disorder overlap to a greater extent compared with other personality disorders and major depressive disorder.

Compared with the proliferation of pharmacological treatment studies, fewer studies have examined electroconvulsive therapy (ECT) in depressed patients with comorbid personality disorder. Two reviews of ECT studies offered consistent evidence that depressed patients with personality disorders, especially borderline personality disorder, have a poorer outcome (De Battista and Mueller 2001; Ilardi and Craighead 1995). One retrospective review of 107 inpatients with a major depressive episode found that those with a personality disorder (particularly Cluster B) had a poorer acute response to ECT than did those without a personality disorder (Sareen et al. 2000). Among responders, a higher relapse rate of depression was seen. However, better-controlled studies provide the weakest evidence that personality disorders adversely affect treatment outcome (Mulder 2002).

As evident from this review, much inconsistency exists in the empirical literature as to whether personality disorders negatively affect treatment of depression. One potential source for the inconsistency is that these studies are often based on varying samples, which greatly limits generalizability. Many clinical trials of depressed patients exclude individuals who are suicidal or self-injuring, and many of the reviewed studies of depression and personality disorders exclude severe personality disorders (typically borderline and antisocial personality disorders). Even studies of one disorder, such as borderline personality disorder, will have great variability in the severity of the illness in the sample population. In a study that included more severely ill patients, dialectical behavior therapy (DBT) treatment was not effective in reducing depressive symptomatology (Linehan et al. 1991). Not surprisingly, when the population is more severely ill, the treatment outcomes tend to be less promising.

Another source of sample inconsistency lies with the unclear distinctions between the personality disorders that occur because studies often collapse multiple disorders into one category, thus possibly obscuring some meaningful effects. Furthermore, issues of measurement remain a major problem because the ways in which personality disorders are diagnosed vary greatly (Mulder 2002). Related to the issue of measurement is the variability in designs; they range from naturalistic observational studies that rely on chart review for diagnoses to controlled studies that use diagnostic structured interviews. Although it has been argued that those with more rigorous designs are preferable to determine whether personality disorders affect treatment of depression (Mulder 2002), it can be similarly argued that controlled trials are much less generalizable than naturalistic conditions in which the treatment provider assigns a clinical diagnosis on the basis of all sources of information. Furthermore, although controlled trials are optimal for measuring treatment outcome and use more valid diagnostic assessments, they are less ideal for examining the process of treatment, including factors that pertain more to personality pathology, such as alliance building and rapport. Regardless, it seems evident from more recent studies that there may be specific interactions between depression, type of personality pathology, and type of treatment that may affect treatment outcome.

Treatment of Depression With Comorbid Personality Disorders

Although treatment outcome for depression may be affected by personality traits or personality disorders, substantial overlap exists among treatment strategies (psychosocial and pharmacological) for depression and personality disorders. Because of the heterogeneity of personality disorders, and the wide spectrum of traits that could potentially affect treatment, it is unlikely that any one medication or treatment could ameliorate the personality dysfunction that is often associated with depression or affects depression. For example, medications cannot address character issues, dysfunctional attitudes, or environmental stressors; these issues are best addressed through psychotherapy, with pharmacotherapy as an adjunctive treatment (Soloff 1998).

Psychosocial treatment is strongly recommended for the depressed patient with personality disorder or extreme personality traits (Oldham et al. 2001). To date, two therapeutic approaches have been found to be effective in randomized, controlled treatment trials for reducing symptoms associated with both depression and borderline personality disorder. Although they were developed from different schools of thought (i.e., behavior therapy and psychoanalytic therapy), they are similar in that they use multiple treatment modalities (individual and group therapy), are of substantial duration (at least 1 year of treatment), and incorporate some form of peer consultation for treatment providers.

Dialectical behavior therapy was developed specifically for the treatment of borderline personality disorder and is largely influenced by principles of behavior therapy and Eastern philosophy (Linehan 1993). Traditional behavioral techniques such as reinforcements, chain analyses, and daily monitoring, in addition to Eastern-influenced techniques of mindfulness and validation, are integral to DBT. Formal DBT involves weekly individual therapy, weekly group sessions focused on teaching specific skill sets, and weekly meetings of therapists who provide consultation to one another, although there have been many adaptations in modality since its inception. A randomized, controlled trial of DBT treatment lasting for 1 year found significant improvements: parasuicidal behavior was reduced, adherence to individual therapy was improved, and the number of inpatient psychiatric days was decreased, compared with a treatment-as-usual regimen. However, no significant differences in depression, hopelessness, or suicidal ideation were found (Linehan et al. 1991). Numerous other empirical studies, with varying degrees of rigor, have supported these initial findings (Koerner and Linehan 2000). One randomized, controlled study found significant improvements in depression, hopelessness, and suicidal ideation among patients after receiving 3 months of DBT (Koons et al. 2001).

The other treatment that has received empirical support for the treatment of symptoms of both borderline personality disorder and depression is a psychoanalytically informed *partial hospitalization* program. Treatment consists of weekly individual psychoanalytic psychotherapy, thrice-weekly group therapy, weekly expressive therapy informed by psychodrama, weekly community meetings, monthly meetings with a case administrator, and monthly medication review with a resident (Bateman and Fonagy 1999, 2001). The average length of stay in the partial hospitalization program was 1.5 years. The comparison group received standard psychiatric care in the community. Those who completed the program reported significantly decreased self-injurious and suicidal behaviors, anxiety, depression, and global symptoms compared with those who received general psychiatric care. However, improvements emerged only after the first 6 months of treatment. The results from this randomized, controlled trial are encouraging, but it remains difficult to ascertain whether the improvements can be attributed to the intensity of treatment and services that were provided, including the structure of community and social support that is inherent in partial hospitalization programs, rather than the specific type of psychosocial intervention. Nonetheless, results from this study and studies of DBT offer support for the notion that intensive psychotherapy involving multiple modalities and of a significant duration can offer significant benefits to patients in reducing symptoms associated with borderline personality disorder and depression.

Aside from these two reviewed treatments, other psychosocial interventions have been developed or adapted for the treatment of depressed patients with personality dysfunction, although currently, none has shown efficacy in a randomized, controlled trial. Furthermore, to date, no published large-scale controlled studies have examined combined pharmacological and psychosocial treatment for personality and depressive symptoms. More research on both somatic and psychosocial treatments of depression and comorbid personality disorders is clearly needed given the high rate of comorbidity between depressive and personality disorders, the difficulty in distinguishing features of these disorders, and what little is currently known about treatments for comorbid depression and personality disorder. At present, it is unclear whether targeting symptoms of one disorder will result in amelioration of symptoms in the other disorder or whether one has a stronger influence on the other.

With regard to psychopharmacology, one approach assumes that certain symptom dimensions crosscut Axis I

and II disorders, thereby sharing a common pathophysiology and possibly a shared responsiveness to medication (Soloff 1998). Some crosscutting dimensions speculated to be mediated by neurotransmitter functioning and to be responsive to medications include cognitive-perceptual, affective, and impulsive-behavioral. Specific algorithms have been developed for each dimension; for example, a low-dose neuroleptic is the suggested first line of treatment for cognitive-perceptual disturbances, whereas selective serotonin reuptake inhibitors (SSRIs) are the suggested first-line treatment for affective dysregulation and impulsive-behavioral dysfunction (Soloff 1998).

Efforts to empirically examine the efficacy of treatments for specific aspects of personality dysfunction have been limited and have focused mainly on borderline personality disorder. According to the American Psychiatric Association "Practice Guideline for the Treatment of Patients With Borderline Personality Disorder," the above-mentioned algorithms also pertain to the treatment of borderline personality disorder symptoms (Oldham et al. 2001). Therefore, SSRIs are often the treatment of choice for both personality disorders (particularly borderline personality disorder) and major depression. However, some have speculated that borderline personality disorder should be conceptualized as being on the same diagnostic spectrum as bipolar disorder (Akiskal 1996) and caution that those patients with borderline personality disorder who also have a subclinical presentation of bipolar disorder may respond negatively to antidepressant treatment, especially SSRIs (Deltito et al. 2001). Finally, despite the recommended guidelines, very few rigorous pharmacological trials (i.e., randomized, double-blind, controlled) have examined both depression and personality disorder features as target outcomes. Among the studies examining the efficacy of SSRIs in borderline personality disorder samples, only fluoxetine has been examined in randomized, double-blind trials. One such study recruited borderline personality disorder (and subthreshold borderline personality disorder) subjects through newspaper advertisement and found that fluoxetine significantly reduced depression and anger (Salzman et al. 1995). However, because potential subjects were excluded if they had recent self-injurious behaviors, other Axis II disorders, or previous psychiatric hospitalizations, the findings may not be representative of borderline personality disorder patients often seen in more acute clinical settings.

Using a more clinically impaired sample, one 12-week randomized, controlled, double-blind study compared combined DBT and fluoxetine to DBT and placebo in women with a diagnosis of borderline personality disorder (including those with self-injurious behaviors, who are often excluded from clinical trials). Combined DBT and fluoxetine treatment was not superior to DBT and placebo in reducing depressive and borderline symptomatology (Simpson et al. 2004). However, although the *difference* between group outcomes was not statistically significant, patients in the DBT and placebo condition had statistically significant improvements in depression and anxiety symptoms, anger, suicidality, and global functioning, unlike their counterparts in the DBT and fluoxetine condition. Specifically, whereas all subjects in the DBT and placebo condition reported a decrease in symptomatology from baseline to 12 weeks posttreatment, a small subset of subjects in the DBT and fluoxetine condition reported worsening of symptoms. The authors speculate that these subjects may have experienced increased agitation, possibly a side effect of the medication or possibly due to an undiagnosed subclinical bipolar disorder that might manifest in ways similar to borderline personality disorder.

Other pilot randomized, controlled, double-blind studies have examined divalproex sodium (Frankenburg and Zanarini 2002; Hollander et al. 2001) and olanzapine (Zanarini and Frankenburg 2001). In a 6-month trial, olanzapine was associated with a greater rate of improvement over placebo in all symptom areas, except for depression. The two studies of divalproex sodium found a reduction in most symptoms, including depression, although high dropout rates in one of these studies limit the extent of conclusions that can be drawn (Hollander et al. 2001). Other treatments for depression, such as tricyclics, monoamine oxidase inhibitors (MAOIs), and ECT, have been examined in nonrandomized trials and have received either inconsistent or insufficient support for the treatment of borderline personality disorder features or depression.

To summarize, adjunctive psychotherapy and symptom-focused psychopharmacology are suggested for the treatment of depression and comorbid personality disorders. These recommendations are based on the best available evidence. However, relatively few controlled studies of the treatment of comorbid depression and personality disorders have been done, and findings in such studies have been inconsistent and of limited comparability because of variations in inclusion and exclusion criteria, target samples, and severity of illness. An apparent need exists for future treatment studies, particularly of combined pharmacological and psychotherapy treatment for comorbid depression and personality disorder in samples representative of clinical outpatient populations.

Clinical and Safety Issues

Establishing a positive and trusting therapeutic relationship is important to a successful treatment outcome. This is often particularly difficult with patients who have personality disorders. Each disorder has its unique set of challenges. Othmer and Othmer (1989), in their text on clinical interviewing, gave advice for establishing rapport with patients who have personality disorders. Bender (2005) also describes the challenges of building treatment alliance with respect to each of the personality disorders. A summary of the above authors' suggestions follows. In short, careful consideration of the patient's characteristic way of relating is necessary.

The Cluster A personality disorders (paranoid, schizoid, and schizotypal) are associated with emotional withdrawal, lack of warmth, and odd or eccentric behavior. Establishing and maintaining rapport with a patient who has paranoid personality disorder may be challenged by the patient's suspiciousness because the patient will likely find it difficult to trust the interviewer's motives and may respond to queries with one- or two-word answers. Schizoid personality disorder patients are marked by extreme withdrawal and social detachment, which can make rapport and reciprocity of communication difficult to establish. They may have flat affect and appear to be lacking in appropriate emotions. Schizotypal personality disorder is marked by unusual or bizarre thought content. Rapport may be challenged to the extent that the clinician may have difficulty appreciating or validating those ideas.

Patients with Cluster B disorders (borderline, antisocial, narcissistic, and histrionic) present quite different problems for rapport than do patients with Cluster A disorders, mostly as a function of the affective instability and impulsivity that underlies these disorders. Borderline personality disorder is one of the more common psychiatric disorders seen in clinical settings for a variety of reasons. Borderline personality disorder is associated with dangerous, life-threatening behaviors such as suicidal and self-injurious behaviors and substance use. Furthermore, it has high rates of comorbidity with several Axis I disorders, such as depression, substance use disorders, and eating disorders, that are often the primary presenting diagnoses. Finally, individuals with borderline personality disorder have higher rates of treatment use compared with those with other personality disorders (Bender et al. 2001). Affective instability, intense anger, the tendency to alternate between idealization and devaluation, and a fear of abandonment are all traits that present treatment challenges with this population. The borderline personality disorder patient may at one moment feel that the clinician is an ally who truly understands him or her and in the next moment feel rage toward the clinician for not being supportive enough. In a treatment setting involving a team of clinicians, it is important to be consistent with an agreed-on treatment plan. In individual treatment, it has been advocated that after life-threatening behaviors, therapy-interfering behaviors should be the next to be targeted in treatment (Linehan 1993).

Patients with antisocial personality disorder rarely seek help from mental health professionals for depression and often arrive through court mandate. The antisocial personality disorder patient may be deceptive or attempt to manipulate the clinician; it is important to set clear limits about acceptable behavior. Histrionic personality disorder is associated with excessive emotionality. Rapport may be hindered by the patient's constant approval seeking. Narcissistic personality disorder is associated with grandiosity, lack of empathy, and sense of entitlement. Individuals with this disorder often have contempt for others while needing constant affirmation, have poor insight, and can seem off-putting.

Patients with Cluster C personality disorders (avoidant, dependent, and obsessive-compulsive) generally have better insight than do patients with Cluster A and B disorders. Patients with avoidant personality disorder present with considerable interpersonal anxiety. The fear of rejection can interfere with rapport because the patient may be hesitant to divulge his or her problems to the clinician and may appear withdrawn. Conversely, patients with dependent personality disorder readily establish rapport. Attempts to explore or challenge the dependency will often engender resistance by the patient.

Clinicians working with depressed patients who also meet criteria for one or more personality disorder diagnoses should be attuned to issues related to patients' safety. High-risk behavior such as *parasuicide* (a term used to denote suicide attempts, suicidal gestures, and self-injurious behavior with or without intention of suicide) (Pirkis et al. 1999; Yen et al. 2003), drug or alcohol abuse (Kokkevi et al. 1998; Skodol et al. 1999), violence (Johnson et al. 2000; Miller et al. 1993), and risky sexual behavior (Lavan and Johnson 2002) occur more frequently among patients meeting criteria for personality disorder (particularly Cluster B diagnoses) than among psychiatric patients without personality disorder. Furthermore, one prospective study found that among patients with comorbid depression and personality disorders, an exacerbation of depressive symptoms significantly increases the likelihood of a suicide attempt in the following month (Yen et al. 2003).

Considerations of risk assessment and management are particularly relevant to clinicians treating borderline personality disorder. This disorder is the most common personality disorder in clinical settings, and it is associated with several high-risk behaviors. The recently published American Psychiatric Association "Practice Guideline for the Treatment of Patients With Borderline Personality Disorder" (Oldham et al. 2001) highlights the importance of ongoing assessment of suicide risk, as well as the value of maintaining collaborative relationships with other clinicians who are treating the same patient. Additionally, the APA Guideline emphasizes the necessity of maintaining clear boundaries. Another resource for strategies for managing high-risk behavior is Linehan's (1993) manual of DBT for borderline personality disorder. Linehan (1993) provides a framework for conceptualizing the disorder and for guiding interventions and pays particular attention to parasuicide.

A thorough assessment of a patient's history of self-harm, suicide attempts, substance abuse, and risky sexual behavior is recommended at the outset of treatment. In addition to the routine assessment of suicidal thoughts or plans and suicide attempts among patients with depressive disorders, clinicians should be alert to other high-risk behavior and to protective factors (e.g., social support) when treating patients with comorbid personality disorder. The problem of impulsive behavior in this population is frequently exacerbated by inadequate social support (Overholser 1996; Pfohl et al. 1984; Tyrer et al. 1994). In addition to being life-threatening, such behavior can be conceptualized as maladaptive coping and, as such, should be understood functionally. That is, clinicians should seek to understand the contexts (e.g., affective states, interpersonal experiences) that give rise to these behaviors, as well as the consequences of maintaining the behavior. Risky behavior should be a focus of intervention, and development of healthy coping skills should be a goal of treatment (Linehan 1993).

Conclusion

Incontrovertible evidence indicates that some personality traits and disorders are related to depression. However, the degree of association between specific traits or disorders and major depression and the specific etiological nature of that relation both remain unclear. For example, is the depression that occurs in the context of a personality disorder qualitatively different from depression without personality pathology? Is either depression or personality disorder more influential or predominant than the other? Or does having both disorders produce a simple additive effect? Are there crosscutting dimensions that underlie mechanisms for both depressive and personality disorders? If so, what is the cause of their different manifestations in Axis I and personality disorders? And if a shared etiology exists, what accounts for the large proportion of independently occurring personality disorders or depression?

Understanding the relation between depression and personality disorders would elucidate treatment implications. Thus, if personality pathology is more prominent and leads to poor interpersonal functioning, limited social supports, increased negative stressful events, and more interpersonal chaos, all of which contribute to increased depressive symptomatology, it would follow that the personality pathology would negatively affect the treatment of depression (e.g., through poor alliance with therapist, less support in sustaining treatment, poor compliance) and should be itself a primary target for treatment—most preferably, cognitive-behavioral therapy based on the cumulative empirical evidence. On the other hand, if the depressive symptomatology is more prominent and leads to avoidance and withdrawal from interpersonal supports and to exacerbation of previous personality tendencies in a maladaptive direction, then it seems warranted to target the depressive symptomatology with combined pharmacological and psychosocial treatment. Clearly, more research is needed to elucidate the relation between depression and personality pathology and disorders and to increase understanding of how comorbidity affects treatment.

References

Akiskal HS: The temperamental borders of affective disorders. Acta Psychiatr Scand Suppl 379:32–37, 1994

Akiskal HS: Prevalent clinical spectrum of bipolar disorder: beyond DSM-IV. J Clin Psychopharmacol 16:4S–14S, 1996

Alnaes R, Torgersen S: Personality and personality disorders predict development and relapses of major depression. Acta Psychiatr Scand 95:336–342, 1997

American Psychiatric Association: Diagnostic and Statistical Manual of Mental Disorders, 3rd Edition. Washington, DC, American Psychiatric Association, 1980

American Psychiatric Association: Diagnostic and Statistical Manual of Mental Disorders, 3rd Edition, Revised. Washington, DC, American Psychiatric Association, 1987

American Psychiatric Association: Diagnostic and Statistical Manual of Mental Disorders, 4th Edition. Washington, DC, American Psychiatric Association, 1994

American Psychiatric Association: Diagnostic and Statistical Manual of Mental Disorders, 4th Edition, Text Revision. Washington, DC, American Psychiatric Association, 2000

Arieti S, Bemporad J: The psychological organization of depression. Am J Psychiatry 136:1360–1365, 1980

Bateman A, Fonagy P: Effectiveness of partial hospitalization in the treatment of borderline personality disorder: a randomized controlled trial. Am J Psychiatry 156:1563–1569, 1999

Bateman A, Fonagy P: Treatment of borderline personality disorder with psychoanalytically oriented partial hospitalization: an 18-month follow-up. Am J Psychiatry 158:36–42, 2001

Beck AT: Cognitive therapy of depression: new perspectives, in Treatment of Depression: Old Controversies and New Approaches. Edited by Clayton PJ, Barrett JE. New York, Raven, 1983, pp 265–290

Bender DS: Therapeutic alliance, in The American Psychiatric Publishing Textbook of Personality Disorders. Edited by Oldham JM, Skodol JM, Skodol AE, et al. Washington, DC, American Psychiatric Publishing, 2005, pp 405–420

Bender DS, Dolan RT, Skodol AE, et al: Treatment utilization by patients with personality disorders. Am J Psychiatry 158:295–302, 2001

Blatt SJ, D'Afflitti JP, Quinlan DM: Experiences of depression in normal adults. J Abnorm Psychol 85:383–389, 1976

Casey P, Birbeck G, McDonagh C, et al: Personality disorder, depression and functioning: results from the ODIN study. J Affect Disord 82:277–283, 2004

Clark LA: Manual for the Schedule for Nonadaptive and Adaptive Personality. Minneapolis, University of Minnesota Press, 1993

Clark LA, Watson D: Tripartite model of anxiety and depression: psychometric evidence and taxonomic implications. J Abnorm Psychol 100:316–336, 1991

Clark LA, Watson D, Mineka S: Temperament, personality, and the mood and anxiety disorders. J Abnorm Psychol 103:103–116, 1994

Cloninger CR: A unified biosocial theory of personality: its role in the development of anxiety states. Psychiatr Dev 3:167–226, 1986

Cloninger CR: A systematic method for clinical description and classification of personality variants. Arch Gen Psychiatry 44:573–588, 1987

Coccaro EF, Siever LJ, Klar HM, et al: Serotonergic studies in patients with affective and personality disorders: correlates with suicidal and impulsive aggressive behavior. Arch Gen Psychiatry 46:587–599, 1989

Corruble E, Ginestet D, Guelfi JD: Comorbidity of personality disorders and unipolar major depression: a review. J Affect Disord 37:157–171, 1996

Costa PT, McCrae RR: NEO PI-R Professional Manual. Odessa, FL, Psychological Assessment Resources, 1992

Cyranowski JM, Frank E, Winter E, et al: Personality pathology and outcome in recurrently depressed women over 2 years of maintenance interpersonal psychotherapy. Psychol Med 34:659–669, 2004

De Battista C, Mueller KM: Is electroconvulsive therapy effective for the depressed patient with comorbid borderline personality disorder? J ECT 17:91–98, 2001

Deltito J, Martin L, Riefkohl J, et al: Do patients with borderline personality disorder belong to the bipolar spectrum? J Affect Disord 67:221–228, 2001

Eysenck HJ: Biological dimensions of personality, in Handbook of Personality: Theory and Research. Edited by Pervin LA. New York, Guilford, 1990, pp 244–276

First MB, Gibbon M, Spitzer RL, et al: Structured Clinical Interview for DSM-IV Axis I Disorders (SCID-I). New York, Biometrics Research, New York State Psychiatric Institute, 1996

First MB, Bell CC, Cuthbert B, et al: Personality disorders and relational disorders: a research agenda for addressing crucial gaps in DSM, in A Research Agenda for DSM-V. Edited by Kupfer DJ, First MB, Regier DA. Washington, DC, American Psychiatric Association, 2002, pp 123–200

Frank E, Kupfer DJ, Jacob M, et al: Personality features and response to acute treatment in recurrent depression. J Personal Disord 1:14–26, 1987

Frankenburg FR, Zanarini MC: Divalproex sodium treatment of women with borderline personality disorder and bipolar II disorder: a double-blind placebo-controlled pilot study. J Clin Psychiatry 63:442–446, 2002

Grant BF, Hasin DS, Stinson FS, et al: Prevalence, correlates, and disability of personality disorders in the United States: results from the National Epidemiological Survey on Alcohol and Related Conditions. J Clin Psychiatry 65:948–958, 2004

Grilo CM, Sanislow CA Shea MT, et al: Two-year prospective naturalistic study of remission from major depressive disorder as a function of personality disorder comorbidity. J Consult Clin Psychol 73:78–85, 2005

Hardy GE, Barkham M, Shapiro DA, et al: Impact of Cluster C personality disorders on outcomes of contrasting brief psychotherapies for depression. J Consult Clin Psychol 6:997–1004, 1995

Hart AB, Craighead WE, Craighead LW: Predicting recurrence of major depressive disorder in young adults: a prospective study. J Abnorm Psychol 110:633–643, 2001

Hirschfeld RMA, Klerman GL, Gough HG, et al: A measure of interpersonal dependency. J Personal Assess 41:610–618, 1977

Hirschfeld R, Klerman GL, Andreasen N, et al: Psycho-social predictors of chronicity in depressed patients. Br J Psychiatry 148:648–654, 1986

Hirschfeld RMA, Klerman GL, Lavori P, et al: Premorbid personality assessments of first onset of major depression. Arch Gen Psychiatry 46:345–350, 1989

Hollander E, Allen A, Lopez RP, et al: A preliminary double-blind, placebo-controlled trial of divalproex sodium in borderline personality disorder. J Clin Psychiatry 62:199–203, 2001

Hyler SE: Personality Diagnostic Questionnaire—4. New York, New York State Psychiatric Institute, 1994

Ilardi S, Craighead W: Personality pathology and response to somatic treatments for major depression: a critical review. Depression 2:200–217, 1995

Ilardi SS, Craighead WE, Evans D: Modeling relapse in unipolar depression: the effects of dysfunctional cognitions and personality disorders. J Consult Clin Psychol 65:381–391, 1997

Jackson HJ, Burgess PM: Personality disorders in the community: a report from the Australia National Survey of Mental Health and Wellbeing. Soc Psychiatry Psychiatr Epidemiol 35:531–538, 2000

Johnson JG, Cohen P, Smailes E, et al: Adolescent personality disorders associated with violence and criminal behavior during adolescence and early adulthood. Am J Psychiatry 157:1406–1412, 2000

Joyce PR, Mulder RT, Luty SE, et al: Borderline personality disorder in major depression: symptomatology, temperament, character, differential drug response, and 6-month outcome. Compr Psychiatry 44:35–43, 2003

Kaye AL, Shea MT: Personality disorders, personality traits, and defense mechanisms measures, in Handbook of Psychiatric Measures. Washington, DC, American Psychiatric Publishing, 2002, pp 713–749

Kendler KS, Neale MC, Kessler RC, et al: A longitudinal twin study of personality and major depression in women. Arch Gen Psychiatry 50:853–862, 1993

Klein MH, Wonderlich S, Shea MT: Models of relationships between personality and depression: toward a framework for theory and research, in Personality and Depression: A Current View. Edited by Klein MH, Kupfer DJ, Shea MT. New York, Guilford, 1993, pp 1–54

Koerner K, Linehan MM: Research on dialectical behavior therapy for patients with borderline personality disorder. Psychiatr Clin North Am 23:151–167, 2000

Kokkevi A, Stefanis N, Anastasopoulou E, et al: Personality disorders in drug abusers: prevalence and their association with Axis I disorders as predictors of treatment retention. Addict Behav 23:841–854, 1998

Kool S, Dekker J, Duijsens IJ, et al: Efficacy of combined therapy and pharmacotherapy for depressed patients with or without personality disorders. Harv Rev Psychiatry 11:133–141, 2003

Koons CR, Robins CJ, Tweed JL, et al: Efficacy of dialectical behavior therapy in women veterans with borderline personality disorder. Behav Ther 32:371–390, 2001

Kraepelin E: Manic-depressive Insanity and Paranoia. Edited by Robertson GM. Translated by Barclay RM. Edinburgh, Scotland, E & S Livingstone, 1921

Lavan H, Johnson JG: The association between Axis I and II psychiatric symptoms and high-risk sexual behavior during adolescence. J Personal Disord 16:73–94, 2002

Linehan MM: Cognitive-Behavioral Treatment of Borderline Personality Disorder. New York, Guilford, 1993

Linehan MM, Armstrong HE, Suarez A, et al: Cognitive-behavioral treatment of chronically parasuicidal borderline patients. Arch Gen Psychiatry 48:1060–1064, 1991

Loranger AW: International Personality Disorder Examination (IPDE): DSM-IV and ICD-10 Modules. Odessa, FL, Psychological Assessment Resources, 1999

Meyers BS, Sirey JA, Bruce M, et al: Predictors of early recovery from major depression among persons admitted to community-based clinics: an observational study. Arch Gen Psychiatry 59:729–735, 2002

Miller RJ, Zadolinnyi K, Hafner RJ: Profiles and predictors of assaultiveness for different psychiatric ward populations. Am J Psychiatry 150:1368–1373, 1993

Millon T, Davis R, Millon C: MCMI-III Manual, 2nd Edition. Minneapolis, MN, National Computer Systems, 1994

Morey LC: Personality Assessment Inventory: Professional Manual. Odessa, FL, Psychological Assessment Resources, 1991

Mulder RT: Personality pathology and treatment outcome in major depression: a review. Am J Psychiatry 159:359–371, 2002

Mulder RT, Joyce PR, Luty SE: The relationship of personality disorders to treatment outcome in depressed outpatients. J Clin Psychiatry 64:259–264, 2003

O'Boyle M, Self D: A comparison of two interviews for DSM-III-R personality disorders. Psychiatry Res 32:85–92, 1990

Oldham JM, Gabbard GO, Goin MK, et al: Practice guideline for the treatment of patients with borderline personality disorder. Am J Psychiatry 158 (suppl):1–52, 2001

Othmer E, Othmer S: The Clinical Interview Using DSM-III-R. Washington, DC, American Psychiatric Press, 1989

Overholser JC: The dependent personality and interpersonal problems. J Nerv Ment Dis 184:8–16, 1996

Perry JC: Problems and considerations in the valid assessment of personality disorders. Am J Psychiatry 149:1645–1653, 1992

Pfohl B, Stangl D, Zimmerman M: The implications of DSM-III personality disorder for patients with major depression. J Affect Disord 7:309–318, 1984

Pfohl B, Blum N, Zimmerman M: Structured Interview for DSM-IV Personality. Washington, DC, American Psychiatric Press, 1997

Pilkonis PA, Frank E: Personality pathology in recurrent depression: nature, prevalence, and relationship to treatment response. Am J Psychiatry 145:435–441, 1988

Pirkis J, Burgess P, Jolley D: Suicide attempts by psychiatric patients in acute inpatient, long-stay inpatient and community care. Soc Psychiatry Psychiatr Epidemiol 34:634–644, 1999

Reich J: The effect of Axis II disorders on the outcome of treatment of anxiety and unipolar depressive disorders: a review. J Personal Disord 17:387–405, 2003

Russell JM, Kornstein SG, Shea MT, et al: Chronic depression and comorbid personality disorders: response to sertraline versus imipramine. J Clin Psychiatry 64:554–561, 2003

Salzman C, Wolfson AN, Schatzberg A, et al: Effects of fluoxetine on anger in symptomatic volunteers with borderline personality disorder. J Clin Psychopharmacol 15:23–29, 1995

Sareen J, Enns MW, Guertin JE: The impact of clinically diagnosed personality disorders on acute and one-year outcomes of electroconvulsive therapy. J ECT 16:43–51, 2000

Schiavone P, Dorz S, Conforti D, et al: Comorbidity of DSM-IV personality disorders in unipolar and bipolar affective disorders: a comparative study. Psychol Rep 95:121–128, 2004

Schneider K: Psychopathic Personalities. Springfield, IL, Charles C Thomas, 1958

Shea MT, Pilkonis PA, Beckham E, et al: Personality disorders and treatment outcome in the NIMH Treatment of Depression Collaborative Research Program. Am J Psychiatry 147:711–718, 1990

Shea MT, Widiger TA, Klein MH: Comorbidity of personality disorders and depression: implications for treatment. J Consult Clin Psychol 60:857–868, 1992

Shea MT, Stout RL, Yen S, et al: Associations in the course of personality disorders and Axis I disorders over time. J Abnorm Psychol 113:499–508, 2004

Siever LJ: Biological markers in schizotypal personality disorder. Schizophr Bull 11:564–575, 1985

Siever LJ, Davis KL: A psychobiological perspective on the personality disorders. Am J Psychiatry 148:1647–1658, 1991

Simpson EB, Yen S, Costello E, et al: Combined dialectical behavior therapy and fluoxetine pharmacotherapy in patients with borderline personality disorder: is there an additive effect? J Clin Psychiatry 65:379–385, 2004

Skodol AE, Oldham JM, Gallaher PE: Axis II comorbidity of substance use disorders among patients referred to treatment of personality disorders. Am J Psychiatry 156:733–738, 1999

Soloff PH: Algorithms for pharmacological treatment of personality dimensions: symptom-specific treatments for cognitive-perceptual, affective, and impulsive-behavioral dysregulation. Bull Menninger Clin 62:195–214, 1998

Tyrer P, Merson S, Onyett S, et al: The effect of personality disorder on clinical outcome, social networks, and adjustment: a controlled clinical trial of psychiatric emergencies. Psychol Med 24:731–740, 1994

Widiger TA: Personality and depression: assessment issues, in Personality and Depression: A Current View: Mental Health and Psychopathology. Edited by Klein MH, Kupfer DJ, Shea MT. New York, Guilford, 1993, pp 77–118

Widiger TA, Frances AJ: Interviews and inventories for the measurement of personality disorders. Clin Psychol Rev 7:49–75, 1987

Widiger TA, Mangine S, Corbitt EM, et al: Personality Disorder Interview-IV: A Semi-Structured Interview for the Assessment of Personality Disorders. Odessa, FL, Psychological Assessment Resources, 1995

World Health Organization: International Classification of Diseases, 9th Revision. Geneva, World Health Organization, 1977

World Health Organization: International Statistical Classification of Diseases and Related Health Problems, 10th Revision. Geneva, World Health Organization, 1992

Yen S, Shea MT, Pagano M, et al: Axis I and Axis II disorders as predictors of prospective suicide attempts: findings from the Collaborative Longitudinal Personality Disorders Study. J Abnorm Psychol 112:375–381, 2003

Zanarini MC, Frankenburg FR: Olanzapine treatment of female borderline personality disorder patients: a double-blind, placebo-controlled pilot study. J Clin Psychiatry 62:849–854, 2001

Zanarini MC, Frankenburg FR, Sickel AE, et al: The Diagnostic Interview for DSM-IV Personality Disorder. Belmont, MA, McLean Hospital, Laboratory for the Study of Adult Development, 1996

Zimmerman M, Coryell W: DSM-III personality diagnoses in a nonpatient sample. Arch Gen Psychiatry 46:682–689, 1989

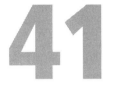

Depression and Gender

SUSAN G. KORNSTEIN, M.D.
DIANE M.E. SLOAN, PHARM.D.

THE PREVALENCE of major depressive disorder (MDD) in women is approximately twice as high as in men, particularly during the childbearing years (Kessler et al. 1993). According to data from the Global Burden of Disease Study (Michaud et al. 2001), unipolar major depression is the leading cause of disease burden in females age 5 and older worldwide. This increased risk for depression in women coupled with the significant individual and societal burden underscore the need for improved detection and management of this debilitating disorder. Until recently, however, women of childbearing age were not routinely included in clinical trials, thus limiting the available evidence specific to depression in women. The inclusion of premenopausal women in contemporary studies and a greater interest in examining the effect of gender on outcome in clinical trials have contributed to a growing body of literature in this area.

At various times throughout the female reproductive life cycle, women may experience depressive disorders with unique clinical considerations. For some women, the luteal phase of the menstrual cycle may be associated with mood and behavioral symptoms or a worsening of preexisting conditions. Likewise, certain women may be at increased risk for new-onset depression or a recurrent depressive episode during pregnancy, the postpartum period, and the menopausal transition.

In this chapter, we review evidence regarding gender differences in depression and approaches to the management of depressive disorders unique to women. Specifically, we examine differences in the prevalence, symptoms, course of illness, and response to treatment for women relative to men. We also review the phenomenology and treatment of premenstrual dysphoric disorder (PMDD) and depression during pregnancy, the postpartum period, and the menopausal transition.

Gender Differences in Depression

Epidemiology

The gender gap in risk for first onset of depression is well documented. Data from large community-based epidemiological surveys in the United States estimate that the cumulative lifetime prevalence of MDD in women is 1.7–2.7 times the rate for men (Kessler 2003; Kessler et al. 1993; Weissman et al. 1993), a difference that begins in adolescence and continues to midlife (Figure 41–1) (Kessler et al. 1993), approximately corresponding to the span of childbearing years in women. Although there is some variation in the magnitude of the difference, cross-national epidemiological studies (Weissman et al. 1996) have documented higher rates of depression in women across multiple countries and most ethnic groups.

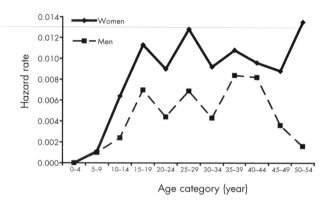

FIGURE 41–1.   Major depression hazard rates by age and gender.

Source.   Kessler et al. 1993. Reprinted with permission from Elsevier.

Etiology

Many theories have been proposed to explain the gender difference in the prevalence of depression (Kornstein and Wojcik 2002). For example, it has been suggested that the greater tendency for women to report symptoms and seek treatment (Kessler et al. 1981) may artifactually inflate the magnitude of gender differences. However, the increased prevalence of depression in women is observed in both clinical and community-based epidemiological studies; thus, differences in help-seeking behavior do not account for the difference in prevalence (Kornstein 1997).

The marked separation in depression risk emerges during a relatively short time span (i.e., 5 years) that is coincident with the onset of puberty. It has been suggested that the heightened risk for onset of depression is likely the result of a complex interaction between psychosocial factors and neuroendocrine changes occurring at this time (Cyranowski et al. 2000). From menarche to menopause, women experience monthly fluctuations of gonadal hormones. Estrogen and progesterone both have central nervous system (CNS) neuromodulatory effects (Rubinow et al. 1998), and changes in these reproductive hormones may directly affect the function of various neurotransmitters (e.g., serotonin, norepinephrine) and, in turn, cerebral functioning (P.J. Schmidt et al. 1997). In particular, changes in estrogen levels have been shown to influence concentrations of serotonin and serotonin receptor subtypes and to modulate response to serotonin agonists (Joffe and Cohen 1998; Rubinow et al. 1998). Although the exact relation between reproductive hormones and depression in women remains unclear, fluctuations in the neuromodulatory effects of the gonadal steroids may

confer an increased risk for mood disorders in women with differential sensitivity to normal hormonal changes (i.e., during the premenstrual period, the puerperium, and the perimenopause) (Joffe and Cohen 1998).

Psychological and social factors also may contribute to an increased risk for depression in women. For example, gender differences in early developmental socialization processes may result in differences in self-concept and vulnerability to depression (Ruble et al. 1993). The self-focused ruminative coping style of women in response to feelings of sadness has been hypothesized to lead to longer and more severe depressive episodes (Nolen-Hoeksema 1995). The lower socioeconomic status of women also may be important; more women than men live in poverty, and many are single mothers (Brown and Moran 1997). Gender differences in major life trauma such as sexual abuse is another factor that may explain, in part, why depression disproportionately affects women (Weiss et al. 1999).

Symptomatology, Comorbidities, and Course of Illness

In addition to the difference in prevalence rates, some evidence supports differences in the nature of depression that women experience compared with men. Women tend to endorse a greater number of depressive symptoms compared with men and, for a particular level of severity, a higher degree of subjective distress (Angst and Dobler-Mikola 1984; Frank et al. 1988; Kornstein et al. 2000a; Perugi et al. 1990). Specific symptoms such as sleep disturbance, psychomotor retardation, feelings of worthlessness or guilt, anxiety, and somatization are endorsed more often by women than by men (Frank et al. 1988; Kornstein et al. 2000a; Perugi et al. 1990), and women more commonly present with atypical or reverse vegetative symptoms of depression, including hypersomnia, hyperphagia, carbohydrate craving, and weight gain (Carter et al. 2000; Frank et al. 1988; Young et al. 1990). Consistent with the higher degree of subjective distress, women attempt suicide approximately three times as often as men, although they are less likely than men to complete the act (Hirschfeld and Russell 1997; Rapaport et al. 1995).

Depressed women are more likely than men to have comorbid anxiety disorders (especially panic and phobic symptoms) and eating disorders, but they are less likely to have comorbid alcoholism and other substance use disorders (Fava et al. 1996; Rapaport et al. 1995).

Although some studies have shown no gender difference in course of depression, others have shown that women may have a more chronic and recurrent course of illness. In addition, evidence indicates that chronic depression may affect women more seriously than men, with an earlier age at onset, greater severity of illness, and more functional impairment, especially in the areas of marital and family adjustment (Kornstein et al. 2000a).

Antidepressant Treatment

Given the differences in symptomatology, comorbid conditions, and course of illness between women and men, it is important to consider the possibility that there may be gender differences in response to antidepressant treatment. Although the exclusion of women of childbearing age from clinical trials in the past has limited evidence in this area, several recent studies have examined this issue. Likewise, because of the variation in hormone levels among premenopausal, perimenopausal, and postmenopausal women and the growing understanding that gonadal hormones have CNS modulatory properties, investigators also have begun to explore whether the efficacy of antidepressant therapy differs among these groups of women.

Several analyses have found that gender, menopausal status, and age can affect response to antidepressants (Hamilton et al. 1996; Kornstein et al. 2000b; Martenyi et al. 2001; Raskin et al. 1974; Thase et al., in press), whereas others have failed to show such differences (Entsuah et al. 2001; Hildebrandt et al. 2003; Quitkin et al. 2002). As a whole, the available data suggest that symptoms in postmenopausal women tend to respond similarly to those in men, whereas symptoms in premenopausal women may respond differently, with higher rates of response to selective serotonin reuptake inhibitors (SSRIs) and monoamine oxidase inhibitors relative to tricyclic antidepressants. These findings may reflect differential efficacy of these agents in treating different subtypes of depression (e.g., atypical vs. melancholic features) commonly presented by women and by men, or differential effects of gonadal hormones on response to these antidepressants. Further research is needed to determine the clinical relevance of the observed differences and the role of menopausal status and gonadal hormones in response to antidepressant treatment.

Premenstrual Dysphoric Disorder

PMDD is characterized by a constellation of affective and somatic symptoms that are manifest during the late luteal phase of the menstrual cycle and resolve shortly after the onset of menses. Unlike other mood disorders, the mood disturbances associated with PMDD are cyclical and tightly linked to the menstrual cycle; hence the occurrence of symptoms ceases during pregnancy and after menopause.

Epidemiology

Premenstrual syndrome (PMS) is a common condition among menstruating women, with prevalence estimates ranging from 30% to more than 60% (Johnson 1987; Logue and Moos 1986; Ramcharan et al. 1992; Stout et al. 1986). PMDD is a severe form or subgroup of PMS that affects only about 3%–9% of women (Halbreich et al. 2003). Although symptoms may appear anytime after menarche, the average age at onset for PMDD is the mid-20s, and women generally do not seek treatment until their 30s. Women commonly report that their symptoms gradually worsen with age until the onset of menopause.

Diagnosis and Clinical Features

PMDD is more strictly defined than PMS, with an emphasis on mood and behavior symptoms and functional impairment (American Psychiatric Association 2000). According to DSM-IV-TR, at least 5 out of a possible 11 symptoms are required, and at least 1 must be a core mood symptom—either irritability/anger, depressed mood, anxiety, or mood swings (Table 41–1). The symptoms must be severe enough to cause impairment in social or occupational functioning. The presence and severity of symptoms and their cyclical relation to the luteal phase must be confirmed by prospective daily ratings for at least two consecutive menstrual cycles.

Prospective documentation of symptoms is a critical step in diagnosis, given that a significant number of women who seek treatment for premenstrual emotional symptoms actually have premenstrual exacerbation of another underlying psychiatric condition—usually, a depressive or an anxiety disorder (Bailey and Cohen 1999). The luteal phase of the menstrual cycle is a period of increased vulnerability in some women for the onset of a new depressive episode or for exacerbation of symptoms of an ongoing episode (Endicott 1993). Premenstrual exacerbation of symptoms also may be seen with a variety of other psychiatric disorders and general medical conditions (e.g., anxiety disorders, eating disorders, substance abuse, migraines, asthma, seizures). The high prevalence of depressive and anxiety disorders found in women thought to have PMS or PMDD highlights the need for clinicians to be aware of this overlap in presenting complaints and hence to be better able to assess patients, clarify the diagnosis, and initiate appropriate treatment.

Etiology

There is no clear evidence of hormonal dysregulation in the etiology of PMDD (Bloch et al. 1998). Rather, PMS

TABLE 41–1. **DSM-IV-TR research criteria for premenstrual dysphoric disorder**

A. In most menstrual cycles during the past year, five (or more) of the following symptoms were present for most of the time during the last week of the luteal phase, began to remit within a few days after the onset of the follicular phase, and were absent in the week postmenses, with at least one of the symptoms being either (1), (2), (3), or (4):

   (1) markedly depressed mood, feelings of hopelessness, or self-deprecating thoughts

   (2) marked anxiety, tension, feelings of being "keyed up," or "on edge"

   (3) marked affective lability (e.g., feeling suddenly sad or tearful or increased sensitivity to rejection)

   (4) persistent and marked anger or irritability or increased interpersonal conflicts

   (5) decreased interest in usual activities (e.g., work, school, friends, hobbies)

   (6) subjective sense of difficulty in concentrating

   (7) lethargy, easy fatigability, or marked lack of energy

   (8) marked change in appetite, overeating, or specific food cravings

   (9) hypersomnia or insomnia

   (10) a subjective sense of being overwhelmed or out of control

   (11) other physical symptoms, such as breast tenderness or swelling, headaches, joint or muscle pain, a sensation of "bloating," weight gain

   Note: In menstruating females, the luteal phase corresponds to the period between ovulation and the onset of menses, and the follicular phase begins with menses. In nonmenstruating females (e.g., those who have had a hysterectomy), the timing of luteal and follicular phases may require measurement of circulating reproductive hormones.

B. The disturbance markedly interferes with work or school or with usual social activities and relationships with others (e.g., avoidance of social activities, decreased productivity and efficiency at work or school).

C. The disturbance is not merely an exacerbation of the symptoms of another disorder, such as Major Depressive Disorder, Panic Disorder, Dysthymic Disorder, or a Personality Disorder (although it may be superimposed on any of these disorders).

D. Criteria A, B, and C must be confirmed by prospective daily ratings during at least two consecutive symptomatic cycles. (The diagnosis may be made provisionally prior to this confirmation.)

Source. Reprinted from American Psychiatric Association: *Diagnostic and Statistical Manual of Mental Disorders,* 4th Edition, Text Revision. Washington, DC, American Psychiatric Association, 2000. Used with permission.

and PMDD appear to represent an abnormal response to normal fluctuations of gonadal steroids (Roca et al. 2003; P.J. Schmidt et al. 1998). Prevention or suppression of cyclic gonadal hormones may relieve symptoms (Hammarback and Backstrom 1988; Muse et al. 1984; P.J. Schmidt et al. 1998), whereas hormone replacement therapy may provoke cyclical dysphoric mood changes in women with a history of PMS or PMDD (P.J. Schmidt et al. 1998).

The role of serotonin and serotonergic systems in the pathogenesis of PMDD has been supported by several findings. Women with PMDD have a blunted prolactin response to buspirone challenge during the follicular phase, which suggests that serotonin type 1A (5-HT$_{1A}$) receptor subsensitivity may be a trait in women with PMDD (Yatham 1993). The prolactin response to L-tryptophan challenge is blunted in the luteal phase compared with the midfollicular phase of the menstrual cycle in women with PMDD, suggesting an altered postsynap-

tic serotonergic responsivity (Halbreich 1990). Significant aggravation of symptoms of PMDD, particularly irritability, can be provoked by tryptophan depletion (Menkes et al. 1994), supporting other evidence implicating the role of serotonin in PMDD. Whole blood serotonin levels and serotonin platelet reuptake have been reported to be decreased in women with PMDD (Ashby et al. 1990; Rapkin et al. 1987; Tam et al. 1985; Taylor et al. 1984). Finally, platelet imipramine binding is lower in women with PMDD, suggesting that vulnerability to PMDD may be associated with impaired gonadal hormone regulation of the serotonergic system (Rojansky et al. 1991).

Treatment

As would be expected given the proposed role of serotonin in PMDD, serotonergic antidepressants have been found to be effective in women with PMDD and are con-

sidered first-line therapy. The efficacy of SSRIs, in particular, has been reported in numerous randomized, controlled trials (see, for example, Dimmock et al. 2000;
Freeman et al. 1999; Steiner et al. 1995; Yonkers et al.
1997). In addition to the SSRIs, clomipramine (Sundblad
et al. 1992, 1993) and venlafaxine (Freeman et al. 2001b)
have been shown to be effective in the treatment of
PMDD. Intermittent dosing of antidepressants during
the luteal phase only (as opposed to daily continuous
treatment throughout the entire menstrual cycle) has
been shown to be effective in several studies (Cohen et al.
2002; Halbreich et al. 2002) and may be an attractive
option for many patients. Intermittent treatment allows
for less exposure to medication and lower costs and may
reduce long-term side effects, such as weight gain and
sexual dysfunction.

Consistent with the theory that fluctuations in ovarian
hormones (such as those occurring around and after ovulation) are a trigger for premenstrual symptoms, agents
that suppress ovulation also have been investigated (see,
for example, Hahn et al. 1995; Hammarback and Backstrom 1988; P.J. Schmidt et al. 1998). Gonadotropin-
releasing hormone agonists and danazol have been associated with improvement of premenstrual symptoms, but
their use is limited by potential side effects, such as increased risk of osteoporosis with gonadotropin-releasing
hormone agonists and weight gain, acne, hot flashes, and
facial hair associated with danazol. Moreover, these
agents have not been tested for PMDD.

Despite widespread belief among clinicians that oral
contraceptives are effective in the management of PMS
and PMDD, very few randomized, placebo-controlled
trials have been conducted, and little evidence suggests
their efficacy in treating premenstrual emotional symptoms. The latest clinical guidelines from the American
College of Obstetricians and Gynecologists (2000) do not
recommend oral contraceptives for the treatment of
PMDD. However, some newer oral contraceptives are
undergoing evaluation and have shown promise in preliminary studies (Freeman et al. 2001a).

Evidence for the role of benzodiazepines, specifically
alprazolam, in the treatment of PMS is mixed (Freeman
et al. 1995; P.J. Schmidt et al. 1993), and no studies have
been conducted for PMDD.

Nonpharmacological approaches also have been studied. Cognitive-behavioral therapy may be an appropriate
option for some patients (Blake et al. 1998; Hunter et al.
2002). Dietary supplements such as calcium, vitamin B_6,
and magnesium have shown some benefit for PMS symptoms (Thys-Jacobs et al. 1998; Walker et al. 1998; Wyatt
et al. 1999), although they have not been studied for
PMDD.

Depression During Pregnancy

Epidemiology

Traditionally, pregnancy was viewed as a time of emotional
well-being in which women were protected from depression
and other psychiatric disorders. However, evidence from the
few controlled trials of depression in pregnancy indicates
that the prevalence of MDD in pregnant women is similar to
that in nongravid women, with rates of MDD ranging from
4% to 16%, depending on the population studied and the
diagnostic criteria used (Evans et al. 2001; Gotlib et al. 1989;
Hobfoll et al. 1995; Kelly et al. 2001; Kumar and Robson
1984; O'Hara 1986). Although the prevalence of major
depression is similar in pregnant and nonpregnant women,
certain factors convey additional risk for some women
(O'Hara 1986; O'Hara et al. 1991). The most well-defined
risk factor for depression during pregnancy is a personal history of mood disorder. Several investigations have explored
the association of various demographic and psychosocial factors with risk for depression during pregnancy; these include
younger age, a greater number of children, living alone,
inadequate social support, marital discord, unwanted pregnancy, and recent adverse life events (Nonacs and Cohen
2003).

Clinical Features

Depressed pregnant women have an increased risk of self-
harm and higher rates of drug, alcohol, and tobacco use
(Zuckerman et al. 1989). Untreated depression during pregnancy is also associated with poor obstetrical outcome,
including an increased risk of preterm delivery (Orr et al.
1995, 2002; Steer et al. 1992) and increased risk of delivering
a low-birth-weight (<2.5 kg) or small-for-gestational-age
(less than tenth percentile) infant (Steer et al. 1992). These
findings may be explained by impaired self-care and failure
to follow prenatal guidelines. Another possible mechanism
by which depression might increase the risk for negative
pregnancy outcome is via alteration of the internal biochemical or hormonal environment (e.g., hypothalamic-pituitary-
adrenal axis hyperactivity) (Lundy et al. 1999). Long-term
physiological and neurobehavioral sequelae (e.g., decreased
activity, lower vagal tone, higher rates of behavior problems)
have been reported in the infants of mothers who were
depressed during pregnancy (Abrams et al. 1995; Brennan et
al. 2000; Jones et al. 1998; Lundy et al. 1999).

Treatment

A diagnosis of depression in a pregnant patient presents a
clinical challenge. An appropriate treatment plan should be

developed in collaboration with the patient, ideally before the pregnancy. Psychiatric history should help to guide decision making. When comparing treatment options (including the option of no treatment), it is important to be aware that every option affords some degree of exposure, either to the treatment or to the illness itself.

For some pregnant women with mild to moderate symptoms, psychotherapy is an appropriate and efficacious option. Structured psychotherapies, including interpersonal psychotherapy and cognitive-behavioral therapy, may be particularly helpful.

If pharmacotherapy is indicated, monotherapy is preferable. The decision to initiate antidepressant treatment during pregnancy should entail thoughtful consideration of the potential risks of treatment to the fetus relative to the known risks of the illness to the mother and fetus. No controlled studies of antidepressants have been done in pregnant women, and the U.S. Food and Drug Administration has not approved any psychotropic drug for use during pregnancy or lactation. Most antidepressants are in the C category, indicating that clinicians must carefully weigh the risks of treatment with the risks associated with no treatment on an individual basis. When making the decision to initiate, discontinue, or maintain antidepressant pharmacotherapy during pregnancy, clinicians should consider the mother's psychiatric history, the wishes of the patient, and the available safety data. Taken as a whole, the safety data for antidepressants in pregnant women published to date (see, for example, Chambers et al. 1996; Ericson et al. 1999; Kulin et al. 1998; McElhatton et al. 1996; Nulman et al. 1997) have not shown evidence of an increased risk of major congenital malformations, spontaneous pregnancy loss, or behavioral teratogenicity relative to the baseline rate in the general population. Transient neonatal distress syndromes have been described in association with antidepressant exposure in utero, although a causal link to particular medications has not been clearly established (Nonacs and Cohen 2003). Although a comprehensive review of the use of antidepressants during pregnancy is beyond the scope of this chapter, many excellent reviews have been published describing this body of evidence (see, for example, Nonacs and Cohen 2003).

Hospitalization and electroconvulsive therapy (ECT) should be considered in patients with severe depression. ECT has been used safely in pregnancy for more than 50 years, with more than 300 cases documented in the literature (Miller 1994).

Postpartum Mood Disturbances

The spectrum of postpartum mood disturbances ranges from the transient, relatively benign postpartum blues to postpartum major depression to postpartum psychosis, which is considered a psychiatric emergency.

Postpartum Blues

Postpartum blues is the most frequently observed postpartum mood disturbance, occurring in up to 70% of women after delivery. Symptoms are generally transient and nonpathological, but the presence of postpartum blues may herald the development of major depression in some patients.

Postpartum Depression

Epidemiology

Depression during the postpartum period affects approximately 10% of patients, which is similar to the risk for depression at other time points in a woman's life (O'Hara et al. 1984). The risk of major depression in the postpartum period is considerably higher, however, among patients with a history of major depression, postpartum depression, or depression during the pregnancy (O'Hara 1995). Additional risk factors for depression at this time include psychosocial factors such as limited social support, marital conflict, and ambivalence about the pregnancy.

Diagnosis and Clinical Features

The signs and symptoms of depression during the postpartum period are essentially indistinguishable from those of MDD during other times in a woman's life, although anxiety about the infant may be prominent. Thus, the diagnosis of postpartum depression is not distinct from a diagnosis of a major depressive episode at another time. The DSM-IV-TR postpartum onset specifier for MDD is restricted to episodes with an onset within 4 weeks of delivery; however, some women develop symptoms more insidiously, weeks or even months later.

Treatment

Psychotherapy is an appropriate option for some postpartum women with mild to moderate symptoms. Interpersonal psychotherapy (O'Hara et al. 2000; Stuart and O'Hara 1995), cognitive-behavioral therapy (Appleby et al. 1997), and counseling sessions with a health nurse (Wickberg and Hwang 1996) have been shown to reduce depressive symptoms significantly in randomized, controlled trials of postpartum depression.

Few well-controlled studies have evaluated the efficacy of pharmacotherapy for the treatment or prevention of depression in the postpartum period. However, no data indicate that approaches shown as clinically efficacious at other times would be less effective during the postpartum period. In a double-blind, placebo-controlled study, 12 weeks of treatment with fluoxetine resulted in a significantly greater reduction of depressive symptoms compared with placebo (Appleby et al. 1997). Open-label treatment with sertraline (Stowe et al. 1995), venlafaxine (Cohen et al. 2001), or fluvoxamine (Suri et al. 2001) also has been shown to be effective in women with postpartum depression.

Prevention studies in women with a history of postpartum depression have had mixed results. In an open study, 23 women with a history of postpartum depression were given the option to receive monitoring alone or monitoring in addition to treatment (beginning within 24 hours of childbirth) with either the antidepressant that had been effective previously or nortriptyline. The proportion of women who experienced recurrence was significantly greater in those who elected monitoring compared with those who elected monitoring plus medication (Wisner and Wheeler 1994). However, a double-blind, randomized study of nortriptyline treatment initiated immediately postpartum in nondepressed women with a history of postpartum depression failed to show a reduction in recurrence risk compared with placebo (Wisner et al. 2001).

Clinical Considerations in Breast-Feeding Women

Treatment decisions for a depressed woman who is breast-feeding should entail a careful risk-benefit assessment in collaboration with the patient. The potential risks of treatment exposure to the infant must be weighed against the risks of untreated illness to the mother and infant. All psychotropic medications are excreted into breast milk, at varying concentrations. The extent of exposure is dependent on the amount of drug in the breast milk, the chemical properties of the drug (e.g., lipid solubility, protein binding, molecular weight), and the neonate's metabolism (Newport et al. 2001). In weighing the risks and benefits of treatment, considerations also should include the severity of the illness, psychiatric history, and available safety data in lactation of previously effective treatments.

The safety database on antidepressants in breast-feeding is rapidly expanding. A review of the literature describing the use of newer antidepressants during breast-feeding identified more than 50 published reports documenting the effects of exposure to antidepressants via breast milk in more than 300 infants (bibliography available from authors on request). Adverse events have been reported in only a handful of cases to date (Brent and Wisner 1998; Chambers et al. 1999; Isenberg 1990; Kristensen et al. 1999; Lester et al. 1993; K. Schmidt et al. 2000; Yapp et al. 2000), with no evidence of serious adverse events or long-term sequelae related to medication exposure.

Postpartum Psychosis

Postpartum psychosis, the most severe form of postpartum psychiatric illness, is a rare condition that typically has a dramatic onset and is characterized by psychotic symptoms, disorientation, and disorganized behavior. Patients may have manic, depressive, or mixed mood (often rapidly shifting) and considerable dysfunction. As with depression in the postpartum period, postpartum psychosis is not a discrete diagnosis separate from psychotic episodes at other times (American Psychiatric Association 2000). Postpartum psychosis is a psychiatric emergency and usually requires hospitalization.

Depression During the Menopausal Transition

Epidemiology and Clinical Features

The perimenopause, or menopausal transition, represents the passage from reproductive to nonreproductive life. The onset of perimenopause is usually in the late 40s, with a mean age of 47.5 years and an average duration of 4–8 years (McKinlay et al. 1992). This process is characterized by marked biological variability, resulting in various endocrinological and clinical changes (e.g., more frequent anovulatory cycles, occurrence of vasomotor symptoms, and other physical complaints). The hormonal fluctuations experienced by some women during the menopausal transition may translate into an increased frequency of depressive symptoms (Avis et al. 1994; Hunter 1990; Joffe et al. 2002; Maartens et al. 2002) or an increased risk of recurrence of depression in women with a history of depression (Hay et al. 1994; Kessler et al. 1993). Some evidence indicates that women with a history of depression may be at risk for an earlier menopausal transition (Harlow et al. 2003). Several studies exploring the relation between depressive symptoms during the menopausal transition and the presence and severity of vasomotor symptoms have found that severe vasomotor symptoms (e.g., hot flushes, night sweats) may particularly increase the risk for depressive symptoms (Avis et al. 2001; Bosworth et al. 2001; Harlow et al. 2003; Joffe et al. 2002).

Treatment

Although treatment studies that have controlled for menopausal status are limited, antidepressants are the treatment of choice for major depression in peri- and postmenopausal women. Because some evidence indicates that patients with marked vasomotor symptoms may be more vulnerable to depression, the adequate management of these symptoms is essential (American College of Obstetricians and Gynecologists 2002; Kaufert et al. 1998). The role of reproductive hormones in response to antidepressant treatment remains to be systematically investigated, but some studies suggest that estradiol or estrogen replacement therapy, with or without concomitant antidepressants, may improve depressive symptoms in peri- and postmenopausal women (Rasgon et al. 2002; P.J. Schmidt et al. 2000; Schneider et al. 1997, 2001; Soares et al. 2001, 2003). The effects of hormone therapy on other medical outcomes in menopausal women remain controversial (Rossouw et al. 2002).

Given the increased risk of negative outcomes in women receiving hormone replacement therapy, antidepressants should be considered the treatment of first choice for depression in peri- and postmenopausal women. The potential benefit of adjunctive treatment with hormone therapy for women who are unresponsive to antidepressants alone must be weighed against the small but potentially serious risks associated with such treatment.

Conclusion

Throughout their childbearing years, women are approximately twice as likely as men to experience an episode of major depression. Both psychosocial and neurobiological factors likely contribute to this observed phenomenon. Gender differences in clinical presentation, comorbidity, course of illness, and response to treatment also have been documented and should be considered when screening for, evaluating, and selecting treatment for depression in women. The menstrual cycle, pregnancy, and menopause may be associated with increased vulnerability to depressive symptoms in certain at-risk women. Treatment of depression in pregnant or breast-feeding women requires unique clinical considerations and careful assessment of the risks and benefits of treatment.

References

Abrams SM, Field T, Scafidi F, et al: Newborns of depressed mothers. Infant Ment Health J 16:233–239, 1995

American College of Obstetricians and Gynecologists: Premenstrual Syndrome. ACOG Practice Bulletin No. 15, April 2000

American College of Obstetricians and Gynecologists, Committee on Gynecologic Practice: ACOG committee opinion: risk of breast cancer with estrogen-progestin replacement therapy. Int J Gynaecol Obstet 76:333–335, 2002

American Psychiatric Association: Diagnostic and Statistical Manual of Mental Disorders, 4th Edition, Text Revision. Washington, DC, American Psychiatric Association, 2000

Angst J, Dobler-Mikola A: Do the diagnostic criteria determine the sex ratio in depression? J Affect Disord 7:189–198, 1984

Appleby L, Warner R, Whitten A, et al: A controlled study of fluoxetine and cognitive-behavioural counselling in the treatment of postnatal depression. BMJ 314:932–936, 1997

Ashby CR Jr, Carr LA, Cook CL, et al: Alteration of 5-HT uptake by plasma fractions in the premenstrual syndrome. J Neural Transm Gen Sect 79:41–50, 1990

Avis NE, Brambilla D, McKinlay SM, et al: A longitudinal analysis of the association between menopause and depression: results from the Massachusetts Women's Health Study. Ann Epidemiol 4:214–220, 1994

Avis NE, Crawford S, Stellato R, et al: Longitudinal study of hormone levels and depression among women transitioning through menopause. Climacteric 4:243–249, 2001

Bailey JW, Cohen LS: Prevalence of mood and anxiety disorders in women who seek treatment for premenstrual syndrome. J Womens Health Gend Based Med 8:1181–1184, 1999

Blake F, Salkovskis P, Gath D, et al: Cognitive therapy for premenstrual syndrome: a controlled trial. J Psychosom Res 45:307–318, 1998

Bloch M, Schmidt PJ, Su TP, et al: Pituitary-adrenal hormones and testosterone across the menstrual cycle in women with premenstrual syndrome and controls. Biol Psychiatry 43:897–903, 1998

Bosworth HB, Bastian LA, Kuchibhatla MN, et al: Depressive symptoms, menopausal status, and climacteric symptoms in women at midlife. Psychosom Med 63:603–608, 2001

Brennan PA, Hammen C, Andersen MJ, et al: Chronicity, severity, and timing of maternal depressive symptoms: relationships with child outcomes at age 5. Dev Psychol 36:759–766, 2000

Brent NB, Wisner KL: Fluoxetine and carbamazepine concentrations in a nursing mother/infant pair. Clin Pediatr 37:41–44, 1998

Brown GW, Moran PM: Single mothers, poverty and depression. Psychol Med 27:21–33, 1997

Carter JD, Joyce PR, Mulder RT, et al: Gender differences in the presentation of depressed outpatients: a comparison of descriptive variables. J Affect Disord 61:59–67, 2000

Chambers CD, Johnson KA, Dick LM, et al: Birth outcomes in pregnant women taking fluoxetine. N Engl J Med 335:1010–1015, 1996

Chambers CD, Anderson PO, Thomas RG, et al: Weight gain in infants breastfed by mothers who take fluoxetine. Pediatrics 104:e61, 1999

Cohen LS, Viguera AC, Bouffard SM, et al: Venlafaxine in the treatment of postpartum depression. J Clin Psychiatry 62:592–596, 2001

Cohen LS, Miner C, Brown EW, et al: Premenstrual daily fluoxetine for premenstrual dysphoric disorder: a placebo-controlled, clinical trial using computerized diaries. Obstet Gynecol 100:435–444, 2002

Cyranowski JM, Frank E, Young E, et al: Adolescent onset of the gender difference in lifetime rates of major depression: a theoretical model. Arch Gen Psychiatry 57:21–27, 2000

Dimmock PW, Wyatt KM, Jones PW, et al: Efficacy of selective serotonin reuptake inhibitors in premenstrual syndrome: a systematic review. Lancet 356:1131–1136, 2000

Endicott J: The menstrual cycle and mood disorders. J Affect Disord 29:193–200, 1993

Entsuah AR, Huang H, Thase ME: Response and remission rates in different subpopulations with major depressive disorder administered venlafaxine, selective serotonin reuptake inhibitors, or placebo. J Clin Psychiatry 62:869–877, 2001

Ericson A, Kallen B, Wiholm B: Delivery outcome after the use of antidepressants in early pregnancy. Eur J Clin Pharmacol 55:503–508, 1999

Evans J, Heron J, Francomb H, et al: Cohort study of depressed mood during pregnancy and after childbirth. BMJ 323:257–260, 2001

Fava M, Abraham M, Alpert J, et al: Gender differences in Axis I comorbidity among depressed outpatients. J Affect Disord 38:129–133, 1996

Frank E, Carpenter LL, Kupfer DJ: Sex differences in recurrent depression: are there any that are significant? Am J Psychiatry 145:41–45, 1988

Freeman EW, Rickels K, Sondheimer SJ, et al: A double-blind trial of oral progesterone, alprazolam, and placebo in treatment of severe premenstrual syndrome. JAMA 274:51–57, 1995

Freeman EW, Rickels K, Sondheimer SJ, et al: Differential response to antidepressants in women with premenstrual syndrome/premenstrual dysphoric disorder: a randomized controlled trial. Arch Gen Psychiatry 56:932–939, 1999

Freeman EW, Kroll R, Rapkin A, et al: Evaluation of a unique oral contraceptive in the treatment of premenstrual dysphoric disorder. J Womens Health Gend Based Med 10:561–569, 2001a

Freeman EW, Rickels K, Yonkers KA, et al: Venlafaxine in the treatment of premenstrual dysphoric disorder. Obstet Gynecol 98:737–744, 2001b

Gotlib IH, Whiffen VE, Mount JH, et al: Prevalence rates and demographic characteristics associated with depression in pregnancy and the postpartum. J Consult Clin Psychol 57:269–274, 1989

Hahn PM, Van Vugt DA, Reid RL: A randomized, placebo-controlled, crossover trial of danazol for the treatment of premenstrual syndrome. Psychoneuroendocrinology 20:193–209, 1995

Halbreich U: Gonadal hormones and antihormones, serotonin and mood. Psychopharmacol Bull 26:291–295, 1990

Halbreich U, Bergeron R, Yonkers KA, et al: Efficacy of intermittent, luteal phase sertraline treatment of premenstrual dysphoric disorder. Obstet Gynecol 100:1219–1229, 2002

Halbreich U, Borenstein J, Pearlstein T, et al: The prevalence, impact, and burden of premenstrual dysphoric disorder. Psychoneuroendocrinology 28 (suppl 3):1–23, 2003

Hamilton JA, Grant M, Jensvold MF: Sex and treatment of depressions: when does it matter? In Psychopharmacology and Women: Sex, Gender, and Hormones. Edited by Jensvold MF, Halbreich U, Hamilton JA. Washington, DC, American Psychiatric Press, 1996, pp 241–257

Hammarback S, Backstrom T: Induced anovulation as treatment of premenstrual tension syndrome: a double-blind cross-over study with GnRH-agonist versus placebo. Acta Obstet Gynecol Scand 67:159–166, 1988

Harlow BL, Wise LA, Otto MW, et al: Depression and its influence on reproductive endocrine and menstrual cycle markers associated with perimenopause: the Harvard Study of Moods and Cycles. Arch Gen Psychiatry 60:29–36, 2003

Hay AG, Bancroft J, Johnstone EC: Affective symptoms in women attending a menopause clinic. Br J Psychiatry 164:513–516, 1994

Hildebrandt MG, Steyerberg EW, Stage KB, et al: Are gender differences important for the clinical effects of antidepressants? Am J Psychiatry 160:1643–1650, 2003

Hirschfeld RMA, Russell JM: Assessment and treatment of suicidal patients. N Engl J Med 337:910–915, 1997

Hobfoll SE, Ritter C, Lavin J, et al: Depression prevalence and incidence among inner-city pregnant and postpartum women. J Consult Clin Psychol 63:445–453, 1995

Hunter MS: Psychological and somatic experience of the menopause: a prospective study. Psychosom Med 52:357–367, 1990

Hunter MS, Ussher JM, Browne SJ, et al: A randomized comparison of psychological (cognitive behavior therapy), medical (fluoxetine) and combined treatment for women with premenstrual dysphoric disorder. J Psychosom Obstet Gynaecol 23:193–199, 2002

Isenberg KE: Excretion of fluoxetine in human breast milk. J Clin Psychiatry 51:169, 1990

Joffe H, Cohen LS: Estrogen, serotonin, and mood disturbance: where is the therapeutic bridge? Biol Psychiatry 44:798–811, 1998

Joffe H, Hall JE, Soares CN, et al: Vasomotor symptoms are associated with depression in perimenopausal women seeking primary care. Menopause 9:392–398, 2002

Johnson SR: The epidemiology and social impact of premenstrual symptoms. Clin Obstet Gynecol 30:367–376, 1987

Jones NA, Field T, Fox NA, et al: Newborns of mothers with depressive symptoms are physiologically less developed. Infant Behav Dev 21:537–541, 1998

Kaufert P, Boggs PP, Ettinger B, et al: Women and menopause: beliefs, attitudes, and behaviors. The North American Menopause Society 1997 Menopause Survey. Menopause 5:197–202, 1998

Kelly R, Zatzick D, Anders T: The detection and treatment of psychiatric disorders and substance use among pregnant women cared for in obstetrics. Am J Psychiatry 158:213–219, 2001

Kessler RC: Epidemiology of women and depression. J Affect Disord 74:5–13, 2003

Kessler RC, Brown RL, Broman CL: Sex differences in psychiatric help-seeking: evidence from four large-scale surveys. J Health Soc Behav 22:49–64, 1981

Kessler RC, McGonagle KA, Swartz M, et al: Sex and depression in the National Comorbidity Survey, I: lifetime prevalence, chronicity and recurrence. J Affect Disord 29:85–96, 1993

Kornstein SG: Gender differences in depression: implications for treatment. J Clin Psychiatry 58 (suppl 15):12–18, 1997

Kornstein SG, Wojcik BA: Depression, in Women's Mental Health: A Comprehensive Textbook. Edited by Kornstein SG, Clayton AH. New York, Guilford, 2002, pp 147–165

Kornstein SG, Schatzberg AF, Thase ME, et al: Gender differences in chronic major and double depression. J Affect Disord 60:1–11, 2000a

Kornstein SG, Schatzberg AF, Thase ME, et al: Gender differences in treatment response to sertraline versus imipramine in chronic depression. Am J Psychiatry 157:1445–1452, 2000b

Kristensen JH, Ilett KF, Hackett LP, et al: Distribution and excretion of fluoxetine and norfluoxetine in human milk. Br J Clin Pharmacol 48:521–527, 1999

Kulin NA, Pastuszak A, Sage SR, et al: Pregnancy outcome following maternal use of the new selective serotonin reuptake inhibitors: a prospective controlled multicenter study. JAMA 279:609–610, 1998

Kumar R, Robson KM: A prospective study of emotional disorders in childbearing women. Br J Psychiatry 144:35–47, 1984

Lester BM, Cucca J, Andreozzi L, et al: Possible association between fluoxetine hydrochloride and colic in an infant. J Am Acad Child Adolesc Psychiatry 32:1253–1255, 1993

Logue CM, Moos RH: Perimenstrual symptoms: prevalence and risk factors. Psychosom Med 48:388–414, 1986

Lundy BL, Jones NA, Field T, et al: Prenatal depression effects on neonates. Infant Behav Dev 22:119–129, 1999

Maartens LW, Knottnerus JA, Pop VJ: Menopausal transition and increased depressive symptomatology: a community based prospective study. Maturitas 42:195–200, 2002

Martenyi F, Dossenbach M, Mraz K, et al: Gender differences in the efficacy of fluoxetine and maprotiline in depressed patients: a double-blind trial of antidepressants with serotonergic or norepinephrinergic reuptake inhibition profile. Eur Neuropsychopharmacol 11:227–232, 2001

McElhatton PR, Garbis HM, Elefant E, et al: The outcome of pregnancy in 689 women exposed to therapeutic doses of antidepressants: a collaborative study of the European Network of Teratology Information Services (ENTIS). Reprod Toxicol 10:285–294, 1996

McKinlay SM, Brambilla DJ, Posner JG: The normal menopause transition. Maturitas 14:103–115, 1992

Menkes DB, Coates DC, Fawcett JP: Acute tryptophan depletion aggravates premenstrual syndrome. J Affect Disord 32:37–44, 1994

Michaud CM, Murray CJ, Bloom BR: Burden of disease—implications for future research. JAMA 285:535–539, 2001

Miller LJ: Use of electroconvulsive therapy during pregnancy. Hosp Community Psychiatry 45:444–450, 1994

Muse KN, Cetel NS, Futterman LA, et al: The premenstrual syndrome: effects of "medical ovariectomy." N Engl J Med 311:1345–1349, 1984

Newport DJ, Wilcox MM, Stowe ZN: Antidepressants during pregnancy and lactation: defining exposure and treatment issues. Semin Perinatol 25:177–190, 2001

Nolen-Hoeksema S: Gender differences in coping with depression across the lifespan. Depression 3:81–90, 1995

Nonacs R, Cohen LS: Assessment and treatment of depression during pregnancy: an update. Psychiatr Clin North Am 26:547–562, 2003

Nulman I, Rovet J, Stewart DE, et al: Neurodevelopment of children exposed in utero to antidepressant drugs. N Engl J Med 336:258–262, 1997

O'Hara MW: Social support, life events, and depression during pregnancy and puerperium. Arch Gen Psychiatry 43:569–573, 1986

O'Hara MW: Postpartum Depression: Causes and Consequences. New York, Springer-Verlag, 1995

O'Hara MW, Neunaber DJ, Zekoski EM: Prospective study of postpartum depression: prevalence, course, and predictive factors. J Abnorm Psychol 93:158–171, 1984

O'Hara MW, Schlechte JA, Lewis DA, et al: Controlled prospective study of postpartum mood disorders: psychological, environmental, and hormonal variables. J Abnorm Psychol 100:63–73, 1991

O'Hara MW, Stuart S, Gorman LL, et al: Efficacy of interpersonal psychotherapy for postpartum depression. Arch Gen Psychiatry 57:1039–1045, 2000

Orr S, Miller C: Maternal depressive symptoms and the risk of poor pregnancy outcome: review of the literature and preliminary findings. Epidemiol Rev 17:165–171, 1995

Orr ST, James SA, Blackmore Prince C: Maternal prenatal depressive symptoms and spontaneous preterm births among African-American women in Baltimore, Maryland. Am J Epidemiol 156:797–802, 2002

Perugi G, Musetti L, Simonini E, et al: Gender-mediated clinical features of depressive illness: the importance of temperamental differences. Br J Psychiatry 157:835–841, 1990

Quitkin FM, Stewart JW, McGrath PJ, et al: Are there differences between women's and men's antidepressant responses? Am J Psychiatry 159:1848–1854, 2002

Ramcharan S, Love EJ, Fick GH, et al: The epidemiology of premenstrual symptoms in a population-based sample of 2650 urban women: attributable risk and risk factors. J Clin Epidemiol 45:377–392, 1992

Rapaport MH, Thompson PM, Kelsoe JR, et al: Gender differences in outpatient research subjects with affective disorders: a comparison of descriptive variables. J Clin Psychiatry 56:67–72, 1995

Rapkin AJ, Edelmuth E, Chang LC, et al: Whole-blood serotonin in premenstrual syndrome. Obstet Gynecol 70:533–537, 1987

Rasgon NL, Altshuler LL, Fairbanks LA, et al.: Estrogen replacement therapy in the treatment of major depressive disorder in perimenopausal women. J Clin Psychiatry 63 (suppl 7):45–48, 2002

Raskin A, Schulterbrandt JG, Reatig N, et al: Depression subtypes and response to phenelzine, diazepam, and a placebo: results of a nine hospital collaborative study. Arch Gen Psychiatry 30:66–75, 1974

Roca CA, Schmidt PJ, Altemus M, et al: Differential menstrual cycle regulation of hypothalamic-pituitary-adrenal axis in women with premenstrual syndrome and controls. J Clin Endocrinol Metab 88:3057–3063, 2003

Rojansky N, Halbreich U, Zander K, et al: Imipramine receptor binding and serotonin uptake in platelets of women with premenstrual changes. Gynecol Obstet Invest 31:146–152, 1991

Rossouw JE, Anderson GL, Prentice RL, et al: Risks and benefits of estrogen plus progestin in healthy postmenopausal women: principal results from the Women's Health Initiative randomized controlled trial. JAMA 288:321–333, 2002

Rubinow DR, Schmidt PJ, Roca CA: Estrogen-serotonin interactions: implications for affective regulation. Biol Psychiatry 44:839–850, 1998

Ruble DN, Greulich F, Pomerantz EM, et al: The role of gender-related processes in the development of sex differences in self-evaluation and depression. J Affect Disord 29:97–128, 1993

Schmidt K, Olesen OV, Jensen PN: Citalopram and breastfeeding: serum concentration and side effects in the infant. Biol Psychiatry 47:164–165, 2000

Schmidt PJ, Grover GN, Rubinow DR: Alprazolam in the treatment of premenstrual syndrome: a double-blind, placebo-controlled trial. Arch Gen Psychiatry 50:467–473, 1993

Schmidt PJ, Roca CA, Bloch M, et al: The perimenopause and affective disorders. Semin Reprod Endocrinol 15:91–100, 1997

Schmidt PJ, Nieman LK, Danaceau MA, et al: Differential behavioral effects of gonadal steroids in women with and in those without premenstrual syndrome. N Engl J Med 338:209–216, 1998

Schmidt PJ, Nieman L, Danaceau MA, et al: Estrogen replacement in perimenopause-related depression: a preliminary report. Am J Obstet Gynecol 183:414–420, 2000

Schneider LS, Small GW, Hamilton SH, et al: Estrogen replacement and response to fluoxetine in a multicenter geriatric depression trial. Fluoxetine Collaborative Study Group. Am J Geriatr Psychiatry 5:97–106, 1997

Schneider LS, Small GW, Clary CM: Estrogen replacement therapy and antidepressant response to sertraline in older depressed women. Am J Geriatr Psychiatry 9:393–399, 2001

Soares CN, Almeida OP, Joffe H, et al: Efficacy of estradiol for the treatment of depressive disorders in perimenopausal women: a double-blind, randomized, placebo-controlled trial. Arch Gen Psychiatry 58:529–534, 2001

Soares CN, Poitras JR, Prouty J, et al: Efficacy of citalopram as a monotherapy or as an adjunctive treatment to estrogen therapy for perimenopausal and postmenopausal women with depression and vasomotor symptoms. J Clin Psychiatry 64:473–479, 2003

Steer RA, Scholl TO, Hediger ML, et al: Self-reported depression and negative pregnancy outcomes. J Clin Epidemiol 5:1093–1099, 1992

Steiner M, Steinberg S, Stewart D, et al: Fluoxetine in the treatment of premenstrual dysphoria. Canadian Fluoxetine/Premenstrual Dysphoria Collaborative Study Group. N Engl J Med 332:1529–1534, 1995

Stout AL, Grady TA, Steege JF, et al: Premenstrual symptoms in black and white community samples. Am J Psychiatry 143:1436–1439, 1986

Stowe ZN, Casarella J, Landry J, et al: Sertraline in the treatment of women with postpartum major depression. Depression 3:49–55, 1995

Stuart S, O'Hara MW: Treatment of postpartum depression with interpersonal psychotherapy. J Psychother Pract Res 4:18–29, 1995

Sundblad C, Modigh K, Andersch B, et al: Clomipramine effectively reduces premenstrual irritability and dysphoria: a placebo-controlled trial. Acta Psychiatr Scand 85:39–47, 1992

Sundblad C, Hedberg MA, Eriksson E: Clomipramine administered during the luteal phase reduces the symptoms of premenstrual syndrome: a placebo-controlled trial. Neuropsychopharmacology 9:133–145, 1993

Suri R, Burt VK, Altshuler LL, et al: Fluvoxamine for postpartum depression. Am J Psychiatry 158:1739–1740, 2001

Tam WY, Chan MY, Lee PH: The menstrual cycle and platelet 5-HT uptake. Psychosom Med 47:352–362, 1985

Taylor DL, Mathew RJ, Ho BT, et al: Serotonin levels and platelet uptake during premenstrual tension. Neuropsychobiology 12:16–18, 1984

Thase ME, Entsuah R, Cantillon M, et al: Relative antidepressant efficacy of venlafaxine and SSRIs: sex–age interactions. J Womens Health (in press)

Thys-Jacobs S, Starkey P, Bernstein D, et al: Calcium carbonate and the premenstrual syndrome: effects on premenstrual and menstrual symptoms. Am J Obstet Gynecol 179:444–452, 1998

Walker AF, De Souza MC, Vickers MF, et al: Magnesium supplementation alleviates premenstrual symptoms of fluid retention. J Womens Health 7:1157–1165, 1998

Weiss EL, Longhurst G, Mazure CM: Childhood sexual abuse as a risk factor for depression in women: psychosocial and neurobiological correlates. Am J Psychiatry 156:816–828, 1999

Weissman MM, Bland R, Joyce PR, et al: Sex differences in rates of depression: cross-national perspectives. J Affect Disord 29:77–84, 1993

Weissman MM, Bland RC, Canino GJ, et al: Cross-national epidemiology of major depression and bipolar disorder. JAMA 276:293–299, 1996

Wickberg B, Hwang CP: Counselling of postnatal depression: a controlled study on a population based Swedish sample. J Affect Disord 39:209–216, 1996

Wisner KL, Wheeler SB: Prevention of recurrent postpartum major depression. Hosp Community Psychiatry 45:1191–1196, 1994

Wisner KL, Perel JM, Peindl KS, et al: Prevention of recurrent postpartum depression: a randomized clinical trial. J Clin Psychiatry 62:82–86, 2001

Wyatt KM, Dimmock PW, Jones PW, et al: Efficacy of vitamin B6 in the treatment of premenstrual syndrome: systematic review. BMJ 318:1375–1381, 1999

Yapp P, Ilett KF, Kristensen JH, et al: Drowsiness and poor feeding in a breast-fed infant: association with nefazodone and its metabolites. Ann Pharmacother 34:1269–1272, 2000

Yatham LN: Is 5HT1A receptor subsensitivity a trait marker for late luteal phase dysphoric disorder? A pilot study. Can J Psychiatry 38:662–664, 1993

Yonkers KA, Halbreich U, Freeman E, et al: Symptomatic improvement of premenstrual dysphoric disorder with sertraline treatment: a randomized controlled trial. Sertraline Premenstrual Dysphoric Collaborative Study Group. JAMA 278:983–988, 1997

Young MA, Scheftner WA, Fawcett J, et al: Gender differences in the clinical features of unipolar major depressive disorder. J Nerv Ment Dis 178:200–203, 1990

Zuckerman B, Amaro H, Bauchner H, et al: Depressive symptoms during pregnancy: relationship to poor health behaviors. Am J Obstet Gynecol 160:1107–1111, 1989

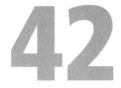

Depression Across Cultures

LAURENCE J. KIRMAYER, M.D.

G. ERIC JARVIS, M.D., M.SC.

DEPRESSION IS NOW recognized as a global health problem, with estimates that it accounts for up to 10% of years lost to disability in developing countries and that this proportion is likely to increase in the decades to come (Desjarlais et al. 1995; Murray and Lopez 1997). Given this widespread prevalence and social effect, a pressing need exists to examine cross-cultural differences in the causes, course, and treatment of depression (Scott and Dickey 2003). At the same time, responding to the health disparities associated with cultural diversity is increasingly recognized as an important issue in high-income countries, creating new challenges for mental health care (U.S. Surgeon General 2002).

Cultural psychiatry is concerned with the effect of variations of ways of life on psychiatric disorders and their treatment (Kleinman 1988). Cultural psychiatry seeks to address the following questions: How does culture shape the experience and expression of human suffering? What are the most effective methods of interpreting and responding to suffering in a given social or clinical context? Are the forms of distress identified in current psychiatric nosology similar around the globe? More specifically, can mood disorders be recognized across diverse cultures, and

do they have similar symptoms, course, treatment response, and outcome? These questions raise complex epistemological and methodological problems for psychiatric research and practice. The answers are crucial to the advance of research, the design of health care systems, and the delivery of clinical care in societies facing increasing cultural diversity (Kirmayer and Minas 2000).

Much of what we know about the role of culture in psychopathology comes from qualitative ethnographic research in clinical settings and in the community (Kirmayer 1989; Kleinman 1988). Conventional psychiatric research is ill suited to explore the cultural meaning of distress because it tends to reduce the complexity of illness narratives to a checklist of symptoms and signs of disorder. However, a growing body of epidemiological research informed by ethnography goes beyond parochial assumptions to identify clinically important cultural variation. In this chapter, we review some of what is known about cultural variations in the prevalence, clinical presentation, mechanisms, and treatment of depressive disorders and address some of the broader conceptual issues that are central to meaningful research and effective clinical intervention.

Defining Culture

Culture encompasses all the forms of knowledge and practices that make up a way of life, with its social roles, values, and institutions. This includes the ways in which social groups are marked off from one another in terms of ethnicity, race, religion, or other social categories. The definition of a group is always vis-à-vis some other group; hence, the meanings of ethnicity, race, and other culturally constructed aspects of identity change depending on the larger social context.

Older notions of cultures as homogeneous, self-contained homeostatic systems have given way to a view of culture as an abstraction based on fluid, ever-changing constructions that emerge from interactions among individuals, communities, and social institutions, which are embedded in global systems (Bibeau 1997; Kirmayer 2002). Individuals use resources available in their local social worlds to construct durable and culturally valued identities and competent selves. At the same time, individuals and groups are constrained by the ways in which culture frames and defines their options and experience. In the contemporary world, migration and electronic communication allow individuals to position themselves within multiple cultural worlds, resulting in cultural hybridization or creolization, the creation of new cultural forms.

Despite this complex reality of culture, most psychiatric research has worked with outmoded concepts of culture. World Health Organization (WHO) studies have used geographic location as a proxy for culture, ignoring local cultural diversity and the sometimes unrepresentative nature of local collaborating centers. In the United States, the vast majority of studies refer to ethnoracial blocs (African American, Asian American, Native American, Hispanic American, white), which are heterogeneous categories constructed by the census. Epidemiological research tends to use these categories, whereas specialized clinical texts offer chapters on specific ethnocultural groups with case studies or rules of thumb that lead to stereotypes. In this chapter, we try to move beyond the data generated with these outmoded notions of culture to consider ways in which culture can be better conceptualized for research and clinical practice.

The Problem of Cross-Cultural Equivalence

Studying any psychiatric disorder across cultures presupposes that we can accurately identify or measure the same construct across different social and cultural contexts. This is not simply a technical problem of determining psychometric equivalence, for which there are established methods (Westermeyer and Janca 1997), but a conceptual problem that involves translating vocabularies of distress and showing that they have similar clinical and pathological significance across cultures. Thus, it may be possible to identify people whose symptoms fit conventional psychiatric criteria for depression in diverse settings, but this may not be the best or only way to understand and describe their problem; and there may be unknown numbers of people with related forms of distress whose symptoms do not fit the conventional categories and criteria of mood disorders. Kleinman (1977) has termed this potentially misleading application of categories across different cultural contexts the *category fallacy*.

One way to avoid the category fallacy is to step back from the received categories of psychiatric nosology and begin with ethnographic research on local ways of expressing distress. This type of research can uncover idioms of distress, which include local cultural models and metaphors for distress that emerge from the interaction of biology and culture-specific understandings of affliction. Such work may identify symptoms and behaviors that are culturally salient and that can be investigated alongside the established symptoms of depression. Standard diagnostic instruments can be used to provide an anchor point for comparison, but they can supplemented with an expanded symptom pool based on ethnographic research. This strategy generates clinical and epidemiological data that may confirm the validity of existing categories and criteria or suggest alternative ways of categorizing distress with greater utility in predicting treatment response and outcome.

There have been several efforts to develop culturally sensitive measures of depression and related forms of demoralization or emotional distress (Abas et al. 1998; Beiser and Fleming 1986; Ebigbo 1982; El-Rufaie et al. 1997; Kinzie et al. 1982; Mollica et al. 1987; Mumford et al. 1991; Patel et al. 1997; Phan et al. 2004; Singh et al. 1974; Sulaiman et al. 2001) (Table 42–1). Most of these measures are self-report scales that tap nonspecific dimensions of depression, anxiety, and common somatic symptoms of distress. For example, Abas and colleagues (1998) developed the Caribbean Culture-Specific Screen questionnaire for emotional distress, which incorporates common expressions for dysphoria and depression among older African-Caribbean people (e.g., "Have you felt pressured, like pressure is rising in your head? Have you had lots of pain or gas in the belly or the pit of your stomach? Have you been feeling empty or spiritless inside?"). A validation study comparing the screening measure with

TABLE 42-1. Some culture-specific measures of depression and related forms of distress

Scale	Target population (language)	Characteristics
Vietnamese Depression Scale (Kinzie et al. 1982)	Vietnamese	15-item scale derived from a clinical sample
Four Measures of Mental Health (Beiser and Fleming 1986)	Vietnamese	15-item depression scale
Indochinese Hopkins Symptom Checklist—25 (Mollica et al. 1987)	Cambodian (Khmer) Laotian Vietnamese	Uses 25 items from the Hopkins Symptom Checklist—58
Phan Vietnamese Psychiatric Scale (Phan et al. 2004)	Vietnamese in Australia	26-item depression subscale (also anxiety and somatization scales); good psychometrics
Bradford Somatic Inventory (Mumford et al. 1991)	Pakistan (Urdu)	44-item scale of common somatic symptoms developed simultaneously in Pakistan and the United Kingdom
Amritsar Depression Inventory (Singh et al. 1974)	Punjabi-speaking patients in India	30-item depression scale
Enugu Somatization Scale (Ebigbo 1982, 1986)	Nigeria	65-item somatic symptom inventory
Shona Symptom Questionnaire (Patel et al. 1997)	Shona-speaking primary health care users in Zimbabwe	14-item common mental disorder scale
Caribbean Culture-Specific Screen (Abas et al. 1998)	Older (>60 years) African-Caribbean primary care users in South London	13-item depression scale
Primary Care Anxiety and Depression Scale (El-Rufaie et al. 1997)	Arabic-speaking primary health care users in United Arab Emirates	12-item anxiety and depression scale
Symptom Checklist for Depression in Dubai (Sulaiman et al. 2001)	Arabic-speaking natives of Dubai	22 aspects of depression comprising 96 expressions; no psychometrics

both standard and culturally adapted diagnostic interviews found that the culture-specific measure did not perform any better than the standard Geriatric Depression Scale (GDS) in identifying clinical depression (Sheikh and Yesavage 1986) but that the sensitivity and overall performance of the GDS could be improved by lowering its cutoff score. Thus, it appeared that African-Caribbean patients might have been significantly depressed even when they reported only a few symptoms of depression.

Notwithstanding these attempts at developing culture-specific measures of distress, most epidemiological research on depression has used only standard instruments constructed and validated with Euro-American and European populations. Moreover, studies published to date do not consider the internal cultural variation of countries and hence cannot determine the significance of cultural variables for the prevalence, course, or outcome of mood disorders. Future research will depend on culturally validated measures and, most importantly, on unpacking the meaning of cultural variation within and across countries in terms of social, psychological, and biological processes that may interact in the cause and course of depression.

Cultural Epidemiology of Depression

International research over the last four decades has found that depression can be identified in all countries, regions, and cultures that have been studied (Sartorius et al. 1980; Weissman et al. 1996). Even with standard epidemiological techniques, depression can be found around the world (World Health Organization 1983) and has an especially high prevalence in some low-income countries (Desjarlais et al. 1995; Orley and Wing 1979; Vorcaro et al. 2001). Despite this apparent universality, wide variations in prevalence, symptomatology, and clinical presentation are evident (Kleinman and Good 1985).

The WHO Collaborative Study on the Standardized Assessment of Depressive Disorders compared patients seeking help for depressive symptoms at clinics in cities from four countries (Canada, Switzerland, Iran, and Japan) with a standardized interview instrument (Sartorius et al. 1980). The most common symptoms across sites were sadness, joylessness, anxiety, tension, and lack of energy (Jablensky et al. 1981). Other common symptoms included loss of interest,

TABLE 42-2. Prevalence of depressive disorder in World Health Organization cross-national study of mental disorders in primary care

Country	City	Point prevalence (%)	Female (%)	Male (%)	Gender ratio (F/M)
Brazil	Rio de Janeiro	15.8	19.6	5.8	3.4
Chile	Santiago	29.5	36.8	11.2	3.3
China	Shanghai	4.0	4.4	3.3	1.3
France	Paris	13.7	18.7	9.3	2.0
Germany	Berlin	6.1	7.7	3.7	2.1
Germany	Mainz	11.2	12.3	9.8	1.3
Greece	Athens	6.4	6.4	6.5	1.0
India	Bangalore	9.1	13.3	4.8	2.8
Italy	Verona	4.7	5.5	3.2	1.7
Japan	Nagasaki	2.6	2.8	2.3	1.2
The Netherlands	Groningen	15.9	17.9	13.0	1.4
Nigeria	Ibadan	4.2	3.8	5.3	0.7
Turkey	Ankara	11.6	12.5	9.8	1.3
United States	Seattle	6.3	6.5	6.0	1.1
United Kingdom	Manchester	16.9	18.3	13.9	1.3

Source. Data from Üstün and Sartorius (1995).

loss of ability to concentrate, and ideas of oneself as insufficient, inadequate, and worthless. Feelings of guilt and self-reproach varied in frequency across sites: 68% in Basel, Switzerland; 58% in Montreal, Quebec; 48% in Tokyo, Japan; 41% in Nagasaki, Japan; and 32% in Tehran, Iran. Suicidal ideation also varied substantially, ranging from 70% in Montreal and Nagasaki to 41% in Tokyo. Somatic symptoms (including vegetative symptoms of anorexia, weight loss, loss of libido, and constipation) were most common in Tehran (57%) and least frequent in Montreal (27%).

More recently, the WHO Cross-National Study of Mental Disorders in Primary Care (Table 42–2) studied clinical samples at 15 centers in 14 countries. In a two-stage design, 25,916 primary care patients were screened with the General Health Questionnaire, and the diagnosis of depression was made by use of the Composite International Diagnostic Interview (CIDI) (Üstün and Sartorius 1995). As summarized in Table 42–2, the prevalence of major depression varied 15-fold across centers. The pattern of symptom co-variation and threshold behavior was similar across sites (Simon et al. 2002). However, at the center with a higher prevalence, depression was associated with lower levels of disability, suggesting that people with milder cases were obtaining help. This may account for some of the variation in prevalence across clinical sites. This study illustrates how identical measures and diagnostic criteria may,

in fact, identify different levels of depression severity in different countries and cultures.

Cross-national comparisons of the community prevalence of mood disorders have been made possible with data from surveys that used the Diagnostic Interview Schedule (DIS) (Robins et al. 1985) in the United States, Canada, Puerto Rico, West Germany, Taiwan, Korea, and New Zealand (Weissman et al. 1996) (Table 42–3). The annual prevalence of depression varied widely—from less than 1% in Taiwan to almost 6% in Christchurch, New Zealand. Lifetime prevalence varied from 1.5% in Taiwan to 11.6% in Christchurch; 12.4% in Florence, Italy; 16.4% in Paris, France; and 19.0% in Beirut, Lebanon. The exceptionally low rates in Taiwan remain unexplained but may reflect both underreporting of distress and positive effects of social support and family function. Lifetime rates of bipolar disorder showed much less variability (from 0.3% to 1.5%) but also were consistently lower in Asian countries.

Cross-national comparisons with the DIS found that the most common symptoms of depression (reported by 60% or more of the patients with major depression) were insomnia, loss of energy, thoughts of death, suicidal ideation, and concentration problems (Weissman et al. 1996). Feelings of worthlessness were less common in Puerto Rico, Beirut, and Taiwan. Poor appetite was common only in Beirut, Taiwan, and Korea.

TABLE 42–3.   Cross-national comparative community studies of depression

Study/Sites	Lifetime prevalence (%)	Annual prevalence (%)	Gender ratio (F/M)
Cross-national comparison with Diagnostic Interview Schedule (Weissman et al. 1996)			
Canada (Edmonton)	9.6	5.2	1.9
France (Paris)	16.4	4.5	2.1
Italy (Florence)	12.4	—	2.0
Korea	2.9	2.3	1.6
Lebanon (Beirut)	19.0	—	1.6
New Zealand (Christchurch)	11.6	5.8	2.1
Puerto Rico	4.3	3.0	1.8
Taiwan	1.5	0.8	1.6
United States	5.2	3.0	2.6
West Germany	9.2	5.0	3.1
International Consortium in Psychiatric Epidemiology Study with Composite International Diagnostic Interview (Andrade et al. 2003)			
Brazil	12.6	5.8	2.1
Canada	8.3	4.3	2.0
Chile	9.0	5.6	2.1
Czech Republic	7.8	2.0	1.2
Germany	11.5	5.2	2.3
Japan	3.0	1.2	2.5
Mexico	8.1	4.5	1.9
The Netherlands	15.7	5.9	1.9
Turkey	6.3	3.5	2.3
United States	16.9	10.0	2.0

New data from comparative studies that used the CIDI (Wittchen et al. 1991) confirm the wide variation found in earlier studies. The International Consortium in Psychiatric Epidemiology compared data from community surveys in 10 different countries (Andrade et al. 2003). As shown in Table 42–3, lifetime rates of depression showed great variability, with Asian countries showing the lowest rates, as in the earlier consortium study (from 3.0% in Japan to 16.9% in the United States). In all countries, women had higher rates than men, and the sex ratio varied only slightly. Comparison of the ratios of 12-month to lifetime prevalence, and 30-day to 12-month, also suggested that there may be differences in the course of depression across countries.

Although these are the best available data for cross-national comparisons, many methodological problems remain. The probe flow sheet of the CIDI, designed to establish the clinical significance of depressive symptoms, relies on a series of criteria for severity, including medical help-seeking, use of medication, and interference with daily activities. Variations in context may render the probes insensitive and hence result in biased estimates of prevalence (Hicks 2002; Van Ommeren et al. 2000). Of course, the diagnostic interviews only canvas symptoms already identified as criteria for depression. Although Simon and colleagues (2002) claimed that their item-response analysis of the CIDI showed that large cross-national variations in depression cannot be attributed to a category fallacy, in fact, the lack of use of locally developed measures means that existing studies cannot resolve basic questions, including 1) Is there further undetected morbidity in the community or in the clinic that is not captured by the category of depression but that is related in some important way (by underlying mechanism, symptomatic overlap, or common predicament)? 2) Can people with mild to moderate depression identified by the CIDI be better understood and treated in terms of different categories?

These broad comparisons across countries also do not address the important issue of variations by ethnocultural groups within each region. For example, in the United States, major depression has been found to be significantly less common among African Americans than among other groups (Kessler et al. 2003; Zhang and Snowden 1999). Depression is less prevalent among Mexican immigrants with indigenous Indian heritage but increases with acculturation to approximate that of the general U.S. population (Alderete et al. 2000; Vega et al. 1998). The reasons for these variations are poorly understood but do not appear to be purely methodological artifact and may be related to cultural differences in values and identity, as well as family and social support.

Studies in the United Kingdom have found that South Asian (i.e., Indian and Pakistani) immigrants had lower rates of depression than the general United Kingdom population (Bhui 1999). However, ethnographic studies found significant levels of distress, suggesting that there was underrecognition of distress in research measures or some form of sampling bias. Surveys in Pakistan that used culturally adapted instruments found high levels of depression (Mumford et al. 1997). Of course, the prevalence of any disorder in immigrant populations need not reflect that of their country of origin because migration itself involves many selection biases. However, a study in the United Kingdom that used a culturally adapted measure found higher levels of depression among Punjabi immigrants, particularly women, compared with their white counterparts in the United Kingdom (Bhui et al. 2004). This underscores the need for culturally adapted measures to tap expressions of distress that may otherwise be unreported or unrecognized.

Cultural Constructions of Affect and Depression

Even though there are cross-cultural concepts of affective meaning (Osgood et al. 1975) and recognition of emotional states in facial expressions (Ekman 1992), these are rudimentary feelings with relatively crude meanings. These basic emotions are built in to more complex or refined feelings that refer to social situations with specific antecedents and consequences. Emotion terms thus reference bodily states, behaviors, feelings, and social situations (Shweder and Haidt 2000). Through the course of development, even the simplest bodily experiences are imbued with specific cultural meanings (Kirmayer 1992). Emotions then can be understood as metaphorical elaborations of bodily feelings and social events, as cognitive schemas or scenarios, and as discursive or rhetorical practices that contribute to the cultural construction of the person and the social world (White 2000).

The etymology of emotion terms in each language reflects a cultural history that centers emotions on prototypical social situations (White 2000). Like other concepts, emotions are based on metaphorical constructs with both universal and culture-specific connotations (Lakoff 1987). Finally, emotions lend rhetorical force to discourse in multiple social contexts. The emotional lexicon therefore encodes the socially and morally significant values of a cultural community (Levy 1978; Lutz 1988; Rosaldo 1980; Shweder and Haidt 2000).

Jackson (1996) traced the history of the emergence of the modern concept of depression. The English term *acedia*, derived from the Latin *accidia* (meaning "heedlessness or torpor"), was used to describe a condition common in medieval monks characterized by "exhaustion, listlessness, sadness or dejection, restlessness, aversion to the cell and the ascetic life, and yearning for family and former life" (Jackson 1996, p. 66). The term *melancholia* (from the Latin for black bile) was invoked in humoral theories of temperament and affliction but by the 1600s came to have positive connotations as an affliction of those with superior intelligence, sensitivity, and refinement (Radden 2000). The term *depression*, which supplanted *melancholia* only in the twentieth century, derives from the verb "to depress" (Latin *de primere*, "to press down"). In the fourteenth century, "to depress" had the meaning "to subjugate," and by the fifteenth century, it also meant "to bring down in vigor or spirits" (Onions 1966).

Although the term *depression* is now readily used in English both as a metaphor for everyday fluctuations in mood and as the diagnostic label for a clinical disorder, the term has not had the same fate in other societies. Around the world, a common way to describe the experiences associated with depression in psychiatric nosology is as an expression of soul loss or spirit loss, the implication being that the person has somehow lost or been abandoned by the indwelling source of energy and vitality that animates the healthy person (Shweder 1985). This loss of spirit can occur in many different ways, and concern may be directed toward the cause that is located in social or other salient events. The anthropologist Robert Desjarlais (1996, p. 146) described this event among the Yolmo of Nepal:

> Although bouts of spirit loss bear a common sensory range, which in many respects compares to what Westerners call "depression," each incident presents a slightly different form and etiology. A middle-aged woman named Nyima lost her spirit while crossing a stream on her way to participate in a funeral rite; she lost the desire to walk, eat, work, and socialize. Yeshi, a young Yolmo bride, also lost her spirit; she displayed a lethargy of body and spirit, a lack of emotionality and a general apathy towards her surroundings.

The metaphorical logic of depression (which makes links between low mood; low spirits; sadness; dejection; and feeling cold, slow, dark, or dry) is intelligible across cultures but is not the most immediate way to describe mood. On the face of it, there is no reason that our English lexicon, freighted as it is with its own particular cultural history, should provide a universally applicable scheme for mapping and articulating distress (Shweder and Haidt 2000). There is something to be learned about the nature of depression from the ways in which each culture interprets the human responses to loss, failure, and despair.

Somatization and Cultural Idioms of Distress

The early WHO studies suggested that the core features of depression are similar in many societies—an impression borne out by many subsequent clinical and epidemiological studies (Abas and Broadhead 1997; Beiser 1985, 1999; Escobar et al. 1983; Gupta et al. 1991; Liu et al. 1997; Weissman et al. 1996). However, it is important to recognize that these core symptoms include many common somatic complaints. Indeed, around the world, most primary care patients with major depression or anxiety disorders (70%–80%) present exclusively with somatic complaints (García-Campayo et al. 1998; Kirmayer et al. 1993; Kroenke et al. 1997; Simon et al. 1999). This behavior has been misleadingly termed *somatization*, with the implication that some specific type of psychopathology is involved (Kirmayer et al. 1998). In epidemiological studies, however, somatic symptoms and emotional distress are highly intercorrelated (Piccinelli and Simon 1997; Simon et al. 1999). The most common somatic symptoms associated with depression are musculoskeletal pain and fatigue.

Most patients with depression experience prominent somatic symptoms, but the number and intensity of somatic symptoms reported by patients are influenced by

cognitive factors that increase attention to and concern about bodily sensations (Sayar et al. 2003). These cognitive-interpretive processes, in turn, are shaped by cultural models of symptoms and illness based on ethnophysiological and ethnopsychological theories (Kirmayer et al. 1994). Style of clinical presentation is largely a matter of symptom attribution and patients' strategic decision as to what aspects of their distress are appropriate and useful to present to the clinician (Araya et al. 2001; Kirmayer and Robbins 1996). Some somatic symptoms may seem bizarre when encountered outside their usual cultural context and may lead clinicians to mistakenly diagnosis a delusional or psychotic disorder. For example, sensations of "heat" or "peppery feeling" in the head are common nonspecific symptoms of depression in equatorial regions of Africa (Ifabumuyi 1981). Dissociative symptoms also may commonly accompany mood disorders and give the impression of psychosis, which, however, may remit rapidly with changes in context or suggestion (Guinness 1992).

The manifestations of depression are understood in terms of available cultural models of the origins and meanings of distress (American Psychiatric Association 1994). These models, in turn, support specific *cultural idioms of distress*—conventional ways of talking about distress that are readily understood by others in the same local world. Some common cultural idioms of distress that may be associated with depression (and other common mental disorders) are listed in Table 42–4.

Cultural idioms not only provide the vocabulary through which depressive experience is expressed; they also define the social matrix in which depression is embedded. In many industrialized countries, for example, "burnout" has become a common way of describing distress related to conditions of stressful, demanding, and unrewarding work, which may include depression (Mausner-Dorsch and Eaton 2000; Tennant 2001). Other examples of the cultural embedding of depressive experience reflected in idioms of distress include *tabanka* in Trinidad, a form of reactive depression in men brought on by the breakup of a relationship (Littlewood 1985); "loneliness" among some American Indian groups, related to social marginalization (O'Nell 1996); and a wide variety of notions of "nerves" in diverse cultures, which link distress to personal hardships and adversity (Lock and Wakewich-Dunk 1990; Low 1994).

Much ethnographic work has documented the prevalence of sociosomatic theories in which a social predicament is understood to give rise to bodily illness (Groleau and Kirmayer 2004; Kirmayer and Young 1998; Kleinman and Becker 1998). For example, *hwa-byung*, a Korean term meaning "fire illness," refers not only to symptoms of epigastric burning and other forms of somatic distress

TABLE 42–4.   Some cultural idioms of distress associated with depression

Area or Population	Idiom	Reference
American Indian	Loneliness	O'Nell 1996
China	*shenjing shuairuo* ("nervous weakness")	Kleinman and Kleinman 1985; Lee 1998
India	Sinking heart, feeling hot, gas, semen loss	Bhugra and Mastrogianni 2004; Mumford 1996; Raguram et al. 1996
Iran	Heavy heart, heart distress, chest tightness	Good et al. 1985
Japan	*futeishuso* (nonspecific symptoms, e.g., shoulder pain) *shinkei suijaku* (neurasthenia) *jibyo* (personal illness)	Kirmayer 2002; Lock 1993
Korea	*hwa-byung* ("fire illness")	Lin et al. 1992; Pang 1990
Latin America	*nervios* ("nerves")	Jenkins and Cofresi 1998; Low 1994
Nigeria	Heat in the head, peppery feeling in the head, heaviness in the head	Ebigbo 1986; Ohaeri and Odejide 1994
Trinidad	*tabanka* (reactive depression)	Littlewood 1985
United States, Canada, France	Burnout	Ehrenberg 1998
Vietnam	Wind illness *phong tap* ("rheumatism") *uat u'c* ("indignation")	Eisenbruch 1983; Groleau and Kirmayer 2004; Phan and Silove 1999

but also to anger resulting from interpersonal conflict and a wider sense of collectively experienced injustice (Lin et al. 1992; Pang 1990). For the clinician knowledgeable about cultural meanings, the somatic symptoms of patients who label their distress *hwa-byung* point to psychological and interpersonal issues.

An individual's awareness of dysphoria and difficult social circumstances may coexist with a reluctance to express depressed mood and to explicitly point to social conflict, particularly in societies influenced by cultural values of social harmony, hierarchy, and equilibrium. In Chinese culture, for example, "affective expressions of depression may be perceived as self-centered, asocial, distancing, and threatening to the social structure. However, the expression of physical suffering and bodily pain, which are amenable to treatment and do not threaten social ties, are much more acceptable" (Yen et al. 2000, p. 998). As a result, Chinese depressed patients may choose to emphasize somatic symptoms, even though they are experiencing affective symptoms of distress as well (Parker et al. 2001). Similar observations have been made of other ethnocultural groups said to somatize (Raguram et al. 1996).

Figure 42–1 summarizes some of the processes involved in the cultural shaping of depressive experience.

The cultural shaping of depressive illness experience implies that clinicians must understand symptoms not simply as indices of disorder or disease but also as interpersonal communications to the clinician and to significant others in the patient's lifeworld (Kirmayer and Young 1998). Patients' initial reticence to disclose or discuss affective symptoms and psychological conflict may diminish as a trusting relationship is established with a clinician who is willing to learn about cultural difference (Tompar-Tiu and Sustento-Seneriches 1995).

Cultural Dynamics of Depression

Mood disorders involve biopsychological amplifying loops between cognitive evaluations and intense affect, as well as interpersonal loops in which the response of others may dampen or aggravate withdrawal, demoralization, and negative self-evaluation (Joiner and Coyne 1999). Cultural concepts of the person influence both cognitive and interpersonal strategies for managing dysphoria. In this way, cultural values and practices may contribute to causing or maintaining depression.

Murphy (1982) surveyed cultural variations in the prevalence of symptoms of guilt in depression and related

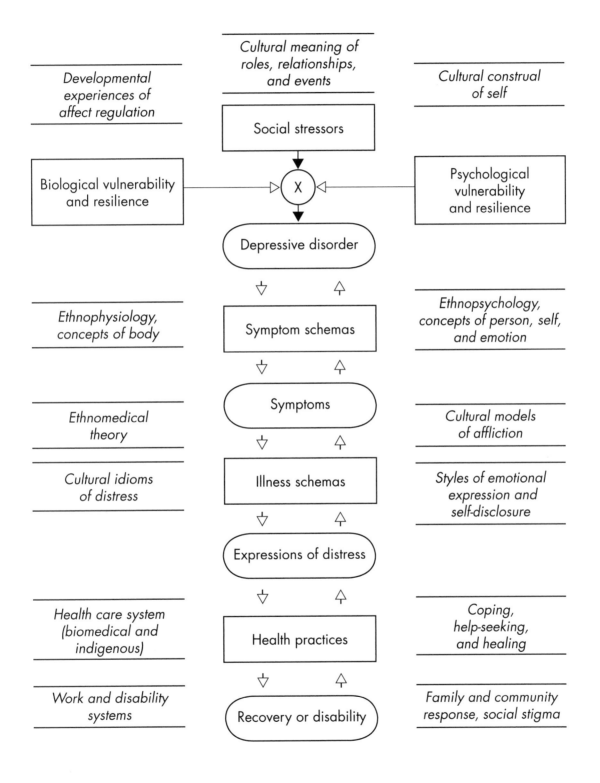

FIGURE 42–1. Cultural matrix of depressive experience.

the symptomatology of depression to the ways in which experiences of personal failure or defeat are interpreted in terms of the conceptual differentiation of self and other within the culture. When little differentiation exists between self and other, identity is construed in terms of group affiliation, and personal loss and failure may be viewed as a threat to group membership. When a sharper distinction between self and other is made, loss and failure are seen in terms of the potential criticism by others (i.e., as shame), and when the boundary between self and other is sharply drawn, loss and failure manifest as self-criticism and guilt.

Marsella (1978) suggested that depression was an expression of a psychologized self, in which the distinction between body and mind leads to a distinction between bodily fatigue, slowing down, lack of energy, and malaise and their mental equivalents. Depression thus comes to be experienced in terms of its interference with mental faculties, and, indeed, the whole process is understood to take place in an inner theater of the mind. The recent tendency to biologize depression, as a state of bodily depletion of energy, moves it out of this mental domain.

In a critique of the assumption of universality, based on ethnographic work in Sri Lanka, Obeyesekere (1985) argued that the affects identified as depression derive from larger sociomoral and religious frames, which differ across cultures. Some of what is considered pathological thought and affect in depression (e.g., denigration of the self and the body) may be given a positive value in the context of a Buddhist society that seeks to understand the illusoriness of the self.

In many Asian societies, influenced by Confucianism and both secular and religious familism, the sense of self is fundamentally relational (Phung 1979; Slote 1986). In general, the boundaries that define the self as separate from others are culturally shaped and negotiated (Hsu 1971). The self may be construed as more or less independent or interdependent (Markus and Kitayama 1991). The independent self is understood in terms of its own achievements and accomplishments, whereas the interdependent self is built on collective ties of mutuality and shared endeavors. For interdependent or relational selves, important decisions are made in a frame defined not by the individual but by the family or larger social unit. Well-being is thus derived from fitting in and the overall harmony and success of the group (Kitayama and Markus 2000; Rothbaum et al. 2000). The independent self aims to feel unique and special by maximizing qualities such as being attractive, interesting, independent, confident, and intelligent. For the interdependent self in the East Asian context, the goals are to fit in and ensure the harmonious functioning of the group. Thus, the most valued personal traits include being cooperative, loyal, considerate, hardworking, and dependable.

Psychological research in the United States suggests that healthy people have a self-enhancing bias in which they tend to view themselves as better than others (Asendorpf and Ostendorf 1998). People who are depressed are less likely to show self-enhancement (Lewinsohn et al. 1980). This self-enhancement bias appears to be one way that people maintain a strong sense of an independent self (Kitayama et al. 1997). However, cross-cultural research shows that people from several Asian cultures are less prone to self-enhance and, instead, tend to be self-critical (Heine et al. 2001). For example, Japanese tend to view themselves self-critically as part of a socially shaped process of self-improvement (Heine et al. 1999). This would suggest that Japanese (and other Asians who do not tend to show the self-enhancement bias) should have higher rates of depression, but as was seen earlier (in the section "Cultural Epidemiology of Depression"), quite the opposite appears to be true. Striving for social harmony and solidarity has its own rewards. Conformity with cultural ideologies of the person also may be as important as any specific attributional pattern for the individual's health and functioning. The sources of well-being lie not simply in success or failure or in the achievement of personal goals but in the fulfillment of larger social and cultural ideals of personhood and morality (Kitayama and Markus 2000; Shweder et al. 1997).

Treating Depression Across Cultures

For many years, people from diverse cultural backgrounds were viewed as not psychological minded and, hence, as unsuitable for psychotherapy (Fernando 2003). In addition, some clinicians who were aware of patients' adverse social circumstances assumed that treatment of depression would be futile as long as their life situation did not change. Increasing evidence, however, indicates that depression can be successfully treated even when people face implacable social problems. Conventional cognitive and interpersonal therapies for depression may be effective across a wide range of contexts if suitable modifications are made to ensure accessibility and participation despite social and economic constraints (Araya et al. 2003; Miranda et al. 2003a, 2003b).

Only a few systematic trials of psychotherapeutic treatment across cultures have been published. A trial of group interpersonal psychotherapy (IPT) in rural Uganda established its effectiveness (Bolton et al. 2003). The research used locally developed measures of depressive symptomatology and functional status. IPT was chosen because its focus on interpersonal situations fit local values and because it had the potential to be cost-effective.

The standard treatment was modified in several ways to take into account local cultural realities, including the interdependent sense of self, strongly differentiated gender roles, concerns about secrecy, and the ubiquity of loss through the ravages of acquired immunodeficiency syndrome (Verdeli et al. 2003).

A currently popular mode of psychotherapy for depression—mindfulness training—is based on Buddhist concepts of mental functioning and meditative practice. Interventions focus on modifying habitual patterns of thinking as a means of preventing responses likely to maintain depression or contribute to relapse (Ma and Teasdale 2004; Teasdale et al. 2000). Obviously, the emphasis on internal self-control fits well with cultures sharing Buddhist values of equanimity and containment of affect, and it should be possible to design culturally consonant interventions for primary care and other settings that build on the insights of these traditions.

Although antidepressant medications are broadly effective, significant variations across cultures in their effectiveness and the incidence and profile of adverse effects of specific medications have been reported. Several studies have found very low rates of treatment compliance among Southeast Asian patients in clinics in the United States (Kinzie et al. 1987; Kroll et al. 1990). Adherence to treatment is strongly affected by the experience of adverse effects and by the cultural meanings of medication. Nonadherence to biomedical or psychiatric treatment also may reflect patients' use of alternative sources of help. Collaboration with traditional healers can be helpful in identifying and reducing potential conflicts between different systems of knowledge and treatment.

Differences across ethnocultural groups in the pharmacokinetics and dynamics of common medications are well documented (Lin 2001). However, it is difficult to derive rules of thumb because the research generally shows that intracultural variation is greater than the variation among groups. Hence, clinicians must monitor and adjust levels carefully, attend closely to side effects, and watch for potential interactions with commonly used herbal remedies and dietary practices.

Before we rush to export various biomedical and psychological treatments of depression, however, it is important to recognize that there are a wide range of potentially effective traditional or indigenous forms of healing (Kirmayer 2004). In some countries, depression may be more prevalent in some traditional health care settings than in primary medical care because of patterns of help-seeking (Ngoma et al. 2003). Many of these healing traditions fit well with local values and resources and may provide cost-effective treatments for depression and related common mental disorders. Their effectiveness needs to be system-atically studied, with culturally appropriate measures of outcome. As illustrated by the adaptation of Buddhist meditative practices in mindfulness therapy, serious attention to the diversity of forms of healing may lead to innovations in clinical practice.

Political Economy of Depression

Depression imposes an enormous and increasing burden in many developing countries, and this can be directly related to economic hardship and oppressive social conditions, especially for women and marginalized groups such as indigenous peoples and some ethnocultural minorities (Desjarlais et al. 1995). The economic importance of depression has made it a major public health concern and the target of commercial activity (Anonymous 1998). Pharmaceutical companies have an interest in encouraging the recognition and treatment of depression, and, in concert with other social forces, this may have led to broadening the definitions of depression to include conditions that involve everyday problems in living (Metzl and Angel 2004).

Not only the prevalence of depression but also the diagnosis and treatment of depression have been increasingly rapidly around the globe. This reflects both the dissemination of biomedical knowledge and wider social forces. For example, Kleinman's (1986) work on neurasthenia and depression in China had a substantial influence on professional diagnostic practices, leading to greater recognition and treatment of major depression (Lee 1998). The process of change in diagnostic practices may continue to accelerate, with changes in public perceptions engineered through advertising, the news media, and the Internet driving professional response (Kirmayer 2002).

The diagnosis of depression suits a society that emphasizes individual responsibility for social and psychological well-being. In its current configuration, a focus on depression tends to shift attention away from social circumstances and toward the resources of the individual. Skultans (2003) described the rapid change in recent years in Latvia, from diagnosing neurasthenia to using the category of depression. Psychological idioms of distress have privatized suffering and increased feelings of guilt and shame among people dealing with personal and economic adversity.

Ironically, there appears to be an ongoing increase in the number of people with depression in urban, industrialized societies (Andrade et al. 2003; Cross-National Collaborative Group 1992; Klerman et al. 1985). This increase may be associated with the effects of urbanization on the family and conditions of work, with unemployment and economic uncertainty (Rodriguez et al. 2001), and with wider forces related to the dissemination of a culture of individualism and material consumption supported by forces of globalization and consumer capitalism (Bauman 1998). Increased material wealth and consumer choice have contributed to escalating expectations and, along with this, to greater risk of a sense of personal limitations and failure (Kasser 2002; Schwartz 2000). A focus on material success may interfere with the cultivation of the bonds of family and community (Nickerson et al. 2003). This lack of bonding may set the stage for greater vulnerability to depression and dysphoria. Although its mandate remains the health of individuals, psychiatry cannot afford to ignore the larger problems of society lest clinical theory and practice become unwitting accomplices to a way of life that undermines health and well-being.

Conclusion

The partitioning of distress into categories of mood, anxiety, somatoform, and dissociative disorders in contemporary nosology does not reflect the natural co-variation of symptoms and syndromes. As a result, local clinical presentations of disorders that are related to major depression or to anxiety disorders may differ substantially from the descriptions in DSM-IV-TR (American Psychiatric Association 2000). Somatic symptoms are a prominent part of the clinical presentation of most patients with depression and anxiety. Dissociative symptoms may further complicate the picture by giving the impression of a psychotic disorder when none is present.

The clinical presentation of depression is a function not only of patients' ethnocultural background but also of the structure of the health care system they find themselves in and the diagnostic categories and concepts they encounter in mass media and in dialogue with family, friends, and clinicians. Bodily idioms of distress are very common in many cultures. In place of psychosomatic theories that emphasize individuals' inner conflict, many traditions of medicine have sociosomatic theories that link bodily and emotional distress to problems in the social world (Kleinman and Becker 1998). This provides a rich language for articulating distress and seeking help. Clinicians who learn to work collaboratively with their patients, as well as with culture brokers and colleagues from other cultural communities, will be better able to identify their patients' problems and to uncover cultural resources that can complement and, at times, supplant conventional psychiatric treatment (Kirmayer et al. 2003).

The clinician's ability to understand local idioms of distress is crucial not only for accurate diagnosis but also for developing the communication necessary for a therapeutic alliance. At the same time, cultural idioms of distress provide a way for patients to safely initiate a therapeutic conversation. To understand this conversation, the clinician must think in terms of both disorders and life predicaments. Feelings of depression and despair may come not only from universally recognized losses or conflicts but also from the failure to achieve or maintain deeply held cultural values.

Future work on culture in depression must advance on multiple fronts. Careful qualitative and ethnographic research on illness experience and the social context of depression is needed to design culturally valid larger-scale longitudinal studies of course and outcome (Alarcón et al. 2002). Such studies must consider alternative configurations of distress that reflect indigenous categories to determine whether these are better predictors of social course and treatment outcome. At the same time, study of indigenous forms of coping with loss, failure, and demoralization may identify new strategies for therapeutic intervention that can be supported locally and adapted for use in other cultural contexts.

Clinicians must develop an ongoing dialogue with patients that acknowledges and works with cultural differences rather than assuming that ethnic matching finesses the issues. There is much to be learned from the models of service developed in different countries (Kirmayer and Minas 2000). In situations with high levels of diversity, a model of cultural consultation that uses multilingual, multicultural clinicians and culture brokers may provide a useful supplement to routine care and improve clinicians' cultural competence (Kirmayer et al. 2003).

In recent years, psychiatry has developed a complex and complicit relationship with the pharmaceutical industry that has undermined professional autonomy. New standards in research, publishing, and the regulation of the profession are emerging to ensure that the evidence on which clinical practice is based is not biased by commercial interests and that clinicians are able to choose from a wide array of interventions on the basis of established efficacy and cost-effectiveness.

Social marketing and media campaigns, as well as the poignant testimonials of writers, artists, and figures of popular culture, can do much to reduce the stigma attached to depression. At the same time, it is important to examine the causes and contexts of depression more critically. Distress may serve as a barometer of wider social problems attached to certain features of modernity—particularly consumerism—that need to be named and confronted, even as clinicians strive to help the afflicted person before them.

References

Abas MA, Broadhead JC: Depression and anxiety amongst women in an urban setting in Zimbabwe. Psychol Med 27:59–71, 1997

Abas MA, Phillips C, Carter J, et al: Culturally sensitive validation of screening questionnaires for depression in older African-Caribbean people living in south London. Br J Psychiatry 173:249–254, 1998

Alarcón RD, Bell CC, Kirmayer LJ, et al: Beyond the funhouse mirrors: research agenda on culture and psychiatric diagnosis, in A Research Agenda for DSM-V. Edited by Kupfer DJ, First MB, Regier DA. Washington, DC, American Psychiatric Publishing, 2002, pp 219–289

Alderete E, Vega WA, Kolody B, et al: Effects of time in the United States and Indian ethnicity on DSM-III-R psychiatric disorders among Mexican Americans in California. J Nerv Ment Dis 188:90–100, 2000

American Psychiatric Association: Diagnostic and Statistical Manual of Mental Disorders, 4th Edition. Washington, DC, American Psychiatric Association, 1994

American Psychiatric Association: Diagnostic and Statistical Manual of Mental Disorders, 4th Edition, Text Revision. Washington, DC, American Psychiatric Association, 2000

Andrade L, Caraveo-Anduaga JJ, Berglund P, et al: The epidemiology of major depressive episodes: results from the International Consortium of Psychiatric Epidemiology (ICPE) Surveys. Int J Methods Psychiatr Res 12:3–21, 2003

Anonymous: Spirit of the age: malignant sadness is the world's great hidden burden. The Economist (London), Dec 19, 1998, pp 115–123

Araya R, Lewis GH, Rojas G, et al: Patient knows best—detection of common mental disorders in Santiago, Chile: cross sectional study. BMJ 322:79–81, 2001

Araya R, Rojas G, Fritsch R, et al: Treating depression in primary care in low-income women in Santiago, Chile: a randomized controlled trial. Lancet 361:995–1000, 2003

Asendorpf JB, Ostendorf F: Is self-enhancement healthy? Conceptual, psychometric, and empirical analysis. J Pers Soc Psychol 74:955–966, 1998

Bauman Z: Globalization: The Human Consequences. New York, Columbia University Press, 1998

Beiser M: A study of depression among traditional Africans, urban North Americans, and Southeast Asian refugees, in Culture and Depression. Edited by Kleinman A, Good B. Berkeley, University of California Press, 1985, pp 272–298

Beiser M: Strangers at the Gate: The "Boat People"'s First Ten Years in Canada. Toronto, Ontario, University of Toronto Press, 1999

Beiser M, Fleming JAE: Measuring psychiatric disorder among Southeast Asian refugees. Psychol Med 16:627–639, 1986

Bhugra D, Mastrogianni A: Globalisation and mental disorders: overview with relation to depression. Br J Psychiatry 184:10–20, 2004

Bhui K: Common mental disorders among people with origins in or immigrant from India and Pakistan. Int Rev Psychiatry 11:136–144, 1999

Bhui K, Bhugra D, Goldberg D, et al: Assessing the prevalence of depression in Punjabi and English primary care attenders: the role of culture, physical illness and somatic symptoms. Transcult Psychiatry 41:307–322, 2004

Bibeau G: Cultural psychiatry in a creolizing world: questions for a new research agenda. Transcult Psychiatry 34:9–41, 1997

Bolton P, Bass J, Neugebauer R, et al: Group interpersonal psychotherapy for depression in rural Uganda: a randomized controlled trial. JAMA 289:3117–3124, 2003

Cross-National Collaborative Group: The changing rate of major depression: cross-national comparisons. JAMA 268:3098–3105, 1992

Desjarlais RR: Presence, in The Performance of Healing. Edited by Laderman C, Roseman M. New York, Routledge, 1996, pp 143–164

Desjarlais R, Eisenberg L, Good B, et al: World Mental Health: Problems and Priorities in Low-Income Countries. New York, Oxford University Press, 1995

Ebigbo PO: Development of a culture specific (Nigeria) screening scale of somatic complaints indicating psychiatric disturbance. Cult Med Psychiatry 6:29–43, 1982

Ebigbo PO: A cross sectional study of somatic complaints of Nigerian females using the Enugu Somatization Scale. Cult Med Psychiatry 10:167–186, 1986

Ehrenberg A: La Fatigue d'etre soi: Dépression et Société [The Fatigue of Being Oneself: Depression and Society]. Paris, France, Éditions Odile Jacob, 1998

Eisenbruch M: "Wind illness" or somatic depression? A case study in psychiatric anthropology. Br J Psychiatry 143:323–326, 1983

Ekman P: An argument for basic emotions. Cognition and Emotion 6(3/4):169–200, 1992

El-Rufaie OEF, Absood GH, Abou-Saleh MT: The Primary Care Anxiety and Depression (PCAD) Scale: a culture-oriented screening scale. Acta Psychiatr Scand 95:119–124, 1997

Escobar JL, Gomez J, Tuason VB: Depressive phenomenology in North and South American patients. Am J Psychiatry 140:47–51, 1983

Fernando S: Cultural Diversity, Mental Health and Psychiatry: The Struggle Against Racism. New York, Brunner/Routledge, 2003

García-Campayo J, Lobo A, Pérez-Echeverría MJ, et al: Three forms of somatization presenting in primary care settings in Spain. J Nerv Ment Dis 186:554–560, 1998

Good BJ, Good MJD, Moradi R: The interpretation of Iranian depressive illness and dysphoric affect, in Culture and Depression. Edited by Kleinman A, Good B. Berkeley, University of California Press, 1985, pp 369–428

Groleau D, Kirmayer LJ: Sociosomatic theory in Vietnamese immigrants' narratives of distress. Anthropology and Medicine 11:117–133, 2004

Guinness EA: Brief reactive psychosis and the major functional psychoses: descriptive case studies in Africa. Br J Psychiatry 160 (suppl 16):24–41, 1992

Gupta R, Singh P, Verma S, et al: Standardized Assessment of Depressive Disorders: a replicated study from northern India. Acta Psychiatr Scand 84:310–312, 1991

Heine SJ, Lehman DR, Markus HR, et al: Is there a universal need for positive self-regard? Psychol Rev 106:766–794, 1999

Heine SJ, Lehman DR, Ide E, et al: Divergent consequences of success and failure in Japan and North America: an investigation of self-improving motivations and malleable selves. J Pers Soc Psychol 81:599–615, 2001

Hicks MH-R: Validity of the CIDI probe flow chart for depression in Chinese American women. Transcult Psychiatry 39:434–451, 2002

Hsu FLK: Psychosocial homeostasis and Jen: conceptual tools for advancing psychological anthropology. Am Anthropol 173:23–44, 1971

Ifabumuyi OI: The dynamics of central heat in depression. Psychopathologie Africaine 17:127–133, 1981

Jablensky A, Sartorius N, Gulbinat W, et al: Characteristics of depressive patients contacting psychiatric services in four cultures. Acta Psychiatr Scand 63:367–383, 1981

Jackson S: Melancholia and Depression: From Hippocratic to Modern Times. New Haven, CT, Yale University Press, 1996

Jenkins JH, Cofresi N: The sociosomatic course of depression and trauma: a cultural analysis of suffering and resilience in the life of a Puerto Rican woman. Psychosom Med 60:439–447, 1998

Joiner T, Coyne JC (eds): The Interactional Nature of Depression. Washington, DC, American Psychological Association, 1999

Kasser T: The High Price of Materialism. Cambridge, MA, MIT Press, 2002

Kessler RC, Berglund P, Demler O, et al: The epidemiology of major depressive disorder: results from the National Comorbidity Survey Replication (NCS-R). JAMA 289:3095–3105, 2003

Kinzie JD, Manson SM, Vinh DT, et al: Development and validation of a Vietnamese-language depression rating scale. Am J Psychiatry 139:1276–1281, 1982

Kinzie JD, Leung P, Boehnlein JK, et al: Antidepressant blood levels in Southeast Asians: clinical and cultural implications. J Nerv Ment Dis 175:480–485, 1987

Kirmayer LJ: Cultural variations in the response to psychiatric disorders and emotional distress. Soc Sci Med 29:327–339, 1989

Kirmayer LJ: The body's insistence on meaning: metaphor as presentation and representation in illness experience. Med Anthropol Q 6:323–346, 1992

Kirmayer LJ: Psychopharmacology in a globalizing world: the use of antidepressants in Japan. Transcult Psychiatry 39:295–312, 2002

Kirmayer LJ: The cultural diversity of healing: meaning, metaphor and mechanism. Br Med Bull 69:33–48, 2004

Kirmayer LJ, Minas H: The future of cultural psychiatry: an international perspective. Can J Psychiatry 45:438–446, 2000

Kirmayer LJ, Robbins JM: Patients who somatize in primary care: a longitudinal study of cognitive and social characteristics. Psychol Med 26:937–951, 1996

Kirmayer LJ, Young A: Culture and somatization: clinical, epidemiological, and ethnographic perspectives. Psychosom Med 60:420–430, 1998

Kirmayer LJ, Robbins JM, Dworkind M, et al: Somatization and the recognition of depression and anxiety in primary care. Am J Psychiatry 150:734–741, 1993

Kirmayer LJ, Young A, Robbins JM: Symptom attribution in cultural perspective. Can J Psychiatry 39:584–595, 1994

Kirmayer LJ, Dao THT, Smith A: Somatization and psychologization: understanding cultural idioms of distress, in Clinical Methods in Transcultural Psychiatry. Edited by Okpaku S. Washington, DC, American Psychiatric Press, 1998, pp 233–265

Kirmayer LJ, Groleau D, Guzder J, et al: Cultural consultation: a model of mental health service for multicultural societies. Can J Psychiatry 48:145–153, 2003

Kitayama S, Markus HR: The pursuit of happiness and the realization of sympathy: cultural patterns of self, social relations, and well-being, in Culture and Subjective Well-Being. Edited by Diener E, Suh EM. Cambridge, MA, MIT Press, 2000, pp 113–161

Kitayama S, Markus HR, Matsumoto H, et al: Individual and collective processes in the construction of the self: self-enhancement in the United States and self-criticism in Japan. J Pers Soc Psychol 72:1245–1267, 1997

Kleinman AM: Depression, somatization and the "new cross-cultural psychiatry." Soc Sci Med 11:3–10, 1977

Kleinman A: Social Origins of Distress and Disease: Depression, Neurasthenia, and Pain in Modern China. New Haven, CT, Yale University Press, 1986

Kleinman A: Rethinking Psychiatry. New York, Free Press, 1988

Kleinman A, Becker AE: Sociosomatics: the contribution of anthropology to psychosomatics. Psychosom Med 60:389–393, 1998

Kleinman AM, Good B (eds): Culture and Depression. Berkeley, University of California Press, 1985

Kleinman A, Kleinman J: Somatization: the interconnections among culture, depressive experiences, and the meanings of pain, a study in Chinese society, in Culture and Depression. Edited by Kleinman A, Good B. Berkeley, University of California Press, 1985, pp 132–167

Klerman GL, Lavori PW, Rice J, et al: Birth cohort trends in rates of major depressive disorder among relatives of patients with affective disorder. Arch Gen Psychiatry 42:689–693, 1985

Kroenke K, Jackson JL, Chamberlin J: Depressive and anxiety disorders in patients presenting with physical complaints: clinical predictors and outcome. Am J Med 103:339–347, 1997

Kroll J, Linde P, Habenicht M, et al: Medication compliance, antidepressant blood levels, and side effects in Southeast Asian patients. J Clin Psychopharmacol 10:279–283, 1990

Lakoff G: Women, Fire, and Dangerous Things. Chicago, IL, University of Chicago Press, 1987

Lee S: Estranged bodies, simulated harmony, and misplaced cultures: neurasthenia in contemporary Chinese society. Psychosom Med 60:448–457, 1998

Levy RI: Tahitians: Mind and Experience in the Society Islands. Chicago, IL, University of Chicago Press, 1978

Lewinsohn PM, Mischel W, Chaplin W, et al: Social competence and depression: the role of illusory self-perceptions. J Abnorm Psychol 89:203–212, 1980

Lin KM: Biological differences in depression and anxiety across races and ethnic groups. J Clin Psychiatry 62:13–21, 2001

Lin K-M, Lau JKC, Yamamoto J, et al: Hwa-byung: a community study of Korean Americans. J Nerv Ment Dis 180:386–391, 1992

Littlewood R: An indigenous conceptualization of reactive depression in Trinidad. Psychol Med 15:275–281, 1985

Liu CY, Wang SJ, Teng EL, et al: Depressive disorders among older residents in a Chinese rural community. Psychol Med 27:943–949, 1997

Lock M: Encounters With Aging: Mythologies of Menopause in Japan and North America. Berkeley, University of California Press, 1993

Lock M, Wakewich-Dunk P: Nerves and nostalgia: expression of loss among Greek immigrants in Montreal. Can Fam Physician 36:253–258, 1990

Low S: Embodied metaphors: nerves as lived experience, in Embodiment and Experience: The Existential Ground of Culture and Self. Edited by Csordas T. Cambridge, MA, Cambridge University Press, 1994, pp 139–162

Lutz CA: Unnatural Emotions. Chicago, IL, University of Chicago Press, 1988

Ma SH, Teasdale JD: Mindfulness-based cognitive therapy for depression: replication and exploration of differential relapse prevention effects. J Consult Clin Psychol 72:31–40, 2004

Markus HR, Kitayama S: Culture and the self: implications for cognition, emotion, and motivation. Psychol Rev 98:224–253, 1991

Marsella AJ: Thoughts on cross-cultural studies on the epidemiology of depression. Cult Med Psychiatry 2:343–357, 1978

Mausner-Dorsch H, Eaton WW: Psychosocial work environment and depression: epidemiologic assessment of the demand-control model. Am J Public Health 90:1765–1770, 2000

Metzl JM, Angel J: Assessing the impact of SSRI antidepressants on popular notions of women's depressive illness. Soc Sci Med 58:577–584, 2004

Miranda J, Azocar F, Organista KC, et al: Treatment of depression among impoverished primary care patients from ethnic minority groups. Psychiatr Serv 54:219–225, 2003a

Miranda J, Chung JY, Green BL, et al: Treating depression in predominantly low-income young minority women: a randomized controlled trial. JAMA 290:57–65, 2003b

Mollica FR, Wyshak G, de Marneffe D, et al: Indochinese version of the Hopkins Symptom Checklist-25: a screening instrument for the psychiatric care of refugees. Am J Psychiatry 144:497–500, 1987

Mumford DB: The "Dhat syndrome": a culturally determined symptom of depression? Acta Psychiatr Scand 94:163–167, 1996

Mumford DB, Bavington JT, Bhatnagar KS, et al: The Bradford Somatic Inventory: a multi-ethnic inventory of somatic symptoms reported by anxious and depressed patients in Britain and the Indo-Pakistan subcontinent. Br J Psychiatry 158:379–386, 1991

Mumford DB, Saeed K, Ahmad I, et al: Stress and psychiatric disorder in rural Punjab. Br J Psychiatry 170:473–478, 1997

Murphy HBM: Comparative Psychiatry: The International and Intercultural Distribution of Mental Illness. New York, Springer-Verlag, 1982

Murray CJ, Lopez AD: Global mortality, disability, and the contribution of risk factors: Global Burden of Disease Study. Lancet 349(9063):1436–1442, 1997

Ngoma MC, Prince M, Mann A: Common mental disorders among those attending primary health clinics and traditional healers in urban Tanzania. Br J Psychiatry 183:349–355, 2003

Nickerson C, Schwarz N, Diener E, et al: Zeroing in on the dark side of the American Dream: a closer look at the negative consequences of the goal for financial success. Psychol Sci 14:531–536, 2003

O'Nell TD: Disciplined Hearts: History, Identity and Depression in an American Indian Community. Berkeley, University of California, 1996

Obeyesekere G: Depression, Buddhism, and the work of culture in Sri Lanka, in Culture and Depression. Edited by Kleinman AM, Good B. Berkeley, University of California Press, 1985, pp 134–152

Ohaeri JU, Odejide OA: Somatization symptoms among patients using primary health care facilities in a rural community in Nigeria. Am J Psychiatry 151:728–731, 1994

Onions CT (ed): The Oxford Dictionary of English Etymology. Oxford, UK, Oxford University Press, 1966

Orley J, Wing JK: Psychiatric disorders in two African villages. Arch Gen Psychiatry 36:513–520, 1979

Osgood CE, May WH, Miron MS: Cross-Cultural Universals of Affective Meaning. Urbana, University of Illinois Press, 1975

Pang KYC: Hwabyung: the construction of a Korean popular illness among Korean elderly immigrant women in the United States. Cult Med Psychiatry 14:495–512, 1990

Parker G, Cheah YC, Roy K: Do the Chinese somatize depression? A cross-cultural study. Soc Psychiatry Psychiatr Epidemiol 36:287–293, 2001

Patel V, Simunyu E, Gwanzura F, et al: The Shona Symptom Questionnaire: the development of an indigenous measure of common mental disorders in Harare. Acta Psychiatr Scand 95:469–475, 1997

Phan T, Silove D: An overview of indigenous descriptions of mental phenomena and the range of traditional healing practices amongst the Vietnamese. Transcult Psychiatry 36:79–94, 1999

Phan T, Steel Z, Silove D: An ethnographically derived measure of anxiety, depression and somatization: the Phan Vietnamese Psychiatric Scale. Transcult Psychiatry 41:200–232, 2004

Phung TH: The family in Vietnam and its social life, in An Introduction to Indo-Chinese History, Culture, Language and Life. Edited by Withmore JK. Ann Arbor, Center for South and Southeast Asian Studies, University of Michigan, 1979, pp 77–84

Piccinelli M, Simon G: Gender and cross-cultural differences in somatic symptoms associated with emotional distress: an international study in primary care. Psychol Med 27:433–444, 1997

Radden J (ed): The Nature of Melancholy: From Aristotle to Kristeva. New York, Oxford University Press, 2000

Raguram R, Weiss M, Channabasavanna SM, et al: Stigma, depression, and somatization in South India. Am J Psychiatry 153:1043–1049, 1996

Robins LN, Helzer JE, Orvaschel H: The Diagnostic Interview Schedule, in Epidemiologic Field Methods in Psychiatry. Edited by Eaton WW, Kessler LG. Orlando, FL, Academic Press, 1985, pp 143–170

Rodriguez E, Frongillo EA, Chandra P: Do social programmes contribute to mental well-being? The long-term impact of unemployment on depression in the United States. Int J Epidemiol 30:163–170, 2001

Rosaldo MZ: Knowledge and Passion: Ilongot Notions of Self and Social Life. Cambridge, MA, Cambridge University Press, 1980

Rothbaum F, Pott M, Azuma H, et al: The development of close relationships in Japan and the United States: paths of symbiotic harmony and generative tension. Child Dev 71:1121–1142, 2000

Sartorius N, Jablensky A, Gulbinat W, et al: Application of WHO scales for the assessment of depressive states in different cultures. Acta Psychiatr Scand 62:204–211, 1980

Sayar K, Kirmayer LJ, Taillefer S: Predictors of somatic symptoms in depressive disorder. Gen Hosp Psychiatry 25:108–114, 2003

Schwartz B: Self-determination: the tyranny of freedom. Am Psychol 55:79–88, 2000

Scott J, Dickey B: Global burden of depression: the intersection of culture and medicine. Br J Psychiatry 183:92–94, 2003

Sheikh JA, Yesavage GA: Geriatric Depression Scale (GDS): recent evidence and development of a shorter version, in Clinical Gerontology: A Guide to Assessment and Intervention. Edited by Brink TL. New York, Haworth, 1986, pp 165–173

Shweder RA: Menstrual pollution, soul loss, and the comparative study of emotions, in Culture and Depression. Edited by Kleinman A, Good B. Berkeley, University of California Press, 1985, pp 182–214

Shweder RA, Haidt J: The cultural psychology of the emotions: ancient and new, in Handbook of Emotions. Edited by Lewis M, Haviland-Jones JM. New York, Guilford, 2000, pp 397–414

Shweder RA, Much NC, Mahapatra M, et al: The "big three" of morality (autonomy, community, divinity) and the "big three" explanations of suffering, in Morality and Health. Edited by Brandt A, Rozin P. New York, Routledge, 1997, pp 119–126

Simon GE, Goldberg DP, Von Korff M, et al: Understanding cross-national differences in depression prevalence. Psychol Med 32:585–594, 2002

Simon GE, VonKorff M, Piccinelli M, et al: An international study of the relation between somatic symptoms and depression. N Engl J Med 341:1329–1336, 1999

Singh G, Verma HC, Kaur H: A new depressive inventory. Indian J Psychiatry 61:183–188, 1974

Skultans V: From damaged nerves to masked depression: inevitability and hope in Latvian psychiatric narratives. Soc Sci Med 56:2421–2431, 2003

Slote WH: The intrapsychic locus of power and personal determination in a Confucian society: the case of Vietnam, in The Psycho-Cultural Dynamics of the Confucian Family: Past and Present. Edited by Slote WH. Seoul, International Cultural Society of Korea, 1986

Sulaiman S, Bhudgra D, de Silva P: The development of a culturally sensitive symptom checklist for depression in Dubai. Transcult Psychiatry 38:219–229, 2001

Teasdale JD, Segal ZV, Williams JM, et al: Prevention of relapse/recurrence in major depression by mindfulness-based cognitive therapy. J Consult Clin Psychol 68:615–623, 2000

Tennant C: Work-related stress and depressive disorders. J Psychosom Res 51:697–704, 2001

Tompar-Tiu A, Sustento-Seneriches J: Depression and Other Mental Health Issues: The Filipino American Experience. San Francisco, CA, Jossey-Bass, 1995

U.S. Surgeon General: Mental Health: Culture, Race, and Ethnicity. Rockville, MD, U.S. Department of Health and Human Services, 2002

Üstün TB, Sartorius N (eds): Mental Illness in General Health Care: An International Study. Chichester, UK, Wiley, 1995

Van Ommeren M, Sharma B, Makaju R, et al: Limited cultural validity of the Composite International Diagnostic Interview's probe flow chart. Transcult Psychiatry 37:119–129, 2000

Vega WA, Kolody B, Aguilar-Gaxiola S, et al: Lifetime prevalence of DSM-III-R psychiatric disorders among urban and rural Mexican Americans in California. Arch Gen Psychiatry 55:771–778, 1998

Verdeli H, Clougherty KF, Bolton P, et al: Adapting group interpersonal psychotherapy for a developing country: experience in rural Uganda. World Psychiatry 2:114–120, 2003

Vorcaro CM, Lima-Costa MF, Barreto SM, et al: Unexpected high prevalence of 1-month depression in a small Brazilian community: the Bambui Study. Acta Psychiatr Scand 104:257–263, 2001

Weissman MM, Bland RC, Canino GJ, et al: Cross-national epidemiology of major depression and bipolar disorder. JAMA 276:293–299, 1996

Westermeyer J, Janca A: Language, culture and psychopathology: conceptual and methodological issues. Transcult Psychiatry 34:291–311, 1997

White GM: Representing emotional meaning: category, metaphor, schema, discourse, in Handbook of Emotions. Edited by Lewis M, Haviland-Jones JM. New York, Guilford, 2000, pp 30–44

Wittchen H-U, Robins LN, Cottler LB, et al: Cross-cultural feasibility, reliability and sources of variance of the Composite International Diagnostic Interview (CIDI). Br J Psychiatry 159:645–653, 1991

World Health Organization (ed): Depressive Disorders in Different Cultures: Report on the WHO Collaborative Study on Standardized Assessment of Depressive Disorders. Geneva, World Health Organization, 1983

Yen S, Robins CJ, Lin N: A cross-cultural comparison of depressive symptom manifestation: China and the United States. J Consult Clin Psychol 68:993–999, 2000

Zhang AY, Snowden LR: Ethnic characteristics of mental disorders in five U.S. communities. Cultur Divers Ethnic Minor Psychol 5:134–146, 1999

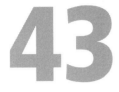

Mood Disorders and Sleep

DANIEL J. BUYSSE, M.D.

ANNE GERMAIN, PH.D.

ERIC A. NOFZINGER, M.D.

DAVID J. KUPFER, M.D.

SLEEP AND MOOD DISORDERS are linked to each other in several fundamental ways. First, sleep disturbances are one of the most consistent symptoms in mood disorders of all types. Although some patients present with insomnia and others with hypersomnia, some type of sleep difficulty is almost universal. Second, a growing body of evidence linking sleep to mood involves risk relationships. Specifically, insomnia confers increased risk for the subsequent onset of mood disorders. Among patients with existing mood disorders, sleep disturbance is a risk factor for worse outcome. Third, disturbances of sleep and mood appear to share fundamental neurobiological relations. For instance, the rapid eye movement (REM) sleep disturbances characteristic of depression may have their basis in abnormal activation patterns in specific brain structures. Finally, the relation between sleep and mood disorders is important because of therapeutic implications. Specific treatment of sleep disturbances alleviates suffering and improves outcomes. In this chapter, we explore each of these relations in greater detail.

Symptom Overlap Between Sleep and Mood Disorders

Sleep symptoms are very common among patients with mood disorders, including depressive and bipolar disorders. Conversely, mood symptoms are common among patients with specific sleep disorders, including insomnia and hypersomnia.

Sleep Symptoms in Mood Disorders

Common sleep symptoms in depression include insomnia, hypersomnia, and dream disturbances, which may exacerbate or maintain disturbances of mood. In mania, severe sleep loss is the most common sleep symptom.

Insomnia

Insomnia is defined as difficulty falling asleep or staying asleep despite adequate opportunity for sleep. More than

80% of depressed individuals complain of insomnia (Reynolds and Kupfer 1987). The incidence is especially high in older patients. Early-morning awakening with the inability to return to sleep may be an especially informative indicator of a current depressive episode. Depression is the most frequent cause of chronic insomnia in both clinical and epidemiological samples (Buysse et al. 1994; Ohayon et al. 1998).

Hypersomnia

Hypersomnia refers to increased sleep duration relative to habitual total sleep time or the presence of excessive daytime sleepiness. Hypersomnia is less frequently reported than insomnia in depressed patients, but young adult patients, patients with seasonal depression, and bipolar depressed patients commonly report hypersomnia rather than insomnia. Across age groups, the lifetime prevalence and incidence of hypersomnia is 7%–8% (Breslau et al. 1996). Depression is among the strongest risk factors for hypersomnia.

Dream Disturbances

Complaints such as disturbing dreams and nocturnal panic attacks are also reported by depressed patients. Suicidal depressed patients appear to have more severe sleep complaints than do nonsuicidal depressed patients, and depressed women who report frequent distressing dreams report more suicidal symptoms than do those without bad dreams (Nowell and Buysse 2001).

Specific Mood Disorders and Subtypes of Depression

Specific mood disorders and subtypes of depression may be associated with specific sleep disturbances. For instance, patients with psychotic depression may report more severe insomnia complaints compared with nonpsychotic depressed patients. Of the patients with seasonal affective disorder, 80% report hypersomnia, which can be reduced by bright light therapy (Levitt et al. 2002). The minority of patients with seasonal affective disorder who report insomnia tend show poorer treatment response to bright light therapy (Terman et al. 1996). Dysthymic patients commonly report hypersomnia.

Reduced Amount of Sleep and Reduced Need for Sleep

Reduced amount of sleep and reduced need for sleep are the most consistent early symptoms of mania (Jackson et al. 2003). Life events that disrupt daily rhythms, particularly sleep-wake rhythms, are associated with the onset of manic episodes in bipolar disorder (Malkoff-Schwartz et

al. 1998). Likewise, short sleep duration is associated with increased severity of mania and longer time to stabilization of mania (Barbini et al. 1996; Leibenluft et al. 1996; Nowlin-Finch et al. 1994). In contrast, both insomnia and hypersomnia are common symptoms during the depressive phase of bipolar disorder (e.g., Jackson et al. 2003; Nofzinger et al. 1991).

Sleep symptoms in mood disorders may be affected by gender, race/ethnicity, and age. In general, women report more sleep complaints than do men. Non-Caucasian women report more severe insomnia complaints than do non-Caucasian men and Caucasian samples (e.g., Bixler et al. 2002; Foley et al. 1999). In the general population and clinical samples, insomnia and hypersomnia complaints increase with age. However, the relation between age and sleep disturbances also may be explained in part by other factors such as medical illnesses.

Mood Symptoms in Sleep Disorders

Insomnia Disorders

The most common insomnia disorder is insomnia related to another mental disorder. Studies in general populations and clinical samples indicate that 35%–70% of the individuals who report insomnia also present with mood, anxiety, or substance use disorders or have psychological characteristics associated with psychopathology (Nowell et al. 1997; Ohayon et al. 1998). Even insomnia patients who do not a have a current mood disorder appear to report more depressed mood than do individuals without insomnia (Moul et al. 2002; Vandeputte and de Weerd 2003).

Obstructive Sleep Apnea Syndrome

Obstructive sleep apnea syndrome refers to repeated episodes of breathing cessation and reduction in airflow for 10 seconds or more, most often caused by the collapse of the upper airway tissues during sleep. These respiratory events are associated with transient arousals from sleep, which result in significant daytime sleepiness and anergia. The sleep disruption, excessive daytime sleepiness, anergia, impaired concentration, and other cognitive difficulties associated with sleep apnea can be mistaken for depressive symptoms. The severity of respiratory events in sleep apneic patients is correlated with depression severity, and treatment of sleep apnea with continuous airway pressure can alleviate depressive symptoms (Means et al. 2003). Given the prevalence of both obstructive sleep apnea syndrome and depression, the two conditions also can be expected to occur together frequently.

Narcolepsy

Narcolepsy is a sleep disorder characterized by chronic extreme daytime sleepiness and unexpected episodes of sleep. Sleep episodes are often accompanied by dreams or dreamlike hallucinations and episodes of cataplexy (sudden episodes of voluntary muscle atonia triggered by emotional stimuli). Approximately 25%–50% of the patients with narcolepsy have experienced a depressive episode or significant depression symptoms (Vandeputte and de Weerd 2003). Daytime sleepiness in narcolepsy may be confused with fatigue and atypical depression.

Circadian Rhythm Sleep Disorders

Circadian rhythm sleep disorders are characterized by abnormal timing of sleep. For instance, in delayed sleep phase syndrome, patients report difficulty falling asleep at the desired bedtime and difficulty waking in the morning but no such difficulties when bedtime and awakening time are delayed. As many as 75% of the patients may have a past or current history of depression (Regestein and Monk 1995). In advanced sleep phase syndrome, the major sleep episode is advanced in relation to the desired clock time, resulting in early evening sleepiness, early sleep onset, and early-morning awakening. Patients with either of these disorders often report mild depression symptoms (Vandeputte and de Weerd 2003).

Other Sleep Disorders

As many as 53% of the patients seen in a sleep clinic with a diagnosis of periodic limb movements or restless legs syndrome have high rates of self-reported depressive symptomatology (Ulfberg et al. 2001; Vandeputte and de Weerd 2003). Data on the prevalence of mood disturbances in patients with parasomnias, such as nightmares, sleep terrors, or somnambulism, are scarce. Frequent nightmares, whether associated with trauma exposure or not, are often associated with moderate to severe depressive symptoms (e.g., Krakow et al. 2001).

Risk Relationships Between Sleep and Mood Disorders

The risk relationship between sleep and mood disorders is bidirectional. Mood disorders and mood disturbances are significant risk factors for both insomnia and hypersomnia. Conversely, several epidemiological studies indicated that symptoms of insomnia are strong risk factors for the subsequent development of mood disorders, even

when baseline mood symptoms are controlled (see Table 43–1). These studies found that individuals with insomnia are at higher risk to develop a psychiatric disorder over follow-up intervals of 1–35 years. This risk relationship has been found in young, middle-aged, and older adults. Patients with mood disorders commonly report retrospectively that insomnia appeared before or at the same time as other mood disorder symptoms rather than after other depressive symptoms (Ohayon and Roth 2003).

Sleep symptoms also interfere with treatment response and maintenance of therapeutic gains in depression across a variety of treatment modalities. Poor subjective sleep quality before initiation of nonpharmacological treatments also may predict reduced treatment response. Depressed women who showed significant improvements in mood with interpersonal therapy reported better sleep quality pretreatment compared with women whose depression did not remit (Buysse et al. 1999). Similar findings have been observed with combined pharmacological and psychological treatments of depression. Specifically, worse subjective sleep quality is associated with worse treatment response (Dew et al. 1997). Improvements in subjective sleep quality following treatment, however, appear to be associated with lower recurrence rates of depression (Buysse et al. 1996). Poor sleep quality is a risk factor for recurrence of depression among recovered depressed patients who do not receive maintenance treatment (Reynolds et al. 1997), and insomnia may be the first symptom to occur prior to a recurrence (Perlis et al. 1997).

Electroencephalogram Sleep Findings in Mood Disorders

Complaints of disturbed sleep in patients with mood disorders have been supported by hundreds of studies over the past 30 years that used electroencephalography or polysomnography (PSG). These studies have examined sleep disturbances at baseline during the course of illness and in response to treatment, during successive episodes of mood disorder, and in affected and unaffected family members. These findings have been reviewed in detail elsewhere (Benca et al. 1992; Buysse and Kupfer 1993) and are summarized here.

Electroencephalogram Sleep Findings in Depressive Disorders

During an acute episode of major depression, electroencephalogram (EEG) sleep studies show a set of abnormal-

TABLE 43–1.   Insomnia as a risk factor for depression

Study	Sample description	Follow-up period (years)	Relevant findings
Ford and Kamerow 1989	N= 7,954 Age>18 years	1	Risk of developing depression over 1 year was higher in individuals with insomnia at baseline and/or at follow-up than in individuals without insomnia (odds ratio [OR]=38.9; 95% confidence interval [CI]=19.8–80.0). For people who had insomnia that resolved over 1 year, the risk of depression was not significantly elevated (OR=1.6; 95% CI=0.5–5.3).
Dryman and Eaton 1991	N=9,295 with no history of disorders Age≥18 years	1	Sleep disturbances at baseline predicted onset of depression at follow-up in women (risk OR=9.4; 95% CI=4.3–20.3).
Livingston et al. 1993	N=524 Age>65 years	2–3	Sleep disturbances at baseline predicted depression at follow-up after adjustment for other risk factors. Individuals with persistent sleep disturbances were more likely to be depressed than individuals with insomnia that resolved or individuals who developed insomnia during follow-up.
Eaton et al. 1995	N=10,009 with no history of affective disorders Age≥18 years	1	Sleep disturbances identified 47% of individuals who develop depression in the following year.
Chang et al. 1997	N=1,053 male medical students	Median=34 (range=1–45)	Men with self-reported insomnia and difficulty sleeping under stress were at greater risk to develop depression and greater psychiatric distress at follow-up.
Weissman et al. 1997	N=7,113 n=533 with insomnia without psychiatric disorder in the past year n=408 with insomnia and psychiatric disorder in the past year n=6,172 with no insomnia and no psychiatric disorder ever	1	Individuals with insomnia and no psychiatric disorders (uncomplicated insomnia) in the year prior to baseline were 4.5 times more likely than those without insomnia to have depressive symptoms during follow-up. Individuals with uncomplicated insomnia were more likely to meet criteria for major depression at follow-up (OR=5.4; 95% CI=2.6–11.3).
Breslau et al. 1998	N=979 Age=21–30 years	3.5	15.9% of the individuals with insomnia at baseline met criteria for major depression at follow-up (OR=2.1; 95% CI=1.1–4.2).
Mallon et al. 2000	N=1,870 at initial assessment N=1,244 at follow-up Age=45–75 years	12	Insomnia at baseline predicted depression at follow-up in women (OR=4.2; 95% CI=2.5–7.3) but not in men (OR=1.3; 95% CI=0.8–2.3).

ities relative to healthy individuals without depression. These are summarized in Table 43–2 and illustrated in Figure 43–1. First, patients with depression show disturbances of *sleep continuity* and *sleep-wake balance*. Specifically, depressed patients have prolonged sleep latency (time to fall asleep), increased wakefulness during the night, decreased sleep time, and decreased "sleep effi-

ciency" (time spent asleep / total time in bed). Several studies also have documented a specific increase in wakefulness in the last third of the sleep period, the PSG correlate of early-morning awakening. Patients with major depression also show abnormalities in the relative amounts of different sleep stages, or *sleep architecture*. In particular, depression is associated with an increase in

Stage 1 non-REM sleep, a decrease in Stage 3/4 non-REM sleep, and an increase in the total amount or percentage of REM sleep. Within this constellation of findings, depressed patients also may show abnormalities of temporal distribution in specific sleep stages. For instance, one of the earliest abnormalities described was a decrease in duration of the first non-REM sleep period, also known as *REM sleep latency* (Kupfer 1976). Depressed patients also have been noted to have longer REM sleep periods in the first part of the night than do age- and sex-matched control subjects, which contrasts with the usual pattern of progressively longer REM periods during the course of sleep.

Another set of abnormalities associated with sleep and depression relies on quantitative analysis of eye movements during REM sleep or specific EEG waveforms during non-REM sleep. *REM density* refers to an estimate of the number of rapid eye movements per minute of REM sleep; it has an analog in computer-based algorithms that detect the number of eye movements. The number of eye movements during REM sleep is often increased among patients with depression, particularly in the first REM period. Quantitative measures of EEG activity have shown a decrease in EEG activity in the 0.5–4.0 Hz range, also known as *slow-wave* or *delta* activity, during non-REM sleep. Once again, abnormal temporal distributions have been described, with depressed patients showing a specific decrease in delta activity during the first non-REM period relative to the second period, an abnormality also known as *decreased delta ratio*. Other quantitative EEG findings in depression include increased higher-frequency EEG activity (Borbély et al. 1984; Kupfer et al. 1986), decreased coherence between different EEG frequencies (intrahemispheric coherence) and between right and left hemispheres (interhemispheric coherence) (Armitage et al. 2000), and greater EEG power in the right hemisphere than in the left hemisphere during REM sleep (Armitage et al. 1992).

Although many EEG sleep disturbances have been reported in depression, these findings are not highly sensitive or specific and cannot be used as diagnostic tests. For instance, studies comparing patients with major depressive disorder with patients with other psychiatric disorders have found a sensitivity of only 60%–75% (Buysse and Kuper 1987). A meta-analysis of PSG findings in patients with different psychiatric disorders (Benca et al. 1992) found that sleep continuity and non-REM sleep measures were not consistently different among patients with depression and patients with other psychiatric disorders. REM sleep findings, including increased amount and percentage of REM sleep and increased phasic REM activity, were the most discriminating features for depression. Several investigators also have used multivariate statistical analyses with combinations of different EEG sleep measures. Such studies have found a sensitivity of approximately 80% for discriminating patients with depression from control subjects and patients with other disorders (Gillin et al. 1979; Kerkhofs et al. 1985; Reynolds et al. 1988; Thase et al. 1996).

EEG sleep findings in depression may be affected by several patient-related characteristics, as described in the following subsections.

Age

In general, differences between depressed and control subjects are less notable in adolescent subjects (Goetz et al. 1987). In adult samples, EEG sleep differences between depressed patients and control subjects become larger as a function of age (Knowles and MacLean 1990). An example of these increasing differences is shown in Figure 43–2.

Sex

Although the same general profile of EEG sleep changes in depression is seen in both men and women, the findings may be more pronounced in men, who have less Stage 3/4 and less delta EEG activity than do women across a range of ages (Reynolds et al. 1990). Other quantitative EEG studies also have shown substantial differences between depressed men and women, with depressed men having less slow EEG activity compared with depressed women, healthy women, and healthy men (Armitage et al. 1995).

Severity

The relation between severity and the degree of disturbance in EEG sleep measures has been inconsistent. Several early studies found more severe disturbances among more severely depressed patients (Giles et al. 1986a; Reynolds et al. 1983), but other studies did not confirm this finding (Ansseau et al. 1985; Kumar et al. 1987). Studies of depressed inpatients compared with outpatients, an approximate surrogate for severity, generally have shown more severe disturbances in inpatient samples (Buysse et al. 1990; Reynolds et al. 1982). Perlis and colleagues (1997) comprehensively examined the general relation between depression symptoms and EEG sleep measures. Canonical correlation showed a single dimension of severity for both EEG sleep and Hamilton Rating Scale for Depression items, indicating that more severe symptoms were indeed related to more severe depression.

Other Clinical Variables

Psychosocial factors such as life stressors and lower social support have been associated with more abnormal EEG

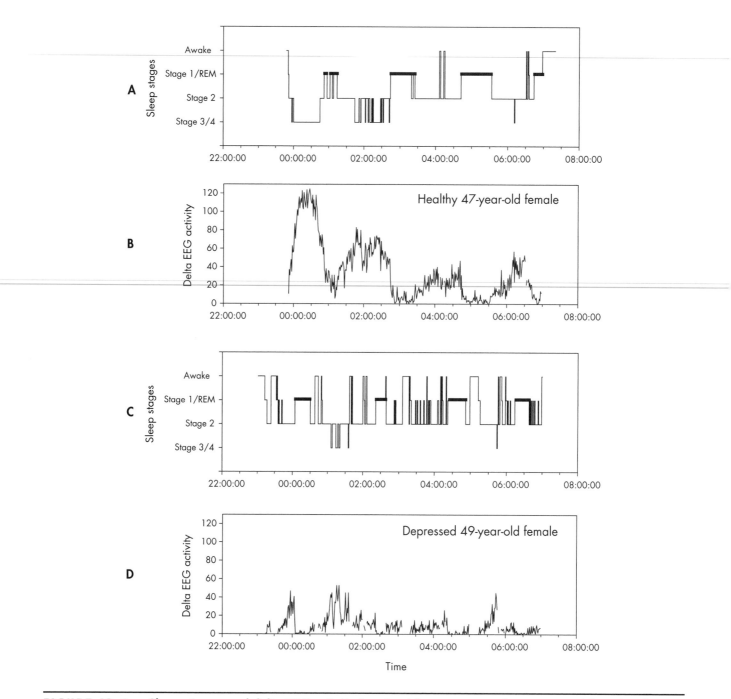

FIGURE 43–1.   Sleep stages and delta EEG activity in a healthy woman and a woman with major depressive disorder.

A: The hypnogram represents the time course of sleep stages across the night. Wakefulness and "lighter" stages of sleep appear at a higher level on the *y* axis, and "deeper stages appear at a lower level. This healthy woman transitions quickly from wakefulness to deep non-REM sleep, then cycles between non-REM and REM across the night. A few brief awakenigs occur in the second half of the night. **B:** Delta EEG activity represents the number of slow, low-frequency EEG waves during non-REM sleep. Higher amounts of delta activity correspond to "deeper" sleep in non-REM Stages 3/4. Delta activity is typically highest in the first non-REM period of the night and declines in subsequent non-REM periods, as shown in this example. **C:** Compared with the healthy subject, the hypnogram from a depressed patient shows greater difficulty in falling asleep, more awakenings during the night, reduced amount of Stage 3/4 non-REM sleep, and a shorter interval between the onset of consolidated sleep and the first episode of REM sleep (reduced "REM latency"). **D:** Overall delta EEG activity is reduced in the depressed subject, and the highest amount of delta activity occurs in the second, rather than the first, non-REM period. EEG=electroencephalogram; REM=rapid eye movement.

TABLE 43–2. Electroencephalogram (EEG) sleep findings in patients with major depression compared with healthy subjects

Type of measure	Usual finding in patients with major depression
Sleep continuity measures	
Sleep latency (time to fall asleep)	Increased
Number of awakenings	Increased
Duration of wakefulness	Increased
Sleep efficiency (total sleep time/time spent in bed)	Decreased
Sleep architecture measures	
Non-REM Stage 1 sleep %	No change or increased
Non-REM Stage 2 sleep %	No change or increased
Non-REM Stage 3/4 sleep %	No change or decreased
REM sleep %	Increased
REM sleep measures	
REM sleep latency (time between sleep onset and first REM period)	Decreased
REM density (number of eye movements per minute of REM sleep)	Increased
Distribution of REM sleep	Shifted toward beginning of sleep period
Quantitative EEG measures	
Delta (0.5–4.0 Hz) activity, power	Decreased
Temporal distribution of delta activity	Shifted from first to second non-REM period (decreased delta ratio)

Note. REM=rapid eye movement.

sleep findings (Dew et al. 1996). However, older individuals who have never sought treatment for depression have been found to have essentially normal EEG sleep profiles (Vitiello et al. 1990).

Subtype of Depression

Objective sleep disturbances, including sleep continuity difficulties and REM sleep disturbances, are more pronounced in depressed patients with endogenous depression (Kupfer et al. 1982) and psychotic depression (Thase et al. 1986). Patients who complain of hypersomnia, typically those with "atypical" depression, have less disturbance of sleep continuity at night but do not show increased objective sleepiness when assessed with daytime sleep latency tests (Nofzinger et al. 1991). Likewise, depressed patients with bipolar disorder tend to have less sleep disturbance and longer nighttime sleep (Giles et al. 1986b). Finally, patients with seasonal affective disorder have EEG sleep findings similar to those of other depressed patients (Anderson et al. 1994).

Findings During the Course of a Depressive Episode

EEG sleep findings also have been examined at various points during the course of a depressive episode. Although medications have prominent effects on EEG sleep, several studies have examined recovered and drug-free patients, and other studies have examined the longitudinal course of EEG sleep findings in patients who received psychotherapy. From these studies, several general conclusions can be drawn.

The most severe sleep abnormalities, including "sleep-onset REM periods," are less likely to be observed in recovered patients than in symptomatic ones (Schulz et al. 1979). Patients very early in an episode of major depression appear to have more severe EEG sleep disturbances (Dew et al. 1996; Kupfer et al. 1991). The amount of REM sleep and the number of eye movements during REM sleep tend to decrease over time during an episode of depression (Coble et al. 1979; Dew et al. 1996; Kupfer et al. 1988). Studies following treatments with medications and psychotherapy also tend to show improvement in sleep continuity and REM sleep measures (Buysse et al. 1992a; Riemann and Berger 1989; Thase et al. 1998) but stability in Stage 3/4 sleep, delta ratio, and REM sleep latency. Sleep continuity measures also show improvements with adequate treatment of depression (Lee et al. 1993). Finally, slow-wave sleep measures appear to show few changes with either psychotherapy or medication (Buysse et al. 1997a). Categorically defined REM sleep latency (e.g., less than 60 minutes vs. greater than 60 minutes) is also stable between symptomatic and recovered periods (Giles et al. 1987). Thus, sleep continuity and REM sleep abnormalities appear to be more state related, whereas slow-wave sleep and REM sleep latency are more traitlike findings in depression (Kupfer and Ehlers 1989).

Family Studies

Family studies also have been conducted with regard to EEG sleep findings in depression. These studies suggest strong familial aggregation of reduced and nonreduced REM sleep latency, as well as risk for subsequent depression (e.g., Giles et al. 1988, 1989; Lauer et al. 1995).

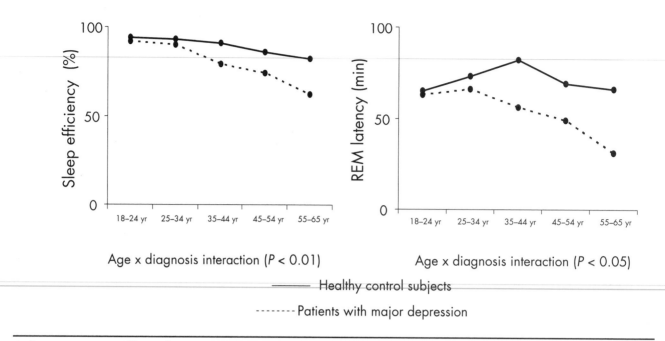

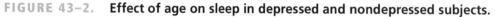

FIGURE 43–2. **Effect of age on sleep in depressed and nondepressed subjects.**

The difference between sleep in healthy subjects and patients with depression becomes larger with increased age. The left panel shows sleep efficiency (total sleep time / time in bed × 100), and the right panel shows rapid eye movement (REM) sleep latency.

Source. Adapted from Lauer CJ, Riemann D, Wiegand M, et al: "From Early to Late Adulthood Changes in EEG Sleep of Depressed Patients and Healthy Volunteers." *Biological Psychiatry* 29:979–993, 1991.

Electroencephalogram Sleep Findings in Depressive Disorders: Relation to Clinical Outcome

Other studies have examined the relation between EEG sleep measures and specific clinical outcomes. Depressed patients with reduced REM sleep latency and those who show prolonged REM sleep latency during initial treatment with tricyclic antidepressants are more likely to show an eventual response to such medications (Kupfer et al. 1981; Rush et al. 1989). Reduced REM sleep latency alone does not seem to be related to treatment outcome with psychotherapy (Buysse et al. 1992a; Jarrett et al. 1990; Thase and Simons 1992). Another study with psychotherapy showed reduced likelihood of response among subjects with increased phasic REM activity (Buysse et al. 1999). An abnormal sleep profile—defined by the combination of REM sleep latency, visually estimated REM number, and sleep deficiency—also was associated with reduced likelihood of response to psychotherapy but not subsequent pharmacotherapy (Thase and Kupfer 1996; Thase et al. 1997). Finally, several studies have linked slow-wave sleep and slow-wave activity to depressive recurrences. Specifically, patients with reduced REM sleep latency and reduced EEG delta activity appear to be at increased risk for recurrences (Buysse et al. 1997a; Giles et al. 1987; Kupfer et al. 1993).

Electroencephalogram Sleep Findings in Mania

Methodological difficulties have made it far more difficult to study EEG sleep during acute manic episodes. The reduced amount of sleep in these patients, as well as their behavioral agitation, makes it difficult to conduct EEG sleep studies. Nevertheless, a few investigations have been conducted (Hudson et al. 1988, 1992; Linkowski et al. 1986). It is not surprising that these studies showed reduced total sleep time and sleep continuity disturbance. It was somewhat more surprising that some studies also showed sleep findings similar to those seen in depression, including reduced REM sleep latency and increased phasic REM activity.

Sleep Deprivation and Mood Disorders

Although depression is associated with reduced sleep and insomnia, a paradoxical relation between depression and sleep has long been recognized. Specifically, intentional sleep deprivation results in short-lived improvement of depressive symptoms in approximately 60% of patients

(Wirz-Justice and Van den Hoofdakker 1999). Relapse of depressive symptoms is commonly observed after even short durations of sleep. Total sleep deprivation, partial sleep deprivation for either half of the night, and specific deprivation of REM sleep all have been observed to show therapeutic effects, but only the last of these has been associated with sustained remission. Some studies also have suggested that sleep deprivation effects may be more sustained when used in combination with antidepressant drugs (Wirz-Justice and Van den Hoofdakker 1999) or that sleep deprivation may accelerate or potentiate the response to antidepressant drugs (Leibenluft and Wehr 1992; Leibenluft et al. 1993). However, such effects have not been consistently observed. Other sleep deprivation strategies have included serial partial sleep deprivation (Holsboer-Trachsler and Ernst 1986) and sleep deprivation followed by phase advance of the sleep-wake schedule (Riemann et al. 1996). Among unipolar depression patients, sleep deprivation appears to have more beneficial effects in those with pronounced diurnal variation of mood (Reinink et al. 1990).

Conversely, sleep deprivation can precipitate mania or hypomania in patients with bipolar disorder. When used in combination with drugs such as lithium or pindolol, however, sleep deprivation has been reported to lead to sustained improvements in bipolar depression (Colombo et al. 2000; Smeraldi et al. 1999). As described later in this chapter (see section "Sleep Deprivation in Depression"), consistent neuroanatomical correlates of sleep deprivation responses in depression also have been identified.

Theoretical Models of Sleep Disturbance in Depression

The finding of characteristic, if not specific, EEG sleep disturbances in depression led to several early neurobiological models of depression. Several investigators (Kripke 1983; Papousek 1975; Wehr and Wirz-Justice 1982) proposed that sleep and mood disturbances in depression might result from abnormalities in biological rhythms. In particular, these theories asserted either a phase advance in REM sleep and body temperature rhythms or abnormalities of internal phase among different rhythms. Further support for these theories came from studies showing that advancing the timing of sleep could have an antidepressant effect in some patients. Subsequently, the "social zeitgeber" hypothesis of depression proposed a link between disturbances in social rhythms and sleep-wake schedules and subsequent biological disturbances, including the EEG sleep abnormalities (Ehlers et al. 1988).

Ultimately, circadian rhythm theories of sleep disturbance in depression have not been consistently supported by empirical evidence. Significant phase advances cannot be identified in most depressed patients, and very few studies in depressed patients have adequately controlled for the "masking effects" of sleep on circadian rhythms. A few studies that used the "constant routine" method to control for such effects in depressed patients failed to show significant abnormalities (Monk et al. 1994). Although some depressed patients may have biological rhythm disturbances, these do not appear to be characteristic of depression in general.

A second hypothesis is that sleep disturbance in depression is caused by a reduction in wake-dependent sleep drive (Borbély and Wirz-Justice 1982). According to this hypothesis, depressed patients have a reduced homeostatic sleep drive that is improved following sleep deprivation. Ultimately, however, this theory does not adequately account for the fact that improvement in mood is seen during sleep deprivation but before the expression of actual non-REM sleep. In fact, subsequent investigators have proposed that sleep itself, either non-REM or REM sleep, may be "depressogenic" (Beersma and Van den Hoofdakker 1992; Vogel et al. 1975; Wu and Bunney 1990).

A third set of theories has considered the neurochemical bases of REM and non-REM sleep and the relation to depression. These theories are based on the "reciprocal interaction" model of non-REM and REM sleep regulation (McCarley and Massaquoi 1992). In this model, REM sleep is promoted when specific cholinergic cell populations of the pedunculopontine tegmentum become active, and non-REM sleep occurs when the cholinergic cells become inactive and serotonergic and noradrenergic brain stem neurons in the raphe nuclei and locus coeruleus become active. Cholinergic and serotonergic or noradrenergic cell groups have mutual negative and positive feedback effects that lead to self-sustaining cycles of non-REM and REM sleep. Neurochemical sleep models of depression suggest that depression is characterized by cholinergic hypersensitivity and/or reduced serotonergic or noradrenergic sensitivity. Evidence in support of this theory comes from studies in which cholinergic drugs were given to depressed patients and control subjects. These studies showed a more rapid induction of REM sleep in depressed patients than in nondepressed control subjects. On the other hand, depressed patients do not have different EEG responses to acute tryptophan depletion, even when they have worsening of mood.

Neurochemical theories of sleep disturbance in depression remain very general and account for subcortical aspects of EEG sleep findings better than they explain the complex cortical processes that also must occur in depression. However, the basic notion of cholinergic and noradrenergic/serotonergic imbalance underlying sleep disturbances in depression remains plausible.

Neurobiology of Sleep in Mood Disorders

Over the past decade, functional neuroimaging studies have identified regional changes in brain activity and function across sleep-wake states in humans. Many of the structures involved in these changes also have been implicated in the neurobiology of depression. In this section, we briefly review functional neuroimaging findings during sleep in healthy subjects and in patients with mood disorders.

Functional Neuroimaging Findings During Sleep in Healthy Subjects

Cerebral blood flow and glucose metabolic activity show broad, reliable changes across the sleep-wake cycle in humans, decreasing during non-REM sleep compared with wakefulness, then increasing to waking or near-waking levels during REM sleep (Braun et al. 1997; Kjaer et al. 2002; Nofzinger et al. 1997, 2002). Non-REM sleep is characterized by functional deafferentation of the cortex at the level of the thalamus and the occurrence of intrinsic thalamocortical electrical oscillations. Imaging studies in humans have reported that, compared with wakefulness, non-REM sleep is associated with reductions in blood flow and metabolism in the thalamus and in heteromodal association cortex of the frontal, parietal, and temporal lobes (Figure 43–3). Thus, the thalamocortical circuits that play an important role in non-REM sleep overlap with regions that support conscious, goal-directed behavior during wakefulness.

REM sleep is associated with an electrophysiological activation of cortex, with selective activation of cholinergic networks that originate in the brain stem and basal forebrain and densely innervate limbic and paralimbic cortices. Consistent with this observation, functional imaging studies in humans show that, compared with wakefulness and non-REM sleep, REM sleep is associated with increased activity in the pontine reticular formation, limbic structures (e.g., amygdala and hypothalamus), and paralimbic cortex (e.g., ventral striatum, anterior cingulate, and medial prefrontal cortex) (see Figure 43–3). Given the involvement of these structures in the regulation of affect and motivated behavior during wakefulness,

sleep neuroimaging findings suggest that REM sleep also may play an important role in emotional regulation or behavior.

Functional Neuroimaging Findings During REM Sleep in Depressed Subjects

As reviewed earlier, increases in the amount of REM sleep and phasic eye movements are among the more reliable and specific EEG sleep findings in patients with mood disorders. Because REM sleep activates limbic and anterior paralimbic cortices in healthy subjects, it seems plausible to hypothesize that increased REM sleep in depression may be associated with greater activation of these structures. A preliminary analysis of fluorine-18 fluorodeoxyglucose positron emission tomography ([18F]-FDG PET) studies in depressed patients (Nofzinger et al. 1999) showed increases in relative metabolism during REM sleep compared with wakefulness in the tectal area and a series of left hemispheric areas, including sensorimotor cortex, inferior temporal cortex, uncal gyrus–amygdala, and subicular complex. Many of these brain stem and limbic regions are involved in the modulation of emotional arousal. Depressed patients did not show increases in relative metabolism in anterior paralimbic structures during REM sleep compared with waking.

Subsequent analyses (Nofzinger et al. 2001) suggested that the absence of an increase in relative metabolism from waking to REM sleep in depressed patients may have been related to hypermetabolism in these structures during wakefulness, which imposed a "ceiling effect" for changes observed between REM sleep and wakefulness. In another analysis that used [18F]-FDG PET, depressed patients had greater increases than healthy subjects in relative metabolism during REM sleep in the midbrain reticular formation, including the pretectal area, and in a larger region of anterior paralimbic cortex (Nofzinger et al. 2004). This is consistent with the hypothesis that depressed patients would show increased activation in limbic and anterior limbic structures during REM sleep compared with wakefulness. Additionally, depressed patients had greater increases in relative metabolism during REM sleep in a broad region of dorsolateral prefrontal, parietal, and temporal cortices, predominantly in the left hemisphere. This area included the dorsolateral prefrontal cortex and the frontal and parietal eye fields. Figure 43–4 illustrates typical REM-related changes in regional glucose metabolism in depressed subjects.

Increased activation of the brain stem reticular formation during REM sleep compared with wakefulness in depressed patients is consistent with the model of altered balance in brain stem monoaminergic and acetylcholine

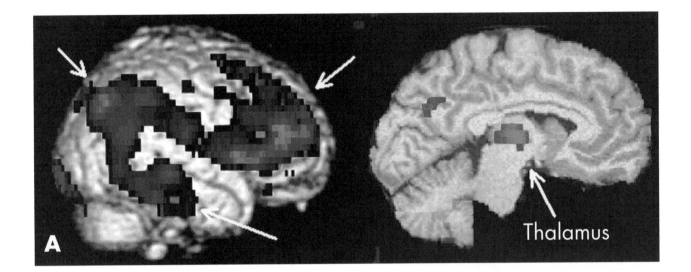

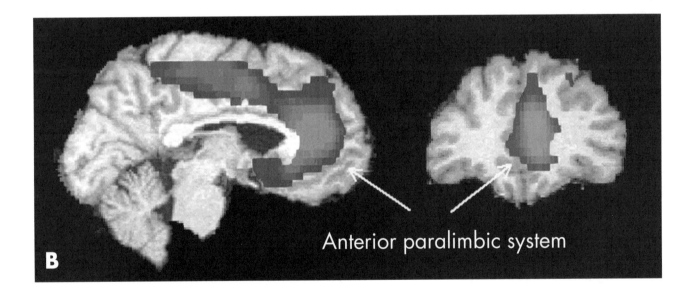

FIGURE 43–3. Relative metabolism during non–rapid eye movement (non-REM) and REM sleep in healthy adults.

A: Dark regions represent those areas where relative metabolism is decreased during non-REM sleep compared with during waking across 28 healthy subjects. The left image shows that broad regions of heteromodal association cortex are involved, and the right image shows that the thalamus is involved. **B:** Dark regions represent those areas where relative metabolism is increased during REM sleep compared with during waking across 38 healthy subjects. The left image shows an anterior paralimbic pattern, and the right image shows that this pattern is midline.

neuronal systems in depressed patients, described in an earlier section. The increased activation of limbic and anterior paralimbic cortices during REM sleep also may reflect underlying neurochemical changes in depressed patients. Limbic structures such as the hippocampus and amygdala have the highest density of cholinergic axons, and limbic and anterior paralimbic cortices also have high densities of inhibitory serotonin type 1A (5-HT$_{1A}$) postsynaptic receptors. Increased REM-related activation of limbic and paralimbic cortices in depressed patients

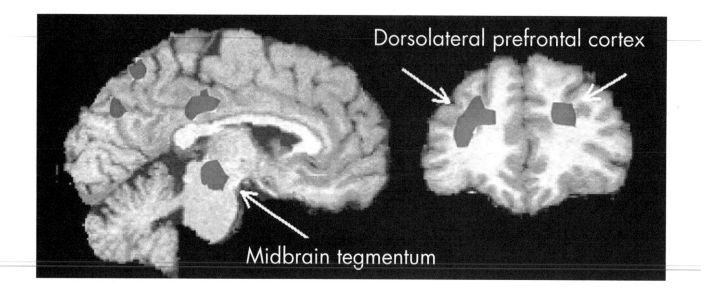

FIGURE 43–4.   **Relative glucose metabolism during REM sleep in depressed patients compared with healthy control subjects.**

Dark regions represent those areas where relative metabolism increases more from waking to rapid eye movement (REM) sleep in depressed patients than in healthy subjects. The left image shows that the midbrain reticular formation is involved, and the right image shows that the dorsolateral prefrontal cortex is also involved bilaterally.

may reflect the experience of stimuli in a more affectively intense, negative context; during wakefulness, these structures show increased activation in response to negatively valenced stimuli or increased affective states. Finally, the relatively greater REM-related activation of cortical regions serving executive functions in depressed patients also may result from the hypothesized monoaminergic–cholinergic imbalance. Greater involvement of executive function during REM sleep in depressed patients could represent a response to the increased activation of limbic and paralimbic cortices during REM sleep.

Functional Neuroimaging Findings During Non-REM Sleep in Depressed Subjects

As reviewed earlier, alterations in sleep continuity and non-REM sleep are also common in patients with depression. An initial study of cerebral metabolism in which [18F]-FDG PET was used found increased whole brain metabolism during the first non-REM period in depressed compared with healthy men. The increases were largest in the posterior cingulate, amygdala, hippocampus, occipital and temporal cortices, and pons. Depressed men also had relative hypofrontality and reduced relative metabolism in the anterior cingulate, caudate, and medial thalamus compared with control sub-

jects. Taken together, these findings suggest hyperarousal during non-REM sleep in depressed subjects.

The hyperarousal hypothesis was further evaluated in a study that assessed the relation between beta EEG power, an electrophysiological marker of cortical arousal, and regional cerebral glucose metabolism during non-REM sleep in healthy subjects and depressed patients (Nofzinger et al. 2000b). Depressed patients had increased beta power and worse sleep quality compared with healthy subjects. In both groups, beta power during non-REM sleep negatively correlated with subjective sleep quality and positively correlated with relative cerebral glucose metabolism in the ventromedial prefrontal cortex. This region is functionally related to other structures that mediate arousal, suggesting that increased activity in depressed patients may contribute to cortical arousal during non-REM sleep.

As noted, sleep in depression is also characterized by reductions in slow-frequency EEG activity, which is most prominent over frontal cortical regions. In healthy adults, non-REM sleep is associated with decreased metabolic activity in frontal, parietal, and temporal cortices compared with wakefulness. Compared with healthy subjects, depressed patients show smaller decreases in relative metabolism during non-REM sleep compared with presleep wakefulness in bilateral laterodorsal frontal gyri, right medial prefrontal cortex, right superior and middle temporal gyri

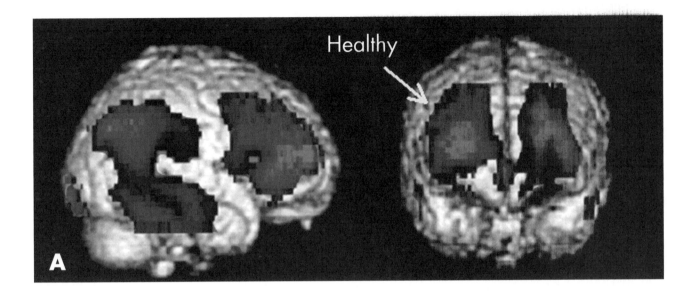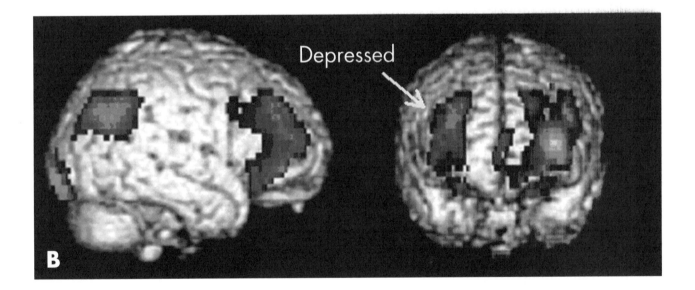

Mood Disorders and Sleep

FIGURE 43–5. **Relative glucose metabolism during non-REM sleep in healthy and depressed subjects.**
Dark regions represent those areas where relative metabolism is less during non-REM sleep than during waking. **A:** Results from 28 healthy subjects. **B:** Results from 29 depressed subjects. Notably, the extent of this decline is less in depressed patients, especially in prefrontal cortex (*arrows*).

and insula, right posterior cingulate cortex, lingual gyrus, striate cortex, cerebellar vermis, and left thalamus (see Figure 43–5) (Germain et al. 2004). These findings suggest that non-REM sleep abnormalities in depressed patients may result from a "blunting" of the normal wake–non-REM deactivation of cortical and thalamic structures.

Sleep Deprivation in Depression

The concept of hyperarousal in paralimbic structures during sleep in depressed patients has received further support from an extensive literature describing the functional neuroanatomical correlates of the antidepressant response to sleep deprivation in depressed patients (Ebert et al. 1991; G.S. Smith et al. 2002; Volk et al. 1997). These studies point to an important role for the anterior cingulate cortex in the response to sleep deprivation. Across studies, patients who have elevated baseline metabolism in the anterior cingulate cortex have more favorable clinical responses to sleep deprivation, accompanied by normalization of increased metabolism following sleep deprivation.

Therapeutic Implications of Sleep Disturbances in Mood Disorders

Depression and other mood disorders have significant effects on subjective and EEG sleep measures. Conversely, treatment of depression can have substantial effects on sleep as well. In the case of antidepressant medication, treatment-related changes in sleep are largely the result of pharmacological actions of the drugs. However, studies of subjective and EEG sleep during psychotherapy indicate that treatment of the depression itself can have beneficial effects on sleep.

Effects of Antidepressant Drugs on Sleep Symptoms and Electroencephalogram Sleep Findings

Antidepressant drugs are pharmacologically heterogeneous and have a wide range of effects on subjective and EEG sleep. The effects of antidepressant drugs on sleep have been reviewed elsewhere (Buysse et al. 2005) and are summarized in Table 43–3.

Tricyclic antidepressants have various effects on neurotransmission and, as a result, have different effects on subjective and EEG sleep. Noradrenergic agents such as desipramine can be associated with subjective reports of insomnia and EEG evidence of increased wakefulness during sleep (Shipley et al. 1985). In contrast, tertiary tricyclic agents such as amitriptyline, doxepin, and trimipramine are associated with subjective sedation. These more-sedating drugs are also associated with EEG evidence of increased sleep continuity, and some evidence indicates increased Stage 3/4 sleep and increased delta activity. Drugs with an "intermediate" profile include imipramine and clomipramine. A feature common to all tricyclic drugs, with the exception of trimipramine, is REM sleep suppression. In particular, tricyclic agents decrease the total number of minutes and percentage of REM sleep but cause little change in phasic eye movement activity. As a result, REM density may actually increase while taking these drugs.

Tricyclic antidepressants also can have adverse effects on sleep. Aside from the insomnia reported with more activating tricyclics, patients can develop symptoms of restless legs syndrome and can evidence increased periodic limb movements during sleep. These effects appear particularly likely with serotonergic drugs such as clomipramine. However, tricyclic drugs have not been observed to impair respiration during sleep and may even be associated with small improvements in sleep apnea (Buysse et al. 1996).

Selective serotonin reuptake inhibitors (SSRIs) have somewhat more consistent effects on sleep than do tricyclics. Although insomnia is a well-recognized side effect of these drugs, dose-related sedation also has been observed. SSRIs also have been associated with subjective complaints of restless legs syndrome and vivid dreaming. Nevertheless, clinical trials with SSRIs have shown improvements in overall scores for sleep disturbance (e.g., for review, see Jindal et al. 2003), which are probably related to nonspecific improvements in depression. SSRIs have variable effects on EEG sleep continuity, but in general, they are associated with no change or an increase in wakefulness (Jindal et al. 2003). SSRIs decrease REM sleep and increase REM sleep latency, although less substantially than tricyclic drugs. SSRI drugs also have been associated with eye movement activity during non-REM sleep, periodic limb movements, and abnormal loss of the usual REM sleep atonia. Conversely, SSRIs may have a small beneficial effect on sleep disorder breathing.

Other antidepressants have distinctive effects on sleep in depression. Bupropion has been associated with insomnia and worsened sleep continuity but also has been associated with a decrease in periodic limb movements (Nofzinger et al. 2000a). Nefazodone is mildly sedating but may actually be associated with insomnia at higher doses; EEG sleep studies show improvement in sleep continuity with little or no suppression of REM sleep (Rush et al. 1998). Trazodone, on the other hand, is associated with subjective and less consistent EEG sleep evidence of improved sleep continuity. Like nefazodone, it causes little or no suppression of REM sleep, and it has been observed to increase the amount of Stage 3/4 non-REM sleep, which is typically associated with subjectively perceived depth of sleep. This profile, together with its relatively short half-life, has made trazodone in low doses a popular hypnotic drug among patients with or without depression. Mirtazapine is also subjectively very sedating, although this effect is primarily observed at lower doses. Objectively, mirtazapine also improves sleep continuity and may increase slow-wave sleep.

TABLE 43–3. Polysomnographic effects of sedating antidepressant drugs on sleep[a]

Drug	Sleep latency	Sleep continuity[b]	Stage 3/4 non-REM sleep amount (%)	REM sleep	Other
Tertiary tricyclic drugs					
Doxepin	↓	↑	↔	↓ Amount, % of REM	*All tricyclics:*
Amitriptyline	↓	↑	↔	↑ Phasic eye movements (REM density)	↓ Sleep apnea (minor effect)
Trimipramine	↓	↑	↔	↓ Amount, % of REM ↑ Phasic eye movements (REM density) ↔ Amount, % of REM	↔ or ↑ Periodic limb movements ↑ Restless legs symptoms May induce eye movements during non-REM sleep
Secondary tricyclic drugs					
Nortriptyline	↔	↑	↔	↓ Amount, % of REM ↑ Phasic eye movements (REM density)	
Desipramine	↔	↔ ↓	↔	↓ Amount, % of REM ↑ Phasic eye movements (REM density) ↔ Amount, % of REM	
SSRI	↔ ↑	↔ ↓	↔ ↓	↓	*SSRIs* **and** *venlafaxine:*
Venlaflaxine	↔ ↑	↔ ↓	↔	↓	↑ Restless legs symptoms May induce eye movements during non-REM sleep ↓ Sleep apnea (minor effect)
Trazodone	↓	↔ to ↑	↑	↔ Amount, % of REM (↓ to ↑ in individual studies)	
Mirtazapine	↓	↑	↔	↔	
Bupropion	↑	↓	↔	↔	

Note. ↑=increase from pretreatment baseline; ↓=decrease from pretreatment baseline; ↔=no change from pretreatment baseline; REM=rapid eye movement; SSRI=selective serotonin reuptake inhibitor.

[a]Reported effects are based on preponderance of evidence from published studies (see text for details). Many effects are inconsistent between individual studies.

[b]Sleep continuity refers to the proportion of sleep relative to wakefulness after sleep onset, as reflected by measures such as sleep efficiency. Other indicators of sleep continuity, such as wakefulness after sleep onset or number of awakenings, would have opposite signs. Thus, ↑ indicates improvement in overall sleep continuity.

Effects of Psychotherapy on Sleep Symptoms and Electroencephalogram Sleep Findings

Although fewer studies have been conducted, successful treatment with psychotherapy also appears to result in sleep changes, as discussed earlier. Psychotherapy, including interpersonal therapy, cognitive-behavioral therapy, and their variants, has been associated with improved sleep following remission of depression (Buysse et al. 1992b; Manber et al. 2000; Thase et al. 1998). The magnitude of subjective improvement may not be as great with psychotherapy alone as with psychotherapy in combination with antidepressant medication such as nefazodone (Manber et al. 2000). Taken together, evidence from sleep studies in which medications and psychotherapy were used suggests that sleep changes during treatment represent the combined effects of specific treatments as well as a general effect of reduction in depression.

Treatment Options for Sleep Disturbances in Mood Disorders

Treatment of mood disorders is addressed in detail in other chapters of this volume. We focus on specific aspects of treatment related to sleep disturbances in mood disorders. These interventions always should be used in combination with adequate treatment of the mood disorder itself.

Treating Sleep Disturbances in Depression

Empirical research and clinical practice suggest four basic strategies for treating insomnia associated with major depression.

1. *Antidepressant medication alone:* As indicated earlier, studies with a wide range of antidepressant drugs, ranging from the relatively alerting SSRIs to the more sedating tricyclic antidepressants, suggest that sleep disturbance in general improves the successful treatment of depression. In patients who do not have a particularly severe sleep disturbance, treatment with an SSRI or a similar antidepressant alone is an appropriate first strategy. In patients with more severe insomnia symptoms, more-sedating drugs such as mirtazapine may be appropriate.
2. *Psychotherapy alone:* On average, patients treated with psychotherapy also show improved sleep when depressive symptoms resolve. Thus, in patients for whom sleep disturbance is not severe, and in whom psychotherapy is otherwise appropriate, this treatment alone is expected to lead to substantial improvements. Additional evidence suggests that behavioral and cognitive-behavioral treatments directed at insomnia itself can be efficacious in patients with comorbid depression (Lichstein et al. 2000).
3. *SSRI plus sedating antidepressant:* In some patients taking an SSRI or other antidepressants such as bupropion, insomnia may be a severe complaint initially, or it may emerge during treatment. In such situations, a low dose of a second, more-sedating antidepressant may be appropriate. The most common drug used as an adjunct is trazodone. In fact, adjunctive use of trazodone appears to be more beneficial than placebo for improving sleep disturbance associated with depression (Nierenberg et al. 1994). Low doses of sedating tricyclic drugs, such as amitriptyline or doxepin, have not been empirically tested as adjunctive treatments. Although combinations of two antidepressants are generally well tolerated, there is theoretical concern that adjunctive use of sedating serotonergic drugs such as trazodone could lead to "serotonin syndrome" (Metz and Shader 1990). However, when trazodone is used in low doses and the SSRI is within the recommended dose range, such cases appear to be rare.
4. *SSRI plus other hypnotic agent:* Although clinicians are sometimes taught that benzodiazepines may worsen depression, evidence from studies of low doses of hypnotic agents does not support this concern. Studies in which benzodiazepines such as lormetazepam, clonazepam, and lorazepam were used showed that patients reported improved sleep with no evidence of worsening of depression (Buysse et al. 1997b; Nolen et al. 1993; W.T. Smith et al. 2002). In fact, each of these studies suggested that adjunctive benzodiazepines may be associated with more rapid response, improved response, greater compliance, or a greater percentage of responders. Zolpidem also has been examined in the treatment of insomnia among patients taking SSRIs and was associated with significantly better self-reported measures of sleep latency and sleep duration.

The use of adjunctive hypnotic drugs, whether a low-dose sedating antidepressant or a benzodiazepine receptor agonist, allows the clinician additional flexibility that is not available with the prescription of a sedating antidepressant alone for both depression and sleep disturbance. That is, if a patient's sleep disturbance improves during the course of depression, adjunctive hypnotic drugs can be discontinued while the SSRI or other antidepressant agent is maintained.

Treating Sleep Disturbances in Mania

Severe sleep disturbance has been associated with worse acute treatment outcomes in mania. Therefore, treatment of insomnia is a priority during treatment of an acute manic episode, and stabilization of sleep-wake schedules to prevent sleep loss may be an important aspect of maintenance treatment (Frank et al. 1997, 2000). Although little empirical research has been conducted in this area, several sleep-focused interventions may be appropriate during acute mania in conjunction with adequate pharmacotherapy for the manic episode and underlying bipolar disorder itself.

Behavioral measures to stabilize sleep. Patients presenting with acute mania may benefit from a quiet environment with low levels of external stimulation (light, noise, social contact, activity options). In addition, being placed on a regular light-dark and sleep-wake schedule may help to stabilize circadian rhythms. A fixed wake-up time is often the most important single element of a regular sleep-wake schedule. Routine "sleep hygiene" measures also include reduction in use of caffeine and alcohol, restriction of strenuous physical activity shortly before bedtime, and limitation of daytime naps.

Pharmacological treatment. For acute treatment, benzodiazepines may be useful both as hypnotics and as nonspecific sedative agents. Rapid-onset drugs such as zolpidem or diazepam given immediately before the desired sleep time may be especially useful. Sedating antipsychotic drugs such as olanzapine or quetiapine given at bedtime can have beneficial effects not only on sleep but also on mania itself. Finally, "loading" doses of sedating mood stabilizers such as lithium, lamotrigine, or carbamazepine at bedtime also may be a useful strategy during acute mania.

Conclusion

Insomnia is intimately related to the mood disorders. Although this has long been recognized, recent evidence has shown new dimensions to these relationships. In particular, accumulating evidence suggests that insomnia and other sleep disturbances are risk factors for the new onset of depression. Once a mood disorder is established, sleep disturbance appears to be a risk factor for adverse outcomes. Direct manipulations of sleep have significant effects on mood symptoms. Finally, sleep and mood regulatory systems appear to share many neurobiological features, suggesting that insomnia and mood disturbances may arise from common neurobiological pathways. Treating sleep disturbances during the course of depression appears to offer substantial benefits in terms of patient well-being and may have small effects in terms of improving overall depression outcome. Future research with tools such as functional imaging with specific receptor ligands will further clarify the neurobiology of sleep and mood disturbances. Additional treatment studies focusing on the co-treatment of sleep and mood symptoms, as well as the effect of insomnia treatment on longer-term mood outcomes, are important avenues of research as well.

References

Anderson JL, Rosen LN, Mendelson WB, et al: Sleep in fall/winter seasonal affective disorder: effects of light and changing seasons. J Psychosom Res 38:323–337, 1994

Ansseau M, Kupfer DJ, Reynolds CF, et al: REM latency distribution in depression: clinical characteristics associated with sleep onset REM. Biol Psychiatry 19:1651–1666, 1985

Armitage R, Roffwarg HP, Rush AJ, et al: Digital period analysis of sleep EEG in depression. Biol Psychiatry 31:52–68, 1992

Armitage R, Hudson A, Trivedi M, et al: Sex differences in the distribution of EEG frequencies during sleep: unipolar depressed outpatients. J Affect Disord 34:121–129, 1995

Armitage R, Hoffmann R, Trivedi M, et al: Slow-wave activity in NREM sleep: sex and age effects in depressed outpatients and healthy controls. Psychiatry Res 95:201–213, 2000

Barbini B, Bertelli S, Colombo C, et al: Sleep loss, a possible factor in augmenting manic episode. Psychiatry Res 65:121–125, 1996

Beersma DGM, Van den Hoofdakker RH: Can non-REM sleep be depressogenic? J Affect Disord 24:101–108, 1992

Benca RM, Obermeyer WH, Thisted RA, et al: Sleep and psychiatric disorders: a meta-analysis. Arch Gen Psychiatry 49:651–668, 1992

Bixler EO, Vgontzas AN, Lin HM, et al: Insomnia in central Pennsylvania. J Psychosom Res 53:589–592, 2002

Borbély AA, Tobler I, Loepfe M, et al: All-night spectral analysis of the sleep EEG in untreated depressives and normal controls. Psychiatry Res 12:27–33, 1984

Borbély AA, Wirz-Justice A: Sleep, sleep deprivation and depression: a hypothesis derived from a model of sleep regulation. Hum Neurobiol 1:205–210, 1982

Braun AR, Balkin TJ, Wesenten NJ, et al: Regional cerebral blood flow throughout the sleep-wake cycle: an H2(15)O PET study. Brain 120:1173–1197, 1997

Breslau N, Roth T, Rosenthal L, et al: Sleep disturbance and psychiatric disorders: a longitudinal epidemiological study of young adults. Biol Psychiatry 39:411–418, 1996

Breslau N, Chilcoat H, Schultz LR: Anxiety disorders and the emergence of sex differences in major depression. J Gend Specif Med 1:33–39, 1998

Buysse DJ, Kupfer DJ: Diagnostic and research applications of electroencephalographic sleep studies in depression: conceptual and methodological issues. J Nerv Ment Dis 178:405–414, 1990

Buysse DJ, Kupfer DJ: Sleep disorders in depressive disorders, in The Biology of Depressive Disorders: An Examination of Illness Subtypes, State Versus Trait and Comorbid Psychiatric Disorders. Edited by Mann JJ, Kupfer DJ. New York, Plenum, 1993, pp 123–153

Buysse DJ, Jarrett DB, Miewald JM, et al: Minute-by-minute analysis of REM sleep timing in major depression. Biol Psychiatry 28:911–925, 1990

Buysse DJ, Kupfer DJ, Frank E, et al: Electroencephalographic sleep studies in depressed patients treated with psychotherapy, I: baseline studies in responders and nonresponders. Psychiatry Res 40:13–26, 1992a

Buysse DJ, Kupfer DJ, Frank E, et al: Electroencephalographic sleep studies in depressed patients treated with psychotherapy, II: longitudinal studies at baseline and recovery. Psychiatry Res 40:27–40, 1992b

Buysse DJ, Reynolds CF, Kupfer DJ, et al: Clinical diagnoses in 216 insomnia patients using ICSD, and proposed DSM-IV and ICD-10 categories: a report from the APA/NIMH DSM-IV field trials. Sleep 17:630–637, 1994

Buysse DJ, Reynolds CF, Hoch CC, et al: Longitudinal effects of nortriptyline on EEG sleep and the likelihood of recurrence in elderly depressed patients. Neuropsychopharmacology 14:243–252, 1996

Buysse DJ, Frank E, Lowe KK, et al: Electroencephalographic sleep correlates of episode and vulnerability to recurrence in depression. Biol Psychiatry 41:406–418, 1997a

Buysse DJ, Reynolds CF, Houck PR, et al: Does lorazepam impair the antidepressant response to nortriptyline and psychotherapy? J Clin Psychiatry 58:426–432, 1997b

Buysse DJ, Tu XM, Cherry CR, et al: Pre-treatment REM sleep and subjective sleep quality distinguish depressed psychotherapy remitters and nonremitters. Biol Psychiatry 45:205–213, 1999

Buysse DJ, Schweitzer PK, Moul DE: Clinical pharmacology of other drugs used as hypnotics, in Principles and Practice of Sleep Medicine, 4th Edition. Edited by Kryger MH, Roth T, Dement W. Philadelphia, PA, Elsevier/Saunders, 2005

Chang PP, Ford DE, Mead LA, et al: Insomnia in young men and subsequent depression. The Johns Hopkins Precursors Study. Am J Epidemiol 146:105–114, 1997

Coble PA, Kupfer DJ, Spiker DG, et al: EEG sleep in primary depression: a longitudinal placebo study. J Affect Disord 1:131–138, 1979

Colombo C, Lucca A, Benedetti F, et al: Total sleep deprivation combined with lithium and light therapy in the treatment of bipolar depression: replication of main effects and interaction. Psychiatry Res 95:43–53, 2000

Dew MA, Reynolds CF, Buysse DJ, et al: Electroencephalographic sleep profiles during depression: effects of episode duration and other clinical and psychosocial factors in older adults. Arch Gen Psychiatry 53:148–156, 1996

Dew MA, Reynolds CF, Houck PR, et al: Temporal profiles of the course of depression during treatment: predictors of pathways toward recovery in the elderly. Arch Gen Psychiatry 54:1016–1024, 1997

Dryman A, Eaton WW: Affective symptoms associated with the onset of major depression in the community: findings from the U.S. National Institute of Mental Health Epidemiologic Catchment Area Program. Acta Psychiatr Scand 84:1–5, 1991

Eaton WW, Badawi M, Melton B: Prodromes and precursors: epidemiologic data for primary prevention of disorders with slow onset. Am J Psychiatry 152:967–972, 1995

Ebert D, Feistel H, Barocka A: Effects of sleep deprivation on the limbic system and the frontal lobes in affective disorders: a study with Tc-99m-HMPAO SPECT. Psychiatry Res 40:247–251, 1991

Ehlers CL, Frank E, Kupfer DJ: Social zeitgebers and biological rhythms: a unified approach to understanding the etiology of depression. Arch Gen Psychiatry 45:948–952, 1988

Foley DJ, Monjan AA, Izmirlian G, et al: Incidence and remission of insomnia among elderly adults in a biracial cohort. Sleep 22:S373–S378, 1999

Ford DE, Kamerow DB: Epidemiologic study of sleep disturbances and psychiatric disorders: an opportunity for prevention. JAMA 262:1479–1484, 1989

Frank E, Hlastala S, Ritenour A, et al: Inducing lifestyle regularity in recovering bipolar disorder patients: results from the maintenance therapies in bipolar disorder protocol. Biol Psychiatry 41:1165–1173, 1997

Frank E, Swartz HA, Kupfer DJ: Interpersonal and social rhythm therapy: managing the chaos of bipolar disorder. Biol Psychiatry 48:593–604, 2000

Germain A, Nofzinger EA, Kupfer DJ, et al: Neurobiology of non-REM sleep in depression: further evidence for hypofrontality and thalamic dysregulation. Am J Psychiatry 161:1856–1863, 2004

Giles DE, Roffwarg HP, Schlesser MA, et al: Which endogenous depressive symptoms relate to REM latency reduction? Biol Psychiatry 21:473–482, 1986a

Giles DE, Rush AJ, Roffwarg HP: Sleep parameters in bipolar I, bipolar II, and unipolar depressions. Biol Psychiatry 21:1340–1343, 1986b

Giles DE, Roffwarg HP, Rush AJ: REM latency concordance in depressed family members. Biol Psychiatry 22:910–914, 1987

Giles DE, Biggs MM, Rush AJ, et al: Risk factors in families of unipolar depression, I: psychiatric illness and reduced REM latency. J Affect Disord 14:51–59, 1988

Giles DE, Kupfer DJ, Roffwarg HP, et al: Polysomnographic parameters in first-degree relatives of unipolar probands. Psychiatry Res 27:127–136, 1989

Gillin JC, Duncan W, Pettigrew KD, et al: Successful separation of depressed, normal, and insomniac subjects by EEG sleep data. Arch Gen Psychiatry 36:85–90, 1979

Goetz RR, Puig-Antich J, Ryan N, et al: Electroencephalographic sleep of adolescents with major depression and normal controls. Arch Gen Psychiatry 44:61–68, 1987

Holsboer-Trachsler E, Ernst K: Sustained antidepressive effect of repeated partial sleep deprivation. Psychopathology 19:172–176, 1986

Hudson JI, Lipinski JF, Frankenburg FR, et al: Electroencephalographic sleep in mania. Arch Gen Psychiatry 45:267–273, 1988

Hudson JI, Lipinski JF, Keck PE, et al: Polysomnographic characteristics of young manic patients: comparison with unipolar depressed patients and normal control subjects. Arch Gen Psychiatry 49:378–383, 1992

Jackson A, Cavanagh J, Scott J: A systematic review of manic and depressive prodromes. J Affect Disord 74:209–217, 2003

Jarrett DB, Greenhouse JB, Miewald JM, et al: A reexamination of the relationship between growth hormone secretion and slow wave sleep using delta wave analysis. Biol Psychiatry 27:497–509, 1990

Jindal RD, Friedman ES, Berman SR, et al: Effects of sertraline on sleep architecture in patients with depression. J Clin Psychopharmacol 23:540–548, 2003

Kerkhofs M, Hoffmann G, DeMartelaere V, et al: Sleep EEG recordings in depressive disorders. J Affect Disord 9:47–53, 1985

Kjaer TW, Law I, Wiltschiotz G, et al: Regional cerebral blood flow during light sleep—a H(2)(15)O-PET study. Sleep Res 11:201–207, 2002

Knowles JB, MacLean AW: Age-related changes in sleep in depressed and healthy subjects: a meta-analysis. Neuropsychopharmacology 3:251–259, 1990

Krakow B, Hollifield M, Johnston L, et al: Imagery rehearsal therapy for chronic nightmares in sexual assault survivors with posttraumatic stress disorder: a randomized controlled trial. JAMA 286:537–545, 2001

Kripke DF: Phase-advance theories for affective illness, in Circadian Rhythms in Psychiatry. Edited by Wehr TA, Goodwin FK. Pacific Grove, CA, Boxwood Press, 1983

Kumar A, Shipley JE, Eiser AS, et al: Clinical correlates of sleep onset REM periods in depression. Biol Psychiatry 22:1473–1477, 1987

Kupfer DJ: REM latency: a psychobiologic marker for primary depressive disease. Biol Psychiatry 11:159–174, 1976

Kupfer DJ, Ehlers CL: Two roads to rapid eye movement latency. Arch Gen Psychiatry 46:945–948, 1989

Kupfer DJ, Spiker DG, Coble PA, et al: Sleep and treatment prediction in endogenous depression. Am J Psychiatry 138:429–434, 1981

Kupfer DJ, Targ E, Stack J: Electroencephalographic sleep in unipolar depressive subtypes: support for a biological and familial classification. J Nerv Ment Dis 170:494–498, 1982

Kupfer DJ, Grochocinski VJ, McEachran AB: Relationship of awakening and delta sleep in depression. Psychiatry Res 19:297–304, 1986

Kupfer DJ, Frank E, Grochocinski VJ, et al: Electroencephalographic sleep profiles in recurrent depression: a longitudinal investigation. Arch Gen Psychiatry 45:678–681, 1988

Kupfer DJ, Ehlers CL, Frank E, et al: EEG sleep profiles and recurrent depression. Biol Psychiatry 30:641–655, 1991

Kupfer DJ, Frank E, McEachran AB, et al: EEG sleep correlates of recurrence of depression on active medication. Depression 1:300–308, 1993

Lauer CJ, Schreiber W, Holsboer F, et al: In quest of identifying vulnerability markers for psychiatric disorders by all-night polysomnography. Arch Gen Psychiatry 52:145–153, 1995

Lee JH, Reynolds CF, Hoch CC, et al: Electroencephalographic sleep in recently remitted, elderly depressed patients in double-blind placebo-maintenance therapy. Neuropsychopharmacology 8:143–150, 1993

Leibenluft E, Wehr TA: Is sleep deprivation useful in the treatment of depression? Am J Psychiatry 149:159–168, 1992

Leibenluft E, Moul DE, Schwartz PJ, et al: A clinical trial of sleep deprivation in combination with antidepressant medication. Psychiatry Res 46:213–227, 1993

Leibenluft E, Albert PS, Rosenthal NE, et al: Relationship between sleep and mood in patients with rapid-cycling bipolar disorder. Psychiatry Res 63:161–168, 1996

Levitt AJ, Lam RW, Levitan R: A comparison of open treatment of seasonal major and minor depression with light therapy. J Affect Disord 71:243–248, 2002

Lichstein KL, Wilson NM, Johnson CT: Psychological treatment of secondary insomnia. Psychol Aging 15:232–240, 2000

Linkowski P, Kerkhofs M, Rielaert C, et al: Sleep during mania in manic-depressive males. Eur Arch Psychiatry Neurol Sci 235:339–341, 1986

Livingston G, Blizard B, Mann A: Does sleep disturbance predict depression in elderly people? A study in inner London. Br J Gen Pract 43:445–448, 1993

Malkoff-Schwartz S, Frank E, Anderson B, et al: Stressful live events and social rhythm disruption in the onset of manic and depressive bipolar episodes: a preliminary investigation. Arch Gen Psychiatry 55:702–707, 1998

Mallon L, Broman JE, Hetta J: Relationship between insomnia, depression, and mortality: a 12-year follow-up of older adults in the community. Int Psychogeriatr 12:295–306, 2000

Manber R, Allen JJ, Burton K, et al: Valence-dependent modulation of psychophysiological measures: is there consistency across repeated testing? Psychophysiology 37:683–692, 2000

McCarley RW, Massaquoi SG: Neurobiological structure of the revised limit cycle reciprocal interaction model of REM cycle control. Sleep Res 1:132–137, 1992

Means MK, Lichstein KL, Edinger JD, et al: Changes in depressive symptoms after continuous positive airway pressure treatment for obstructive sleep apnea. Sleep Breath 7:31–42, 2003

Metz A, Shader RI: Adverse interactions encountered when using trazodone to treat insomnia associated with fluoxetine. Int Clin Psychopharmacol 5:191–194, 1990

Monk TH, Petrie SR, Hayes AJ, et al: Regularity of daily life in relation to personality, age, gender, sleep quality and circadian rhythms. J Sleep Res 3:196–205, 1994

Moul DE, Buysse DJ, Nofzinger EA, et al: Symptoms reports in severe chronic insomnia. Sleep 25:553–563, 2002

Nierenberg AA, Adler LA, Peselow E, et al: Trazodone for antidepressant-associated insomnia. Am J Psychiatry 151:1069–1072, 1994

Nofzinger EA, Thase ME, Reynolds CF, et al: Hypersomnia in bipolar depression: a comparison with narcolepsy using the Multiple Sleep Latency Test. Am J Psychiatry 148:1177–1181, 1991

Nofzinger EA, Mintun MA, Wiseman MB, et al: Forebrain activation in REM sleep: an FDG PET study. Brain Res 770:192–201, 1997

Nofzinger EA, Nichols TE, Meltzer CC, et al: Changes in forebrain function from waking to REM sleep in depression: preliminary analyses of [18F]FDG PET studies. Psychiatry Res 91:59–78, 1999

Nofzinger EA, Fasiczka A, Berman S, et al: Bupropion SR reduces periodic limb movements that are associated with arousals from sleep in depressed patients with periodic limb movement disorder. J Clin Psychiatry 61:858–862, 2000a

Nofzinger EA, Price JC, Meltzer CC, et al: Towards a neurobiology of dysfunctional arousal in depression: the relationship between beta EEG power and regional cerebral glucose metabolism during NREM sleep. Psychiatry Res 98:71–91, 2000b

Nofzinger EA, Berman S, Fasiczka A, et al: Effects of bupropion SR on anterior paralimbic function during waking and REM sleep in depression: preliminary findings using [18F]-FDG PET. Psychiatry Res 106:95–111, 2001

Nofzinger EA, Buysse DJ, Miewald JM, et al: Human regional cerebral glucose metabolism during non-rapid eye movement sleep in relation to waking. Brain 125:1105–1115, 2002

Nofzinger EA, Buysse DJ, Germain A, et al: Increased activation of anterior paralimbic and executive cortex from waking to rapid eye movement sleep in depression. Arch Gen Psychiatry 61:695–702, 2004

Nolen WA, Haffmans PMJ, Bouvy PF, et al: Hypnotics as concurrent medication in depression: a placebo-controlled, double-blind comparison of flunitrazepam and lormetazepam in patients with major depression, treated with a (tri)cyclic antidepressant. J Affect Disord 28:179–188, 1993

Nowell PD, Buysse DJ: Treatment of insomnia in patients with mood disorders. Depress Anxiety 14:7–18, 2001

Nowell PD, Buysse DJ, Reynolds CF, et al: Clinical factors contributing to the differential diagnosis of primary insomnia and insomnia related to mental disorders. Am J Psychiatry 154:1412–1415, 1997

Nowlin-Finch NL, Altshuler LL, Szuba MP, et al: Rapid resolution of first episodes of mania: sleep related? J Clin Psychiatry 55:26–29, 1994

Ohayon MM, Roth T: Place of chronic insomnia in the course of depressive and anxiety disorders. J Psychiatr Res 37:9–15, 2003

Ohayon MM, Caulet M, Lemoine P: Comorbidity of mental and insomnia disorders in the general population. Compr Psychiatry 39:185–197, 1998

Papousek M: [Chronobiological aspects of cyclothymia] (German; author's translation). Fortschr Neurol Psychiatr Grenzgeb 43:381–440, 1975

Perlis ML, Giles DE, Buysse DJ, et al: Which depressive symptoms are related to which sleep EEG variables? Biol Psychiatry 42:904–913, 1997

Regestein QR, Monk TH: Delayed sleep phase syndrome: a review of its clinical aspects [review]. Am J Psychiatry 152:602–608, 1995

Reinink E, Bouhuys N, Wirz-Justice A, et al: Prediction of the antidepressant response to total sleep deprivation by diurnal variation of mood. Psychiatry Res 32:113–124, 1990

Reynolds CF, Kupfer DJ: Sleep research in affective illness: state of the art circa 1987 (state-of-the-art review). Sleep 10:199–215, 1987

Reynolds CF, Newton TF, Shaw DH, et al: Electroencephalographic sleep findings in depressed outpatients. Psychiatry Res 6:65–75, 1982

Reynolds CF, Shaw DH, Newton TF, et al: EEG sleep in outpatients with generalized anxiety: a preliminary comparison with depressed outpatients. Psychiatry Res 8:81–89, 1983

Reynolds CF, Kupfer DJ, Houck PR, et al: Reliable discrimination of elderly depressed and demented patients by EEG sleep data. Arch Gen Psychiatry 45:258–264, 1988

Reynolds CF, Kupfer DJ, Thase ME, et al: Sleep, gender, and depression: an analysis of gender effects on the electroencephalographic sleep of 302 depressed outpatients. Biol Psychiatry 28:673–684, 1990

Reynolds CF, Buysse DJ, Brunner D, et al: Maintenance nortriptyline effects on homeostatic control of sleep in elders with recurrent major depression: double-blind, placebo- and plasma-level controlled evaluation. Biol Psychiatry 42:560–567, 1997

Riemann D, Berger M: EEG sleep in depression and in remission and the REM sleep response to the cholinergic agonist RS 86. Neuropsychopharmacology 2:145–152, 1989

Riemann D, Hohagen F, Konig A, et al: Advanced vs. normal sleep timing: effects on depressed mood after response to sleep deprivation in patients with a major depressive disorder. J Affect Disord 37:121–128, 1996

Rush AJ, Giles DE, Jarrett RB, et al: Reduced REM latency predicts response to tricyclic medication in depressed outpatients. Biol Psychiatry 26:61–72, 1989

Rush AJ, Armitage R, Gillin JC, et al: Comparative effects of nefazodone and fluoxetine on sleep in outpatients with major depressive disorder. Biol Psychiatry 44:3–14, 1998

Schulz H, Lund R, Cording C, et al: Bimodal distribution of REM sleep latencies in depression. Biol Psychiatry 14:595–600, 1979

Shipley JE, Kupfer DJ, Griffin SJ, et al: Comparison of effects of desipramine and amitriptyline on EEG sleep of depressed patients. Psychopharmacology 85:14–22, 1985

Smeraldi E, Benedetti F, Barbini B, et al: Sustained antidepressant effect of sleep deprivation combined with pindolol in bipolar depression: a placebo-controlled trial. Neuropsychopharmacology 20:380–385, 1999

Smith GS, Reynolds CF, Houck PR, et al: Glucose metabolic response to total sleep deprivation, recovery sleep and acute antidepressant treatment as functional neuroanatomic correlates of treatment outcome in geriatric depression. Am J Geriatr Psychiatry 10:561–567, 2002

Smith WT, Londborg PD, Glaudin V, et al: Is extended clonazepam cotherapy of fluoxetine effective for outpatients with major depression? J Affect Disord 70:251–259, 2002

Terman M, Amira L, Terman JS, et al: Predictors of response and nonresponse to light treatment for winter depression. Am J Psychiatry 153:1423–1429, 1996

Thase ME, Kupfer DJ: Recent developments in the pharmacotherapy of mood disorders. J Consult Clin Psychol 64:646–659, 1996

Thase ME, Simons AD: The applied use of psychotherapy in the study of the psychobiology of depression. J Psychother Pract Res 1:72–80, 1992

Thase ME, Kupfer DJ, Ulrich RF: Electroencephalographic sleep in psychotic depression: a valid subtype? Arch Gen Psychiatry 43:886–893, 1986

Thase ME, Simons AD, Reynolds CF: Abnormal electroencephalographic sleep profiles in major depression: association with response to cognitive behavior therapy. Arch Gen Psychiatry 53:99–108, 1996

Thase ME, Buysse DJ, Frank E, et al: Which depressed patients will respond to interpersonal psychotherapy? The role of abnormal electroencephalographic sleep profiles. Am J Psychiatry 154:502–509, 1997

Thase ME, Fasiczka AL, Berman SR, et al: Electroencephalographic sleep profiles before and after cognitive behavior therapy of depression. Arch Gen Psychiatry 55:138–144, 1998

Ulfberg J, Nystrom B, Carter N, et al: Prevalence of restless legs syndrome among men aged 18 to 64 years: an association with somatic disease and neuropsychiatric symptoms. Mov Disord 16:1159–1163, 2001

Vandeputte M, de Weerd A: Sleep disorders and depressive feelings: a global survey with the Beck depression scale. Sleep Med 4:343–345, 2003

Vitiello MV, Prinz PN, Avery DH, et al: Sleep is undisturbed in elderly, depressed individuals who have not sought health care. Biol Psychiatry 27:431–440, 1990

Vogel GW, Thurmond A, Gibbons P, et al: REM sleep reduction effects on depression syndromes. Arch Gen Psychiatry 32:765–777, 1975

Volk SA, Kaendler SH, Hertel A, et al: Can response to partial sleep deprivation in depressed patients be predicted by regional changes of cerebral blood flow? Psychiatry Res 75:67–74, 1997

Wehr TA, Wirz-Justice A: Circadian rhythm mechanism in affective illness and in antidepressant drug action. Pharmacopsychiatry 15:31–39, 1982

Weissman MM, Greenwald S, Nino-Murcia G, et al: The morbidity of insomnia uncomplicated by psychiatric disorders. Gen Hosp Psychiatry 19:245–250, 1997

Wirz-Justice A, Van den Hoofdakker RH: Sleep deprivation in depression: what do we know, where do we go? Biol Psychiatry 46:445–453, 1999

Wu JC, Bunney WE: The biological basis of an antidepressant response to sleep deprivation and relapse: review and hypothesis. Am J Psychiatry 147:14–21, 1990

Index

*Page numbers printed in **boldface** type refer to tables or figures.*